OTOLOGIC SURGERY

OTOLOGIC SURGERY

SECOND EDITION

Editor

Derald E. Brackmann, MD, FACS

Clinical Professor of Otolaryngology–Head and Neck Surgery
Clinical Professor of Neurosurgery
University of Southern California School of Medicine
President, House Ear Clinic
Board of Directors, House Ear Institute
Los Angeles, California

Associate Editor

Clough Shelton, MD, FACS

Professor
Otology, Neuro-Otology and Skull Base Surgery
The University of Utah School of Medicine
Salt Lake City, Utah

Associate Editor

Moisés A. Arriaga, MD

Clinical Associate Professor of Otolaryngology
University of Pittsburgh
Adjunct Associate Professor of Otolaryngology and Neurosurgery
Hahnemann Medical School and Medical College of Pennsylvania
Pittsburgh Ear Associates
Director, Hearing and Balance Center
Allegheny General Hospital
Pittsburgh, Pennsylvania

Illustrated by

Anthony Pazos

W.B. SAUNDERS COMPANY
A Harcourt Health Sciences Company
Philadelphia London New York St. Louis Sydney Toronto

W.B. SAUNDERS COMPANY
A Harcourt Health Sciences Company

The Curtis Center
Independence Square West
Philadelphia, Pennsylvania 19106

Library of Congress Cataloging-in-Publication Data

Otologic surgery / [edited by] Derald E. Brackmann, Clough Shelton, Moisés A. Arriaga.—2nd ed.

p.   cm.

ISBN 0–7216–8976–0

1. Ear—Surgery.   I. Brackmann, Derald E.   II. Shelton, Clough. III. Arriaga, Moisés A. [DNLM: 1. Ear—surgery.   2. Otologic Surgical Procedures. WV 200 O878 2001]

RF126.O87 2001   617.8′059–dc21

DNLM/DLC   00–049256

Acquisitions Editor: Stephanie Smith Donley
Production Editor: Edna Dick
Production Manager: Norman Stellander
Illustration Specialist: Rita Martello
Illustrator: Anthony Pazos

OTOLOGIC SURGERY   ISBN 0–7216–8976–0

Printed in the United States of America

Last digit is the print number: 9   8   7   6   5   4   3   2   1

Dedication

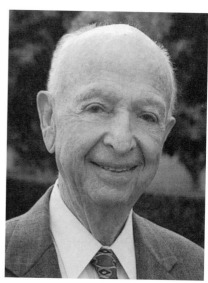

Howard P. House

This book is dedicated to our mentors and teachers, Drs. Howard P. House, William F. House, and James L. Sheehy. Each of these outstanding physicians has special talents and characteristics that, when melded together, resulted in an outstanding clinical, research, and educational facility, The House Ear Clinic and Institute.

Howard House, the founder of our Institutions, was among the first to concentrate his activities in the field of otology. He has devoted his career to the treatment of otosclerosis. In addition to his surgical genius, Howard is recognized as an outstanding statesman and fundraiser. Without him the House Ear Institute, which has provided so many opportunities for all of us, would not exist.

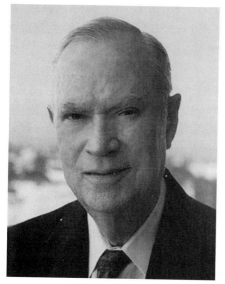

William F. House

William F. House joined his brother in practice after completing his residency. A creative genius, Bill recognized that the future of otology lay in the diagnosis and treatment of diseases of the inner ear. He introduced the operating microscope and microsurgical techniques to the field of neurosurgery and revolutionized the treatment of acoustic tumors and other neurotologic problems. Bill is also recognized as instrumental in bringing the cochlear implant to the state of a practical clinical device that is now widely applied.

The final link in the chain that resulted in the success of the House Ear Clinic and Institute is Dr. James L. Sheehy. His special interest is in the field of chronic otitis media. In addition to his outstanding surgical ability, Jim possesses exceptional talent in organizational ability and teaching. Jim was responsible for developing all the patient educational materials as well as serving as the editor for all of the many publications produced by members of the House Ear Clinic. His course development, panel discussions, and slide preparation techniques became standards for our specialty.

It was our great privilege to be under the personal tutelage of each of these outstanding men. In addition to all the attributes enumerated above, first and foremost each is an outstanding physician. They practice the art and science of surgery in the finest fashion, making it most appropriate that this book on surgical technique be dedicated to them.

DERALD E. BRACKMANN, M.D.
CLOUGH SHELTON, M.D.
MOISÉS A. ARRIAGA, M.D.

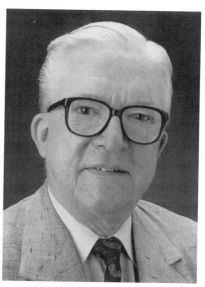

James L. Sheehy

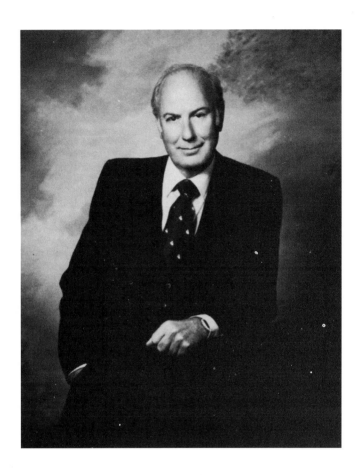

In Memoriam

Harold Frederick Schuknecht
(February 10, 1917 to October 19, 1996)

On October 19, 1996, the field of otology lost one of its most influential leaders of modern times. Harold Frederick Schuknecht, M.D., Professor Emeritus of the Department of Otology and Laryngology at the Harvard Medical School and Chief Emeritus of the Department of Otolaryngology at the Massachusetts Eye and Ear Infirmary, was a world-renowned clinical otologist, otopathologist, teacher, and scholar. His contribution to human otopathology is unparalleled. His book, *Pathology of the Ear,* which he solely authored, is without question the most complete and comprehensive thesis on the subject. His clinical approach and technical innovations were based on scientific principle, and he unabashedly held others to the same standard. His influence as a teacher and role model is evidenced by the unprecedented number of his students who have followed in his footsteps and have risen as leaders in our specialty. Through his life's work and through the lives of those he has touched, his influence lives on.

Contributors

Sean R. Althaus, M.D., F.A.C.S.
Associate Clinical Professor, Otolaryngology–Head and
Neck Surgery, University of California San Francisco
School of Medicine; California Ear Institute at Stanford,
Palo Alto; Active Staff, San Ramon Regional Medical
Center, San Ramon, California
*Traumatic Perforation—Office Treatment of the
Chronically Draining Ear*

Moisés A. Arriaga, M.D.
Clinical Associate Professor of Otolaryngology,
University of Pittsburgh; Adjunct Associate Professor of
Otolaryngology and Neurosurgery, Hahnemann Medical
School and Medical College of Pennsylvania; Pittsburgh
Ear Associates; Director, Hearing and Balance Center,
Allegheny General Hospital, Pittsburgh, Pennsylvania
*Mastoidectomy: The Canal Wall Down Procedure;
Overview of Transtemporal Skull Base Surgery; Surgery
for Glomus and Jugular Foramen Tumors; Anterior and
Subtemporal Approaches to the Infratemporal Fossa*

Gregory A. Ator, M.D.
Associate Professor, Department of Otolaryngology, and
Director of Otology–Neurotology Division, University of
Kansas Medical Center, Kansas City, Kansas
Traumatic Facial Paralysis

R. Stanley Baker, M.D.
Clinical Assistant Professor of Otolaryngology, University
of Oklahoma College of Medicine; Chairman, Department
of Otolaryngology, Integris–Baptist Medical Center,
Oklahoma City, Oklahoma
Stapedectomy: Use of Natural Material

George P. Bauer, M.D.
Private Practice, Attending Staff, Mercy Franciscan
Hospital, Cincinnati, Ohio
Management of Complications of Chronic Otitis Media

James E. Benecke, Jr., M.D., F.A.C.S.
Private Practice, Ear and Hearing Specialists, St. Louis,
Missouri
Otologic Instrumentation

Leonard P. Berenholz, M.D., F.A.C.S.
Lecturer in Otolaryngology, Tel Aviv University; Senior
Otolaryngology Surgeon, Wolfson Hospital, Holon, Israel
Special Problems of Otologic Surgery

Charles D. Bluestone, M.D.
Eberly Professor of Pediatric Otolaryngology, University
of Pittsburgh School of Medicine; Director, Department of
Pediatric Otolaryngology, Children's Hospital of
Pittsburgh, Pittsburgh, Pennsylvania
The Abnormally Patulous Eustachian Tube

K. Paul Boyev, M.D.
Assistant Professor, Department of Otolaryngology–Head
and Neck Surgery, Director, Division of Otology/
Neurotology, and Director, Hearing and Balance Center,
University of South Florida College of Medicine;
University of South Florida Physicians Group, Tampa,
Florida
Cochleosacculotomy

Derald E. Brackmann, M.D., F.A.C.S.
Clinical Professor of Otolaryngology–Head and Neck
Surgery, Clinical Professor of Neurosurgery, University of
Southern California School of Medicine; President, House
Ear Clinic; Board of Directors, House Ear Institute, Los
Angeles, California
*Drainage Procedures for Petrous Apex Lesions; Surgery
for Glomus and Jugular Foramen Tumors; Middle Fossa
Approach; Auditory Brainstem Implant; Management of
Postoperative Cerebrospinal Fluid Leaks*

Graham Bryce, M.D.
Clinical Associate Professor, Division of Otolaryngology,
University of British Columbia; Director, Division of
Otolaryngology, St. Paul's Hospital, Vancouver, B.C.,
Canada
Stapedectomy: Use of Natural Material

Robert L. Campbell, M.D.
Betsy Barton Professor of Neurosurgery, Indiana
University School of Medicine, Indianapolis, Indiana
Treatment of Bilateral Acoustic Neuromas

Ricardo L. Carrau, M.D.
Associate Professor, Department of Otolaryngology–Head
and Neck Surgery, University of Pittsburgh, Pittsburgh,
Pennsylvania
*Anterior and Subtemporal Approaches to the
Infratemporal Fossa*

Stephen P. Cass, M.D., M.P.H.
Associate Professor, Department of Otolaryngology,
University of Colorado Health Sciences Center, Denver,
Colorado
Chemical Treatment of the Labyrinth

Sujana S. Chandrasekhar, M.D.
Associate Professor of Surgery, Division of
Otolaryngology/Head and Neck Surgery, University of
Medicine and Dentistry of New Jersey, New Jersey
Medical School; Director of Otology/Neurotology,
Medical Director of the Cochlear Implant Center of New
Jersey, UMDNJ–University Hospital, Newark, New Jersey
*Congenital Malformation of the Temporal Bone;
Transcochlear Approach to Cerebellopontine Angle
Lesions*

Joseph M. Chen, M.D., F.R.C.S.(C)
Associate Professor, Department of Otolaryngology,
University of Toronto; Staff Surgeon, Sunnybrook and
Women's College Health Science Center, Toronto,
Ontario, Canada
*Middle Cranial Fossa: Vestibular Neurectomy; Transotic
Approach*

C. Philip Daspit, M.D.
Clinical Professor, Department of Surgery, University of
Arizona Health Sciences Center, Tucson; Chief, Section
of Neurotology, Department of Neurosurgery, Barrow
Neurological Institute, Phoenix, Arizona
Petrosal Approach

Antonio De la Cruz, M.D.
Clinical Professor, Otolaryngology/Head and Neck
Surgery, University of Southern California School of
Medicine; Active Staff, St. Vincent Medical Center, USC
University Hospital, LAC–University of Southern
California Medical Center, Los Angeles, California
*Congenital Malformation of the Temporal Bone;
Transcochlear Approach to Cerebellopontine Angle
Lesions*

Paul W. Detwiler, M.D.
Tyler Neurosurgical Group, Tyler, Texas
Petrosal Approach

Jose N. Fayad, M.D.
Assistant Professor, Department of Otolaryngology/Head
and Neck Surgery, Columbia University College of
Physicians and Surgeons; Director of Otology,
Department of Otolaryngology–Head and Neck Surgery,
Columbia Presbyterian Medical Center, New York, New
York
*Congenital Malformation of the Temporal Bone;
Transcochlear Approach to Cerebellopontine Angle
Lesions*

Ugo Fisch, M.D.
Professor Emeritus of ENT, University of Zurich; Head of
ENT and Skull Base Surgery, University Hospital, Zurich,
Switzerland
*Middle Cranial Fossa: Vestibular Neurectomy; Transotic
Approach*

Rick A. Friedman, M.D., Ph.D.
Clinical Assistant Professor of Otolaryngology, University
of Southern California School of Medicine; Associate,
House Ear Clinic, Los Angeles, California
*Surgery of Ventilation and Mucosal Disease;
Translabyrinthine Approach*

Lendra M. Friesen, M.S.
Research Audiologist, House Ear Institute, Los Angeles,
California
Auditory Brainstem Implant

Mark R. Gacek, M.D.
Clinical Assistant Professor, Department of Neurology,
University of South Alabama College of Medicine,
Mobile, Alabama
*Posterior Ampullary Nerve Section for Benign
Paroxysmal Positional Vertigo*

Richard R. Gacek, M.D.
Professor of Otolaryngology–Head and Neck Surgery,
University of South Alabama College of Medicine; Chief,
Division of Otolaryngology–Head and Neck Surgery,
University of South Alabama Medical Center, Mobile,
Alabama
*Posterior Ampullary Nerve Section for Benign
Paroxysmal Positional Vertigo*

Bruce J. Gantz, M.D.
Professor and Head, Brian F. McCabe Distinguished Chair
in Otolaryngology–Head and Neck Surgery, University of
Iowa Hospitals and Clinics, Iowa City, Iowa
Management of Bell's Palsy and Ramsay Hunt Syndrome

Neil A. Giddings, M.D.
Sacred Heart Medical Center, and Deaconess Medical
Center, Spokane, Washington
Drainage Procedures for Petrous Apex Lesions

Michael E. Glasscock, III, M.D.
Formerly Clinical Professor, Department of
Otolaryngology (Head and Neck Surgery), Georgetown
University Medical Center, Washington, DC; Consultant
in Neurotology, The Otology Group, Nashville, Tennessee
*Tympanoplasty: The Undersurface Graft
Technique—Postauricular Approach*

Malcolm D. Graham, M.D., F.R.C.S.(C), F.A.C.S.
Clinical Professor, Department of Surgery, Division of
Otolaryngology–Head and Neck Surgery, University of
North Carolina at Chapel Hill, Chapel Hill, North
Carolina; Medical Director, Georgia Ear Institute,
Savannah, Georgia
Dural Herniation and Cerebrospinal Fluid Leaks

Jan J. Grote, M.D., Ph.D.
Professor, and Chairman, ENT Department, Leiden
University Medical Center, Leiden, The Netherlands
Biocompatible Materials in Chronic Ear Surgery

Hal L. Hankinson, M.D.
Neurosurgeon, Albuquerque, New Mexico
*Middle Fossa Transpetrous Approach for Access to the
Petroclival Region (Extended Middle Fossa Approach)*

Steven A. Harvey, M.D.
Clinical Assistant Professor, Department of
Otolaryngology, Medical College of Wisconsin; Attending
Staff, St. Luke's Medical Center, Children's Hospital of
Wisconsin, Milwaukee, Wisconsin
Management of Complications of Chronic Otitis Media

William E. Hitselberger, M.D.
Neurosurgeon, Los Angeles, California
Middle Fossa Transpetrous Approach for Access to the Petroclival Region (Extended Middle Fossa Approach); Auditory Brainstem Implant

Dieter F. Hoffmann, M.D.
Assistant Clinical Professor, Oregon Health Sciences University, Portland; Otolaryngologist/Head and Neck Surgeon, Kaiser Sunnyside Medical Center, Clackamas, Oregon
Facial Reanimation Techniques

Karl L. Horn, M.D.
Medical Director, Presbyterian Ear Institute; Associate Clinical Professor, University of New Mexico Medical School; Presbyterian Hospital, St. Joseph's Hospital, University of New Mexico Hospital, Albuquerque, New Mexico
Middle Fossa Transpetrous Approach for Access to the Petroclival Region (Extended Middle Fossa Approach)

J.V.D. Hough, M.D.
Clinical Professor, Otorhinolaryngology–Head and Neck Surgery, University of Oklahoma College of Medicine; Founder and Chairman of the Board, Hough Ear Institute, Oklahoma City, Oklahoma
Stapedectomy: Use of Natural Material

Howard P. House, M.D.
Professor Emeritus, University of Southern California; Founder and Chairman Emeritus, House Ear Institute, St. Vincent Medical Center; LAC–University of Southern California Medical Center, Hospital of The Good Samaritan, Children's Hospital of Los Angeles, Los Angeles, California
Total Stapedectomy

James R. House III, M.D.
Associate Professor of Surgery, Department of Surgery, Division of Otolaryngology, University of Mississippi School of Medicine, Jackson, Mississippi
Hypoglossal Facial Anastomosis

John W. House, M.D.
Clinical Professor, Department of Otolaryngology–Head and Neck Surgery, University of Southern California School of Medicine, Los Angeles, California
Translabyrinthine Approach

William F. House, M.D.
Hoog Hospital, Newport Beach, California
Middle Fossa Approach

Robert K. Jackler, M.D.
Professor of Otolaryngology and Neurological Surgery, University of California San Francisco, San Francisco, California
Retrosigmoid Approach to Tumors of the Cerebellopontine Angle

C. Gary Jackson, M.D., F.A.C.S.
Clinical Professor, Department of Surgery, University of North Carolina School of Medicine, Chapel Hill, North Carolina; Clinical Professor, Department of Otolaryngology (Head and Neck Surgery), Georgetown University Medical Center, Washington, DC; President, Otology Group, and The Ear Foundation, Nashville, Tennessee
Tympanoplasty: The Undersurface Graft Technique—Postauricular Approach

Ivo P. Janecka, M.D., F.A.C.S.
Professor, Harvard Medical School; Director, Skull Base International; Staff, Children's Hospital, Brigham and Women's Hospital, Boston, Massachusetts
Malignancies of the Temporal Bone—Radical Temporal Bone Resection

Peter J. Jannetta, M.D.
Vice Chairman and Professor of Otolaryngology and Neurological Surgery, University of Pittsburgh; Allegheny General Hospital, Pittsburgh, Pennsylvania
Operations for Vascular Compressive Syndromes

Herman A. Jenkins, M.D.
Professor and Chairman, Department of Otolaryngology, University of Colorado Health Sciences Center; Chief, Otolaryngology Service, University of Colorado Hospital, Denver, Colorado
Traumatic Facial Paralysis

Amin Kassam, M.D.
Assistant Professor, Department of Neurological Surgery, University of Pittsburgh Medical Center, Pittsburgh, Pennsylvania
Anterior and Subtemporal Approaches to the Infratemporal Fossa

Bradley W. Kesser, M.D.
Private practice, Piedmont Ear, Nose and Throat Associates, Atlanta, Georgia
Surgery of Ventilation and Mucosal Disease

Sam E. Kinney, M.D.
Clinical Associate Professor of Otolaryngology, Head and Neck Surgery, Case Western Reserve School of Medicine; Head, Section of Otology and Neurotology, Department of Otolaryngology and Communicative Disorders, Cleveland Clinic Foundation, Cleveland, Ohio
Malignancies of the Temporal Bone: Limited Temporal Bone Resection

Jed A. Kwartler, M.D.
Clinical Associate Professor, Division of Otolaryngology, University of Medicine and Dentistry of New Jersey, Newark; Ear Specialty Group, Springfield, New Jersey
Total Stapedectomy

Robert E. Levine, M.D.
Clinical Professor, Department of Ophthalmology, University of Southern California School of Medicine; Cofounder and Codirector, Facial Nerve Disorders Center, House Ear Clinic, Los Angeles, California
Care of the Eye in Facial Paralysis

Elad I. Levy, M.D.
Resident, Department of Neurosurgery, University of
Pittsburgh, Pittsburgh, Pennsylvania
Operations for Vascular Compressive Syndromes

William H. Lippy, M.D.
Clinical Professor, Ohio State University, Columbus,
Ohio; Clinical Assistant Professor, University of Eastern
Virginia, Norfolk, Virginia; Chief of Otology, Warren
General Hospital, Attending Staff, Trumbull Memorial
Hospital, Warren, Ohio
Special Problems of Otologic Surgery

Larry B. Lundy, M.D.
Consultant in Otology/Neuro-otology, Mayo Clinic
Jacksonville, Jacksonville, Florida
*Dural Herniation and Cerebrospinal Fluid Leaks; Laser
Revision Stapedectomy*

William M. Luxford, M.D.
Associate, House Ear Clinic, Associate Clinical Professor
of Otolaryngology, University of Southern California
Medical School; Attending Physician, St. Vincent Medical
Center, Los Angeles, California
*Surgery for Cochlear Implantation; Hypoglossal Facial
Anastomosis*

Anthony E. Magit, M.D.
Assistant Professor of Otolaryngology and Pediatrics,
University of California at San Diego School of
Medicine; Children's Associated Medical Group, Inc., San
Diego, California
The Abnormally Patulous Eustachian Tube

Mark May, M.D.
Clinical Professor Emeritus, Department of
Otolaryngology/Head and Neck Surgery, University of
Pittsburgh, Pittsburgh, Pennsylvania
Facial Reanimation Techniques

Michael McGee, M.D.
Clinical Assistant Professor of Otolaryngology, University
of Oklahoma College of Medicine; President, Hough Ear
Institute, Oklahoma City, Oklahoma
Stapedectomy: Use of Natural Material

Michael J. McKenna, M.D.
Associate Professor, Department of Otology and
Laryngology, Harvard Medical School; Associate
Surgeon, Department of Otolaryngology, Massachusetts
Eye and Ear Infirmary, Boston, Massachusetts
Cochleosacculotomy; Transcanal Labyrinthectomy

Richard T. Miyamoto, M.D., F.A.C.S., F.A.A.P.
Arilla Spence DeVault Professor and Chairman,
Department of Otolaryngology–Head and Neck Surgery,
Indiana University School of Medicine; Medical Director
of Audiology and Speech/Language Pathology, Indiana
University Hospitals, Indianapolis, Indiana
Treatment of Bilateral Acoustic Neuromas

Aage R. Møller, Ph.D. (D.Med.Sci.)
Professor, The University of Texas at Dallas, Dallas,
Texas
Intraoperative Neurophysiologic Monitoring

Edwin M. Monsell, M.D., Ph.D.
Professor and Director of Otology and Neurotological
Skull Base Surgery, Department of Otolaryngology—
Head and Neck Surgery, Wayne State University School
of Medicine, Detroit, Michigan
Chemical Treatment of the Labyrinth

Joseph B. Nadol, Jr., M.D.
Walter Augustus Lecompte Professor and Chairman,
Department of Otology and Laryngology, Harvard
Medical School; Chief of Otolaryngology, Massachusetts
Eye and Ear Infirmary, Boston, Massachusetts
Transcanal Labyrinthectomy

Julian M. Nedzelski, M.D., F.R.C.S.(C)
Professor and Chair, Department of Otolaryngology,
University of Toronto; Otolaryngologist-in-Chief
Sunnybrook and Women's College Health Sciences
Center, Toronto, Ontario, Canada
Chemical Treatment of the Labyrinth

J. Gail Neely, M.D., F.A.C.S.
Professor and Director, Otology/Neurotology/Base of
Skull Surgery, Washington University School of
Medicine; Attending Physician, Barnes–Jewish Hospital,
St. Louis Children's Hospital, Veterans Affairs Medical
Center, St. Louis, Missouri
Surgery of Acute Infections and Their Complications

Ralph A. Nelson, M.D., M.S.
Professor, University of Southern California, Los Angeles,
Los Angeles, California
Translabyrinthine Vestibular Neurectomy

James L. Netterville, M.D.
Professor, Department of Otolaryngology, Head and Neck
Surgery, Vanderbilt University Medical Center, Nashville,
Tennessee
*Rehabilitation of Lower Cranial Nerve Deficits After
Neurotologic Skull Base Surgery*

Steven R. Otto, M.A.
Advanced Research Associate, House Ear Institute, Los
Angeles, California
Auditory Brainstem Implant

Michael M. Paparella, M.D.
Clinical Professor and Chairman Emeritus, Department of
Otolaryngology, University of Minnesota; President,
Minnesota Ear, Head and Neck Clinic, Minneapolis,
Minnesota
Endolymphatic Sac Procedures

Lorne S. Parnes, M.D., F.R.C.S.C.
Professor, Departments of Otolaryngology and Clinical Neurological Sciences, University of Western Ontario; Associate Chair/Chief, Department of Otolaryngology, London Health Sciences Centre, London, Ontario, Canada
Posterior Semicircular Canal Occlusion for Benign Paroxysmal Positional Vertigo

Rodney Perkins, M.D.
Professor of Surgery, Stanford University, California Ear Institute at Stanford, Palo Alto, California
Canalplasty for Exostoses of the External Auditory Canal and Miscellaneous Auditory Canal Problems; Laser Stapedotomy

Brian P. Perry, M.D.
Clinical Assistant Professor, University of Texas–Health Science Center; The Otology Group of Texas, San Antonio, Texas
Management of Bell's Palsy and Ramsay Hunt Syndrome

Sanjay Prasad, M.D.
Clinical Assistant Professor, Department of Otolaryngology, Head and Neck Surgery, Georgetown University Medical Center, Washington, DC; President and Founder, Metropolitan Ear Group, Bethesda, Maryland
Malignancies of the Temporal Bone—Radical Temporal Bone Resection

Miriam I. Redleaf, M.D.
Assistant Professor, University of Chicago; Clinical Associate, University of Chicago, Chicago, Illinois
Management of Bell's Palsy and Ramsay Hunt Syndrome

Joseph B. Roberson, Jr., M.D.
Clinical Assistant Professor and Director, Education and Fellowship Programs, Stanford University, California Ear Institute at Stanford, Palo Alto; Medical Staff, San Ramon Regional Medical Center, San Ramon; Medical Staff, Children's Hospital Oakland, Oakland, California
Canalplasty for Exostoses of the External Auditory Canal and Miscellaneous Auditory Canal Problems; Avoidance and Management of Complications of Otosclerosis Surgery

Mendell Robinson, M.D., F.A.C.S.
Clinical Associate Professor, Brown University School of Medicine; Senior Surgeon, Miriam Hospital, Rhode Island Hospital, Providence, Rhode Island
Partial Stapedectomy

Grayson K. Rodgers, M.D.
Birmingham Hearing and Balance Center, Birmingham, Alabama
Management of Postoperative Cerebrospinal Fluid Leaks

Karen L. Roos, M.D.
Professor of Neurology, Indiana University School of Medicine, Indianapolis, Indiana
Treatment of Bilateral Acoustic Neuromas

Seth I. Rosenberg, M.D., F.A.C.S.
Clinical Assistant Professor, University of Pennsylvania School of Medicine, Philadelphia, Pennsylvania; Ear Research Foundation, Sarasota, Florida
Retrolabyrinthine/Retrosigmoid Vestibular Neurectomy

Leonard P. Rybak, M.D., Ph.D.
Professor of Surgery, Southern Illinois University School of Medicine; Memorial Medical Center and St. John's Hospital, Springfield, Illinois
Chemical Treatment of the Labyrinth

Harold F. Schuknecht, M.D.†
Was Professor and Chairman Emeritus, Department of Otology and Laryngology, Harvard Medical School; Emeritus Chief of Otolaryngology, Department of Otolaryngology, Massachusetts Eye and Ear Infirmary, Boston, Massachusetts
Cochleosacculotomy

M. Coyle Shea, Jr., M.D.
Associate Clinical Professor, Department of Otolaryngology–Head and Neck Surgery, University of Tennessee Center for the Health Sciences; Active Staff, Baptist Memorial Hospitals, Associate Staff, City of Memphis Hospitals, Courtesy Staff, Methodist Hospitals, St. Francis Hospital, Memphis, Tennessee
Tympanoplasty: The Undersurface Graft Technique—Transcanal Approach

James L. Sheehy, M.D.
Clinical Professor of Surgery and Otolaryngology, University of Southern California School of Medicine, Los Angeles, California
Tympanoplasty: The Outer Surface Grafting Technique; Tympanoplasty: Cartilage and Porous Polyethylene; Mastoidectomy: The Intact Canal Wall Procedure; Tympanoplasty: Staging and Use of Plastic

Clough Shelton, M.D., F.A.C.S.
Professor, Otology, Neuro-otology and Skull Base Surgery, The University of Utah School of Medicine, Salt Lake City, Utah
Facial Nerve Tumors; Middle Fossa Approach

Herbert Silverstein, M.D., F.A.C.S.
Clinical Professor, University of Pennsylvania School of Medicine, Philadelphia, Pennsylvania; President, Ear Research Foundation, Sarasota, Florida
Retrolabyrinthine/Retrosigmoid Vestibular Neurectomy

David W. Sim, F.R.C.S. Ed. (URL)
Clinical Tutor, University of Edinburgh, Scotland
Retrosigmoid Approach to Tumors of the Cerebellopontine Angle

George T. Singleton, M.D.
Professor of Otolaryngology, University of Florida College of Medicine; Attending Staff, Shands Hospital; Chief of Otolaryngology, VA Hospital, Gainesville, Florida
Perilymphatic Fistula

---

†Dr. Schuknecht is deceased.

William H. Slattery III, M.D.
Associate Clinical Professor, University of Southern California Los Angeles; Director, Clinical Studies Department, House Ear Institute, Associate, House Ear Clinic, Los Angeles, California
Perilymphatic Fistula; Implantable Hearing Devices

Sigfrid D. Soli, Ph.D.
Vice President, Technology Transfer and Director of Hearing Aid Research, House Ear Institute, Los Angeles, California
Implantable Hearing Devices

Robert F. Spetzler, M.D.
Tenured Professor, Section of Neurosurgery, University of Arizona School of Medicine, Tucson; Director, Barrow Neurological Institute, St. Joseph's Hospital and Medical Center, Phoenix, Arizona
Petrosal Approach

Barbara A. Stahl, R.N.
Self-employed Registered Nurse; Surgical Assistant, Dr. W.E. Hitselberger (Neurosurgeon); St. Vincent Medical Center, Doheny Operating Room, Los Angeles, California
Otologic Instrumentation

Katrina R. Stidham, M.D.
Clinical Faculty, California Ear Institute at Stanford; Active Staff, San Ramon Regional Medical Center, San Ramon, Community Physicians Stanford Hospital, Palo Alto, California
Traumatic Perforation—Office Treatment of the Chronically Draining Ear

Barry Strasnick, M.D.
Professor and Chairman, Department of Otolaryngology—Head and Neck Surgery, Eastern Virginia Medical School; Active Staff, Sentara Norfolk General Hospital, Children's Hospital of the King's Daughters, DePaul Medical Center, Sentara Leigh Hospital, Norfolk, Virginia
Tympanoplasty: The Undersurface Graft Technique—Postauricular Approach

Christopher A. Sullivan, M.D.
Assistant Surgeon, Division of Otolaryngology, Head and Neck Surgery, Brigham and Women's Hospital, Boston, Massachusetts
Rehabilitation of Lower Cranial Nerve Deficits After Neurotologic Skull Base Surgery

Fred F. Telischi, M.E.E., M.D.
Associate Professor, University of Miami School of Medicine; Jackson Memorial Hospital; Chief of Otolaryngology, Veterans Administration Hospital, Miami, Florida
Auditory Brainstem Implant

Anders Tjellström, M.D., Ph.D.
Associate Professor, Department of Otolaryngology, Sahlgren University Hospital, Göteborg, Sweden
The Bone-Anchored Hearing Aid

Mark S. Wallace, M.D., F.A.C.S.
Assistant Professor, Department of Otolaryngology–Head and Neck Surgery, Washington University School of Medicine; Attending Physician, Barnes–Jewish Hospital, St. Louis Children's Hospital, St. Louis, Missouri
Surgery of Acute Infections and Their Complications

Roger E. Wehrs, M.D.
Clincal Professor, University of Oklahoma College of Medicine; Active Staff, Saint Francis Hospital, Tulsa, Oklahoma
Tympanoplasty: Ossicular Tissue, Hydroxyapatite, and HAPEX

Richard J. Wiet, M.D.
Professor and Section Chief, Neurotology, Northwestern University Medical School, Chicago; Chief, Division of ENT, Evanston Hospital, Evanston, Illinois
Management of Complications of Chronic Otitis Media

Preface

The First Edition of *Otologic Surgery* published in 1994 was extremely well received by the otolaryngology community. We have received innumerable favorable comments from residents in training, as well as our colleagues in practice. The format of the book describing the various surgical techniques has proven to be very useful in day-to-day practice.

Since the publication of the First Edition, numerous changes have occurred in the field of otology. New instruments have been introduced, and surgical techniques have evolved. There has been expansion in the field with inclusion of skull base surgery.

With the rapidly evolving changes in the field, a revised edition of the text was necessary. The entire text has been updated and new chapters have been added to detail surgical procedures in our expanded field.

We are grateful for the acceptance of the First Edition of *Otologic Surgery* and hope that the Second Edition again meets your expectations.

Acknowledgments

Publication of a book of this scope requires a tremendous effort on the part of many, all of whom I wish to sincerely thank.

First, my thanks to my lovely wife, Charlotte, who supports all my efforts and forgave my absence for the time devoted to this project. No less supportive are our four sons, David, Douglas, Mark, and Steven, who provide diversion and pleasure by taking me hunting and fishing.

Since the publication of the first edition, two grandchildren, Lauren and Nicholas, have blessed Charlotte and me. What we have been told about the joy of grandparenting was underemphasized.

My associate editors, Dr. Shelton and Dr. Arriaga, worked tirelessly to bring this volume to fruition.

Anthony Pazos deserves special recognition. He spent countless hours in the temporal bone laboratory learning at first hand the various operations that he then illustrated. All the authors have appreciated his attention to detail and willingness to work with them until everything was "just right."

The publishers have been extremely supportive throughout the development of this book. From the beginning they made a major commitment to ensure that this volume was of the highest quality. I wish to thank particularly Stephanie Smith Donley.

Finally, I wish to thank our office staff, who work tirelessly on behalf of our patients and us. I would particularly like to thank Rita Koechowski, my surgery counselor, who not only schedules my surgery but also offers tremendous encouragement and support to all my patients. Her assistant, Robin Griffin, has been a tremendous help to both of us in supporting our patients.

I have recently been saddened by the untimely death of my secretary of seventeen years, Carol O'Reilly, who was great help to me in putting together the first edition of this text as well as this revision. She is sorely missed.

DERALD E. BRACKMANN, M.D.

I would like to thank my wife, Kay, and my children, Jordan and Bill, for their support and encouragement during my career development as well as their understanding regarding the demands of my profession.

I would also like to take this opportunity to thank my teachers, friends, and associates at the House Ear Clinic, and my teachers at Stanford, all of whom gave me the skills necessary to practice otologic surgery.

Special gratitude goes to Jim Sheehy and Blair Simmons, both of whom spent much time and effort teaching me to write scientific papers.

CLOUGH SHELTON, M.D.

I am particularly grateful to Derald Brackmann for the opportunity to participate in this book; his rational approach to patient care, incomparable surgical skills, innovations, patience as a teacher, and genuine personal warmth make him a role model to all young otologists.

Rosie, Becca, Moi-Moi, and Toby are continuing sources of encouragement and support. Thanks to Moisés Agusto and Leticia for their personal sacrifices and conviction that education is the only permanent gift from a parent to a child.

MOISÉS A. ARRIAGA, M.D.

Contents

†Deceased.

1

Otologic Instrumentation

James E. Benecke, Jr., M.D., F.A.C.S. ▪ Barbara A. Stahl, R.N.

Sophisticated micro-otosurgical techniques mandate that the otologic surgeon and surgical team have an in-depth understanding of the operating room (OR) layout and surgical instrumentation. This chapter provides a detailed description of different surgical procedures. The OR setup and instruments necessary for the various types of otologic procedures are described. The Appendix provides a comprehensive list of instruments and equipment.

THE OPERATING ROOM

The operating theater for otologic surgery requires features that differ from ORs that are used for nonotologic surgery. The following sections elaborate on the general environment of the OR designed for ear surgery. A word about the sterile field is in order. Respecting the sterile field is vital during routine otologic surgery and takes on special significance during neurotologic procedures. Maintaining the proper environment means limiting traffic through the OR and keeping the number of visitors to a minimum. It is preferable for observers to be in a remote room watching the procedures on video. Those allowed in the OR should be experienced in sterile technique and should wear jackets over scrubs so that all skin surfaces are covered. Some surgeons prefer that observers be "mummified" (Fig. 1–1).

The psychologic environment of the OR must be respected since many otologic procedures are performed on awake patients under local anesthesia. Members of the surgical team and visitors must use discretion when making comments during surgery.

The first piece of OR equipment to be discussed is the operating table. The surgeon must be comfortable while performing microsurgery. Adequate legroom under the table can be achieved with older OR tables by placing the patient 180 degrees opposite the usual position; in other words, the patient's head is where the feet would normally be (Fig. 1–2). Newer electric tables easily accommodate the patient and surgeon. Since most otologists spin the OR table 180 degrees after the induction of anesthesia, the new tables allow for spinning the table without unlocking it. Nonetheless, once the patient is properly positioned, the table must be firmly locked in place.

All ORs are equipped with wall suction. Standard suction devices are acceptable for otologic surgery. However, it is preferable to use a multiple-canister suction setup, minimizing the number of times the bottles must be emptied (Fig. 1–3). Suction systems have several locations

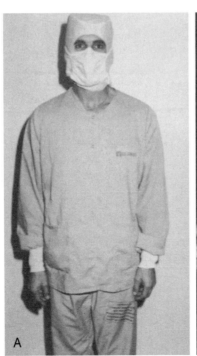
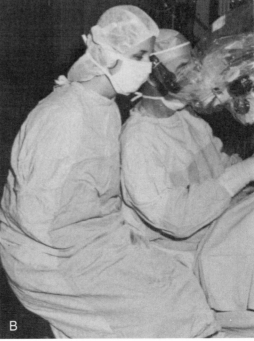

FIGURE 1–1. *A,* Observer in jacket. *B,* Observer mummified.

A

B

1

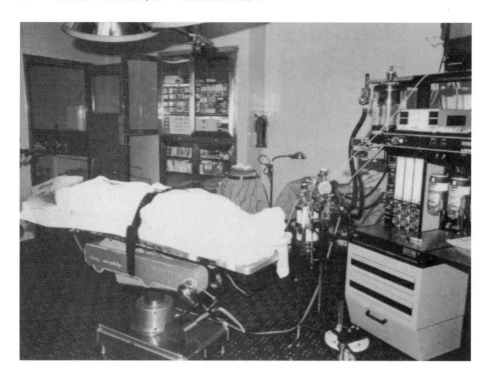

FIGURE 1–2. Operating table with patient's head at foot of bed.

where the amount of suction can be varied, but the surgeon should also employ a control clamp on the suction tubing on the sterile field (Fig. 1–4).

The tubing that is attached to the suction tips and suction irrigators should be highly flexible. The readily available disposable tubing is not flexible enough for microsurgery and places awkward torque on the surgeon's hands. Suction setup problems are common in every OR. The prudent team will troubleshoot the system in advance and have access to backup equipment.

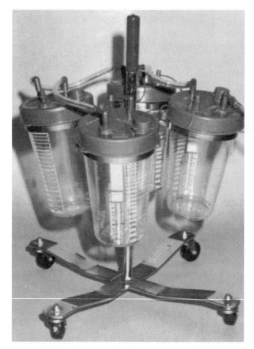

FIGURE 1–3. Multiple-canister suction setup.

Electrocautery equipment should be in a ready-to-use state on all procedures, except, perhaps, stapes surgery. The patient must be properly grounded. It is advantageous to have both unipolar and bipolar cautery on the field for all chronic ear and neurotologic procedures. Teflon tips are available for most cautery devices and are desirable. Surgeons are fortunate to have at their disposal a wide array of safe cautery devices, but they must be thoroughly familiar with these electrical instruments prior to use.

The surgical drill is another essential piece of equipment for otologic surgery. The vast array of available drills precludes an in-depth discussion of each system. In general, otologic drills fall into two categories: air driven and electrical. There are advantages and disadvantages to each type, and most surgeons have a distinct preference based on training and experience. For those using air-driven drills, it is preferable to use a central source of nitrogen to power the drill, instead of using room tanks of the gas. This eliminates the need for changing tanks during long cases.

High-speed drills capable of doing most of the bone work in the temporal bone include the Osteon, Fisch, Midas Rex, and Med-next drill systems. These drills, in general are not suitable for work in the middle ear, especially around the stapes footplate. For the latter purposes, a microdrill, such as the Skeeter drill, is suitable (Fig. 1–5). Whatever drill is used in the middle ear, it must have a variable speed control and a wide array of drill bits.

Most larger otologic drills are equipped with both straight and angled handpieces. Most surgeons prefer the straight handpieces for early gross removal of the mastoid cortex, switching to the angled handpiece for working deeper in the temporal bone. Midas Rex has a handpiece that can be converted from straight to angled simply by rotating the connection. A full complement of cutting and diamond burrs is mandatory. Space does not permit a detailed discussion of all available burrs and dissecting

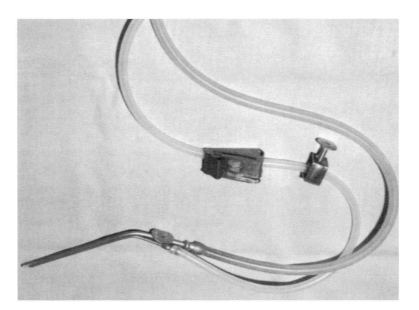

FIGURE 1–4. Suction tubing with control clamp.

tools for systems such as the Midas Rex and Med-next. Figures 1–6 and 1–7 show the two different drills and a sample of burrs. Most drill systems have attachments that vary in shape, diameter, and length. Needless to say, it is the surgeon's responsibility to be intimately familiar with the drill system and to have all of the attachments and burrs that might be needed.

The otologic drill should be held in the hand like a pencil, with the hand resting comfortably on the sterile field. The side of the burr should be utilized to provide maximum contract between the bone and the flutes of the burr, affording safer and more efficient drilling (Fig. 1–8). The newer drills are remarkably reliable, but, like other tools, may malfunction. Drill systems require proper care and inspection prior to use. A backup system should be readily available.

The introduction of the operating microscope revolutionized otologic surgery. Most otolaryngologists are familiar with the use of the microscope. Several brands of optically superior instruments are available, most sufficiently similar to share the same general principles.

The otologic surgeon must be familiar with the adjustments on the microscope and also must be prepared to troubleshoot the problems that may arise with the scope. The focal length of the objective lens is a matter of personal preference. Most otologists use a 200 mm or 250 mm objective. If a laser is attached to the microscope, one might even consider a 300 mm objective. The objective lens should be selected, confirmed, and properly mounted prior to draping the microscope. Other adjustments, such as the most comfortable interpupillary distance, should also be done before the scope is draped. Par focal vision should

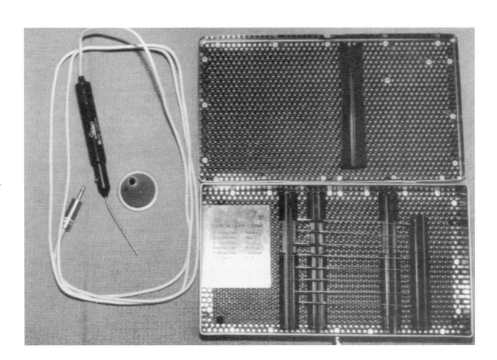

FIGURE 1–5. Skeeter microdrill for footplate work.

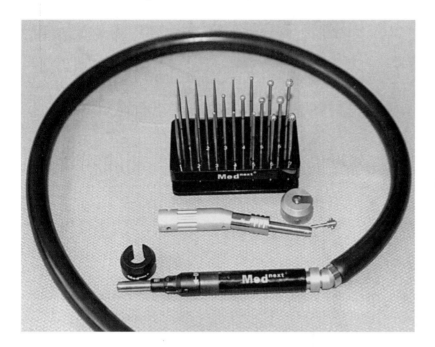

FIGURE 1–6. Med-next drill system.

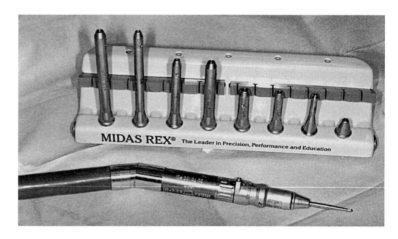

FIGURE 1–7. Midas Rex drill system.

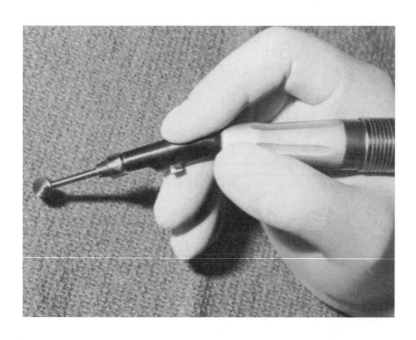

FIGURE 1–8. Proper holding of the drill.

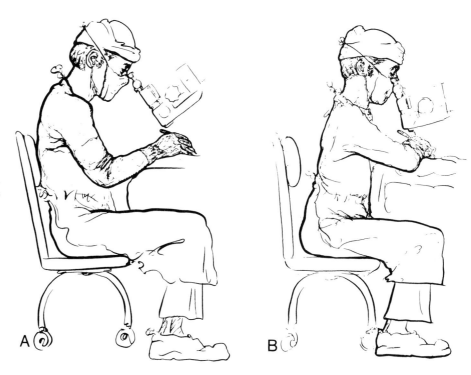

FIGURE 1–9. *A,* Proper posture for the surgeon. *B,* Wrong posture for the surgeon.

be established so that the surgeon can change magnification without having to change focus. This is accomplished by first setting the diopter setting of both eyepieces to zero. The 40× magnification (or highest available setting) is selected. The locked microscope is focused on a towel using the focus knob only. Without disturbing any of the settings, the magnification is now set at 6 × (or the lowest available setting). The eyepieces are then individually adjusted to obtain the sharpest possible image. The diopter readings are recorded for future use. The surgeon should have par focal vision when these appropriate eyepieces are used.

The microscope should move easily. All connections should be adjusted so that the microscope will not wander by itself yet permit movement to any position with minimal effort. Wrestling with the microscope during microsurgery is an extreme distraction.

Proper posture at the operating table is crucial. To perform microsurgical procedures, rule number one is that the surgeon must be comfortable. One should be seated comfortably in a proper chair with the back support at the correct height. Both feet should be resting comfortably on the floor. Fatigue is avoided by assuming a restful position in the chair rather than a rigid upright posture (Fig. 1–9).

The overall OR setup for routine otologic surgery is shown in Figure 1–10. For neurotologic surgery, more space must be available for additional equipment. Middle cranial fossa procedures require some modifications to the OR setup (Fig. 1–11). Basically, the surgeon and the microscope trade places such that the surgeon is seated at the

FIGURE 1–10. Usual otologic/neurotologic operating room setup.

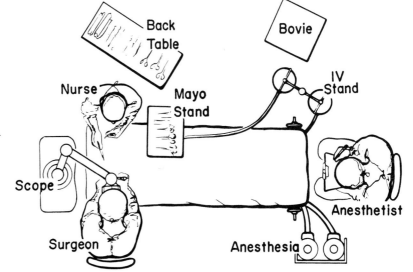

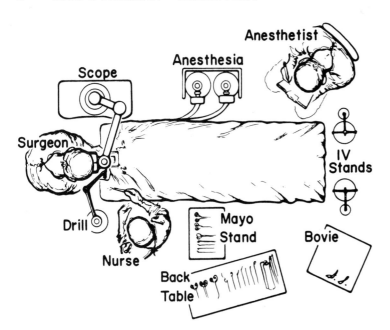

FIGURE 1–11. Operating room layout for middle fossa surgery.

head of the table. Cooperation and careful orchestration between surgeon, nursing personnel, and anesthesiologist are required for otologic surgery. The needs of the otologist are best served by having the anesthesiologist at the foot of the bed and the scrub nurse opposite the surgeon.

STAPES SURGERY

The following description of the instrumentation and operative setup for stapes surgery also provide information useful for other middle ear procedures. Under most circumstances, it is preferable to perform stapes surgery under local anesthesia, and surgeons who do so usually employ some type of preoperative sedation. Numerous regimens are available and are beyond the scope of this text. If sedation is administered by the surgeon or nursing personnel, without the assistance of an anesthetist or anesthesiologist, the agents used should be short acting and reversible.

It is far safer for the patient to be psychologically prepared for the procedure than to be oversedated. The author (JEB) prefers to perform all local anesthesia cases (including stapes surgery) under what is commonly known as MAC, or, monitored anesthesia care. This requires the presence of anesthesia personnel in the OR to sedate the patient, as is required for the operation, and also to monitor vital functions. This relieves the surgeon from this duty, allowing total concentration on the microsurgery.

About 30 minutes prior to the operation, the patient is brought to the preoperative holding area. If the surgeon routinely harvests a postauricular graft, this area is now shaved. A plastic aperture drape is applied to the operative site and trimmed so as not to cover the patient's face (Fig. 1–12). An intravenous (IV) line is started and the patient is now ready to go to the OR. Once the patient is on the OR table, the monitors are placed on the patient by the nursing or anesthesia staff. Minimal monitoring includes pulse oximetry, automatic blood pressure cuff, and electro-

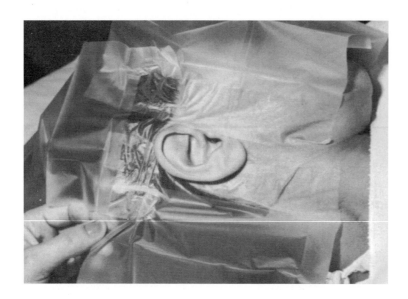

FIGURE 1–12. Plastic drape (3M) applied for stapes surgery.

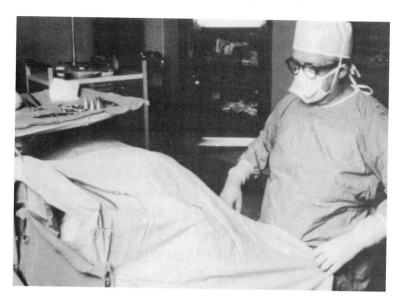

FIGURE 1–13. Patient draped in the operating room for stapes surgery.

cardiogram electrodes. The ear and plastic drape are scrubbed with an iodine-containing solution, unless the patient is allergic to iodine. A head drape is applied, and the ear is draped with sterile towels so as not to cover the patient's face. This can be facilitated by supporting the drapes with a metal bar attached to the OR table or by fixing the drapes to the scrub nurse's Mayo stand (Fig. 1–13).

The patient's head is now gently rotated as far away from the ipsilateral shoulder as possible, and the table is placed in slight Trendelenburg position. These maneuvers increase the surgeon's working room and help to straighten the external auditory canal (EAC). The EAC is gently irrigated with body-temperature saline. Vigorous cleaning of the canal is avoided until the ear is anesthetized. The local anesthesia is administered with a plastic Luer-Lok–type syringe that has finger and thumb control holes. A 1½ inch, 27-gauge needle is firmly attached to the syringe. If the ear is injected slowly and strategically, excellent anesthesia and hemostasis can be achieved with a solution of 1 per cent lidocaine with 1:100,000 epinephrine. Some surgeons prefer stronger concentrations of epinephrine, such as 1:40,000. When using stronger concentrations of epinephrine, the patient's blood pressure and cardiac status must be considered, in addition to the possibility of mixing errors.

The canal is injected slowly in four quadrants starting lateral to the bony-cartilaginous junction. The final injection is in the vascular strip. If one routinely harvests fascia or tragal perichondrium, these areas are now injected.

Before describing stapes surgical instruments, a few general comments are in order. All microsurgical instruments should be periodically inspected to ensure sharp points and cutting surfaces. The instruments for delicate work should have malleable shanks, enabling the surgeon to bend the instrument to meet the demands of the situation.

If the surgeon prefers a total stapedectomy over the small fenestra technique, an oval window seal must be selected. If fascia is used, the tissue is harvested prior to exposing the middle ear. The tissue is then placed on a Teflon block or fascia press to dry. If perichondrium is

preferred, this may be harvested immediately prior to footplate removal. For the small fenestra technique, a small sample of venous blood is obtained when the IV is started. This is passed to the scrub nurse and placed in a vial on the sterile field.

A variety of ear specula should be available in both oval and round configurations. Sizes typically range from 4.5 to 6.5 mm (Fig. 1–14). It is desirable to always work through the largest speculum that the meatus will permit, without lacerating canal skin. Some surgeons prefer to use a speculum holder for stapes and other middle ear procedures. The tympanomeatal flap is started with incisions made at the 6 and 12 o'clock positions with the No. 1, or sickle, knife. These incisions are united with the No. 2, or lancet, knife. This instrument actually undermines the vascular strip instead of cutting it. The strip is then cut with the Bellucci scissors. The defined flap is elevated to the tympanic annulus with the large round knife, known as the large "weapon." Once properly identified, the annulus is elevated superiorly with the Rosen needle, and inferiorly with the annulus elevator, or gimmick. Figure 1–15 shows a typical set of stapes instruments, including suction tips.

Adequate exposure usually requires removal of the bony

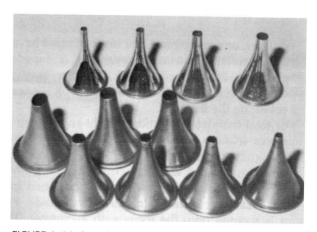

FIGURE 1–14. Speculum array.

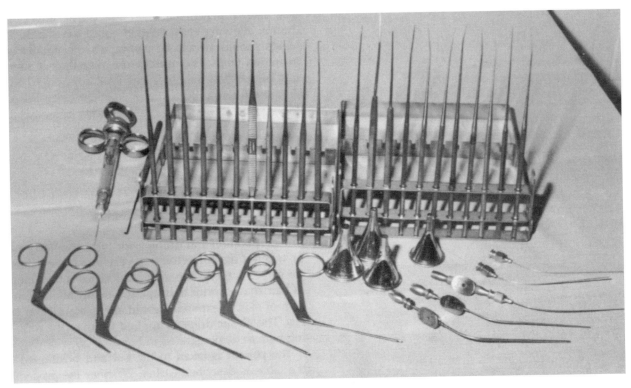

FIGURE 1–15. Stapes instruments.

ledge in the posterosuperior quadrant. This can be initiated with the Skeeter microdrill and completed with a stapes curette (Fig. 1–16).

From this point on, the steps differ depending on the technique preferred by the surgeon. The diagnosis of otosclerosis should be confirmed on entering the middle ear, and a measurement should be taken from the long process of the incus to the stapes footplate with a measuring stick. The next step is to make a control hole in the footplate with a sharp pick/needle (Barbara needle) or the laser. The incudostapedial joint is separated with the joint knife, the tendon is cut with scissors or laser, and the superstructure is fractured inferiorly and extracted.

For work on the footplate, the surgeon must have a variety of suitable instruments available. A stapedotomy can be created with a microdrill, laser, or needles and hooks. The 0.3-mm obtuse hook is useful for enlarging the fenestra.

For total footplate extraction, a right-angle hook or excavator (Hough hoe) is used. The harvested graft is guided into place with a footplate chisel. The prosthesis is grasped with a smooth alligator or strut forceps and placed on the incus. It is positioned on the graft, or into the fenestra, with a strut guide. The wire is secured onto the incus with a crimper, or wire-closing forceps. The McGee crimper is useful, especially if followed by a fine alligator forceps for the last gentle squeeze. A small right-angle hook may be necessary to fine-tune the position of the prosthesis (Fig. 1–17).

Suction tubes for stapes surgery include Nos. 3 to 7 Fr Baron suctions plus Rosen needle suction tips (18 to 24 gauge) with the House adapter (Fig. 1–18). The Rosen tips are useful when working near the oval window, with the surgeon's thumb off the thumb port.

Ear packing following stapes surgery is accomplished with an antibiotic ointment to hold the flap in place. A piece of cotton suffices as a dressing unless a postauricular incision has been made, in which case a mastoid dressing is applied.

For all middle ear procedures, the surgeon should hold the instruments properly. The instrument should rest, like a pencil, between the index finger and thumb, allowing easy rotation about the shank. The hands should always be resting on the patient and the OR table. The middle and ring fingers should rest on the speculum, so that the hand moves as a unit with the patient. Proper hand position

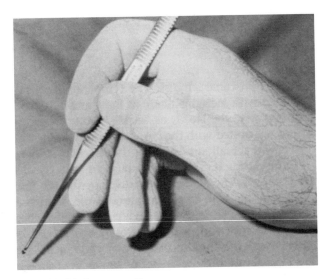

FIGURE 1–16. Stapes curette.

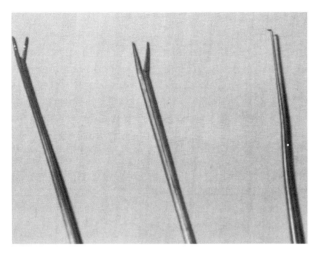

FIGURE 1–17. Crimpers and footplate hook.

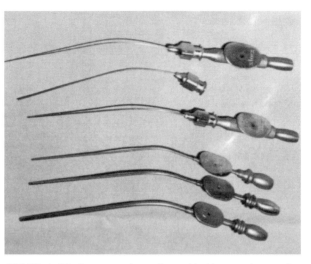

FIGURE 1–18. Rosen suction tubes with House adapter; Baron tubes.

and holding of instruments should afford the surgeon an unimpeded view (Fig. 1–19).

TYMPANOPLASTY AND TYMPANOPLASTY WITH MASTOIDECTOMY

The preparation and draping for tympanoplasty with or without mastoidectomy are much the same as for stapes surgery. The major difference is the amount of hair shaved prior to draping. Usually, enough hair is shaved to expose about 3 to 4 cm of skin behind the postauricular sulcus. The plastic drape is applied to cover the remaining hair, as seen in Figure 1–20.

The patient is positioned on the OR table as described earlier. Whether the procedure is performed under local or general anesthesia depends on the extent of the surgery, the surgeon's preference, and, of course, the desire of the patient. After appropriate sedation or induction of anesthesia, the ear and plastic drape are scrubbed with the proper

soap or solution. Some surgeons place a cotton ball in the meatus if a perforation exists, preferring not to allow the prep solution to enter the middle ear. The field is draped as described earlier, the head is rotated toward the contralateral shoulder, and the table is placed in slight Trendelenburg (Fig. 1–21). The postauricular area, canal, and tragus (if necessary) are injected with 1 per cent lidocaine with 1:100,000 epinephrine for both local and general anesthesia cases.

Most chronic ear procedures begin in a similar fashion. Through an ear speculum, vascular strip incisions are made with the sickle or Robinson knife and united along the annulus with the lancet knife. The vascular strip incisions are completed with a No. 64 or 67 Beaver blade. This same blade can be used to transect the anterior canal skin just medial to the bony-cartilaginous junction. The postauricular incision is then made with a No. 15 Bard-Parker blade behind the sulcus. The level of the temporalis fascia is identified, and a small self-retaining (Weitlaner) retractor is inserted. The fascia is cleared of areolar tissue

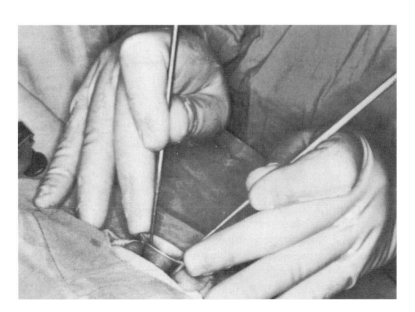

FIGURE 1–19. Proper holding of instruments.

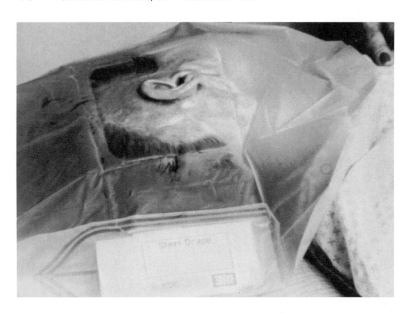

FIGURE 1–20. Drape (3M 1020) applied for chronic ear surgery.

and incised. A generous area of fascia is undermined and removed with Metzenbaum scissors. The scrub nurse can assist by using a Senn retractor to elevate skin and soft tissues away from the fascia. The fascia is thinned on the Teflon block and dehydrated by placing it under an incandescent bulb, carefully monitoring its progress. The fascia may also be dehydrated by placing it on a large piece of Gelfoam and compressing this complex in a fascia press. Figure 1–22 shows the instruments used in the initial stages of chronic ear surgery.

Continued postauricular exposure is obtained by incising along the linea temporalis with a knife or with the electrocautery. A perpendicular incision is then made down to the mastoid tip. Soft tissues and periosteum are elevated with a Lempert elevator (Fig. 1–23, *upper*), the vascular strip is identified, and a large self-retaining retractor is inserted. A very large retractor, such as an Adson cerebellar retractor with sharp prongs, is preferred. The retractors can be modified as shown in Figure 1–24. Rings have been attached so that a small oxygen catheter can be threaded and attached to suction. This acts as a sump in the most dependent portion of the wound.

Next, under the microscope, the anterior canal skin is removed down to the level of the annulus with the large weapon. The plane between the fibrous layer of the drum remnant and the epithelium is developed with a sickle knife, and the skin is pulled free with a cup forceps. The anterior canal skin is placed in saline for later use as a free graft. The ear canal is then enlarged with the drill and suction-irrigators. An angled handpiced and medium to small cutting burr are used. Irrigation through the suction-irrigators is done with a physiologic solution such as Tis-U-Sol, lactated Ringer's, or saline. Two large (3000 ml) bags of irrigant are hung and connected by way of a three-way stopcock to the delivery system (Fig. 1–25).

For mastoidectomy surgery, the surgeon must have a full array of cutting and diamond burrs, as well as a complete set of suction-irrigators. It is advisable to have bone wax and Surgical readily available. Cholesteatoma removal can be accomplished with middle ear instruments such as the gimmick, weapon, and fine scissors.

Although the setup for closing and packing following chronic ear surgery varies with the specifics of the situation, a few generalities should cover most situations en-

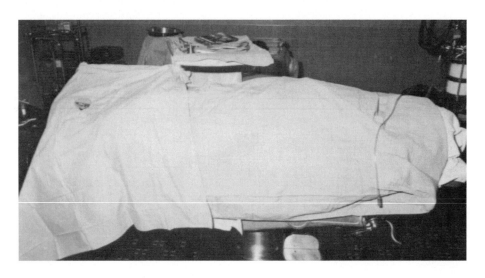

FIGURE 1–21. Chronic ear surgery draping for local anesthesia.

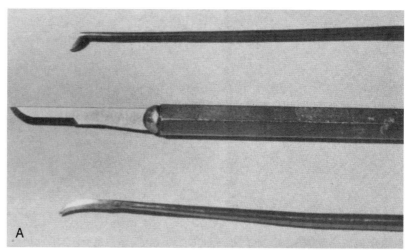

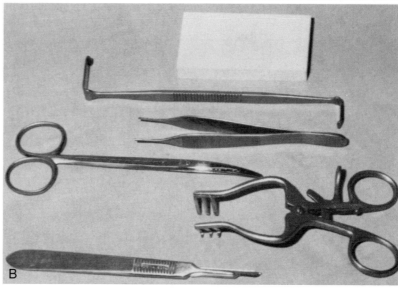

FIGURE 1–22. *A*, Instruments for making canal incisions. *B*, Instruments for handling fascia.

countered by the otologist. To maintain the middle ear space, Silastic sheeting works well and is still readily available. This comes in various thicknesses, with and without reinforcement. For middle ear packing, Gelfoam is the usual choice, soaked in saline or an antibiotic otic preparation. The same Gelfoam is used to pack the EAC, through some surgeons prefer an antibiotic ointment, as described in the section on stapes surgery. For meatoplasty packing, 1-inch Adaptic or nasal packing gauze is saturated with an antibiotic ointment and rolled around the tip of a

bayonet forceps. This creates a plug that conforms to the new meatus and is easily removed (Fig. 1–26).

Wound closure is accomplished in two layers with absorbable sutures. The skin is closed with a running intradermal suture of 4-0 Vicryl or Dexon on a cutting needle. Steri-Strips are applied, and the wound covered with a standard mastoid dressing.

There are some additional instruments that prove to be handy in many chronic ear procedures. These include an ossicle holder, Crabtree dissectors, Zini mirrors, right-angle

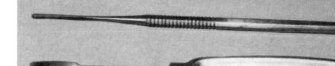

FIGURE 1–23. Periosteal elevators.

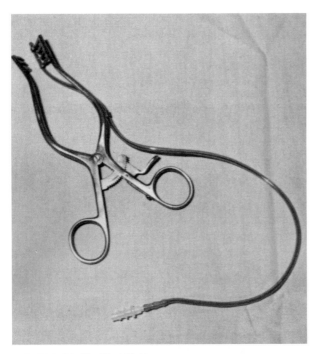

FIGURE 1–24. Modified Weitlaner retractor.

hooks, and the House-Dieter malleus nipper (Fig. 1–27). It is impossible to describe instruments for every conceivable situation, but the foregoing should cover most of the needs of the otologist.

ENDOLYMPHATIC SAC SURGERY

There are many well-described procedures on the endolymphatic sac (ELS). It is not the purpose of this chapter to outline the surgical options but rather to discuss the methodology for performing sac surgery. The preparation and draping of the patient for ELS surgery are essentially the same as for tympanoplasty with mastoidectomy surgery. In the preoperative holding area the postauricular area is shaved, exposing at least 4 cm of skin behind the sulcus. Plastic adhesive drapes are applied and the patient is transported to the OR. ELS surgery is performed under general anesthesia. The field is scrubbed in the usual manner, and the patient is positioned as described for chronic ear surgery.

This would be a good time to briefly mention the use of intraoperative facial nerve monitoring (FNM) and other forms of physiologic monitoring, including eighth nerve and cochlear potentials. Suffice it to say that many surgeons use FNM whenever the facial nerve might be in jeopardy. Electrodes for FNM or other forms of monitoring should be positioned prior to the prep.

After the prep for ELS surgery, the planned incision is injected with 1 per cent lidocaine with 1:100,000 epinephrine. The incision is made 2 to 3 cm behind the sulcus. Periosteal incisions are made sharply or with the electrocautery. A Lempert elevator elevates soft tissues and periosteum up to the level of the spine of Henle. A House narrow (canal) elevator is used to delineate the EAC, and a large self-retaining retractor inserted. With drill and suc-

tion-irrigator, a complete mastoidectomy is performed. The antrum is *not* widely opened but is instead blocked with a large piece of Gelfoam to prevent bone debris from entering the middle ear.

Bone over the sigmoid sinus and posterior fossa dura is thinned with diamond burrs. The retrofacial air tract is opened widely to locate the ELS. The sac is decompressed with a diamond burr. A stapes currette can be used to remove bone over the proximal sac. The occasional bleeding that occurs over the surface of the sac or surrounding dura is best controlled with bipolar cautery. Alternatively, unipolar cautery at a very low setting can be used. The cautery tip is touched to an insulated Rosen or gimmick that is in contact with the offending vessel (Fig. 1–28). Another method used to control small areas of bleeding in ELS and chronic ear surgery is to cover the area with pledgets of Gelforms that have been soaked in topical thrombin.

Prior to opening the sac, the wound is copiously irrigated with saline or bacitracin solution. Fresh towels are placed around the field. The sac is opened with a disposable Beaver ophthalmic blade (No. 59S, 5910, or 5920). The lumen is probed with a blund hook or gimmick. The shunt tube preferred by the surgeon is now inserted. Thin Silastic sheeting (0.005 inch) can be used to fashion a shunt. Figure 1–29 shows the materials for the latter steps of ELS surgery. As with chronic ear procedures, the wound is closed in layers, usually beginning with 2-0 chromic and finishing with 4-0 Vicryl or Dexon. A standard mastoid

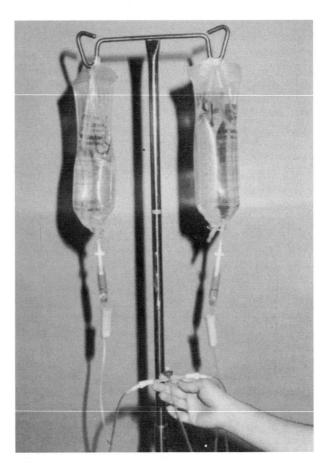

FIGURE 1–25. Irrigation setup with three-way stopcock.

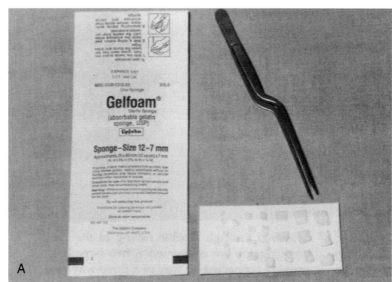

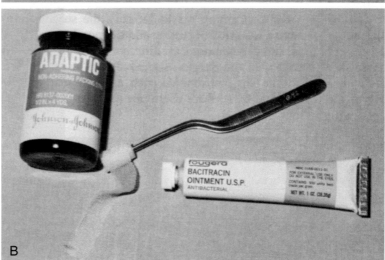

FIGURE 1–26. *A,* Gelfoam packing. *B,* Adaptic meatoplasty packing.

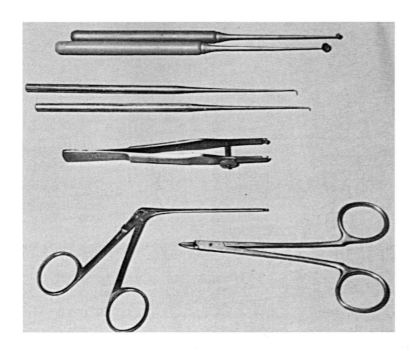

FIGURE 1–27. Additional instruments used in chronic ear procedures (see text).

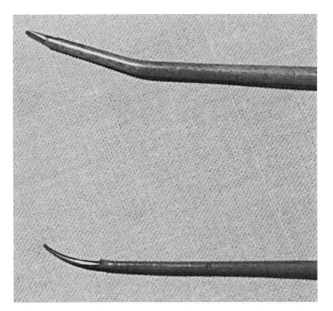

FIGURE 1–28. Insulated gimmick *(top)* and Rosen *(bottom)*.

dressing is applied. This is either manufactured in the OR or is obtained as a prepackaged dressing (e.g., Glasscock dressing).

NEUROTOLOGIC PROCEDURES

This section describes the OR layout for neurotologic procedures, the only exception being middle fossa surgery, which is discussed separately. For procedures involving intracranial structures, extraordinarily meticulous attention to detail is mandatory. The preparation for neurotologic surgery may begin the evening prior to surgery by having the patient wash his or her hair and scalp with an antiseptic

shampoo. The day of surgery, the patient is seen by the surgeon in the holding area so that the ear to be operated on is positively identified. The surgical site is shaved so that at least 6 cm of postauricular scalp is exposed. The area is sprayed with an adhesive and the plastic drapes are applied (Fig. 1–30). At the same time, the abdomen is shaved from below the umbilicus to the inguinal ligaments, in preparation for harvesting a fat graft. The fat donor site is surrounded by plastic drapes (Fig. 1–31).

After anesthetic induction, a catheter is inserted and, when indicated, arterial and central venous lines are placed. Electrodes for monitoring cranial nerves VII and VIII (and possibly other nerves) are positioned. The patient's head is supported on towels or a "donut" as needed and rotated toward the contralateral shoulder. The surgical sites are scrubbed, then blotted dry with a sterile towel. The areas are draped off with towels and then covered with plastic adhesive drapes (e.g., Steri-Drape, Ioban, Cranial-Incise). Some surgeons prefer to next include another layer of towels around the cranial site, followed by either sheets or a disposable split sheet. It is important to have several layers of draping to prevent saturation of the drapes with fluids down to level of the patient (Fig. 1–32).

Because the scrub nurse must handle a number of items attached to tubes and cords, it is helpful to have fastened to the field a plastic pouch into which the drill, suction, and cautery tips can be placed (Fig. 1–33). Two Mayo stands are kept near the field: one for the neurotologic instruments and the other for the fat-harvesting tools (Fig. 1–34).

The postauricular area is injected with the usual local anesthetic, and the plastic drape is then cut away with scissors to expose the mastoid and lateral subocciput. As with other procedures, a skin incision is made, hemostasis is obtained, soft tissues and periosteum are elevated, and a large self-retaining retractor is inserted. Bone removal is accomplished using a drill and suction-irrigation. For neu-

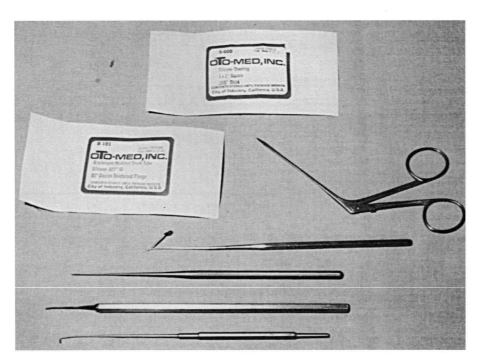

FIGURE 1–29. Endolymphatic sac instruments and materials.

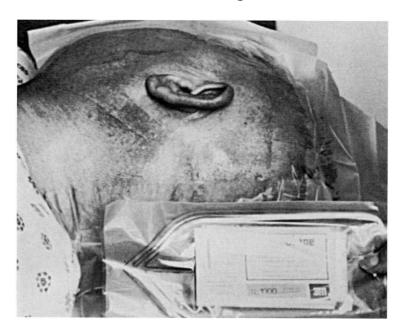

FIGURE 1–30. Drapes (3M 1000) applied for neurotologic surgery.

rotologic cases, bone removal is more extensive, exposing
the sigmoid sinus and a considerable amount of posterior
fossa dura behind the sigmoid. It is imperative that the
surgeon have immediate access to bone wax and Surgicel.
Hemoclips and thrombin-soaked Gelfoam are other items
that many surgeons insist on having immediate access to.

The extent of bone removal varies depending on the
surgeon's preference and the nature of the procedure. Some
surgeons completely decompress the sigmoid, whereas others leave a thin shell of bone over the sinus (Bill's island).
After appropriate bone removal, the retractor is removed
and the field is vigorously irrigated with bacitracin solution.
Bacitracin solution can be prepared by dissolving 50,000
U of bacitracin in 1 L of normal saline. After wound
irrigation, fresh towels are placed around the field.

With a wound free of bone dust and debris, the dura can
now be opened. This can be accomplished with a No. 11
Bard-Parker scalpel blade or with the tips of the Jacobson
scissors. The dura can be pulled away from underlying

structures by using a corkscrew-like instrument, included
in some neurotologic instrument sets (Fig. 1–35). The
subdural space is entered, taking care not to violate the
arachnoid. This helps to avoid injury to vessels prior to
adequate exposure. The dural flap is carefully developed
with Jacobson scissors. Hemostasis is controlled with bipolar cautery. The arachnoid is carefully opened with a sharp
hook or the tips of the scissors, allowing the egress of
cerebrospinal fluid (CSF). Figure 1–35 shows the instruments for dural and arachnoid opening. After opening the
arachnoid, one should switch to fenestrated (Brackmann)
suction tips (Fig. 1–36). The cerebellum and other intracranial structures should be protected with moist neurosurgical cottonoids. A variety of cottonoids should always be
on the field.

For vestibular neurectomy procedures, the plane between
the cochlear and vestibular nerves can be developed with
a blunt hook, or the gimmick. The nerve section itself can
be completed with a sharp hook or microscissors (Fig.

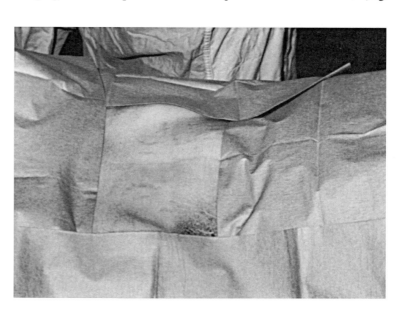

FIGURE 1–31. Abdominal area prepared.

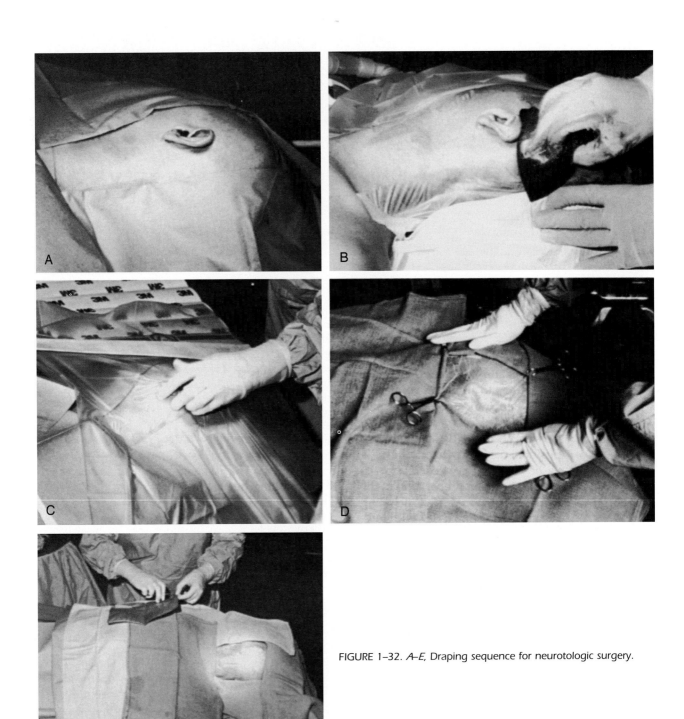

FIGURE 1–32. *A–E*, Draping sequence for neurotologic surgery.

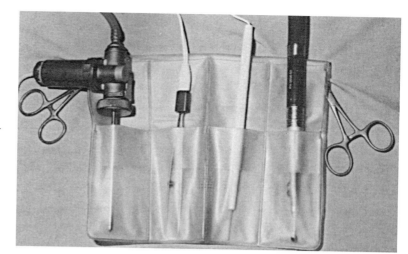

FIGURE 1–33. SK-100 Surgi-kit for holding instruments.

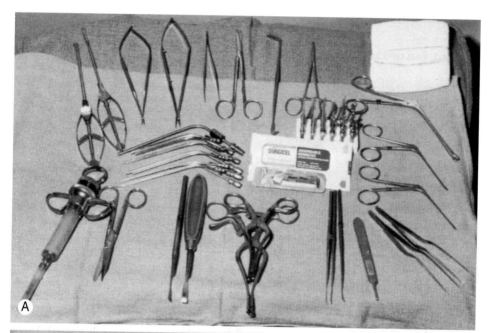

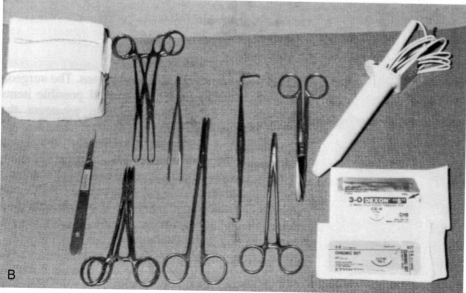

FIGURE 1–34. *A,* Mayo stand setup for tumor. *B,* Mayo stand setup for fat graft.

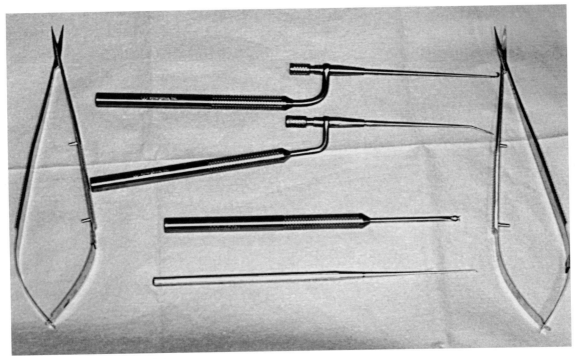

FIGURE 1–35. Benecke neurotologic instruments.

1–37). The same instruments can be used to define the plane between an acoustic neuroma and the facial nerve. A sharp right-angle hook palpates Bill's bar and sections the superior vestibular nerve fibers along with the vestibulofacial fibers. After establishing the proper plane between the tumor and facial nerve, a blunt hook is used to continue the dissection, taking care not to stretch the facial nerve. FNM has greatly facilitated this part of the dissection. For small tumors, the previously mentioned technique might suffice for total tumor removal. Larger tumors are removed by gutting the tumor extensively, mobilizing the capsule, and then removing the capsule in a piecemeal fashion. This

is accomplished by morselizing the tumor with a large crushing forceps, such as the Decker. The Urban rotary suction-dissector is used to extract the pieces (Fig. 1–38). Bayonet forceps direct the tumor into the suction port of the Urban. As the tumor is gutted, the capsule collapses and can be dissected from the brainstem.

The Cavitron ultrasonic aspirator is another instrument that some surgeons prefer for gutting the tumor. Whatever tool is used, proper use of these sophisticated, and potentially dangerous, instruments must be learned from user manuals and appropriate inservices and courses.

Hemostasis is vital during neurotologic surgery, and the surgeon must have immediate access to all possible items necessary to control bleeding from whatever the source. In addition to unipolar and bipolar cautery, bone wax and precut pieces of Surgicel should be on the Mayo stand. Microfibrillar collagen (Avitene) is another preferred hemostatic agent to have available. Pledgets of Gelfoam soaked in topical thrombin are quite useful. Vascular clips and a reliable clip applicator are useful for controlling bleeding from the petrosal vein and its tributaries (Fig. 1–39).

Infratemporal fossa and other approaches to the skull base are set up in much the same manner as has already been discussed. Incisions are generally longer and may even extend into the upper cervical region to access major neurovascular structures. Silastic vessel loops should be placed around these structures for control and easy identification. Ligatures of 0 silk and transfixion sutures of 2-0 silk need to be available for jugular vein ligation. Cardiovascular sutures (e.g., 5-0 and 6-0 Prolene) should also be close by.

The self-retaining retractors described earlier are usually insufficient for skull base surgery. The Fisch infratemporal retractor or a pediatric rib retractor are better suited to these tasks, which often include anterior displacement of

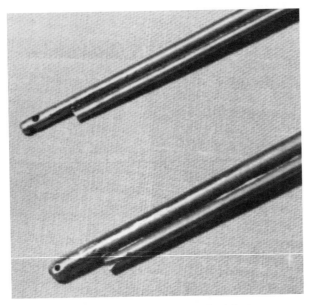

FIGURE 1–36. Brackmann fenestrated suction-irrigators.

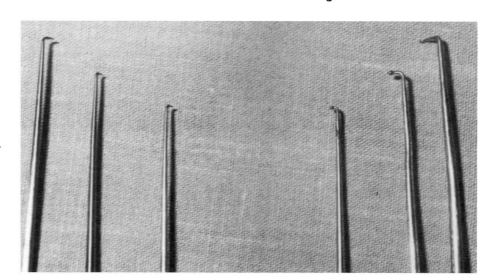

FIGURE 1–37. Hooks for neurectomy and tumor dissection.

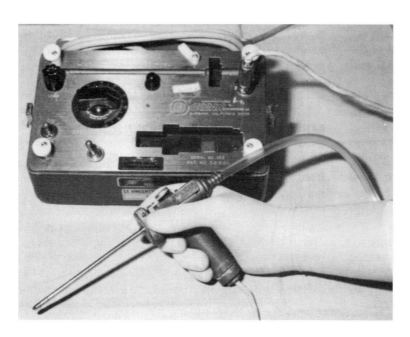

FIGURE 1–38. Urban dissector.

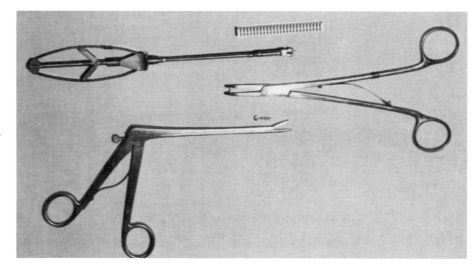

FIGURE 1–39. Clips and clip applicators.

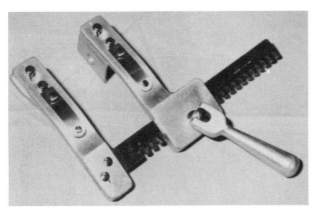

FIGURE 1–40. Rib retractor for infratemporal fossa surgery.

the mandible (Fig. 1–40). If mandibulotomy is indicated, the appropriate oscillating saw will need to be available.

There are some instruments that facilitate work on or near the facial nerve. For rerouting the facial nerve, bone is removed with a drill until an eggshell thickness remains. The remaining bone is gently removed with a stapes curette. The nerve can be mobilized with a dental excavator or microraspatory. If a segment of the nerve is to be excised, as in a facial neuroma, this should be done sharply with a fresh knife blade. Likewise, prior to any neurorrhaphy, the ends of the nerve and graft should be freshened. A 9-0 monofilament suture is used for nerve anastomosis. Appropriate needle holders and forceps must be available (Fig. 1–41).

Prior to closing neurotologic and skull base wounds, abdominal fat is removed from the left lower quadrant, most of the dissection being done with electrocautery. The abdominal wound is closed (over a drain if necessary) in layers, with the skin being approximated with a running intradermal 4-0 Vicryl or Dexon. The fat is cut into strips and insinuated into the dural defect. Continuous lumbar drainage is rarely necessary to prevent CSF leakage, except in extensive intracranial-extracranial resections. If the neck is opened, a suction drain is inserted into the depths of the

wound prior to closure. Wounds are closed as in other otologic procedures and dressed with a standard mastoid dressing.

Also under the rubric of neurotologic surgery is cochlear implant surgery. Each presently available cochlear implant device has its own unique set of requirements and, possibly, instruments. The surgeon must have proper training and experience to perform cochlear implant procedures. He or she must have all of the necessary special equipment for electrode placement and internal receiver fixation (Fig. 1–42).

MIDDLE CRANIAL FOSSA SURGERY

Middle fossa procedures are discussed separately from other neurotologic procedures because they involve a different OR setup and some different instruments. The most obvious deviation from other procedures is the position from which the surgeon operates. The surgeon and the microscope trade locations, so that the surgeon operates from the head of the bed facing caudally (see Fig. 1–11).

As with other neurotologic procedures, middle fossa surgery is performed under general anesthesia. In the preoperative holding area, the ipsilateral scalp is shaved to a distance of 6 cm postauricularly and nearly to the midline of the head above the ear in the temporal fossa. Plastic adhesive drapes are applied and the patient is taken to the OR. After anesthesia, the surgical site and plastic drapes are scrubbed and blotted dry. The area is covered with another plastic adhesive drape. Towels are positioned to block off the entire temporoparietal scalp, including the auricle and zygomatic arch. Sterile sheets complete the draping (Fig. 1–43). The abdomen is usually prepared as in other neurotologic surgeries.

The incision is planned so that it begins in the preauricular incisura below the root of the zygoma. It extends cephalad to the area just above the superficial temporal line. A gentle curve facilitates exposure. Prior to the incision, as in other cases, the area is infiltrated with local anesthesia.

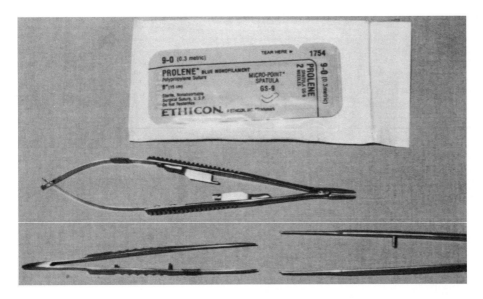

FIGURE 1–41. Nerve anastomosis equipment.

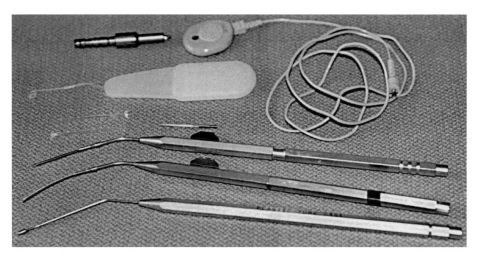

FIGURE 1–42. Cochlear implant tools.

The plastic drape is cut away to expose the skin. After the skin incision is made, the superficial temporal vessels are identified and ligated. After the temporalis fascia is identified, it is recommended that an inferiorly based temporalis muscle flap be created, instead of splitting the muscle. This flap is centered over the zygoma, is elevated from the calvarium, and is reflected caudally by suturing the end of the flap to the drapes. Preserving the muscle with its neurovascular bundle does not limit the surgeon's exposure and allows the use of this muscle if facial reanimation surgery should ever be necessary. The remaining temporalis muscle is reflected laterally and a self-retaining retractor is inserted. A craniotomy is then performed. The size of the bone flap removed is dictated by the amount of exposure necessary. For tumor removal, it is wise to err on the large side.

The bone flap is carefully removed from the dura with an Adson periosteal elevator, or "joker" (Fig. 1–44). The bone flap is then placed in bacitracin solution. The craniotomy edges are smoothed with a rongeur and bleeding is controlled with bone wax.

The joker is used to dissect the dura from the floor of the middle fossa. The surgeon is now ready to insert the House-Urban middle fossa retractor. The surgeon must be familiar with the mechanical workings of this device (Fig. 1–45). The retractor is locked under the bony edges of the craniotomy. The blade housing is positioned so that it allows good visualization of the field without placing excessive traction on the temporal lobe. This usually requires repositioning the retractor several times during the early stages of the dissection. Next, the retractor blade is inserted and the extradural dissection proceeds. The blade can be tilted with the hand and advanced with the thumb, leaving the other hand free for suctioning. Bleeding can be troublesome from the floor of the middle fossa, especially near the middle meningeal artery. Bipolar cautery, bone wax, Surgicel, and other hemostatic agents should be readily available.

The surgeon elevates the dura and temporal lobe until the arcuate eminence, superior petrosal sinus, and greater superficial petrosal nerve are visible. Bone over the internal auditory canal (IAC) and geniculate ganglion is removed with a large diamond burr. When the dura over the IAC has been completely skeletonized as far medially as the porus, the wound is irrigated with bacitracin solution and fresh towels are placed around the field. The dura over the IAC is opened posteriorly (away from the facial nerve) with a sharp hook. For vestibular neurectomy, Bill's bar is palpated with the same sharp hook that then transects the superior vestibular nerve. Fine microscissors (e.g., Malis, Jacobson) are used to remove a segment of the nerve in continuity with Scarpa's ganglion. In a likewise fashion, the inferior vestibular and singular nerves are sectioned.

For acoustic tumor removal, significantly more bone removal is required. Having established adequate exposure, the plane between the facial nerve and tumor is developed as in the translabyrinthine approach.

At the conclusion of the procedure, the defect over the IAC can be reconstructed by filling it with small pieces of

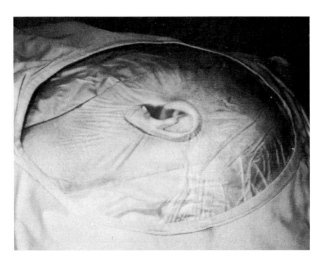

FIGURE 1–43. Patient draped for middle fossa surgery.

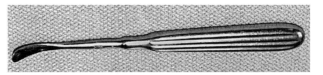

FIGURE 1–44. Adson periosteal elevator ("joker").

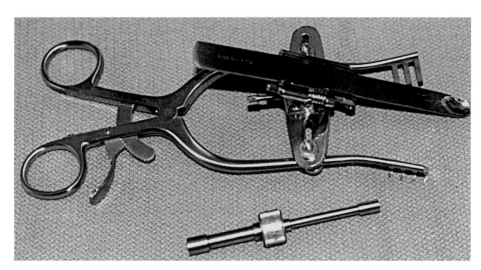

FIGURE 1–45. House-Urban middle fossa retractor.

muscle or abdominal fat and covering it with a small piece of the bone flap that has been cut and trimmed to an appropriate size. The field is inspected for hemostasis and the middle fossa retractor is removed, allowing the brain to re-expand. The wound is once again irrigated with bacitracin. The bone flap is sutured in place with Vicryl sutures and the wound is closed in layers, suturing the temporalis flap back to its normal anatomic position. Some surgeons close the skin over a Penrose drain, which is removed the day following surgery. A mastoid dressing completes the closure.

CONCLUSION

This chapter has provided a detailed description of the OR environment and instrumentation for the majority of procedures that the otologist is likely to encounter. Although these descriptions by no means exhaust all possibilities, they have proved to be satisfactory for many otologists. The Appendix contains the lists of instruments and equipment that have been presented in the text.

Appendix

INSTRUMENTS AND EQUIPMENT FOR OTOLOGIC SURGERY

General Operating Room Equipment

1. 3M 1000 plastic aperture drapes
2. 3M 1020 aperture drapes
3. 3M Steri-Drape, Ioban drape, or Cranial-Incise drape
4. Pharmaseal preoperative skin preparation tray, No. 4480
5. Dow-Corning flexible surgical tubing
6. Suction canisters
7. Electrocautery unit
8. Skytron operating table

Stapes Surgery

1. Assorted Farrior specula
2. Finger-control Luer-Lok syringe
3. 1½ inch, 25- or 27-gauge needle
4. Small Weitlaner retractor
5. Sheehy fascia press
6. House cutting block
7. Scalpel, No. 15 Bard-Parker blade
8. Adson tissue forceps
9. Iris scissors
10. House-Baron suction tubes, No. 3–7 Fr
11. House suction tube adapter
12. Rosen suction tubes, 18–24 gauge
13. Sickle knife (No. 1 knife)
14. Lancet knife (No. 2 knife)
15. Robinson knife
16. Sheehy-House weapon (large and small)
17. Rosen needle
18. House elevator
19. Gimmick annulus elevator
20. House stapes curette
21. Incudostapedial joint knife
22. Bellucci scissors
23. Straight Barbara pick
24. Measuring struts, 4.0–5.0 mm
25. Measuring disk, 0.6 mm
26. Hough hoe
27. Obtuse, 30-degree, 0.25-mm hook
28. Pick, 0.3 mm, 90 degree
29. Strut guide
30. Footplate chisel
31. Skeeter drill; 1.0-, 0.7-, and 0.6-mm burrs
32. House strut forceps (nonserrated)
33. McGee wire closing forceps (crimper)
34. Antibiotic ointment
35. Cotton balls, Band-Aids, mastoid dressing
36. Speculum holder

Chronic Ear Surgery

1. Assorted Farrior specula
2. Finger-control syringe
3. 1½-inch, 25- or 27-gauge needle
4. Small Weitlaner retractor
5. Large self-retaining retractor (Weitlaner, Adson cerebellar)
6. Scalpel, No. 15 Bard-Parker blade
7. No. 64 or 67 Beaver blade
8. House cutting block
9. Sheehy fascia press
10. House-Baron suction tubes, No. 3–7 Fr
11. Adson forceps
12. Iris scissors
13. Small Metzenbaum scissors
14. Sickle knife
15. Lancet knife
16. Robinson knife
17. Sheehy-House weapon (large and small)
18. Rosen needle
19. Gimmick
20. Crabtree dissector (large and small)
21. Lempert elevator
22. House narrow elevator
23. Pick, right angle, 0.6 mm
24. Pick, right angle, 1.5 mm
25. Pick, right angle, 3 mm
26. Bellucci scissors
27. Hartmann forceps
28. House alligator forceps
29. House cup forceps
30. House-Dieter malleus nipper
31. Zini mirrors
32. Sheehy ossicle holder
33. Speculum, endaural (or nasal)
34. Drill with cutting and diamond burrs
35. House suction-irrigators, No. 2.5 × 4 Fr through No. 8 × 12 Fr
36. Needle holder, Webster
37. Suture scissors
38. Suture, 2-0 chromic and 4-0 Vicryl (or Dexon)
39. Gelfoam (saline- and antibiotic-soaked)
40. Adaptic gauze
41. Silastic sheeting
42. Gelfilm
43. Steri-Strips
44. Mastoid dressing
45. Bone wax
46. Surgicel
47. Sheehy bone pate collector

Endolymphatic Sac Surgery

1. Finger-control syringe
2. 1½ inch, 25- or 27-gauge needle
3. Scalpel, No. 15 Bard-Parker blade
4. Large self-retaining retractor
5. Lempert elevator
6. House narrow elevator
7. Drill and burrs
8. House suction-irrigators (assortment)
9. Brackmann suction-irrigators, No. 4 × 5 Fr, No. 5 × 7 Fr
10. Stapes curette
11. Gimmick
12. Insulated gimmick
13. Bone wax
14. Surgicel
15. Bipolar cautery

16. Bacitracin irrigation solution
17. Beaver ophthalmic blade (No. 59S, 5910, or 5920)
18. Pick, right angle, 1.5 mm
19. Hook, right angle, blunt
20. Rosen needle
21. House alligator forceps
22. Shunt tube or material
23. Suture, 2-0 chromic and 4-0 Vicryl (or Dexon)
24. Steri-Strips
25. Mastoid dressing
26. Cranial nerve monitoring equipment

Neurotologic Surgery

1. Finger-control syringe
2. 1½ inch, 25- or 27-gauge needle
3. Scalpel, No. 15 Bard-Parker blade
4. Large self-retaining retractor
5. Lempert elevator
6. House narrow elevator
7. Drill and burrs
8. Assorted House suction-irrigators
9. Assorted Brackmann suction-irrigators
10. Stapes curette
11. Gimmick
12. Insulated gimmick
13. Bone wax
14. Surgicel
15. Bipolar cautery
16. Bacitracin irrigation
17. SK-100 Surgi-Kit (Ethox Corp.)
18. Suture scissors
19. House-Urban dissector
20. Pick, right angle, 1 mm
21. Pick, right angle, 1.5 mm
22. Hook, right angle, blunt, 1.5 mm
23. Bellucci scissors
24. House cup forceps
25. Blakesley nasal forceps (No. 1)
26. House alligator forceps
27. Myringoplasty knife
28. Jacobson scissors
29. Malis scissors
30. Allis forceps
31. Bayonet forceps
32. Adson tissue forceps
33. Microclip applicator
34. Assorted hemostats
35. Metzenbaum scissors
36. Senn retractor
37. U.S. Army retractor
38. Pediatric rib retractor
39. Fisch infratemporal fossa retractor
40. Woodson elevator
41. Fisch microraspatory
42. Sagittal saw
43. Needle holder, Castroviejo

44. Needle holder, Crile-Wood
45. Needle holder, Webster
46. Avitene
47. Drains, Penrose and Jackson-Pratt
48. Vessel loops
49. Suture, 5-0 and 6-0 vascular Prolene
50. Suture, 0 and 2-0 chromic
51. Suture, 0 and 2-0 silk
52. Suture, 9-0 nylon or Prolene
53. Suture, 4-0 Dexon or Vicryl
54. Neurosurgical cottonoids
55. Steri-Strips
56. Mastoid dressing
57. Topical thrombin
58. Gelfoam
59. Special neurotologic instrument sets (e.g., Kartush, Benecke)
60. Cranial nerve monitoring equipment

Middle Cranial Fossa Surgery

1. Finger-control syringe
2. 1½ inch, 25- or 27-gauge needle
3. Scalpel, No. 15 Bard-Parker blade
4. Large self-retaining retractor
5. Lempert elevator
6. House narrow elevator
7. Drill and burrs
8. Assorted House suction-irrigators
9. Brackmann suction-irrigators
10. Stapes curette
11. Gimmick
12. Insulated gimmick
13. Bone wax
14. Surgicel
15. Bipolar cautery
16. Bacitracin irrigation
17. SK-100 Surgi-Kit
18. Pick, right angle, 1 mm
19. Pick, right angle 1.5 mm
20. Hook, right angle, blunt, 1.5 mm
21. Bellucci scissors
22. House cup forceps
23. Metzenbaum scissors
24. House-Urban middle fossa retractor
25. Rongeur, Leksell
26. Adson tissue forceps
27. Microclip applicator
28. Assorted hemostats
29. Avitene
30. Cottonoids
31. Gelfoam
32. Suture, 0 and 2-0 chromic
33. Suture, 4-0 Vicryl (or Dexon)
34. Topical thrombin
35. Mastoid dressing
36. Special neurotologic instrument sets
37. Cranial nerve monitoring equipment

2

Canalplasty for Exostoses of the External Auditory Canal and Miscellaneous Auditory Canal Problems

Rodney Perkins, M.D. ▪ Joseph B. Roberson, Jr., M.D.

Although the clinical disease caused by exostoses of the external auditory canal is not frequent, it occurs often enough to warrant that a method of surgical management be in the armamentarium of the otologic surgeon. Because it is not a high-incidence problem or one that is life threatening, most otolaryngologists use a variety of independent approaches that, by and large, result in elimination of or damage to the canal skin. Unfortunately, these procedures frequently produce less than optimal results. A well-conceived approach addresses the problem of exostoses' removal while maintaining the valuable residual skin of the external auditory canal. This chapter begins with clinical observations regarding this condition and then describes an operative procedure that has been very successful in its management.

The etiology of these benign growths of the tympanic bone is not completely understood. A widely held belief based on clinical information is that they occur primarily during the years of growth, their proliferation being enhanced or perhaps even caused by exposure to cold water during this period. This tends to be supported by historical information from patients with exostoses, who almost always indicate that they swam in cold water during their youth.[1-3] This is strongly corroborated by the high incidence of the problem in avid surfers who spend hours in the water almost daily. In our clinical experience, this problem occurs almost exclusively in males, who are more likely than females of the same age to have had frequent cold water exposure during their youth.

Most exostoses do not develop to a degree sufficient to cause clinical symptoms. Patients are frequently referred to otologists because the growths are observed, and not understood, by primary care physicians. This is particularly true with those that have a more pedunculated form than the more subtle sessile configuration. However, when exostoses become more marked, they obstruct the natural elimination of desquamated epithelium from the ear canal, and patients usually present with recurrent episodes of external otitis. In their most prolific expression, exostoses can lead to hearing impairment by causing the collection of epithelial debris that tamponades tympanic membrane movement, by impinging on and limiting the mobility of the malleus, or by markedly narrowing the aperture of the canal. These conditions may appear as a conductive hearing impairment on audiometric examination.

The external auditory canal is part of the hearing pathway. Essentially, it is a tube with resonant characteristics that amplify the incoming sound. The degree of amplification and the frequency at which it occurs are a function of the diameter and the length of the canal. When the diameter becomes small, it can interfere with the passage of sound and cause a hearing impairment. However, this effect does not become significant until the aperture becomes very small. With apertures under 3 mm, high-frequency sounds begin to diminish, and further compromise of the channel diameter results in increased impairment and lower-frequency loss.

EXOSTOSES OF THE EXTERNAL AUDITORY CANAL

Surgical Indications

Surgery is indicated when chronic or recurrent external otitis exists or a conductive hearing impairment develops. The presence of chronic and recurrent infection over an extended period seems to debilitate the canal skin and can compromise the skin's ability to re-epithelialize in a robust and healthy manner in the postoperative period. For this reason, surgical therapy should be considered once a pattern of recurrent external otitis has been established in these patients. Patients who have significant external canal exostoses without recurrent infection or hearing impairment should be observed periodically, and surgery should be avoided until these symptoms occur.

Preoperative Preparation

Patient Preparation

There are two components of patient preparation for otologic surgery performed under local anesthesia: psychologic and pharmacologic.

Psychologic. To reduce anxiety and create rapport, the surgeon should provide the patient with a full explanation of the procedure and its objectives, benefits, and risks. In addition, a surgical nurse or medical assistant should explain what will happen to the patient in the operating room by describing such things as the operating room environment, use of an intravenous line for medication delivery, placement of monitor electrodes, and draping. By informing the patient of these things and making him or her part of the process, the clinician reduces the patient's anxiety, encourages cooperation, and reduces bleeding. Beyond the technical advantages achieved by such preparation, there is an ethical responsibility to inform the patient. In addition, the likelihood of the patient's becoming litigious because of a poor result is markedly reduced if he or she has been informed about the procedure and its risks and benefits and has had an opportunity to discuss them with the surgeon prior to the surgery.

Pharmacologic. The chemical preparation of the patient can be achieved in many ways. In the average adult, we give fentanyl 50 to 100 μg and midazolam (Versed) 5 to 10 mg intramuscularly 1 hour prior to the surgical incision. An intravenous catheter is started in the arm opposite the ear to be operated on before the patient arrives in the operating room, and 5 per cent dextrose in Ringer's solution is started with a Volutrol. Unless the patient appears very sedated, an additional 50- to 100-μg dose of fentanyl is placed in the Volutrol and infused slowly over 30 to 45 minutes. As the surgery proceeds, alternating supplements of intravenous midazolam and fentanyl are infused as needed to maintain sedation. In addition, patients receive cefazolin 1 g intravenously or another appropriate antibiotic 1 hour before surgery.

Site Preparation

The hair is shaved behind the ear to a distance of approximately 1.5 inches posterior to the postauricular fold. The auricle and the periauricular and postauricular areas are scrubbed with povidone-iodine (Betadine) solution. A plastic drape is placed over the area with the auricle and the postauricular area exteriorized through the opening in the drape. This drape is placed over an L-shaped bar that is fixed in the rail attachment of the operating table (Fig. 2–1). Attached to the bar is a small, low-volume office fan that provides a gentle cooling breeze to the patient's face during the procedure. The plastic drape forms a canopy, allowing the patient to see from under the drape and reducing the feeling of claustrophobia. In addition, a foam earpiece from an insert speaker is put into the opposite ear. The earpiece is connected to a compact disk player and input microphone that allows the patient to listen to relaxing music and provides a pathway to converse with the patient, if desired.

Analgesia

It is important not only to achieve analgesia but also to maximize canal hemostasis with injections into the external auditory meatus. Using 2 per cent lidocaine (Xylocaine) with 1:20,000 epinephrine solution in a ringed syringe with a 27-gauge needle, a classic quadratic injection is made such that each injection falls within the wheal of the previous injection. Another useful injection is an anterior canal injection, which is made with the bevel of the needle parallel to the bony wall of the external meatus (Fig. 2–2). In the patient with extensive exostoses, this injection is usually made into the lateral base of a large anterior sessile osteoma. After insinuation of the needle, it is advanced a few millimeters, and a few drops are injected extremely slowly. The solution infiltrates medially along the anterior canal wall and provides some analgesia to the auriculotemporal branch of cranial nerve V, which is usually unaffected by the quadratic injection and adds to the hemostasis anteriorly. The postauricular area is infiltrated with 2 per cent lidocaine with 1:100,000 epinephrine solution mixed with equal parts of 0.5 per cent bupivacaine.

Surgical Technique

Most surgical approaches for removal of external canal exostoses are done through the transmeatal route.[4–6] This approach has two distinct disadvantages. It usually results in significant loss of the remaining canal wall skin through damage by the drill, and it does not allow adequate visibility or instrument and drill access to safely remove the medial portion of the exostotic mass near the tympanic membrane. A large sessile anterior exostosis is almost uniformly present in these patients (Fig. 2–3). The approach described here is primarily postauricular and one that maximizes conservation of the canal wall skin and facilitates careful removal of the anterior exostosis, which is usually extremely close to the tympanic membrane.

A curvilinear postauricular incision is made approximately 1 cm behind the postauricular fold (Fig. 2–4). The skin and subcutaneous tissues are elevated anteriorly to the area of the spine of Henle and the bony posterior canal, and a toothed, self-retaining retractor is placed (Fig. 2–5). Locating this area is facilitated by finding the plane of the lateral surface of the inferior border of the temporalis muscle and dissecting in this plane anteriorly to reach the meatus. Once this area is reached, the skin overlying the lateral slope of the posterior exostosis is elevated from its surface, and a Perkins bladed tympanoplasty retractor is inserted such that it holds elevated skin off the surface of the lateral portion of the bony mass (Fig. 2–6). Although there may be more than one posterior and anterior exostosis, predominant anterior and posterior exostoses are usually present along with others of lesser mass. These secondary masses may be handled similarly to the primary exostoses or may be removed directly. However, to simplify the description, this operation is divided into two major segments: removal of the posterior exostosis and removal of the anterior exostosis.

Removal of Posterior Exostosis

By use of medium-sized cutting burr and an appropriately scaled suction-irrigator, the posterior exostosis is entered along its lateral sloping edge, and the bony removal is progressed medially, keeping a shell of bone over the area being burred anteriorly (Fig. 2–7). Thus, the remaining skin over the exostosis medial to that elevated earlier is protected from the burr. As this shell becomes thinner, it is advisable to switch to a diamond burr to prevent a sudden breakthrough to the skin that might occur if one continues with the cutting burr on the excessively thinned bone. The bone removal is continued medially and posteriorly until the estimated normal posterior canal contour and dimension is achieved. As one approaches a medial depth

FIGURE 2-1

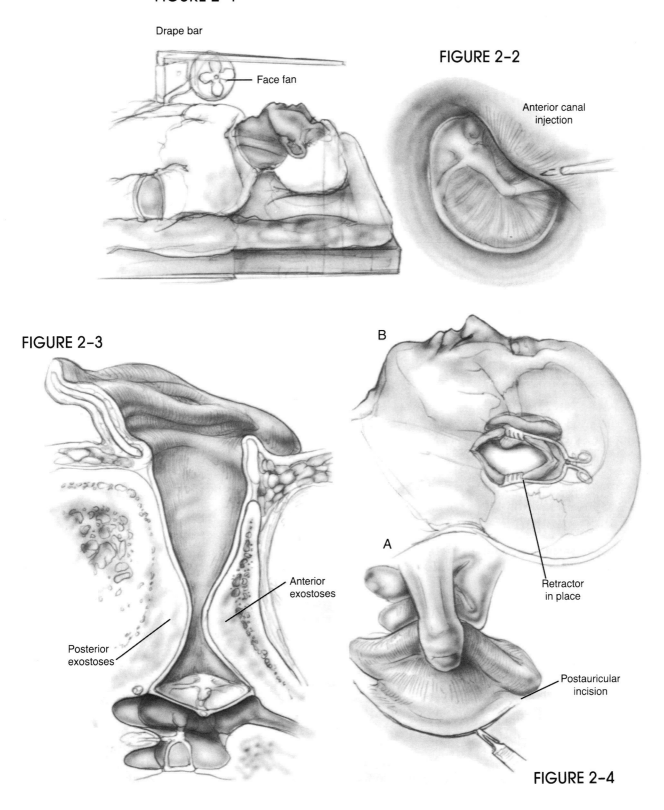

Drape bar

Face fan

FIGURE 2-2

Anterior canal injection

FIGURE 2-3

Anterior exostoses

Posterior exostoses

B

A

Retractor in place

Postauricular incision

FIGURE 2-4

consistent with the posterior annulus of the tympanic membrane (which usually cannot be seen directly at this point), care must be taken to avoid damage to the chorda tympani nerve and the posterior aspect of the tympanic membrane. It should also remain in the surgeon's mind that some

patients' facial nerve exists lateral to the tympanic annulus at its posteroinferior border. Facial nerve monitoring reduces the possibility of injury to the nerve in the patient unable to tolerate local anesthesia. The thinned bony shell is collapsed, and a small elevator reveals the inside surface

FIGURE 2–5

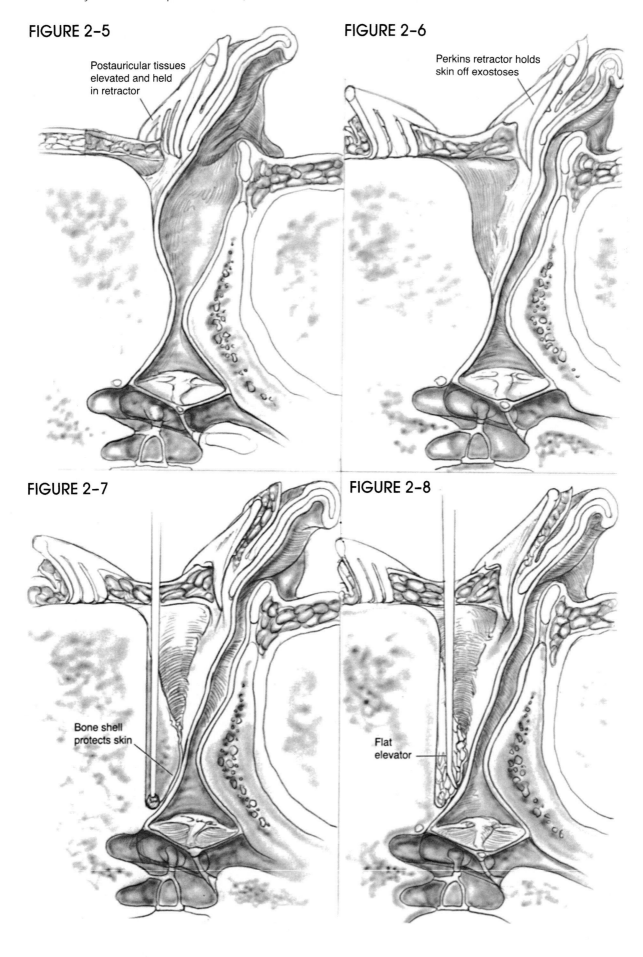

Postauricular tissues elevated and held in retractor

FIGURE 2–6

Perkins retractor holds skin off exostoses

FIGURE 2–7

Bone shell protects skin

FIGURE 2–8

Flat elevator

of the posterior canal skin that was over the exostosis (Fig. 2–8).

An incision is made midway along the posterior canal skin perpendicular to the long axis of the external auditory canal. (Fig. 2–9). The posterior canal skin medial to this incision is then positioned onto the new contour of the posterior canal wall (Fig. 2–10). Then, the transmeatal approach is taken, and incisions are made with a sickle knife superiorly and inferiorly in the canal, extending from the ends of this previous incision laterally to the meatus and creating a laterally based posterior canal skin flap. This flap is then involuted back into the meatal portion of the canal and held there with the Perkins retractor (Fig. 2–11). Attention is then turned to the anterior exostosis, which has now been revealed.

Removal of Anterior Exostosis

By use of a round knife, an incision is made in the skin overlying the anterior exostosis from superior to inferior over the dome of the exostosis and as far medially as can be seen. This incision is connected to the incisions previously made superiorly and inferiorly in the canal that defined the posterior canal skin flap, and this anterior canal flap is elevated laterally (Fig. 2–12). Frequently, the skin of the vascular strip can be left intact if the exostoses do not involve this portion of the canal. By use of a back-angled Perkins tympanoplasty elevator, this laterally based anterior canal skin flap is elevated further to the cartilaginous portion of the anterior canal and is then smoothed so as to lie laterally near the posterior canal flap under the retractor (Fig. 2–13).

With a cutting burr and small suction-irrigator, the anterior exostosis is removed in a manner similar to that of the posterior one, and a thin shell of bone that protects the canal skin is left over the anteromedial portion of the exostosis from the burr (Fig. 2–14). This bone removal is continued to the area of the anterior annulus of the tympanic membrane. The bony shell is then collapsed and removed, leaving the intact anterior canal skin (Fig. 2–15). Usually, it is necessary to finish up and smooth an edge of bone that remains at the anterior extent of this dissection to have a smooth contour near the annulus area. To protect the elevated anterior sulcus skin from the burr, a small tympanic membrane–sized piece of silicone sheeting (Silastic) is placed on the inside surface of the anterior canal skin to hold it against the tympanic membrane during drilling. This prevents the skin flap from getting involved with the burr and also prevents damage to the tympanic membrane that might occur with the burr being used in such close proximity to the membrane. Subsequently, the Silastic is removed, the medial anterior canal skin is placed on the bone, and all skin flaps are folded back into position on the new contours of the bony canal (Fig. 2–16). The medial flaps are packed into place with chloramphenicol (Chloromycetin)–soaked absorbable gelatin sponge (Gelfoam) pledgets, and the postauricular incision is closed with interrupted subcuticular 4-0 Vicryl suture.

Through the transmeatal route the laterally based canal skin flaps are packed into place with gelatin sponge pledgets. A cotton ball is placed in the meatus, and a mastoid dressing is applied. The patient is returned to the outpatient recovery area and discharged 2 hours later.

Postoperative Care

The patient is placed on prophylactic antibiotics for 5 days and is instructed to remove the mastoid dressing the next morning. The gelatin sponge packing is removed using the stereo microscope on the first office visit 1 week later. Antibiotic-steroid ear drops are prescribed for use twice daily for 1 week and once every 3 days for another 3 weeks. The second postoperative visit is at 1 month. If there is no evidence of infection, no additional drops are recommended. Because most of the patients in whom this procedure is done have had recurrent external otitis, and because time is needed for epithelialization of uncovered bone, the ear canal may remain moist for a longer period than in a typical tympanoplasty. Until the ear canal is completely dry and healed, the patient should be seen every few weeks to inspect and clean debris from the canal as needed.

It should be remembered that the canal skin has usually been exposed to numerous infections and has been stretched over the exostoses; therefore, it may not be as resilient as normal canal skin. Return to water exposure should be avoided until 2 months after complete healing has occurred. Frequently, however, avid surfers return to the water much sooner than instructed. Antibiotic drops given after water exposure reduce the risk of early postoperative infection. If the patient is still in the growth years, further repeated exposure of the ear to cold water should be moderated. The bone may reproliferate under these conditions, and further surgery may become necessary. In patients who want to return to frequent surfing or similar water exposure, earplugs should be worn to prevent water entrance. This problem lessens in older surfers because they may be beyond their rapid growth phase, and the economic exigencies of life tend to decrease their frequency of exposure. It is advisable to see the patient annually for 2 years to assess the tendency for the problem to recur, although recurrence is infrequent.

Problems and Complications

Although this procedure is not fraught with serious complications, complications can occur during several aspects of the operation. As the medial extent of the canal is approached in the removal of the posterior exostosis, the course of the chorda tympani nerve must be kept in mind. This portion of the bone removal is done largely without definite landmarks: the surgeon must rely on mental estimation of the distances in arriving at the posterior annulus. The chorda tympani nerve is beneath the bone near this field of dissection and could suffer damage. Also, it is important to remember the course of the facial nerve, which passes posterior and inferior to the canal, although this area is farther from the immediate area of dissection than is the chorda tympani nerve. When a burr is used very near the tympanic membrane and the malleus, a diamond

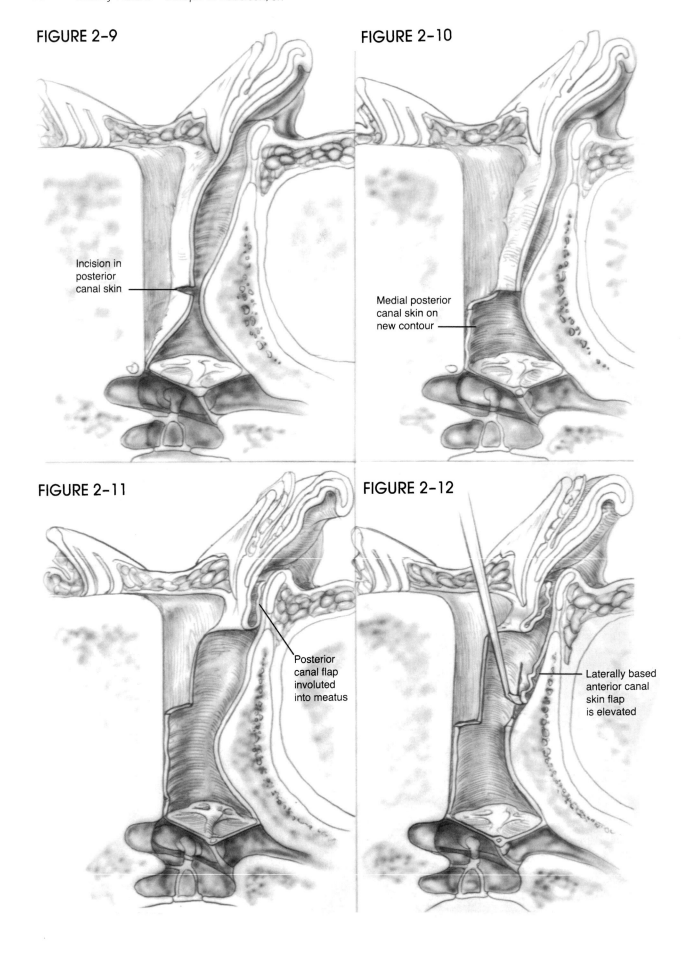

FIGURE 2-9

Incision in posterior canal skin

FIGURE 2-10

Medial posterior canal skin on new contour

FIGURE 2-11

Posterior canal flap involuted into meatus

FIGURE 2-12

Laterally based anterior canal skin flap is elevated

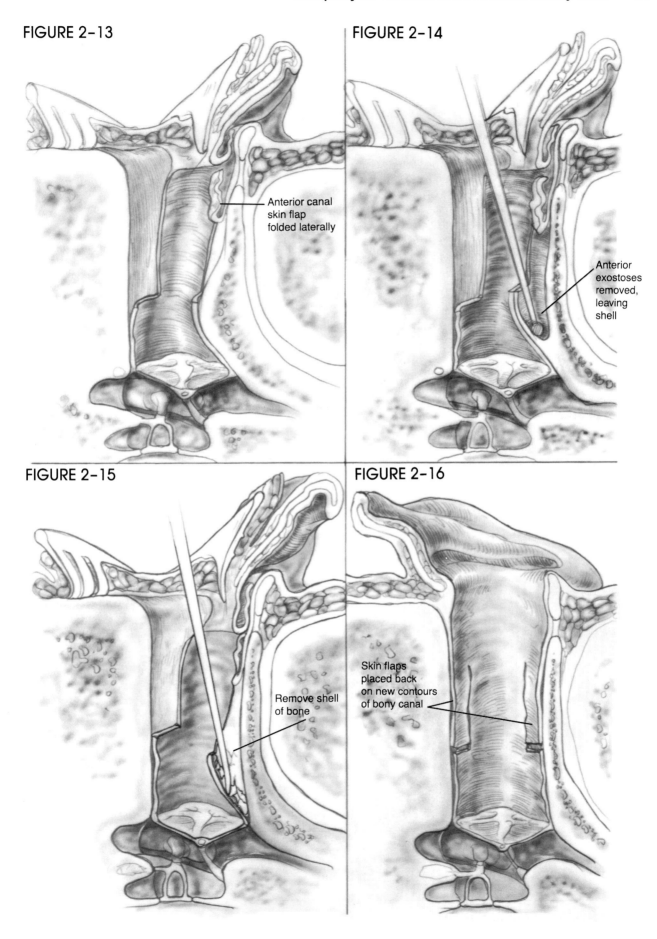

FIGURE 2–13

Anterior canal skin flap folded laterally

FIGURE 2–14

Anterior exostoses removed, leaving shell

FIGURE 2–15

Remove shell of bone

FIGURE 2–16

Skin flaps placed back on new contours of bony canal

burr should be used because it is less likely to run erratically than is the cutting burr.

Summary

Exostoses of the external auditory canal usually present without attendant compromise in function or clinical disease. However, when recurrent external otitis or hearing impairment results, surgical removal is indicated. Canalplasty has significant advantages over commonly employed transmeatal approaches by maximizing conservation of canal skin and providing surgical access to the anterior medial zone of the canal. Complications are infrequent, but attention to the anatomy of the chorda tympani and facial nerve pathways and careful drill technique in the area of the tympanic membrane are important.

Although surgical techniques involving the external auditory canal have had little attention compared with other reconstructive procedures, they should be in the armamentarium of all otologic surgeons. This technique has proved to be effective for the management of exostoses of the external auditory canal.

MISCELLANEOUS EXTERNAL AUDITORY CANAL CONDITIONS

Medial Third Stenosis

For unknown reasons, some patients develop weeping epitheliitis over the medial third of the external auditory canal. Treatment consists of antibiotic-steroid ear drops that supply broad-spectrum bacterial coverage. Intense treatment, including débridement in addition to the use of topical agents, is usually necessary to bring the process under control. Despite attempts at treatment, progression of the condition may follow a relentless course, resulting in dense fibrosis of the medial segment of the external auditory canal with conductive hearing loss. The mesotympanum and ossicular chain are characteristically spared.

Surgical repair may be necessary when conductive hearing loss produces a functionally significant deficit for the patient. Successful repair is frequently possible, although restenosis may occur and should be included in the informed consent. Technically, a postauricular approach is used to allow complete resection of the fibrotic segment medial to noninvolved external auditory canal skin where an incision has been previously created working through a transcanal route (Fig. 2–17). Removal of most of the fibrous layer of the tympanic membrane appears to lower the chance of postoperative restenosis. Tympanoplasty is performed with a lateral graft or Fasciaform technique. Coverage of the resultant exposed bone is mandatory and is provided with a free split-thickness skin graft. The skin of the posterior surface of the pinna provides skin of appropriate character within the operative field and can be taken with a No. 10 blade. Skin grafts should overlap the fascia used for tympanic membrane replacement but should not extend to cover the lateral surface of the reconstructed drum. Antibiotic-containing absorbable packing is removed 7 to 14 days later and antibiotic-steroid ear drops are continued for 2 weeks beyond healing to be tapered over time. Close observation postoperatively is necessary to intervene with any signs of restenosis. Recurrent epitheliitis may occur months or years following successful repair.

Collapsing Canal

Stenosis of the cartilaginous portion of the lateral external auditory canal may produce symptoms for some patients. In severe cases, conductive hearing loss may result when closure to less than 2 mm occurs. More commonly, accumulation of debri and a warm, moist environment lead to recurrent external otitis. Although this condition occurs naturally, an iatrogenic component is frequently present.

FIGURE 2-17

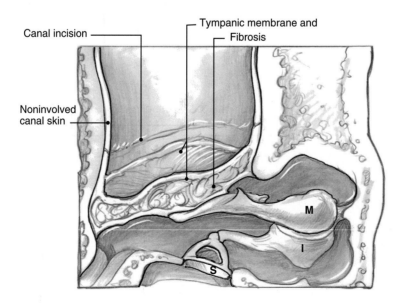

Canal incision

Tympanic membrane and Fibrosis

Noninvolved canal skin

M

I

S

FIGURE 2-18

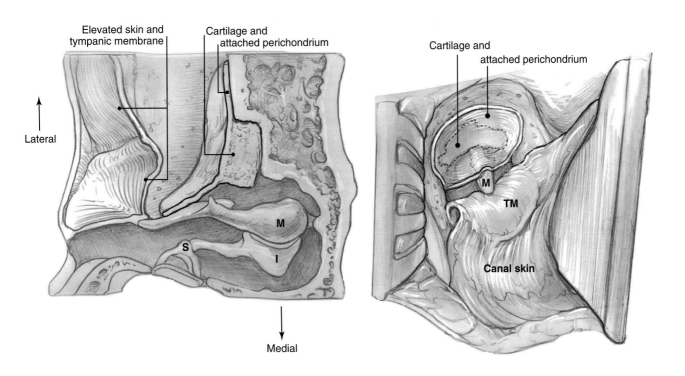

FIGURE 2-19

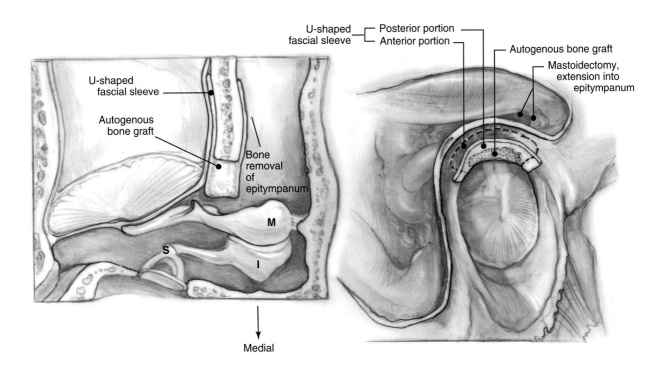

Following a postauricular incision, the natural tension of the cartilaginous canal may be unopposed by inadequately reapproximated deep layers such as the mastoid periosteum. Gradual stenosis may occur until symptoms become evident. Operative repair includes removal of cartilage from the anterior concha and posterior cartilaginous canal from the postauricular area with imbrication of the deep tissue layers overlying the mastoid cortex similar to imbrication of the subcutaneous musculoaponeurotic system in a facelift. The skin of the ear canal need not be violated in such a procedure. Postoperative stenting for 2 weeks also is helpful in restoring a normal contour to the canal.

Keratosis Obturans

Exuberant accumulation of desquamated skin may produce bony erosion and gradual expansion of the bony external auditory canal.[7] The process may progress to the point of erosion into structures adjacent to the canal such as the temporomandibular joint or mastoid. Erosion lateral to the eardrum may cause loss of support of the fibrous annulus of the tympanic membrane and a characteristic "jump rope sign" inferiorly (which can also be seen following curetting for a stapes procedure more superiorly). Poor epithelial migration has been proposed as the cause of the disorder. Frequent cleaning may retard the process. Cleaning may be much easier if the typically inspissated and adherent material is softened with mineral oil for several days before the clinical appointment. Surgical intervention is rarely indicated unless severe erosion exposes vital structures.

Osteonecrosis and Osteoradionecrosis of the Tympanic Bone

Radiation and occasionally chronic vasculitis devascularize a portion of the tympanic bone, producing skin loss and bone exposure. The low-grade osteomyelitis can be managed conservatively with topical antimicrobials and mild débridement. Addition of oral antibiotics may improve the chance of healing lesions in the early phases. Frequently, however, bone involvement progresses and can lead to further skin loss. A culture and sensitivity test is indicated before institution of topicals and later with deterioration of healing to look for resistant organisms.

Operative repair is indicated for progression of bone exposure and/or associated cellulitis. Removal of all devitalized bone with the postauricular approach is necessary. The margins of the canal skin are freshened similar to what is performed in a tympanoplasty. Autogenous fascia is placed directly on the freshly drilled bone and the skin is returned to anatomic position overlying it. The external canal is packed with antibiotic-containing absorbable sponge, which is removed in 7 to 10 days when antibiotic drops are initiated and then continued until complete healing occurs.

Scutum Defects

Cholesteatoma of the pars flaccida produces bone erosion in a significant number of patients. Repair of the external auditory canal is necessary to prevent re-retraction and cholesteatoma formation through the canal defect. Small defects (<2 mm) may be repaired with double-layered fascia. Large defects must be addressed for best long-term patient outcome. Repair may be accomplished with a composite cartilage graft or a fascial sleeve and bone pate.

Cartilagenous repair is possible with cartilage harvested from the base of the tragus. The perichondrium is left attached to one side of the cartilage, which is carved to match the bony defect like the piece of a puzzle. The composite graft is inserted in the defect after elevation of the canal skin and eardrum from the lateral surface of the handle of the malleus. The graft is positioned such that the perichondrium faces the elevated skin and eardrum and the cartilage extends into the defect (Fig. 2–18).

Alternatively, bone formation may be stimulated with placement of autogenous bone chips (bone pate harvested with a microdrill and mixed with antibiotic) within a U-shaped fascial sleeve.[8] This technique requires removal of bone lateral to the heads of the ossicles in the epitympanum and sculpting of the posterior surface of the bony external canal to allow placement of the fascia (Fig. 2–19).

Post-Traumatic Suture Dehiscence

Temporal bone trauma may produce partial dislocation of either the temporosquamous or the temporomastoid suture lines. When visible on examination, these signs indicate a temporal bone fracture. Rarely, surgical intervention is necessary for entrapped epithelium.

References

1. Adams W: The aetiology of swimmer's exostoses of the external auditory canals and of associated changes in hearing: I. J Laryngol 65: 133–153, 1951.
2. Harrison D: Exostosis of the external auditory meatus. J Laryngol 65: 704–714, 1951.
3. Fowler EP Jr, Osmun PM: New bone growth due to cold water in the ears. Arch Otolaryngol Head Neck Surg 36: 455–466, 1942.
4. Rauch SD: Management of soft tissue and osseous stenosis of the ear canal and canalplasty. In Nadol JB Jr, Schuknecht HF (eds): Surgery of the Ear and Temporal Bone. New York, Raven Press, 1993, pp 117–125.
5. Shambaugh GE Jr, Glasscock ME III: Operations on the auricle, external meatus, and tympanic membrane. In Shambaugh GE Jr, Glasscock ME III (eds): Surgery of the Ear. Philadelphia, WB Saunders, 1980, pp 194–215.
6. Dibartolomeo JR: Exostoses of the external auditory canal. Ann Otol Rhinol Laryngol 88(Suppl 61): 2–20, 1979.
7. Piepergerdes JC, Kramer BM, Behnke EE: Keratosis obturans and external auditory canal cholesteatoma. Laryngoscope 90: 383–390, 1980.
8. Althaus SR: Tympanomastoid surgery: A technique for repairing posterior osseous canal wall defects with autologous temporalis fascia and bone pate. Otolaryngol Head Neck Surg 93: 529–535, 1985.

3

Malignancies of the Temporal Bone: Limited Temporal Bone Resection

Sam E. Kinney, M.D.

Malignant tumors involving the external auditory canal and temporal bone present a unique challenge to otologic and head and neck oncology surgeons. The most common primary lesion involving the temporal bone is squamous cell carcinoma originating in the skin of the external auditory canal. The lesion may remain confined to this anatomic area; however, it may extend medially through the tympanic membrane and into the various recesses of the middle ear and temporal bone and petrous apex. The origin of this tumor remains a mystery, for cutaneous squamous cell carcinoma most frequently results from the effect of solar ultraviolet radiation.

In addition to squamous cell carcinoma, there are lesions involving the auricle, such as basal cell carcinoma, which may extend to the bony portion of the external auditory canal and into the temporal bone. This tumor presents unique challenges that are discussed further.

Rhabdomyosarcoma, aggressive middle ear adenoma, and adenocarcinoma of the endolymphatic sac are rare and require individualized treatment.

Early diagnosis of a malignancy of the external auditory ear canal will result in the best therapeutic outcome. External ear canal infections respond to local treatment within 7 to 10 days. Otolaryngology–head and neck surgeons must continue to encourage their primary care colleagues to be suspicious of an ear canal lesion that does not respond to local treatment and to biopsy the tissue. A second biopsy may be necessary.

A complete otolaryngology–head and neck examination follows the diagnosis. The canal lesion is evaluated with all adjacent structures such as the parotid gland, postauricular area, upper jugular digastric area, and all cranial nerves.

Imaging studies are performed including computed tomographic (CT) scans of the temporal bone, temporal mandibular joint, and neck. Magnetic resonance imaging (MRI) scans are helpful if middle or posterior fossa involvement is suspected. Arteriograms with temporary balloon occlusion may be helpful for carotid artery involvement.

Using primarily the CT scan, the lesion may be staged according to the TNM system described by Arriaga. T1 lesions are limited to the external auditory canal without bone erosion or soft tissue extension. T2 lesions would have limited bone erosion of the external bony canal and has less than 5 mm of soft tissue extension. T3 lesions would demonstrate full-thickness erosion of the bony external auditory meatus with less than 5 mm of soft tissue extension. This would also include tumors in the middle ear mastoid and facial nerve paralysis. T4 lesions would include extension to the cochlea, petrous apex, carotid canal, jugular foramen, or dura with greater than 5 mm soft tissue extension.

Preoperative imaging studies are still unable to identify malignancy in some areas of the temporal bone. When attempting en bloc tumor removal, the tumor is often violated in one of the planes of resection. It is for this reason that most tumors are treated with limited temporal bone resection and aggressive piecemeal removal of all gross tumor. This is followed by full therapy, that is, high-dose targeted irradiation delivered to the tumor bed with sparing of adjacent neural structures.

PATIENT SELECTION

The average age of patients who develop squamous cell carcinoma of the external auditory canal is 62 years. These individuals may also have other medical conditions that may make a major surgical procedure more complicated; these conditions need to be evaluated in the process of patient selection. The patients most frequently experience severe pain that is not well controlled with medical treatment. Therefore, surgery becomes necessary both to control the lesion and to improve the patient's quality of life. Radiation therapy as the primary method of treatment may be effective temporarily in controlling pain; however, its long-term control of the primary neoplasm has not been found to be satisfactory.

There are specific lesions for which an attempt at formal temporal bone resection may be the only surgical option. Patients with such lesions include those who have residual disease following full radiation therapy as well as some in whom the disease has developed in a previous modified or radical mastoidectomy cavity. The attempt to remove these lesions without formal temporal bone resection would be unsatisfactory. If the lesion is identified early and confined to the external auditory canal without involvement of the tympanic membrane and middle ear or without extensive bone involvement of the external auditory canal, a lateral temporal bone resection or external auditory canal resection may be curative.

The limited temporal bone resection of squamous cell carcinoma of the external auditory canal and middle ear involves removal of all gross tumor identified intraoperatively. This may include complete resection of the glenoid fossa, condyle of the mandible, base of the skull, the floor of the middle fossa, the middle meningeal artery, and the third division of the fifth cranial nerve. It may involve removal of the entire jugular bulb, carotid jugular spine, and, in some instances, the carotid artery itself preceded by balloon occlusion by interventional radiography. Resection of the entire skull base of the occiput to the foramen magnum may be necessary in an attempt to control spread of the tumor. Following total gross tumor resection, the operative field is covered with a vascularized tissue flap (either muscle or free flap). Approximately 6 weeks after surgery, full-therapy radiation is administered to the involved field.

The lateral temporal bone or external auditory canal resection can be used as an important adjunct in managing other lesions that may not have their primary origin in the external auditory canal but that may originate either on the auricle or in the parotid gland and extend to the external canal. The external canal resection becomes a margin of normal tissue resection to control the lesion.

Basal cell carcinomas that have extended into the external auditory canal may best be controlled by resection of the bony portion of the canal with the tympanic membrane, malleus, and incus to provide a medial margin for these often difficult lesions. In all instances the extent of the resection is controlled by intraoperative frozen-section margin control.

Adenomatous tumors of the middle ear are quite rare. The patient presents with a blocked feeling in the ear and a conductive hearing loss; on examination, a mass is identified behind the eardrum. A mass that does not have the appearance of a cholesteatoma or the pulsatile character of a typical glomus tumor should be considered in the differential diagnosis to be an adenomatous tumor of the middle ear. A search of the literature suggests that opinions regarding the nature of this tumor have varied over time. Most pathologists propose that it is a benign tumor that can have aggressive local invasion. There have been suggestions that it is a low-grade adenocarcinoma. Most often, adenomatous tumors of the middle ear can be controlled with conservative therapy. This includes an intact canal wall tympanoplasty with mastoidectomy performed in such a way that all reaches of the middle ear mastoid epitympanum and eustachian tube can be examined; this may require resection of the malleus and incus. In most instances the tumor can be carefully dissected away from the stapes. This tumor has a high incidence of residual disease; therefore, the preoperative counseling of the patient should indicate the need for a planned second-stage evaluation of the middle ear and mastoid to make sure that no disease remains. The planned second-stage procedure can be performed approximately 1 year following the initial procedure. If no evidence of residual disease is detected, a reconstruction of the middle ear transformer mechanism can be performed at that time.

PREOPERATIVE EVALUATION AND PATIENT COUNSELING

Preoperative staging of the lesion, based on imaging studies, has been outlined previously. Findings at surgery often change the preoperative plan into a different level of intraoperative staging, with significant change of prognosis based on these findings.

It is important to counsel the patient as to the nature of the lesion and the necessity for surgical resection followed by planned postoperative radiation therapy. The emphasis is placed on planned postoperative radiation therapy, for experience has shown that if the radiation therapy is not given in a planned postoperative course or if it is delayed until residual or recurrent disease becomes evident, its effectiveness in the patient with recurrent disease is very slight. In T1 disease, with the tumor limited to the external auditory canal without extensive bone invasion, an external auditory resection with skin grafting of the resultant cavity produced a 5-year survival rate of better than 90 per cent.

T2 disease with limited extension into the bone of the external auditory canal and limited extension into the middle ear, treated with a lateral temporal bone resection followed by a full course of radiation therapy, results in survival rate at 5 years of approximately 90 per cent. T3 and T4 disease with involvement of the medial wall of the middle ear, middle fossa dura, jugular bulb, and carotid artery, have a 5-year survival of less than 50 per cent. Experience has shown that if a T3 or T4 squamous cell carcinoma of the external auditory canal and middle ear is not controlled by surgery combined with radiation therapy, the patient's survival will be less than 6 months.

SURGICAL TECHNIQUE

Although the surgical team may have only a head and neck surgeon with otologic surgical experience, it may include an otologist-neurotologist, head and neck surgeon, and, in some instances, a neurosurgeon. The operative procedure is performed under general anesthesia. The anesthesiologist most often chooses to place monitoring lines, including central venous catheters as well as arterial catheters, to observe the patient carefully throughout the procedure. This is particularly important in older patients and in those in whom major vascular structures are thought to be at risk as the result of the operative procedure.

The patient is placed on the operating table in the supine position as for otologic surgery, with foot-to-head reversed so that circulating nurses can have access to the controls of the table without disturbing the operative field. This position also allows the otologic portion of the procedure to be performed with the surgeon seated while having access to equipment under the end of the table. An indwelling bladder catheter is used to allow anesthesia personnel to monitor fluid balance. This also allows the intraoperative use of urea or mannitol to give greater intracranial access, should this become necessary as part of the surgery.

Facial nerve monitoring may be performed during the procedure. This procedure requires careful anatomic identification of the facial nerve in both the temporal bone and the parotid gland. The potential risk to the facial nerve will have been described previously to the patient during preoperative counseling. In some instances, facial nerve alteration is to be expected as a result of the surgery. Perioperative antibiotics may be used. The use of steroids and diuretics would depend on the need to perform extensive intracranial surgery to resect the limits of the lesion.

The patient's head is rotated away from the involved ear toward the anesthesia personnel, who are positioned at the side of the table approximately two thirds of the way down from the head. The otologic nurse can sit directly in front of the patient's face. The patient's head may be placed in point fixation. The patient's head is extended, possibly with a roll under the shoulders, to expose the superior portion of the jugular digastric lymph nodes. The patient's head is prepared to include potential extension of the incision into the middle and posterior fossa as well as extension of the incision across the mastoid tip along the anterior border of the sternocleidomastoid muscle to expose the superior cervical lymph nodes. If a preoperative physical examination has suggested positive lymph nodes, the entire neck is exposed for the possibility of a formal radical neck dissection. The draping is also carried forward to the lateral canthus of the eye so that the flap elevation can include the entire parotid gland.

If it is anticipated that a regional flap, such as a pectoralis myocutaneous flap, will be necessary to cover the surgical site, this area is also included in the preoperative preparation. An area of the lower abdomen to obtain fat to obliterate dead space may also be prepared as may a site for a free microvascular flap positioned to obliterate a large surgical defect.

Instrumentation for this procedure is similar to that for otologic surgery, in addition to the instruments for radical neck dissection and possible free flap transfer. An oval burr approximately 4 mm in diameter may be useful in expediting the epitympanic dissection over the ossicles into the temporomandibular joint and eustachian tube. The operative plan is determined by the surgical team. The head and neck surgeon begins the procedure so that the operative field is clean and not involved with the bone dust.

A wide postauricular incision is performed as shown in Figure 3–1. This incision is carried approximately 3 fingerbreadths posterior to the auricle and approximately 3 or 4 fingerbreadths superior to the auricle, giving a wide base to the anterior portion of the flap. Care is taken not to limit the vascular pedicles anteriorly because there will be a hole in the center of the flap as the result of the tragal-conchal incisions on the lateral aspect of the external auditory canal. The incision is carried to the mastoid tip inferiorly so that it may be extended down along the anterior border of the sternocleidomastoid muscle to identify the structures in the superior neck.

The incision is carried down through the skin and subcutaneous tissues. If violation of cerebrospinal fluid (CSF) is anticipated, the incision should be made in two separate layers to include the deep layer of fascia and periosteum; a watertight seal can be accomplished when the wound is closed. The temporalis muscle is left in place with its blood supply originating underneath the zygomatic arch so that it may be used as a rotational flap at the conclusion of the procedure. A separate incision is made to outline the resection of the tragus and a portion of the conchal cartilage (see Fig. 3–1). This incision is carried down to the bone of the external auditory canal. On completion of this incision, the external canal can be oversewn so that no spillage of cancer cells occurs. If the entire auricle is involved and a complete auriculectomy is anticipated, the incisions may be modified to a preauricular and postauricular Y-type

incision or a circumferential incision, which must be closed with regional or distant vascularized flaps.

The postauricular flap is then elevated across the mastoid. On reaching the external auditory canal, it is elevated away from the tragal-conchal incision. The flap is elevated forward across the surface of the superficial lobe of the parotid gland. Approaching the mastoid tip from inferiorly, the facial nerve may be identified as it exits the temporal bone and may be traced out into the substance of the parotid gland for later removal of the superficial lobe of the parotid gland.

The ear canal resection portion of the procedure is performed next by the otologic surgeon. A complete mastoidectomy is performed as shown in Figure 3–2, *left*). The lateral dural sinus and middle fossa tegmen are identified. All the air cells in the mastoid down to the labyrinth are removed. The retrofacial air cells are opened primarily to examine this area for gross tumor. The external auditory canal is thinned, and the facial nerve is identified just inferior to the horizontal semicircular canal and traced to the stylomastoid foramen.

Figure 3–2, *right* is a close-up view of the major portion of the bony resection of the external auditory canal. The facial recess is opened widely, identifying the annulus of the tympanic membrane as well as the chorda tympani nerve. Facial recess dissection is carried inferiorly and anteriorly to the facial nerve, sacrificing the chorda tympani nerve. Care is taken to recognize that the narrowest space in the facial recess is between the facial nerve and the annulus at the most posterior portion of the annular ring. From that point inferiorly, the annulus will be moving medially at a rapid pace and dissection must be carried significantly more medially to stay posterior to the tympanic annulus.

Using larger cutting burrs, the entire tympanic bone lateral to the facial nerve and inferior to the residual external auditory canal is removed. This dissection is carried forward into the temporomandibular joint. The hypotympanic dissection is then performed by continuing to follow the annulus around inferiorly, remaining medial to the annulus and removing all bone of the inferior portion of the tympanic bone. As the surgeon proceeds medially, the jugular bulb may become apparent; as the surgeon moves forward, the carotid artery will be identified. The dissection is carried forward along the external auditory canal until it completely joins the soft tissues of the temporomandibular joint. The dissection is carried medially through the hypotympanum to the anterior wall of the mesotympanum medial to the bony annulus and the carotid artery. This portion of the dissection is important to obtain complete removal of the bony annulus at the time that it is fractured across the anterior wall of the middle ear.

The epitympanic resection is performed by removing the bone between the dura of the middle fossa and the retained external auditory canal. Dissection is carried lateral to the body of the incus and the head of the malleus. As the dissection is carried forward, the dura tends to dip inferiorly; therefore, the dissection must stay close to the curvature of the external auditory canal. The dissection is carried forward inferiorly until it again joins the soft tissues of the temporomandibular joint. Anterior to the head of the malleus, the dissection is carried medially into the anterior

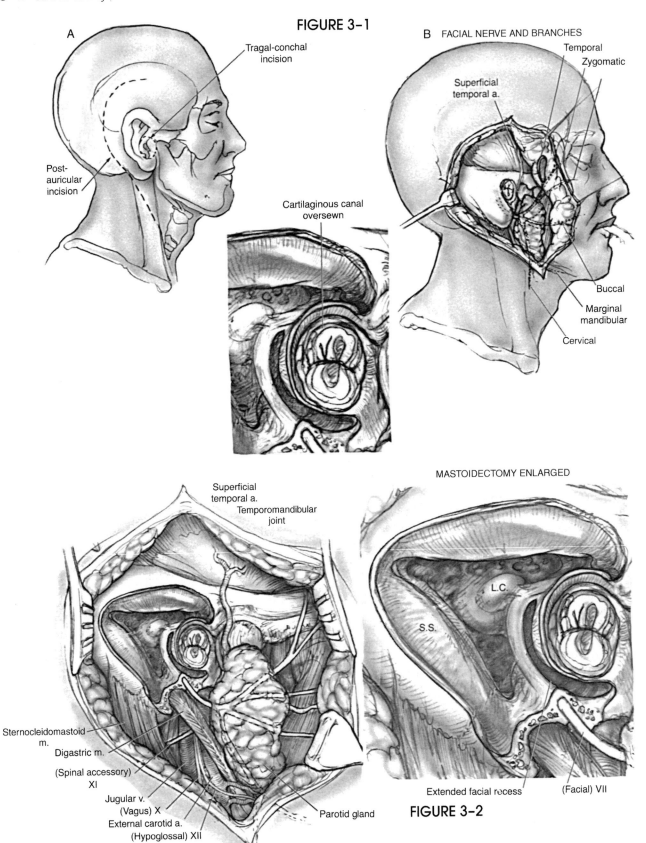

FIGURE 3-1

A

Tragal-conchal
incision

Post-
auricular
incision

Cartilaginous canal
oversewn

B   FACIAL NERVE AND BRANCHES

Temporal
Zygomatic

Superficial
temporal a.

Buccal

Marginal
mandibular

Cervical

Superficial
temporal a.
Temporomandibular
joint

MASTOIDECTOMY ENLARGED

L.C.

S.S.

Sternocleidomastoid
m.
Digastric m.
(Spinal accessory)
XI
Jugular v.
(Vagus) X
External carotid a.
(Hypoglossal) XII

Parotid gland

Extended facial recess

(Facial) VII

FIGURE 3-2

epitympanum and forward from the anterior epitympanum until it joins the eustachian tube medial to the tympanic annulus. In this dissection, care must be taken not to drop too far medially, for the geniculate ganglion lies in the floor of the anterior epitympanum and can be inadvertently injured at that point.

With completion of both the hypotympanic and the epitympanic dissections, the final bar of bone separating the facial recess from the fossa incudis is carefully removed. The incudostapedial joint is separated, the tensor tympani tendon is cut, and the superior ligamentous attachments of the body of the incus and the head of the malleus and the anterior mallear ligament are cut. Gentle pressure is then placed with the thumb against the bony external auditory canal. If the hypotympanic and epitympanic dissections have been completed accurately and with minimal pressure, the anterior wall of the middle ear will fracture across the carotid artery, thus releasing the entire external auditory canal, tympanic membrane, malleus, and incus. The bony portion of the external auditory canal is then carefully separated from the soft tissues of the temporomandibular joint using heavy Mayo scissors. There is often brisk bleeding from the parotid gland that can be controlled using bipolar coagulation. The external canal resection is then left attached to the superficial lobe of the parotid gland.

The entire bony tip of the mastoid has been removed in this procedure. The facial nerve can be traced out of the stylomastoid foramen into the parotid gland. The external canal and superficial lobe of the parotid gland can then be elevated off the facial nerve (Fig. 3–3). The specimen is removed with the external canal attached to the superficial lobe of the parotid gland.

Throughout the external canal resection, the surgeon observes carefully for potential extension of the tumor outside the external canal. Particular notice is taken as the fissures of Santorini are approached anteriorly, because this may be a route of growth of the tumor. If the tumor has extended anteriorly, the soft tissues of the temporomandibular joint, including the articular cartilage disk, are removed. The condyle of the mandible may be removed as an anterior margin of the tumor. If the tumor extends into the glenoid fossa, the middle fossa dura is followed forward, removing the bone of the glenoid fossa and sacrificing the middle meningeal artery and the third division of the fifth cranial nerve as necessary. If the tumor has extended to the middle fossa dura, the neurosurgeon can perform a bone flap craniectomy of the middle fossa. The dura of the middle fossa is then elevated until the tumor is encountered. The dura is further elevated in an attempt to identify a free margin of uninvolved dura medially. It may be necessary to resect the superior petrosal sinus to obtain a free tumor margin.

On occasion, the tumor will extend along the middle fossa dura deep to the petrous apex toward the clivus. In this case, the chances of completely removing the tumor begin to diminish significantly. If the tumor has extended to the posterior fossa dura, the entire lateral sinus can be uncovered of bone and the posterior fossa dura resected away from the tumor, again searching for a medial free margin of dura with which to attach a dural graft. If there is direct invasion of the cochlea or semicircular canals, these can be removed using the otologic drills until normal

bone has been identified. If the facial nerve has been involved by the tumor, it can be resected segmentally, and a nerve graft from the great auricular or sural nerve may be placed from the tympanic bone segment to the parotid gland. If the tumor involves the stylomastoid foramen, the surgeon must have a high suspicion that this tumor will extend along the periosteum of the skull base. The tumor may extend into the plane between the outer and inner tables of the calvarium over the occiput. The tumor resection continues until the surgeon believes that no gross tumor remains. If the tumor extends into the carotid jugular spine, a decision may be made to sacrifice the jugular vein and jugular bulb. This would imply involvement of the carotid artery and a decision to occlude it; resection of the carotid artery may be made in specific cases. The principle remains constant: *total removal of all gross tumor.*

If the tumor appears to be confined to the external auditory canal, but the lesion was tightly packed into the anterior sulcus against the tympanic membrane, a decision may be made to perform a deep lobe parotidectomy as shown in Figure 3–4. The facial nerve may be completely mobilized off the deep lobe and the deep lobe dissected free off the masseter muscles as a second specimen.

Following the total removal of tumor, the incision can be extended along the anterior border of the sternocleidomastoid muscle to expose the high jugular digastric chain of lymph nodes. If nodes are identified, they may be sent for frozen-section sampling (Fig. 3–5). The head and neck surgeon decides whether microscopic involvement of lymph nodes needs to be controlled with a radical neck dissection or by full-therapy irradiation. If the lesion in the external auditory canal was located on the posterior and inferior canal wall, the surgeon must examine the area posterior to the mastoid tip and attempt to identify microscopic involvement of lymph nodes so that this area can be included in the radiation therapy field. If there are grossly positive lymph nodes in the neck, the incisions may be extended further inferiorly and a modified or formal radical neck dissection performed.

With the exception of limited T1 lesions, all patients with squamous cell carcinoma of the external auditory canal and middle ear are given full-therapy postoperative irradiation. To avoid osteoradionecrosis, the middle ear transformer is sacrificed and the temporal bone is covered by vascularized tissue.

As shown in Figure 3–6, the temporalis muscle may be mobilized from its attachments along the linea temporalis and the superior temporal line and left attached at its insertion under the root of the zygoma with its associated blood supply. This flap can be rotated down to obliterate the mastoid cavity in the area of the tragal-conchal incision. The incision can then be covered with a split-thickness skin graft. A pectoralis myocutaneous flap may reach the area of the temporal bone as well as a trapezius flap rotated from posteriorly. If the soft tissue loss in the dead space obliteration seems to be extensive, a microvascular free flap from the rectus abdominis may be used to obliterate this space. It is important that viable tissue be used to cover the temporal bone in patients in whom postoperative irradiation therapy is to be delivered. If the CSF space has not been entered, positive suction drain catheters are placed

FIGURE 3–3

Ear canal and superficial
parotid gland removed

FIGURE 3–4

Muscle graft sutured
to perichondrium

Deep lobe
of parotid
removed

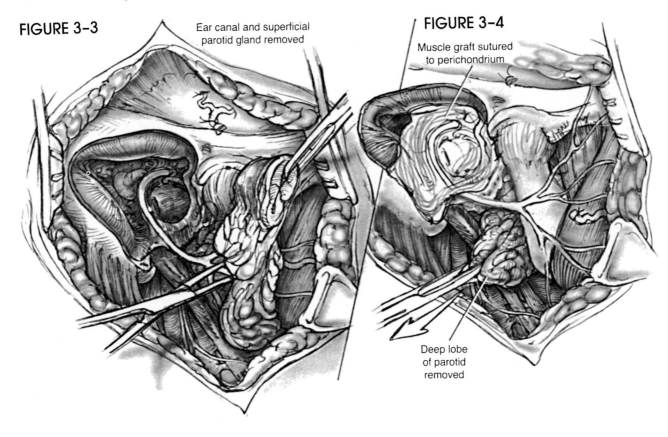

FIGURE 3–5

FIGURE 3–6

Sample taken
of lymph nodes

Temporalis
muscle flap
in defect

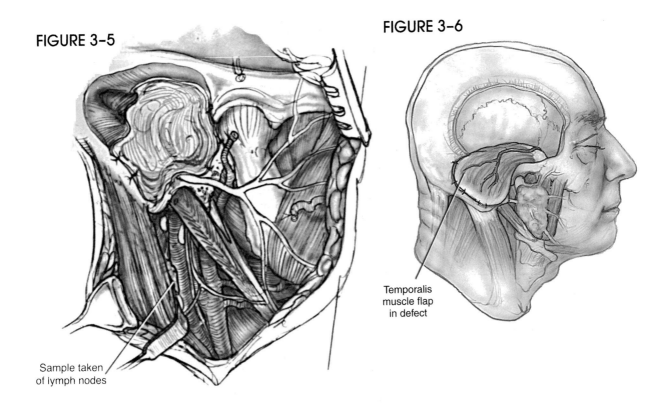

dependently in the wound to remove accumulated tissue fluids.

Once the wounds are closed and flaps placed into position, a formal mastoid dressing (or possibly other forms of dressings that would allow inspection and protection of a flap) may be chosen based on the recommendations of the head and neck surgeon. If there has been entrance into the CSF space, it is important that the eustachian tube be completely obliterated by removing the mucosa and tightly packing the eustachian tube with a free muscle graft. In these circumstances, it is often important to use tissue to fill an opening into the dura. This may be abdominal fat or muscle or a free flap. Gentle pressure over the wound for a minimum of 3 days using a mastoid dressing may help prevent CSF from forming a pseudomeningocele under the flap.

Postoperative care of patients with lateral temporal bone resection is structured. If there has been involvement of the facial nerve, immediate eye care must be instituted. This may include patching of the eye and use of artificial tears and ointments. If the facial nerve has been resected and not regrafted, a decision to provide eye care (such as the implantation of a gold weight in the upper eyelid and a tensing of the lower eyelid by shortening at the lateral canthus) may be carried out, most often by an occuloplastic surgeon. The combination of the gold weight implant and tensing of the lower eyelid provides better protection as well as a better cosmetic result than the standard lateral tarsorrhaphy. If there is extensive involvement of the tumor in the jugular foramen, paresis or paralysis of the ninth or tenth cranial nerve may occur. Care must be taken to protect the airway and also provide nutrition, most often temporarily, through a nasogastric tube or possibly a longer-term nutritional line through a percutaneous endoscopic gastrostomy, as determined in the postoperative period.

The greatest problem in surgery for squamous cell carcinoma of the external auditory canal and middle ear is removal of all gross tumor. In difficult cases with involvement of the deep petrous apex, the skills of the otologic surgeon, head and neck surgeon, and neurosurgeon must be brought to bear for complete removal of gross tumor. If the surgical team cannot remove all the gross tumor at the time of surgery, the patient's prognosis for survival with radiation therapy is very grave.

The results of lateral temporal bone resection followed by total gross removal of all tumor and full-therapy irradiation have been encouraging; however, they are not always successful.

T1 lesions of the external auditory canal treated with a canal resection without postoperative radiation therapy have approximately a 95 per cent 5-year survival rate. The T2 and some T3 lesions, in which total tumor removal has been obtained and the patient is given full-therapy irradiation, have approximately an 85 per cent 5-year survival. For more extensive T3 and T4 lesions, the 5-year survival drops below 50 per cent to approximately 43 per cent. Survival may also be altered by the histology of the tumor. Rare examples of verrucous carcinoma and carcinoma in situ may be staged as T3 or T4 lesions preoperatively. With total tumor removal followed by postoperative irradiation therapy, however, the prognosis may

be quite good. Undifferentiated squamous cell carcinoma that has reached the dura, the carotid jugular spine, or the periosteum of the skull base will have limited potential for cure and survivability.

Patients with a T4 lesion by imaging studies preoperatively have a poor prognosis. However, palliative surgery using the lateral bone resection approach, without the associated morbidity and mortality of a formal temporal bone resection, may be indicated. This may offer the patient a significant period of pain relief. Survival in these cases is often less than 6 months.

Postoperative irradiation is planned in conjunction with the radiotherapist. As noted earlier, the operative plan should include covering of the temporal bony by viable vascularized tissue to avoid potential for osteoradionecrosis in long-term survival cases. Radiation is usually given in divided doses with portals to avoid injury to the central nervous system (CNS) structures. Newer radiotherapy systems such as the gamma knife, Peacock system, and cyberknife may be used to target the therapy, giving high doses to the tumor while preserving important neural structures. On occasion, in a younger person with an aggressive undifferentiated squamous cell carcinoma, the treatment plan may include consultation with an oncologic physician for the purpose of giving chemotherapy. The role of chemotherapy in controlling squamous cell carcinoma of the temporal bone has not been determined. The incidence of the lesion is sufficiently small that the entering of these patients into a protocol that might help determine the effectiveness of chemotherapy has not been possible.

The lateral temporal bone resection associated with total gross tumor removal followed by irradiation therapy as a treatment for squamous cell carcinoma has been chosen for the following reasons. The imaging studies available have not yet been able to accurately diagnose the extent of tumor. The studies are not able to differentiate neoplasm from an inflammatory reaction resulting from infection associated with the neoplasm. The lateral temporal bone resection with total gross tumor removal violates standard oncologic principles of en bloc resection. However, attempts at total temporal bone resection with en bloc tumor resection have a high incidence of transgression of the tumor, a situation that is based on the inability to accurately determine the extent of tumor with preoperative evaluation. Total temporal bone resection may once again become the procedure of choice if advances in imaging technology make possible the differentiation of tissue types. The surgical techniques for performing temporal bone resection are improving at a rapid pace. The time may come when total temporal bone resection can be performed with a level of morbidity and mortality acceptable and comparable to lateral temporal bone resection, followed by gross tumor removal and postoperative irradiation therapy.

Bibliography

Arena S: Tumor surgery of the temporal bone. Laryngoscope 84: 615–670, 1974.

Arena S, Keen M: Carcinoma of the middle ear and temporal bone. Am J Otol 9: 351–356, 1988.

Arriaga M, Curtin H, Takahashi, H, et al: Staging proposal for external auditory meatus carcinoma based on preoperative clinical examination and computed tomography findings. Ann Otol Rhinol Laryngol 99: 714–721, 1990.

Batsakis JG: Adenomatous tumors of the middle ear. Ann Otol Rhinolo Laryngol 98: 749–752, 1989.

Benecke JE Jr, Noel FL, Carberry JN, et al: Adenomatous tumors of the middle ear and mastoid. Am J Otol 11: 20–26, 1990.

Boland J: The management of carcinoma of the middle ear. Radiology 80: 285, 1963.

Conley J: Cancer of the middle ear. Ann Otol Rhinol Laryngol 74: 555–572, 1965.

Crabtree JA, Britton BH, Pierce MK: Carcinoma of the external auditory canal. Laryngoscope 86: 405–415, 1976.

Eby TL, Makek MS, Fisch U: Adenomas of the temporal bone. Ann Otol Rhinol Laryngol 97: 605–612, 1988.

Go KG, Annyas AA, Vermey A, et al: Evaluation of results of temporal bone resection. Acta Neurochir (Wien) 110: 110–115, 1991.

Goodwin WJ, Jesse RH: Malignant neoplasms of the external auditory canal and temporal bone. Arch Otolaryngol 106: 675–679, 1980.

Graham MD, Sataloff RT, Kemink JL, et al: Total en bloc resection of the temporal bone and carotid artery for malignant tumors of the ear and temporal bone. Laryngoscope 94: 528–533, 1984.

Howard JD, Elster AD, May JS: Temporal bone: Three-dimensional CT: II. Pathologic alterations. Radiology 177: 427–430, 1990.

Kinney SE: Squamous cell carcinoma of the external auditory canal. Am J Otol 10: 111–116, 1989.

Kinney SE, Wood BG: Malignancies of the external ear canal and temporal bone: Surgical techniques and results. Laryngoscope 97: 158–164, 1987.

Kinney SE, Wood BG: Surgical treatment of skull base malignancy. Otolaryngol Head Neck Surg 92: 94–99, 1984.

Lewis JS: Surgical management of tumors of the middle ear and mastoid. J Laryngol Otol 97: 299–311, 1983.

Lewis JS: Temporal bone resection. Arch Otolaryngol 101: 23–25, 1975.

Li JC, Brackman DE, Lo WWM, et al: The reclassification of aggressive adenomatous mastoid neoplasms as endolymphatic sac tumors. Laryngoscope 103: 1342–1348, 1993.

Mafee MF, Valvassori GE, Kumar A, et al: Tumors and tumor-like conditions of the middle ear and mastoid: Role of CT and MRI—an analysis of 100 cases. Otolaryngol Clin North Am 21: 349–375, 1988.

Manolidis S, Pappas D, Von Doersten P, et al: Temporal bone and lateral skull base malignancy: Experience and results with 81 patients. Am J Otol 19:S_1–S_{15}, 1998.

Meyerhoff WL, Mickey BE, Roland PS, Drummond JE: Magnetic resonance imaging in the diagnosis of temporal bone and skull base lesions. Am J Otol 10: 121–137, 1989.

Neely JG, Forrester M: Anatomic considerations of the medial cuts in subtotal temporal bone resection. Otolaryngol Head Neck Surg 90: 641–645, 1982.

Sataloff RT, Myers DL, Lowry LD, et al: Total temporal bone resection for squamous cell carcinoma. Otolaryngol Head Neck Surg 96: 4–14, 1987.

Sataloff RT, Roberts BR, Myers DL, Spiegel JR: Total temporal bone resection—a radical but life-saving procedure. AORN J 48: 932–948, 1988.

Wang CL: Radiation therapy in the management of carcinoma of the external canal, middle ear, of mastoid. Radiology 116: 713–715, 1975.

Wang CL, Doppke K: Osteoradionecrosis of the temporal bone: Considerations of national standard dose. Int J Radiat Oncol Biol Phys 1: 881–883, 1976.

Wiatrak BJ, Pensak ML: Rhabdomyosarcoma of the ear and temporal bone. Laryngoscope 99: 1188–1192, 1989.

Willging JP, Pensak ML: Temporal bone resection. Ear Nose Throat J 70: 612–617, 1991.

4

Malignancies of the Temporal Bone—Radical Temporal Bone Resection

Sanjay Prasad, M.D. ▪ Ivo P. Janecka, M.D.

Primary malignancies of the temporal bone were first recognized in the late eighteenth century and histologically first confirmed in the 1850s. These lesions are uncommon, with only 250 cases having been reported in the English literature by 1974.[1] The overall prevalence in the general population is six cases per million.[2] Because of their infrequent occurrence, these tumors are often misdiagnosed and treated as chronic external otitis or chronic mastoiditis. They are usually discovered at a later stage, when more radical treatment is required. The infrequent occurrence of the disease poses a challenging obstacle to any attempt at a clinical study regarding treatment.

Secondary malignancies of the temporal bone from regional spread of parotid cancers appear far more commonly. The fissures of Santorini provide a conduit for regional spread through the anterior cartilaginous ear canal.

Basal cell carcinoma and squamous cell carcinoma are the more common malignancies to affect the temporal bone. Basal cell carcinoma is thought to occur secondary to actinic exposure and commonly involves the external ear and/or ear canal. Squamous cell carcinoma can arise primarily from the external canal and/or middle ear or spread into the temporal bone from a primary lesion in the parotid gland. Unlike squamous cell carcinoma of the upper aerodigestive tract, squamous cell carcinoma of the temporal bone is not related to tobacco or alcohol use. Predisposing factors to these lesions are few. Chronic infection within the temporal bone is the most commonly cited factor.

Adenoid cystic carcinoma can arise either from the ear canal and middle ear or from the parotid gland and spread secondarily into the temporal bone. These lesions have a tendency toward perineural spread. Ceruminous adenoma, adenocarcinoma, and mucoepidermoid carcinoma are other lesions that can affect the temporal bone.

Regional spread to cervical nodes and distant metastases are uncommon. Depending on the extent of the disease, radical resection coupled with radiation treatment offers the best treatment. The efficacy of chemotherapy has not been clearly established, and it may play a role only in recalcitrant disease.

Radical temporal bone resection refers to one of three operations that can be offered to patients with this disease. A lateral temporal bone resection (LTBR) implies the removal of the external auditory canal, tympanic membrane, malleus, and incus. Subtotal temporal bone resection (STBR) refers to the additional removal of the otic capsule, and total temporal bone resection (TTBR) implies the additional removal of the petrous apex with or without the carotid artery.

LTBR is well accepted for lesions that involve the external auditory canal and/or tympanic membrane. Controversy arises in defining the optimal management of neoplasms that invade the mesotympanum. Some authors advocate LTBR with gross removal of middle ear disease followed by radiation therapy, whereas others prefer more radical surgery (namely STBR or TTBR), followed by radiation therapy. Once the tumor has invaded the petrous apex, involvement of either dura mater, brain parenchyma, and/or internal carotid artery (ICA) is usually present.

This chapter focuses on preoperative diagnostic evaluation, the surgical techniques of STBR and TTBR, postoperative management, and potential complications. Rehabilitation and adjuvant treatment for recalcitrant disease are briefly discussed. At the conclusion, we present a literature review of squamous cell carcinoma of the temporal bone in an effort to define the optimal management for middle ear disease and discuss the prognostic significance of dural, brain, and ICA involvement.

DIAGNOSTIC EVALUATION

The diagnostic evaluation begins with a thorough history and physical examination, with special emphasis on the chronology of developing cranioneuropathies. The pathway of tumor spread can occasionally be deduced from a careful history. Facial nerve function, hearing, and balance function should be carefully documented. Examination includes palpation of the parotid gland and cervical lymph glands for the presence of local spread and regional metastases, respectively. Patients should be questioned and tested for temporal lobe signs (e.g., memory loss, dysphasia, left-sided neglect, hemiparesis, and olfactory hallucinations) and cerebellar signs (e.g., ocular dysmetria, truncal ataxia, nystagmus, and dysdiadochokinesia).

Imaging allows determination of the extent of tumor involvement. High-resolution axial and coronal computed tomographic (CT) imaging at 1.5-mm thickness can identify areas of bony involvement. Enhanced and unenhanced magnetic resonance imaging (MRI) can determine intracranial involvement.

Histologic confirmation of the lesion is essential in further treatment planning. Lesions involving the external canal or periauricular skin can be easily biopsied. Needle aspiration biopsy of parotid lesions can also be performed.

Angiography is used when involvement of the major vessels is suspected on preoperative imaging, or when surgical exposure of the petrous carotid artery is anticipated. The venous phase of the study can provide important information regarding blood flow through the dural venous sinuses. Embolization of feeding vessels is rarely required because most lesions are relatively avascular.

Cerebral blood flow evaluation is indicated when involvement of the ICA is present. Patency of the anterior and posterior communicating arteries on angiography is an inadequate evaluation for collateral flow. Our current method of preoperative carotid artery testing is described.[3] A 30-minute temporary balloon occlusion of the ICA allows identification of patients who will most likely tolerate carotid artery sacrifice. Transfemoral introduction of a nondetachable intravascular balloon, inflated in the ICA, is performed in the patient while sensory, motor, and higher cortical functions are assessed.

Patients who develop a neurologic deficit during temporary occlusion are at high risk for stroke following carotid sacrifice. Preoperative or intraoperative extracranial-to-intracranial arterial bypass should be considered. Repeating the temporary balloon occlusion prior to surgical extirpation should also be considered. Conservative treatment options should also be discussed with these patients.

Patients who tolerate a 30-minute balloon occlusion of the ICA are at low risk for development of a stroke provided that a long "distal" stump is avoided. Permanent ICA occlusion can be performed angiographically. Hypotension and hypovolemia in the perioperative period should be avoided if permanent ICA occlusion is performed.

PREOPERATIVE PREPARATION

Preoperative preparation sets the stage for the operative and postoperative course. The evening before surgery, the operative site is shampooed and scrubbed with hexachlorophene. Intravenous phenytoin or phenobarbital and cefuroxime are used for prophylactic anticonvulsant and antibiotic coverage, respectively. To facilitate intraoperative cranial nerve monitoring, short-acting neuromuscular blocking agents are used only for the induction of anesthesia and not during the operation.

On the morning of the operation, sequential compression stockings are placed on both legs to help decrease the incidence of thromboembolic disease. Following insertion of a central venous catheter and an arterial line, the patient is intubated, and the endotracheal tube is secured. The operating table is then turned 90 degrees from the anesthesiologist, giving him or her access to the contralateral arm. The head is positioned on a horseshoe (Mayfield) head holder to allow repositioning during the course of the operation. Temporary bilateral tarsorrhaphies are placed to prevent corneal abrasions. The operative site, which includes the temporal fossa, lateral half of the face, postauricular area, neck, and ipsilateral thigh and lower leg (for the potential use of tensor fascia lata, and sural nerve), is shaved and scrubbed with an iodine-based solution. Bipolar facial electromyographic electrodes are placed in areas where facial function exists.

SURGICAL PROCEDURE

Incisions vary according to the extent of the tumor (Fig. 4–1). For lesions contained within the temporal bone, a C-shaped incision extending from the temporal fossa postauricularly into the neck is used. A blind-sac closure of the external auditory canal helps contain the specimen. When tumor invasion of the conchal cartilage or periauricular skin is suspected, an appropriate skin island is incorporated into the overall design. The external auditory canal skin is then sutured shut to avoid tumor spillage. The outline of the incisions should preserve the blood supply to the remaining auricle. The anterior and posterior skin flaps are elevated (Fig. 4–2A). The superficial temporal fat pad is elevated with the anterior skin flap in a subperiosteal plane over the zygomatic arch. The superficial temporal and middle temporal arteries are ligated.

The facial nerve can be handled differently, depending on tumor invasion of the parotid gland. When the gland is involved, peripheral branches of the facial nerve are identified with the help of the facial nerve monitor and then divided. The stumps of the anterior segments are secured to the anterior skin flap. The entire parotid gland is then dissected off the masseteric fascia, provided that the latter is free of disease, and mobilized posteriorly while the attachment to the external auditory canal is maintained. When the parotid gland is suspected to be free of tumor, the facial nerve trunk is located in the usual manner at the tympanomastoid suture and divided. The parotid gland, along with the distal stump of the facial nerve, is dissected free of the external auditory canal and mobilized anteriorly off the masseteric fascia.

The jugulodigastric region is then explored, and cervical lymph nodes are sent for frozen section pathologic analysis. Regional metastases determine the need for a formal cervical lymphadenectomy. Cranial nerve XI, the greater auricular nerve, or cervical cutaneous nerves can be used as cable grafts for facial nerve reconstruction. Cranial nerves IX, X, XI, and XII, the internal jugular vein, and the external and ICAs are dissected in an infero–superior direction toward the temporal bone. The sternocleidomastoid and digastric muscles are detached from their attachment to the mastoid.

The masseter is then detached from the zygomatic arch, allowing exposure of the zygoma and mandible. Zygomatic and mandibular osteotomies (see Fig. 4–2A) can then be performed. The meniscus of the temporomandibular joint is separated from the glenoid fossa, and the chorda tympani nerve emerging from the petrotympanic fissure is divided. The stylomandibular and sphenomandibular ligaments are divided and allow removal of the mandibular segment (Fig. 4–2B). The temporalis muscle is then elevated in a subperiosteal fashion and reflected inferiorly. The temporalis muscle must be separated from the lateral pterygoid muscle, and care should be taken not to injure the deep temporal arteries supplying blood to the temporalis muscle. The lateral and medial pterygoid muscles are then resected either en bloc with the specimen or separately, depending on tumor invasion.

In a subperiosteal manner, the contents of the infratemporal fossa are elevated off the floor of the middle fossa to expose the middle meningeal artery and vein in the foramen spinosum and the mandibular division of the trigemi-

FIGURE 4-2

FIGURE 4-1

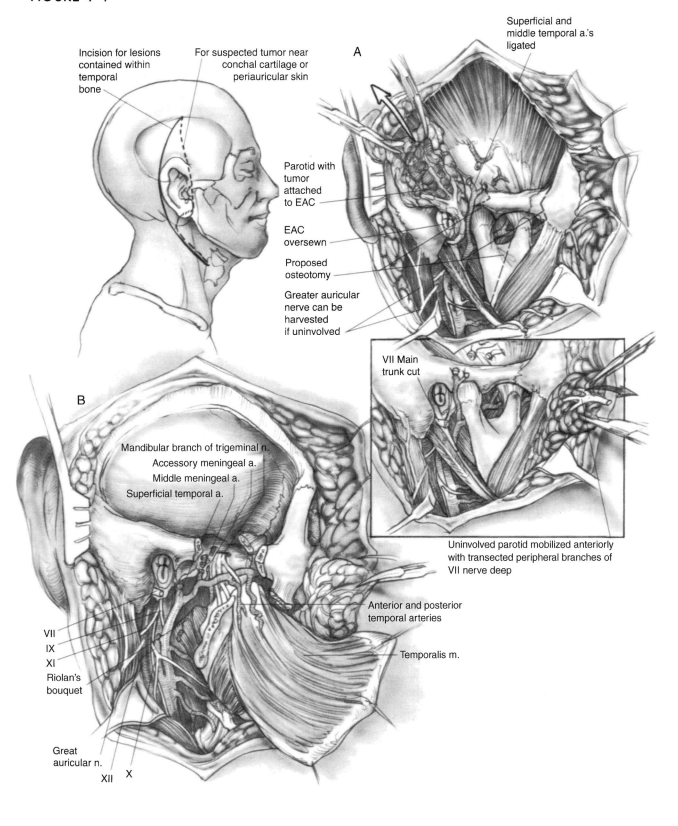

FIGURE 4–1. Incisions vary according to whether the tumor is contained in the temporal bone.

FIGURE 4–2. *A,* The facial nerve can be divided peripherally at the distal branches or centrally at the facial nerve trunk, depending on involvement of the parotid gland. *B,* Following osteotomies and removal of the zygomatic arch and mandibular segments, dissection in the infratemporal fossa continues. EAC, external auditory canal.

nal nerve in the foramen ovale. The contents of the foramen spinosum are bipolarly coagulated and divided. Frequently, the venous plexus of the foramen ovale requires bipolar coagulation and packing with oxidized cellulose. The lesser petrosal nerve can be seen emerging from the innominate canal, on its way to the otic ganglion.

The stylohyoid, stylopharyngeus, and styloglossus muscles (Riolan's bouquet) are detached from the styloid process, which is then rongeured away. The branches of the external carotid artery are then dissected in the infratemporal fossa. The anterior tympanic and deep auricular branches of the internal maxillary artery are often divided before identification and may require bipolar coagulation. The internal maxillary artery is preserved up to the branches of the deep temporal artery. When the internal maxillary artery must be sacrificed, brisk backflow from the anterior stump indicates that the temporalis muscle may derive its blood supply from reversed flow via the pterygoid system. If brisk backflow is not observed, the temporalis muscle cannot be relied on to reconstruct the surgical defect, and microvascular free flap options must be considered. The cartilaginous eustachian tube is divided and the anterior end sutured closed to prevent postoperative cerebrospinal fluid rhinorrhea (Fig. 4–3*A*).

The ICA is then dissected toward the carotid canal, and care is taken not to injure cranial nerve IX, which crosses its anterior surface. Kerrison rongeurs are used to uncover the vertical and horizontal petrous segments of the carotid artery (Fig. 4–3*B*). Occasionally, bleeding from the pericarotid venous plexus requires bipolar coagulation. The caroticotympanic artery is also divided when the petrous carotid artery is separated from the specimen. The extent of petrous carotid mobilization depends on whether an STBR or a TTBR is performed. When an STBR is performed, the vertical petrous carotid artery is mobilized from the carotid foramen and canal. When a TTBR is performed, the vertical and horizontal petrous carotid artery is mobilized out of the carotid canal to the foramen ovale.

A temporal craniectomy is then performed, and the intracranial portion of the middle meningeal vessels is coagulated (Fig. 4–3*B*). The patient is hyperventilated to keep the PCO_2 at 25 mm Hg for adequate brain relaxation. Mannitol and furosemide can improve brain relaxation. Subtemporal dural elevation proceeds in a postero–anterior direction. The greater superficial petrosal nerve and accompanying petrosal artery are coagulated and divided to lessen traction on the geniculate ganglion. Similarly, the lesser petrosal nerve and superior tympanic artery are also divided. Subtemporal dural elevation then proceeds as far medially as possible to expose the superior petrosal sinus. When carcinomatous involvement of the middle fossa dura is suspected, an intradural approach keeps the involved dura attached to the specimen.

The extent of the mastoidectomy depends on whether tumor is present in the mastoid air cells. Care is taken to avoid exposure of tumor in the mastoid. In this case, the confluence of the transverse, sigmoid, and superior petrosal sinuses are decorticated to expose posterior fossa dura on either side of the sigmoid sinus. When posterior fossa dural involvement is suspected, a presigmoid intradural approach with gentle retraction of the cerebellum (Fig. 4–4*A*) allows exposure of the vessels and nerves in the cerebellopontine

angle that are keeping the involved dura attached to the specimen. When the mastoid air cells are thought to be free of tumor, a translabyrinthine approach to the IAC is used (Fig. 4–4*B*). The anterior inferior cerebellar artery is retracted after the labyrinthine artery is bipolarly coagulated and divided. The superior and inferior vestibular nerves, cochlear nerve, facial nerve, and nervus intermedius (nerve of Wrisberg) are divided. A segment of the proximal facial nerve stump can be sent for frozen section pathologic examination if it is suspicious for carcinoma. The dome of the jugular bulb must be separated from the specimen when the dural venous sinuses are spared.

The surgical technique from here varies according to whether the dural venous sinuses or the ICA is preserved. When both are preserved and an STBR is being performed, the bone between the bony canal of the carotid artery at the junction of the vertical and horizontal segments (Fig. 4–5*A*) and the fundus of the IAC is removed with a high-powered drill. Separation of the petro-occipital synchondrosis sometimes requires insertion of an osteotome just above the jugular bulb. This step releases the specimen en bloc from attachment to the clivus. Packing oxidized cellulose intraluminally toward the cavernous sinus controls bleeding from the inferior petrosal sinus.

When both vascular structures are preserved and a TTBR is being performed, the bone between the posterior edge of the foramen ovale and spheno-occipital synchondrosis is removed (Fig. 4–5*B*). The petro-occipital synchondrosis may require an additional osteotomy before the specimen is delivered.

When the dural venous sinuses are sacrificed, the internal jugular vein is double ligated in the upper cervical area and mobilized toward the jugular bulb (Fig. 4–6). The superior petrosal sinus and sigmoid sinus are divided and intraluminally packed with oxidized cellulose. Care is taken not to overpack the sigmoid sinus proximally to avoid obstruction of the vein of Labbe. This can cause hemorrhagic necrosis of the temporal lobe. Similarly, excessive packing of the inferior petrosal sinus can lead to cavernous sinus thrombosis. The sigmoid sinus is then opened toward the jugular bulb and resected. Intraluminal rather than extraluminal packing of the inferior petrosal sinus is preferred to avoid injury to cranial nerves traversing the jugular foramen.

The results of the temporary balloon occlusion determine whether the ICA can be safely resected. When the patient is at high risk for stroke following sacrifice of the ICA, the patient will require revascularization to ensure adequate cerebral blood flow. An extracranial-to-intracranial arterial bypass, such as a superficial temporal artery to middle cerebral artery bypass, must be considered.

The middle and posterior fossa dura is then inspected for carcinomatous involvement. Any involved areas are resected, and margins are sent for frozen section pathologic examination. The temporal lobe and cerebellum are also examined, and limited involvement of the inferior temporal gyrus and cerebellum can be resected. Once intradural hemostasis is achieved, the dura is then closed in a watertight manner using pericranium, fascia lata, or cadaveric dura.

Reconstruction includes restoration of facial nerve continuity and closing the dead space following tumor resection.

FIGURE 4-3

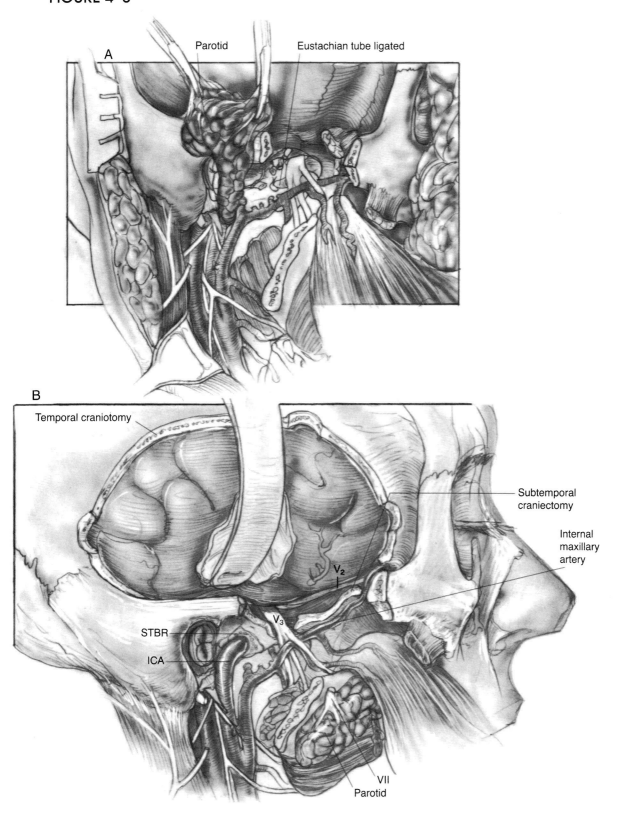

FIGURE 4-3. *A,* Further dissection in the infratemporal fossa allows division and ligation of the eustachian tube and exposure of the petrous carotid artery. *B,* The petrous carotid artery is further dissected according to whether a subtotal or total temporal bone resection is performed. STBR, subtotal temporal bone resection; ICA, internal carotid artery.

PRESIGMOID INTRADURAL APPROACH

FIGURE 4-4

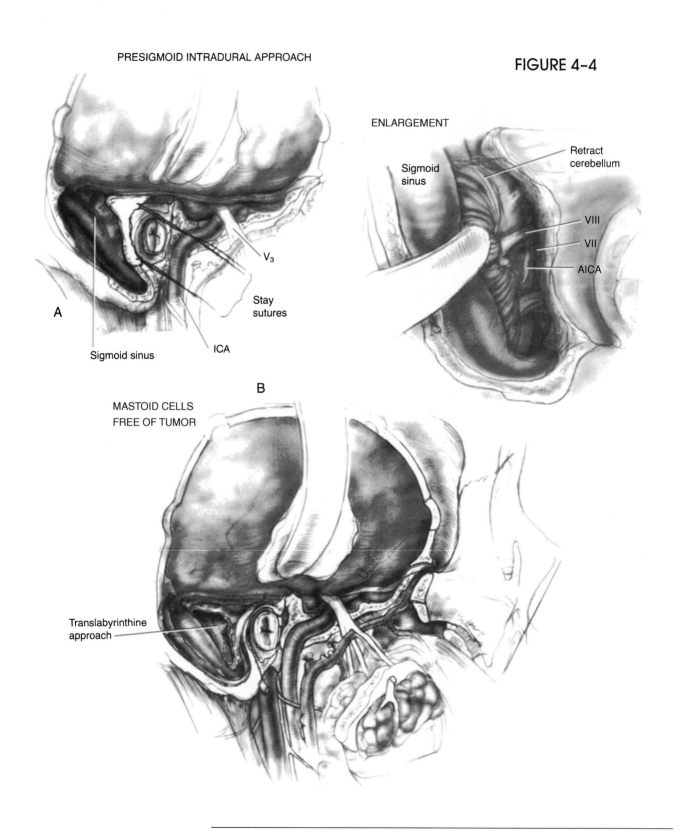

ENLARGEMENT

Sigmoid sinus

Retract cerebellum

VIII

VII

AICA

A

Sigmoid sinus

ICA

V_3

Stay sutures

B

MASTOID CELLS FREE OF TUMOR

Translabyrinthine approach

FIGURE 4–4. *A (left* and *right)*, When tumor is thought to be present in the mastoid, a presigmoid intradural approach (enlarged view on the right) to the porus acusticus is used. *B*, When the mastoid is thought to be free of tumor, a translabyrinthine approach allows exposure of the internal auditory canal. ICA, internal carotid artery; AICA, anteroinferior cerebellar artery.

FIGURE 4-5

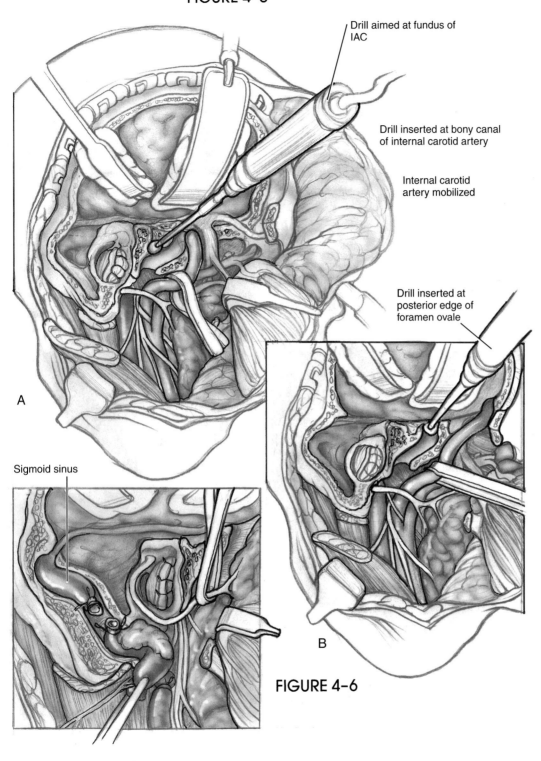

Drill aimed at fundus of IAC

Drill inserted at bony canal of internal carotid artery

Internal carotid artery mobilized

Drill inserted at posterior edge of foramen ovale

Sigmoid sinus

A

B

FIGURE 4-6

FIGURE 4–5. *A*, A drill, inserted at the junction of the vertical and horizontal petrous carotid canal, is aimed toward the fundus of the internal auditory canal (IAC) to allow removal of the subtotal temporal bone specimen. *B*, A drill, inserted at the horizontal petrous carotid canal just posterior to the foramen ovale, is directed slightly posteriorly to avoid entry into the foramen lacerum. This releases the total temporal bone specimen.

FIGURE 4–6. When the dural venous sinus is sacrificed, the internal jugular vein is mobilized toward the cranial base as the sigmoid sinus is intraluminally packed.

The greater auricular nerve, cervical cutaneous nerve, or eleventh cranial nerve can be used as a cable graft from the facial nerve in the IAC to the peripheral branches. When greater length is required, the sural nerve can be harvested from the lower leg. Use of vascularized tissue, rather than autogenous fat, is preferred to fill in the surgical defect. The temporalis muscle can be rotated into the defect. Split-thickness skin grafts can be used for cutaneous defects. A small bolus dressing is placed to ensure adequate adhesion. When the temporalis is not available, plastic surgery teams can harvest microvascular free flaps. Jackson-Pratt drains are installed under the neck and scalp skin flaps to ensure tissue coaptation.

POSTOPERATIVE CARE

Following extubation in the operating room, the patient is examined for neurologic deficits. Unanticipated neurologic deficits are further studied by noncontrast CT imaging to evaluate the presence of intracranial edema or bleeding. Antibiotics are continued postoperatively until the drains are removed or if an infectious process dictates otherwise. Dexamethasone is continued for 48 hours and then tapered over 5 days.

When the ICA has been sacrificed, great care is taken to avoid even minor hypotensive and hypovolemic periods. These events can reduce the cerebral blood flow through the remaining contralateral carotid artery and lead to cerebral ischemia.

Intermittent spinal drainage, through a lumbar drain installed at the end of the procedure, reduces the pressure in the subarachnoid space and accelerates healing of dural defects. Continuous spinal drainage can cause overdrainage and pneumocephalus and is not used. Depending on patient tolerance, 35 to 50 ml of spinal fluid is drained every 8 hours for 48 hours. The drain is then clamped for 24 hours and removed.

POTENTIAL COMPLICATIONS

Inadvertent carotid artery injury can be managed initially by local pressure to the site of entry and placement of temporary clips on either side. After systemic heparinization, the tear is examined, irrigated with heparinized saline, and repaired using 8-0 Novofil suture. Prior to placement of the last suture, the lumen is irrigated with heparinized saline to clear any clots. The hemoclips are then released, and any minor leaks are managed with oxidized cellulose. If the tear is beyond repair, then the results of the preoperative temporary balloon occlusion dictate further management.

ADJUVANT TREATMENT

Treatment of temporal bone malignancies extending into the middle ear should consist of surgical resection of all visible disease followed by external-beam radiotherapy. Occasionally, large, aggressive tumors invading brain parenchyma, the dominant carotid artery, or dural venous sinus are encountered, and total tumor removal is not possible without serious neurologic deficits. In these instances, brachytherapy catheters can be inserted and used.

REHABILITATION

Facial palsy following temporal bone resection requires careful assessment and treatment. A temporary tarsorrhaphy at the conclusion of the operation affords early corneal protection. Once the periorbital edema subsides, a gold-weight implant in the upper eyelid can offer long-term corneal protection. Elderly patients may also require lower eyelid tightening procedures. Facial nerve recovery can be expected at 12 to 18 months. The best facial function a patient can expect with a cable graft, in our hands, is House-Brackmann grade III.

Excessive packing of the inferior petrosal sinus can lead to lower cranial nerve dysfunction (IX, X, XI) that can be a debilitating disability. Some patients require temporary tracheostomy and gastrostomy, and others suffice with Teflon injection of the vocal fold or an Isshiki thyroplasty.[4]

FOLLOW-UP

Patients are seen every month for the first year, and repeat imaging (CT and MRI) is obtained at 6 months and yearly thereafter. Enhancing tumors are best visualized by contrast-enhanced fat-suppression MRI that helps differentiate transposed flaps from tumor recurrence. Any suspicious areas require biopsies either directly or by needle aspiration techniques with or without CT guidance.

RESULTS

Temporal bone neoplasms occur infrequently. The limited experience makes analysis of treatment difficult. Because of this difficulty, we reviewed the literature for all cases of squamous cell carcinoma of the temporal bone,[5] analyzed the extent of disease present, studied the different treatment strategies employed, and reported on outcome. Our findings are presented.

All publications in the English language from 1915 to 1992 dealing with the treatment of squamous cell carcinoma of the temporal bone were reviewed. Ninety-six publications[1, 6–100] were encountered, of which 26 articles[75–100] contained enough information on 144 patients. Various parameters were then analyzed. The major reason for exclusion of a study was the lack of a descriptive table in which the extent of disease, type of treatment, and follow-up for each patient was carefully documented.

Several conclusions about overall survival could be made. When disease was confined to the external auditory canal, no statistically significant difference in 5-year survival was found between patients treated with LTBR (48.6 per cent) and those treated with STBR (50 per cent). When disease extended into the middle ear, patients who had STBR had better 5-year survival (41.7 per cent) than those who had LTBR (28.6 per cent) (Fig. 4–7). The experience with carcinoma that invaded the petrous apex was limited.

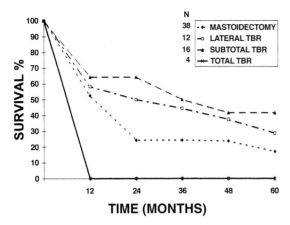

FIGURE 4–7. Treatment-specific survival for patients with carcinoma extending to the middle ear. TBR, temporal bone resection. (From Prasad S, Janecka IP: Efficacy of surgical treatments for squamous cell carcinoma of the temporal bone. Otol Head Neck Surg 110: 270–280, 1994.)

Four patients treated with TTBR had a 50 per cent 1-year survival and zero per cent 2-year survival. One patient treated with STBR was dead of disease at 1 year.

The value of preoperative or postoperative radiation therapy was also analyzed. When disease was confined to the external auditory canal, the addition of either preoperative or postoperative radiation therapy to LTBR did not significantly improve 5-year survival (48.0 per cent with radiation therapy, 44.4 per cent without radiation therapy) (Fig. 4–8). This was the only group in which a conclusion regarding radiation treatment could be made.

The prognostic value of dural involvement was also studied. Resection of involved dura mater, surprisingly, did not improve overall 5-year survival (11.1 per cent with or without resection). It must also be remembered that margin status was not always reported.

Four patients had extension of disease to involve the ICA. Of the two patients treated with TTBR and ICA sacrifice, one died from postoperative cerebral ischemia

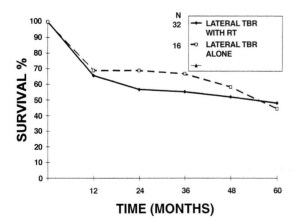

FIGURE 4–8. Survival of patients with carcinoma confined to the external auditory canal treated with lateral temporal bone resection (TBR) with or without preoperative or postoperative radiation therapy (RT). (From Prasad S, Janecka IP: Efficacy of surgical treatments for squamous cell carcinoma of the temporal bone. Otol Head Neck Surg 110: 270–280, 1994.)

and the other died from disease at 14 months of regional and distant failure. The other two patients who were treated in a method that spared the ICA died from disease shortly after resection.

Two patients with carcinomatous invasion of the temporal lobe treated with limited resection also died from disease shortly after resection. No patient was encountered who had resection of involved cerebral or cerebellar tissue.

Site of failure was also studied. Of 54 patients who died from their disease, 45 had local failure, 5 had locoregional failure, 3 had regional failure alone, and 1 had regional-distant failure.

Several other aspects of this disease could not be studied because of the lack of information provided by the authors. First, the histologic differentiation of the tumor and its relationship to overall survival could not be analyzed. Second, the method of temporal bone removal, whether by en bloc resection, piecemeal resection or a drillout, and its relationship to survival could not be ascertained. The status of the margins of resection and relationship to overall survival remains to be studied.

SUMMARY

Radical resection of the temporal bone requires thorough knowledge of the intricate anatomy of the temporal bone and surrounding structures. There is no substitute for laboratory dissection prior to embarking on such an endeavor. Thorough preoperative imaging, delineation of the extent of tumor involvement, and preoperative carotid artery testing are imperative.

The indications for the operation are slowly evolving as we gain experience and collate data for analysis. From our literature review regarding squamous cell carcinoma,[5] it appears that cancerous involvement of the middle ear is best treated by STBR rather than LTBR and gross removal of middle ear disease. Once the tumor involves the petrous apex, we believe that TTBR can allow total tumor extirpation and possibly prolonged survival, although the latter remains to be proved. Prospective, randomized studies are needed to define the value of margin-free dural, carotid artery, and brain parenchymal resection. The value of adjunctive radiation therapy for extensive lesions also requires further study.

References

1. Johns ME, Headington JT: Squamous cell carcinoma of the external auditory canal: A clinicopathologic study of 20 cases. Arch Otolaryngol Head Neck Surg 100: 45–49, 1974.
2. Kinney SE: Tumors of the external auditory canal, middle ear, mastoid, and temporal bone. *In* Thawley SE, Panje WR, Batsakis JG, Lindberg RD (eds): Comprehensive Management of Head and Neck Tumors. Philadelphia, WB Saunders, 1987, p 182.
3. Janecka IP, Sekhar LN, Horton JA, Yonas H: Cerebral blood flow evaluation. *In* Cummings CW, Frederickson JM, Harlor LA, et al (eds): Otolaryngology Head and Neck Surgery: Update II. St. Louis, Mosby–Year Book, 1990, pp 54–63.
4. Sasaki CT, Leder SB, Petcu L, Freidman CD: Longitudinal voice quality changes following Isshiki thyroplasty type I: The Yale experience. Laryngoscope 100: 849–852, 1990.
5. Prasad S, Janecka IP: Efficacy of surgical treatments for squamous cell carcinoma of the temporal bone. Otol Head Neck Surg 110: 270–280, 1994.

6. Campbell E, Volk BM, Burkland CW: Total resection of the temporal bone for malignancy of the middle ear. Ann Surg 134: 397–404, 1951.

7. Coleman CC, Khuri A: A rational treatment for advanced cancer of the external ear and temporal bone. VA Med Monthly 86: 21–24, 1959.

8. Hutcheon JR: Experiences with aural carcinoma over the past six years. Med J Aust 2: 406–407, 1966.

9. Figi FA, Weisman PA: Cancer and chemodectoma in the middle ear and mastoid. JAMA 156: 1157–1162, 1954.

10. Wang CC: Radiation therapy in the management of carcinoma of the external auditory canal, middle ear, or mastoid. Ther Rad 116: 713–715, 1975.

11. Sinha PP, Aziz HI: Treatment of carcinoma of the middle ear. Ther Rad 126: 485–487, 1978.

12. Boland J: The management of carcinomas of the middle ear. Radiology 80: 285, 1963.

13. Holmes KS: The treatment of carcinoma of the middle ear by the 4-MV linear accelerator. Proc R Soc Med 53: 242–244, 1960.

14. Yamada S, Schuh FD, Harvin JS, Perot PL: En bloc subtotal temporal bone resection for cancer of the external ear. J Neurosurg 39: 370–379, 1973.

15. Hahn SS, Kim JA, Goodchild N, Constable WC: Carcinoma of the middle ear and external auditory canal. Int J Rad Oncol Biol Phys 9: 1003–1007, 1983.

16. Sorenson H: Cancer of the middle ear and mastoid. Acta Radiol 54: 460–468, 1960.

17. Frazer JS: Malignant disease of the external acoustic meatus and middle ear. Proc R Soc Med 23: 1235–1244, 1930.

18. Barnes EB: Carcinoma of the ear. Proc R Soc Med 23: 1231–1234, 1930.

19. Conley JS: Cancer of the middle ear and temporal bone. NY State J Med 74: 1575–1579, 1974.

20. Kinney SE, Wood BG: Malignancies of the external ear canal and temporal bone: Surgical techniques and results. Laryngoscope 97: 158–164, 1987.

21. Kinney SE: Squamous cell carcinoma of the external auditory canal. Am J Otol 10: 111–116, 1989.

22. Graham MD, Sataloff RT, Kemink J, McGillicuddy JF: En bloc resection of the temporal bone and carotid artery for malignant tumors of the ear and temporal bone. Laryngoscope 94: 528–533, 1984.

23. Clark LJ, Narola AA, Morgan DAL, Bradley PJ: Squamous carcinoma of the temporal bone: A revised staging. J Laryngol Otol 105: 346–348, 1991.

24. Corey JP, Nelson E, Crawford M, et al: Metastatic vaginal carcinoma to the temporal bone. Am J Otol 12: 128–131, 1991.

25. Hiraide F, Inonye T, Ishii T: Primary squamous cell carcinoma of the middle ear invading the cochlea: A histopathologic case report. Ann Otol Rhinol Laryngol 92: 290–294, 1983.

26. Schusterman MA, Kroll SS: Reconstruction strategy for temporal bone and lateral facial defects. Ann Plastic Surg 26: 233–294, 1983.

27. Haughey BH, Gates GA, Skerhut HE, Brown WE: Cerebral shift after lateral craniofacial resection and flap reconstruction. Otolaryngol Head Neck Surg 101: 79–86, 1989.

28. Bergetedt HF, Lind MG: Temporal bone scintigraphy. Acta Otolaryngol (Stockh) 89: 465–473, 1980.

29. Jahn AF, Farkashidy J, Berman JM: Metastatic tumors in the temporal bone—a pathophysiologic study. J Otolaryngol 8: 85–95, 1979.

30. Ruben RJ, Thaler SU, Holzer N: Radiation-induced carcinoma of the temporal bone. Laryngoscope 87: 1613–1621, 1977.

31. Katsarkas A, Seemayer TA: Bilateral temporal bone metastases of a uterine cervix carcinoma. J Otolaryngol 5: 315–318, 1976.

32. Ramsden RT, Bulman CH, Lorigan BP: Osteoradionecrosis of the temporal bone. J Laryngol Otol 89: 941–955, 1975.

33. Vize G: Laryngeal metastasis to the temporal bone causing facial paralysis. J Laryngol Otol 88: 175–177, 1974.

34. Schuknecht HF, Allam AF, Murakami Y: Pathology of secondary malignant tumors of the temporal bone. Ann Otol Rhinol Laryngol 77: 5–22, 1968.

35. Lewis JS: Temporal bone resection: Review of 100 cases. Arch Otolaryogol Head Neck Surg 101: 23–25, 1975.

36. Arriaga M, Curtin H, Takahashi H, et al: Staging proposal for external auditory meatus carcinoma based on preoperative clinical examination and computed tomography findings. Ann Otol Rhinol Laryngol 99: 714–721, 1990.

37. Adams WS, Morrison R: On primary carcinoma of the middle ear and mastoid. J Laryngol Otol 69: 115–131, 1955.

38. Gacek RR: Management of temporal bone carcinoma. Trans Penn Acad Otolaryngol Ophthalmol 32: 67–71, 1978.

39. Conley J, Schuller DE: Malignancies of the ear. Laryngoscope 86: 1147–1163, 1976.

40. Greer JA, Body DTR, Weiland LH: Neoplasms of the temporal bone. J Otolaryngol 5: 391–398, 1978.

41. Goodman ML: Middle ear and mastoid neoplasms. Ann Otol Rhinol Laryngol 80: 419–424, 1971.

42. Arena S, Keen M: Carcinoma of the middle ear and temporal bone. Am J Otol 9: 351–356, 1988.

43. Hilding DA, Selker R: Total resection of the temporal bone for carcinoma. Arch Otolaryngol Head Neck Surg 89: 98–107, 1969.

44. Cundy RL, Sando I, Hemenway WG: Middle ear extension of nasopharyngeal carcinoma via the eustachian tube. Arch Otolaryngol Head Neck Surg 98: 131–133, 1973.

45. Lewis JS: Squamous carcinoma of the ear. Arch Otolaryogol Head Neck Surg 97: 41–42, 1973.

46. Sekhar LN, Pomeranz S, Janecka IP, et al: Temporal bone neoplasms: A report on 20 surgically treated cases. J Neurosurg 76: 578–587, 1992.

47. Lessor RW, Spector GJ, Divinens VR: Malignant tumors of the middle ear and external auditory canal: A 20-year review. Otolaryngol Head Neck Surg 96: 43–47, 1987.

48. Kenyon GS, Marks PV, Scholtz CL, Dhillon R: Squamous cell carcinoma of the middle ear: A 25-year retrospective study. Ann Otol Rhinol Laryngol 94: 273–277, 1985.

49. Arthur K: Radiotherapy in carcinoma of the middle ear and auditory canal. J Laryngol Otol 90: 753–762, 1976.

50. Tucker WN: Cancer of the middle ear. Cancer 16: 642–650, 1965.

51. Conley JJ, Novack AJ: The surgical treatment of malignant tumors of the ear and temporal bone. Arch Otolaryngol Head Neck Surg 71: 635–652, 1960.

52. Conley JJ, Novack AJ: Surgical treatment of cancer of the ear and temporal bone. Trans Am Acad Ophthalmol Otolaryngol 64: 83–92, 1960.

53. Wagenfield DJH, Keane T, Norstrand AWP, Bryce DP: Primary carcinoma involving the temporal bone: Analysis of 25 cases. Laryngoscope 90: 912–919, 1980.

54. Lewis JS, Parsons H: Surgery for advanced ear cancer. Ann Otol Rhinol Laryngol 67: 364–399, 1958.

55. Lewis JS, Page R: Radical surgery for malignant tumors of the ear. Arch Otolaryngol Head Neck Surg 83: 56–61, 1966.

56. Lewis JS: Surgical management of tumors of the middle ear and mastoid. J Laryngol Otol 97: 299–311, 1983.

57. Lederman M: Malignant tumors of the ear. J Laryngol Otol 79: 85–119, 1965.

58. Frew I, Finney R: Neoplasms of the middle ear. J Laryngol Otol 77: 415–421, 1963.

59. Goodwin WJ, Jesse RH: Malignant neoplasms of the external auditory canal and temporal bone. Arch Otolaryngol Head Neck Surg 106: 675–679, 1980.

60. Lindahl JWS: Carcinoma of the middle ear and meatus. J Laryngol Otol 69: 457–467, 1955.

61. Bradley WH, Maxwell JH: Neoplasms of the middle ear and mastoid: Report of 54 cases. Laryngoscope 54: 533–556, 1954.

62. Miller D: Cancer of the external auditory meatus. Laryngoscope 65: 448–461, 1955.

63. Colledge L: Two cases of malignant disease of the temporal bone. J Laryngol Otol 58: 251–254, 1943.

64. Peele JC, Hauser GH: Primary carcinoma of the external auditory canal and middle ear. Arch Otolaryngol Head Neck Surg 34: 254–266, 1941.

65. Garnett-Passe ER: Primary carcinoma of the eustachian tube. J Laryngol Otol 62: 314–315, 1948.

66. Spencer FR: Malignant disease of the ear. Arch Otolaryngol Head Neck Surg 28: 916–940, 1938.

67. Means RG, Gersten J: Primary carcinoma of the mastoid process. Ann Otol Rhinol Laryngol 62: 93–100, 1953.

68. Spector JG: Management of temporal bone carcinomas: A therapeutic analysis of two groups of patients and long-term follow-up. Otolaryngol Head Neck Surg 104: 58–66, 1991.

69. Ariyan S, Sasaki CT, Spencer D: Radical en bloc resection of the temporal bone. Am J Surg 142: 443–447, 1981.

70. Arena S: Tumor surgery of the temporal bone. Laryngoscope 84: 645–670, 1974.
71. Brooker GB: Bilateral middle ear carcinomas associated with Waldenström's macroglobulinemia. Ann Otol Rhinol Laryngol 91: 299–303, 1982.
72. Towson CE, Shofstall WH: Carcinoma of the ear. Arch Otolaryngol Head Neck Surg 51: 724–738, 1950.
73. Robinson GA: Malignant tumors of the ear. Laryngoscope 41: 467–473, 1931.
74. Kinney SE, Wood BG: Malignancies of the external ear canal and temporal bone: Surgical techniques and results. Laryngoscope 97: 158–164, 1987.
75. Buckmann LT, Barre W: Carcinoma of the middle ear and mastoid. Ann Otol Rhinol Laryngol 52: 194–201, 1943.
76. Liebeskind MM: Primary carcinoma of the external auditory canal, middle ear, and mastoid. Laryngoscope 61: 1173–1187, 1951.
77. Stokes HB: Primary malignant tumors of the temporal bone. Arch Otolaryngol Head Neck Surg 32: 1023–1030, 1990.
78. Rosenwasser H: Neoplasms involving the middle ear. Arch Otolaryngol Head Neck Surg 32: 38–53, 1940.
79. Grossman AA, Donnelly WA, Smithman MF: Carcinoma of the middle ear and mastoid process. Ann Otol Rhinol Laryngol 56: 709–721, 1947.
80. Mattick WL, Mattick JW: Some experience in management of cancer of the middle ear and mastoid. Arch Otolaryngol Head Neck Surg 53: 610–621, 1951.
81. Wahl JW, Gromet MT: Carcinoma of the middle ear and mastoid. Arch Otolaryngol Head Neck Surg 58: 121–126, 1953.
82. Crabtree JA, Britton BH, Pierce MK: Carcinoma of the external auditory canal. Laryngoscope 86: 405–415, 1976.
83. Hanna DC, Richardson GS, Gaisford JC: A suggested technique for resection of the temporal bone. Am J Surg 114: 553–558, 1967.
84. Adams GL, Paparella MM, Fiky FM: Primary and metastatic tumors of the temporal bone. Laryngoscope 81: 1273–1285, 1971.
85. Sataloff RT, Myers DL, Lowry LD, Spiegel JR: Total temporal bone resection for squamous cell carcinoma. Otolaryngol Head Neck Surg 96: 4–14, 1987.
86. Nadol JB, Schoknecht HF: Obliteration of the mastoid in the treatment of tumors of the temporal bone. Ann Otol Rhinol Laryngol 93: 6–12, 1984.
87. Arriaga M, Hirsch BE, Kamerer DB, Myers EN: Squamous cell carcinoma of the external auditory meatus (canal). Otolaryngol Head Neck Surg 101: 330–337, 1989.
88. Michaels L, Wells M: Squamous cell carcinomas of the middle ear. Clin Otolaryngol 5: 235–248, 1980.
89. McCrea RS: Radical surgery for carcinoma of the middle ear. Laryngoscope 82: 1514–1523, 1972.
90. Gacek RR, Goodman M: Management of malignancy of the temporal bone. Laryngoscope 87: 1622–1634, 1977.
91. Scholl LA: Neoplasms involving the middle ear. Arch Otolaryngol Head Neck Surg 22: 548–553, 1935.
92. Clairmont AA, Conley JJ: Primary carcinoma of the mastoid bone. Ann Otol Rhinol Laryngol 86: 306–309, 1977.
93. Beal DD, Lindsay JR, Ward PH: Radiation-induced carcinoma of the mastoid. Arch Otolaryngol Head Neck Surg 81: 9–16, 1965.
94. Coleman CC: Removal of the temporal bone for cancer. Am J Surg 112: 583–590, 1966.
95. Parsons H, Lewis JS: Subtotal resection of the temporal bone for cancer of the ear. Cancer 7: 995–1001, 1954.
96. Miller D, Silverstein H, Gacek RR: Cryosurgical treatment of carcinoma of the ear. Trans Am Acad Ophthalmol Otolaryngol 76: 1363–1367, 1972.
97. Tabb HG, Komet H, McLaurin JW: Cancer of the external auditory canal: Treatment with radical mastoidectomy and irradiation. Laryngoscope 74: 634–643, 1964.
98. Lodge WO, Jones HM, Smith MEN: Malignant tumors of the temporal bone. Arch Otolaryngol Head Neck Surg 61: 535–541, 1955.
99. Ward GE, Loch WE, Lawrence W: Radical operation for carcinoma of the external auditory canal and middle ear. Am J Surg 82: 169–178, 1951.
100. Newhart H: Primary carcinoma of the middle ear: Report of a case. Laryngoscope 27: 543–555, 1917.

5

Congenital Malformation of the Temporal Bone

Antonio De la Cruz, M.D. ▪ Sujana S. Chandrasekhar, M.D.
▪ Jose N. Fayad, M.D.

Congenital malformation of the temporal bone is characterized by aplasia or hypoplasia of the external auditory canal (EAC), often associated with absence or deformity of the auricle (microtia) and the middle ear, with occasional inner ear abnormalities. Aural atresia occurs in 1 in 10,000 to 20,000 live births,[1-5] with unilateral atresia being three times more common than bilateral atresia. This disorder occurs more commonly in males and on the right side.[1] The EAC atresia is more often bony rather than membranous, and bony atresia is regularly accompanied by malformation of the middle ear cavity and structures of the middle ear.[6-9] More severe forms of congenital microtia are usually associated with EAC atresia; in rare instances, canal atresia may be seen in patients with a normal pinna.[10] In general, a more severe external deformity implies a more severe middle ear abnormality.[11-12]

Kiesselbach, in 1883, is credited with the first deep operation attempting to correct this malformation.[8] More recently, Lascaratos and Assimakopoulos credit the Byzantine physician Paul d'Egine with the use of a straight–sharp-pointed bistouri (Scolopomachairion) in the treatment of congenital aural atresia.[13-14] Unfortunately, the procedure done by Kiesselbach resulted in facial paralysis. Due to the lack of middle ear microsurgery and the high complication rate, congenital aural atresia surgery was considered dangerous and to be avoided for the most part. In 1914, Page reported hearing improvement in five of eight patients.[15] In 1917, Dean and Gittens reported excellent hearing result in a patient and reviewed the various types of operations that had been tried by other surgeons.[16] The prevailing attitude toward surgical correction in these cases remained generally pessimistic, despite these and other occasional reports of successful operations, until 1947. That year, Ombredanne in France and Pattee in the United States each reported a series of patients successfully operated on to improve the hearing.[17, 18] Pattee's technique included removal of the incus to "mobilize" the stapes; Ombredanne added fenestration of the lateral semicircular canal (LSCC).

With the advent of tympanoplasty techniques in the 1950s, interest in atresiaplasty rose as the teachings of Wullstein and Zollner carried over into surgery of the congenital ear.[8] Larger series with greater success rates were reported as surgeons attempted to improve their results, using ossiculoplasty, mastoidectomy, and differing degrees of bone removal and different types and techniques of graft placement.[2, 4, 17, 19-26] Ombredanne went on to report on more than 600 aplasia cases by 1971 and 1600 cases with major and minor malformations by 1976.[8, 27] Gill's series of 83 cases is a landmark paper.[2] In the last two decades, Crabtree,[28] Jahrsdoerfer,[8, 29, 30] Marquet,[31, 32] and De la Cruz[6, 33] have reported on large surgical series, with modifications of classification and operative techniques.

Although techniques of canalplasty, meatoplasty, tympanoplasty, and ossiculoplasty have improved considerably, surgical correction of congenital aural atresia remains one of the most challenging operations performed by otologists. This is a complex surgical problem, requiring application of all modern tympanoplasty techniques and a thorough knowledge of the surgical anatomy of the facial nerve, oval window, and inner ear as well as their congenital variants.[1, 6, 8, 17, 21, 26, 27, 29-31, 33-40] The temporomandibular joint is displaced posteriorly by the lack of development of the EAC, narrowing the distance between the glenoid fossa and the anterior wall of the mastoid tip.[19, 41] Fusion of the incus and malleus is common, but due to its dual origin, the stapes footplate is usually normal.[4, 42]

The timing of repair must take into account any planned auricular reconstruction procedures.[6] Criteria for patient selection must be stringent when attempting to achieve closure of the air-bone gap to within 20 to 30 dB. Preoperative counseling and several postoperative visits are essential for optimal results. In this chapter, we discuss these issues and provide guidelines for patient evaluation and selection, surgical techniques, and postoperative management.

EMBRYOLOGY

A review of the normal embryologic development of the ear will aid in understanding the myriad of possible combinations of malformations encountered in congenital aural atresia. The inner ear, middle ear, and external ear develop independently and in such a way that deformity of one does not necessarily presuppose deformity of another.[9, 43] Most frequently, abnormalities of the outer and middle ear are encountered in combination with a normal inner ear structure.[44, 45]

Microtia is a result of first and second branchial arches anomalies. Growth of mesenchymal tissue from the first and second branchial arches forms six hillocks around the primitive meatus that fuse to form the auricle (Table 5–1). By the end of the third month, the primitive auricle has

TABLE 5–1. Development of the Auricle

FIRST BRANCHIAL ARCH	SECOND BRANCHIAL ARCH
First hillock—tragus	Fourth hillock—antihelix
Second hillock—helical crus	Fifth hillock—antitragus
Third hillock—helix	Sixth hillock—lobule and lower helix

been completed. The external auditory meatus develops from the first branchial groove. During the second month, a solid core of epithelium migrates inward from the rudimentary pinna toward the first branchial pouch. This core, the precursor of the EAC, starts to hollow out and take shape in the sixth month. It canalizes in the seventh month, causing the developing mastoid to become separated from the mandible. Its subsequent posterior and inferior development carries the middle ear and facial nerve to their normal positions.[1, 43, 46–48] Some of the literature supports the notion that microtia grade can indicate the status of middle ear development in aural atresia. Thus, the better developed the external ear, the better developed will be the middle ear.

The first branchial pouch grows outward to form the middle ear cleft. The plaque of tissue where this meets the epithelium of the EAC forms the tympanic membrane (TM). While the pouch is forming the eustachian tube, tympanic cavity, and mastoid air cells, Meckel's cartilage (first branchial arch) is forming the neck and head of the malleus and incus body. Reichert's cartilage (second branchial arch) forms the remainder of the first two ossicles' long processes and the stapes superstructure. The footplate has a dual origin from the second arch and the otic capsule. The ossicles attain their final shape by the fourth month. By the end of the seventh to eighth month, the expanding middle ear cleft surrounds the ossicles and covers them with a mucous membrane.[1, 45, 49]

The facial nerve is the nerve of the second branchial arch. At 4.5 weeks, this developing nerve divides the blastema, which is the condensation of the second arch mesenchymal cells, into the stapes, the interhyale (stapedius muscle precursor), and the laterohyale (precursor of the posterior wall of the middle ear). The nerve's intraosseous course is dependent on this bony expansion.[45, 47] The membranous portion of the inner ear develops during the third to the sixth week from an auditory placode on the lateral surface of the hindbrain. The surrounding mesenchyme transforms into the bony otic capsule.[50]

Congenital aural atresia can, therefore, range in severity from a thin membranous canal atresia to complete lack of tympanic bone, depending on the time of arrest of intrauterine development.[1, 51, 52] The usual finding of a normal inner ear is explained, as the inner ear is formed by the time of external/middle ear development arrest. Facial nerve course abnormalities are often seen. Only 4 per cent of congenital malformations of the external and middle ear are associated with inner ear deformities.

CLASSIFICATION SYSTEMS

Of historical significance is a classification in congenital aural atresia developed in 1955 by Altmann.[51] In this system, atresias are categorized into three groups:

Group 1 (mild): Some part of the EAC, although hypoplastic, is present. The tympanic bone is hypoplastic and the ear drum is small. The tympanic cavity is either normal in size or hypoplastic.
Group 2 (moderate): The EAC is completely absent, the tympanic cavity is small and its content deformed, and the "atresia plate" is partially or completely osseous.
Group 3 (severe): The EAC is absent and the tympanic cavity is markedly hypoplastic or missing.

Altmann's classification system is purely descriptive, and most surgical candidates fall into groups 2 and 3.

The *De la Cruz classification* involves only advanced Altmann groups 2 and 3 and divides abnormalities into "minor" and "major" categories.[6] Minor malformations consist of

1. Normal mastoid pneumatization
2. Normal oval window footplate
3. Reasonable facial nerve-footplate relationship
4. Normal inner ear

Major malformations are

1. Poor pneumatization
2. Abnormal or absent oval window/footplate
3. Abnormal course of the facial nerve
4. Abnormalities of the inner ear

The clinical importance of this classification is that surgery in cases of minor malformations has a good possibility of yielding serviceable hearing, whereas cases of major malformations are frequently inoperable but treatable with the bone-anchored hearing aid (BAHA) system.[3]

A widely used point-grading system to guide surgeons in their preoperative assessment of the best candidates for hearing improvement has been developed by Jahrsdoerfer[53] (Table 5–2). This takes into account the parameters of mastoid pneumatization, presence of the oval and round windows, facial nerve course, status of the ossicles, and

TABLE 5–2. Jahrsdoerfer's Grading System of Candidacy for Surgery of Congenital Aural Atresia

PARAMETER	POINTS
Stapes present	2
Oval window open	1
Middle ear space	1
Facial nerve normal	1
Malleus-incus complex present	1
Mastoid well pneumatized	1
Incus-stapes connection	1
Round window normal	1
Appearance of external ear	1
Total available points	10

RATING	TYPE OF CANDIDATE
10	Excellent
9	Very good
8	Good
7	Fair
6	Marginal
≤5	Poor

From Jahrsdoerfer RA, Yeakley JW, Aguilar EA, et al: Grading system for the selection of patients with congenital aural atresia. Am J Otol 13:6–12, 1992.

external appearance. Point allocation is based primarily on the findings on high-resolution computed tomography (HRCT). Jahrsdoerfer proposes that when the preoperative evaluation of the patient is itemized into this grading system, the best results (>80 per cent success) will be achieved with a score of 8 or better. A score of 7 implies a fair chance, 6 is marginal, and below this the patient becomes a poor candidate.

Schuknecht's system of classification of congenital aural atresia is based on a combination of clinical and primarily surgical observations.[54] Type A (meatal) atresia is limited to the fibrocartilaginous part of the EAC. Meatoplasty is the surgical procedure of choice and, when performed in a timely fashion, will prevent formation of canal cholesteatoma and conductive hearing loss. In type B (partial) atresia, there is narrowing of both the fibrocartilaginous and bony EAC, but a patent dermal tract allows partial inspection of the TM. The TM is small and partly replaced by a bony septum. Minor ossicular malformations exist, and hearing loss may be mild to severe. Type C (total) atresia includes all cases with a totally atretic ear canal but a well-pneumatized tympanic cavity. There is a partial or total bony atretic plate, the TM is absent, the heads of the ossicles are fused, there may be no connection to a possibly malformed stapes, and the facial nerve is more likely to have an aberrant course over the oval window. Type D (hypopneumatic total) atresia is a total atresia with poor pneumatization, common in dysplasias such as Treacher Collins syndrome. There are abnormalities of the facial nerve canal and the bony labyrinth. These patients are poor candidates for hearing improvement surgery.

Chiossone, in 1983, presented a classification scheme based primarily on the location of the glenoid fossa.[55] In type I the fossa is in the normal position; in type II it is moderately displaced; in type III the fossa overlaps the middle ear; and in type IV, in addition to the fossa overlapping the middle ear, there is lack of mastoid pneumatization. Types I and II are ideal surgical candidates. Type III cases have a tendency toward graft lateralization. Type IV is not a surgical candidate.

In atresiaplasty surgery, a classification scheme is useful for surgical planning, patient counseling, and comparison of outcomes.

INITIAL EVALUATION AND PATIENT SELECTION

When aural atresia is noted in a newborn, several issues must be addressed. Where one congenital abnormality is found, others must be sought. A high-risk registry for deafness is helpful in this regard.[56] After the degree of aural deformity is assessed by physical examination, evaluation of auditory function in both unilateral and bilateral atresia should be performed using auditory brainstem response (ABR) audiometry within the first few days of life. There is an 11 to 47 per cent incidence of inner ear abnormality associated with congenital aural atresia.[12] Occasionally, in unilateral cases, there is a total sensorineural hearing loss (SNHL) on the side of the normal-appearing ear, which might otherwise be missed.[6, 33]

In bilateral cases, a bone conduction hearing aid should

be applied as soon as possible, ideally in the third or fourth week of life. In unilateral cases in which the opposite ear hears normally, a hearing aid is not necessary. The syndromic child with aural atresia and associated cephalic abnormalities (e.g., hemifacial microsomia and Treacher Collins, Crouzon, Pierre Robin syndrome) should be recognized.[56–60] In this subset, surgical correction has poor results,[54] and long-term bone-conduction aiding is indicated or BAHA in these nonoperable bilateral congenital aural atresia situations is beneficial.[3] This is discussed in more detail later in the chapter.

Prompt and careful counseling of the parents of a child with sporadic (nonsyndromal) congenital aural atresia is necessary to alleviate concerns regarding possible occurrence in their subsequent children (no more than the general population), to answer questions regarding future auricular reconstruction, and, most important, to ensure that proper hearing amplification is instituted in a timely fashion. The child should be enrolled in special education at an early age to maximize speech and language acquisition, in preparation for "mainstreaming" at the preschool age. Radiologic and surgical evaluations are deferred until the child reaches 5 or 6 years of age and are discussed later in this chapter.

In the initial evaluation of an older individual with congenital aural atresia, the most crucial elements remain the functional and anatomic integrity of the inner ear. Audiometry and HRCT in coronal and axial views are necessary. Prognosis for hearing improvement is dependent on the presence and degree of malformations. Auricular reconstruction must be addressed prior to undertaking hearing restorative surgery to avoid alterations in the blood supply to the surrounding soft tissue that may compromise microtia repair.

A patient with congenital aural atresia may present with an infected or draining ear or acute facial palsy; 14 per cent have congenital cholesteatoma.[6] The priority in these cases is removal of the cholesteatoma and resolution of the infection; however, preoperative audiometry and HRCT scanning may be necessary at an earlier age.[6, 54, 61]

There are two requirements for planning surgery in congenital aural atresia: radiographic evidence of an inner ear and audiometric evidence of cochlear function.[8, 62] Other conditions mandating prompt surgical intervention are congenital cholesteatoma, a draining postoperative atretic ear, or acute facial palsy. The CT scan should always be reviewed for cholesteatoma, which necessitates surgery at any age.[54, 61, 63] It is not included in any of the grading systems because these are used only for predicting hearing results in elective atresiaplasty surgery.

TIMING OF AURICULAR RECONSTRUCTION AND ATRESIAPLASTY

In binaural atresia, auricular reconstruction and atresiaplasty are recommended at 6 years of age. By this time, the costal cartilage has developed sufficiently to allow for harvesting and transplantation to the auricle, and the mastoid has become as pneumatized as possible. The microtia repair should be done first, because the complex flaps and use of autologous rib graft demand excellent blood supply.[64, 65] Notably, many surgeons will not perform atresiaplasty on an ear with previous reconstruction attempts.[63] The hearing restoration surgery is then performed 2 months following the microtia repair. Rehabilitation of severe auricular defects using tissue-integrated percutaneous mastoid implant prostheses with and without bone conduction aids has also been described in the literature.[3, 48, 66–68]

In unilateral atresia cases, atresiaplasty surgery may be delayed until the patient is old enough to understand the significant risks to the cochlea, vestibular system, and facial nerve. The exception to this is the individual who has a "minor" unilateral atresia with excellent pneumatization and normal middle ear, ossicles, and facial nerve. This deformity is a "minor" atresia. In these cases, surgery can be performed in childhood with the parents' consent.[33] We often see older adults with unilateral atresia who request surgery when their normal ear begins having high-frequency hearing loss (presbycusis).

Bone-Anchored Hearing Aids

Implantable bone aids available for clinical use were introduced in 1977 in Sweden. Surgery for the BAHA is a two-stage procedure with an interval of 3 to 4 months, allowing for osseointegration to start before a load is applied. The first stage is implantation of the fixture into the mastoid cortex. Following implantation, the skin flap is replaced and healing is allowed to take place. At the second stage, a skin-penetrating abutment is secured to the fixture, reducing the amount of subcutaneous tissue and eliminating hair follicles in the site. Often this necessitates a hairless skin transplant. The aid is first useable 3 to 5 weeks following this second stage. Clinical trials are at present under way to convert the insertion of the BAHA into a one-stage procedure. Other implants are discussed in detail elsewhere in this textbook.[3, 48, 69]

In general, we do not recommend implantable hearing aids in children, because the surgical scars may preclude any future microtia repair. However, the BAHA titanium implant is ideally placed 5 to 6 cm behind and 3 cm above the ear canal in a hair-bearing area. This placement seems to allow for the possibility of transplanting costal cartilage to an area with unscarred skin for future microtia repair. On the other hand, the titanium implants for a bone-anchored epithesis for a cosmetic ear are ideally placed 18 to 20 mm behind the (future) ear canal. This interferes with the skin of a future auricle, if reconstruction is contemplated.[69]

Granstrom and associates[3] reviewed their experience with BAHA and bone-anchored epithesis in 101 patients with atresia and microtia. Plastic surgery—rib graft or, less commonly, Silastic implant—was performed on 47 ears. The number of procedures ranged from 1 to 35, with a mean of 8.4 operations. The authors report astonishingly poor aesthetic outcomes. On 73 auricles in 62 patients, surgery for bone-anchored epithesis was performed; 25 of these patients had had prior microtia surgery. The results are nearly universally excellent. The authors point out that their patient population is selected because of referrals of operative failures or difficult cases.[3, 48, 69]

The same series compared 45 atresiaplasty surgeries with 39 BAHA surgeries. Of 44 postatresiaplasty ears followed for more than 2 years, hearing gain was less than 10 dB in 24 ears, 10 to 30 dB in 19 ears, and more than 30 dB in only 5 ears: The worse the Altmann classification stage, the worse was the surgical outcome. Twenty-four ears were reoperated on within 5 years. Despite reoperation, final outcome was not good in general, with 10 ears undergoing restenosis, 6 ears with continuous or sporadic otorrhea, and 1 patient with continuous vertigo. Of the 39 patients supplied with a BAHA, 16 had had prior atresiaplasty work. The youngest patients were 2 years old, and in this younger age group there was a significant incidence of dural contact and sigmoid sinus contact by the titanium implant. All BAHA patients in the series considered the implant to be superior to conventional bone conduction hearing aids and also superior to hearing improvement obtained surgically. Again, the population is selected out for difficult cases.

Van der Pouw and colleagues[70] described the experience of bilateral BAHA in four patients with bilateral inoperable congenital aural atresia, three of whom had Treacher Collins syndrome. Bilateral BAHA application resulted in better performance in all tested audiologic parameters, including sound localization, speech recognition in quiet, speech recognition in noise, and cued listening task. This appears to be a good option for children with bilateral inoperable atresia.[70]

Implantable hearing aids, therefore, appear to offer a good alternative for patients with inoperable atresia and for patients in whom the operative prognosis is poor.

PREOPERATIVE EVALUATION AND PATIENT COUNSELING

Early diagnosis with ABR and auditory enhancement with bone conduction hearing aid(s) in bilateral cases should be done in the first weeks of life.[71] Corrective surgery begins at 6 years of age. Imaging is deferred until the child reaches this age. Microtia repair is performed prior to atresiaplasty. An estimate of the size of the mastoid on physical examination can be determined by palpation of the mastoid tip, suprameatal spine of Henle (if present), condyle, and zygomatic arch. This is a useful measure because the new ear canal will be constructed at the expense of the mastoid air-cell system.

The only imaging acceptable today for preoperative evaluation is HRCT scanning in both axial and coronal planes (Fig. 5–1).[5, 12, 62, 72] The CT scan must be examined carefully by the otologic surgeon, together with the otoradiologist, because one interpretation often does not provide all of the information necessary for operative planning.[41, 73] The four important imaging elements that are most helpful to the surgeon planning reconstruction of a congenitally malformed ear are (1) the degree of pneumatization of the temporal bone; (2) the course of the facial nerve, both the relationship of the horizontal portion to the footplate, as well as the location of the mastoid segment; (3) the existence of the oval window and stapes footplate; and (4) the status of the inner ear.[5, 6, 62] CT also provides information on thickness and form of the bony atretic plate, size and status of the middle ear cavity, existence of congenital

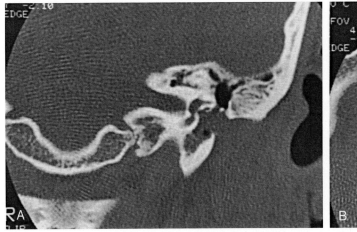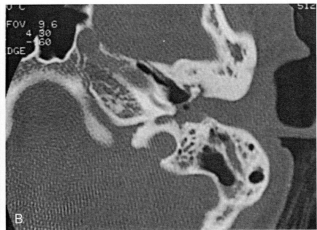

FIGURE 5–1. Congenital aural atresia, left ear. *A,* Coronal HRCT demonstrates atretic external auditory canal and underdeveloped mastoid system, with normal inner ear. *B,* Axial HRCT of the same case.

cholesteatoma, and soft tissue contribution to the atresia,[6] but these are less critical for the repair.

The use of three-dimensional reconstruction CT for preoperative evaluation has been interesting, but it has not been of practical use (Fig. 5–2). Proponents of this technique believe that three-dimensional imaging clearly shows the relationships between the condyle, the zygomatic arch, the temporal bone, and the temporomandibular joint.

Lack of pneumatization is the major cause of inoperability in congenital aural atresia.[6, 33] Fortunately, normal pneumatization is present in the majority of cases. The facial nerve over the oval window may prevent ossiculoplasty and hearing improvement. If the oval window is absent, surgery with fenestration of the lateral semicircular canal or placement of a hearing aid is indicated. There is potential for facial nerve injury in atresia surgery.[74] The nerve may describe a more acute angle rather than its usual 120 degrees at the mastoid genu and often lies more lateral than usual[75] (Fig. 5–3). On HRCT, it is important not to mistakenly "identify" the vertical lie of the facial nerve in the marrow bone leading to the styloid process and the hypoplastic mastoid process[76] (Fig. 5–4). Even in atretic ears in which the facial nerve does not have an abnormal course, a significantly reduced distance is found between the facial canal and the temporomandibular joint[41] and the facial canal and the posterior wall of the cavum tympani.[47]

To be considered a surgical candidate, the patient must have sufficient cochlear function as determined by ABR or on routine audiometry, a normal-appearing inner ear on CT scan, and, preferably, a well-developed mastoid and a good oval window/footplate–facial nerve relationship.

Patient counseling integrates all of the aforementioned issues. Those with a degree of malformation equivalent to a 7 or better on the Jahrsdoerfer grading scale are given a greater than 75 per cent chance of hearing improvement. The risk to the facial nerve is small, made more so by the use of the facial nerve monitor intraoperatively.[33, 75] Patients are informed that a split-thickness skin graft from the hypogastrium will be used to line the new EAC. Initially, frequent postoperative visits are necessary. The risk of graft lateralization is 26 to 28 per cent, the risk of SNHL is 2 per cent, and the risk of facial nerve palsy is 1 per cent. Otherwise, the risks and complications are similar to those for other mastoidectomy procedures.

SURGICAL TECHNIQUE

The first atresiaplasty operations failed because of poor tympanoplasty, large mastoidectomies, and faulty skin grafting techniques[18]; as this was improved, hearing restoration was added using LSCC fenestration.[19, 26, 51] Simultaneously, advances in meatoplasty added to the success rate of atresiaplasty surgery.[19, 77] Although fenestration remains a rare option in bilateral congenital absence of the oval window, modern methods of ossiculoplasty are used preferentially and yield superior results.[6, 8, 19, 23, 26, 28, 31, 34–36, 78–80]

General endotracheal anesthesia is used; muscle relaxants are avoided. Facial nerve monitoring is used in all cases. The patient is in the otologic position and the head is turned away. A large shave of the postauricular area is done, and the auricle and postauricular area are prepared

FIGURE 5–2. *A,* Three-dimensional CT imaging of normal ear demonstrating complete tympanic ring, normal mastoid development, and normal location of glenoid fossa. *B,* Three-dimensional CT image of opposite atretic ear shows only partial development of the tympanic ring and mastoid, with poor pneumatization, and posterior positioning of the glenoid fossa.

FIGURE 5–3. The facial nerve in congenital aural atresia. *A,* Normal intratemporal facial nerve anatomy. *B,* Intratemporal facial nerve anatomy in congenital aural atresia.

FIGURE 5–4. Pitfalls in congenital aural atresia surgery: facial nerve on coronal HRCT. *A, Arrows* point to marrow of the styloid process in an atretic ear. *B, Arrows* point to a vertical segment of the facial nerve in the same ear.

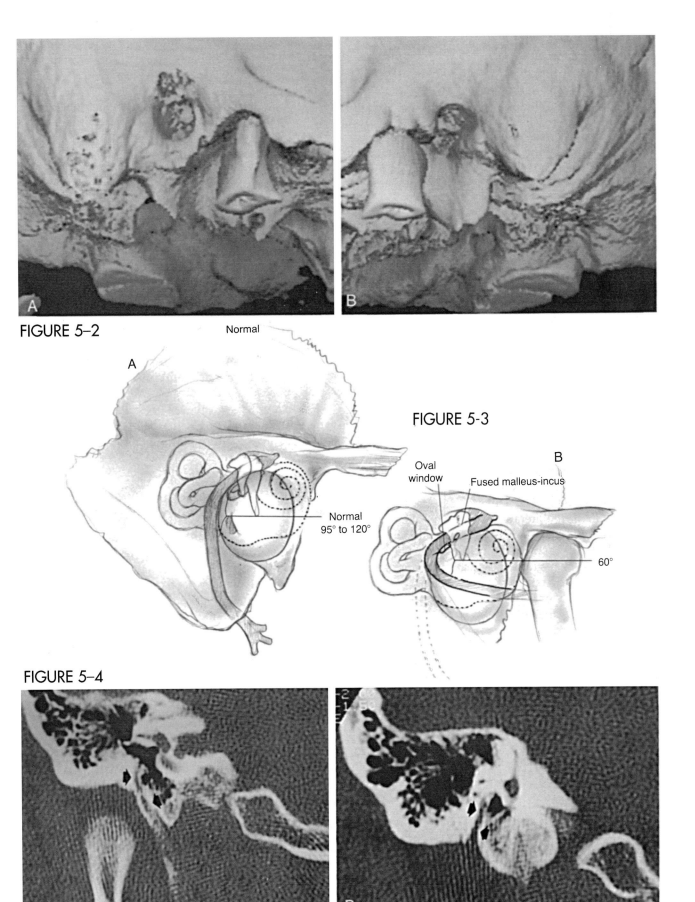

FIGURE 5–2

FIGURE 5-3

Normal

A

Normal
95° to 120°

B

Oval
window

Fused malleus-incus

60°

FIGURE 5–4

FIGURE 5–6

ANTERIOR APPROACH

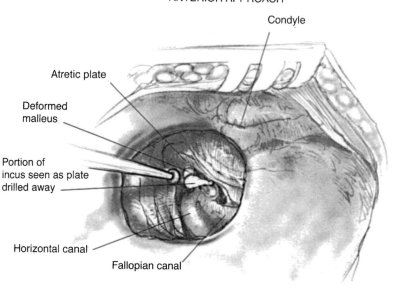

Condyle

Atretic plate

Deformed malleus

Portion of incus seen as plate drilled away

Horizontal canal

Fallopian canal

FIGURE 5–5

FIGURE 5–7

FIGURE 5–8

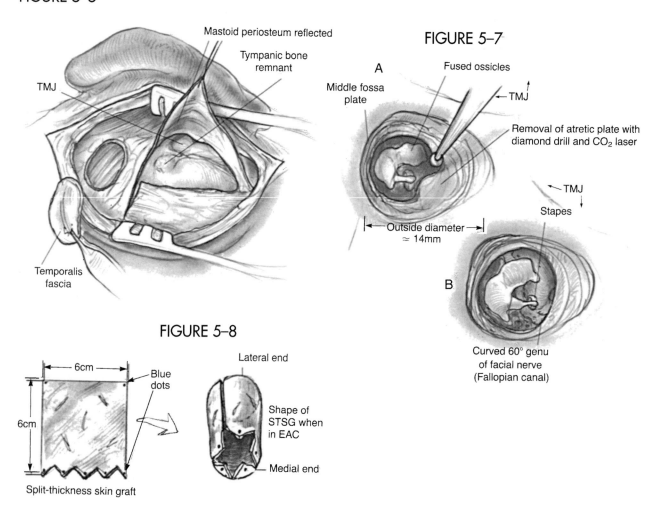

Mastoid periosteum reflected

Tympanic bone remnant

TMJ

Temporalis fascia

A

Middle fossa plate

Fused ossicles

←TMJ

Removal of atretic plate with diamond drill and CO_2 laser

←TMJ

Stapes

Outside diameter ≃ 14mm

B

Curved 60° genu of facial nerve (Fallopian canal)

6cm

Blue dots

6cm

Split-thickness skin graft

Lateral end

Shape of STSG when in EAC

Medial end

FIGURES 5–5 to 5–8. *See legends on opposite page*

with povidone-iodine and draped. Additionally, the lower abdomen is shaved, aseptically prepared, and draped for the skin graft donor site.

A postauricular temporo-occipital incision is made. In cases in which microtia repair has been done, care is taken not to expose the grafted costal cartilage. Subcutaneous tissue is elevated anteriorly to the temporomandibular joint. A T-shaped incision is made in the periosteum, which is elevated exposing the mastoid cortex and, anteriorly, the temporomandibular joint space (Fig. 5–5). Care is taken to avoid injury to an anomalous facial nerve exiting the temporal bone in this area. A large piece of temporalis fascia is harvested, trimmed of excess soft tissue if needed, and placed aside to dry. The temporomandibular joint space is explored to verify that the facial nerve or tympanic bone is not lying within it.

The literature has fostered the belief that there are separate and distinct approaches to the bony work necessary in atresiaplasty: the anterior approach, the transmastoid approach, and modification of the anterior approach.[6, 8, 24, 33, 35, 56, 63] We believe that strict distinction between these surgical approaches is unnecessary because each can be used alone or in combination to facilitate the atresiaplasty. For purposes of discussion, however, each technique in elucidated in detail.

Standard Surgical Approach

If a remnant of tympanic bone is present, the new 11 mm cylindrical ear canal is begun at the cribiform area. If no such remnant is present, drilling begins at the level of the linea temporalis, just posterior to the glenoid fossa. Using cutting and diamond burrs, the dissection is carried anteriorly and medially. The middle fossa plate (mastoid tegmen) is identified and followed to the epitympanum, where the fused malleus head/incus body mass is identified (Fig. 5–6). Care is taken not to drill on the ossicular mass, because the incudostapedial joint is usually intact, and transmission of high-speed drill energy to the inner ear can result in high-tone SNHL. The ossicular mass in the epitympanum is meticulously dissected free of the atresia plate and is left intact. This protects the horizontal facial nerve, because it always lies medial to these structures.

The atresia bone is removed with diamond microdrills and curettes to completely expose the ossicles (Fig. 5–7A). While dissecting the inferior and posterior aspect, an aberrant facial nerve can be encountered as it passes laterally through the atretic bone in this area. Although deformed, if the ossicular chain is believed to be complete, it is left in place. The ever-present fibrous ligaments and bony adhesions are better vaporized with a laser in the final

phases of ossicular dissection to avoid delayed refixation of the ossicles. (Fig. 5–7B) Ossicular reconstruction with the patient's intact ossicular chain is preferred to the use of prostheses. When the ossicular chain is not complete, ossiculoplasty is performed using a total or partial ossicular reconstruction prosthesis to either a mobile footplate or the stapes head. The prosthesis is covered with cartilage prior to grafting the new drum. On occasion, the stapes footplate may not be seen well because of anomalous facial nerve anatomy, making placement of an ossicular prosthesis difficult or dangerous. In these instances, gentle transposition of the facial nerve has been described, but more commonly hearing restoration can be accomplished with LSCC fenestration or the patient can be counseled to use a hearing aid only.[4, 8, 17, 26, 31, 36, 42]

Drilling is continued to create a new ear canal measuring about 1.3 times the normal size, being careful not to expose the temporomandibular joint space or to open an excessive number of mastoid air cells.

The previously prepared skin graft donor site in the hypogastrium is exposed. A 0.09-inch thick, 6 × 6 cm split-thickness graft is obtained using a dermatome. Hemostasis of the donor site is accomplished by pressure with a gauze sponge wet with 1 per cent lidocaine with epinephrine 1:100,000 and thrombin solution. When the donor site is dry, a sterile Tegaderm dressing is applied.[81] One edge of the skin graft is cut in a zigzag fashion such that four or five triangular points are created (Fig. 5–8). The points of the zigzag are colored with a skin marker, as are the two points on the other edge. This allows for easy inspection in the final stages of the procedure. The skin graft is kept moist and set aside.

The now-dry temporalis fascia is inspected and trimmed to size, ideally a 20 × 15-mm oval. Steps must be taken to prevent lateralization of this graft by cutting small 3 × 6 mm "tabs" into the anterior and superior aspects of the graft, because it will be used for TM grafting.[82] Lateralization is the most common delayed cause of a poor hearing outcome, occurring in 22 per cent of patients.[6, 33] Nitrous oxide, if used by the anesthesiologist, must be discontinued 30 minutes before grafting begins. The fascia is placed over the ossicular chain, medial to the malleus if available (Fig. 5–9A), or, when ossicular reconstruction is needed, over the cartilage covering the prosthesis (Fig. 5–9B). The tabs are placed medially into the protympanum in an attempt to prevent lateralization of the new TM.

The new ear canal is circumferentially lined with the split-thickness skin. The zigzags are placed medially and partially overlap the fascia. All bone of the EAC is covered.[8, 29] The colored points allow the surgeon to be sure that no skin lies folded on itself and that the entire width of the graft is being used (the number of points seen

---

FIGURE 5–5. Incision, harvesting temporalis fascia, T-incision, and elevation of periosteum.

FIGURE 5–6. Anterior approach: mastoidectomy completed, demonstrating the lateral semicircular canal, fallopian canal, atresia plate, and ossicles.

FIGURE 5–7. A and B, Anterior approach: removal of atretic plate and adhesions, exposing the ossicles.

FIGURE 5–8. Split-thickness skin graft (STSG) used to line new external auditory canal (EAC).

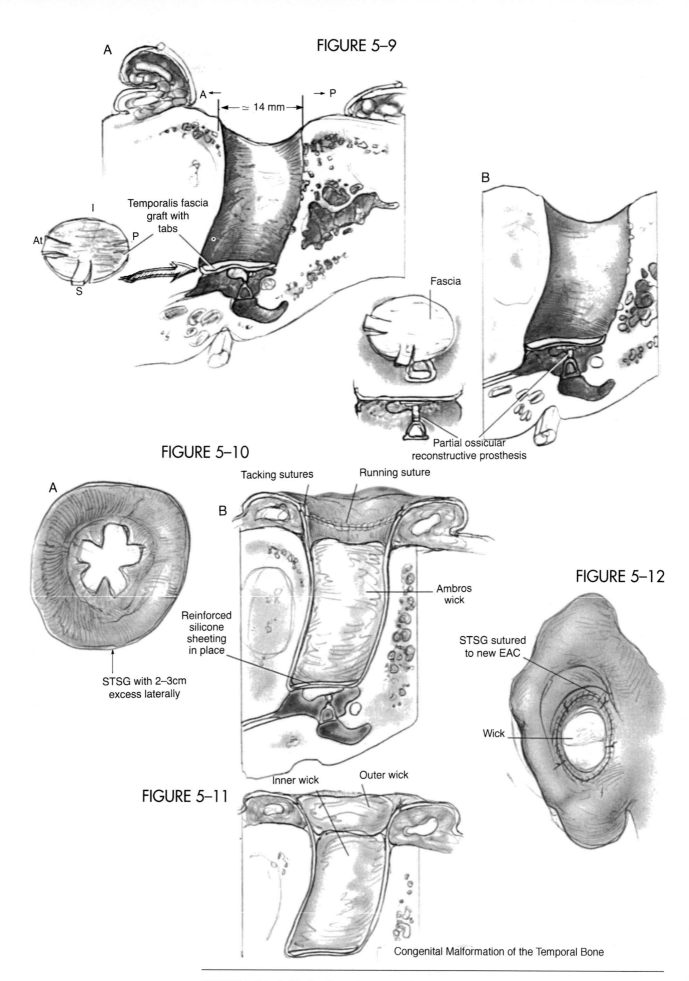

FIGURE 5–9

A

A ← ≃ 14 mm → P

Temporalis fascia
graft with
tabs

I
At
P
S

B

Fascia

Partial ossicular
reconstructive prosthesis

FIGURE 5–10

A

STSG with 2–3cm
excess laterally

B

Tacking sutures   Running suture

Reinforced
silicone
sheeting
in place

Ambros
wick

FIGURE 5–12

STSG sutured
to new EAC

Wick

Inner wick   Outer wick

FIGURE 5–11

Congenital Malformation of the Temporal Bone

matches the number of points created) (Fig. 5–10). A single layer of antibiotic-soaked Gelfoam is used to hold the fascia and skin of the new eardrum in place. A disc of Gelfilm is placed over the TM to reproduce the anterior tympanomeatal angle (Fig. 5–11). Thin Silastic 0.005 lines the skin before a large Ambros Merocel wick is placed over this medial canal wall packing while attention is then turned to meatoplasty.

An 11-mm meatus is created, because 30 per cent of the diameter will reduce eventually due to the normal healing process. It is important to avoid denuding or otherwise damaging the cartilage of the microtia repair. Skin, subcutaneous tissue, and cartilage are removed in a 1.4-cm-diameter core over the new meatus. The ear is turned and the excess canal skin graft is brought through the meatoplasty. With one or two absorbable sutures bringing the periosteum back in place over the mastoid cortex, the pinna and meatus are stabilized. Five tacking sutures of 5-0 Ti-Cron attach the lateral edge of the skin graft circumferentially to the meatal skin. Next, absorbable suture (6-0 fast-absorbing plain gut) is used in a running manner between each Ti-Cron suture. The lateral portion of the EAC and the meatus are packed. We prefer to use the large Ambros Merocel ear wick, divided longitudinally as necessary, for diffuse pressure over the entire lateral skin graft and for wide packing of the meatus (Fig. 5–12).

The periosteum is sutured back into position. This allows additional comfort that the meatus will heal wide open. The postauricular incision is closed using absorbable sutures (3-0 Dexon). Steri-Strips cover the incision, a mastoid dressing is applied, anesthesia is reversed, monitoring equipment is removed, and the patient leaves the operating room.

"Modified Anterior" Approach

In patients with thick, atretic bone, orientation may be difficult during the medial dissection. Dissection too far in either the inferior or posterior direction risks inadvertent carotid, lateral canal, or facial nerve injury. Orientation can be achieved in these cases with initial posterior dissection and limited posterior antrotomy at the sinodural angle only, enabling identification of the levels of the LSCC and the ossicular mass. A new ear canal is then created similarly to the anterior approach by drilling just posterior to the glenoid fossa and following an intact canal wall mastoidectomy approach. The lateral canal can be used repeatedly as a landmark to indicate depth and anteroposterior and superoinferior directionality, thus making the dissection safer. An "intact canal wall"–like procedure is carried out.

The remainder of the surgery proceeds as described earlier. The posterior (radical mastoidectomy–like approach) has not been used for more than 20 years.

POSTOPERATIVE CARE

The mastoid dressing is removed on the first postoperative day. The Steri-Strips are left in place over the postauricular incision for 7 days. The patient is counseled to keep the operative site dry and to change the cotton ball over the canal/meatus packing once or twice daily. The Tegaderm over the skin graft donor site is left on for at least 3 weeks and requires no special attention. Epithelialization occurs under the plastic, and the typical pain associated with older methods of donor site dressing is absent.[81]

The patient is seen 1 week after surgery, at which time the postauricular strips are removed, the tacking Ti-Cron sutures at the meatus are removed, and the dried and crusted lateral end of the meatus pack is trimmed off. The donor site is inspected. The postauricular site can now be washed, but water precautions continue to apply to the canal. We see the patient again weekly. At 3 weeks, the Merocel pack and Silastic are removed. The meatus is repacked with antibiotic-soaked Gelfoam. At this point, the patient is instructed to begin applying antibiotic suspension to the packing in the EAC twice a day. By this time, also, the Tegaderm has peeled off and the donor site has completed the initial healing phase. At the third postoperative week, the Gelfoam and the Gelfilm disc are removed. The patient continues to use eardrops for 8 to 12 weeks.

The first postoperative audiogram is obtained at 6 to 8 weeks, when nearly all of the Gelfoam is gone and the canal is healing well. Audiograms are then obtained at 6 months, 1 year, and yearly thereafter.

PITFALLS

In all cases, we prefer, and often begin with, a standard "anterior" approach; however, in atretic bone there are often no clearly identifiable landmarks. Clear communication between the surgeon and the anesthesiologist will ensure that the patient is not paralyzed during the procedure, because facial nerve monitoring is essential in these cases. When the monitor is off transiently due to the use of electrocautery, we monitor the facial nerve manually with a hand on the patient's face. In poorly pneumatized mastoids, the otic capsule may be difficult to distinguish, resulting in blue lining or worse of the semicircular canals.

Postoperative office care is important. Patients should

FIGURE 5–9. *A* and *B*, Temporalis fascia graft with tabs used over an ossicular mass or a partial ossicular replacement prosthesis and cartilage.

FIGURE 5–10. *A* and *B*, Split-thickness skin graft (STSG) in place over fascia, lining new EAC (two views).

FIGURE 5–11. Split-thickness skin graft with ear wicks to maintain contact with bony external auditory canal, and wide meatus.

FIGURE 5–12. Skin graft sutured into place at meatus.

know beforehand that they must follow the instructions given "to the letter" and that they must keep all scheduled postoperative office visits. We recommend checking the circumference of the pack each week to ensure that there is no ingrowth of grafted skin into the pack, although we have not seen this problem with the Ambros packs. If it appears that the meatus is narrowing, usually at the third month, it should be dilated every 2 weeks and restented effectively with the large Merocel wick, for a period of 12 to 24 months.

RESULTS

At the House Ear Clinic, a review of 302 atretic ears in 239 patients was done by De la Cruz and colleagues in 1985.[6] All of the cases were classified under major and minor malformation categories using the De la Cruz classification; 141 (59 per cent) of the patients were male. The right ear was involved in 108 (64 per cent) of 169 unilateral cases. There were 70 bilateral cases. Thirty patients had associated anomalies: cleft palate ($n = 5$), Treacher Collins syndrome ($n = 6$), Mondini's inner ear deformity ($n = 7$), stenotic internal auditory canal ($n = 1$), and congenital ipsilateral facial anomaly—either microtia or paralysis. There were two "dead ears" before surgery. Of the unilateral patients, five had either dead ears or cholesteatoma in the normal-appearing ear. Nine atretic ears had cholesteatoma, usually lateral to the atretic plate.

A primary atresiaplasty was performed on 65 ears. Hearing results were excellent, with 16 per cent having a conductive deficit of less than 10 dB, 53 per cent under 20 dB, and 73 per cent under 30 dB. Of the patients with poorer auditory outcomes, one developed a high-frequency SNHL but the low tones were preserved and one developed a dead ear following a planned LSCC fenestration procedure. In six bilaterally atretic patients, the operated ear was so poorly pneumatized and the deformity so severe that the surgeon attempting the repair elected to close the ear without hearing restoration (before CT scan and facial nerve monitoring). No patient had postoperative facial palsy. Two cases of transient facial palsy were seen in 18 ears operated on elsewhere. Fourteen per cent had cholesteatoma.

Twenty patients needed revision surgery. The most common reason for failure was lateralization of the TM, which occurred in 14 cases (22 per cent). This usually occurs within 12 months. Five patients had canal stenoses and required reoperation. The other reason for revision surgery was persistent drainage. Eighteen of the 20 revision cases, including all 5 stenosis cases, had had full-thickness skin graft used to line the EAC initially. The change to split-thickness skin grafting has reduced the incidence of stenosis and the need for revision surgery. Hearing results following revision surgery have been very good: 10 per cent closed the air-bone gap to within 10 dB, and 60 per cent did so to within 20 dB. One patient had a profound SNHL following a drill-out for an absent oval window. There were no facial nerve injuries. Our revisions of two cases initially operated on elsewhere resulted in hearing within 20 dB.

Molony and De la Cruz's review of 24 atresiaplasties from the House Ear Clinic in 1988[33] revealed similar rates

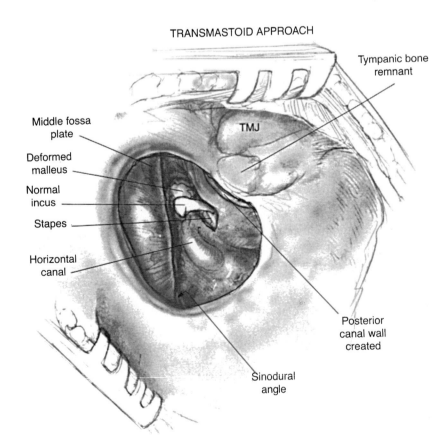

TRANSMASTOID APPROACH

Tympanic bone remnant

Middle fossa plate

Deformed malleus

Normal incus

Stapes

Horizontal canal

Sinodural angle

TMJ

Posterior canal wall created

FIGURE 5–13.
Transmastoid approach.

of air-bone gap closure and no SNHL. Four of the seven failures in this series were from the transmastoid approach, which also had the only instances of recurrent drainage. This approach has therefore gone into disuse.

In 1995, Chandrasekhar and coworkers reviewed the experience of another 92 atresiaplasty surgeries performed at the House Ear Clinic.[83] With long-term follow-up, closure of the air-bone gap to within 30 dB was seen in 59.5 per cent of primary surgeries and 53.8 per cent of revision surgeries. The most common complications were soft tissue and bony EAC stenosis, seen in 22 per cent of primary cases and 15 per cent of revision cases, and lateralization of the TM, seen in 9 per cent and 15 per cent, respectively. Over time, hearing deterioration was demonstrated in 19 per cent.

Shih and Crabtree reviewed long-term surgical results for 39 ears.[84] Hearing averages of 25 dB were achieved for mild atresia, 40 dB for moderate atresia, and 46 dB for severe atresia. Serviceable hearing was achieved in 64 per cent; 33 per cent had some restenosis; and 31 per cent had recurrent cavity/canal skin infections. This was reduced with the use of split-thickness skin grafting.

COMPLICATIONS AND THEIR MANAGEMENT

Complications of atresiaplasty include lateralization of the TM in up to 26 per cent, stenosis of the external auditory meatus in 8 per cent, SNHL in 2 per cent, and facial nerve palsy in 1 per cent. Care taken at the time of surgery can help minimize the incidence of lateralization. The anesthesiologist should be alerted to shut off any nitrous oxide 30 minutes before grafting is begun. The graft should be anchored medially to the malleus and the tabs should be placed into the hypotympanum and epitympanum. Use of an accurately sized Gelfilm disc helps re-form an anterior tympanomeatal angle and keep the graft in position. The patient must be followed carefully for at least 24 months, because lateralization has been known to occur up to 12 months postoperatively.

The incidence of stenosis has been reduced with the use of large split-thickness skin grafts. Careful inspection of the meatus at frequent intervals and early stenting with Merocel wicks can obviate the need for reoperation. The importance of early identification and treatment of infection to prevent graft failure and stenosis cannot be overemphasized.

High-tone SNHL occurs in 5 per cent of the cases. The laser is used to minimize manipulation when trying to free the ossicles from the EAC. Care is taken not to manipulate the ossicular chain when dissecting it away from the atretic bone.

With better imaging techniques, oval window problems can be identified preoperatively and problems of SNHL due to oval window drill-out can be avoided. Likewise, patients with CT evidence of severe malformations in whom surgery would be fraught with problems can be counseled against surgical intervention and fitted with hearing aids instead. Intraoperative facial nerve electromyographic monitoring serves to reduce even further the incidence of facial nerve injury of less than 1 per cent.

SUMMARY

The treatment of congenital aural atresia poses a challenging, complex problem.[85, 86] Early identification, amplification, and speech and language therapy are crucial in bilateral cases.[87] Cooperation with the auricular reconstruction surgeon will allow for better aesthetic and functional success. The use of strict radiologic and clinical criteria for operative candidates is necessary. Patients classified into categories of minor and major malformations should understand the prognosis for hearing improvement and the risks and results of surgery. A thorough understanding of the embryologic maldevelopment and rigorous adherence to the surgical principles of mastoidectomy, facial nerve dissection, and tympanoplasty will enable us to offer our patients optimal hearing restoration.[88, 89] Diligent postoperative office care is vital to maintaining the good results obtained at surgery.

References

1. Federspil P, Delb W: Treatment of congenital malformations of the external and middle ear. *In* Ars B (ed): Congenital External and Middle Ear Malformations: Management. Amsterdam, Kugler Publications, 1992, pp 47–70.
2. Gill NW: Congenital atresia of the ear: A review of the surgical findings in 83 cases. J Laryngol Otol 83: 551–587, 1969.
3. Granstrom G, Bergstrom K, Tjellstrom A: The bone-anchored hearing aid and bone-anchored epithesis for congenital ear malformations. Otolaryngol Head Neck Surg 109: 46–53, 1993.
4. House HP: Management of congenital ear canal atresia. Laryngoscope 63: 916–946, 1953.
5. Mehra YN, Dubey SP, Mann SBS, Suri S: Correlation between high-resolution computed tomography and surgical findings in congenital aural atresia. Arch Otolaryngol Head Neck Surg 114: 137–141, 1988.
6. De la Cruz A, Linthicum FH Jr, Luxford WM: Congenital atresia of the external auditory canal. Laryngoscope 95: 421–427, 1985.
7. Hiraide F, Nomura Y, Nakamura K: Histopathology of atresia auris congenita. J Laryngol Otol 88: 1249–1256, 1974.
8. Jahrsdoerfer RA: Congenital atresia of the ear. Laryngoscope 88 (Suppl 13): 1–48, 1978.
9. Kelemen GD: Aural participation in congenital malformations of the organism. Acta Otolaryngol Suppl 321: 1–35, 1974.
10. Grundfast KM, Camilon F: External auditory canal stenosis and partial atresia without associated anomalies. Ann Otol Rhinol Laryngol 95: 505–509, 1986.
11. Harada O, Ishii H: The condition of the auditory ossicles in microtia: Findings in 57 middle ear operations. Plast Reconstr Surg 50: 48–53, 1972.
12. Hasso AN, Broadwell RA: Congenital anomalies. *In* Som PM, Bergeron RT (eds): Head and Neck Imaging. St. Louis, CV Mosby, 1991, pp 960–966.
13. Lascaratos J, Assimakopoulos D: From the roots of otology: Diseases of the ear and their treatment in Byzantine times (324–1453 A.D.). Am J Otol 20: 397–402, 1999.
14. Briau R: Chirurgie de Paul d'Egine. Paris, Masson, 1855.
15. Page JR: Congenital bilateral microtia with total osseous atresia of the external auditory canals: Operation and report of cases. Trans Am Otol Soc 13: 376–390, 1914.
16. Dean LW, Gittens TR: Report of a case of bilateral, congenital osseous atresia of the external auditory canal with an exceptionally good functional result following operation. Trans Am Laryngol Rhinol Otol Soc 23:296–309, 1917.
17. Ombredanne M: Chirurgie de la surdité: Fenestration dans les aplasies de l'oreille avec imperforation du conduit: Resultats. Otorhinolaryngol Int 31: 229–236, 1947.
18. Pattee GL: An operation to improve hearing in cases of congenital atresia of the external auditory meatus. Arch Otolaryngol Head Neck Surg 45: 568–580, 1947.
19. Bellucci RJ: The problem of congenital auricular malformation: I.

Construction of the external auditory canal. Trans Am Acad Ophth Otolaryngol. 64: 840–852, 1960.

20. Meurman Y: Congenital microtia and meatal atresia. Arch Otolaryngol 66: 443–463, 1957.

21. Nager GT: Aural atresia: Anatomy and surgery. Postgrad Med 29: 529–541, 1961.

22. Ombredanne M: Malformations des Osselets dans les Embryopathies de L'oreille. Acta Otorhinolaryngol (Belg) 20: 623–652, 1965.

23. Ruedi L: The surgical treatment of the atresia auris congenita: A clinical and histological report. Laryngoscope 64: 666–684, 1954.

24. Scheer AA: Correction of congenital middle ear deformities. Arch Otolaryngol 85: 269–277, 1967.

25. Shambaugh GE Jr: Developmental anomalies of the sound conducting apparatus and their surgical correction. Ann Otol 74: 873–887, 1952.

26. Woodman DG: Congenital atresia of the auditory canal. Arch Otolaryngol 55: 172–181, 1952.

27. Ombredanne M: Chirurgie des surdites congenitales par malformations ossiculaires. Acta Otorhinolaryngol Belg 25: 837–869, 1971.

28. Crabtree JA: Congenital atresia: Case selection, complications, and prevention. Otolaryngol Clin North Am 15: 755–762, 1982.

29. Jahrsdoerfer RA, Cole RR, Gray LE: Advances in congenital aural atresia. Adv Otolaryngol Head Neck Surg 5: 1–15, 1991.

30. Jahrsdoerfer RA: Clinical aspects of temporal bone anomalies. AJNR Am J Neuroradiol 13: 821–825, 1992.

31. Marquet J: Homogreffes Tympano-ossiculaires dans Le Traitement Chirurgical de L'agenesie de Woreille: Rapport Preliminaire. Acta Otorhinolaryngol Belg 25: 885–897, 1971.

32. Marquet JE, Declau F, De Cock M, et al: Congenital middle ear malformations. Acta Otorhinolaryngol Belg 42: 117–302, 1988.

33. Molony TB, De la Cruz A: Surgical approaches to congenital atresia of the external auditory canal. Otolaryngol Head Neck Surg 103: 991–1001, 1990.

34. Crabtree JA: Tympanoplastic techniques in congenital atresia. Arch Otolaryngol 88: 89–96, 1968.

35. Minatogawa T, Nishimura Y, Inamori T, Kumoi T: Results of tympanoplasty for congenital aural atresia and stenosis, with special reference to fascia and homograft as the graft material of the tympanic membrane. Laryngoscope 99: 632–638, 1989.

36. Schuknecht HF: Reconstructive procedures for congenital aural atresia. Arch Otolaryngol 101: 170–172, 1975.

37. Bellucci RJ: Congenital auricular malformations: Indications, contraindications, and timing of middle ear surgery. Ann Otol Rhinol Laryngol 81: 659–663, 1972.

38. Linthicum FH Jr: Surgery of congenital deafness. Otolaryngol Clin North Am 4: 401–409, 1971.

39. Patterson ME, Linthicum FH Jr: Congenital hearing impairment. Otolaryngol Clin North Am 3: 201–219, 1970.

40. Ruben RJ: Management and therapy of congenital malformations of the external and middle ears. In Alberti PW, Ruben RJ (eds): Otologic Medicine and Surgery. New York, Churchill Livingstone, 1988, pp 1135–1154.

41. Jahrsdoerfer RA, Garcia ET, Yeakley JW, Jacobson JT: Surface contour three-dimensional imaging in congenital aural atresia. Arch Otolaryngol Head Neck Surg 119: 95–99, 1993.

42. Ombredanne M: Absence Congenitale de Fenetre Ronde dans Certaines Aplasies Mineures. Ann Otolaryngol (Paris) 85: 369–378, 1968.

43. Aase JM: Microtia: Clinical observations. Birth Defects 16: 289–297, 1980.

44. Sando I, Shibahara Y, Takagi A, et al: Congenital middle and inner ear anomalies. Acta Otolaryngol (Stockh) Suppl 458: 76–78, 1988.

45. Van de Water TR, Maderson PF, Jaskoll TF: The morphogenesis of the middle and external ear. Birth Defects 16: 147–180, 1980.

46. Barrios-Montes JM: Malformaciones auriculares. Acta Otorrhinolaryngol Esp 27: 17–46, 1976.

47. Savic D, Jasovic A, Djeric D: The relations of the mastoid segment of the facial canal to surrounding structures in congenital middle ear malformations. Int J Pediatr Otorhinolaryngol 18: 13–19, 1989.

48. Tjellstrom A, Bergstrom K: Bone-anchored hearing aids and prostheses. In Ars B (ed): Congenital External and Middle Ear Malformations: Management. Amsterdam, Kugler Publications, 1992, pp 1–9.

49. Gill NW: Congenital atresia of the ear. J Laryngol Otol 85: 1251–1254, 1971.

50. Melnick M: The etiology of external ear malformations and its relation to abnormalities of the middle ear, inner ear, and other organ systems. Birth Defects 16: 303–331, 1980.

51. Altmann F: Congenital atresia of the ear in man and animals. Ann Otol Rhinol Laryngol 64: 824–858, 1955.

52. Bellucci RJ: Congenital aural malformations: Diagnosis and treatment. Otolaryngol Clin North Am 14: 95–124, 1981.

53. Jahrsdoerfer RA, Yeakley JW, Aguilar EA, et al: Grading system for the selection of patients with congenital aural atresia. Am J Otol 1992; 13: 6–12, 1992.

54. Schuknecht HF: Congenital aural atresia and congenital middle ear cholesteatoma. In Nadol JB Jr, Schuknecht HF (eds): Surgery of the Ear and Temporal Bone. New York, Raven Press, 1993, pp 263–274.

55. Chiossone E: Surgical management of major congenital malformations of the ear. Am J Otol 6: 237–242, 1985.

56. Sando I, Suehiro S, Wood RP II: Congenital anomalies of the external and middle ear. In Bluestone CD, Stool SE (eds): Pediatric Otology. Philadelphia, WB Saunders, 1983, pp 263–274.

57. Fernandez AO, Ronis ML: The Treacher Collins Syndrome. Arch Otolaryngol 80: 505–520, 1964.

58. Rapin I, Ruben RJ: Patterns of anomalies in children with malformed ears. Laryngoscope 86: 1469–1502, 1976.

59. Ruben RJ, Toriyama M, Dische MR, et al: External and middle ear malformations associated with mandibulo facial dysostosis and renal abnormalities: A case report. Ann Otol Rhinol Laryngol 78: 605–624, 1969.

60. Sanchez-Corona J, Garcia-Cruz D, Ruenes R, Cantu JM: A distinct dominant form of microtia and conductive hearing loss. Birth Defects 18: 211–216, 1982.

61. Miyamoto RT, Fairchild TH, Daugherty HS: Primary cholesteatoma in the congenitally atretic ear. Am J Otol 5: 283–285, 1984.

62. Jahrsdoerfer RA, Yeakley JW, Hall JW III, et al: High-resolution CT scanning and auditory brain stem response in congenital aural atresia: Patient selection and surgical correlation. Otolaryngol Head Neck Surg 93: 292–298, 1985.

63. Jahrsdoerfer RA, Hall JW: Congenital malformations of the ear. Am J Otol 7: 267–269, 1986.

64. Brent B: The correction of microtia with autogenous cartilage grafts: I. The classic deformity. Plast Reconstr Surg 66: 1–12, 1980.

65. Brent B: Auricular repair with autogenous rib cartilage grafts: Two decades of experience with 600 cases. Plast Reconstr Surg 90: 355–374; discussion 375–376, 1995.

66. Gates GA, Hough JV, Gatti WM, Bradley WH: The safety and effectiveness of an implanted electromagnetic hearing device. Arch Otolaryngol 115: 924–930, 1989.

67. Hakansson B, Liden G, Tjellstrom A, et al: Ten years of experience with the Swedish bone-anchored hearing system. Ann Otol Rhinol Laryngol Suppl 151: 1–16, 1990.

68. Niparko JK, Langman AW, Cutler DS, Carroll WR: Tissue-integrated prostheses in the rehabilitation of auricular defects: Results with percutaneous mastoid implants. Am J Otol 14: 343–348, 1993.

69. Tjellstrom A, Hakansson B: The bone-anchored hearing aid (BAHA) design: Principles, indications and long-term clinical results. Otolaryngol Clin North Am 115: 1–20, 1995.

70. van der Pouw KTM, Snik AFM, Cremers CWRJ: Audiometric results of bilateral bone-anchored hearing aid application in patients with bilateral congenital aural atresia. Laryngoscope 108: 548–553, 1998.

71. Sortini AJ: Hearing aids for children with bilateral congenital ear canal atresia. Hear Instrument 6: 20–23, 1981.

72. Zalzal GH, Shott SR, Towbin R, Cotton RT: Value of CT scan in the diagnosis of temporal bone diseases in children. Laryngoscope 96: 27–32, 1986.

73. Andrews JC, Anzai Y, Mankovich NJ, et al: Three-dimensional CT scan reconstruction for the assessment of congenital aural atresia. Am J Otol 13: 236–240, 1992.

74. Crabtree JA: The facial nerve in congenital ear surgery. Otolaryngol Clin North Am 7: 505–510, 1974.

75. Linstrom CI, Meiteles LZ: Facial nerve monitoring in surgery for congenital auricular atresia. Laryngoscope 103: 406–415, 1993.

76. Chandrasekhar SS, De La Cruz A, Lo WWM, Telischi FJ: Imaging of the facial nerve. In Jackler RA, Brackmann DE (eds): Neurotology. St. Louis, Mosby–Year Book, 1993, pp 341–359.

77. Chole RA: Meatoplasty using inferiorly based island pedicle flap for congenital aural atresia. Laryngoscope 93: 954–955, 1983.

78. Colman BH: Congenital malformations of the ear—aspects of management. J Otolaryngol Soc Austral 4: 197–200, 1978.

79. Wigand ME: Tympano-Meatoplastie Endurale Pour Les Atresies Congenitales Severes De L'oreille. Rev Laryngol 99: 14–28, 1978.

80. Ombredanne M: Transposition des osselets dans certaines "Aplasies Mineures." Ann Otolaryngol (Paris) 83: 273–280, 1966.
81. Weymuller EA Jr: Dressings for split-thickness skin graft donor sites. Laryngoscope 91: 652–653, 1981.
82. Sheehy JL: Surgery of Chronic Otitis Media. English GE (ed): Otolaryngology, Vol 1. Hagerstown, MD, Harper & Row, 1977.
83. Chandrasekhar SS, De la Cruz A, Garrido E: Surgery of congenital aural atresia. Am J Otol 16: 713–717, 1995.
84. Shih L, Crabtree JA: Long-term surgical results for congenital aural atresia. Laryngoscope 103: 1097–1102, 1993.
85. Schuknecht HF: Congenital aural atresia. Laryngoscope 99: 908, 1989.
86. Bellucci RJ: Congenital aural malformations: Diagnosis and treatment. Otolaryngol Clin North Am 15: 95, 1981.
87. Trigg DJ, Applebaum EL: Indications for the surgical repair of unilateral aural atresia in children. Am J Otol 19: 679, 1998.
88. Jahrsdoerfer RA, Lambert PR: Facial nerve injury in congenital aural atresia surgery. Am J Otol 19: 283–287, 1998.
89. Lambert PR: Long-term hearing results in congenital aural atresia surgery. Laryngoscope 108: 1801, 1998.

6

Surgery of Ventilation and Mucosal Disease

Rick A. Friedman, M.D., Ph.D. ▪ Bradley W. Kesser, M.D.

Bilateral myringotomy with placement of ventilation tubes is the most common surgical procedure performed in the United States. An estimated 1.05 million tympanostomy tube procedures are performed annually in the United States.[1] In addition, otitis media is the most common diagnosis of patients who make office visits to physicians in the United States—the diagnosis increased from about 10 million visits in 1975 to 25 million in 1990.[2] The annual visit rate for children younger than 2 years of age statistically increased by 224 per cent during one study period.[3] Otitis media with effusion (OME) incurs approximately $5 billion annually in direct and indirect costs.[1] Given the magnitude of the disease and its impact on our society as well as conflicting reports over the most appropriate and cost-effective management of the problem,[1, 3–5] consensus on the treatment of OME has been difficult to achieve. Attempts have been made to devise an algorithm for the management of OME in young children,[6] but even these guidelines have been met with criticism (see later).

This chapter briefly reviews the terminology, epidemiology, pathophysiology, and treatment—medical and surgical—of OME.

TERMINOLOGY

Otitis media, in its broadest sense, refers to any inflammatory process in the middle ear. The etiology of the inflammation can (and usually is) infectious in nature, but it can also involve rarer systemic inflammatory diseases (e.g., Wegener's granulomatosis). The inflammation can be marked by the presence or absence of an effusion, or fluid in the middle ear space. The fluid can be serous (thin, watery, often golden), purulent (pus), or mucoid (thick, viscid, "glue").

Acute Otitis Media Without Effusion

Acute otitis media without effusion is characterized by an inflamed middle ear mucosa and tympanic membrane in the absence of an effusion. This can be seen in the early stages of acute otitis media or during its resolution. The tympanic membrane appears dull, erythematous, and inflamed; normal landmarks are often lost. In infants and children, acute otitis media without effusion is usually caused by the same organisms that are isolated from acute OME.[7] Treatment principles are the same and are discussed later.

Acute Otitis Media with Effusion

Acute OME occurs most frequently in infants. Redness with or without bulging of the tympanic membrane, fever, irritability, and pain are the hallmark signs and symptoms. The older child with acute OME has a red tympanic membrane and middle ear effusion but may not have pain or fever. The middle ear effusion is generally purulent. Casselbrant and associates reported a cumulative incidence of acute OME of 43 per cent in a study of 198 newborns followed monthly until the age of 2 years.[8] In the Greater Boston Otitis Media Study Group, infants had an average of 1.2 and 1.1 episodes per year, with 46 per cent of children having had 3 or more episodes by the age of 3 years.[9]

Recurrent acute otitis media refers to frequent bouts of acute otitis media. The child most likely has intercurrent, persistent (chronic) OME (COME). The effusion becomes infected, and the child develops acute otitis media. Recurrent acute otitis media is an indication for surgical intervention (see later).

Otitis Media with Effusion

OME simply refers to fluid in the middle ear without signs or symptoms of ear infection. Asymptomatic OME can be classified as acute (<3 weeks), subacute (3 weeks to 3 months), or chronic (>3 months).[10] Note that *acute* and *chronic* refer to the temporal course of the disease, not to severity. Synonyms of OME include secretory otitis media, nonsuppurative otitis media, or serous otitis media; the most commonly used is OME.

Chronic Suppurative Otitis Media

Chronic suppurative otitis media (CSOM) is a stage of ear disease in which there is chronic infection of the middle ear and mastoid and in which a central perforation of the tympanic membrane (or a patent tympanostomy tube) and discharge (otorrhea) are present.[11] To meet the requirement for "chronic," the otorrhea should be present for 6 weeks or longer. The infection involves both the mastoid and middle ear and usually drains through a central perforation. Chronic otorrhea through a nonintact tympanic membrane (perforation or ventilation tube) may or may not be accompanied by cholesteatoma. Cholesteatoma may or may not result in CSOM. CSOM should not be confused with COME; in the latter, no perforation is present, and the fluid is not purulent.

Idiopathic Hemotympanum

The clinical hallmark of idiopathic hemotympanum (IH) is the dark blue–appearing tympanic membrane. There is usually no antecedent history of trauma, but trauma can induce this condition. IH represents a tissue response of the temporal bone to the presence of a foreign body—cholesterol crystals. Three etiologic factors are thought to be responsible: interference with drainage, hemorrhage, and obstruction of ventilation. COME is the principal precursor. Cholesterol granuloma is the histopathologic correlate.

These cholesterol cysts can take an aggressive course with bone erosion and osteitis. Treatment is generally surgical drainage (see later).

EPIDEMIOLOGY

Studies by Teele and colleagues[9, 12, 13] have found that 13 per cent of children in their study groups had at least one episode of acute otitis media by age 3 months; that percentage increased to 67 per cent by 12 months. By age 3 years, 46 per cent of children had three or more episodes of acute otitis media. The highest incidence of acute otitis media was found in children 6 to 11 months of age. The majority of children with multiple recurrences of otitis media have their first episode before the age of 12 months.

An episode of acute otitis media is a significant risk factor for the development of OME. A number of investigators have documented persistent middle ear effusion following a single episode of acute otitis media.[12–15] Middle ear effusion has been shown to persist following an episode of acute otitis media for 1 month in 40 per cent of children, 2 months in 20 per cent, and 3 or more months in 10 per cent.[13]

Risk Factors

Risk factors for OME include male gender, recent upper respiratory infection (URI), bottle feeding, cigarette smoke in the house, increased number of siblings in the house, and probably the most important—day care. Children in a public day-care facility have a fivefold increase in otitis media at age 2 years compared with children in home care.[16] Whites and Hispanics are more susceptible than African Americans; Native Americans and Inuit are at greater risk.

Skeletal and anatomic factors also predispose to OME. Cleft palate—either overt or submucous—is a significant risk factor. Other craniofacial anomalies including Treacher Collins, Apert's, and Down syndrome and the mucopolysaccharidoses put children at greater susceptibility to middle ear disease, presumably due to immaturity, dysfunction, and anatomic course of the eustachian tube.

Children with immunodeficiencies are also at greater risk. IgG subclass deficiencies, acquired immunodeficiency syndrome, complement deficiencies, and immunosuppression secondary to medication all predispose to otitis media. Ciliary dysfunction and cystic fibrosis are also known risk factors.

Microbiology

Bluestone and coworkers obtained aspirates of middle ear effusions by tympanocentesis in infants and children with acute otitis media or OME. Thirty-five per cent of aspirates from ears with acute otitis media grew *Streptococcus pneumoniae*, 23 per cent grew *Haemophilus influenzae*, and 14 per cent grew *Moraxella catarrhalis*.[17] *S. pneumoniae* remains the most common bacteria causing acute otitis media.[18–20] Introduction of the pneumococcal vaccine may significantly reduce the incidence of pneumococcal disease, including otitis media.

The asymptomatic middle ear effusion (OME) had been previously thought to be sterile. Newer, more sensitive cultures as well as the introduction of polymerase chain reaction (PCR) testing have shown bacteria and bacterial DNA in asymptomatic middle ear effusions.[21] These investigators found that 77 per cent of middle ear effusions had evidence of the three major organisms by PCR (with or without being culture positive), whereas only 28 per cent were culture positive. The most common bacteria were *H. influenzae* (54.5 per cent), *M. catarrhalis* (46.4 per cent), and *S. pneumoniae* (29.9 per cent).[21] By comparison, in an earlier study of ears with OME, 30 per cent of aspirates did not grow bacteria, 45 per cent grew "other" strains, 15 per cent had *H. influenzae*, 10 per cent had *M. catarrhalis*, and 7 per cent grew *S. pneumoniae*.[17] Other bacteria include *Staphylococcus aureus* and gram-negative enteric bacilli. In infants younger than 6 weeks of age, gram-negative bacilli cause about 20 per cent of acute otitis media episodes.[18] The incidence of β-lactamase–producing bacteria *(H. influenzae)* is on the rise.[17]

The bacteriology of CSOM with or without cholesteatoma is different. Most frequently isolated bacteria include *Pseudomonas aeruginosa* (most common), *S. aureus*, *Corynebacterium*, *Klebsiella pneumoniae*, and anaerobes.[20] Given better culture techniques, anaerobes have been increasingly isolated from chronic suppurating ears; these organisms include *Bacteroides* spp., *Peptococcus* spp., *Peptostreptococcus* spp., and *Propionibacterium acnes*.[20]

PATHOPHYSIOLOGY

Acute Otitis Media

Retrograde reflux of material from the nasopharynx through the eustachian tube is thought to account for the introduction of microorganisms into the middle ear. Bacteria colonize the nasopharynx but infect the host as a result of a breakdown in barrier or protective factors in the nasopharynx, eustachian tube, and middle ear. Acute otitis media is principally a sequela of a viral URI. The URI impairs ciliary motility and breaks down mucosal barriers that prevent bacterial adherence and growth. Poor clearance of secretions results in stasis and allows bacteria to infect the host. Pathogenic bacteria that appear in the nasopharynx following a URI are the same as those cultured from middle ear effusions (*S. pneumoniae* and *H. influenzae*).[22] The adenoid appears to be the source of infecting bacteria in middle ear disease; Pillsbury and associates demonstrated higher bacterial colony counts in the adenoids of children with recurrent otitis media than in those undergoing adenoidectomy for adenoid hypertrophy without otitis media.[23]

During a URI, sneezing, blowing the nose, and swallowing in the presence of nasal obstruction may create a pressure differential between the nasopharynx and middle ear, forcing bacteria through the eustachian tube into the middle ear.

Finally, eustachian tube dysfunction is held accountable for OME. The eustachian tube has three functions: (1) clearance of secretions from the middle ear into the nasopharynx; (2) protection of the middle ear from nasopharyngeal pathogens; and (3) equalization of pressure between the atmospheric pressure (in the nose) and middle ear pressure. The middle ear is an aerated "sinus." It too must be ventilated and cleared of secretions—the eustachian tube serves this capacity.

In children, the tube is short, horizontal, and relatively flaccid. As a result, the protective function of the tube is compromised, and retrograde reflux of secretions into the middle ear occurs. During an acute infection, ciliary function is also compromised, further leading to stasis of secretions and persistence of effusion (see next section).

Chronic Otitis Media with Effusion

Two theories have been proposed to account for the persistence of middle ear effusion in the absence of acute infection. As demonstrated by the Boston Collaborative Group, persistent effusion is a natural sequela of acute middle ear infection.[13] Effusion persists for 1 month in 40 per cent of children after an episode of acute otitis media, 2 months in 20 per cent, and 3 or more months in 10 per cent.[13] Since pathogenic bacteria and bacterial DNA have been recovered from "nonacutely infected" fluid in the middle ear, [21, 25] it therefore appears that eustachian tube obstruction and retained secretions in these cases are the *result* of the acute infection rather than the cause.

On the other hand, eustachian tube dysfunction may be a primary disorder that *causes* acute and chronic OME. Primary eustachian tube dysfunction results in underaeration and poor ventilation of the middle ear space. This leads to negative pressure in the middle ear with resultant transudation of fluid. Negative middle ear pressure also causes hypoxia and hypercapnia of the middle ear mucosa, resulting in goblet cell hyperplasia and hypersecretion.[26, 27] The result is a sterile fluid that becomes secondarily infected. The fluid resolves only after adequate ventilation is restored, either by return of eustachian tube function or by placement of alternative ventilation, such as a ventilation tube.

According to Gates,[28] the available evidence lends support to the theory that the secretory changes in the middle ear that exist in cases of COME are the histologic sequelae of chronic infection, rather than a separate pathologic disor-

der. The majority of cases of COME begin as acute infection of the middle ear; postinflammatory alterations in the mucosa of the middle ear and eustachian tube lead to persistent effusion. Obstruction of the eustachian tube is therefore secondary to the infection and not the cause of it. Of course, eustachian tube obstruction then prevents clearance of secretions, impedes ventilation and drainage, and perpetuates the inflammatory process.

Idiopathic Hemotympanum

Long-standing cases of COME that develop granulomatous deposits in the middle ear and mastoid can lead to IH. Symptoms of IH are those of OME—hearing loss with a plugged or pressure sensation in the ear. IH is more common in adults. It is characterized by a dark blue–appearing tympanic membrane—fluid at myringotomy is dark brown and syrupy in consistency. Histologically, cholesterol crystals are seen, hence the pathologic term *cholesterol granuloma*. It is theorized that a small mucosal hemorrhage in the absence of adequate ventilation and drainage results in deposition of hemosiderin, iron, and blood breakdown products into the submucosa. The contents can be walled off, with resultant cyst development. The cyst then slowly expands, causing bone thinning and erosion.

TREATMENT AND PATIENT SELECTION

Acute Otitis Media and Recurrent Acute Otitis Media

For the single episode of acute otitis media, antimicrobial therapy targets the most common offending pathogens: *S. pneumoniae*, *H. influenzae*, and *M. catarrhalis*. We recommend a 10-day course of amoxicillin as first-line empiric therapy. Studies have shown a rise in the β-lactamase–producing organisms, *H. influenzae* and *M. catarrhalis*.[17, 29] β-Lactamase renders the organism that produces it resistant to penicillin (and ampicillin). Persistent or recurrent acute otitis media may be secondary to a β-lactamase–producing organism and requires a broader spectrum antibiotic[30]; good choices in this setting include cefuroxime, erythromycin-sulfisoxazole, trimethoprim-sulfamethoxazole, amoxicillin, or cefaclor. Antipyretics (but not aspirin) are also indicated for children with acute otitis media.

A child (or adult) with an infectious complication of otitis media demands more aggressive therapy, including intravenous antibiotics and possible surgical intervention. This subject is beyond the scope of this chapter and is covered in Chapter 19.

Children with recurrent acute otitis media may exhibit normal middle ear examinations between episodes or may retain persistent effusions and also fall into the category of COME. The goal of any treatment of the patient with recurrent acute otitis media is the long-term prevention of further episodes of otitis media. Two modalities have been proposed: (1) antimicrobial prophylaxis and (2) ventilation tube placement. Antimicrobial prophylaxis involves placing the patient on a low-dose daily antibiotic to prevent further infections. Many trials using many different regimens have shown efficacy in the prevention of recurrent acute otitis media.[31–35] Children with multiple episodes of acute otitis media can be treated with long-term, low-dose chemoprophylaxis before surgical therapy is considered. Antibiotic prophylaxis has especially been recommended for high-risk children during the winter season and/or during a URI (amoxicillin 20 mg/kg at bedtime or sulfisoxazole 50 to 75 mg/kg at bedtime.)

Placement of tympanostomy tubes is also effective treatment in the prevention of recurrent otitis media. Many authorities accept four episodes of acute otitis media in 6 months as a criterion for tympanostomy tube placement. Failure of antibiotic prophylaxis is also a clear indication. Gebhart was the first to demonstrate a reduction in the number of new episodes of acute otitis media following the insertion of tympanostomy tubes.[36] Casselbrant and colleagues studied 264 children younger than 3 years of age with a history of recurrent acute otitis media. At 2 years, episodes of acute otitis media were 44 per cent lower in both the tube and prophylaxis patients.[37]

Parents often tire of frequent courses of antibiotics (or the daily use of prophylaxis) and may favor surgical treatment. The child who develops acute otitis media after withdrawal of prophylaxis is also a surgical candidate. Any child who fails antibiotic prophylaxis (i.e., develops infection while on prophylaxis) should undergo placement of tympanostomy tubes.

The role of adenoidectomy in the treatment of recurrent acute otitis media is controversial. Although Paradise and coworkers found a significant reduction (28 and 35 per cent) in the incidence of acute otitis media in the first and second years, respectively, following adenoidectomy,[38] a formal study examining the role of adenoidectomy in the treatment of recurrent acute otitis media has not been done. Results of studies of COME and adenoidectomy may or may not be applicable for patients with recurrent acute otitis media. On the other hand, for patients with recurrent acute otitis media and persistent effusion, adenoidectomy is an appropriate surgical treatment (see the following section on COME).

Chronic Otitis Media with Effusion

As mentioned, 10 per cent of children with acute otitis media have persistent middle ear effusion 3 or more months after resolution of the acute infection.[13] Since most children clear their effusion within 1 to 2 months, these patients need no further therapy. The minority who retain fluid in the middle ear longer than 3 months, however, are at risk for other sequelae, including hearing loss, language delay, vertigo or unsteadiness, tympanic membrane changes (including atelectasis and/or retraction pockets), further middle ear pathology (including ossicular problems and adhesive otitis), and discomfort with night-time wakefulness and irritability.

A number of treatment strategies have been proposed for COME: antimicrobial therapy, antihistamines/decongestants, corticosteroids, tympanostomy tubes with or without adenoidectomy, and mastoidectomy.

Antimicrobial Therapy. More sensitive techniques (e.g., PCR) have demonstrated bacterial DNA in middle ear effusions once thought to be "sterile" or culture negative. Prolonged antibiotic therapy theoretically eradicates the organism and eliminates the chronic source of effusion. Studies have shown the efficacy of antibiotics in OME.[18, 39] According to the Clinical Practice Guideline, "Managing Otitis Media with Effusion in Young Children,"[6] antimicrobial therapy is an appropriate treatment option in the child (aged 1 to 3 years) with OME up to 3 months after documentation of effusion. The patient with persistent effusion at 3 months should then undergo hearing evaluation; 20 dB or worse bilateral hearing level is then an indication for tympanostomy tube insertion. Antibiotics are also an option.

Despite studies showing the efficacy of antibiotics in OME, both theoretical and practical arguments can be made against their use in COME. Clinical experience indicates that the utility of antibiotics is reduced as the number of treatment courses increases. Children receiving four or more courses of antibiotics over a 3- to 4-month period are most likely not going to resolve their effusion with medical management. Other adverse effects of prolonged antimicrobial therapy include development of anaphylaxis and allergic reactions, hematologic disorders, and the emergence of resistant organisms, a serious worldwide problem best demonstrated by the development of resistance to penicillin by *S. pneumoniae*.[44] Finally, Rosenfeld and Post found through a large meta-analysis of existing studies that the benefit of antimicrobial therapy in COME is slight.[40]

Antihistamines/Decongestant Therapy. Antihistamine/decongestant combinations or monotherapy have not been shown to be of benefit in the treatment of COME.[39] The Agency for Health Care Policy and Research (AHCPR) guideline does not recommend these agents for COME.[6]

Corticosteroid Therapy. Steroid therapy for COME has been controversial. Lambert[41] found no difference in outcomes between the steroid group and the control group with COME. At this time, the AHCPR guideline does not recommend steroid therapy for COME.[6, 42]

Surgical Therapy. Armstrong introduced ventilation tube placement in 1954 as a treatment for OME.[43] The ventilation tube acts as an artificial eustachian tube, aerating the middle ear and equilibrating middle ear pressure with atmospheric pressure. The pathophysiology of COME involves both eustachian tube dysfunction and reflux of nasopharyngeal organisms. Ventilation tubes are aimed at correcting the former. Children with tubes in place can still get otitis media—the acute infection will not be painful, because the infected effusion is allowed to pass through the tube and out of the middle ear. The effusion will also not be associated with hearing loss; correction of hearing loss is one of the most important goals of surgical therapy. Tube insertion with or without adenoidectomy has been shown to improve conductive hearing loss secondary to OME and to decrease the amount of time spent with middle ear effusion.[18] The AHCPR guideline recommends tube insertion for the 1- to 3-year-old child with a 3-month or longer history of OME and a 20 dB or worse bilateral hearing loss.[6] In practice, however, tube insertion is performed on a more frequent basis than the recommendations would allow; the guideline has a "serious bias toward nonsurgical treatment."[44] Placement of tubes is often a clinical judgment based on experience and is addressed on a case-by-case basis.

Adenoidectomy. Nasopharyngeal reflux of secretions and microorganisms into the middle ear plays a large role in the pathophysiology of COME. As such, adenoidectomy is designed to remove the source of the infecting microorganisms. Three landmark studies have demonstrated the efficacy and low morbidity associated with adenoidectomy for COME.[4, 38, 45] Adenoidectomy is effective treatment for COME and significantly reduces its morbidity. Its effect is independent of adenoid size. In fact, it is argued that the small, "smoldering" adenoid chronically harbors bacteria and is a major contributor to OME. The decision for adenoidectomy should be based on the severity and persistence of the middle ear disease, not the size of the adenoid. Of course, nasal obstruction with adenoid hypertrophy stands alone as an indication. Given the increased cost and slightly increased risk to the patient, Paradise and Bluestone have argued for adenoidectomy only in recurrent cases.[46]

The AHCPR guideline addresses children 1 to 3 years old and does not recommend adenoidectomy in these patients. Most of the literature published on the role of adenoidectomy in OME has been in children 4 to 8 years of age.[8] Nevertheless, adenoidectomy has been shown to be safe in children older than 18 months[47] and may be effective in younger, high-risk children. In the San Antonio study, the effect of adenoidectomy was greater for the younger children.[4] We recommend adenoidectomy for recurrent cases—cases in which the child (>4 years of age) needs a second set of tubes.

Mastoidectomy. Rarely, mastoidectomy is required for COME. The continuously draining ear with secretory tissue in the mastoid (serous mastoiditis) benefits most from opening the aditus ad antrum and facial recess to increase aeration of the middle ear/mastoid air cell system. Removal of secretory tissue or granulation tissue also improves symptoms. Because of the rare necessity for mastoidectomy in COME, no systematic study has been undertaken to prove its efficacy. Decision to proceed with mastoid surgery is based on clinical experience and judgment. We have often left a small Penrose drain in the mastoid and carried it out through the postauricular incision. The drain is removed once the drainage has stopped. Mastoidectomy should be reserved for those cases with abnormal mucosa or cholesterol granuloma in the mastoid; it is more commonly indicated for IH.

PATIENT COUNSELING

Benefits, limitations, and risks and complications all should be addressed preoperatively with the patient and/or the parents.

Benefits

Hearing improvement and reduction in the number of subsequent episodes of ear infections stand as the chief benefits of tympanostomy tube placement. Certainly hearing improvement will speed and sharpen language and devel-

opmental maturation. If the child develops otitis media, tympanostomy tubes will also eliminate pain, because the infected fluid is allowed to drain out of the middle ear space. Studies have also demonstrated improvement in vestibular function following tympanostomy tube placement.[48–50] Finally, reducing the number of secondary problems of recurrent ear infections means less time lost from work for the parents, fewer (if any) courses of antibiotics, and reduction in the cost to the parents of multiple courses of antibiotics. Surgery has been shown to be a cost-effective treatment for children in whom medical therapy fails.[1]

Benefits of adenoidectomy include improved nasal airway and breathing and removal of the probable source of the offending pathogens causing middle ear infection. It is associated with a reduction in the number of new episodes of otitis media. It can also improve sleep, especially in the child with obstructive sleep apnea. As discussed, size of the adenoid has no influence on the incidence of COME; it is theorized that the smaller, chronically infected adenoid may lead to more middle ear problems.

Limitations

Tympanostomy tube placement is only a temporizing measure—the tube ventilates the middle ear but eventually extrudes. The goal is that the tube will serve as an artificial eustachian tube until the child's own eustachian tube matures and functions properly. Some children need a second and even third set of tubes before their own eustachian tube functions well enough to ventilate the middle ear. Some, of course, never work well and the child may develop further ear disease. Nevertheless, parents should know that tubes are placed to buy time for their child's own eustachian tube to function normally. Tubes can also become obstructed.

Adenoidectomy certainly does not sterilize the nasopharynx, and it does not prevent otitis media. It can improve the nasal airway but may not cure obstructive sleep apnea.

Risks and Complications

All potential risks and complications, including the risk of anesthesia, should be explained to the parents. Risks of tympanostomy tube insertion include persistent otorrhea, tympanic membrane perforation, and hearing loss. We do advise water precautions in children with tubes in place. Eardrum perforation is related to bore of the tube, length of time in place, number of intercurrent infections, and previous history of tubes. Incidence of perforation can be from 1 to 15 per cent.

Bleeding occurs in fewer than 1 per cent of cases of adenoidectomy. It can require a trip back to the operating room. Temporary velopharyngeal insufficiency (VPI) has been reported in less than 5 per cent, but permanent disability is rare in the absence of problems with palatal clefting (must check for submucous cleft palate by palpation and inspection before proceeding with adenoidectomy). Nasopharyngeal stenosis with subsequent nasal airway and speech problems is a rare complication but should be mentioned preoperatively.

Idiopathic Hemotympanum. We generally recommend tympanostomy tube placement as first-line treatment for IH. Unfortunately, this usually falls short, and the patient requires mastoidectomy. Preoperatively, we order a high-resolution temporal bone computed tomography scan to examine the air cell pattern, evidence of erosion, and extension of the cholesterol granuloma. Intact canal wall mastoidectomy with removal of diseased mucosa aerates the mastoid and middle ear; aeration is the goal of surgery. The greatest limitation is the risk of recurrence, which is reported to be as high as 50 per cent. Risks of hearing loss, facial nerve injury, and dizziness are low but are also discussed with the patient.

SURGICAL TECHNIQUE

Preoperative Preparation

The child is kept NPO after midnight the night before surgery. As a consequence, surgery on children should be the first cases when possible. NPO status 4 to 6 hours prior to the administration of anesthesia is generally adequate. We do not use perioperative antibiotics for tubes or mastoidectomy. We attempt to keep the child with the parent as long as possible, depending on the child's age, the anesthesiologist, and hospital policy. Anesthesia is delivered via mask induction and maintenance.

A general history and physical examination with screening for anesthetic risks is done for patients needing mastoidectomy. This is done in concert with the anesthesiologist and hospital policy. Mastoidectomy usually requires a general anesthetic.

Surgical Site Preparation and Draping

Tympanostomy Tubes

Sterilization of the external auditory canal is not necessary; thorough cleaning of the canal is important, however, for visualization of the tympanic membrane and for postoperative care. The child lies in the supine position with the anesthesiologist delivering anesthetic by holding the mask over the face. The head can be turned to gain optimal visualization. A drape is placed over the child's body but not over the head. The operating microscope is then brought into position directly below (inferior to) the surgeon, next to the patient bed.

Mastoidectomy

The patient is placed in the supine position with the head at the foot end of the table. The table is turned such that the anesthesiologist and equipment are located at the patient's feet. Long tubing is used to span the distance. The head is turned away from the affected side; a shoulder roll is placed under the child to improve the surgeon's angle of view. Straps or heavy tape across the chest and pelvis are used to avoid patient sliding as the table is rotated.

The postauricular area is shaved, and clear plastic drapes with sticky edges are applied to the skin edges after the skin is dried and coated with tincture of benzoin. These drapes keep unwanted hair out of the wound and blood and bone dust out of the hair. An antibacterial soap followed by povidone-iodine is used to scrub the ear, postauricular area, and sticky drapes.

A second layer of sticky blue drapes or blue towels is placed around the postauricular area, followed by a standard ENT split sheet that is placed in such a way as to frame the operative site. A trough is created with the split sheet and clips to catch the irrigant and direct it away from the field and into a floor trash can.

Adenoidectomy

For adenoidectomy, we turn the table 90 degrees from the anesthesiologist. The patient is placed in the Rose position with shoulder roll. The head is brought to the edge of the table. A towel wrap is placed around the head and secured with a towel clip. This wrap leaves the nose and mouth exposed. Care is taken to ensure that the eyes are closed and taped shut properly before the head wrap is placed. A body drape is placed at the level of the shoulders and unfolded down over the body. A single Mayo stand with all necessary instruments is used over the body.

Instruments

Tympanostomy Tubes

A set of metal speculums, cerumen curettes, and several sizes of suction cannulas (Baron Nos. 3, 5, and 7) are necessary. The operating microscope is also essential. Sterile myringotomy knives come in various shapes and angles. It is useful to choose a knife with a blade width the size of the tube to aid in making the correct dimensions of the incision. Tubes are placed with a cup or alligator forceps and positioned with a Rosen needle. Placement of long-stemmed T-tubes is facilitated by the use of an inserter in which the tube is positioned with the short arms of the tube folded forward (Fig. 6–1*B*). Care is taken to minimize trauma to the external canal, drum, or ossicles.

The tremendous variety of tube shapes and sizes is testament to the success of the operation. Choice of tube is dictated by surgeon preference on a case-by-case basis. The following basic principles guide tube choice:

1. Short, wide-bore tubes offer little resistance to water entry into the middle ear compared with the longer shaft tubes.

2. Longer shaft tubes can be more easily removed in the office; removal of short tubes with rigid flanges may require an anesthetic.

3. For longer middle ear intubation, long-stemmed T-tubes are preferred.

4. The Richards T-tube with flanges that rest against the middle ear side of the tympanic membrane stay in longest and can be permanent.

5. Risk of perforation increases with increasing duration of intubation, increasing number of infections, and increasing size of the tube.

For short-term intubation, short grommets are the best

FIGURE 6-1

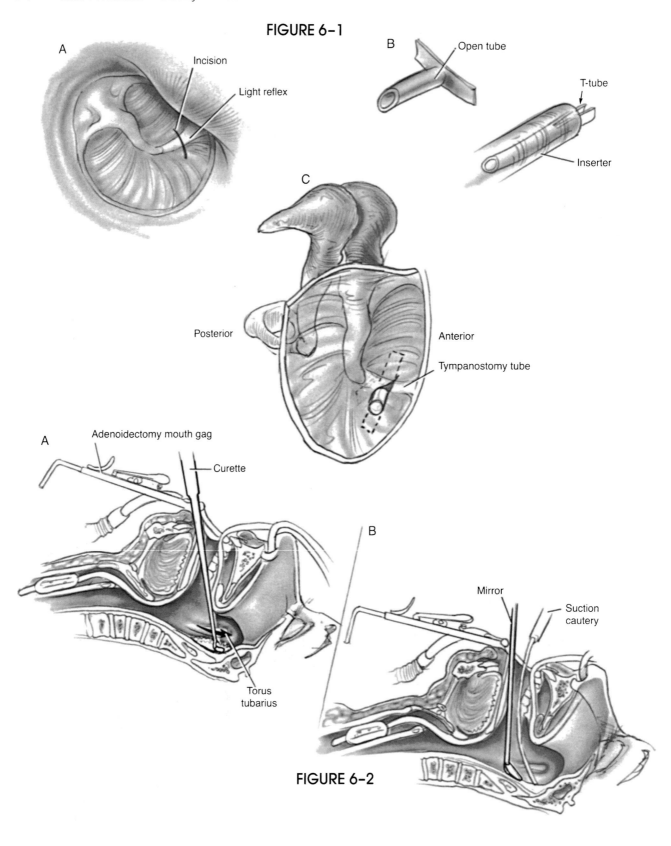

FIGURE 6–1. *A,* The incision in tympanic membrane. *B,* The placement of the T-tube within the inserter. *C,* The proper position of the tube.

FIGURE 6–2. *A,* The technique of adenoidectomy using the curette. It is important to keep the handle in the sagittal or parasagittal plane to prevent injury to the torus tubarius. *B,* The use of the suction cautery with mirror for hemostasis.

choice—they can last anywhere from several months to 2 years. For long-term intubation, T-tubes are preferred.

Adenoidectomy

Any of the available mouth gags/retractors is adequate with proper technique. Adenoid curettes are available in several sizes and configurations. Angled instruments are easier to use than straight ones. Red rubber catheters placed through the nares and brought out the mouth are used to retract the soft palate. Laryngeal mirrors are useful to inspect the adenoid pad, any residual adenoid tissue, bleeding sites, and final operative site. Tonsil packs are used to pack the nasopharynx for hemostasis. A malleable suction cautery can also be helpful for hemostasis; we urge caution using this device, however, because it can lead to nasopharyngeal stenosis. A bulb irrigator and suction are also used to flush the nose and nasopharynx.

Mastoidectomy

The ideal operating room table has motorized controls for adjustment of height and side-to-side rotation. The surgeon's stool has castors, easy height adjustment, and a flexible back support that permits the surgeon to lean backward as necessary while still receiving full back support. The operating microscope should be adjusted to the surgeon's refraction and interpupillary distance. A standard set of ear instruments is necessary, including Rosen needle, annulus elevator, round knives, flat knives, and right-angle dissectors. Bovie electrocautery can be used in the subcutaneous tissue of the postauricular incision, but it is not recommended around the middle or inner ear. Drill systems (Ototome, Midas Rex, Med-Next, Anspach) with various sizes of cutting and diamond burrs and suction irrigators are also necessary. Finally, facial nerve monitoring may be necessary. There are several facial nerve monitors available; the device should have the capacity for continuous monitoring and for stimulating the nerve for localization during the case.

Technical Details

Tympanostomy Tube Insertion

The ear canal is gently cleaned of all wax and debris. Contact with the anterior bony canal wall is avoided because of risk of bleeding. The tympanic membrane is inspected and the short process of the malleus is identified. This is a constant landmark and may be the only one available in cases of acute infection. The tympanic membrane is incised anteroinferiorly by using an incision that parallels the fibrous annulus (see Fig. 6–1). Use of a radial incision is satisfactory but may be limited by an overhanging anterior canal wall. Posterior incisions should be avoided because they place the ossicles at risk. The incision is gently spread open. Care is taken to avoid any major vessel in the tympanic membrane to prevent hemorrhage into the layers of the eardrum. This bleeding into the drum is thought to predispose to tympanosclerosis.

The middle ear should be evacuated by using a small-diameter (5 Fr) suction cannula. Occasionally, gluey material is too viscous to pass through the cannula. We do not recommend using anything larger than the 5 Fr. In these cases, the middle ear and ear canal can be irrigated with warm sterile saline. This usually breaks the viscous material up enough to pass through the cannula. Not all of the effusion needs to be evacuated; as long as the middle ear has a near-normal air space to place the tube, the remainder of the effusion will be carried into the eustachian tube or will drain out the tube. Culture of the effusion is done rarely.

It is important to position the tube such that the lumen is in line with the surgeon's line of sight, thereby facilitating postoperative examination of the middle ear mucosa in the office and also cleaning of the tube should it become plugged later on. When using T-tubes, the surgeon should assure that the short arms of the tube are completely unfolded. Ototopical drops are placed if there is an acute infection. A small cotton ball is placed in the meatus.

Laser Myringotomy

The laser has become a useful, albeit expensive, tool in the management of COME. Advantages of the laser include office-based application, ease of use, and the ability to place a controlled perforation in the tympanic membrane that will stay open for a medium length of time (2 to 6 weeks). Using the CO_2 laser at 12 W with a single 100-msec pulse through a 200 mm objective, Goode[51] reliably placed 1.5- to 2.0-mm perforations in the tympanic membranes of 10 subjects. Ten of the 11 ears healed within 6 weeks. Tube placement was avoided.

Marchant[52] performed 20 consecutive CO_2 laser myringotomies on ears with COME; all myringotomies closed within 4 weeks, with an average closing time of 17 days; 60 per cent of cases of COME were cured after 3 months. CO_2 laser myringotomy has application in clinical situations when middle ear ventilation is needed for a medium length of time (weeks) without having to place a ventilation tube. Disadvantages include cost, need for extra machinery that can be bulky, required maintenance, instruction on use and technique, and office space. Local anesthesia (iontophoresis or topical phenol application) is still required. Most otologists prefer simple cold-steel myringotomy with or without tube placement, but CO_2 myringotomy is an alternative; only time and experience will tell whether this technique will have widespread application and use.

Adenoidectomy

For an adenoidectomy, the patient is given a general anesthetic and the airway is secured via endotracheal intubation. The patient is placed in the Rose position with the neck extended over a shoulder roll and draped, as described earlier. The mouth gag is inserted and suspended from the Mayo stand located over the body of the patient. The soft palate is retracted with red rubber catheters. The hard and soft palates are palpated for the presence of a submucous cleft. The adenoid pad is inspected with the curved laryngeal mirror. The adenoid is then excised with curved curettes of various sizes (Fig. 6–2A). The curette is seated high in the nasopharynx, and the adenoid pad is resected

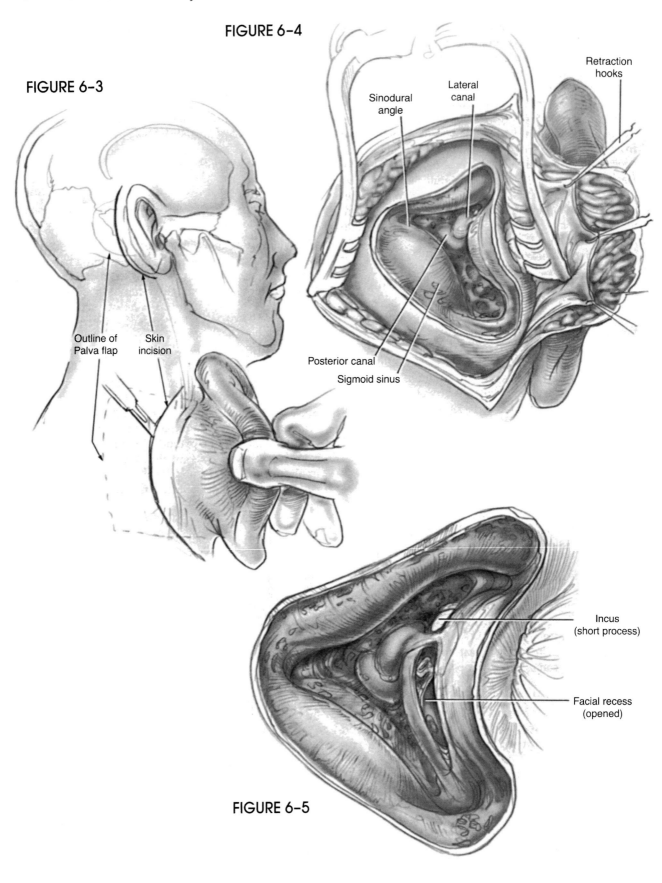

FIGURE 6-3

FIGURE 6-4

Outline of
Palva flap

Skin
incision

Sinodural
angle

Lateral
canal

Retraction
hooks

Posterior canal

Sigmoid sinus

Incus
(short process)

Facial recess
(opened)

FIGURE 6-5

FIGURES 6–3 to 6–5. *See legends on opposite page*

with a downsweeping motion on the curette. Care must be taken to avoid injury to the prevertebral fascia and muscles, which may cause excessive bleeding. The nasopharynx is palpated for residual adenoid tissue; a second or third pass may be necessary. Curved biting forceps are useful to remove tissue not accessible by the curette. The mirror is again used to inspect the site. Curettage of the tissue in the fossa of Rosenmüller is not done because it may lead to scar tissue formation and contracture that might result in stenosis and/or eustachian tube reflux. Direct injury to the eustachian tube is also avoided. The goal of surgery is the complete removal of the midline adenoid pad to achieve smooth re-epithelialization of the nasopharynx.

Bleeding usually stops quickly; tonsil sponges are used to pack the nasopharynx for hemostasis. The nasal cavities and nasopharynx are irrigated with warm saline. A malleable suction cautery can be used for precise coagulation, but its use is cautioned due to the risk of stenosis (Fig. 6–2*B*).

Mastoidectomy

The ear canal and postauricular areas are initially injected with 1 per cent lidocaine with 1:100,000 concentration of epinephrine. Vascular strip incisions are started medially at the fibrous annulus and carried laterally along the tympano-mastoid and tympanosquamous suture lines (approximately 12 and 8 o'clock for a right ear and 12 and 4 o'clock for a left ear). The incisions should come over the bony-cartilaginous junction laterally. The incisions are connected medially around the annulus with the round knife, and the vascular strip is elevated from medial to lateral. A cotton ball soaked in a 1:100,000 epinephrine solution (with or without lidocaine) is placed in the canal, and attention is turned to the postauricular area.

The postauricular incision is based about 1 fingerbreadth behind the postauricular crease, roughly paralleling the free margin of the helix (Fig. 6–3). The further posterior the incision, the greater the ease of inspecting the middle ear and eustachian tube through the facial recess. The incision is carried slightly anterior in its inferior dimension to allow the ear to be retracted forward easily. In the child, care is taken not to extend the incision beyond the mastoid tip, which is more superior than in the adult. Carrying the incision more inferior or anterior puts the facial nerve at risk. Superiorly, the temporalis fascia is identified, and a piece of fascia is harvested if needed. The fascia identifies the plane of dissection. The ear is held forward with a self-retaining retractor. The linea temporalis is palpated, and an incision is made down to the bone along this line from anterior to posterior. A second incision is made perpendicu-

lar to the first in a curvilinear fashion down to the mastoid tip. The Lempert elevator is used to elevate the periosteum to identify the cribriform area and posterior canal wall. A small elevator is next used to elevate the vascular strip out of the canal. The vascular strip is held forward with the ear under the self-retaining retractor. The tympanic membrane is next carefully elevated and the middle ear inspected.

A large cutting burr and continuous-suction-irrigation are now used to remove the lateral mastoid cortex. Important landmarks to identify include the posterior bony canal wall anteriorly, the tegmen mastoideum superiorly, the sigmoid sinus posteriorly, and the digastric ridge inferiorly. Care is taken not to expose the dura of the middle cranial fossa or the sigmoid sinus. Once these lateral landmarks have been identified, the dissection is continued medially under the microscope. Koerner's septum is opened medially and the mastoid antrum is identified. This dissection is carried anteriorly to open the aditus ad antrum and attic. The fossa incudis and short process of incus are carefully uncovered. The short process of the incus should be seen refracted through water. The short process marks the level of the facial recess. All air cells of the mastoid cortex should be taken down to reduce the surface area of the system. The bony plates over the posterior and middle fossa dura are skeletonized to form a smooth surface (Fig. 6–4). Care is taken to avoid exposing dura. The epithelium will regenerate into a single large cavity.

The descending segment of the facial nerve is identified (utilizing a diamond burr and copious suction-irrigation) by gentle dissection from superior to inferior using the fossa incudis, lateral semicircular canal, and digastric ridge as essential landmarks. The nerve and blood vessels on the nerve can be seen through bone. Care is taken not to expose the nerve.

The facial recess is opened into the middle ear by the use of progressively smaller diamond burrs. The plane of the short process of the incus leads to the facial recess (Fig. 6–5). Once the fallopian canal and chorda tympani nerve are identified, the dissection is carried between them medially to open into the middle ear. Coupled with the tympanotomy, all parts of the mesotympanum can be inspected. The ossicular chain is palpated, and any hyperplastic mucosa, granulation tissue, or secretory tissue is removed. If bone of the middle ear/promontory is exposed, a piece of absorbable gelatin film (Gelfilm) is placed through the facial recess and across the promontory toward the eustachian tube at the end of the case to prevent adhesions and to keep the recess open.

Once all hyperplastic mucosa has been removed, the

FIGURE 6–3. *The skin incision and the second incision for the Palva flap.*

FIGURE 6–4. *The mastoidectomy in progress. The sigmoid plate is skeletonized, and the bulge of the lateral semicircular canal in the antrum is visible. Note the positioning of the large retractor and dural hooks to keep the Palva flap rotated forward.*

FIGURE 6–5. *The completed mastoidectomy in the right ear with the facial recess opened. The dimensions of the facial recess are exaggerated by the artist to display the middle ear structures that may be seen by the surgeon after multiple repositionings of the viewing angle of the microscope.*

tympanic membrane is folded down back over the bony annulus and grafted if necessary. Cortisporin-soaked Gelfoam packing is placed in the medial canal. The vascular strip is returned to the posterior canal wall, and the periosteal flap is resutured to the native periosteum with 2-0 chromic suture. The vascular strip is inspected transcanal and carefully placed back so that no edges are rolled under. The remainder of the canal is packed with Cortisporin-soaked Gelfoam. The postauricular incision is closed meticulously with 3-0 undyed Vicryl in the subcutaneous layer, avoiding the need for skin sutures. A small Penrose drain can be placed in the mastoid and carried out through the inferior aspect of the incision if the mastoid is very weepy. The drain is removed when the mastoid no longer drains. A cotton ball is placed in the meatus, Steri-Strips are applied to the postauricular incision, and a sterile dressing consisting of Telfa, gauze, fluffs, and a mastoid (or cup) wrap is placed.

Postoperative Care and Follow-Up

Tympanostomy Tubes

A cotton ball is inserted into the ear canal to absorb any drainage. Parents are asked to change the cotton ball once or twice daily for a couple of days, until the drainage stops. If the ear was acutely infected at the time of surgery, a topical antibiotic/steroid suspension is used twice a day for 5 days. The first follow-up visit is done at 10 to 14 days to ensure tube placement and resolution of infection. Children are seen every 6 months for tube check thereafter. Water precautions are instituted. Parents are instructed to treat any new otorrhea with the antibiotic/steroid suspension. If the drops do not clear the infection in 2 to 3 days, an oral antibiotic is prescribed. Should this fail, the child is seen in the office for aural hygiene and cleaning and possibly intravenous antibiotics if the infection fails to resolve. Occasionally, the tube will elicit an allergic reaction with granulation tissue; removal of the tube will often calm the ear down in these situations. Tubes generally extrude within 1 to 2 years.

Adenoidectomy

Otalgia is common after adenoidectomy, and the parents should be counselled as such. Acetaminophen is usually adequate. The child should be started on a liquid diet initially, and if tolerated, advanced. Transient nasal speech may occur in a small percentage of cases, but regurgitation of liquids through the nose is rare. Palatal and pharyngeal wall compensation occurs quickly. If the child is old enough, chewing gum may speed the process and strengthen the pharyngeal and palatal musculature. Children return to the office 10 to 14 days after surgery for a checkup.

Mastoidectomy

Mastoidectomy is generally well tolerated. Patients receive pain medication; antibiotics are given in cases of acute infection. If a drain was placed, it is removed when the drainage has ceased—usually on the first or second postoperative day. The vast majority of patients do not require drains and are discharged the evening after surgery. Some require overnight observation for prolonged recovery from general anesthesia. We advise patients not to lift anything heavier than 5 to 10 pounds and not to blow their nose. The postauricular area should be kept dry. Patients return to the office 7 to 10 days after surgery for wound and canal-packing inspection. Drops are started 3 weeks after surgery to dissolve the packing; patients return again 8 weeks after surgery to check and clean the canal and for a postoperative audiogram. Drops can be started earlier if drainage or infection develop.

Surgical Pitfalls

Tympanostomy Tubes

Great care should be taken to avoid trauma to the external auditory canal during tube insertion. The resultant bleeding, although minor in amount, obscures vision and leads to a clot that is difficult to remove and obscures vision in the office. Irrigation with saline and application of a topical vasoconstrictor such as phenylephrine or oxymetazoline usually bring this under control.

Bleeding within the tympanic membrane is commonly seen when a vessel is included in the incision. Such bleeding will dissect between the layers of the drum and may result in the formation of a tympanosclerotic plaque. Careful placement of the incision avoids this potential problem.

Dislodgement of the tube into the middle ear may be a problem with a large myringotomy incision and small tube, or too small a myringotomy where the tube is pushed through. Tubes usually fall toward the eustachian tube orifice; widening a small myringotomy will allow the surgeon to retrieve the tube. Early extrusion of the tube usually occurs because the incision is too large or the tube is only partially inserted. Placement of a tube in an atelectatic ear can be difficult. The best area to place the tube is around the eustachian tube orifice (anterior) because this area usually contains the most aeration and will allow tube placement. Ossicular injury is rare if the incision is kept anterior and tube manipulation is gentle.

Adenoidectomy

The chief surgical pitfalls to avoid during adenoidectomy are trauma to the torus tubarius, which protects the opening of the eustachian tube, and deep removal of the posterior wall of the nasopharynx, which leads to excessive bleeding. Palpation and careful inspection of the nasopharynx with a mirror avoid inadequate removal of adenoid tissue. Bleeding usually can be controlled with packing of the nasopharynx and saline irrigation. Bleeding is usually from residual adenoid tissue—mirror examination can be helpful to identify the source and apply precise suction cautery or to remove adenoid remnants.

Before placing a patient with Down syndrome in the Rose position with the neck extended, the cervical spine should be cleared.

Mastoidectomy

The chief pitfall of mastoidectomy is injury to the facial nerve when opening the facial recess. This trauma is rare in experienced hands, especially with continuous monitoring of the nerve during the procedure. Dural exposure in the tegmen mastoideum should be avoided due to the risk of later encephalocele. Care should also be taken around the sigmoid sinus; opening of the sinus can usually be controlled with precise Surgicel packing.

Contact of the drill with the incus may result in mild to moderate high-frequency sensorineural hearing loss due to vibratory energy transmitted to the cochlea. Drill contact should also be minimized on labyrinthine bone. Blue lining or opening a semicircular canal should be addressed immediately by gently closing the opening with bone wax. A blue-lined canal should be recognized and avoided. Wound infection is uncommon; copious irrigation during and after the procedure aids in removal of unwanted debris and/or bone dust that might serve as a nidus for infection.

Results

Goals of surgery include hearing improvement, reducing the time spent with middle ear effusion, and reducing the number of recurrences of middle ear effusion. Tube insertion with and without adenoidectomy has been shown to improve conductive hearing loss secondary to COME and to decrease the amount of time spent with effusion.[18]

Gates and colleagues assigned 491 children, 4 to 9 years old, with OME persisting 60 days or more after repeated medical therapy, to various combinations of myringotomy, tympanostomy tube insertion, and adenoidectomy for COME.[4] They found that time with recurrent middle ear effusion was decreased by 29 per cent in the tympanostomy tubes–only group, by 38 per cent in the adenoidectomy-plus-myringotomy group, and by 47 per cent in the adenoidectomy-plus–tympanostomy tubes group. Hearing was equivalent in all groups except the myringotomy-alone group; hearing in this group was significantly worse. Surgical re-treatments were necessary more often in children initially treated with myringotomy alone (36 per cent) or tympanostomy tubes alone (20 per cent) than in those treated by adenoidectomy and myringotomy (10 per cent) or adenoidectomy plus tympanostomy tubes (10 per cent). The number of repeat operations in the two adenoidectomy groups was significantly less than in the two nonadenoidectomy groups ($P < 0.001$).[4]

Paradise and associates randomly placed patients who had previously undergone tympanostomy tube placement and had recurrent middle ear disease into either an adenoidectomy or control group. During the first and second years of follow-up, the adenoidectomy group had 47 and 37 per cent less time with otitis media than the control patients.[38]

Although most cases of IH resolve satisfactorily, surgical management (tube placement and/or mastoidectomy) is generally successful. Often it takes months for the ear to aerate and for satisfactory hearing to return. Nonetheless, persistence and patience are often rewarded.

Complications and Management

Tympanostomy Tubes

Otorrhea. The most common sequela of tympanostomy tubes is purulent otorrhea. In the Gates study,[4] otorrhea occurred one or more times in 22 per cent of the myringotomy-alone group, 29 per cent of the tympanostomy tube group, 11 per cent of the adenoidectomy-myringotomy group, and 24 per cent of the adenoidectomy–tympanostomy tube group. Some cases of otorrhea are due to water contamination; others are the result of acute otitis media. Some cases also involve an allergy to the tube itself. Treatment is the same: a topical polymicrobial-steroid suspension with or without an oral antibiotic, along with aural hygiene in the office. Most cases clear quickly. In the recalcitrant case, the tube is removed and cultures are done. Failure to clear persistent otorrhea after maximal medical therapy is an indication for tympanoplasty with mastoidectomy.

Persistent Perforation. Tympanostomy tubes extrude within 1 to 2 years of insertion. Depending on the tube, 1 to 15 per cent of cases will result in a persistent perforation. Older children may be able to tolerate attempts to close the perforation in the office with freshening of the edges and placement of a paper patch. Other children will be good candidates for a fat plug myringoplasty[53] or more formal myringoplasty/tympanoplasty under anesthesia.

Adenoidectomy

Bleeding. The most common complication of adenoidectomy is postoperative bleeding. However, the incidence is low: of 250 cases done by 13 surgeons, only one child required operative treatment for bleeding, and none needed transfusion.[4] Helmus and colleagues noted that only four patients in 1000 (0.4 per cent) bled after outpatient adenoidectomy; all instances occurred in the first 6 postoperative hours and were managed without transfusion.[54] Return trip to the OR for bleeding involves the same positioning as for routine adenoidectomy. Irrigation with suction cautery generally will control bleeding.

Velopharyngeal Insufficiency. Other less common complications include nasopharyngeal stenosis and VPI. Stenosis results from excessive tissue destruction, including excessive use of cautery, excessive curettage of the fossa of Rosenmüller, and removal of the lateral pharyngeal bands. Stenosis can require reoperation for scar tissue removal or pharyngeal flap reconstruction. The best treatment is prevention.

Transient VPI may occur after removal of a large adenoid but resolves quickly in the majority of cases. If the child is old enough, gum chewing will strengthen and recondition the injured pharyngeal musculature. Persistent VPI is the most feared complication because it requires either a prosthesis or a secondary procedure (pharyngeal flap) for reconstruction. The majority of cases are due to an undetected submucous cleft palate. Preoperative palpation and inspection (note bifid uvula) will identify patients at risk.

Mastoidectomy

Facial Paralysis. Complications following mastoidectomy are rare. Facial paresis occurs rarely in experienced

hands. Intraoperative facial nerve monitoring has further
decreased this complication. Heat injury should not occur
if continuous irrigation is used. Intimate knowledge of the
anatomy and anatomic relationships is the best prevention
of facial nerve injury. Injury, if it involves more than 25
per cent of the nerve, has historically been repaired with
direct anastomosis after mild decompression and freshening
of the edges. However, review of our results reveals that
recovery to a maximum House-Brackmann grade III was
similar for primary anastomosis and cable graft.[55]

Hearing Loss. High-frequency sensorineural hearing
loss may be caused by drill trauma around the ossicles,
especially the incus. Careful inspection of the aditus
through water will identify the incus and minimize drill
trauma. Drilling on labyrinthine bone should be kept to a
minimum. Inadvertent opening of a semicircular canal
should be sealed with bone wax with no suctioning around
the fistula.

Recurrent Hemotympanum. Recurrent IH is common.
Treatment should be with a large-bore tympanostomy tube.
Occasionally, a second-look mastoid operation is indicated.
Hearing amplification helps with hearing loss.

ALTERNATIVE TECHNIQUES

Children with persistent effusion for whom both medical
and surgical treatment have failed should be evaluated for
auditory trainer, hearing aid use, or other form of hearing
rehabilitation, especially when the child is in school. Pref-
erential seating in class is strongly encouraged.

ALLERGY TREATMENT

Children with symptomatic food or inhalant allergy deserve
therapy whether they have OME or not. Given that the
majority of cases of OME have had prior nasal infection
and that children with nasal allergy have a higher prevalence of infection, allergy evaluation is appropriate for
children with OME who also have nasal symptoms. However, Gates and colleagues found a lower incidence of
allergy in their subjects with OME than in the general
population.[4] Although a cause-effect relationship between
nasal allergy and OME has not been shown, the surgeon
should inquire about allergic symptoms to provide proper
therapy to those patients with dual problems.

ACKNOWLEDGMENT

We would like to thank George A. Gates, M.D., author of
this chapter in the previous edition.

References

1. Gates GA: Cost-effectiveness considerations in otitis media treatment. Otolaryngol Head Neck Surg 114: 525–530, 1996.
2. Schappert SM: Office visits for otitis media: United States, 1975–90. Adv Data 214: 1–19, 1992.
3. Kleinman LC, Kosecoff J, Dubois RW, Brook RH: The medical appropriateness of tympanostomy tubes proposed for children younger than 16 years in the United States. JAMA 271: 1250–1255, 1994.
4. Gates GA, Avery CA, Prihoda TJ, Cooper JC: Effectiveness of adenoidectomy and tympanostomy tubes in the treatment of otitis media with effusion. N Engl J Med 317: 1444–1451, 1987.
5. Gates GA, Muntz HR, Gaylis B: Adenoidectomy and otitis media. Ann Otol Rhinol Laryngol 101: 24–32, 1992.
6. Stool SE, Berg AO, Berman S, et al: Managing otitis media with effusion in young children: Quick reference guide for clinicians. AHCPR Publication No. 94-0623. Rockville, MD, Agency for Health Care Policy and Research, Public Health Service, U.S. Department of Health and Human Services, July 1994.
7. Bluestone CD: Otitis media: A spectrum of diseases. In Lalwani AK, Grundfast KM (eds): Pediatric Otology and Neurotology. Philadelphia, Lippincott-Raven, 1998, pp 233–240.
8. Casselbrant ML, Mandel EM, Kurs-Lasky M, et al: Otitis media in a population of black American and white American infants, 0–2 years of age. Int J Pediatr Otorhinolaryngol 33: 1–16, 1995.
9. Teele DW, Klein JO, Rosner BA, and the Greater Boston Otitis Media Study Group: Epidemiology of otitis media during the first seven years of life in children in Greater Boston: A prospective cohort study. J Infect Dis 160: 83–94, 1989.
10. Senturia BH, Bluestone CD, Klein JO, et al: Report of the Ad Hoc Committee on Definition and Classification of Otitis Media and Otitis Media with Effusion. Ann Otol Rhinol Laryngol 89(Suppl 68): 3–4, 1980.
11. Kenna MA: Otitis media with effusion. In Bailey BJ (ed): Head and Neck Surgery—Otolaryngology. Philadelphia, JB Lippincott, 1993, pp 1592–1606.
12. Teele DW, Klein JO, Rosner B, and the Greater Boston Otitis Media Study Group: Middle ear disease in the practice of pediatrics: Burden during the first five years of life. JAMA 249: 1026–1029, 1983.
13. Teele DW, Klein JO, Rosner B: Epidemiology of otitis media in children. Ann Otol Rhinol Laryngol 89(Suppl 68): 5–6, 1980.
14. Schwartz RH, Rodriguez WJ, Grundfast KM: Duration of middle ear effusion after acute otitis media. Pediatr Inf Dis J 3: 204–207, 1984.
15. Shurin PA, Pelton SI, Turczyk VA, et al: Persistence of middle ear effusion after acute otitis media. N Engl J Med 300: 1121–1123, 1979.
16. Henderson FW, Giebink GS: Otitis media among children in day care: Epidemiology and pathogenesis. Rev Infect Dis 8: 533–538, 1986.
17. Bluestone CD, Stephenson JS, Martin LM: Ten-year review of otitis media pathogens. Pediatr Infect Dis J 11(8 Suppl): S7–11, 1992.
18. Bluestone CD, Klein JO: Otitis media, atelectasis, and eustachian tube dysfunction. In Bluestone CD, Stool SE (eds): Pediatric Otolaryngology, 3rd ed. Philadelphia, WB Saunders, 1996, pp 388–582.
19. Kenna MA, Bluestone CD: Microbiology of chronic suppurative otitis media. Pediatr Infect Dis J 5: 223–225, 1986.
20. Papastavros T, Giamarellou H, Varlejides S: Role of aerobic and anaerobic microorganisms in chronic suppurative otitis media. Laryngoscope 96: 438–442, 1986.
21. Post JC, Preston RA, Aul JJ, et al: Molecular analysis of bacterial pathogens in otitis media with effusion. JAMA 273: 1598–1604, 1995.
22. Howie VM, Ploussard JH: Simultaneous nasopharyngeal and middle ear exudate cultures in otitis media. Pediatr Digest 13: 31–35, 1971.
23. Pillsbury HC III, Kveton JF, Sasaki CT, Frazier W: Quantitative bacteriology in adenoid tissue. Otolaryngol Head Neck Surg 89: 355–363, 1981.
24. Bluestone CD, Paradise JL, Beery QC: Physiology of the eustachian tube in the pathogenesis and management of middle ear effusions. Laryngoscope 82: 1654–1670, 1972.
25. Liu YS, Lang RW, Lim DJ: Microorganisms in chronic otitis media with effusion. Ann Otol Rhinol Laryngol 85: 245–249, 1976.
26. Sade J: The natural history of the secretory otitis media syndrome. In Sade J (ed): Secretory Otitis Media and Its Sequelae. New York, Churchill Livingstone, 1979, pp 89–101.
27. Tos M: Production of mucus in the middle ear and eustachian tube: Embryology, anatomy, and pathology of the mucous glands and goblet cells in the eustachian tube and middle ear. Ann Otol Rhinol Laryngol 83(Suppl 11): 44–58, 1974.
28. Gates GA: Surgery of ventilation and mucosal disease. In Brackmann DE, Shelton C, Arriaga MA (eds): Otologic Surgery. Philadelphia, WB Saunders, 1994, p 86.
29. Kovatch AL, Wald ER, Michaels RH: β-Lactamase–producing Branhamella catarrhalis causing otitis media in children. J Pediatr 102: 261–264, 1983.
30. McCracken GH: Management of acute otitis media with effusion. Pediatr Infect Dis J 7: 442–445, 1988.

31. Karma PH, Penttila MA, Sipila MM, Kataja MJ: Otoscopic diagnosis of middle ear effusion in acute and non-acute otitis media. Int J Pediatr Otorhinolaryngol 17: 37–49, 1989.
32. Varsano I, Volovitz B, Mimouni F: Sulfisoxazole prophylaxis of middle ear effusion and recurrent acute otitis media. Am J Dis Child 139: 632–635, 1985.
33. Perrin JM, Charney E, MacWhinney JB Jr, et al: Sulfisoxazole as chemoprophylaxis for recurrent otitis media. N Engl J Med 291: 664–667, 1974.
34. Maynard JE, Fleshman JK, Tschopp CR: Otitis media in Alaskan Eskimo children: Prospective evaluation of chemoprophylaxis. JAMA 219: 597–599, 1972.
35. Principi N, Marchisio P, Massironi E, et al: Prophylaxis of recurrent acute otitis media and middle ear effusion: Comparison of amoxicillin with sulfamethoxazole and trimethoprim. Am J Dis Child 143: 1414–1418, 1989.
36. Gebhart DE: Tympanostomy tubes in the otitis media–prone child. Laryngoscope 91: 849–866, 1981.
37. Casselbrant ML, Kaleida PH, Rockette HE, et al: Efficacy of antimicrobial prophylaxis and of tympanostomy tube insertion for prevention of recurrent otitis media: Results of a randomized clinical trial. Pediatr Infect Dis J 11: 278–286, 1992.
38. Paradise JL, Bluestone CD, Rogers KD, et al: Efficacy of adenoidectomy for recurrent otitis media in children previously treated with tympanostomy tube placement. JAMA 263: 2066–2073, 1990.
39. Mandel EM, Rockette HE, Bluestone CD, et al: Efficacy of amoxicillin with and without decongestant-antihistamine for otitis media with effusion in children. N Engl J Med 316: 432–437, 1987.
40. Rosenfeld RM, Post JC: Meta-analysis of antibiotics for treatment of otitis media with effusion. Otolaryngol Head Neck Surg 106: 378–386, 1992.
41. Lambert PR: Oral steroid therapy for chronic middle ear effusion: A double-blind crossover study. Otolaryngol Head Neck Surg 95: 193–199, 1986.
42. Grundfast KM: Management of otitis media and the new Agency for Health Care Policy and Research Guideline. Arch Otolaryngol 120: 797–798, 1994.
43. Armstrong BW: A new treatment for chronic secretory otitis media. Arch Otolaryngol 69: 653–654, 1954.
44. Healy GB: Managing otitis media with effusion in young children: A commentary. Arch Otolaryngol 120: 1049–1050, 1994.
45. Maw AR: Chronic otitis media with effusion (glue ear) and adenotonsillectomy: A prospective randomized controlled study. BMJ 287: 1586–1588, 1983.
46. Paradise JL, Bluestone CD: Adenoidectomy and chronic otitis media (letter). N Engl J Med 318: 1470–1471, 1988.
47. Gates GA, Muntz H, Gaylis B: Adenoidectomy. Ann Otol Rhinol Laryngol Suppl 155: 24–32, 1992.
48. Koyuncu M, Saka MM, Tanyeri Y, et al: Effects of otitis media with effusion on the vestibular system in children. Otolaryngol Head Neck Surg 120: 117–121, 1999.
49. Golz A, Westerman T, Gilbert LM, et al: Effect of middle ear effusion on the vestibular labyrinth. J Laryngol Otol 105: 987–989, 1991.
50. Jones NS, Radomsky P, Princhard ANJ, Snashell SE: Imbalance and chronic secretory otitis media in children: Effect of myringotomy and insertion of ventilation tubes on body sway. Ann Otol Rhinol Laryngol 99: 477–481, 1990.
51. Goode RL: CO_2 laser myringotomy. Laryngoscope 92:420–423, 1982.
52. Marchant H, Bisschop P: Value of laser CO_2 myringotomy in the treatment of seromucous otitis: Annales d' Oto-Laryngologie et de Chirurgie Cervico-Faciale 115:347–351, 1998.
53. Gross CG, Bessila M, Lazar RH, et al: Adipose plug myringoplasty: An alternative to formal myringoplasty techniques in children. Otolaryngol Head Neck Surg 101: 617–620, 1989.
54. Helmus C, Grin M, Westfall R: Same-day-stay adenotonsillectomy. Laryngoscope 100: 593–596, 1990.
55. Green JD Jr, Shelton C, Brackmann DE: Surgical management of iatrogenic facial nerve injuries. Otolaryngol Head Neck Surg 111: 606–610, 1994.

7

The Abnormally Patulous Eustachian Tube

Charles D. Bluestone, M.D. ▪ Anthony E. Magit, M.D.

The abnormally patulous eustachian tube presents as a spectrum of clinical signs and symptoms. Patient presentations range from subclinical disturbances to debilitating symptoms leading to significant psychologic impairment. The eustachian tube is closed in the normal physiologic state, with brief open periods primarily resulting from activity of the tensor veli palatini muscle. The eustachian tube has at least three physiologic functions with respect to the middle ear: (1) pressure regulation (i.e., ventilatory function) of the middle ear to equilibrate pressure in the middle ear with atmospheric pressure; (2) protection from nasopharyngeal sound pressure and secretions; and (3) clearance (and drainage) of secretions produced within the middle ear into the nasopharynx. The abnormally patulous eustachian tube is permanently open. Patients with a patulous tube have abnormal gas flow from the nasopharynx to the middle ear throughout all phases of respiration and swallowing.

HISTORY AND PATHOPHYSIOLOGY OF PATULOUS EUSTACHIAN TUBE

Schwartze was the first to describe the patulous eustachian tube with the report of a scarred atrophic eardrum moving synchronously with respiration.[1] In 1867, Jago reported having this affliction himself.[2] Zollner[3] and Shambaugh[4] noted that patients with abnormally patulous eustachian tubes complain of autophony. The abnormally patulous eustachian tube is not a rare condition. However, as noted by Rumbolt in 1873[5] and Bull in 1976,[6] the diagnosis requires constant awareness and clinical vigilance. Heightened awareness is an important component to the increased frequency of the diagnosis. From 1940 to 1959, the diagnosis of a patulous eustachian tube was made 41 times at the Mayo Clinic. The diagnosis was made 95 times at the Mayo Clinic in the 7-year period from 1960 to 1966.[7] Zollner cited an incidence of 0.3 per cent in the general population.[3] Munker diagnosed an abnormally patulous eustachian tube in 6.6 per cent of 100 women who had normal results on otoscopic examination.[8]

The diagnosis of an abnormally patulous eustachian tube necessitates an intensive search for an etiology in each patient because of the possibility of a serious underlying disease. Weight loss is the most common etiology and the one most easily treated. As little as 6 pounds of weight loss may lead to sufficient atrophy of soft tissue in the

peritubal area to result in a patulous tube.[7, 9] Atrophy and scarring of the nasopharyngeal muscles secondary to a cerebral vascular accident, poliomyelitis, multiple sclerosis, radiotherapy, and iatrogenic and traumatic injuries to the fifth cranial nerve may result in a functionally patulous eustachian tube.[4, 10–12] Muscular dysfunction secondary to direct damage to the tensor veli palatini muscle during cleft palate surgery, combined with postoperative nasopharyngeal adhesions and fibrosis, may cause a patulous tube.[13] Shambaugh[4] and Pulec and Simonton[14] proposed that repeated tonsillar and pharyngeal infections can alter pharyngeal function to the point of causing a patulous eustachian tube. Palatal myoclonus has also been associated with this disorder.

Pregnancy and supplemental estrogen are implicated in the etiology of a patulous eustachian tube.[11, 14–16] High levels of estrogen may lead to thinning of intraluminal eustachian tube secretions or an increase in relaxin, a hormone known to increase ligamentous relaxation in the pelvis.[17] Estrogen also affects prostaglandin E levels, with a subsequent effect on surfactant levels.[18] Elevated surfactant levels may decrease the intraluminal surface tension, with the development of a more patulous eustachian tube.

Less common conditions associated with a patulous eustachian tube are chronic gum chewing, dental malocclusion, continued voluntary or involuntary subluxation of the temporomandibular joint, and skull dysmorphology, such as brachycephaly.

DIAGNOSIS OF PATULOUS EUSTACHIAN TUBE

The most frequent symptom associated with an abnormally patulous eustachian tube is autophony, the awareness of hearing one's own voice.[13] Autophony may also be described as a roaring sound in the ear synchronous with respiration, fluctuating fullness, and "blockage" in the ear—a feeling of talking into a barrel, or such loud perception of one's voice that normal conversation is impossible.[19, 20] Autophony is usually fluctuant and does not become apparent until the patient has been erect for several minutes. Relief comes from assuming a supine position, sniffing, or by placing one's head between the knees.[21] These maneuvers effectively increase venous congestion in the peritubal area. Acute rhinitis or any increase in edema of the nasal mucosa and postnasal space is usually associated with an improvement in symptoms.[13] Symptoms may be exacerbated by topical or systemic decongestants, exercise, fatigue, or nervousness.[19]

Patients with an abnormally patulous eustachian tube may present with an apparent psychoneurotic condition.[20, 22] Manipulation of the mandible as a means of closing off the eustachian tube may give the appearance of a tic or manifestation of neurotic behavior. Hyponasality and hyporhinolalia secondary to the attempt to close the eustachian tube is a less common presentation of a patulous eustachian tube.[13, 23] Ringing tinnitus, conductive hearing loss, and vestibular symptoms are uncommon characteristics of a patulous eustachian tube. Robinson and Hazell reported an association between patulous eustachian tubes and sensorineural hearing loss.[24]

The diagnostic evaluation of the patient suspected of having a patulous eustachian tube starts with a comprehensive history. Symptoms of autophony as previously described are the hallmark of the patulous eustachian tube. Autophony improves when the patient is supine or when the head is in a dependent position, and the onset of symptoms develops within minutes or hours of assuming an upright position.[21] Otoscopic results may be normal; however, tympanic membrane findings may include atrophic changes. Synchronous movement of the tympanic membrane with respiration has been documented by Schwartze,[1] Harman,[25] and Voltolini.[26] Otoscopy should be performed using a microscope with the patient in the upright position.[24] Movement of the tympanic membrane is enhanced by occlusion of the naris and closure of the mouth during forced inspiration and expiration, or by using the Toynbee or Valsalva maneuver. Gentle pneumatic pressure in the external auditory canal may give the appearance of a flail tympanic membrane. Rarely, respiration and speech may be heard by using a microphone placed in the external auditory canal.

In addition to video documentation of a flail tympanic membrane, objective evidence of a patulous eustachian tube is possible with tympanometry.[27] Two tympanograms are obtained while the patient is in the upright position. The first is done with the patient breathing normally, and the second, during breath holding. Fluctuations in the tympanometry tracing coincide with respiration. Fluctuations are enhanced by occluding one nostril and closing the mouth, or by the Toynbee maneuver. More detailed characterization of a patulous eustachian tube is possible after determination of the passive eustachian tube opening pressure when the tympanic membrane has a tube or perforation present. The patulous eustachian tube and middle ear will not maintain applied positive middle ear pressure, or the opening pressure is extremely low, such as 50 to 100 mm H_2O. An intact tympanic membrane can be evaluated by performing the "nine-step" test.[27, 28] Virtanen is a proponent of sonotubometry for diagnosing the abnormally patulous eustachian tube.[29]

An audiogram should be obtained as a part of the evaluation, because hearing loss is often a part of the constellation of complaints associated with a patulous eustachian tube. Although some reports describe a unilateral sensorineural hearing loss of unknown etiology on the same side as a patulous eustachian tube, no clear association has been established between a patulous eustachian tube and sensorineural hearing loss.

Imaging studies may be useful in patients when a central nervous system etiology or base of skull neoplasm is suspected as the etiology of a patulous eustachian tube. Tolley and Phelps presented clinical cases in which computed tomography scans confirmed the diagnosis of a patulous eustachian tube.[30]

TREATMENT

Once the diagnosis of a patulous eustachian tube has been established, an underlying cause should be sought. Initial therapy involves addressing the underlying cause, if found. When a clear etiology is not apparent, medical and surgical therapies are instituted and are aimed at ultimately decreasing patency of the eustachian tube lumen. The severity of symptoms dictates the urgency with which treatment is implemented.

Children and adolescents rarely present with a patulous eustachian tube. In this population, therapy is usually not indicated, because the symptoms are self-limited. Minimal symptoms of a patulous tube may initially be treated with reassurance and an explanation of the benign nature of the affliction.[7] Weight loss is the most obvious etiology of a patulous eustachian tube and the most responsive to nonsurgical therapy. Weight gain usually results in resolution of symptoms.

Elevated estrogen levels may lead to a patulous condition, as previously described. Pregnant women can be assured that completion of the pregnancy will lead to stabilization of estrogen fluxes and a return to normal eustachian tube function.[11, 14–16] Derkay presented a study of patulous eustachian tubes in pregnant women and showed that when three symptomatic pregnant women were retested in the postpartum period, all three were asymptomatic and no longer had patulous tubes.[31] Prior to the introduction of low-dose estrogen birth control pills, patients complained more frequently of patulous symptoms. Nonetheless, birth control pills may still be responsible for abnormal eustachian tube function.

When an etiology for the patulous eustachian tube condition is not found, or the contributing condition cannot be effectively treated, for example, emaciation due to terminal cancer, medical or surgical therapy is indicated.

Medical therapy intended to decrease eustachian tube patency may be started as an initial course of therapy for patients with moderate symptoms. The oral administration of a saturated solution of potassium iodide (SSKI), 10 drops in a glass of juice three times a day, has been reported to be efficacious in some patients. This may be combined with the use of conjugated estrogens (Premarin) nasal drops, 25 mg in 30 ml of normal saline solution, 3 drops three times a day.[32] The combination of potassium iodide and Premarin drops, with the addition of reserpine chlorothiazide has also been useful but may be associated with lightheadedness. Medical therapy may be tried for 1 month in patients with moderate symptoms before surgery is recommended. Experimentally, atropine has been shown to reduce the inflation pressure and initial opening pressure of a patulous eustachian tube.[33] Medical therapy may not be a plausible first-line management for patients with grossly abnormal results on otoscopic examination and debilitating symptoms and is rarely successful in the long term when the condition is chronic.

Procedures intended to cause irritation and inflammation of the eustachian tube orifice provide transient relief from patulous symptoms. Although not widely used in contemporary practice, several means of creating eustachian tube inflammation are available: eustachian tube catheterization and insufflation with a salicylic acid–boric acid solution in a 1:4 ratio,[34] eustachian tube diathermy,[24, 35] silver nitrate cautery,[13, 36] and the application of nitric acid and phenol.[37] These procedures have variable rates of success, and patients may require re-treatment.

Surgical therapy is an alternative when less invasive methods of treatment have failed. Although the abnormally patulous eustachian tube allows abnormal air flow to the middle ear cleft, some physicians report success with myringotomy and tympanostomy tube placement.[14, 38, 39] Despite the lack of theoretical basis for the success of this procedure, myringotomy with tube placement continues to be used to treat this condition.

Surgical reconstruction of the eustachian tube orifice is one treatment option for a patulous eustachian tube. Closure of the eustachian tube orifice involving the removal of cartilage is one method.[40] This procedure either has been unsuccessful in alleviating the symptoms or has led to complete stenosis of the eustachian tube and refractory middle ear effusion. Transposition of the tendon of the tensor veli palatini muscle with and without hamulotomy has been reported in several small series.[21, 41] With limited follow-up, this procedure has been successful in approximately 70 per cent of cases; long-term follow-up of patients treated with this method has not been reported.

Various methods of blocking the pharyngeal opening of the eustachian tube have been reported. Zollner infiltrated paraffin around the eustachian tube orifice and saw transient improvement in patulous symptoms.[3] Ogawa and associates infused an absorbable gelatin sponge–glycerin mixture into the eustachian tube and found a high recurrence rate within 1 month of the procedure.[42] O'Connor and Shea introduced polytetrafluoroethylene (Teflon) paste into the eustachian tube orifice and saw transient relief.[13] Pulec succeeded in resolving patulous symptoms in 19 of 26 patients after an injection of polytetrafluoroethylene at the anteroinferior margin of the pharyngeal eustachian tube orifice.[7] Polytetrafluoroethylene injection has been associated with serious complications, including cerebral thrombosis and death.

Because the authors have had limited success with either the nonsurgical or the surgical methods reported in the past, we prefer surgically treating the chronically abnormal patulous eustachian tube by inserting an indwelling catheter into the protympanic portion of the eustachian tube.[43] This procedure is combined with myringotomy and tympanostomy tube placement in anticipation of a middle ear effusion forming after the eustachian tube is obstructed. Patients are told that following surgery, water must be kept out of the ear because of the tympanostomy tube. No other limitation of activity is necessary. A tympanostomy tube placed in the anteroinferior portion of the tympanic membrane will not cause hearing loss. The patients should be seen at least twice a year to assess the status of their symptoms and that of the tympanostomy tubes. Some patients will spontaneously extrude the tympanostomy tube and not develop middle ear effusion. Presumably, there is enough gas exchange from the nasopharynx into the middle ear to effectively ventilate the middle ear. However, if middle ear negative pressure or effusion develops, then a tympanostomy tube must be reinserted. With this procedure, removing the indwelling catheter can reverse eustachian tube obstruction if the patient desires it to be removed, or if there are postoperative complications or sequelae.

CATHETER OCCLUSION OF THE PATULOUS EUSTACHIAN TUBE

Catheter occlusion of a patulous eustachian tube is a surgical procedure that may be performed with local anesthesia supplemented with systemic analgesia or under general anesthesia. The type of anesthetic is based on the patient's preference. Advantages of local anesthesia include the safety of the anesthetic and a reduced recovery time. Local anesthetic infiltration is used whether the procedure is performed under mild intravenous sedation or general anesthesia. A standard four-quadrant injection is made at the bony-cartilaginous junction of the external auditory canal by using a solution of 1 per cent lidocaine and 1:100,000 epinephrine injected from a 25-gauge needle. A significant blanching of the anterior canal wall may not be possible because of the thinness of the skin in this area.

Following injection of the ear canal, the ear is prepared with a povidone-iodide solution. If a tympanostomy tube is present, a piece of cotton is placed in the external auditory canal to prevent flow of the solution through the tube. The ear canal is irrigated with a sterile solution prior to beginning the surgical procedure.

Perioperative antibiotics are not used. Any sign or symptom of infection in the external auditory canal or middle ear is a contraindication to surgery until the condition is resolved.

The surgical procedure is performed with the aid of an operating microscope. Using a Rosen knife, or "round knife," an anterior circumferential incision is made 8 mm from the annulus extending from 12 to 6 o'clock (Fig. 7–1). The initial elevation of the anterior tympanomeatal flap is done with a Moon elevator (Fig. 7–2). A No. 3 Fr suction is positioned behind the elevator to prevent trauma to the flap. If the patient has a large anterior bony overhang, it may require drilling with a Skeeter drill to provide adequate exposure. Caution must be exercised during any drilling of the anterior canal to avoid entrance into the temporomandibular joint. Once the level of the annulus is reached, a cotton pledget soaked with 1:100,000 adrenaline may be placed between the flap and anterior canal wall to prevent bleeding prior to entering the middle ear. The anterior annulus is drawn out of the sulcus with a Rosen needle or a gently curved instrument. Once the middle ear is entered, the flap is further elevated with an annulus elevator, or gimmick. The flap is elevated to the malleus. Care must be taken not to traumatize the ossicles; however, this does not usually pose a problem.

A modification of the anterior tympanomeatal flap approach to the middle ear involves using a large anterior

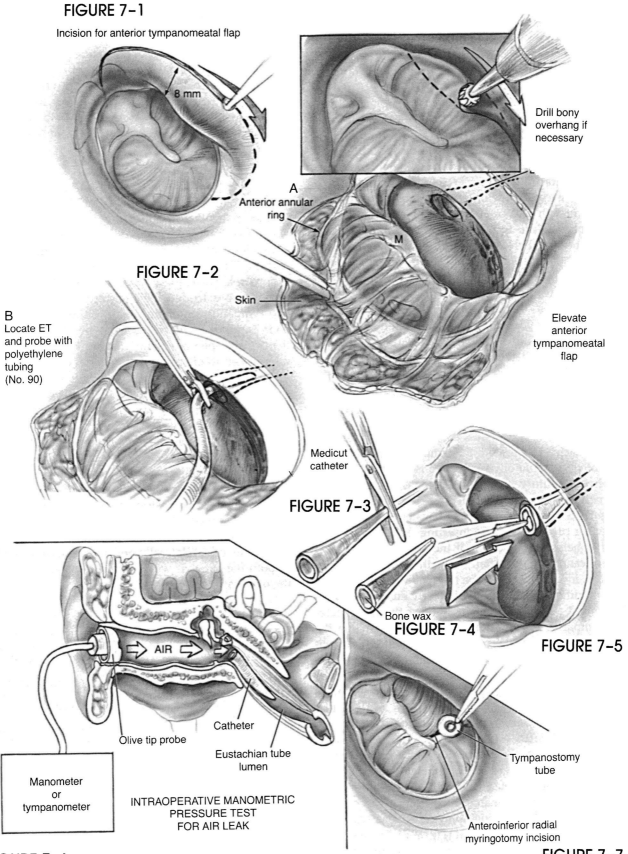

FIGURE 7-1

Incision for anterior tympanomeatal flap

8 mm

Drill bony overhang if necessary

A
Anterior annular ring

M

Skin

Elevate anterior tympanomeatal flap

FIGURE 7-2

B
Locate ET and probe with polyethylene tubing (No. 90)

Medicut catheter

FIGURE 7-3

Bone wax

FIGURE 7-4

FIGURE 7-5

AIR

Catheter

Olive tip probe

Eustachian tube lumen

Manometer or tympanometer

INTRAOPERATIVE MANOMETRIC PRESSURE TEST FOR AIR LEAK

Tympanostomy tube

Anteroinferior radial myringotomy incision

FIGURE 7-6

FIGURE 7-7

myringotomy for access to the middle ear.[32] This method has been reported to be successful in a small series of patients, although operative exposure may not be adequate through a myringotomy for all patients.

The eustachian tube orifice is identified with direct vision or with a piece of No. 90 polyethylene tubing. The polyethylene tubing is helpful in assessing the orientation of the eustachian tube lumen. The eustachian tube catheter is fashioned using an 18-gauge Medicut angiocatheter. The narrowed end of the catheter is cut to leave a total catheter length of approximately 2 cm (Fig. 7–3). The flared end of the catheter is occluded with bone wax (Fig. 7–4). The narrowed end of the catheter is introduced into the eustachian tube orifice using a forceps or large alligator (Fig. 7–5). Sufficient pressure is used to obtain a tight fit.

Once the catheter is secured, a manometer or tympanometer is used to assess the degree of occlusion of the eustachian tube. With the tympanomeatal flap still elevated, a sterile olive-tip probe is inserted into the external auditory canal (Fig. 7–6). Using either the manometer or tympanometer, the pressure is slowly raised to 400 to 600 mm H_2O. Obtaining an opening pressure prior to inserting the Medicut catheter is helpful in assessing if the opening pressure is significantly higher after the catheter has been inserted; ideally, there will be no opening pressure and the middle ear and the obstructed eustachian tube will hold air pressure to the limit of the manometer or tympanometer. It should be noted that when the patient is in the supine position, there will be an opening pressure, albeit lower that normal, prior to inserting the Medicut catheter, because the eustachian tube is engorged in this position. Any leak of air below this level is considered an inadequate seal, and the catheter placement is reassessed. If the Medicut catheter appears to be in place and there is a leak of air, bone pate (taken from the anterior auditory canal) can be used around the edges of the catheter. After the pressure test is completed, the tympanomeatal flap is placed back into its anatomic position. At this point, an anterior radial myringotomy is performed, and a tympanostomy tube is placed (Fig. 7–7). The ear canal is filled with an antibiotic ointment to secure the flap. A cotton ball is then placed in the external meatus and serves as the only necessary dressing.

Postoperative Care

The patient is instructed to limit physical activity for 4 weeks to allow for healing of the tympanomeatal flap. Postoperative antibiotics are not routinely used. Patients are instructed to keep water out of their ears by using an earplug and by avoiding submerging their heads. Earplugs are not used until the patient is seen at the postoperative visit to ensure that the canal incisions are well healed.

Results of Catheter Occlusion of the Eustachian Tube

Of 12 patients with follow-up of 2 to 17 years, half have had significant, long-lasting relief of their symptoms and have not had complications related to the tympanostomy

tubes. Two patients have extruded their eustachian tube catheters and tympanostomy tubes with continued relief from patulous eustachian tube symptoms. These patients apparently developed adequate scarring of the eustachian tube lumen to effectively eliminate the patulous condition. Two patients with catheters in place and extruded tympanostomy tubes and intact tympanic membranes have not experienced any episodes of middle ear effusion. These cases support the concept that in some patients, there is gas exchange around the Medicut catheter. One patient complained of postoperative tinnitus and requested removal of the catheter. The catheter was removed without any complication. This patient still has symptoms of a patulous tube bilaterally and has persistent tinnitus in the previously operated ear as well as in the unoperated ear.

Intraoperative assessment of eustachian tube function with manometry to determine the degree of occlusion of the eustachian tube by the catheter has improved the success of the operation. Patients with intraoperative assessment of eustachian tube occlusion have been more successfully treated than those patients treated prior to the use of intraoperative manometry.

References

1. Schwartze H, as cited in Ogawa S, et al: Arch Otolaryngol 102: 276–280, 1976.
2. Jago J: Functions of the tympanum. Br For Med Chir Rev 39: 496–520, 1867.
3. Zollner R, as cited in Ogawa S, et al: Arch Otolaryngol 102: 276–280, 1976.
4. Shambaugh GE Jr: Continuously open eustachian tube. Arch Otolaryngol 27: 420–425, 1938.
5. Rumbolt TF: The Functions of the Eustachian Tube. St. Louis, South Western, 1873, p 98.
6. Bull TR: Abnormal patency of the eustachian tube (letter). BMJ 283: 1390, 1976.
7. Pulec JL: Abnormally patent eustachian tubes: Treatment with injection of polytetrafluoroethylene (Teflon) paste. Laryngoscope 77: 1543–1554, 1967.
8. Munker GA: The patulous eustachian tube. In Munker GA, Arnold W (eds): Physiology and Pathophysiology of Eustachian Tube and Middle Ear. New York, Thieme-Stratton, 1980, pp 113–117.
9. Perlman HB: The eustachian tube. Arch Otolaryngol 73: 310–321, 1961.
10. Virtanen H: Patulous eustachian tube. Arch Otolaryngol 86: 401–407, 1978.
11. Pulec JL, Horowitz MJ: Diseases of the eustachian tube. In Paparella MM, Shumrick PA (eds): Otolaryngology, Vol 2. Philadelphia, WB Saunders, 1973, pp 275–290.
12. Bluestone CD, Cantekin EI, Beery Q: Certain effects of adenoidectomy on eustachian tube ventilatory function. Laryngoscope 85: 113–127, 1975.
13. O'Connor AF, Shea JJ: Autophony and the patulous eustachian tube. Laryngoscope 91: 1427–1435, 1981.
14. Pulec JL, Simonton KM: Abnormal patency of the eustachian tube. Laryngoscope 74: 267–271, 1964.
15. Suehs GW: The abnormally open eustachian tube. Laryngoscope 70: 1418–1426, 1960.
16. Allen GW: Abnormal patency of the eustachian tube. JAMA 200: 412–413, 1967.
17. Flisberg K, Inglestet S: Middle ear mechanics in patulous eustachian tube cases. Acta Otolaryngol 263: 18–22, 1969.
18. Davis LJ, Sheffield PA, Jackson RT: Drug-induced patency changes in the eustachian tube. Arch Otolaryngol 92: 325–328, 1970.
19. Miller JB: Patulous eustachian tube: Report of 30 cases. Arch Otolaryngol 73: 310–321, 1961.
20. Moore PM, Miller JB: Patulous eustachian tube. Arch Otolaryngol 54: 643–650, 1951.

21. Stroud MH, Spector GT, Maisel RH: Patulous eustachian tube syndrome. Arch Otolaryngol 99: 419–421, 1974.
22. Perlman HB: The eustachian tube: Abnormal patency and normal physiologic state. Arch Otolaryngol 30: 212–238, 1939.
23. Landes BA: Hyporhinolalia associated with eustachian tube dysfunction. Laryngoscope 77:244–246, 1967.
24. Robinson PJ, Hazell JWP: Patulous eustachian tube syndrome: The relationship with sensorineural hearing loss. Treatment with eustachian tube diathermy. J Laryngol Otol 103: 739–742, 1989.
25. Harman A: Experimentelle Studien über die Function der Eustachischen Rhohre. Veit Comp, 1879.
26. Voltolini R: Zwei eigenthumliche Ohrenkrenkheiten. Monatsschr Ohrenheilkd. 17: 1–6, 1883.
27. Bluestone CD: Otitis media, atelectasis, and eustachian tube dysfunction. In Bluestone CD, Stool SE (eds): Pediatric Otolaryngology. Philadelphia, WB Saunders, 1990, pp 350–356, 360–362, 416–418.
28. Bluestone CD: Assessment of eustachian tube function. In Jerger J, Northern J (eds): Clinical Impedance Audiometry. Acton, MA, American Electromedics, 1980, pp 83–108.
29. Virtanen H: Patulous eustachian tube: Diagnostic evaluation by sonotubometry. Acta Otolryngol 86: 401–417, 1978.
30. Tolley NS, Phelps P: Patulous eustachian tube: A radiological perspective. J Laryngol Otol 104: 291–293, 1990.
31. Derkay CS: Eustachian tube and nasal function during pregnancy: A prospective study. Otolaryngol Head Neck Surg 99: 558, 1988.
32. Dyer RK, McElveen JT: The patulous eustachian tube: Management options. Otolaryngol Head Neck Surg 105: 832–835, 1991.
33. Morita M, Matsunaga T: Effects of an anticholinergic on the function of the patulous eustachian tube. Acta Otolaryngol (Stockh) 458: 63–66, 1988.
34. Bezold F, Siebenman F: Textbook of Otology for Physicians and Students (Translated by J. Holinger). Chicago, EH Colgrove, 1908, pp 154–155.
35. Halstead TH: Pathology and surgery of the eustachian tube. Arch Otolaryngol 4: 189–195, 1926.
36. Eisner MF, Alexander MH: Silver nitrate cautery. In Coates GM, Schenck MF (eds): Otolaryngology, Vol 1. Hagerstown, MD, Prior, 1957, pp 17–19.
37. McAliffe GB: Dilatation and stenosis of the eustachian tube. N Y Eye Ear Infirm Rep 6: 116–118, 1898.
38. Thaler S, Yamagisawa E: The abnormally patent eustachian tube. Arch Otolaryngol 84: 418–421, 1966.
39. Chen DA, Luxford WM: Myringotomy and tube for relief of patulous eustachian tube symptoms. Am J Otol 11: 272–273, 1990.
40. Simonton KM: Abnormal patency of the eustachian tube: Surgical treatment. Laryngoscope 67: 342–359, 1957.
41. Virtanen H, Palva T: Surgical treatment for patulous eustachian tube. Arch Otolaryngol 108: 735–739, 1982.
42. Ogawa S, Satoh I, Tanaka H: Patulous eustachian tube: A new treatment with infusion of absorbable gelatin sponge solution. Arch Otolaryngol 102: 276–280, 1980.
43. Bluestone CD, Cantekin EI: Management of the patulous eustachian tube. Laryngoscope 91: 149–152, 1981.

Traumatic Perforation—Office Treatment of the Chronically Draining Ear

Sean R. Althaus, M.D., F.A.C.S. ▪ Katrina R. Stidham, M.D.

TYMPANIC MEMBRANE PERFORATIONS, CHRONIC OTITIS MEDIA, AND CHOLESTEATOMA

Tympanic membrane perforations result from various pathologic conditions. Trauma, inflammatory disease within the middle ear and temporal bone, cholesteatoma, and, rarely, neoplastic disease can interrupt the interface between the external auditory canal and the middle ear cleft. These perforations are generally described as central, marginal, or epitympanic (attic retraction pocket) (Fig. 8–1).

The most common cause of persistent tympanic membrane perforation is suppurative or nonsuppurative chronic otitis media. Additionally, cholesteatoma, although less common now than in the past, continues to represent a significant problem in otologic practice.

A cholesteatoma, or keratoma, is defined as "an accumulation of exfoliated keratin in the middle ear or other pneumatized areas of the temporal bone arising from keratinizing squamous epithelium."[1] Generally, these lesions have a sac-like structure, occur in conjunction with a tympanic membrane perforation, and contain whitish debris composed of cholesterol crystals, hence the term *cholesteatoma*.[2] Cholesteatomas typically expand over time, resulting from the continuing process of desquamation and entrapment of epithelial debris within the sac, or from epithelial migration.[3, 4] The expansion process is thought to be due to a combination of erosive pressure on surrounding structures as the lesion grows in bulk, and a localized destruction of bone from pyogenic osteitis, enzymatic collagenolysis, and osteoclastic bone resorption.[5, 6] In addition to causing both conductive and sensorineural hearing loss, bone erosion from the expanding cholesteatoma may invade the bony covering of the facial nerve, semicircular canals, cochlea, dura, or sigmoid sinus, leading to the feared complications of facial paralysis, labyrinthitis, sensorineural hearing loss, brain abscess, meningitis, or thrombophlebitis of the sigmoid sinus.[7]

Generally, three types of cholesteatoma are recognized: attic retraction cholesteatoma, secondary acquired cholesteatoma, and congenital cholesteatoma. Attic retraction cholesteatoma represents the most common form of cholesteatoma and is generally believed to result from an invagination of the pars flaccida portion of the tympanic membrane, usually caused by chronic eustachian tubal dysfunction and negative middle ear pressures.[8, 9] Attic retraction cholesteatomas may be indolent and hidden beneath a small crust of epithelial debris or cerumen. Meticu-

lous cleaning of the ear, preferably under the otomicroscope, will detect such a lesion. Typically, one will encounter a fairly small erosion of the superior osseous canal wall, just above the malleus short process, that yields moist epithelial debris on cleaning. On the other hand, the patient may present with a chronically discharging ear and the diagnosis, after the ear is cleaned, should be relatively easy.

Secondary acquired cholesteatomas typically arise through an existing posterior marginal tympanic membrane perforation, as squamous epithelium from the external auditory canal and lateral tympanic membrane surface migrates over the edges of the perforation, entering the middle ear cleft. In these cases, the posterior annular ligament of the tympanic membrane is usually attenuated or missing, favoring epithelial migration over the edge of the perforation. Skin ingrowth can involve the middle ear extensively and enter the epitympanic space and mastoid antrum.[10] Eventually, the epithelial contents of most cholesteatomas become contaminated by microbial organisms, leading to otorrhea, which may be foul smelling. The clinical diagnosis of secondary acquired cholesteatoma usually poses little difficulty for the otologist, because layers or accumulations of moist, whitish epithelial debris are found to occupy the involved portions of the middle ear on physical examination.

Congenital cholesteatomas of the temporal bone were first described in 1938.[11] They are thought to be caused by epithelial rests of embryonal origin or through basal cell papillary proliferation and ingrowth and may occur anywhere within the temporal bone.[12, 13] They are relatively rare and develop behind an intact ear drum, frequently in patients with no history of ear disease. Typically, a whitish globular mass is seen behind the anterior portion of the drum on otoscopy adjacent to the malleus handle. Often, an alert pediatrician will spot the problem and request clarification from the otologist. On the other hand, congenital cholesteatomas deep within the temporal bone may remain silent for years until progressive hearing loss, facial paresis, or disequilibrium alerts the clinician to the possibility of such a lesion.

The diagnosis of cholesteatoma is generally made on clinical grounds. Imaging studies, such as computed tomographic scans or mastoid radiographs, are not obtained routinely in the preoperative assessment unless an unusual situation or threatening complication is suspected. The treatment of cholesteatoma is surgical and is detailed in other chapters.

OFFICE TREATMENT OF THE CHRONICALLY DRAINING EAR

Obtaining a dry ear prior to surgery is an important and desirable goal in the surgical treatment of chronic otitis media. This objective can be achieved in the majority of "wet" ears through thorough evaluation and meticulous medical management in the preoperative period. Careful and repeated cleaning of the middle ear and ear canal, the topical use of antimicrobial medications, and the creation of an unfavorable environment for bacterial and fungal growth are essential for achieving the goal of a dry ear preoperatively. On the other hand, in ears not selected for surgery, gaining a dry ear may improve the quality of life for the elderly or poor-risk surgical patient. In some ears, and in particular, some cholesteatoma cases, no amount of preoperative effort will lead to a dry ear, and the surgery itself must be relied on to achieve this goal.

Access to an otomicroscope is a basic requirement for cleaning of a wet ear, as is adequate suction equipment. A head mirror or hand-held otoscope simply does not provide the otologist with the necessary technical help to properly clean an ear.

Most chronic ear drainage results from mixed infections of aerobic and anaerobic pathogens, typically *Pseudomonas aeruginosa, Staphylococcus aureus, Proteus* species, *Escherichia coli*, and anaerobic streptococci.[14, 15] Fungal infections are also significant causes of otorrhea, with *Aspergillus* and *Candida* species being the primary offenders.[16, 17] Often, these otomycoses are combined bacterial and fungal infections. Rarely, uncommon pathogens, such as *Mycobacterium* species, are responsible for chronic resistant otorrhea.

The use of ototopical solutions has been a topic of controversy for several years due to the theoretical ototoxicity of many of the agents used. However, to date, there have been no controlled studies demonstrating definitive ototoxicity and some recent studies have refuted significant ototoxic effects.[18, 19] Widespread clinical usage of these medications for several years supports a wide margin of safety. Otic drops remain a highly effective method of treating the chronic draining ear.

Otic drop solutions include old standards in use for several years and newer solutions for both bacterial and fungal infections with increased efficacy against resistant organisms. Many commonly used preparations contain neomycin or polymyxin, individually or in combination. These agents are active against the majority of middle ear bacterial pathogens. Aminoglycoside topical solutions containing tobramycin or gentamicin are also commonly used. The newest generations of otic drop solutions are the fluoroquinolones and include ofloxacin and ciprofloxacin. These newest agents have been shown to have a high clinical efficacy with decreased microbial resistance and less potential risk for ototoxicity.[20–22] Several antifungal agents have been in use for many years including gentian violet, 1 per cent thymol–95 per cent isopropyl alcohol, cresylate, Castellani Paint, and merthiolate. Topical counterparts to systemic antifungal medications are now available with clotrimazole and nystatin ointment and drops.[16, 23] Many combinations of otic drops also contain corticosteroids, which act to reduce itching and inflammation while decreasing mucosal and canal edema, allowing better penetration of the antibiotic.

Antimicrobial dusting powders offer an effective alternative to otic drops in many instances, particularly in the presence of neomycin sensitivity or pain associated with the application of drops. Although some ears respond nicely to a regimen of boric acid, 95 per cent/salicylic acid 5 per cent, three times a day, the majority of wet ears are truly suppurating, and antibacterial or antifungal preparations are necessary. With a combination of chloramphenicol (Chloromycetin), *p*-aminobenzenesulfonamide (sulfanilamide), and amphotericin B–thimerosal–titanium dioxide (Fungizone) powder delivered through an insufflator twice a day, it is not unusual to see a chronically wet, noncholesteatomatous ear that is unresponsive to topical otic drops dry up quickly. The pharmacist is asked to compound chloramphenicol, 50 mg, *p*-aminobenzenesulfonamide, 50 mg, and amphotericin B, 5 mg, in a No. 4 gel capsule and dispense a suitable starter supply with an Oto-Med Powder Insufflator and instructions for use. Hydrocortisone, 1 mg, can be added to this preparation if desired, and the *p*-aminobenzenesulfonamide can be removed for patients allergic to it.

Measures aimed at promoting an undesirable environment for antimicrobial proliferation are important in the effective medical management of the chronically draining middle ear. Avoiding water contact is mandatory. The patient is instructed in dry ear precautions and is advised to use a silicone ear plug or cotton–petroleum jelly dam when showering or shampooing. Swimming is discouraged. The careful use of a hand-held hair dryer after showering can facilitate drying of the ear and ear canal. Microbial growth is inhibited in an acidic medium, and steps are taken to lower the pH of the ear canal and middle ear. Irrigation of the canal with a diluted white vinegar solution can accomplish this goal while it cleans the canal of debris, which is also a desirable component of effective medical management. Many topical otic preparations contain acetic acid to acidify the pH.

The following approach in the office treatment of the chronically draining ear, in the authors' experience, works well. At the first office visit, a history is obtained, and the ear is carefully examined under the otomicroscope and cleaned. A culture and sensitivity specimen of the drainage is not obtained routinely, unless the patient has been on prolonged systemic antibiotic therapy, or an unusual problem is suspected. Plans are made to obtain an audiogram at some point during the preoperative evaluation period. Instructions are given for cleaning the ear twice daily with a diluted acetic acid and water solution (half-strength white vinegar) using a medicine dropper or small bulb syringe. The patient is seen 7 to 10 days later, and the ear is re-examined. At this point, the ear usually looks less inflamed, with a minimal amount of debris in the canal. If the ear is not better, culture and sensitivity specimen is obtained, and culture-specific oral antibiotic therapy is initiated. Ciprofloxacin use in the pediatric population has been restricted due to animal studies finding erosion of cartilage in weight-bearing joints in immature animals.[24] However, more recent clinical studies have shown extended usage of ciprofloxacin in children without undue side effects.[25–27] In cases where systemic antipseudomonal coverage is needed

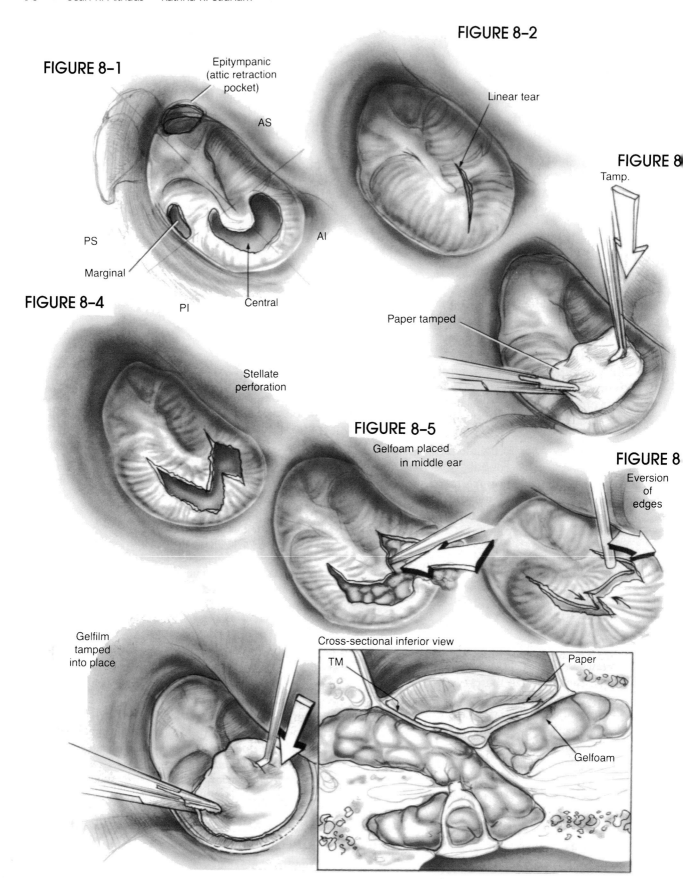

FIGURE 8-1

Epitympanic (attic retraction pocket)

AS

PS

Marginal

PI

Central

AI

FIGURE 8-2

Linear tear

FIGURE 8

Tamp.

Paper tamped

FIGURE 8-4

Stellate perforation

FIGURE 8-5

Gelfoam placed in middle ear

FIGURE 8

Eversion of edges

Gelfilm tamped into place

Cross-sectional inferior view

TM

Paper

Gelfoam

FIGURE 8-7

in a pediatric patient, an infectious disease specialist or pediatrician should be consulted prior to administration of fluoroquinolones.

At this point, if the patient is a child, the parent is instructed to continue the vinegar rinses and to begin using an antibiotic-steroid–containing ear drop twice daily following vinegar cleaning of the ear. This regimen is continued for 10 days and is then discontinued. The ear is examined 3 to 4 days after the drops are completed. If it is dry, surgery can be scheduled. If not, an antibiotic-antifungal powder insufflation regimen is initiated twice daily, following the vinegar rinse. This "dry program" will dry up a significant number of these wet ears. If the ear fails to clear on this regimen a culture and sensitivity specimen is obtained, surgery is scheduled, and the parent is advised that mastoid disease is contributing to the problem and that mastoid surgery will be required.

In adults, dry treatment is usually initiated at the second office visit, and the patient is instructed to clean the ear twice a day, before insufflating the powder, with a cotton-tipped wire applicator, which is supplied by the physician's office. This regimen is continued until maximum improvement has been obtained, and surgery is then scheduled. Once again, not all discharging ears will dry on this regimen, and if the ear remains wet, the patient is advised that mastoid surgery will be required.

OFFICE TREATMENT OF THE DRAINING MASTOID CAVITY

The most common causes for a draining mastoid cavity are (1) inadequate or poorly performed surgery; (2) failure to seal the middle ear from the mastoid cavity at surgery; (3) suboptimal postoperative care; (4) neglect of the cavity; and (5) persistent suppurative disease in the temporal bone.

The principles of well-done canal wall down (CWD) tympanomastoid surgery include beveling the edges of the mastoid cavity and removing all bone overhang, sealing off the middle ear space, obliterating mucosa containing cell tracts, lowering the facial ridge and removing the anterior buttress, taking care of the large mastoid tip, and performing a generous meatoplasty. Details and surgical technique are thoroughly described in Chapter 17.

When the original surgery has been inadequate, leaving a high facial ridge, or when a small meatoplasty prevents adequate aeration and good access to the cavity for cleaning, cavity moisture may become a problem. With moisture due to a troublesome large mastoid tip, or failure to seal the middle ear space at surgery, a revision operation will generally prove necessary, with correction of these causative problems. Adequate and aggressive postoperative care is a requirement for obtaining a dry cavity. Following discharge from the surgical facility, the patient is seen weekly for cleaning and painting of granulation tissue with 1 per cent aqueous gentian violet or cauterization of granulations with silver nitrate. Subsequently, monthly visits are schedule until the mastoid cavity is dry and completely skin lined. The need for annual or semiannual inspection and cleaning of the mastoid cavity throughout life is emphasized.

The presence of a mucosal-skin interface in the mastoid cavity is a frequent reason for a chronically wet cavity. This abnormal relationship was never intended by nature and commonly results when the middle ear cleft is left open at CWD tympanomastoid surgery. On inspection under the otomicroscope, the nature of the problem becomes apparent, as the mastoid cavity is generally well lined with squamous epithelium, and the moisture comes from the middle ear space. Revisionary surgery, with placement of a fascia graft over the middle ear cleft, will usually lead to a dry ear and affords the possibility of ossicular reconstruction for hearing improvement. Occasionally, mucosalization of the cavity occurs, and this problem can be prevented by obliterating mucosa containing cell tracts at the initial surgery with fibromuscular tissue.

Cavity neglect leads to the build-up of cerumen and epithelial debris, then secondary moisture and suppuration beneath the debris. A thorough cleaning under the otomicroscope, followed by a 5-day course of topical antibiotic drops or powder, will usually dry the cavity promptly. Persistent suppurative disease of the temporal bone will require further evaluation and, in most cases, secondary surgery.

From a practical standpoint, the following products have been found useful in the office management of the chronic mastoid cavity:

Nonspecific Agents

1. Vinegar swishes
2. Acetic acid, 2 per cent, and aluminum acetate otic solution
3. Silver nitrate
4. Povidone-iodine, 10 per cent
5. Five per cent boric acid–95 per cent isopropyl alcohol drops
6. Five per cent salicylic–95 per cent boric acid powder

Antibacterial Agents

1. Neomycin-polymyxin–containing otic drops
2. Aminoglycoside containing otic drops (tobramycin, gentamicin)
3. Chloramphenicol otic drops (for patients allergic to neomycin or polymyxin)
4. Chloramphenicol, p-aminobenzenesulfonamide and amphotericin B powder (or chloramphenicol–amphotericin B powder in p-aminobenzenesulfonamide–sensitive patients)
5. Fluoroquinolone otic drops (ofloxacin, ciprofloxacin)

Antifungal Agents

1. Gentian violet (aqueous)
2. One per cent thymol–95 per cent isopropyl alcohol drops
3. Cresylate (a solution containing thimerosal (merthiolate), m-cresyl acetate, propylene glycol, and boric acid)
4. Castellani Paint (a nonspecific antifungal agent whose active ingredients are fuchsin, phenol, resorcinol (paraben) acetone, and 70 per cent isopropyl alcohol)
5. Merthiolate
6. Clotrimazole (Lotrimin, Mycelex), the most effective antifungal agent in in vitro studies of common otomycotic pathogens[23]
7. Nystatin

OTHER CONSIDERATIONS

1. EUSTACHIAN TUBE FUNCTION.

The evaluation of eustachian tube function in the office management of the chronically wet ear is unnecessary in our experience. Significant eustachian tubal dysfunction usually clears by age 6 and is rarely a persistent problem beyond childhood. Localized obstruction of the tubal orifice in the middle ear from inflammatory tissue or cholesteatoma does occur and can be corrected at the time of surgery.

2. ADENOIDECTOMY.

The child presenting with a chronically draining ear with or without cholesteatoma, with persistent middle ear effusion in the contralateral ear, and a history of previous myringotomies with tubes is a candidate for adenoidectomy prior to definitive ear surgery. Chronically infected adenoids, large or small, have been shown to contribute to persistent middle ear effusion, with drastic improvement in symptoms following adenoidectomy.[28] No significant benefit has been proven in removing the tonsils, and tonsillectomy should be performed only when otherwise medically indicated (i.e., recurrent tonsillitis). On the other hand, if the contralateral ear is normal, and the discharging ear clears on medical management, the adenoids are probably not playing a major role in the chronic middle ear problem and surgery can proceed.

3. NASAL PROBLEMS.

Structural problems within the nose rarely contribute to chronic middle ear disease and generally need not be considered in the genesis of chronic middle ear drainage.

4. ALLERGY.

The role of allergy in chronic middle ear disease remains controversial. The assistance of a competent allergist can optimize the preoperative status of the severely allergic individual, particularly in the presence of lower respiratory tract disease. Allergy management alone, however, rarely resolves long-standing otorrhea.

5. GENERAL HEALTH.

The general health of the patient can alter not only the underlying diagnoses of otorrhea but also the patient's response to treatment. Patients with significant compromise in immune function, including those with leukemia, lymphoma, diabetes, neutropenia secondary to chemotherapy, and human immunodeficiency virus, are at risk for more severe and potentially life-threatening infections. The majority of infections are bacterial, with the same pathogenic organisms as identified in nonimmunocompromised individuals.[29] However, immunosuppressed patients are more likely to become susceptible to unusual bacterial infections, invasive fungal infections, and even parasitic infections not seen in the healthy population.[30, 31] These individuals require aggressive therapy because an otherwise benign infection can quickly turn fatal. Consultation with the patient's internist or an infectious disease specialist should be made to determine the best medical regimen with early institution of systemic therapy. Prolonged treatment with intravenous antibiotics and even surgical débridement may be required to definitively treat the infection.

TRAUMATIC TYMPANIC MEMBRANE PERFORATIONS

Traumatic tympanic membrane perforations represent a fairly common problem for the otologist. Hand slaps, water skiing falls, cotton-tipped swab injuries, blast trauma, and penetrating injuries caused by high-velocity missiles are some of the more common causative factors.

Typically, the patient presents acutely with a linear tear in the drum or a stellate opening of variable size, with some fresh blood at the margins. Complaints of aural fullness, tinnitus, altered hearing, and mild dysequilibrium are common. After 72 hours, the perforation tends to become circular as the drum attempts to heal itself. A significant conductive hearing loss or mixed loss with persistent vertigo should alert the physician to the possibility of inner ear damage and the need for formal surgical exploration of the middle ear for possible perilymph fistula. Retained foreign body fragments in the middle ear must be considered if the ear begins to suppurate.

The initial evaluation of the patient consists of a complete ear, nose, and throat history, followed by a head and neck examination, which includes micro-otoscopic evaluation of the tympanic membranes. Debris and clots are carefully cleaned from the ear canal, and an initial assessment of the perforation is completed. If the injury is acute (within 48 to 72 hours), and the ear is uninfected, tympanic membrane patching is undertaken in the office in the following way: For a linear tear (Fig. 8–2) or a small circular defect, a piece of cigarette paper is trimmed to an appropriate shape, and antibiotic ointment is applied to its undersurface for adherence. The patch is applied to the surface of the tympanic membrane with alligator microforceps or suction tip and is gently tamped into place with a blunt hook (Fig. 8–3). No ear canal packing is used, and broad-spectrum oral antibiotic coverage is not started unless there has been water entry into the ear canal. On the other hand, if the ear is suppurating when the patient is first seen, gentle cleaning is carried out, and broad-spectrum antibiotic overage is started. A culture specimen is not obtained routinely. The perforation is left to heal secondarily, and if it does not within 4 to 6 weeks, a formal myringoplasty is recommended.

With a stellate perforation (Fig. 8–4), when the patient is seen acutely without evidence of infection, local anesthesia is applied to the external auditory meatus in circumferential fashion, and the ear is carefully cleaned under the otomicroscope. A sterile piece of dry crushed absorbable gelatin sponge (Gelfoam) is moistened with normal saline and gently placed into the middle ear through the perforation (Fig. 8–5). The edges of the perforation are carefully everted with a No. 3 or 5 Baron suction tip and arranged in proper position (Fig. 8–6). Once this step has been completed, a piece of absorbable gelatin film (Gelfilm) or cigarette paper trimmed to an appropriate shape with antibiotic ointment applied to its undersurface as an adhesive is

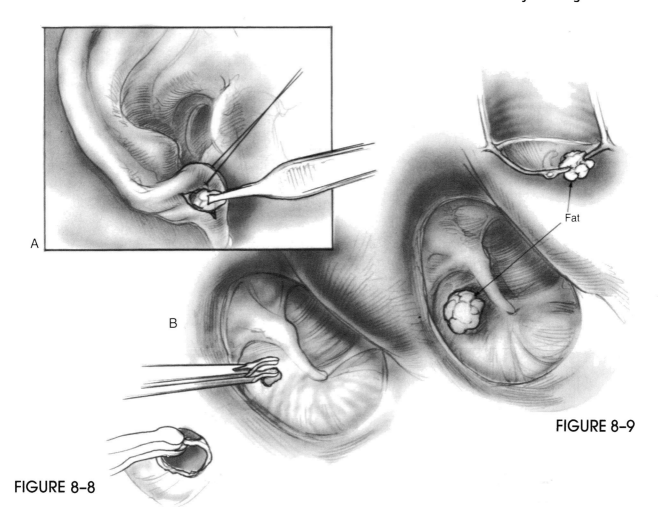

FIGURE 8-8

FIGURE 8-9

positioned over the lateral tympanic membrane surface and gently tamped into place (Fig. 8–7). No canal packing or dressing is used, and broad-spectrum antibiotic coverage is started if there has been water entry or other foreign material into the middle ear space. Antibiotic therapy is continued for 7 to 10 days.

The patient is advised to keep the ear dry and to not blow his or her nose or disturb the area in any other way and is seen in the office 1 week later. If the patch is in place and dry, it is not disturbed. At a secondary visit 4 to 6 weeks later, the patch is carefully removed and the drum is inspected. If healing is complete, the patient is advised to keep the ear dry for another 2 weeks and to then resume full activities. An audiogram is generally obtained at this point. If a persistent perforation is noted, however, formal repair is advised. In our experience, approximately 95 per cent of perforations handled in this fashion will heal, and the patient is so advised before treatment is undertaken. The option of no treatment is examined, because some authorities do not recommend patching traumatic tympanic membrane perforations.[32, 33] When the patient is seen more than 72 hours following a traumatic tympanic membrane perforation, office patching is generally not recommended, and the drum is allowed to heal secondarily. In these subacute cases, antibiotics are not used unless the ear is suppurating. Patients with subacute perforations are told

that the ear has an 85 to 90 per cent chance of healing within 4 to 6 weeks and that formal repair will be recommended if healing has not occurred by then. Once again, water entry into the ear canal and vigorous nose blowing are avoided until healing is complete.

FAT GRAFT MYRINGOPLASTY

Fat graft myringoplasty is the procedure of choice for the repair of persistent small tympanic membrane perforations. This technique is well suited to the repair of small perforations due to chronic otitis media, myringoplasty failure, or following tympanostomy tube extrusion. The procedure represents a cost-effective alternative to standard tympanic membrane grafting techniques in such cases. In most cases, surgery is performed under local anesthesia in the office or outpatient surgery center and requires approximately 15 minutes of operating time. Within 12 to 16 weeks, the grafted tympanic membrane is fully healed and of normal thickness and appearance.

Surgical Technique. Following premedication with agents of the surgeon's choice and the establishment of an intravenous line, the ear is prepared and draped in standard fashion. Local anesthesia is injected circumferentially at the external auditory meatus and into the posteromedial surface of the ear lobe. Through a 5- to 8-mm incision made on the posterior surface of the lobe, a small portion of adipose tissue is removed and placed in sterile normal saline. After hemostasis is achieved, the incision is closed with two or three 5-0 nylon sutures.

Under the otomicroscope, squamous epithelium is carefully removed from the margins of the tympanic membrane perforation with the microsurgical argon laser or a small cupped forceps (Fig. 8–8). A piece of adipose tissue approximately four times the diameter of the defect is inserted through the perforation, leaving one half of its bulk medial and one half lateral to the ear drum (Fig. 8–9). The ear canal is then packed with absorbable gelatin foam containing an antibiotic-steroid suspension, and a mastoid dressing is applied. Actually, the mastoid dressing is placed only to minimize postoperative earlobe swelling or seepage. The dressing is removed the following day, and the ear lobe sutures are removed on the fifth postoperative day. The patient then begins using otic drops to soften the packing, which is removed at 3 weeks after surgery. Instructions are given to avoid vigorous nose blowing for 3 weeks following the surgery and to keep water out of the ear until healing is complete.

Over the years, numerous materials and techniques for myringoplasty have found favor among otologic surgeons. In experienced hands, both lateral and medial surface grafting procedures have been highly successful. Various graft materials have been used, including canal skin, temporalis fascia and prefascia, tragal perichondrium, and vein.[34] Adipose tissue has been used in other forms of otologic surgery, particularly stapedectomy, perilymph fistula repair,[35, 36] and mastoid obliteration following translabyrinthine operations.[37] Additionally, the use of fat tissue to repair small defects of the tympanic membrane has been previously reported by one of us (S.R.A.)[38] and others.[39–45] When used to repair a tympanic membrane perforation, fat functions as both a lateral and a medial surface graft, and this flexibility may in part account for its high success rate.

In selecting cases suitable for this technique, the perforation should be less than 2 mm in diameter, central, and dry and should present without signs of healing for at least 6 to 8 weeks. A wet ear would indicate the probability of more extensive middle ear or mastoid pathology requiring formal surgical intervention. The technique can be modified to permit repair of a posterior or anterior marginal perforation, provided that a tympanomeatal flap is turned before placement of the fat plug to ensure that there has been no growth of squamous epithelium into the middle ear. If such growth is found, it must obviously be removed.

When an ear with a small perforation and significant conductive hearing loss is encountered, the perforation can be repaired first, using the technique described, followed by the raising of a tympanomeatal flap to address the ossicular problem. Repairing the perforation first allows the surgeon to de-epithelialize the margins of the defect and place the graft while working on a stable and secure drum remnant, greatly facilitating the procedure.

The classic technique for repairing small tympanic membrane perforations has been fascia or perichondrial grafting. These more formal techniques are time consuming and carry a small potential for complications, such as graft lateralization. The success rate is certainly no higher. On the other hand, other limited procedures have been described, including paper graft patching of the drum,[46–49] absorbable gelatin film patch,[50] absorbable gelatin sponge plugs, and other materials.[51, 52]

One of us (S.R.A.) has found adipose tissue an ideal material with which to repair small tympanic membrane perforations. This technique has yielded a success rate of 97 per cent in a series of 61 cases over the past 26 years. At 12 to 16 weeks after surgery, the graft site is of normal thickness and appearance and resembles the surrounding tympanic membrane. Postoperative hearing loss has not been encountered to date.

References

1. Schuknecht H: Pathology of the Ear. Cambridge, MA, Harvard University Press, 1974, p 228.
2. Glasscock ME, Shambaugh GE: Surgery of the Ear. Philadelphia, WB Saunders, 1990, p 187.
3. Abramson M, Gantz B, Asarch R, et al: Cholesteatoma pathogenesis: Evidence for the migration theory. *In* McCabe B, Sade J, Abramson M (eds): Cholesteatoma: First International Conference. Birmingham, AL, Aesculapius, 1977, pp 176–186.
4. Litton WB: Epidermal migration patterns in the ear and possible relationship to cholesteatoma genesis. *In* McCabe B, Sade J, Abramson M (eds): Cholesteatoma: First International Conference. Birmingham, AL, Aesculapius, 1977, pp 90–91.
5. Abramson M, Huang CC: Cholesteatoma and bone resorption. *In* McCabe B, Sade J, Abramson M (eds): Cholesteatoma: First International Conference. Birmingham, AL, Aesculapius, 1977, pp 162–166.
6. Gantz B, Clancy C, Abramson M: Decalcification factors in granulation tissue and ear canal skin. *In* McCabe B, Sade J, Abramson M (eds): Cholesteatoma: First International Conference. Birmingham, AL, Aesculapius, 1977, pp 167–169.
7. Glasscock ME, Shambaugh GE: Surgery of the Ear. Philadelphia, WB Saunders, 1990.
8. Bezold F: Cholesteatom, Perforation der membrana flaccida shrapnelli und tubenverschluss. Z Ohrenh 20: 5, 1890.
9. Wittmaack K: Wie entsteht ein genuines cholesteatom? Arch Ohren-Nasen-n Kehlkopfh 137: 306, 1933.
10. Jackler RK: The surgical anatomy of cholesteatoma. Otolaryngol Clin North Am 22: 883–896, 1989.
11. Jefferson C, Smalley AA: Progressive facial palsy produced by intratemporal epidermoids. J Laryngol Otol 53: 417–443, 1938.
12. Cawthorne T: Congenital cholesteatoma. Arch Otolaryngol 78: 248–252, 1963.
13. House JW, Sheehy JL: Cholesteatoma with intact tympanic membrane: A report of 41 cases. Laryngoscope 90: 70–75, 1980.
14. Glasscock ME, Shambaugh GE: Surgery of the Ear. Philadelphia, WB Saunders, 1990.
15. Hughes GB: Textbook of Clinical Otology. New York, Thieme-Stratton, 1985, p 306.
16. Chander J, Maini S, Subrahmanyan S, Handa A: Otomycosis: A clinico-mycological study and efficacy of mercurochrome in its treatment. Mycopathologia 135: 9–12, 1996.
17. Lucente FE: Fungal infections of the external ear. Otolaryngol Clin North Am 26:995–1006, 1993.
18. Merifield DO, Parker NJ, Nicholson NC: Therapeutic management of chronic suppurative otitis media with otic drops. Otolaryngol Head Neck Surg 109: 77–82, 1993.
19. Pickett BP, Shinn JB, Smith MFW: Ear drop ototoxicity: Reality or myth. Am J Otol 18: 782–791, 1997.
20. Tutkun A, Ozagar A, Koc A, et al: Treatment of chronic ear disease: Topical ciprofloxacin versus topical gentamicin. Arch Otolaryngol Head Neck Surg 121: 1414–1416, 1995.
21. Tong MCF, Woo JKS, Van Hasselt A: A double-blind comparative study of ofloxacin otic drops versus neomycin–polymyxin B–hydrocortisone otic drops in the medical treatment of chronic suppurative otitis media. J Laryngol Otol 110: 309–314, 1996.
22. Aslan A, Altuntas A, Titiz A, et al: A new dosage regimen for topical application of ciprofloxacin in the management of chronic suppurative otitis media. Otolaryngol Head Neck Surg 188: 883–885, 1998.

23. Stern JC, Shah MK, Lucente FE: In vitro effectiveness of 13 agents in otomycosis and review of the literature. Laryngoscope 98: 1173–1177, 1988.

24. Physician's Desk Reference. Montvale, NJ, Medical Economics, 1998, pp 607–610.

25. Jick S: Ciprofloxacin safety in a pediatric population. Pediatr Infect Dis J 16: 130–133, 1997.

26. Warren RW: Rheumatologic aspects of pediatric cystic fibrosis patients treated with fluoroquinolones. Pediatr Infect Dis J 16: 118–122, 1997.

27. Heggers JP, Villarreal C, Edgar P, et al: Ciprofloxacin as a therapeutic modality in pediatric burn wound infections: Efficacious or contraindicated? Arch Surg 133: 1247–1250, 1998.

28. Gates GA, Muntz HR, Gaylis B: Adenoidectomy and otitis media. Ann Otol Rhinol Laryngol 101: 24–32, 1992.

29. Shapiro NL, Novell V: Otitis media in children with vertically acquired HIV infection: The Great Ormond Street Hospital experience. Int J Pediatr Otorhinolaryngol 45: 69–75, 1998.

30. Sack CL, Watson DW, Abzug MJ, et al: Fungal mastoiditis in immunocompromised children. Arch Otolaryngol Head Neck Surg 125: 73–75, 1999.

31. Dunand VA, Hammer SM, Rossi R, et al: Parasitic sinusitis and otitis in patients infected with human immunodeficiency virus: Report of five cases and review. Clin Infect Dis 25: 267–272, 1997.

32. Lindeman P, Edstrom S, Granstrom G, et al: Acute traumatic tympanic membrane perforations: Cover or observe? Arch Otolaryngol Head Neck Surg 113: 1285–1287, 1987.

33. Kristensen S, Juul A, Gammelgaard NP, et al: Traumatic tympanic membrane perforations: Complications and management. Ear Nose Throat J 68: 503–516, 1989.

34. Sheehy JL: Surgery of Chronic Otitis Media, Vol 2. Hagerstown, MD, Harper & Row, 1972, p 15.

35. Althaus SR: Spontaneous and traumatic perilymph fistulas. Laryngoscope 87: 361–371, 1977.

36. Althaus SR: Perilymph fistulas. Laryngoscope 91: 538–562, 1981.

37. House JL, Hitselberger WE, House WF: Wound closure and cerebrospinal fluid leak after translabyrinthe surgery. Am J Otol 4: 126–128, 1982.

38. Althaus SR: "Fat plug" myringoplasty: A technique for repairing small tympanic membrane perforations. Same-Day Surg 10: 88–89, 1986.

39. Ringenberg JC: Closure of tympanic membrane perforations by the use of fat. Laryngoscope 88: 982–993, 1978.

40. Terry RM, Bellini Ml, Clayton Ml, et al: Fat graft myringoplasty—a prospective trial. Clin Otolaryngol 13: 227–229, 1988.

41. Gold SR, Chaffoo RAK: Fat myringoplasty in the guinea pig. Laryngoscope 101: 1–5, 1991.

42. Gross CW, Bassila M, Lazar RH, et al: Adipose plug myringoplasty: An alternative to formal myringoplasty techniques in children. Otolaryngol Head Neck Surg 101: 617–620, 1989.

43. Mitchell RB, Pereira KD, Younis RT, Lazar RH: Bilateral fat graft myringoplasty in children. Ear Nose Throat J 75: 652–656, 1996.

44. Terry RM, Bellini MJ, Clayton MI, Gandhi AG: Fat graft myringoplasty—a prospective trial. Clin Otolaryngol 13: 227–229, 1988.

45. Gross CW, Bassila M, Lazar RH, et al: Adipose plug myringoplasty: An alternative to formal myringoplasty techniques in children. Otolaryngol Head Neck Surg 101: 617–620, 1989.

46. Camniitz PS, Bost WS: Traumatic perforations of the tympanic membrane: Early closure with paper patching. Otolaryngol Head Neck Surg 93: 220–223, 1985.

47. Kitchens CC: Theta myringoplasty. Laryngoscope 102: 588–589, 1992.

48. Laurent C, Soderberg O, Anniko M, et al: Repair of chronic tympanic membrane perforations using applications of hyaluronate or rice paper prostheses: ORL J Otorhinolaryngol Relat Spec 53: 37–40, 1991.

49. Merwin GE, Boies LR Jr: Paper patch repair of blast rupture of the tympanic membrane. Laryngoscope 90: 853–860, 1980.

50. Baldwin RL, Loftin L: Gelfilm myringoplasty: A technique for residual perforations. Laryngoscope 102: 340–342, 1992.

51. Saito H, Kazama Y, Yazawa Y: Simple maneuver for closing traumatic ear drum perforation by microscope strip tape patching. Am J Otol 11: 427–430, 1990.

52. Stenfors LE: Repair of tympanic membrane perforations using hyaluronic acid: An alternative to myringoplasty. J Laryngol Otol 103: 39–40, 1989.

9

Tympanoplasty: The Outer Surface Grafting Technique

James L. Sheehy, M.D.

Elimination of disease and restoration of function are the aims of tympanoplasty. Restoration of function requires a tympanic membrane, an air-containing, mucosal-lined middle ear (so that the membrane will vibrate), and a secure connection between the tympanic membrane and the inner ear fluids.

Presented here is one of the three major techniques of tympanic membrane grafting: the outer surface, or onlay, procedure, the technique used with rare exceptions by doctors of the House Ear Clinic (HEC). Before describing the surgical procedure, comments will be made on the evolution of tympanic grafting techniques, patient selection, and evaluation and counseling prior to surgery.

HISTORICAL ASPECTS

Systematic reconstruction of the tympanic membrane, the sine qua non of the modern era of reconstructive ear surgery, had its beginning with reports of Wullstein[1] and Zollner.[2] Split-thickness or full-thickness skin was placed over the de-epithelized tympanic membrane remnant. The initial results were very encouraging, but unfortunately, graft eczema, inflammation, and finally, perforation were common.

As a result of these experiences, most surgeons had begun changing to undersurface (underlay) connective tissue grafts by the late 1950s (see Chapters 10 and 11). The HEC physicians continued using an onlay technique but changed to "canal skin,"[3, 4] which actually was periosteum graft, covered by canal skin.

This change was made in 1958 and resulted in an immediate improvement in results. But draining ears and total perforations continued to have a failure rate as high as 40 per cent.

In 1961, Storrs[5] published the results of a small series of cases in which temporalis fascia had been used as an outer surface graft. Changing to this technique resulted in a dramatic improvement in results over the next 3 years: over 90 per cent graft take.[6–8]

PATIENT SELECTION AND EVALUATION

The patient with chronic otitis media may consult a physician because of a hearing impairment or because of discharge from the ear. Occasionally, the patient may have symptoms of more advanced chronic ear pathology, such as pain, vertigo, or facial nerve paralysis.

Careful evaluation of the symptoms and findings allows the otologist to determine the need for surgery, its urgency, and the anticipated result. Only by so doing can the patient be advised properly. A good surgical result should not be a disappointment to the patient if there is proper counseling.

Let us assume, for purposes of this chapter, that the patient has a dry central perforation. The ear may drain briefly with upper respiratory infections or if water is allowed to get into the ear. This discharge responds promptly to local medication. The preoperative treatment of the draining ear will be discussed in depth in Chapter 16.

When one is dealing with a dry central perforation, or inactive disease, surgery is elective, and the patient (or family) should be so informed. Assuming that the problem is unilateral, with only a mild hearing impairment, the only indication for surgery is to avoid further episodes of otorrhea.

In children, it is best (from the psychologic standpoint) to avoid elective surgery of any type between the ages of 4 and 7 years. Certainly, in ear surgery, it is wise to wait until after the age of 7 years so as not to lay the groundwork for serous otitis media. If the problem is bilateral, there is a hearing problem, and the ears do not drain often, fitting with hearing aids in each ear may be preferable for children younger than 8 years of age; however, the parents have to make the decision. At age 8 years and thereafter, the patient (child) should be allowed to make the decision.

What about eustachian tube function: When contemplating tympanoplasty, the HEC physicians do not usually test to determine the status of the eustachian tube.[9] The philosophy has been that tubal malfunction per se is no contraindication to tympanoplasty but that the operation will not be successful unless tubal function is re-established.

Many persons showing no tubal function by various available tests used in the past have been operated on to eliminate a chronic drainage problem. Surprisingly, when the ear heals, the drum is usually mobile. Re-exploration in some of these patients has demonstrated normal mucosa in the tubotympanum, where before surgery the mucosa was of a very poor quality. It would appear that surgery, in eliminating infection and sealing the ear, is in itself the best treatment for the obstructed tube.

PATIENT COUNSELING

What is the outlook with surgery, and what are the risks and complications? A surgeon must relate his or her own experience. HEC physicians explain that the likelihood of obtaining a permanently healed, dry ear, which may be treated normally, is better than 90 per cent. "The only complication that happens with any degree of regularity, and is serious, is a total loss of hearing in the operated ear. That likelihood is no more than 1 per cent. All of the other things listed here are either very remote or are temporary." ["Listed here" refers to the Risk and Complications section of a Patient Discussion Booklet. The actual Risk and Complications Sheet is given to the patient at the time the surgery is scheduled, which allows the patient to review the sheet leisurely. The Risk and Complications Sheet appears as Appendix 1.]

PREOPERATIVE PREPARATION

If the patient is a child, the preoperative visit occurs the day before surgery. Surgery is under general anesthesia the following morning, and the child is released to the parents' care in the afternoon.

For adults, the preoperative visit is often the morning of surgery. The patient goes to the hospital for afternoon surgery, which will occur under local anesthesia. The patient may be kept in the hospital overnight, depending on many circumstances.

PREPARATION IN SURGERY

The smoothness with which the operation proceeds depends not only on the ability of the surgeon but also on the organization of the team (anesthesiologist and surgical nurse) and arrangements in the operating room.

The patient's hair is shaved 3 cm above and behind the ear. The skin is cleansed with an iodine-based soap, rinsed with water, and sprayed with tincture of benzoin. A sterile plastic adhesive drape is applied.

The mattress of the operating table is taped securely to the table to prevent it from slipping when the table is tipped from side to side or into the Trendelenburg position. The patient is placed on the table with his or her head at the *foot* of the table, which allows the circulating nurse or anesthesiologist free access to the table controls, which are then at the feet of the patient. The patient's head and shoulders should be as near to the surgeon's side of the table as possible. A pillow is placed under the patient's knees. The Bovie plate goes under the patient's buttocks.

Anesthesia

Ear surgery can be performed with the patient under local anesthesia in most cases. The decision on this depends on the age of the patient and other factors.

Lidocaine with 1:100,000 epinephrine is used for post-auricular and meatal incisions. Some of the injection material should find its way under the skin of the posterior superior wall of the canal (the vascular strip) and into the middle ear.

General anesthesia is used in children, in most mastoid surgery, and in procedures that require more than 1 1/2

hours of operating time. The anesthetist should be at the feet of the patient (which is actually the head of the table) to allow the surgeon and scrub nurse complete freedom at the patient's head.

A few useful suggestions for the anesthesiologist are as follows:

1. Have extra-long tubing for the gas machine to allow seating at the foot of the patient.
2. Start the intravenous infusion in the forearm and extend the tubing to the foot of the table.
3. The blood pressure cuff belongs on the arm *opposite* the ear to be operated on.
4. Be certain that the patient is secured to the table with wide adhesive tape. The eyes should be taped shut.

Arrangement and Instrumentation

Particular attention should be paid to operating room arrangement (Fig. 9–1). The anesthesiologist is at the patient's feet, far removed from the operating field, and the scrub nurse is directly across from the surgeon, where the nurse may be of the most assistance. The same arrangement, minus the anesthesiologist, is used for procedures occurring with the patient under local anesthesia.

It is important for the comfort of the surgeon that the patient be in a satisfactory position. The table is usually placed in a few degrees of Trendelenburg position and rolled slightly toward the surgeon. The patient's head is adjusted as necessary, usually flexed slightly onto the opposite shoulder.

The surgeon should be comfortably seated on a chair with a back support. The surgeon should use the back support and be in a comfortable position so that all back and arm muscles are relaxed.

SURGICAL TECHNIQUE

The lateral-surface grafting technique involves eight steps: transmeatal canal incisions and elevations of the vascular strip; postauricular exposure and removal and dehydration of the temporalis fascia; removal of canal skin; enlargement of the ear canal by removal of the anterior (and inferior) canal bulge; de-epithelization of the tympanic membrane remnant; placement of the rehydrated fascia on the outer surface of the remnant, but under the manubrium; replacement of canal skin; and closure of the postauricular incision and replacement of the vascular strip transmeatally.[10]

Transmeatal Incisions

Incisions are made along the tympanomastoid and tympanosquamous suture lines, demarcating the vascular strip, with a No. 1 (sickle) knife (Fig. 9–2). The vascular strip is the area of the canal skin that covers the superior and posterior portions of the ear canal between these two suture lines. It is easily demarcated from the skin of the remainder of the ear canal because of its thickness and the fact that it balloons up when local anesthesia is injected into the

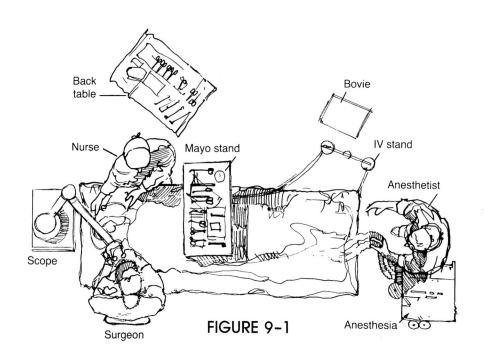

Back table

Bovie

Nurse Mayo stand

IV stand

Anesthetist

Scope

FIGURE 9-1

Surgeon

Anesthesia

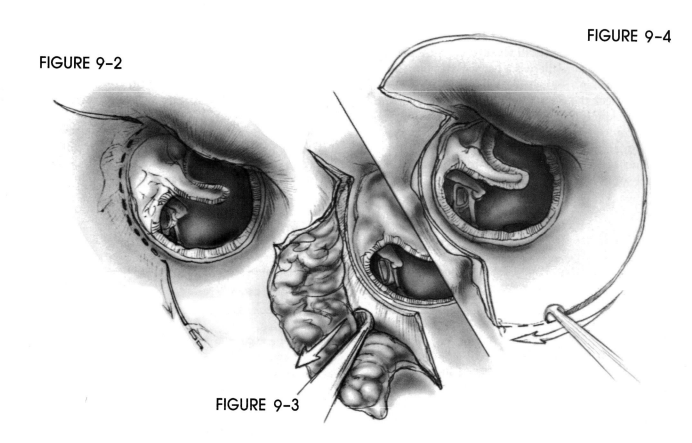

FIGURE 9-4

FIGURE 9-2

FIGURE 9-3

area. The vascular strip is elevated from the bone, from within outward using a round knife (Fig. 9–3).

A semilunar incision is made in the outer third of the ear canal, using a Beaver knife with a No. 64 blade, connecting the two incisions already made along the border of the vascular strip (Fig. 9–4). The knife blade is angled toward the bone to thin the 1- or 2-mm section of the membranous canal included.

Postauricular Exposure and Removal of Fascia

The skin incision must provide adequate exposure for the operative field. It should extend far enough forward, both superiorly and inferiorly, to allow adequate exposure of the bony meatus when the ear is retracted forward. Failure to do this may result in difficulty seeing structures in the posterior part of the middle ear.

The superior portion of the incision begins at the most anterior extent of, and 1 cm above, the postauricular fold. It is then continued into the postauricular fold at the level of the lower border of the muscle and extends inferiorly under the lobule of the ear.

Exposure of the temporalis fascia is facilitated if ample local anesthetic has been injected to balloon the area. A retractor is inserted to retract the skin margins in this area and to obtain hemostasis. By lifting up on the retractor, one may pull the areolar tissue away from the fascia, facilitating the dissection and ensuring that all loose areolar tissue is lifted off the fascia prior to the fascia's removal.

Local anesthesia is injected under the fascia to elevate it slightly from the underlying muscle. A 2 × 2-cm piece of fascia is removed.

The fascia is spread on a polytetrafluoroethylene (Teflon) block, undersurface upward, and any adherent muscle is removed. The fascia is then placed on a fascia press, absorbable gelatin sponge (Gelfoam) is placed on the fascia, and the press is closed. The press is opened after 5 minutes, and the gelatin sponge is removed; the fascia, now smooth and partially dehydrated, is left attached to the press. The press, with the attached fascia, is placed under an electric lamp to complete the dehydration process.

An incision is made through the soft tissue above the meatus, from the root of the zygoma, horizontally, along the linea temporalis. This horizontal incision is extended posteriorly to the level of the skin incision. The incision is then extended inferiorly, below the linea temporalis, following the postauricular incision, incising the periosteum until the incision curves forward, down to the level of the floor of the ear canal.

The periosteum is elevated superiorly (under the temporalis muscle), posteriorly and anteriorly, using a Lempert elevator, to obtain adequate exposure of the mastoid cortex. A self-retaining retractor is inserted to retract the auricle and vascular strip forward, exposing the ear canal.

Removal of the Canal Skin

The periosteum and canal skin are elevated from the bone as far as the annular ligament (Fig. 9–5). Care should be taken not to elevate the ligament and the remnant of the middle fibrous layer. The dissection is superficial to the fibrous layer of the remnant in such a way that the remnant is de-epithelized in continuity with the canal skin, if possible. It is often easier to begin the final removal and de-epithelization by starting anterosuperiorly, using a cup forceps (Fig. 9–6). Removal of the canal skin and de-epithelization are continued inferiorly and posteriorly. The periosteum and canal skin are removed from the ear and kept moist in Tis-U-Sol irrigating solution.

In elevating the periosteum and the canal skin, one should remember to work perpendicular to the annular ligament and remnant, keeping the instrument on the bone at all times, until the dissection is completed to the level of the remnant. The dissection is then continued parallel to the annular ligament to avoid elevating it and the remnant (Fig. 9–7).

Enlargement of the Ear Canal

Through the use of a drill and continuous suction-irrigation, the ear canal is enlarged by removal of the anterior and inferior canal bulges (Fig. 9–8).

The importance of this step in the lateral-surface grafting technique must be emphasized. Removal of this bone enlarges the field of surgery. The anterior and inferior sulci are thoroughly exposed to allow de-epithelization and satisfactory graft placement. The acute angle that exists anteriorly is opened, helping to prevent postoperative blunting. There is no area hidden from postoperative observation. Enlarging the ear canal is routine in all lateral-surface grafting procedures and is the main reason for removal of canal skin.

De-epithelization of the Tympanic Membrane Remnant

The lateral-surface grafting technique demands a complete de-epithelization of the remnant. Although the graft may take without all the skin having been removed, postoperative epithelial cysts may develop.

Direct your attention first to the ear canal bone immediately adjacent to the bony annulus. Pay particular attention to the anteroinferior bone 1-mm lateral to the annulus, where a small vessel and nerve perforate the bone and where there is a particularly tight attachment to the skin.

Next, check the tympanic membrane remnant carefully for skin. If there is a question about whether de-epithelization has been thorough, remove a portion of the remnant to be certain. The size of the perforation is of no consequence in regard to graft take in the lateral-surface technique.

Preparation of Packing

The surgical nurse should have begun preparing absorbable gelatin sponge packing prior to or shortly after the beginning of the operation. Uncompressed gelatin sponge is cut into an ample number of various-sized pieces and then

FIGURE 9-5

FIGURE 9-6

FIGURE 9-7

FIGURE 9-8

FIGURE 9-9

FIGURE 9-11

FIGURE 9-10

FIGURE 9-13

FIGURE 9-12

soaked in antibiotic-cortisone solution. Pieces of gelatin sponge are then removed from the solution and compressed (on a tongue blade or a paper gelatin sponge packet) until most of the solution has been removed. The gelatin sponge is put aside and allowed to dry more until needed by the surgeon.

Placement of Fascia

When the perforation is large, or the fascia is unusually thin, it is helpful to fill the middle ear with gelatin sponge packing prior to placing the graft. The gelatin sponge serves as an artificial remnant and facilitates graft placement. The fascia will be placed under the malleus handle. When the manubrium is surrounded by remnant (small perforation), the remnant is separated from the malleus handle to allow proper placement of the fascia.

The dehydrated fascia is trimmed to an oval shape measuring approximately 1.3 × 1.5 cm. A slit is cut in the fascia to allow placement under the manubrium (Fig. 9–9); the two cut ends are grasped with the forceps, and then the fascia is immersed for a few seconds in Tis-U-Sol irrigating solution to dehydrate it.

The fascia is placed over the perforation and immediately slipped under the manubrium (Fig. 9–10). Be certain that the apex of the slit in the fascia comes into contact with the tensor tendon.

The fascia is then adjusted to the remnant anteriorly and inferiorly, with care being taken that it does not extend onto the bony wall anteriorly, unless there is no remnant at all, then only for a millimeter at the most. The anterior flap is turned back over the exposed manubrium, resulting in a better appearance of the membrane when healed (Fig. 9–11).

When the malleus is absent and there is only a small remnant present, it is necessary to insert the fascia in a different way to result in the stabilized graft (Fig. 9–12). The fascia is cut twice, creating a flap that can then be tucked under the lateral wall of the epitympanum. The anterosuperior edge of the fascia is then swung posteriorly to overlap the upper edge of the graft and secure the seal of the middle ear (Fig. 9–13).

Replacement of Canal Skin

The canal skin is replaced to cover the bone from which it was removed. It is positioned only slightly more medially, allowing it to overlap the fascia by a millimeter (Fig. 9–14), which helps promote rapid epithelization. Epithelization is particularly important in preventing blunting in the anterosuperior sulcus. There must be no edges of epithelium turned under, or small epithelial cysts may develop on the surface of the fascia during healing.

The first piece of packing is a small, dry, rolled up, (cigar-shaped) tightly compressed piece of absorbable gelatin sponge, placed in the sulcus anteriorly. The canal is packed tightly with pledgets of slightly moist gelatin sponge, leaving room posterosuperiorly for the vascular strip.

Closure and Replacement of the Vascular Strip

The retractors are released, and the vascular strip is pushed anteriorly to lie over the packing. One suture is placed subcutaneously postauricularly to stabilize the auricle.

Transmeatally, the vascular strip is lifted up, some packing is removed, and the vascular strip is then replaced in the ear canal in the exact position from which it came (Fig. 9–15). Gelatin sponge packing in the canal is then completed, and a plug of cotton is placed in the outer meatus. The postauricular incision is closed with subcutaneous sutures, and a mastoid dressing is applied.

POSTOPERATIVE CARE

The mastoid dressing is removed the day following surgery. The patient is given a postoperative instruction card (Appendix 2) just before entering the hospital. It is important to review some aspects of this information with the patient. The patient should be reminded not to blow the nose and not to get water in the ear. An antibiotic has been prescribed and should be taken as directed on the prescription label. There will be discomfort for a few days, and the patient should take aspirin or acetaminophen four times a day regularly for the first few days just to keep the pain under control. Nothing need be done with the cotton in the ear, but it may be changed if it becomes terribly soiled.

The patient should be asked to touch the edge of the auricle. Point out that the ear is numb and that it is going to take a few months for that numbness to go away. There is also tenderness on the incision behind the ear. This will diminish rapidly, but it may be 6 months before it is totally gone. Finally, the patient should be reminded of the first postoperative appointment, which should occur 7 to 10 days later in the physician's office.

At the first postoperative visit, the cotton plug in the ear canal is removed and the ear is inspected. The gelatin sponge should appear firm. Remove a piece of this to show to the patient so that the patient understands that it will eventually turn to a liquid and will run out of the ear. The patient is instructed to begin using ear drops (of one type or another) 3 weeks following the date of surgery, twice daily. The drops may be started sooner should the ear begin to drain, an indication of liquefaction of the gelatin sponge.

The second postoperative visit is scheduled for 6 to 8 weeks following the date of surgery. Eighty to 90 per cent of the ear will be totally healed at this point.

PROS AND CONS OF THE OUTER SURFACE TECHNIQUE

One of the problems faced by the novice is that there are many techniques and prostheses recommended as "the best—it always works well." Of course, how well a technique or prosthesis works for the individual depends on the technical ability of that individual—the person's judgment and manual dexterity.[11]

The outer surface grafting technique has numerous ad-

FIGURE 9-14

FIGURE 9-15

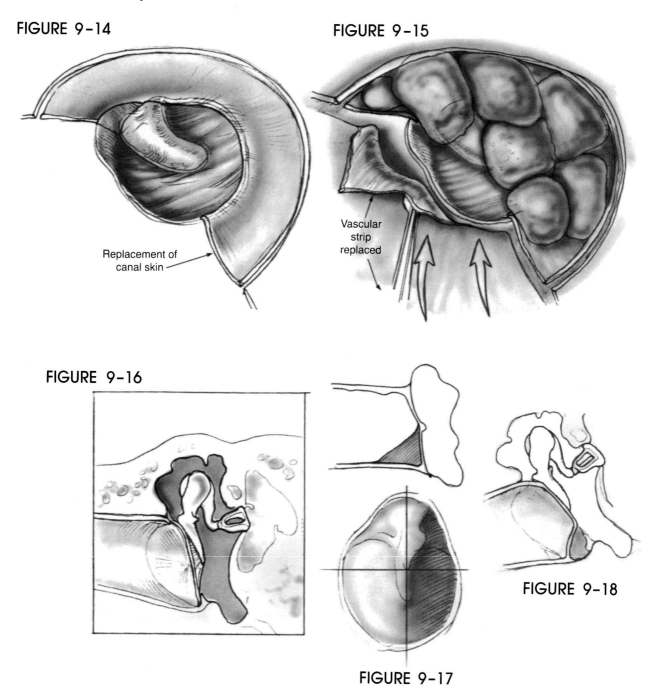

Replacement of canal skin

Vascular strip replaced

FIGURE 9-16

FIGURE 9-18

FIGURE 9-17

vantages and disadvantages. The advantages are well known to all who have used the technique. The exposure is excellent—one can see everything necessary without moving the microscope. Secondly, one may remove as much remnant as necessary to eliminate the disease. There is no need to scrape in many different places. Certainly, the graft rate take is high. Finally, it is one technique that can be used in all cases.

However, there are disadvantages that may outweigh the advantages for some individuals. The technique requires very precise surgery to avoid problems. The healing time is longer than with the undersurface technique. Finally, if the operation is not done extremely skillfully, one may develop either blunting in the anterior sulcus or lateral

healing, both of which may result in a healed ear with worse hearing.

Healing Problems

One of the disadvantages of the outer surface grafting technique, as already noted, is that although there is a very high graft take rate regardless of how the operation is performed, there are healing problems. These healing problems may outweigh the advantages for some individuals.[10]

These healing problems became evident soon after the technique was started in the early 1960s: lateralization of the graft, blunting in the anterior sulcus, excessive membrane thickness, epithelial cysts between the remnant and the fascia, and epithelial pearls on the drum surface and ear canal. Most of these have ceased to be major problems, but they still occur in a small percentage of cases.

Lateralization of the Tympanic Membrane

The very first problem that was noticed with this technique was lateralization of the membrane (Fig. 9–16). This usually did not become apparent until 6 to 12 months following surgery and resulted from the fascia not being placed under the malleus handle when the technique was first introduced (see Fig. 9–10).

When lateralization has occurred, the patient's hearing will be reduced, but often not as much as anticipated. The appearance is of a smaller-than-normal-sized eardrum, mobile, and at a direct right angle to the line of vision. Treatment of this problem (if needed) requires reoperation and the placement of the new graft underneath the malleus handle.

Blunting in the Anterior Sulcus

Blunting in the anterior sulcus, particularly anterosuperiorly, occurs to a minor degree in most lateral surface cases but is of no consequence and results from the formation of excess fibrous tissue. Blunting is probably the most common healing problem encountered by the novice surgeon. It can interfere greatly with the hearing result if it is great enough to involve the malleus handle when the ossicular chain is intact (Fig. 9–17).

To prevent blunting, one should remove the anterior canal bulge so that the anterior angle is open. One should not place the fascia onto the anterior canal bone unless there is no alternative. Finally, one should make sure that the replaced canal skin overlaps the graft slightly anterosuperiorly. Finally, placing the rolled-up piece of dried gelatin foam in the anterior sulcus as the first piece of packing also helps prevent blunting.

When severe blunting occurs, the manubrium becomes indistinguishable, and the anterior half of the tympanic membrane is immobile and takes on a concave appearance with no clear-cut distinction between the edge of the membrane and the bony wall. The posterior half of the membrane may show fair mobility. Should this appearance persist after 6 months, and should there be a hearing problem, reoperation would be required to correct it.

Other Problems

Two varieties of epithelial cysts may be noted. One of these is common and appears as a small pearl on the tympanic membrane or ear canal. It is the result of turning under the skin edges when replacing the canal skin. Spontaneous rupture and healing are common. The cyst might be marsupialized under the microscope in the office if desired.

An epithelial cyst may occur between the remnant and the fascia and enlarge slowly over 1 to 2 years (Fig. 9–18). This is an uncommon problem that results from inadequate de-epithelization of bone and the remnant adjacent to the bone. The only place where this is likely to occur is anterioinferiorly where the small vessel and nerve enter the ear canal a millimeter lateral to the drum. As opposed to blunting, where there is a concave appearance, the appearance here is convex, and it occurs anteroinferiorly. Once it is recognized, it can be corrected by merely incising the cyst and evacuating it.

ACKNOWLEDGMENT

Many of the illustrations are modified from *Otolaryngology*, Vol. 1, published by J. B. Lippincott Company.

References

1. Wullstein H: Theory and practice of tympanoplasty. Laryngoscope 66: 1076–1093, 1956.
2. Zollner F: Principles of plastic surgery of the sound-conducting apparatus. J Laryngol Otol 69: 637–652, 1955.
3. House WF, Sheehy JL: Myringoplasty: Use of ear canal skin compared with other techniques. Arch Otolaryngol Head Neck Surg 73: 407–415, 1961.
4. Plester D: Skin and mucous membrane grafts in middle ear surgery. Arch Otolaryngol Head Neck Surg 72: 718–721, 1960.
5. Storrs LA: Myringoplasty with use of fascia graft. Arch Otolaryngol Head Neck Surg 74: 45–49, 1961.
6. Sheehy JL: Tympanic membrane grafting: Early and long-term results. Laryngoscope 74: 985–988, 1964.
7. Sheehy JL, Glasscock ME: Tympanic membrane grafting with temporalis fascia: A report of four years' experience. Arch Otolaryngol Head Neck Surg 86: 391–402, 1967.
8. Sheehy JL, Anderson RG: Myringoplasty: A review of 472 cases. Ann Otol Rhinol Laryngol 89: 331–334, 1980.
9. Sheehy JL: Testing eustachian tube function. Ann Otol Rhinol Laryngol 90: 562–564, 1981.
10. Sheehy JL, Brackmann DE: Surgery of chronic otitis media. *In* English GM (ed): Otolaryngology. Philadelphia, JB Lippincott, 1994.
11. Sheehy JL, Brackmann DE: Surgery of Chronic Ear Disease: What We Do and Why We Do It. *In* Instructional Courses, Vol 6. St. Louis, CV Mosby, 1993.

Appendix 1

RISKS AND COMPLICATIONS OF
MYRINGOPLASTY, TYMPANOPLASTY,
MASTOID SURGERY, AND OTHER
OPERATIONS FOR CORRECTION OF
CHRONIC EAR INFECTIONS

(Operations to eliminate middle ear or mastoid infection, to repair the eardrum or the sound transmission mechanism)

Ear Infection

Ear infection with drainage, swelling, and pain may persist following surgery or, on rare occasions, may develop following surgery because of poor healing of the ear tissue. If this is the case, additional surgery may be necessary to control the infection.

Loss of Hearing

Further permanent impairment of hearing develops in 3 per cent of patients because of problems in the healing process. In 2 per cent this loss of hearing may be severe or total in the ear that was operated on. Nothing further can be done in these instances.

When a two-stage operation is necessary, the hearing is usually worse after the first operation.

Tinnitus

Should the hearing be worse following surgery, tinnitus (head noises) likewise may be more pronounced.

Dizziness

Dizziness may occur immediately following surgery because of irritation of the inner ear structures. Some unsteadiness may persist for a week postoperatively. Prolonged dizziness is rare unless there was dizziness prior to surgery.

Taste Disturbance and Mouth Dryness

Taste disturbance and mouth dryness are common for a few weeks following surgery. In some patients, this disturbance is prolonged.

Facial Paralysis

A rare postoperative complication of ear surgery is temporary paralysis of one side of the face. This may occur as a result of an abnormality or a swelling of the nerve and usually subsides spontaneously.

On very rare occasions, the nerve may be injured at the time of surgery or it may be necessary to excise it in order to eradicate infection. When this happens, a skin sensation nerve is removed from the upper part of the neck to replace the facial nerve. Paralysis of the face under these circumstances lasts 6 months to a year, and there would be a permanent residual weakness. Eye complications requiring treatment by a specialist could develop.

Hematoma

A hematoma (collection of blood) develops in a small percentage of cases, prolonging healing. Reoperation to remove the clot may be necessary if this complication occurs.

General Anesthesia Complications

Anesthetic complications are very rare but can be serious. You may discuss these with the anesthesiologist if you desire.

Complications Related to Mastoid Surgery

A cerebrospinal fluid leak (leak of fluid surrounding the brain) is a very rare complication. Reoperation may be necessary to stop the leak.

Intracranial (brain) complications, such as meningitis or brain abscess, or even paralysis, were common in cases of chronic otitis media prior to the antibiotic era. Fortunately, these now are extremely rare complications.

Appendix 2

POSTOPERATIVE INSTRUCTION FOLDER: MYRINGOPLASTY, TYMPANOPLASTY, AND MASTOIDECTOMY

Precautions

1. *Do not* blow your nose until your doctor has indicated that your ear is healed. Any accumulated secretions in the nose may be drawn back into the throat and expectorated if desired. This is particularly important if you develop a cold.

2. *Do not* "pop" your ears by holding your nose and blowing air through the eustachian tube into the ear. If it is necessary to sneeze, do so with your mouth open.

3. *Do not* allow water to enter the ear until advised by your doctor that the ear is healed. Until such time, when showering or washing your hair, lambswool or cotton may be placed in the outer ear opening and covered with Vaseline. If an incision was made in the skin behind your ear, water should be kept away from this area for 1 week.

4. *Do not* take an unnecessary chance of catching cold. Avoid undue exposure or fatigue. Should you catch a cold, treat it in your usual way, reporting to us if you develop ear symptoms.

5. You may anticipate a certain amount of pulsation, popping, clicking, and other sounds in the ear, and also a feeling of fullness in the ear. Occasional sharp shooting pains are not unusual. At times, it may feel as if there is liquid in the ear.

6. *Do not* plan to drive a car home from the hospital. Air travel is permissible 2 days following surgery. When changing altitude, you should remain awake and chew gum to stimulate swallowing.

Dizziness

Minor degrees of dizziness may be present on head motion and need not concern you unless it increases.

Hearing

Rarely is a hearing improvement noted immediately following surgery. It may even be worse temporarily because of swelling of the ear tissues and packing in the ear canal. Six to 8 weeks after surgery, an improvement may be noted. Maximum improvement may require 4 to 6 months.

Discharge

A bloody or watery discharge may occur during the healing period. The outer ear cotton may be changed if necessary, but in general, the less done to the ear the better.

A yellow (infected) discharge at any time is an indication to call the appointment desk and arrange to see your doctor. Discharge with foul odor should also be reported.

Pain

Mild, intermittent ear pain is not unusual during the first 2 weeks. Pain above or in front of the ear is common when chewing. If you have persistent ear pain, not relieved by a few aspirins, call the appointment desk and arrange to see your doctor.

Ear Drops

If you were given a prescription for ear drops, begin using these 3 weeks after surgery. Place a few drops in the ear twice daily to loosen the packing, which will run out of the ear as a liquid. Tip the head to the side, place two drops in the ear, and allow them to remain for 5 minutes. Then tip the head in the opposite direction to allow the ear drops to run out. Continue doing this twice daily until you have finished the drops or until advised otherwise by your doctor.

10

Tympanoplasty: The Undersurface Graft Technique—Transcanal Approach

M. Coyle Shea, Jr., M.D.

Many otologic surgeons prefer placing the connective tissue graft medial to the tympanic membrane remnant. This can be accomplished through either the transcanal or postauricular approach. In this chapter, the transcanal technique is described in detail.

In transcanal tympanoplasty using the underlay technique, the grafting material may be any type of autogenous connective tissue, such as vein, fascia, or perichondrium. In 1957, Shea,[1] using vein, was the first to use the underlay grafting technique. Tabb,[2] Austin and Shea,[3] and others soon recognized the superiority of this method over onlay skin grafting and followed Shea's lead. The use of fascia as an underlay graft was first reported by Storrs.[4] Tragal perichondrium was first used in tympanoplasty by Goodhill and associates[5] as an onlay graft, and it is the material I prefer. It is in the immediate surgical field, is extremely durable and, when pressed, is very easy to handle. Vein also is easy to position and, if large enough (as from the antecubital fossa), can be used to repair perforations of any size. Our primary objection to the use of vein grafts is that in the event of a serious future illness, the large vein could be an important means of administering parenteral medications. Temporalis fascia, its overlying areolar tissue, or even scar tissue from the vicinity of a previous postauricular incision can be used with the transcanal undersurface technique, but it is not as easy to handle as vein or perichondrium. Pressing the fascia in a vein or fascia press makes it much more manageable by eliminating the tenacious loose strands and at the same time preventing the stiffness that occurs with drying. We do not recommend pressing vein for tympanoplasty (as done in stapedectomy) because it results in excessive thinning. Instead, we trim away the adventitia and stretch the vessel between the blades of a vein scissors before opening it.

PREOPERATIVE EVALUATION AND PATIENT SELECTION

If the canal is of adequate size, this technique is suitable for any tympanic membrane perforation in which tympanoplasty is indicated, regardless of size or location. If the canal is not large enough to accommodate a 5-mm or larger ear speculum, this procedure may not be technically feasible.

The usual indications for closure of a tympanic membrane perforation are to reduce the incidence of middle ear infection and to improve hearing. Not every perforation

needs to be or should be, closed. Each patient must be evaluated on the basis of what would be best for that individual. An elderly or debilitated patient with an asymptomatic perforation or a patient for which the ear under evaluation is the only hearing ear is usually not a good surgical candidate. In the case of a young child who developed a perforation from a ventilation tube that was initially inserted because the child could not ventilate the ear, it would be unwise to repair the tympanic membrane until it is apparent that eustachian tube function has significantly improved, lest the pathologic process repeat itself.

There is no infallible test of tubal function, but it is reasonable to assume that if the patient can autoinflate by the Valsalva maneuver preoperatively, he or she will be able to ventilate the ear by this method, if necessary, postoperatively. Consequently, the patient is instructed in this procedure before surgery.

SURGICAL TECHNIQUE

Local anesthesia using 1 to 2 per cent lidocaine with 1:100,000 epinephrine is employed in combination with either a general endotracheal anesthetic or an intravenous sedation. The local anesthetic is administered at the time of the immediate preoperative preparation of the surgical area to ensure adequate vasoconstriction by the time the actual surgical procedure is begun. Perioperative antibiotics are rarely used. The hair and skin surrounding the ear are cleansed with 70 per cent alcohol. No hair is shaved unless fascia is to be taken, but it is combed away from the ear and sprayed with liquid spray bandage. The head is secured with tape in a standard foam headrest in the position most conducive to good visibility for the surgeon. This usually involves tilting the head back and the chin up slightly (Fig. 10–1). For this reason, the surgeon rather than a nursing assistant should prepare and position the patient. The ear canal, auricle, and surrounding skin are cleansed with povidone-iodine scrub and then painted with povidone-iodine solution. The field is then draped in a sterile manner.

The sine qua non for successful transcanal surgery is adequate exposure. Inadequate visibility is probably the primary objection to this technique, but there are several moves that can significantly improve it. The external auditory meatus can be enlarged somewhat by making a small slit in the superior aspect of its lateral end with a No. 15 scalpel blade and stretching it with a nasal speculum. The largest-sized ear speculum that can be atraumatically

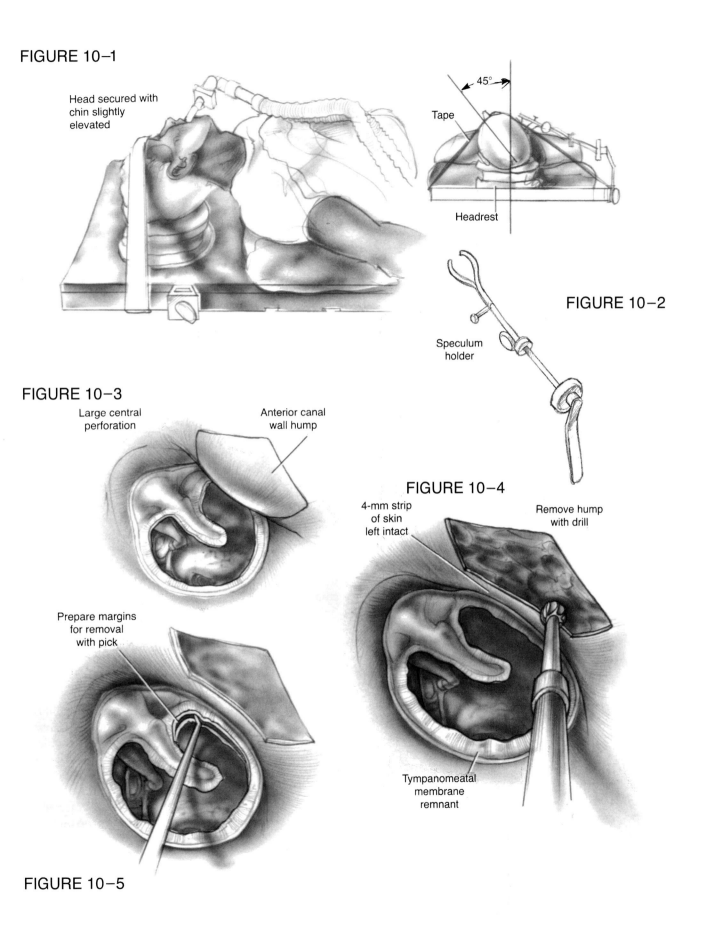

FIGURE 10-1

Head secured with
chin slightly
elevated

45°

Tape

Headrest

FIGURE 10-2

Speculum
holder

FIGURE 10-3

Large central
perforation

Anterior canal
wall hump

FIGURE 10-4

4-mm strip
of skin
left intact

Remove hump
with drill

Prepare margins
for removal
with pick

Tympanomeatal
membrane
remnant

FIGURE 10-5

FIGURE 10–6

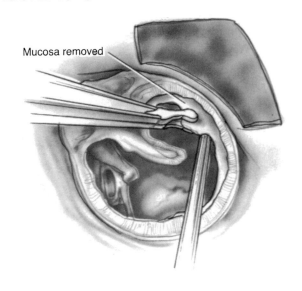

Mucosa removed

FIGURE 10–7

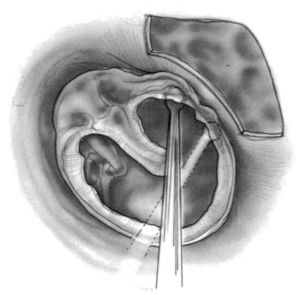

FIGURE 10–8

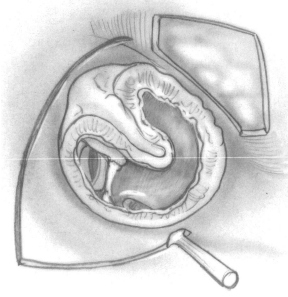

FIGURE 10–9

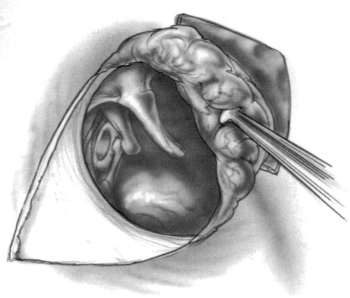

inserted is used and secured with a speculum holder (Fig. 10–2). The speculum holder is essential because it allows the use of both hands and serves as a support for the surgeon's fingers. The holder is quite mobile and allows the speculum to be placed and secured in the optimal position. It should be repositioned as needed throughout the procedure. The microscope head should also be moved about frequently to provide an unobstructed view of the operative field. In general, the less complex the microscope, the more mobile it is and the easier it is to use. Another item that is extremely helpful in improving visibility is the hydraulic chair. Because it can be lowered or raised in a matter of seconds, it rapidly allows the surgeon to change position in relation to the patient's ear without the need for a circulating nurse to tilt the operating table back and forth.

In anterior perforations and large central perforations, the anterior margin frequently cannot be seen because of a bulging anterior canal wall (Fig. 10–3). This problem can easily be remedied in 99 per cent of the cases by removing the hump. Sometimes the removal of a "dog-house" segment of anterior canal wall skin is all that is necessary. Frequently, the bony hump must also be removed, and this can be quickly done with a curette or small cutting burr (Fig 10–4). In the removal of this bony hump, one must be aware of the proximity of the temporomandibular joint and avoid penetration into it. It is important to leave a 2- to 3-mm strip of skin intact between the annulus and the medial end of the resected skin. The excised skin is preserved in physiologic solution until the end of the procedure, at which time it is replaced. Once the margins of the perforation can be adequately visualized, they are prepared by incising the edge with a sharp, slightly angulated pick (Fig. 10–5), removing the rim and about 1 or 2 mm of the mucosa with a cup forceps (Fig. 10–6).

If the anterior perforation is marginal, the Austin "reverse elevator" (Fig. 10–7) is used to elevate the annulus and the 1 to 2 mm of the canal wall skin to provide a larger raw surface area for graft attachment. This elevated area gradually retracts into its normal position as the ear heals. It is an extremely important maneuver in the successful repair of the anterior perforation.

A posterior tympanomeatal incision is then made with the superior limb beginning 2 to 3 mm anterior to the malleus neck (Fig. 10–8). This makes it possible to completely elevate the drumhead remnant off the malleus handle (Fig. 10–9). Removal of the drumhead remnant from the malleus handle is performed in most situations except those in which the perforation is in an inferior or extremely posterior position. The three most important things facilitated by this elevation are the removal of any squamous epithelial ingrowth along the medial aspect of the malleus handle, the ossicular chain reconstruction, and the placement of the graft along the lateral aspect of the malleus.

Some surgeons prefer to place the graft medial to the malleus handle.[6] If there is extreme medial retraction of the malleus handle so that the umbo is touching the promontory, the handle can be slowly elevated laterally with a right-angle pick to release the accompanying contracture of the tensor tympani tendon. When the mucosa is badly diseased or eroded, the medial wall of the middle ear can be lined with absorbable gelatin film (Gelfilm) cut to the

desired size and shape. Because of the potential for delayed reaction, we do not use Silastic sheeting unless a second stage is planned, at which time the Silastic sheeting is removed.

Next, the tragal perichondrial graft is taken. If the perforation involves 60 per cent of the surface of the drumhead or less, the graft may usually be obtained from the posterior aspect of the tragus through an incision immediately posterior to the free border without removal of the cartilage itself (Fig. 10–10). If the perforation involves more than 60 per cent of the drumhead, the entire tragus with its perichondrium is removed through an incision along the free border. The excess soft tissue is removed from the perichondrium overlying the anterior surface of the tragus, and the entire perichondrium is removed from both sides of the cartilage and over the free border with a duckbill or Freer elevator and thumb forceps (Fig. 10–11). The cartilage is reinserted into the wound in its normal position to preserve the tragal contour, and the incision is closed with fine absorbable suture. The perichondrium is pressed with a vein or fascia press (Fig. 10–12). This process thins the graft for easier handling and enlarges it so that any size perforation can be closed.

The middle ear is then filled with gelatin sponge (Gelfoam) soaked in a physiologic solution, such as lactated Ringer's or Tis-U-Sol (Fig. 10–13). It is imperative that the tympanic cavity be filled with the gelatin sponge, especially in the anterior part at the eustachian tube orifice, to prevent medial displacement of the graft. The central part of the middle ear, however, should not be filled lateral to the umbo. If it is overfilled at this point, lateralization and loss of the conical contour of the drumhead may result.

For medium-sized or large perforations, the graft is then advanced under the tympanomeatal flap and over the malleus handle to the anteriormost extent of the perforation with the edges tucked under the margins of the drum remnant (Fig. 10–14). With smaller, inferior perforations, the graft may be inserted through the perforation and smoothed out posteriorly by elevating the tympanomeatal flap.

When using a perichondrial graft, the surface that was in contact with the cartilage should be positioned toward the middle ear. With a vein graft, the intimal surface should be medially placed. After the graft has been roughly positioned, the edges of the perforation are then carefully everted bimanually with a 20-gauge suction tip and a 90-degree pick to prevent the ingrowth of squamous epithelium. If the graft does not appear to be adequately supported by gelatin sponge, it can be reflected back and more gelatin sponge inserted.

If the anterior canal wall skin has been removed, it should now be replaced. Small pledgets of moist gelatin sponge are then used to overlap the junction of rim and graft circumferentially and over the canal incisions for further stabilization (Figs. 10–15 and 10–16).

Finally, the external canal is filled with an antibiotic ointment, such as polymyxin. In the event of antibiotic sensitivity, povidone-iodine ointment may be substituted.

POSTOPERATIVE CARE

The only dressing that is used is a small, sterile, cotton ball that is loosely placed in the conchal cavity to absorb

FIGURE 10–10

FIGURE 10–11

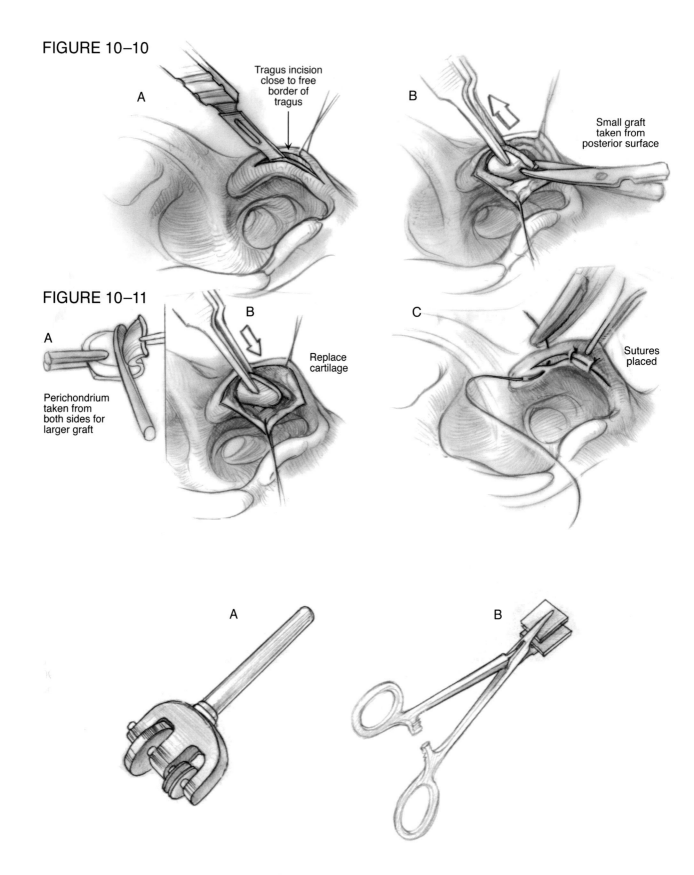

FIGURE 10–12

FIGURE 10-13

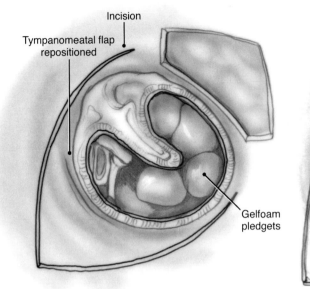

FIGURE 10-14

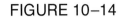
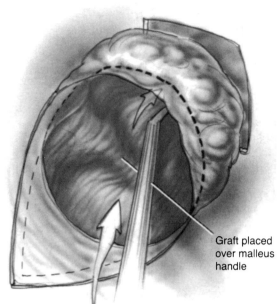

Graft placed over malleus handle

FIGURE 10-15

FIGURE 10-16

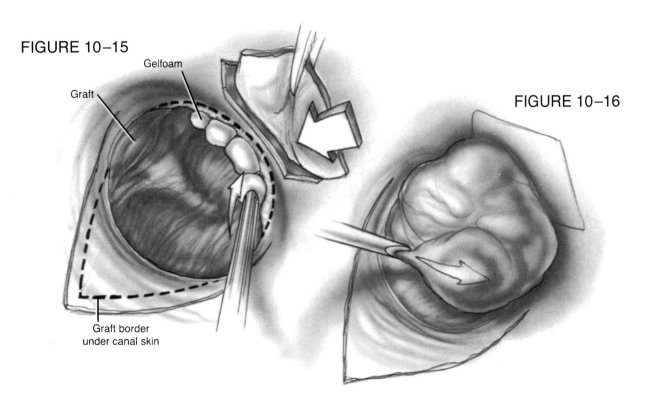

drainage. Once the drainage stops, the cotton is discontinued, and the ear is allowed to ventilate. In the event that purulent discharge occurs, antibiotic otic drops are started and continued until the first postoperative visit. The patient is instructed to avoid getting water in the affected ear or blowing the nose until the first postoperative visit at 3 weeks. At that time, the ear is cleaned using the operating microscope, and the graft is inspected. Approximately 95 per cent of the time, the graft will have taken, and the drumhead will be intact. Autoinflation is now begun using the Valsalva maneuver. If the patient is unable to ventilate the middle ear within a week or 10 days, a small ventilation tube is inserted in the drumhead.

If the graft is intact but not completely epithelialized at the time of the first postoperative visit, antimicrobial drops or a vinegar-alcohol solution should be used for 1 to 3 weeks to promote healing.

Although frank graft failure is a rarity, a small area of residual perforation will occasionally be found. If this occurs, the edges can be cauterized with trichloroacetic acid and then covered with a cigarette paper patch impregnated with povidone-iodine solution. The area is re-examined in 2 to 3 weeks, at which time it is usually healed. If revision surgery is necessary, it should be delayed for at least 3 months to allow for resolution of postoperative inflammatory changes.

References

1. Shea JJ Jr: Vein graft closure of eardrum perforations. J Laryngol Otol 74: 358, 1960.
2. Tabb HG: Closure of perforations of the tympanic membrane by vein grafts: A preliminary report of twenty cases. Laryngoscope 70: 271, 1960.
3. Austin DF, Shea JJ Jr: A new system of tympanoplasty using vein graft. Laryngoscope 71: 596, 1961.
4. Storrs LA: Myringoplasty with the use of fascia grafts. Arch Otolaryngol Head Neck Surg 74: 45, 1961.
5. Goodhill V, Harris I, Brockman SJ: Tympanoplasty with perichondrial graft. Arch Otolaryngol Head Neck Surg 79: 131, 1964.
6. Hough JVD: Tympanoplasty with the interior fascial graft technique and ossicular reconstruction. Laryngoscope 80: 1385, 1970.

11

Tympanoplasty: The Undersurface Graft Technique—Postauricular Approach

C. Gary Jackson, M.D., F.A.C.S.
- Michael E. Glasscock, III, M.D., F.A.C.S.
- Barry Strasnick, M.D.

Since the fundamental principles of tympanoplasty were first introduced by Wullstein[1] and Zollner,[2] there has been great diversity in the accepted surgical techniques used for repair of the tympanic membrane. The multitude of graft materials employed is a testimony to the difficulty of middle ear reconstruction. However, with advanced microsurgical techniques, the state of the art has now developed to the extent that graft success rates on the order of 90 to 97 per cent are to be expected.[3–5]

Over the years, two basic grafting techniques have evolved based on where the graft material is placed in relation to the drum remnant (overlay vs. underlay techniques). In this chapter, a method of undersurface grafting is presented. Detailed surgical techniques along with appropriate preoperative and postoperative care are presented.

HISTORICAL ASPECTS

Modern middle ear reconstructive surgery represents a culmination of more than a century of contributions by numerous dedicated and innovative otologic surgeons. The term *tympanoplasty* was originally defined in 1964 by what was then known as The American Academy of Ophthalmology and Otolaryngology's Committee on Conservation of Hearing as "an operation to eradicate disease in the middle ear and to reconstruct the hearing mechanism without mastoid surgery, with or without tympanic membrane grafting."[6] Should a mastoid procedure be included, the term *tympanoplasty with mastoidectomy* is used.

The era of surgical repair of the tympanic membrane dates as far back as the nineteenth century. In 1853, Toynbee described closure of a perforation of the tympanic membrane using a small rubber disk attached to a silver wire.[7] Ten years later, Yearsley advocated placing a cotton ball over the perforation, whereas in 1887, Blake introduced the concept of placing a thin paper patch over the membrane.[8, 9] The use of cautery to promote spontaneous healing of tympanic membrane perforations was introduced by Roosa in 1876; he used silver nitrate.[10] Later, Joynt,[11] Linn,[12] and Derlacki[13] would describe modifications of this technique using various forms of cautery and patches. However, closure of tympanic membrane perforations was considered appropriate only for dry central perforations. At this point, no one advocated the use of drum closure for the chronically draining ear.

It was not until 1952 that Wullstein[1] and Zollner[2] revolutionized middle ear surgery by advocating reconstructive grafting of the chronically diseased ear through the use of full- or split-thickness skin grafts. House and Sheehy[14] and Plester[15] later used canal skin, believing that it more closely resembled the squamous layer of the tympanic membrane. However, the overall poor success rates of these grafts along with the development of iatrogenic cholesteatomas prompted the search for alternative grafting materials.

Shea[16] and Tabb,[17] working independently, described the use of autogenous vein to close the tympanic membrane. Goodhill advocated tragal perichondrium in the mid 1960s, and tympanic membrane homografts became popular a few years later. The first sizable series of homograft tympanic membrane transplants were reported by Glasscock and House in 1968.[19] However, over the years, interest in homografts has waned largely because of the fear of transmission of infectious diseases.

Storrs is credited with performing the first fascia graft in the United States.[20] Although vein, perichondrium, and homografts still have their advocates, autogenous fascia has now become the standard by which all other grafting materials are measured.

The use of skin grafts required that the tympanic membrane perforation be repaired by laying the graft on top of the denuded drum remnant. This method of repair eventually became known as the overlay technique and was carried over to other forms of grafting material. With the use of connective tissue grafts, the graft material could be placed medial to the tympanic membrane remnant. The success of this approach eventually gave rise to the underlay technique of tympanic membrane grafting of which a large series was reported by Austin and Shea.[3] Proponents of the underlay procedure submit that it eliminates many of the problems associated with overlay grafts, such as anterior blunting, epithelial pearl formation, and lateralization of the new drum.

In 1973, Glasscock described an underlay grafting technique that relied on a postauricular approach.[4] With minor modifications, this approach continues to be the preferred method of dealing with disorders of the tympanic membrane and the middle ear.

PREOPERATIVE FUNDAMENTAL PRINCIPLES

Regardless of the grafting technique chosen, the preoperative evaluation and management of the patient with a tympanic membrane perforation remain the same. A complete clinical history along with a comprehensive head and neck examination is performed. Particular attention is, as well, addressed to the nasopharynx. Otoscopic examination is performed with the aid of an operating microscope. All findings are diagrammed on the patient's chart. All patients receive a pure-tone air and bone conduction audiogram along with speech discrimination testing. Tuning fork tests should be done on all patients to confirm the audiologic findings.

FUNDAMENTALS

Traditional Objectives

As with any surgical task, successful outcomes result from mastery of both understanding and execution of each elemental component of the process as a whole. It is useful to distill the task of tympanoplasty into its important fundamentals.

The traditional objectives of tympanoplasty have not changed in 50 years

▪ Eradication of disease
▪ Closure of the ear by grafting
▪ Hearing rehabilitation

In this priority, reasonable expectations must be established as functional goals.

Predisposing Conditions

Tympanoplasty is successful in the short term. To ensure long-term success, conditions predisposing to failure must be prospectively managed. In general, the status of the upper respiratory tract influences eustachian tube function and, consequently, the long-term success of tympanoplasty.

Adenoidal Hypertrophy and Adenoidectomy

Excessive adenoidal hypertrophy is regarded, by consensus, to influence the success of tympanic membrane grafting. Adenoidectomy should be done prospectively. To perform adenoidectomy, with its significant effects on the nasopharynx in the short term, simultaneously with tympanic membrane grafting seems illogical. The patient is referred to an otolaryngologic colleague; tympanic membrane grafting then scheduled, as a separate procedure, 4 weeks later. Tonsillectomy is performed as an independently indicated consideration. Its effect on tympanoplasty is negligible. The clinical setting in which this occurs in generally in children younger than 10 years of age.

Nasal or Sinus Condition

Like nasopharyngeal disease, significant nasal septal deformity, polyposis, or acute sinusitis should be managed prior to grafting an ear. Acute sinusitis would warrant cancellation of tympanoplasty.

Lesser degrees of nasal obstruction or chronic sinusitis are addressed as logically dictated by the clinical circumstances prior to or at some time after tympanoplasty.

Allergy

Allergic disease is an inexorable detriment to the long-term success of tympanic membrane grafting. In endemic areas it should not be disregarded. At some time in the perioperative period the tympanoplasty patient is referred for comprehensive allergy diagnosis and management. Desensitization is fundamental to long-term outcome. Acute exacerbations, often seasonal, are managed pharmacologically.

Rare Disorders

Particularly in residivistic disease, the presence of rare associated diseases must be kept in mind. Tuberculosis, sarcoidosis, diabetes mellitus, hematologic disorders, the histiocytoses, immunodeficiency syndromes, and, in recurrent adult disease, neoplasm should not be disregarded.

PREOPERATIVE PREPARATION

Otorrhea

Every attempt is made to operate on dry ears. Preoperative infection control in the involved ear is useful but not essential. At the initial evaluation the draining ear is otomicroscopically evacuated. Instructions are then given to irrigate the ear thrice daily with sterile 1.5 per cent acetic acid solution followed immediately by the installation of steroid-containing antibiotic drops. Bulb syringe irrigation of the ear with solution of room temperature evacuates debris from the middle and external ear as well as reinstates more normal pH levels. Drop installation to the infected ear affords minimal ototoxicity risk. Pain on administration constitutes an end point. Associated disorders or unusually significant infection may rarely warrant oral antibiotics. In the absence of any immunocompromising accompaniment, cultures are not routinely done. Contemporary masking of the traditional signs and symptoms of intratemporal or extratemporal complication must always be considered. Surgery is scheduled and the ear is operated on, draining or not.

Eustachian Tubal Tests

There exists no clinical test of eustachian tubal physiology. Eustachian tubal patency is testable via methods such as the Valsalva maneuver and the Toynbee test, but it is not important in the grand schematic of tympanoplasty. Eustachian tubal physiology tests exist (such as the Flisberg) but are clinically impractical. Eustachian tubal testing is not done. A statement attributed to James Sheehy, M.D., is true: "Sometimes the best test of eustachian tubal function is a tympanoplasty."

Eustachian tube function is, nonetheless, important to tympanic membrane grafting success. Status of the contralateral ear often predicts the eustachian tubal capacity of the involved ear. Apparent current eustachian tubal dysfunction may be a consequence of active infections unilaterally or the aftermath of a lifetime of chronic otitis media. Tympanoplasty is not contraindicated. In fact, postoperatively, once the ear is restored to a more normal state, so might its eustachian tubal function. In the difficult situation of cleft palate where eustachian tube function is obviously compromised or when effusion or retraction afflicts the successful graft, the ear can be ventilated in the office. Ventilation tubes should not be placed in tympanic membrane grafts because they promptly extrude. Tube placement can be performed in the first month postprocedure in the office because the tympanic membrane is still anesthetic.

The atelectatic ear should not preclude tympanoplasty. It is rather a perfect indication for cartilage tympanoplasty.

Imaging

The imaging standard for chronic otitis media is now high-resolution temporal bone detail using computed tomography (CT). Contrast medium is also employed to evaluate clinically silent peridural, intracranial, or lateral sinus abscess. Plain mastoid radiographs have been abandoned, as has polytomography.

All ears for grafting are not imaged. Only hearing ears and disease in adult long-standing chronic otitis media are ideal candidates. Revision surgery is imaged. Selected cholesteatomas may be studied.

The current state of magnetic resonance imaging precludes its routine use in ear imaging of chronic otitis media. It is useful when CT suggests an intracranial complication or brain hernia. Magnetic resonance angiography is useful in venous phase to assess the lateral venous sinus.

Complications

Polypharmacy and accessible medical care have changed the face of temporal bone and intracranial complication diagnosis in chronic otitis media. Pain, focal neurology, headache, vertigo, particularly noisome (anaerobic) otorrhea, cephalgia, and sensorineural hearing loss all should elicit the applicable cliche: "high index of suspicion."

Informed Consent

Preoperative counseling as to the nature and extent of the problem, treatment options, surgical details, surgical staging, reasonable expectations, and risks and complications is comprehensive. This discussion is interpersonal as well as reviewed in professionally prepared videotapes. The consent as well as preoperative and postoperative instructions are provided in written form that the patient is asked to execute by signature in the presence of a neutral witness. Common complications discussed include, but are not limited to, hearing loss, infection, graft failure, and facial nerve paralysis. Disorder-focused brochures are also given to the patient.

BASIC TECHNICAL PRINCIPLES

For some reason, the basic surgical principles we all learn as surgical interns are inclined to desert us when the operating microscope is introduced as a surgical tool. They are as important here as ever.

Infection Control

Chronic ear surgery is clean-contaminated or contaminated. As such, 90% of otologic wounds are colonized at the time of surgery. The general surgical principle of infection control seeks to minimize colony counts so host defense mechanisms are not overwhelmed. Whether or not surgeons can accomplish this in ear surgery is highly debated. Otologists seeking higher graft take rates and fewer complications often resort to prophylactic antibiotics as a "protective umbrella."

In the only study of statistical power on this subject, Jackson[23] concluded that prophylactic antibiotics are harmless yet, in point of fact, useless. In common uncomplicated tympanoplasty, antimicrobial prophylaxis is unwarranted. An indication for prophylaxis exists in the draining ear, which, intuitively, has a high postinfection rate with graft failure. This notwithstanding, no protocol exists to prevent such an outcome. This is an ideal indication for intraoperative irrigation, yet ototoxicity and medical legal concerns have impeded human study design to address this issue.

There are indications for antimicrobial prophylaxis in the ear surgery. Violation of the dural integrity with or without cerebrospinal fluid leakage, violation of the labyrinth, acknowledged aseptic technique breaks, only hearing ears, and in implantation of indwelling devices such as cochlear implants all serve as valid indications.

"The secret to pollution is dilution." Aggressive irrigation throughout the procedure theoretically clears devitalized debris and clots and is thought to reduce colony counts. Normal saline is used.

The surgical prep is described in the section on technique.

Hemostasis

Prior injection of the surgical field with 2 per cent lidocaine (Xylocaine) and 1:100,000 epinephrine helps secure a bloodless field essential to microsurgery. These solutions are contained in dental carpules so that loose solutions with their attendant risks are not on the surgical table to be confused.

Electromicrobipolar cautery, adapted from neurotology, is useful in eliminating bleeding from the lateral venous sinus, the dura, facial nerve, and delicate external auditory canal flaps.

Excessive bleeding from infected areas granulating can be difficult. Gelfoam soaked in straight epinephrine placed on the involved site while surgical attention is directed elsewhere is efficient hemostasis. Aggressive irrigation is again thought to help control blood loss and affect hemostasis.

Graft placement of any variety cannot be efficient under water. A bloodless field to identify all margins is essential. While preparing the graft, the operative field is filled with epinephrine-soaked Gelfoam until graft placement is imminent.

Grafting Techniques and Exposure

Two approaches to tympanic membrane grafting have evolved over the years. The overlay technique was once popular owing to its high success rate and reproducibility.[24] Experience, however, has recognized recurring downsides. Blunting of the anterior sulcus, when significant, can result in conductive hearing loss by malleus fixation, as can lateralization of the graft away from the malleus. Inability to completely denude the drum of epithelium could and has resulted in epithelial pearls and/or cholesteatoma. Furthermore, because the external auditory canal skin is removed and replaced, delays in healing occur.

The undersurface graft placement technique has been propelled by the adoption of connective tissue as a grafting material. Because this surgery was commonly performed transcanal through a speculum, underlay grafting was regarded as more technically difficult. Irregular graft placement, hence failure, often resulted. Variations in size and contour of the external auditory canal and operator experience using a speculum impaired visualization of the entire tympanic membrane remnant and anterior sulcus, making graft placement particularly challenging. Adequate exposure of the middle ear and eustachian tubal orifice was rare.

The postauricular approach obviated all of these problems using the vascular strip access. Anterior external auditory canal wall bulges could be easily managed and no speculum was needed. Overall exposure was enhanced, allowing luxurious middle ear exposure and precise graft placement. All the complications of the overlay strategy are avoided.

For the experienced ear surgeon either placement strategy will produce the desired outcome in well over 90 per cent of grafts. For the occasional ear surgeon the postauricular undersurface technique will afford higher take rates with fewer complications.

Mastoidectomy

Tympanic membrane perforation with cholesteatoma virtually mandates clear indication to perform mastoidectomy. Data do not exist to guide the ear surgeon as to mastoidectomy or not when tympanic membrane perforation exists. In uncomplicated tympanic membrane rupture, such as in trauma, mastoidectomy is rarely indicated.

Tympanic membrane grafts fail most commonly because of infection in the middle ear or mastoid. We readily assess and manage middle ear infection at the time of tympanoplasty. In any suggestion of mastoid infection, recent otorrhea, refractory or recurrent disease, difficult

aeration occasions such as tracheostomy, if it seems appropriate, mastoidectomy is executed.

Ossicular Reconstruction

The key to successful ossicular reconstruction is understanding the healing concept of changing anatomic relationships. When anatomic relationships in the middle ear are minimal and/or stabilized, ossicular reconstruction is unstaged. When anatomic relationships are expected to change, such as in the most diseased ears due to complicated tympanic membrane pathology, extensive mucosal disease, extensive ossicular pathology, a fixed footplate or extensive tympanosclerosis or healing biology, ossicular reconstruction is staged.

Autogenous cartilage is always interposed between nonhydroxylapatite platforms and tympanic membrane graft undersurfaces. Cartilage is not interposed for hydroxylapatite. If possible, autogenous material is preferred.

Facial Nerve Monitoring

Neural integrity monitoring of the facial nerve is used for *all* otologic cases. Paralyzing agents are not used in ear surgery anaesthesia. Nerve monitoring educates technique relative to the facial nerve. Monitoring is no substitute for knowledge of the anatomy, sound tissue technique, or surgical instinct.

SURGICAL TECHNIQUE

Surgical Preparation

A 2-cm-wide area of hair is shaved above and behind the auricle. Skin degreaser is applied to the shaved area, followed by tincture of benzoin. Nonsterile 3M (No. 1010) plastic towel drapes are then placed on the skin to cover the hair. Intraoperative facial nerve monitoring electrode insertion occurs prior to the surgical preparation. An iodine soap solution is used to wash the auricle and the skin around it, which is then blotted dry with a sterile towel. The ear itself is bathed in an iodine prep solution for 3 minutes. The solution is allowed to enter the external auditory canal. Finally, the area about the ear is prepared with an alcohol-based solution (DuraPrep).

The circulating nurse injects the postauricular region and the tragus with a 2 per cent lidocaine and 1:100,000 epinephrine solution. Following injection, the scrub nurse drapes the auricle with three layers of sterile sheets. The first layer consists of four paper adhesive sheets placed in a squared-off fashion about the auricle. This is followed by a 3M plastic ear drape (No. 1030). This waterproof sheet effectively isolates the patient and prevents contamination should the paper drapes become soaked with irrigation solution. Finally, a custom-designed paper otologic drape and a plastic drainage bag are applied (Fig. 11–1).

Irrigation and suction tubing and cautery lines are secured to the field using Velcro adhesive pads. The scrub

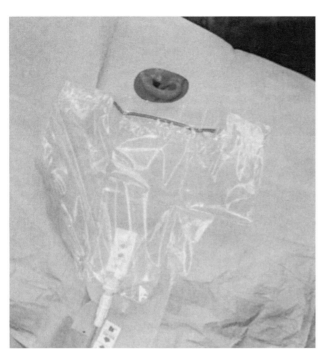

FIGURE 11–1. *The ear and postauricular area are prepared and draped in a sterile fashion.*

nurse attaches a compartmentalized plastic pouch to the Mayo stand to hold suction tips and electrocauteries.

Anesthesia

All patients undergo general endotracheal anesthesia with an epinephrine-compatible anesthetic agent. Long circuits are used on the anesthesia machine to enable the anesthesiologist to be seated at the foot of the table, opposite the surgeon (Fig. 11–2). The scrub nurse is positioned at the head of the table across from the surgeon.

The vascular strip and four quadrants of the ear canal are injected with the 2 per cent lidocaine and 1:100,000 epinephrine solution. The local anesthetic reduces pain and

allows the patient to be kept relatively "light" during the procedure. No limitations on the use of nitrous oxide during graft placement are required. This is because the undersurface placement of the graft, along with packing of the eustachian tube orifice, precludes the graft being elevated off the drum remnant. Rather, the nitrous oxide bubbles escape harmlessly up the posterior canal wall.

Every attempt is made to extubate the patient deeply to avoid straining and potentially detrimental Valsalva efforts. Intravenous antiemetics are given in an attempt to reduce postsurgical nausea and vomiting.

Incisions

The vascular strip is outlined by making incisions at the tympanosquamous and tympanomastoid suture lines using a No. 67 Beaver knife blade. In addition, small inferiorly and superiorly based flaps are created by making right-angle incisions to the vascular strip incisions. The medial end of the vascular strip is formed by connecting the two primary incisions with a No. 72 Beaver blade approximately 2 mm lateral to the annulus (Fig. 11–3).

A postauricular incision approximately 5 mm behind the postauricular crease (Fig. 11–4) is executed. The surgeon firmly grasps the auricle in the left hand and forcefully pulls forward and outward. Constant tension allows identification of the loose areolar tissue overlying the temporalis fascia and creates a bloodless surgical plane. Incisional bleeding is controlled with electrical cautery.

Harvesting Fascia

Once hemostasis is achieved, a small Weitlaner retractor is positioned to hold the auricle forward. The scrub nurse places a small Senn retractor under the upper part of the incision and pulls laterally, exposing the temporalis fascia. The loose areolar tissue overlying the temporalis fascia is then ballooned up with a local anesthetic to facilitate its removal. An incision is made at the level of the linea temporalis and the areolar tissue is dissected free from the

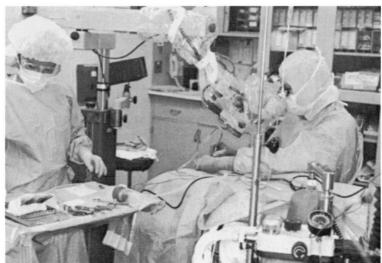

FIGURE 11–2. *Operating room arrangement. The scrub nurse is located directly across from the surgeon, and the anesthesiologist (not shown) is seated at the foot of the table.*

FIGURE 11–3

FIGURE 11–4

FIGURE 11–5

FIGURE 11–6

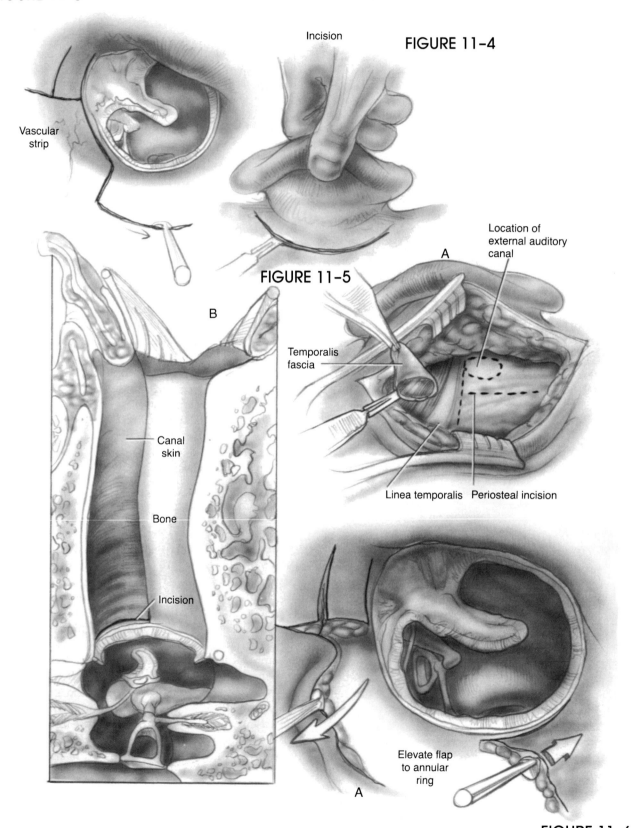

Incision

Vascular strip

Location of external auditory canal

A

B

Temporalis fascia

Canal skin

Bone

Incision

Linea temporalis   Periosteal incision

A

Elevate flap to annular ring

A

FIGURE 11–3 to 11–6. *See legends on opposite page*

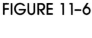

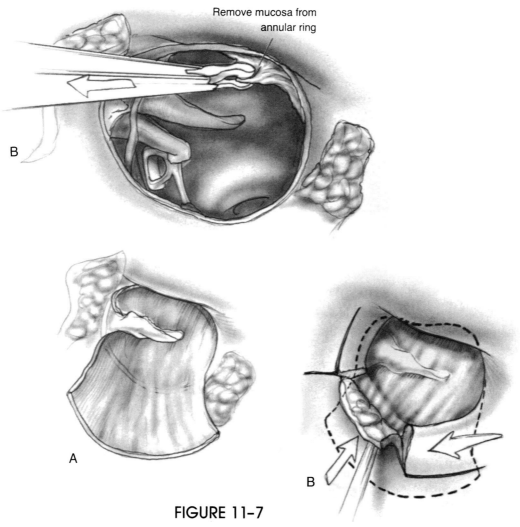

FIGURE 11-7

FIGURE 11-3. The vascular strip is outlined with a No. 67 and No. 72 Beaver blade.

FIGURE 11-4. A standard postauricular incision is fashioned approximately 5 mm behind the postauricular crease.

FIGURE 11-5. *A,* The loose areolar tissue overlying the temporalis fascia is harvested as a free graft. Note the T incision through the mastoid periosteum used to expose the external auditory canal. *B,* The vascular strip is held forward along with the auricle.

FIGURE 11-6. *A,* The inferior canal flap is elevated to the level of the fibrous annulus. *B,* The malleus is denuded and the undersurface of the drum remnant or annulus is abraded, while diseased mucosa is removed.

FIGURE 11-7. *A,* The fascia graft is directed under the fibrous annulus and malleus handle. *B,* The superior and inferior canal flaps are replaced over the fascia graft.

temporalis fascia using Metzenbaum scissors (Fig. 11–5). This tissue is then pressed onto a polytetrafluoroethylene (Teflon) block and placed on the back table under a gooseneck lamp to dehydrate it.

Exposing the Middle Ear

The retractor is removed and an incision is made along the linea temporalis extending anterior and superior to the external auditory canal. A T-shaped incision is then created by dropping a vertical limb from the midpoint of the linea temporalis to the mastoid tip (see Fig. 11–5). A Lempert elevator is used to mobilize the periosteum to the level of the ear canal. The vascular strip is then identified from posteriorly, grasped with Adson forceps and held forward in the blade of a Weitlaner retractor along with the auricle (see Fig. 11–5). A second Weitlaner retractor is placed between the temporalis muscle and the mastoid tip at right angles to the first retractor.

The ear canal is copiously irrigated with a physiologic saline solution to remove blood debris. With a 20-gauge needle suction in the left hand and a House No. 2 lancet knife in the right, the skin of the inferior ear canal is elevated down to the fibrous annulus (Fig. 11–6), creating an inferiorly based flap. Next, a House No. 1 sickle knife is used to develop a superior flap just above the short process of the malleus. The fibrous annulus is mobilized out of its sulcus anterior to the malleus.

If the operating table is rotated away from the surgeon, the anterior drum remnant and annulus are easily seen. Should a bony overhang obscure complete vision, the canal skin can be reflected laterally, the bone removed with a small diamond burr and the skin reflected downward. Care must be taken to protect the anterior annulus and adjacent canal skin.

Eradication of Disease

With the middle ear now well exposed, the primary disease process can be addressed logically. Cholesteatoma, granulation tissue, or polypoid disease can be removed through the middle ear itself or in conjunction with a mastoidectomy if indicated. For better exposure of the middle ear, the facial recess or posterior tympanotomy is opened, leaving the posterior canal wall intact.

Preparation of the Tympanic Membrane Remnant

Once the disease of the middle ear and mastoid has been eradicated, the drum remnant is prepared for grafting. Small attic, marginal, or central perforations are prepared so as to preserve the normal drum remnant. In the case of an extensive perforation of a severely diseased membrane, the entire drum remnant is removed to the level of the annulus. The manubrium of the malleus is denuded, preserving the fibrous annulus. The mucosa of the undersurface of the drum remnant or annulus is then abraded through the use of a House No. 1 sickle knife and cup

forceps to further ensure an adequate recipient surface for the graft (see Fig. 11–6).

Placement of the Graft

It is imperative that excellent hemostasis be achieved prior to graft placement. Absorbable gelatin sponge saturated in 1:1000 epinephrine is packed into the middle ear space while the graft is being fashioned. A dried areolar tissue graft is then removed from the polytetrafluoroethylene block and trimmed to size (approximately 2.5 × 1.5 cm). A slit is made toward the superior aspect of the graft to accommodate placement medial to the malleus handle.

If mucosa has been removed from the middle ear, a sheet of absorbable gelatin film (Gelfilm) is trimmed and placed onto the promontory to prevent adhesions. The epinephrine-soaked gelatin sponge is removed and the middle ear is packed with saline-moistened gelatin sponge starting from the eustachian tube and working posteriorly.

The graft is grasped using cup forceps, rehydrated in a physiologic saline solution, such as Tis-U-Sol, and placed in the middle ear. With a 22-gauge suction in the left hand and a right-angle hook in the other, the graft is slid under the manubrium of the malleus onto the lateral attic wall. A House annulus elevator is used to tuck the fascia under the drum remnant anteriorly and inferiorly (Fig. 11–7).

With this technique, there is a point in the inferior canal at approximately 6 o'clock where the graft makes a transition from lying medial to the annulus to being lateral to it. The remaining graft is draped along the posterior canal wall and the inferior canal flap with attached annulus is repositioned over the graft. Similarly, the superior flap is placed, covering the fascia lying anterior to the malleus (see Fig. 11–7). A gimmick is used to even all edges of the annulus and smooth out the graft. Flap margins must be assured flat because buried skin may result in "pearl" formation. Polysporin ointment is then placed over the fascia graft filling the anterior sulcus. The retractors are removed and the vascular strip is carefully replaced to its original position. The mastoid periosteum incision is closed with 3-0 Vicryl suture in interrupted fashion.

The postauricular incision is then closed with the same 4-0 suture in a subcuticular fashion. No skin sutures are used, obviating later removal. Proper position of the vascular strip is once again confirmed under direct vision through an ear speculum, and the remainder of the ear canal is filled with antibiotic ointment. A cotton ball is placed in the meatus, and a sterile, prepackaged plastic mastoid bubble dressing is applied (Fig. 11–8).

POSTOPERATIVE CARE

Before discharge the mastoid dressing is removed. A sterile, prepackaged postauricular dressing is applied behind the ear and a fresh cotton ball is placed in the meatus of the ear canal to absorb the ointment as it liquifies. Patients are instructed to change the cotton ball at least three times per day and whenever it becomes soiled. A 3-week follow-up appointment is arranged. Each individual is counseled as to the warning signs of infection and instructed to

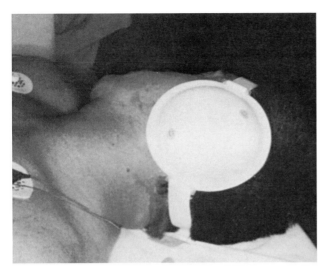

FIGURE 11–8. A sterile prepackaged mastoid dressing is applied.

contact the office immediately should these occur. A prescription for analgesics is given. Patients are asked to keep the ear dry and to avoid nose blowing.

By the first postoperative visit, the postauricular wound should be well healed, the ear canal free of ointment, and the tympanic membrane epithelialized. All tympanoplasty patients undergo a pure-tone audiogram at this visit. By 6 weeks, the grafted eardrum has thinned considerably and takes on an appearance of a normal tympanic membrane. Follow-up visits are arranged at 6 and 12 months and, thereafter, yearly.

RESULTS

In 1982, Glasscock and associates reported their experience in 1556 cases of tympanic membrane repair using the herein described postauricular undersurface grafting technique.[5] Of these cases, 663 were simple tympanoplasties, 687 involved a mastoidectomy, 54 were performed to repair a graft failure at a second stage, 38 involved a tympanoplasty with mastoid revision, and 114 were canal wall down mastoidectomies in which the tympanic membrane was grafted. Four hundred sixty-three ears (34 percent) had undergone at least one previous surgery. All tympanic membranes were repaired using areolar tissue, temporalis fascia, or tragal perichondrium.

Of the 1556 ears, there were a total of 110 failures, for an overall graft success rate of 93 per cent. Of the failures, 19 occurred within 3 weeks of surgery, 31 at 3 months, 19 at 6 months, and 41 after 1 year. Successful grafting occurred in 91.5 per cent of patients younger than 12 years of age as compared with 93.3 per cent of patients older than 12 years. Similarly, the graft success rate was 92.7 per cent in draining ears and 93.1 per cent in dry ears. The presence of cholesteatoma had no apparent effect on success. Ears with cholesteatoma had a 92 per cent success rate; those without averaged 93.2 per cent.

Complications were minimal in this series. Postoperative otorrhea occurred in 6 per cent, varying from a mild otitis externa to a severe middle ear infection promoting loss of the graft. True wound infections were seen in fewer than 0.5 per cent. Sensorineural hearing loss occurred in fewer than 1 per cent of the cases. There were five cases of delayed facial paralysis, all of which recovered completely within 2 to 3 weeks. Serous otitis media occurred in 2 per cent, whereas perichondritis, stenosis of the external auditory canal, and epithelial pearls occurred in fewer than 0.5 per cent.

CARTILAGE GRAFT TYMPANOPLASTY

In cases of severe atelectasis of the tympanic membrane, a cartilage tympanoplasty is often indicated. Cartilage autografts have long been used in repair of canal wall defects as well as ossiculoplasty.[25–28] In 1982, Glasscock and associates first described the successful use of cartilage-perichondral autografts for severe atelectasis, attic cholesteatoma, and posterior retraction pockets.[5] Since that time, others have reported their results with this technique.[29–31]

The goal of cartilage tympanoplasty is to prevent recurrent retraction along with their long-term sequelae including cholesteatoma formation, ossicular erosion, and progressive hearing loss. Incorporation of cartilage in the repair of the eardrum provides sufficient structural integrity to resist recurrent retraction yet imparts minimal impedance. This technique is ideally suited for patients who demonstrate persistent eustachian tubal dysfunction, including cleft palate patients or those with recurrent atelectasis following standard fascia graft tympanoplasty.

Surgical Techniques

Once exposure of the middle ear is obtained, the next step is to excise all diseased and atelectatic tympanic membrane. The posterior fibrous annulus is elevated from its bony sulcus with a House No. 2 lancet knife. Careful dissection is required to avoid tearing the atelectatic drum to ensure that no epithelium will be left in the middle ear. To verify complete removal of an attic retraction, it is often necessary to perform mastoidectomy. Posterosuperior retractions must be elevated in continuity with the remainder of the tympanic membrane. When elevating the drum off the lenticular process and the stapes suprastructure, applying force in the posterior-to-anterior direction will allow the stapedius tendon to provide countertraction, thereby preventing inadvertent stapes subluxation. A House No. 1 sickle knife is used to elevate the diseased membrane off the manubrium and lateral process of the malleus. Fibrous adhesions are lysed and diseased middle ear mucosa is removed with cup forceps (Fig. 11–9).

To harvest the cartilage perichondrial graft, an incision is made on the posteromedial surface of the tragus (Fig. 11–10). This incision is actually carried through the tragal cartilage, and, in so doing, preserving the dome of the tragal cartilage for cosmesis. A House No. 2 lancet elevator is used to elevate the perichondrium from one surface of the cartilage, leaving it hinged on the other side, like a book cover. The cartilage is trimmed to the proper dimensions, depending on the degree of disease present. A posterosup-

FIGURE 11-9

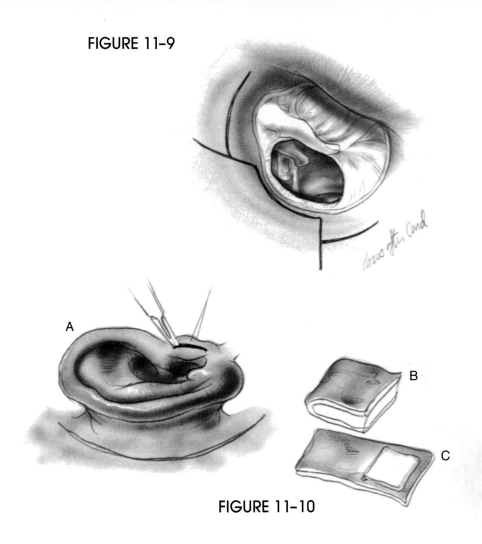

FIGURE 11-10

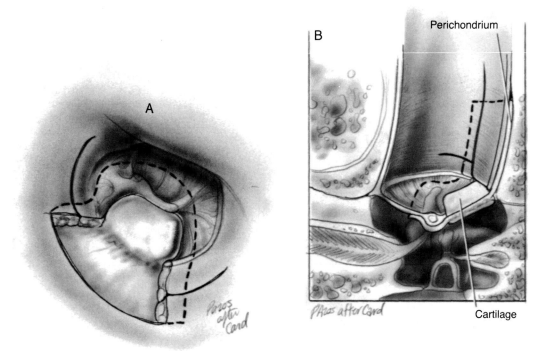

FIGURE 11-11

FIGURE 11–9 to 11–11. *See legends on opposite page*

erior quadrant retraction often requires a cartilage graft of approximately 4 mm in diameter. For cases of atelectasis of the entire tympanic membrane, the cartilage can be incorporated into the entire pars tensa. In this situation, a wedge-shaped area of cartilage is accessed to accommodate the manubrium, if present. When using large cartilage grafts not likely to move in healing, perichondrium is not necessarily needed and is detached.

Once the middle ear has been packed with moistened absorbable gelatin sponge, the cartilage-perichondrial graft is placed with the perichondrium side facing laterally. The perichondrium is then tucked under the manubrium and draped over the ear canal posteriorly. The cartilage should not overlap the posterior canal wall. The areolar tissue graft is then trimmed to size and placed lateral to the cartilage perichondrial graft and medial to the fibrous annulus and manubrium (Fig. 11–11). This areolar graft serves to cover any remaining defects in the tympanic membrane or exposed bone in the external canal. When perichondrium is not used, the cartilage graft is placed atop the middle ear Gelfoam and the tympanic membrane graft lateral. The cartilage is ultimately enveloped by the neo–tympanic membrane. The superior- and inferior-based canal flaps are then returned to their original positions, covering the grafts as they extend onto the posterior canal wall. The external canal is then filled with Polysporin ointment and closure proceeds in the manner previously described.

Results

Results in 100 ears using cartilage tympanoplasty were recently reported.[32] The retracted portion of the tympanic membrane was in the posterosuperior quadrant in 37 per cent, the entire drum in 34 per cent, the posterior half in 18 per cent, the pars flaccida alone in 16 per cent, the pars flaccida and pars tensa combined in 4 per cent, and the anterior half in 1 per cent. Thirty-three ears had cholesteatoma present. Fifty-two ears required ossicular reconstruction, of which 31 were performed simultaneously with the cartilage tympanoplasty. Twenty-one were staged.

Hearing results were reported in 79 ears by calculating the postoperative average air-bone gap for the speech frequencies (500, 1000, and 2000 Hz) in 10-dB increments. On these 79 cases, 38 per cent achieved closure of the air-bone gap to within 10 dB, whereas 39 per cent closed within 20 dB. Eighteen percent closed within 30 dB. Five per cent of the patients failed to demonstrate closure to less than 30 dB.

Of the 100 ears, there were four failures (4 per cent) in terms of the technique itself. There were two recurrent cholesteatomas, one perforation, and one recurrent retraction. Six patients (6 per cent) developed serous otitis media postoperatively. Of these six patients, three eventually required ventilation tubes. Fifteen patients had mild retractions that were easily controlled with modified Valsalva exercises. There were two wound infections and six cases of external auditory canal infections. Perichondritis and external canal stenosis did not occur in this series.

SUMMARY

The major objectives of tympanoplasty may be prioritized as follows: (1) control of infection, (2) creation of an air-containing middle ear space, and (3) hearing rehabilitation. To accomplish these goals, it is imperative that the otologic surgeon exercise sound clinical judgment in terms of selection of patients as well as surgical approach. The fundamental components of the surgery must be understood and assiduously executed. Success should be achievable in well over 90 per cent patients.

For the average surgeon, the postauricular undersurface graft technique of myringoplasty will yield consistently superior functional results with fewer complications than those seen with classic transcanal undersurface procedures or overlay techniques.

References

1. Wullstein H: Funktionelle Operationen im Mittelokr mit Hilfe des Freven Spalthappen-Transplantes. Arch Ohr Nas Kehlhopfheilk 161: 422, 1952.
2. Zollner F: The principles of plastic surgery of the sound-conducting apparatus. J Laryngol Otol 69: 637, 1955.
3. Austin DF, Shea JJ: A new system of tympanoplasty using vein graft. Laryngoscope 71: 596, 1961.
4. Glasscock ME: Tympanic membrane grafting with fascia: Overlay versus underlay technique. Laryngoscope 5: 754, 1973.
5. Glasscock ME, Jackson CJ, Nissen AJ, et al: Postauricular undersurface tympanic membrane grafting: A follow-up report. Laryngoscope 92: 718, 1982.
6. Committee on Conservation of Hearing of the American Academy of Ophthalmology and Otolaryngology: Standard Classification for Surgery of Chronic Ear Infection. Arch Otolaryngol Head Neck Surg 81: 204, 1964.
7. Toynbee J: On the Use of an Artificial Membrane Tympanic in Cases of Deafness Dependent Upon Perforations or Destruction of the Natural Organ. London, J. Churchill and Sons, 1853.
8. Yearsley J: Deafness, Practically Illustrated. Ecl. 6, London, J. Churchill and Sons, 1863.
9. Blake CJ: Transactions of the First Congress of the International Otological Society. New York, D. Appleton, 1887, p 125.
10. Roosa DB St. J: Disease of the Ear, 3rd ed. New York, William Wood, 1876.

FIGURE 11–9. Standard vascular strip incisions are made. A House sickle knife opens the middle ear and elevates the atelectic drum.

FIGURE 11–10. A, The tragal cartilage perichondrial graft is harvested by means of an incision on the posteromedial aspect of the tragus. B, The tragal perichondrium is elevated off the surface of the cartilage. C, The cartilage is trimmed to the desired size.

FIGURE 11–11. A, The cartilage perichondrial graft is positioned medial to the manubrium and fibrous annulus. The areolar tissue graft is then positioned lateral to the cartilage perichondrial graft but medial to the annulus and manubrium. B, Lateral view demonstrating the cartilage perichondrial graft in place. Ossiculoplasty is typically performed at a second stage.

11. Joynt JA: Repair of the drum. J Iowa Med Soc 9: 51, 1919.
12. Linn EG: Closure of tympanic membrane perforations. Arch Otolaryngol Head Neck Surg 58: 405, 1953.
13. Derlacki EL: Repair of central perforations of the tympanic membrane. Arch Otolaryngol Head Neck Surg 58: 405, 1953.
14. House WF, Sheehy JL: Myringoplasty. Arch Otolaryngol 73: 407, 1961.
15. Plester D: Myringoplasty methods. Arch Otolaryngol 78: 310, 1963.
16. Shea JJ: Vein graft closure of eardrum perforations. J Otolaryngol 74: 358, 1960.
17. Tabb HG: Closure of perforations of the tympanic membrane by vein grafts: A preliminary report of 20 cases. Laryngoscope 70: 271, 1960.
18. Goodhill V: Tragal perichondrium and cartilage in tympanoplasty. Arch Otolaryngol 85: 480, 1967.
19. Glasscock ME, House WF: Homograft reconstruction of the middle ear. Laryngoscope 78: 1219, 1968.
20. Storrs LA: Myringoplasty with the use of fascia grafts. Arch Otolaryngol 74: 65, 1961.
21. Gates GA, Avery CA, Prihoda TJ, Cooper JC Jr: Effectiveness of adenoidectomy and tympanostomy tubes in treatment of chronic otitis media with effusion. N Engl J Med 317: 1444–1451, 1987.
22. Fry TL, Pillsbury HC: The implications of controlled studies of tonsillectomy and adenoidectomy. Otolaryngol Clin North Am 20: 409–413, 1987.
23. Jackson CG: Antimicrobial prophylaxis in ear surgery. Laryngoscope 98: 1116–1123, 1988.
24. Sheehy JL, Glasscock ME: Tympanic membrane grafting with temporalis fascia. Arch Otolaryngol 86: 391, 1967.
25. Donald FJ, McCabe BF, Loevy SS, et al: Atticotomy: A neglected otosurgical technique. Ann Otol Rhinol Laryngol 83: 652, 1974.
26. McCleve DE: Repair of bony canal wall defects in tympanomastoid surgery. Am J Otol 6: 76, 1985.
27. McCleve DE: Tragal reconstruction of the auditory canal. Arch Otolaryngol 90: 35, 1969.
28. Linda RE: The cartilage-perichondrium graft in the treatment of posterior tympanic membrane retraction pockets. Laryngoscope 83: 747, 1973.
29. Schwaber MK: Postauricular undersurface tympanic membrane grafting: Some modifications of the "swinging door" technique. Arch Otolaryngol Head Neck Surg 95: 182, 1986.
30. Levenson RM: Cartilage-perichondrial composite graft tympanoplasty in the treatment of posterior marginal and attic retraction pockets. Laryngoscope 97: 1069, 1987.
31. Adkins W: Composite autograft for tympanoplasty and tympanomastoid surgery. Laryngoscope 100: 244, 1990.
32. Glasscock ME, Hart MJ: Surgical treatment of the atelectatic ear. Otolaryngol Head Neck Surg 3: 15, 1992.

12

Tympanoplasty: Ossicular Tissue, Hydroxyapatite, and HAPEX

Roger E. Wehrs, M.D.

In the early and mid 1960s, repositioning of the patient's incus fragment emerged as the most reliable method of ossicular reconstruction in tympanoplasty.[1] In 1967, I published an article suggesting the substitution of homograft incudes when the patient's incus was unusable.[2] These ossicles were first used as wedges between the patient's stapes and malleus in the same way that the autograft incus had been employed. They functioned well, with no tendency to extrude, and were invaded by blood vessels and covered with mucous membrane to become living tissue.

To improve their stability and improve hearing, prostheses were sculptured from these homograft incudes.[3] Two primary prostheses emerged: the notched incus with short process and the notched incus with long process. The first replaced the patient's incus and carried the sound pressure from the malleus to the intact stapes. The second replaced not only the incus but also the stapedial superstructure and carried sound directly to the stapedial footplate (Fig. 12–1A and B).[4] Because two-point fixation occurred between the notch under the malleus handle and the stapedial head or footplate, these prostheses locked in place.

They were stable because the notch under the malleus prevented dislocation either forward or backward. The prostheses would not be displaced inferiorly because of the spring of the malleus, or superiorly, because of the tensor tympani tendon. Furthermore, sound pressure was thus carried to the fluids of the inner ear by direct columellar pressure. This design, therefore, produced excellent hearing and anatomic results.[5] However, there are disadvantages with the use of the human tissue: It can be difficult or impossible to obtain, has a limited shelf life, and carries the remote danger of disease transmission. Also, there cannot be any mass production of a standardized sterile prosthesis that would meet definite criteria.

It was deemed prudent and necessary, therefore, to develop an acceptable alternative for the homograft ossicles that would be biocompatible, similar to bone in weight and physical characteristics, and able to be made into the same dimensions and shape as prostheses derived from homograft ossicles. The rationale for the design was that the notched incus homografts with long and short processes had evolved over time into prostheses of proven reliability. They had consistently produced good anatomic and functional results with a minimum of complications. Hydroxyapatite most nearly met these specifications. It had a long history of excellent biocompatibility, including use in the middle ear.[6] It had the same color and approximate appearance as bone. Furthermore, it could easily be shaped with

a diamond burr into prostheses. The bony prostheses known as *notched incudes with short and long processes* were used as patterns. Prostheses of hydroxyapatite were sculptured to have the same size and characteristics as those of bone (Fig. 12–2A and B). The early prostheses were square and boxy and had sharp edges. Furthermore, their surfaces were smooth and slick, so that they could not be picked up with a suction tip, as was done with their bony counterparts. These first prototypes functioned satisfactorily and proved that the concept of replacing a familiar and time-proven prosthesis with an identical one of a different material was valid.

The early prostheses were modified to make them thinner with rounded contours, even more like their predecessors of bone. By a process similar to sandblasting, the surfaces were satinized so that they could be picked up with suction tips and maneuvered into position.

Further modification, again learned from the homograft prosthesis, consisted of extra notches in the short process to accommodate an anteriorly placed malleus (Fig. 12–3A and B). There is also variation in the height of the stapes and the distance from the footplate to the graft. Therefore, prostheses of different heights were developed.

The most recent innovation occurred in 1996. This involved the attachment of a hydroxyapatite-reinforced polyethylene composite (HAPEX) cuff or shaft to the dense hydroxyapatite body. In this way the portion of the prosthesis that contacted the malleus and tympanic membrane preserved the biocompatible hydroxyapatite body, while the middle ear part that was in contact with the stapes and stapedial footplate was composed of HAPEX, which could be cut to length with a knife. This arose out of the fact that even though the eardrum and ossicles are completely formed at birth and are remarkably similar in size and shape, numerous variations occur, especially in the relationship of the stapes to the eardrum and malleus. To meet these situations it had been necessary to create 16 different shapes and sizes of the solid hydroxyapatite prostheses. Furthermore, it was often necessary to round the square shaft or shorten and modify the prosthesis with a diamond burr. Although this was not difficult, it was problematic and time consuming.

Advantages of these innovations are that it is necessary to maintain only four basic types of prostheses: the incus and the incus-stapes, each with a single or double notch. The rounded cuff of HAPEX on the stapes prosthesis is made slightly larger than the previous hole drilled in the dense hydroxyapatite body and can be cut to the exact

FIGURE 12-1

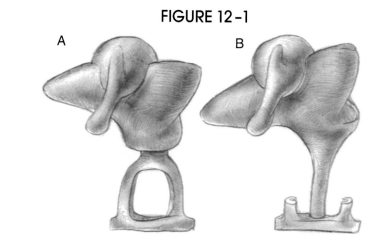

A   B

FIGURE 12-2

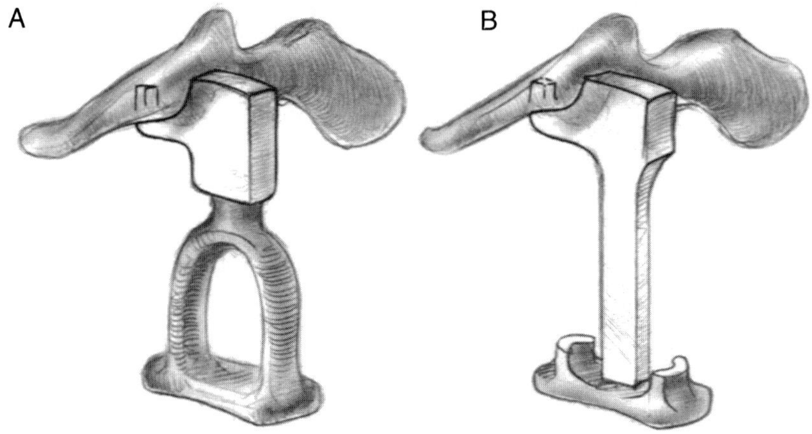

A   B

FIGURE 12-3

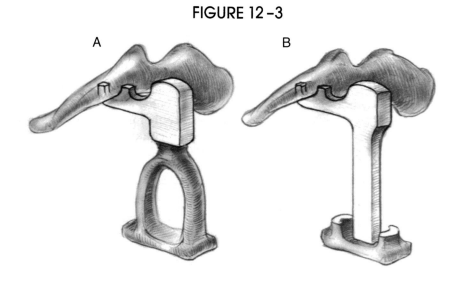

A   B

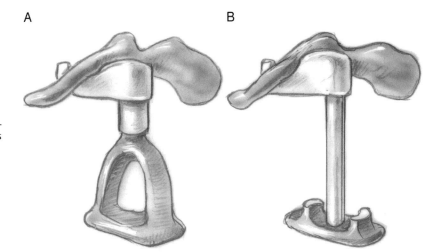

FIGURE 12–4. HAPEX prostheses. *A*, Incus replacement prosthesis of HAPEX. *B*, Incus-stapes replacement prosthesis of HAPEX.

length and the interior of the cuff may be reamed out to more easily engage a large stapedial head.

The original solid incus-stapes prosthesis had a square shaft that fit poorly to the stapedial footplate and occasionally touched the edges of the oval window area. It was often necessary to drill off the square corners and round this shaft with a diamond burr; also, the dense hydroxyapatite shaft was stiff and inflexible. The HAPEX shaft on the other hand is smaller, round, and flexible so that it would fit between the crura of an intact stapes.

HAPEX is a homogeneous osteoconductive biomaterial that is composed of 40 per cent hydroxyapatite and 60 per cent polyethylene (by volume). This material approximates the mechanical strength of bone yet is soft enough to be cut with a knife.

This new design preserves the classic size and shape of the original bony prostheses that carried the time-tested proof of function and reliability. They are inserted and utilized exactly as were their predecessors, but because of their simplicity and ease of use, they have almost completely replaced the homograft and solid dense hydroxyapatite prostheses (Fig. 12–4*A* and *B*).

PATIENT SELECTION

All patients with a perforated eardrum are potential candidates for tympanoplasty with ossicular reconstruction. During the initial or preoperative examination, a significant conductive loss may be discovered. Erosion of the long process of the incus may also be seen. These findings indicate that the patient will require ossicular reconstruction. However, there may be only a slight retraction pocket over the long process of the incus with little conductive component to the hearing loss. Not until the time of surgery is the long process of the incus discovered to be friable or stiff, necessitating reconstruction.

Other candidates for the procedure may present with an intact eardrum but a significant conductive component to their hearing loss. These may represent a congenital malformation of the ossicles or cases of revision, in which the reconstruction was delayed to a second stage.

A history of head injury, especially correlated to distortion of the eardrum or healed fracture of the bony ear canal, may indicate ossicular discontinuity and the need for reconstruction.

Patients with cholesteatoma are prime candidates for ossicular reconstruction, because the incus and head of the malleus usually need to be removed even if the ossicular chain is intact and there was a minimal air-bone gap before surgery.

Surgery is recommended when the ear is dry and clean, often at the initial visit if no cholesteatoma or infection is present. As a general rule the type of prosthesis that will be used and its composition are determined at the time of surgery. Occasionally, a patient will express a specific desire for either artificial material or the homograft transplant, and these wishes are respected as much as possible.

Preoperative Evaluation and Counseling

The patient is informed and brought into the surgical planning as much as possible. Today, most patients are sophisticated and well informed. They need to understand the rationale for as well as the advantages and disadvantages

FIGURE 12–1. Homograft incus prostheses. *A*, Notched incus with short process. *B*, Notched incus with long process.

FIGURE 12–2. Hydroxyapatite prostheses. *A*, Incus replacement prosthesis. *B*, Incus-stapes replacement prosthesis.

FIGURE 12–3. Hydroxyapatite prostheses with double notch. *A*, Incus replacement prosthesis. *B*, Incus-stapes replacement prosthesis.

of the procedure. This is especially true of the patients who have had one or more failures with previous ear surgery.

When patients present with a dry perforation and obvious ossicular discontinuity, they are informed that they have a 90 per cent chance of improved hearing with a dry and grafted eardrum. They are further told that in some instances the hearing may not improve but may actually get worse. In most instances, this loss would be conductive in nature, and a revision would be indicated. However, in rare instances (usually fewer than 1 per cent) the hearing could become worse as a result of deterioration of the nerve of hearing, and in extreme cases the patient could lose all hearing in that ear.

Because most surgery that I perform is through the ear canal, pain is usually controllable with acetaminophen or mild analgesics. Also, bleeding is not a problem, and antibiotics are not used routinely.

The return of hearing acuity varies among patients and depends on several factors. If they have bilateral middle ear disease and a large conductive component in each ear, they may notice some improvement at the first postoperative visit 2 weeks following surgery; however, if the opposite ear exhibits normal hearing, patients are not aware of much improvement until 4 to 6 weeks following the reconstruction. The first postoperative hearing test is obtained when the ear is healed, approximately 6 to 8 weeks after surgery.

PREOPERATIVE EVALUATION

It is my firm opinion that any type of ear surgery is more successful if the ear is dry or at least not infected at the time of surgery. When a patient is initially seen seeking relief from infection and hearing loss, the ear must first be treated medically.

Medical Treatment

The first priority is to carefully clean the ear under microscopic vision so that the pathology can be more accurately evaluated and the proper medications can reach the skin of the ear canal and mucous membrane lining of the middle ear and mastoid. By means of a small suction, exudate is removed from the ear canal, as well as through the perforation. Following this procedure, the ear is carefully wiped with small cotton-tipped wire applicators dipped in a corticosteroid otic suspension, such as Cortisporin. All exfoliated skin and debris are removed by wiping the ear canal. Also, by wiping the ear canal, the medication is applied to the skin of the ear canal. Following this step, chloramphenicol (Chloromycetin) powder is gently insufflated into the ear canal and through the perforation. The patient is then instructed on aural hygiene, which consists of the following regimen.

The patient is instructed not to rub or press on the ear or to clean it with cotton-tipped applicators. After the physician has cleaned the ear, the itching is usually less of a problem and may be controlled with acetaminophen or diphenhydramine (Benadryl). Also, rubbing the ear has often become a habit and part of a vicious circle of itching, rubbing, and drainage. Once patients realize the importance of aural hygiene, they can leave the ear alone.

The only way patients should clean the ear is with a finger in a damp wash cloth with the head tipped toward the affected side. They should also not wash their hair in a shower: They should use a cotton ball saturated in white petroleum jelly in the outer ear when washing hair over a sink or tub.

Most people with a draining ear believe they should sleep on the ear so that it can "drain better." In my opinion, this is exactly the wrong thing to do, because the exudate should drain down the eustachian tube and not onto the external ear, where it causes irritation and crusting. The patient is instructed to place a large spiny hair curler in the hair just above the affected ear. This will remind him or her not to lie on the ear with the perforation.

Careful follow-up is essential, and the patient is asked to return in a few days to 2 weeks, depending on the severity of the infection. On returning, the ear is usually dry and clean. If it is not, the reason for the persistent discharge must be ascertained. Often, this persistence is due to a mucous plug in the eustachian tube. If this condition is suspected, the ear should again be suctioned to remove all excess mucus and debris. The patient then lies with the affected ear up, and the canal is filled with a corticosteroid drop, preferably Neodecadron, because it is less viscid than Cortisporin. A pneumatic otoscope is then used to apply pressure and force the drops through the eustachian tube. One often feels a sudden release of pressure as the eustachian tube opens and the medication flows into the patient's nasopharynx. If the tube will not open easily, excess pressure should be avoided, because it may cause vertigo, and there is also a rare possibility of rupturing the dura over a dehiscent mastoid tegmen and producing meningitis or a brain abscess.

The eustachian tube blockage may be due to mucosal edema or scar tissue from previous surgery. The occasional patient may also develop an allergy to certain medications, often the neomycin present in almost all otic drops. If an allergy is suspected, an ophthalmologic medication, such as Decadron ophthalmic solution, is substituted.

Systemic antibiotics are of limited benefit in a chronically draining ear; however, on the first visit, the ear discharge should be cultured and the appropriate systemic antibiotic administered.

PREOPERATIVE PREPARATION

Before the actual surgery, the patient is positioned on the operating table. Because great variation exists in the size and inclination of the external auditory meatus and the corpus of the patient, a few minutes spent in positioning the patient at the beginning of the procedure is saved many times over by allowing the surgeon to work in a relaxed manner.

Following routine prepping and draping of the ear and immediately prior to the first incision, the ear is copiously irrigated with 70 per cent ethyl alcohol through the ear speculum, with constant irrigation to remove all wax and debris and to further sterilize the ear canal and drum.

After repeated washings, the alcohol is removed with

repeated irrigations and suction with Ringer's lactated solution. The alcohol irrigation is used regardless of an open perforation and is in fact used to remove the mucus and debris from the middle ear and margins of the perforation. If the perforation is dry and clean, Ringer's lactate is used alone.

SPECIAL INSTRUMENTS

Because the canal skin tympanoplasty is often used to prepare the ear for ossicular reconstruction, special instruments are used in this procedure. These consist of canal skin knives, in which the blade is oval and longer than the 2- or 3-mm one usually employed. The blades are approximately 4 and 5 mm in length and are used to elevate the canal skin from under the bony overhang of the anterior bony canal wall. Special diamond burrs, 3 to 4 mm in diameter, have also been designed for the Skeeter drill to remove the bony overhang of the anterior canal wall after the canal skin has been removed.

Another valuable instrument is the Posigator forceps, which is an alligator forceps with a spring design that keeps the jaws closed until they are opened by the surgeon. In this way, the prosthesis may be picked up by the scrub nurse and handed to the surgeon, who can place it in position without the danger of it being released by the forceps and dropping on the floor.

SURGICAL TECHNIQUE

Most cases of ossicular reconstruction are approached through the ear canal. It is important to use a speculum holder so that both hands are free to hold the suction device and instruments. Tapered speculums should also be employed; they hold the vascular strip out of the way, providing good anterior and inferior views.

Dry central perforations, retracted perforations, congenital ear problems with ossicular discontinuity, second-stage tympanoplasties, and cases of ossicular discontinuity due to trauma may be approached in this manner. Infected ears with mastoid disease or squamous ingrowth or cholesteatoma should be approached through a postauricular incision. Regardless of the approach used, the actual ossicular reconstruction is identical and is described in detail.

OSSICULAR RECONSTRUCTION

Three main categories of ossicular defects prevent the transmission of sound pressure across the middle ear: loss of ossicular continuity, (2) fixation of the ossicles, and (3) a combination of the two.

As described previously, sculptured prostheses made from homograft ossicles were used exclusively for many years. However, from 1986 to 1996 clones made of hydroxyapatite played a prominent role in ossicular reconstruction. Since their introduction in 1996 the HAPEX modifications of the prostheses have been used almost exclusively. This has been because of their versatility and ease of use combined with the tried and true design of their predecessors. They are completely interchangeable with the bony or dense hydroxyapatite prostheses, and the following details of technique apply equally to all materials.

INCUS REPLACEMENT PROSTHESIS

The incus replacement prosthesis is used to correct a break in the ossicular chain caused by a defect of the incus. It rebuilds the hearing mechanism between an intact and mobile stapes and the manubrium of the malleus.

The lenticular process of the incus usually remains attached to the head of the stapes. If possible, the incudostapedial joint is separated and the lenticular process is removed. In this way, any squamous epithelium on the tip of the long process or lenticular process is removed. The normal-sized head ensures that the hole in the prosthesis will fit over the capitulum of the stapes. If the incudostapedial joint is fused and replaced by bone, or if the stapes is extremely mobile, the lenticular process should not be removed, because the manipulations required could produce trauma to the inner ear, dislocation of the stapedial footplate, or both. Therefore, if the joint does not separate easily, it should be left attached. It is important, however, to remove all squamous epithelium, scar tissue, or mucous membrane from the lenticular process. Because the attached lenticular process makes the stapes higher, a shorter prosthesis will be required.

The distance between the head of the stapes and the malleus is evaluated. Unless the malleus appears to be directly over the stapes or extremely far forward, the single-notch HAPEX prosthesis is chosen. Next, the height of the stapes to the malleus and posterior annulus is evaluated. In 80 per cent of the cases the stapes head will be 2 to 3 mm below the malleus handle, and the HAPEX cuff of the incus replacement prosthesis is cut just below its attachment to the hydroxyapatite body to create a short prosthesis. Occasionally it is necessary to make the cut higher and next to the body of the prosthesis or to remove the HAPEX cuff completely. If the latter is the case, then the hole in the hydroxyapatite prosthesis becomes larger and will often fit over the fused lenticular process of the incus and capitulum of the stapes, which is an added advantage.

The prosthesis is then introduced lying on its side on the promontory with the notch just off the tip of the malleus and the hole in the base near the stapes head (Fig. 12–5A). By means of a right-angle pick, the manubrium of the malleus is elevated, and the body of the prosthesis is engaged with a slightly curved pick and the notch slid up along the undersurface of the malleus (Fig. 12–5B). The hole in the prosthesis should then engage the stapedial head (Fig. 12–5C). The prosthesis is adjusted until it is vertical to the stapes and appears stable. It should be stable but loose. It should not be wedged tightly in place, because there may be insufficient movement, and the hearing results will not be as good. Also, there is danger of dislocation of the stapedial footplate and inner ear damage.

Gentle pressure on the body of the prosthesis should produce motion of the stapes (Fig. 12–5D). Motion can be

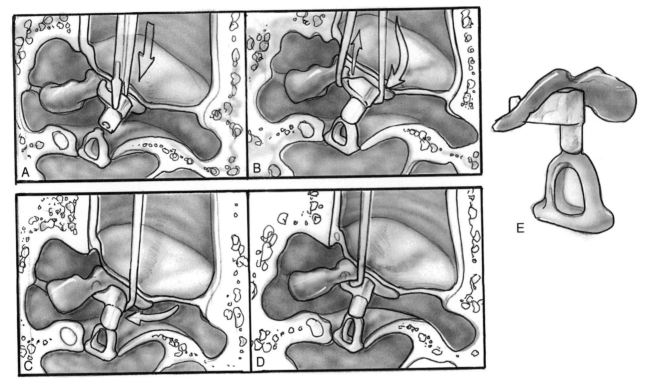

FIGURE 12–5. *A,* Introducing the HAPEX incus replacement prosthesis onto the promontory. *B,* Manipulating the incus prosthesis up under the malleus. *C,* The hole in the prosthesis fits over the stapes capitulum, and it is brought up to a vertical and stable position. *D,* The motion of the stapes is tested by gentle pressure on the prosthesis with a right-angle pick. *E,* Cutaway view of the final placement of HAPEX incus prosthesis.

determined by observing the stapedial footplate or tendon. Occasionally, a round window reflex can be obtained.

INCUS-STAPES PROSTHESIS

The incus-stapes prosthesis is used to reconstruct the hearing mechanisms when the stapes superstructure is absent. Reconstruction is carried out between the stapedial footplate and the malleus handle.

The footplate should be evaluated to determine if it is mobile. If it is covered by thick mucosa or scar tissue, this should be removed prior to reconstruction. The mucosa should also be removed from the undersurface of the malleus handle.

When the ear is prepared, the relationship of the malleus to the stapedial footplate is evaluated. The height from the stapedial footplate to the malleus determines the length of the prosthesis, whereas the distance from the center of the stapes footplate to the malleus determines the position of the notch. In my experience, the short, single-notch prosthesis is suitable in 80 per cent of the cases.

The prosthesis is placed on the promontory with the shaft of the implant on the stapedial footplate and the notch off the tip of the malleus (Fig. 12–6*A*). With a right-angle pick, the manubrium of the malleus is elevated, and a slightly curved pick is placed under the implant (Fig. 12–6*B*). The notch is slid up on the malleus (Fig. 12–6*C*). One should be careful not to exert undue pressure on the stapedial footplate or to wedge the prosthesis tightly in place. It

should fit loosely but not fall over without support. The round HAPEX shaft should be centered on the stapedial footplate by advancing it toward the anterior crus (Fig. 12–6*D*). This maneuver has the effect of increasing the height of the prosthesis and making a loose fit more secure. On the other hand, if the prosthesis is slightly too long, it will tend to tip forward, and the shaft will be at the posterior part of the footplate. If this is the case, the prosthesis should not be forced into place, because this could result in fracture or dislocation of the footplate and inner ear damage. The prosthesis should be pushed back down the malleus and removed. The HAPEX shaft is then shortened by cutting off the tip until it stands upright at the center of the stapedial footplate.

Occasionally, the tip of the malleus is very close to the promontory. In these cases, the prosthesis fits tightly under the tip as it is elevated, but once in an upright position, it appears too loose. It may be tipped slightly toward the promontory and slid down the malleus to a point where it is more stable. Absorbable gelatin sponge (Gelfoam) may be packed around the long process and body to stabilize it in position until healing has taken place.

MALLEAR DEFECTS

The malleus head may be fixed in the epitympanum by a bony bridge or direct attachment. The ossicular chain is usually intact but moves poorly, if at all.

Management of these cases consists of first separating

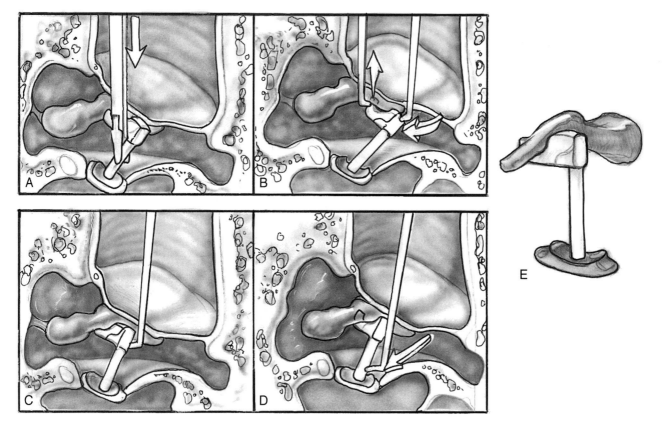

FIGURE 12–6. *A,* Placing the HAPEX incus-stapes prosthesis in the middle ear. *B,* The implant is manipulated with the notch under the malleus handle. *C,* The notch slides up the malleus to a vertical and stable position. *D,* Adjustment of the shaft so that the HAPEX shaft is centered on the stapedial footplate. *E,* Cutaway view demonstrates the final placement of HAPEX incus-stapes prosthesis.

the incudostapedial joint to prevent any injury to the inner ear when the malleus is manipulated. Next, the mobility of the stapes is ascertained to be sure it was not the culprit producing the fixation. The incudomallear joint is engaged with a right-angle pick, and the incus is mobilized and removed. The malleus head is then exposed by curetting some of the bone over the epitympanum. Now the malleus head is engaged with a House-Dieter malleus nipper just above the short process, and the mallear head is mobilized and removed. Although this usually is not difficult, on occasion the bony connection is massive and cannot be fractured without damage to the surgical instruments. When this is the case, the lower part of the head may be drilled or curetted away, and silicone sheeting may be placed in the defect to prevent any reattachment of the neck to the head. The ossicular chain is rebuilt with an incus replacement prosthesis of hydroxyapatite, as described under incus defects.

Another mallear defect is erosion and shortening of the manubrium of the malleus. Often, the incus is present and the remaining ossicular chain intact and mobile. In this instance, I recommend removal of the incus and the remaining head and neck of the malleus. Reconstruction is carried out with a homograft tympanic membrane and malleus. The head of the homograft malleus is placed into the epitympanum, into the space previously occupied by the patient's mallear head. The ossicular chain is rebuilt with the incus replacement prosthesis made of hydroxyapa-

tite and HAPEX. This may be carried out in a single stage; however, because the tensor tympani tendon is no longer present to stabilize the malleus, it is a good idea to postpone the reconstruction until a later date. At this time, the malleus has stabilized, and the reconstruction is easier and more likely to be successful.

If in the situations described earlier the stapedial crura are also absent, the reconstruction is carried out in a similar manner, but with the shaft of the incus-stapes prosthesis centered on the stapedial footplate.

COMBINED DEFECTS OF MALLEUS AND OSSICLES

Erosion of the incus with loss of the stapes superstructure constitutes the most common multiple defect of the ossicular chain. This defect is corrected by removal of the incus and reconstruction with the incus-stapes prosthesis of hydroxyapatite and HAPEX in the manner previously described.

Another combination defect is constituted by an intact but fixed ossicular chain. The first step in this case would be separation of the incudostapedial joint. If the stapes is then found to be fixed but the incus and malleus are mobile, a stapedectomy is indicated. If the tympanic membrane is intact, stapedectomy should be performed immediately. However, if there is a drum defect, it should be repaired first and the stapedectomy should be reserved for a second stage. When the stapes is mobile, the incus should be removed and the mobility of the malleus ascertained. If the malleus is found to be freely mobile, reconstruction should proceed with an incus replacement prosthesis as previously described. However, if the malleus head is fixed, it must be dealt with in the manner described under mallear defects.

The ultimate combination defect consists of loss of all ossicular tissue except the stapedial footplate. This may occur when there is a total perforation or extensive cholesteatoma or when the ossicles have been removed and the drum grafted without any ossicular reconstruction. These defects are rebuilt with the homograft tympanic membrane and malleus as the main building block. The homograft eardrum maintains the malleus in anatomic position as well as reinforces the graft. If the malleus head fits well in the epitympanum and there is good middle ear mucosa, the reconstruction may be carried out in a single stage. However, if the head of the malleus must be amputated or if poor mucosa is present, the reconstruction to the footplate should be reserved for a second stage.

DRESSING

For the procedures performed transmeatally, the dressing consists of a strip of 1/4-inch selvage edge gauze approximately 2 inches in length placed in the outer ear canal. A cotton ball is then used in the concha. When a postauricular incision has been employed, the incision is closed with a subcuticular suture of 4-0 plain catgut; then a standard mastoid dressing secured by 3-inch Kling bandage is applied. The patients are usually discharged the morning following the surgery. The mastoid dressing is removed at this time.

POSTOPERATIVE CARE

Patients are instructed to change the cotton in the external ear approximately three times a day for a few days. When there is no more bleeding, they should leave the cotton out altogether. Scratching or rubbing the ear is forbidden, and patients are instructed to clean it by putting a damp wash cloth over the index finger and tipping the head toward the affected ear, then gently cleaning the outer ear. Ear drops are not used routinely, but if the healing is slow or if there is surface irritation, then Cortisporin otic drops are recommended. The drops are used in a decreasing dosage regimen, usually beginning at two drops three time a day for 3 days, twice a day for 2 days, and at bedtime for a week. Patients should not wash their hair for approximately 5 days after surgery and then not in a shower but rather over a tub or sink. Cotton saturated in white petroleum jelly is used in the outer ear to prevent contamination with water. The patient is seen back for the first postoperative check approximately 2 weeks following the surgery. At this time, any remaining gelatin sponge packing is removed with gentle suction. The patient then returns at 2-week intervals until the ear is healed, usually 6 weeks postoperatively. At that time, a postoperative audiogram may be obtained.

PITFALLS AND COMPLICATIONS

To date, there have been no serious complications with the use of these prostheses; however, as with any device, there are potential complications.

Intraoperative immediate complications would consist of using a prosthesis with too much height and forcing it into place. Fortunately the use of the HAPEX prostheses has reduced this risk because they are much softer and pliable than the dense hydroxyapatite. In the case of the incus prosthesis, this could result in fracture of the crura, dislocation of the stapes, or tear of the annular ligament with a resultant perilymph fistula and severe or total sensorineural hearing loss. In the case of the incus-stapes prosthesis, it could fracture the stapedial footplate and be pushed into the vestibule, with similar results. To prevent these complications, the prostheses must be handled gently, and sudden undue pressure must be avoided. If the prosthesis does not slip into place easily, it should be removed and the HAPEX cuff shortened.

If there is a tear of the annular ligament or a crack in the stapedial footplate, then a tissue seal of fat or fascia should be placed over the affected area. Attempts at ossicular reconstruction should be postponed and the ear closed or grafted. At a second stage, definitive reconstruction could be instituted.

An immediate postoperative complication could be vertigo, which could be related to unrecognized trauma, as previously described. If the reconstruction was difficult, then the possibility of perilymph fistula should be considered. Exploration may be necessary if the patient does not respond to conservative therapy, such as antibiotics and antivertigo drugs. If one is sure that no excess force was used in the reconstruction, the patient's ear should not be re-explored but only observed.

The anatomic results following use of these prostheses have been good. The outline of the prosthesis is often seen through the graft. There has been minimal crusting but no extrusions in the first several years of use. However, in the past year, there have been cases in which the tissue has thinned and crusted over the prosthesis, with resultant granulation tissue formation and breakdown with exposure of the prosthesis. In one instance, the patient underwent a revision with a canal skin tympanoplasty and ossicular reconstruction with a homograft ossicle. In another, a recurrent cholesteatoma was found at revision but the implant was not removed and has continued to function well. In two cases, the prosthesis was removed through the perforation, and the ears subsequently healed and became dry. When a conductive component remains, revision surgery should be carried out. If the prosthesis is exposed but the hearing remains good, one may elevate a tympanomeatal flap and carry the elevation over the prosthesis. There would then be a perforation of the flap where the prosthesis had been. Fascia, homograft dura, or another tissue graft, such as perichondrium, should be placed over the prosthesis. Then, the tympanomeatal flap is replaced in the same manner as that used in an underlay tympanoplasty. If the hearing is poor, the prosthesis should be removed and replaced with a prosthesis that would correct the hearing problem.

If the graft is normal and the ear healed but there has been no improvement in hearing, a revision is usually not recommended until 6 months following the surgery. The reason for this delay is twofold. First, the hearing in many of these ears will improve after 3 to 4 months. Also, it is much better to allow the graft to thin, the ear to become completely healed, and the middle ear to become less vascular before a revision is attempted. At the time of revision, the incisions for the tympanomeatal flap are more lateral than for a virgin ear, because the grafted flap, although thicker than the original canal skin, tends to shrink and may not close the defect. The flap is dissected off the prosthesis and folded forward on the malleus. One usually finds a good mucosal envelope formed around the hydroxyapatite prosthesis similar to those found around the bony prostheses. Once the flap has been elevated, the cause of the hearing failure should be determined: It may be simple dislocation of the prosthesis from the stapes head or malleus. Alternatively, Silastic sheeting may be present between the stapes head and the prosthesis, or the prosthesis may be not be making contact for another reason. If a incus-stapes type of prosthesis had been used in the reconstruction, the footplate area should be inspected. Occasionally, the shaft has been dislocated from the stapedial footplate or is too short to make good contact. The shaft may not have been rounded, and the old square shafts tend to become hung up on the margins of the oval window.

After the cause of the failure has been determined, it is almost always necessary to completely remove the prosthesis from the ear and either modify it or use a new and different prosthesis. If the dislocation occurred because the prosthesis was too loose, a larger size would be indicated. If the stapedial head was eroded or absent, one may elect to rebuild directly to the stapedial footplate with an incus-stapes prosthesis. This may be accomplished without removing the superstructure of the stapes if it is leaning toward the promontory or is partially dislocated with an intact annular ligament. Here, one would place the rounded shaft of the incus-stapes prosthesis between the crura and on the footplate. This placement cannot be accomplished unless the stapes is already displaced. Another solution is removal of the stapedial crura to expose the footplate. When the stapes is intact and normal, it is difficult to remove the crura without dislocating the footplate. However, with use of a laser, this can be more easily accomplished. Following vaporization and removal of the stapes superstructure, reconstruction would proceed in the usual fashion.

HEARING RESULTS

The hearing results have been good. In a study based on the hearing results of 86 patients operated on over a 3-year period, 85 per cent of the incus replacement cases and 65 per cent of the incus-stapes replacement cases closed the air-bone gap to within 20 dB of the preoperative bone conduction.

HISTORY OF OSSICULOPLASTY

Following the introduction of tympanoplasty by Wullstein[7] in the 1950s and proof that a perforation of the tympanic membrane could be closed, attention turned to defects of the ossicular chain. At this point in history no one had heard of biocompatibility; therefore, the early attempts at ossicular reconstruction utilized the materials available at the time. These were the so-called inert materials such as stainless steel, tantalum, polyethylene, and Teflon. The initial hearing success of these materials was often dramatic, proving that by reconnecting the continuity of the ossicular chain the potential of normal hearing could be realized. Unfortunately the initial success of a grafted eardrum and excellent hearing was followed in a few weeks by a gradual diminution of hearing due to erosion of the foreign material through the eardrum. This was soon accompanied by extrusion of the prosthesis from the middle ear and through the eardrum.

This dilemma was solved by the introduction of the concept of utilizing living tissue such as the remains of the patient's incus as an autograft prosthesis.[8] Because this was a biocompatible material, there was no tendency for the prosthesis to erode and the hearing results were not only good but permanent. In the next few years other autograft tissues such as the malleus head, bony chips from the annulus, and sculptured ossicles from the mastoid cortex made their appearance. This was followed by the homograft ossicle, and in 1967 I reported on that technique.[2]

All of these bony tissues were found to be biocompatible and were well tolerated by the middle ear. At this time only the body and short process of the incus were being used; if the stapes was intact and mobile, the resulting prosthesis was wedged between the stapes head and the malleus handle. When the superstructure of the incus was also absent, the short process of the incus fragment could be put directly on the stapedial footplate. The hearing results were good; however, problems included slippage or dislocation of the ossicles and loss of the good hearing result. Also, the short process on the footplate did not reach the tympanic membrane. By taking advantage of the homograft incus and placing the long process rather than the short process on the stapedial footplate, the problem of length was solved. To prevent slippage or dislocation, a notch was created in the short process of the incus body, and this notch was positioned under the handle of the patient's malleus (see Fig. 12–1). This locked the prosthesis in position, producing excellent, consistent, and long-lasting hearing results.

A long-term advocate of the use of homograft ossicles, Chiossone in 1987[9] published his observations on the results of allograft prostheses. He discussed the idea of an ear bank and advocated the use of presculptured prostheses that he modeled from homograft incudes and mallei, preserved in Cialit. His studies were carried out over a period of 13 years and involved 411 implants. Histologic study of homograft ossicles removed five, six, and seven years after implantation showed no signs of absorption or remodeling. The surface was covered with good mucous membrane. The hearing outcomes for his patients were good and compared favorably with similar studies.

There followed numerous variations and modifications of sculpturing both autograft and homograft ossicles, such as drilling a hole in the short process for the stapedial head or attaching a stainless-steel cup prosthesis between the stapes and eardrum.

These bony prostheses were employed successfully for a number of years and are still in use today. A variety of external factors led to their demise. Foremost among these was the acquired immunodeficiency syndrome epidemic, which rendered all transplant material suspect, although no proven case of transmission from an otologic case was reported to my knowledge. Next was the timely development of biocompatible materials, especially hydroxyapatite. These factors combined with the convenience and standardization of artificial materials rendered the ossicular prostheses obsolete.

ALLOPLASTIC PROSTHESES

In the mid 1970s the first artificial materials were introduced as prostheses for ossicular reconstruction. They were called PORPs for partial ossicular replacement prostheses and TORPs for total ossicular replacement prostheses. An early entry was high-density polyethylene introduced under the name of *Plastipore*.[10] Although polyethylene tubing had been tried earlier with disastrous results and early extrusion, this new material was accepted by human tissue. These prostheses were readily available commercially and could easily be cut and shaped with a knife. The tendency to erode the tympanic membrane was avoided by placing a cartilage interface between the implant and the eardrum. According to Chuden[11] the tissue tolerance could be further enhanced by a process of thermal fusion resulting in a new material called *Polycel*. The TORP also had a stainless-steel core in the form of a wire, which was inserted into the prosthesis to increase its strength but still allow elasticity of movement and the ability to be bent into various shapes.[12]

In 1979, various ceramics were recommended for use as implant material and were described as being bioinactive or bioinert. Reck and Helms[13] described the use of a bioactive glass ceramic called *Ceravital*. This material is a nonporous dense material derived from glass and was found to be biocompatible. Because it is glass, it was difficult to handle and shape. It shattered easily but could be trimmed by using a diamond burr and held either by hand or by special silicon-armed metal clamps and low pressure. An advantage of the Ceravital was that it could be used without the interposition of cartilage. The extrusion rate was said to be no greater than with alloplastic ossicles, and the hearing results were also comparable with those obtained with ossicles.

An interesting article by Podoshin and associates[14] in 1988 described the use a of carbon-carbon ossicular replacement prosthesis experimentally in guinea pigs and a short preliminary study in humans. It appeared to be accepted by the tissues.

OTHER HYDROXYAPATITE PROSTHESES

Following the introduction of hydroxyapatite for ear surgery by Grote[6] in 1984 and its proven biocompatibility, this material has been adapted to a variety of uses and designs. It is now used alone or in combination for most ossicular replacement prostheses that contact the tympanic membrane. The dense hydroxyapatite has been machined to the dimensions of the classic PORP and TORP design. Black[15] employs it with his modified round-top prostheses. Brackmann and colleagues[16] have utilized a thin coating of hydroxyapatite on the surface of their prostheses, usually Plastipore, where they interface with tissue, cartilage, or bone.

Prostheses utilizing a hydroxyapatite body combined with a malleable material for the middle ear portion have been designed by several surgeons. Teflon, Plastipore, Fluoroplastic, Polycel, and titanium have been used for the middle ear shaft that contacts the ossicle. Lesinski (personal communication, 1998) states that for the past decade he has used Flex hydroxyapatite for the shaft with a body of hydroxyapatite. Recently, he has employed an all-titanium prosthesis.

A combination prosthesis designed by Goldenberg[17] and labeled as a hybrid utilizes a hydroxyapatite body that extends anteriorly under the malleus and contacts it by a notch or hook. The shaft is made of Plastipore or Fluoroplastic, which is malleable and may be cut to the correct length. In the case of the incus-stapes prosthesis, the shaft to the stapedial footplate is reinforced by a stainless-steel wire embedded in its center. This wire must also be cut when sizing the prosthesis and may be cut short so that it does not contact the footplate or, as I prefer, left slightly longer than the flexible shaft to better stabilize the prosthesis on the footplate.

Another combination prosthetic design has been introduced by Dornhoffer[18] and bears his name. These prostheses have a hydroxyapatite body, a notch for the malleus handle, and a shaft of HAPEX to the stapes capitulum or the stapedial footplate. He states that he chose HAPEX over Plastipore because it has greater rigidity, which facilitates achieving the proper tension between the malleus and stapes, thereby obtaining the optimal sound transmission. He has designated these as HAPEX PORP and HAPEX TORP prostheses. The hearing results are good and compare favorably with similar studies.

The Smith Nephew company has also introduced a classic PORP and TORP design made entirely of HAPEX.

References

1. House WF, Sheehy JL: Functional restoration in tympanoplasty. Arch Otolaryngol Head Neck Surg 78: 304–309, 1963.
2. Wehrs RE: The borrowed incus in tympanoplasty. Arch Otolaryngol Head Neck Surg 85: 371–379, 1967.
3. Wehrs RE: The notched incus in tympanoplasty. Arch Otolaryngol Head Neck Surg 100: 251–255, 1974.
4. Wehrs RE: Incus replacement prostheses of hydroxyapatite in middle ear reconstruction. Am J Otol 10: 181–182, 1989.
5. Wehrs RE: Hearing results in tympanoplasty. Laryngoscope 95: 1301–1306, 1985.

6. Grote JJ: Tympanoplasty with calcium phosphate. Arch Otolaryngol Head Neck Surg 110: 197–199, 1984.
7. Wullstein H: Theory and practice of tympanoplasty. Laryngoscope 66: 1076–1093, 1956.
8. Hall A, Rytzner C: Vitality of autotransplanted ossicles. Acta Otolaryngol 158 (Suppl): 335–340, 1960.
9. Chiossone E: Homograft ossiculoplasty: Long-term results. Am J Otol 8: 545–550, 1987.
10. Shea J, Emmett JR: Biocompatible ossicular implants. Arch Otolaryngol 104: 191–196, 1978.
11. Chuden HG: Total ossicular replacement with a porous ultra-high molecular weight prosthesis. Am J Otol 6: 461–463, 1985.
12. Sheehy J: Personal experience with TORP and PORP: A report on 455 operations. Am J Otol 6: 80–83, 1985.
13. Beck R, Helms J: The bioglass ceramic Ceravital in ear surgery: Five years' experience. Am J Otol 6: 280–283, 1985.
14. Fodoshin L, Nodar R, Hughes G, et al: Long-term histologic study of a new carbon-carbon ossicular replacement prosthesis. Am J Otol 9: 366–374, 1988.
15. Black B: Design and development of a contoured ossicular replacement prosthesis: Clinical trials of 25 cases. Am J Otol 11: 85–89, 1990.
16. Brackmann DE, Sheehy JL, Laxford WM: TORP and PORP in tympanoplasty: A review of 1042 operations. Otolaryngol Head Neck Surg 92: 32–37, 1984.
17. Goldenberg RA: Reconstruction of the middle ear using hydroxylapatite hybrid prostheses. Oper Tech Head Neck Surg 3: 225–231, 1992.
18. Dornhoffer JL: Hearing results with the Dornhoffer ossicular replacement prostheses. Laryngoscope 108: 531–536, 1998.

13

Tympanoplasty: Cartilage and Porous Polyethylene

James L. Sheehy, M.D.

Restoration of function in tympanoplasty requires an intact tympanic membrane, an air-containing mucosa-lined middle ear space, and a connection between the mobile tympanic membrane and the inner ear fluids. Obtaining this connection with porous polyethylene and cartilage, or cartilage alone, is the subject of this chapter.

It is difficult to consider management of ossicular problems separately from management of the mastoid, staging the operation, and use of plastic in the middle ear. In order not to confuse the issue, however, this chapter discusses only the ossicular problem. Each of the other items are considered elsewhere in this book.

HISTORICAL ASPECTS

When tympanoplastic surgery was introduced by Wullstein[1] and Zollner,[2] little attempt was made to reconstruct the ossicular chain. They established a sound pressure differential between the oval and round windows by adapting the operation to the ossicular problem encountered. If the incus was missing, the graft was placed on the stapes capitulum (type III or columellar tympanoplasty). If both the incus and stapes crura were missing, the graft was laid on the promontory, leaving a mobile footplate exposed (type IV, oval window, or cavum minor tympanoplasty), thereby producing sound protection for the round window.

In most instances, the tympanoplasty resulted in a mastoid cavity and, as a result of the aforementioned surgical approach, a shallow middle ear space. With more experience it became apparent that routinely creating a mastoid cavity was a drawback and that the results were better when the middle ear space was not narrowed. If a cavity was to be avoided and the eardrum reconstructed in its natural position, it became necessary to perform some type of reconstruction of the sound pressure transfer mechanism.

Many prostheses and techniques were used at the House Ear Clinic (HEC) beginning in the late 1950s, only to be discarded as better methods evolved. It became apparent that to obtain satisfactory long-term results, the middle ear space should not be narrowed and that whatever connection was used for sound pressure transfer, this connection should be under adequate tension. One also had to take steps to prevent extrusion.

The first prosthesis (used at HEC) was polyethylene tubing connected to the capitulum of the stapes or the mobile footplate.[3] In due time, one of two things happened: extrusion (if under tension) or separation from the stapes (if not under tension). The interposition of soft tissue between the polyethylene tubing and the tympanic membrane only delayed extrusion. Unfortunately, no one (at HEC) thought of using cartilage, as is done now.

In the early 1960s, ossicular transposition was used, and later, the fitted ossicular prosthesis.[4–7] The most common cause of failure there was separation of the ossicle from the stapes. A completely stable malleus and tympanic membrane were therefore a necessity, and this goal frequently required a two-staged procedure when it might not otherwise have been indicated. The use of a homograft tympanic membrane with a malleus attached resolved some of those problems, but the homograft tympanic membrane did not have a satisfactory graft take rate in the hands of the HEC physicians.[8]

The incus replacement prosthesis, developed successfully for use in stapedectomy in the fenestrated ear, was tried but quickly abandoned.[9] It often pulled off the mobile footplate or extruded. Homograft tympanic membrane with en bloc ossicles was also tried.[8] The conclusion reached was that other methods were simpler and usually yielded as good, if not better, results.

In 1967, the HEC physicians began using cartilage alone as a prothesis, following some thoughts by Shea and Glasscock.[10] Tragal cartilage had one significant advantage: it could be applied under tension without fear of extrusion. When cartilage was used as a block to the capitulum of the stapes, the hearing results were stable. This technique is still used regularly in canal wall down procedures so that the middle ear space is not narrowed by placing the graft on the capitulum.[11] When cartilage was used as a strut to the footplate, the results were less stable because of the lack of stiffness of the cartilage; as a result, cartilage is no longer used as a strut to the footplate.[12, 13]

Porous polyethylene prostheses (total ossicular replacement prostheses [TORPs] and partial ossicular replacement prostheses [PORPs]) were introduced by John Shea in 1974.[14] Because of the extrusion experience with polyethylene tubes, these prostheses were not used at HEC. Then, in a 1976 personal communication, Coyle Shea suggested using tragal cartilage interposed between the platform and the tympanic membrane graft. Shortly thereafter, use of porous polyethylene with tragal cartilage became routine at HEC.[15]

PATIENT SELECTION, EVALUATION, AND COUNSELING

Patient selection, evaluation, and counseling were covered in detail in Chapter 9 (tympanic membrane grafting). Most of what was said on this subject in Chapter 9 applies equally here. The main difference is in regard to the hearing results. (Assume that this is a dry central perforation with good mucosa.)

In most cases, it is possible to know ahead of time that ossicular reconstruction will be necessary. One can see that the incus, the stapes, or both, are diseased or missing, or one concludes that there must be an ossicular problem based on a conductive deficit of greater than 25 dB.

When a problem is suspected but cannot be specifically identified, tell the patient merely that the second ear bone will probably need to be replaced. The final outcome from surgery depends on how much of a conductive deficit exists preoperatively and the surgeon's personal experience.

If the bone-air deficit is 45 dB or greater, the patient is told that there are seven out of ten chances that the hearing result will "make both of us happy." If loss is in both ears, one is justified in saying eight chances out of ten. Err on the conservative side.

If the deficit is 40 dB or less, tell the patient that there are six chances out of ten for a good result. Again, if the other ear is similarly involved, "three chances out of four" is a reasonable estimate. Achievement of results satisfactory to both patient and surgeon depends on the overall situation, including the other ear, the bone conduction level, and whether the patient wears hearing aids already. A technical success may not be judged as a success by the patient, and this fact must be remembered when outlook is discussed.

SURGICAL TECHNIQUE

Management in the office, preoperatively, and in surgery are the same as presented in Chapter 9.

TORPs and PORPs were used initially. The platform was modified to 3 mm early on ("Sheehy's modification"). In the mid 1980s, total ossicular prostheses (TOPs) and partial ossicular prostheses (POPs) were developed. These have a rounded platform to better conform to the tenting of the tympanic membrane brought about by putting the prosthesis under slight tension. In addition, the stem of the TOP is oval (0.8 × 1.0 mm) to facilitate bypassing the stapedial crura when necessary.[16, 17]

The basic technique for using a TOP or a POP (or various individual variations of these) is the same.[11] Discussed here (and illustrated) is use of the TOP. To facilitate presentation, a planned second-stage procedure is described; that is, the tympanic membrane is intact, and no ossicles are present.

Exposure

A semilunar incision is made at the junction of the outer and middle thirds of the ear canal. Flap elevation is from posteroinferiorly to anterosuperiorly (Fig. 13–1).

The reason for this type of incision and exposure is to keep the tympanic membrane stable in the area where the prosthesis and cartilage will contact the membrane and to avoid incisions near the bony annulus. One may better judge the proper prosthesis length to maintain slight tension and not have any tension to distract incision edges at the annulus.

Preparation of Cartilage

After any plastic material placed in the middle ear at the first stage is removed and the ear is inspected for residual disease, the middle ear and canal are packed temporarily to keep blood out of the middle ear.

An incision is made on the posterior surface of the tragus (to avoid retracted scars, which may develop if the incision is made over the dome), and a large piece of cartilage is removed. The perichondrium is removed by blunt dissection, using a Bard-Parker knife handle and holding the cartilage on a piece of gauze.

The cartilage is then placed on a moist tongue blade, trimmed to the appropriate size (about 5 × 5 mm), and thinned with a No. 11 Bard-Parker blade. This thinning process, particularly on the edges, results in cartilage that has a slight dome shape. Having this shape, the cartilage will conform more easily to the contours of the tympanic membrane when the prosthesis and cartilage are placed under slight tension.

Preparation of Prosthesis

Trimming the stem to the appropriate size is a matter of judgment and experience. No measuring device has been satisfactory. In cases with an intact canal wall and without a malleus handle, a 5-mm length is usually correct for the TOP (and a 2-mm length for a POP). If the manubrium is present, a 4-mm length may be correct. In open-cavity cases, 3.5 mm is usually the correct length.

Wet the prosthesis and cut it on a moist tongue blade using a No. 11 Bard-Parker blade. By having both the tongue blade and the prosthesis moist, one will find that the prosthesis tends to adhere to the tongue blade.

Placement of Prosthesis

After temporary packing is removed from the middle ear and canal, the middle ear is filled lightly with pieces of slightly moistened absorbable gelatin sponge (Gelfoam). This moistened gelatin sponge is placed to facilitate placement of the prosthesis and cartilage, to stabilize them temporarily, and to act as counterpacking for the packing that will be placed in the canal after replacement of the tympanomeatal flap. A small piece of perichondrium may be placed on the mobile footplate and will be commented on later.

The moistened TOP is most easily placed in position in the middle ear by using a No. 3 Barron suction on the platform as a prosthesis guide and holder. The prosthesis should fit perfectly without tension prior to placement of

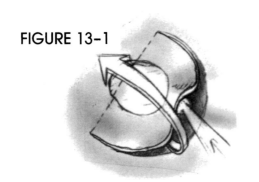

FIGURE 13-1

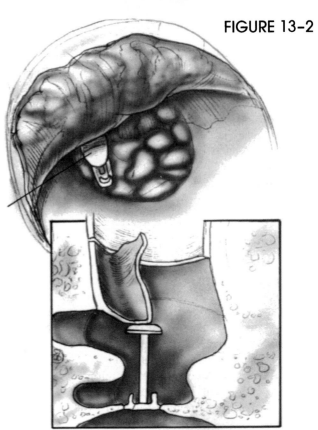

FIGURE 13-2

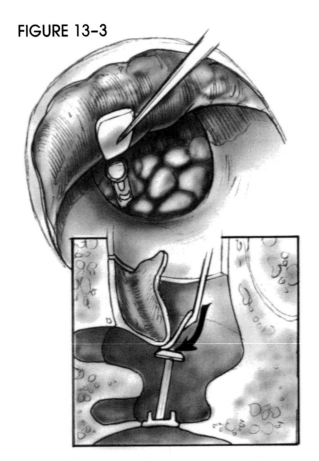

FIGURE 13-3

FIGURE 13-4

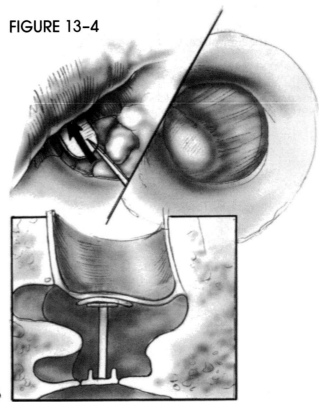

FIGURE 13-5

FIGURES 13–1 to 13–5. *See legends on opposite page*

the cartilage (Fig. 13–2). If the prosthesis is slightly short, the length may be corrected later by adding an additional piece of cartilage.

Because it may be difficult to slide the cartilage across the prosthesis without displacing it, the TOP is tipped posteroinferiorly first. The cartilage is placed on the flap, slid into the proper position, and then flipped onto the platform (Fig. 13–3). Then the assembly is moved into position (Fig. 13–4). There should be slight tension on, or tenting of, the tympanic membrane (Fig. 13–5). The flap is replaced, and gelatin sponge packing is used with a plug of cotton in the outer meatus. A mastoid dressing is not necessary.

Management of Ossicular Chain Fixation

Tympanosclerosis

Tympanosclerosis is a term used to describe a sclerotic or a hyalin change of the submucosal tissue of the middle ear. It appears to be an end product of recurrent acute or chronic ear infection. Hyalinized connective tissue develops under the mucous membrane, superficial to the bone. Calcification and ossification may occur.[11]

Tympanosclerosis is clinically significant only when it impedes motion of the ossicular chain. Plaques in the tympanic membrane remnant are not of significance but are usually removed at the time of grafting. Fixation of the malleus or incus, however, is of significance, and is usually a phenomenon that results from massive involvement in the epitympanum. It is best to remove the malleus and incus, bypassing the chain rather than trying to mobilize it.

Tympanosclerotic fixation of the stapes may be due to involvement of the tendon, to pressure on the crura from lesions on the fallopian canal and promontory, or to diffuse involvement of the oval window niche. Mobilization of the stapes by removal of the lesions is possible two thirds of the time. When the involvement is diffuse, it is best to graft the drum and perform a stapedectomy as a second-stage procedure.

Otosclerosis

Otosclerotic fixation of the stapes should, likewise, be corrected in a secondary procedure after the ear is free of infection and the perforation closed. When fixation is due to either tympanosclerosis or otosclerosis, a stapedectomy may be performed as a planned second stage. If the lateral chain is not available for use, we use a TOP, after covering the oval window with perichondrium.

POSTOPERATIVE CARE

The patient is given a postoperative instruction card just before entering the hospital. This is reviewed with the patient, and appears as Appendix 2 in Chapter 9.

The patient is seen in the office in 7 to 10 days. The cotton plug is removed and the gelatin sponge packing is aspirated. The patient is told that blowing the nose is permitted but that no water should be allowed into the ear. A second postoperative visit is scheduled for a month postoperatively, at which time the hearing is tested. It may take 3 months for the hearing to increase to its maximum, and the patient is told this at the first postoperative visit.

POTENTIAL PROBLEMS

An early-recognized problem was displacement of the lateral (platform) end of the TOP or POP, particularly in ears with a normal malleus. This normal malleus maintains a cone shape to the tympanic membrane, even when the perforation grafted was a total one. This tends to force displacement of the lateral end of the prosthesis, despite the presence of a piece of cartilage. Dislocation outward of the malleus handle is advisable at the time of surgery to prevent this problem and to produce a *flat* tympanic membrane.

Stabilizing the stem of the TOP (or TORP) on the mobile stapes footplate can be a problem. Covering the footplate with tissue (perichondrium or fascia) facilitates stability. It also prevents direct contact of the porous polyethylene with the footplate. There have been a few instances of resorption of the bone in the area of contact without any slippage into the vestibule.

The main concern of ear surgeons is prosthesis extrusion. This problem was common early on, before cartilage was used over the prosthesis platform. But it continued to occur in 5 per cent of cases, even with cartilage use. With the use of larger pieces of cartilage on a 3-mm platform, and with rounded platforms, the incidence has been reduced further. Staging the operation is also important if there is a major mucous membrane problem, to prevent adhesions (see Chapter 18).

Despite all precautions, extrusion continues in a small percentage of cases. When this problem is analyzed, it appears to most often be related to middle ear space and mucous membrane problems: it occurs much more often in cases requiring a two-stage procedure in the first place, the "bad ears."[18]

ACKNOWLEDGMENT

Many of the illustrations are modified from *Otolaryngology*, Vol. 1, published by J. B. Lippincott Company.

FIGURE 13–1. Elevation of tympanomeatal flap after semilunar incision at junction of outer and middle thirds.

FIGURE 13–2. Total ossicular prosthesis between footplate and tympanic membrane, without tension.

FIGURE 13–3. Sliding cartilage into position.

FIGURE 13–4. Shifting of prosthesis and cartilage into position.

FIGURE 13–5. Final position, with slight tension.

References

1. Wullstein H: Theory and practice of tympanoplasty. Laryngoscope 66: 1076–1093, 1956.
2. Zollner F: Principles of plastic surgery of the sound conducting apparatus. J Laryngol Otol 69: 637–652, 1955.
3. House WF, Sheehy JL: Functional restoration in tympanoplasty. Arch Otolaryngol Head Neck Surg 78: 304–309, 1963.
4. Sheehy JL: Ossicular problems in tympanoplasty. Arch Otolaryngol Head Neck Surg 81: 115–122, 1965.
5. Farrior JB: Ossicular repositioning and ossicular prostheses in tympanoplasty. Arch Otolaryngol Head Neck Surg 69: 661–666, 1959.
6. Hall A, Rytzner C: Autotransplantation of ossicles: Stapedectomy and biological reconstruction of the ossicular chain mechanism. Arch Otolaryngol Head Neck Surg 74: 22–26, 1961.
7. House WF, Patterson ME, Linthicum FH: Incus homografts in chronic ear surgery. Arch Otolaryngol Head Neck Surg 84: 148–153, 1966.
8. House WF, Glasscock ME, Sheehy JL: Homograft transplants of the middle ear. Trans Am Acad Ophthalmol Otolaryngol 873: 836–841, 1969.
9. Sheehy JL: Stapedectomy with incus replacement prosthesis: Report of 50 cases. Laryngoscope 76: 1165–1180, 1966.
10. Shea MC, Glasscock ME: Tragal cartilage as an ossicular substitute. Arch Otolaryngol Head Neck Surg 86: 308–317, 1967.
11. Sheehy JL, Brackmann DE: Surgery of Chronic Ear Disease: What We Do and Why We Do It. Instructional Courses, Vol. 6. St. Louis, CV Mosby, 1993.
12. Pulec JL, Sheehy JL: Tympanoplasty: Ossicular chain reconstruction. Laryngoscope 83: 448–465, 1973.
13. Sheehy JL, Altenau MM: Tympanoplasty: Cartilage prosthesis. Laryngoscope 88: 895–904, 1978.
14. Shea JJ, Emmett JB, Smyth GDL: Biocompatible implants in otology. ORL Digest 39: 9–15, 1977.
15. Sheehy JL, Brackmann DE: Tympanoplasty: TORPs and PORPs. Laryngoscope 89: 108–114, 1979.
16. Sheehy JL: Personal experiences with TORPs and PORPs: A report on 455 operations. Am J Otol 6: 80–83, 1985.
17. Brackmann DE, Sheehy JL, Luxford WM: TORPs and PORPs in tympanoplasty: A review of 1042 operations. Otolaryngol Head Neck Surg 92: 32–37, 1984.
18. Sheehy JL: TORPs and PORPs: Causes of failure. Otolaryngol Head Neck Surg 92: 583–587, 1984.

14

Biocompatible Materials in Chronic Ear Surgery

Jan J. Grote, M.D., Ph.D.

Since the introduction of closed techniques for the eradication of chronic middle ear disease and the use of homologous middle ear implants, we thought that the problems of cholesteatoma surgery were solved.[1] It was possible to remove the diseased tissue and preserve or restore the anatomy of the middle ear while avoiding the problems of a cavity. With homologous ossicles and even a total homologous middle ear, including ossicular chain and tympanic membrane, it was possible to reconstruct a sound-conducting system with a normal anatomic structure.[2] At the end of the 1970s, an increasing number of recurrent and residual cholesteatomas were reported,[3] and it was demonstrated that cholesteatoma microscopically invaded the ossicles and the surrounding bone, leading to residual disease. The defects in the bony annulus had to be reconstructed to avoid recurrent cholesteatoma. Also, in many cases because of the local anatomy, a proper and safe way to eradicate cholesteatoma via a combined approach was not possible.

Because of the repeated interventions required, the possibilities of physiologic reconstruction diminished. During the first operation, the stapes superstructure was often present, but during a second look, resorption by the recurrent cholesteatoma was observed, indicating that the best chance for reconstruction is a cholesteatoma-free middle ear. However, the problems of an open cavity and the uncertain results of tympanoplasties in these cavities are well known.

In addition to the controversy over closed versus open techniques for eradication, the use of homologous implants led to new doubts in the 1980s. The preservation of these implants was solved, but a major problem with these implants came with the possibility of virus inclusion and transplantation. However, there is no proof that human immunodeficiency virus (HIV) can be transferred via these implants. In many countries, using these implants is not allowed if they are not proved to be from HIV-free donors. Also, slow virus inclusions, such as Jakob-Creutzfeldt disease, entered the otologic discussion. Therefore, it looked as if we had to start again to find solutions in chronic otitis media surgery. "Once a cholesteatoma always a cholesteatoma" is more true now than ever. In the 1970s, new developments in material science, cell biology, and reconstructive surgery gave rise to new implant materials and a better understanding of the interaction between these implant materials and the body. Biomaterial science became important for middle ear reconstruction.

For reconstructive surgery with biomaterials, the surgeon must combine surgical with biomaterial criteria. Only if a good combination of these criteria is made can reconstructive surgery be successful. The combination of criteria is necessary because of the different tissues involved in the wound healing. The demands for reconstructive surgery performed by an orthopedic surgeon are clearly different from those performed by an otologist. Even in the middle ear, different materials must be used.

SURGICAL CRITERIA

The most important criterion in middle ear surgery for cholesteatoma is radical eradication of the disease. All the tissue that has been in contact with the cholesteatoma, whether the ossicular chain, the canal wall, or the mucosa of the middle ear and mastoid, must be totally removed and in continuity with a safe margin, without consideration of reconstruction. Definitive eradication of cholesteatoma is more possible with an open technique. Many patients with cholesteatoma have a sclerotic mastoid, and if it is eradicated by open technique, the patient is left with a small mastoid cavity. A tympanoplasty type III in this cavity often leads to good function, and the patient is well off with one operation. If indicated, reconstruction can be done in a second stage.

For the reconstruction of a functioning middle ear, a wide middle ear–mastoid cleft must be made. This is possible if the annulus of the middle ear is more lateral than in the often narrow ears of patients with cholesteatoma. The function of a reconstructed middle ear chain must be comparable to that achieved with a normal ossicular chain; that is, the ossicular chain must have a lever mechanism and must have contact with the tympanic membrane by the handle of the malleus. The ossicular chain also must have a good contact with the footplate or the stapes and the tympanic membrane. The ossicles must stay mobile and not be resorbed or extruded, even in an infected middle ear. For a lasting reconstruction of the canal wall, the new canal wall must be bone, or it must become bone.

BIOMATERIAL AND BIOCOMPATIBILITY CRITERIA

The selection of materials for reconstructive surgery is based on information derived from physical, chemical, biochemical, and surgical concepts. With the increasing number of implants on the market, it is essential that the otolaryngologist have a fundamental knowledge of biomaterial science, which can be related to his or her surgical aims.

The interaction of the human body and the implant is studied in terms of local and general reactions. The implant material must have no cytotoxicity. The influence of the body on the prosthesis is also important because these reactions can lead to degradation. The biocompatibility of an implant material determines the interface of the implant with the body, which ultimately leads to a good, permanent integration. This integration is dependent on the surface of the implant material and on the breakdown and remodeling of the implant by the body.

SURFACE ACTIVITY

An implant material is regarded as *bioinert* if the body does not react at all with the implant material, as *biotolerated* if the body regards the implant material as a foreign body but does not extrude the implant, and as *bioactive* if the body has an active surface integration with the implant material, which leads to a firm integration between the body and the implant. An implant material is always placed in a wound, and the normal wound reactions take place. A foreign body is encapsulated by a fibrous capsule with a varying number of reactive cells, particularly foreign body giant cells. In case of a bioinert material, no significant reactions occur on the surface, and although bone may be in contact with the implant, a bond does not occur. With a biotolerated material, a fibrous capsule forms between the implant material and the bone. Cellular activity in the form of giant cell reactions can be present, even after longer postoperative periods, but the integration is stable. Bioactive material achieves a real bond with the surface of the surrounding bone tissue, which takes place via an active ion exchange, leading to a firm bond between the implant and the body.

STRUCTURE

In the 1970s, porous implant materials were developed.[4] This advance enabled the host tissue to grow into the porous part of the implants, resulting in better integration with the body. Macropores of 100 μm allowed the ingrowth of fibrous and bone tissue if they were adjacent to the implant material. Micropores of several micrometers seemed to be essential, especially if the implant material had to be resorbed and remodeled in living tissue. These pores can be a problem in materials that are not meant for degradation. The body always reacts at the surface with the implant, and the material is resorbed to some degree, depending on the surface activity. If the surface area is large, the response of the body to the implant material will be more extensive, with the production of large numbers of macrophages and giant cells. With this degradation, inclusions of toxic substances can be harmful for the body, and therefore a good understanding of the type of implant material is necessary to avoid long-term problems, either locally or systemically. These problems of structure are comparable to those occurring with the homologous implant materials in which, in the case of bone chips or cartilage, resorption can take place before remodeling occurs. Also, the use of mixtures of granules with blood or fibrinogen glue gives a large surface area, which can lead to a resorption before remodeling occurs. This is the reason why initially good anatomic results are achieved, but after longer postoperative periods, resorption takes place, especially if an infection occurs. Therefore, the behavior of the implant material in infected surroundings should be taken into account. With the newer biomaterials, regulating the surface activity and the structure is possible.

Many implants are labeled with trade names that give no information on the capacity of the material. Therefore, the generic names of the material must be used and indicated. In addition to the generic names of the materials, the additives, which might be part of the implant materials and the trace elements present, should be noted.

In otology, three classes of biomaterials are used: metals, polymers, and ceramics. These different classes of biomaterials have advantages and disadvantages with regard to biocompatibility, integration capacity, and surgical application.

CLASSES OF BIOMATERIALS

Metals

Metals are used only in reconstruction of the middle ear in otosclerosis. Integrated into a mobile middle ear chain in a healthy middle ear, these implants are reliable. If mechanically fixed, they will not extrude, but if they are in contact with a mobile tympanic membrane, they will extrude.

Although metals such as stainless steel, gold, and platinum have been used for decades in otosclerosis surgery, in chronic ear surgery, gold has been introduced in ossiculoplasty in recent years. Gold implants have exhibited good biocompatibility, but extrusion occurs if they are exposed to the tympanic membrane.[5]

Polymers

In 1952, Wullstein was the first to use a biomaterial in reconstructive middle ear surgery. He implanted a columella of Palavit in the middle ear for the reconstruction of the middle ear chain, and although the initial hearing results were good, the implants extruded. Then different polymers, such as polyethylene, polytetrafluorethylene (Teflon), and silicon rubber (Silastic) were used,[6] but at the end of the 1960s, the use of polymer implant materials in reconstructive middle ear surgery was abandoned because of their high extrusion rate. Silicone sheeting and Teflon are still used as a plastic sheeting, and Teflon is used in otosclerosis surgery. The concept of porous implant materials was applied to these polymers. The advantage of the pores was better integration in the body, and porous polyethylene has been especially widely used as a total and partial ossicular replacement prosthesis (columella between the footplate and tympanic membrane or between the stapes superstructure and tympanic membrane).[7] The surface activity of the first porous plastic implants was biotolerated, but the surface activity was not favorable for integration, and an interface was necessary between the tympanic membrane and the implants. Even then, an increasing extrusion rate was reported.

Plastipore, a high-density polyethylene sponge, has been used for 20 years and is still used as a total or partial ossicular replacement prosthesis or as part of ossicular prostheses in composites with ceramic. If it is placed under the tympanic membrane, cartilage is used as interface.[8]

Ceramics

For the reconstruction of bone defects, especially in the middle ear, ceramic is the material of choice. Biologically, ceramics can be classified as bioinert materials (most oxide ceramics) and reactive materials (glass ceramics and calcium phosphate ceramics).

Aluminum oxide ceramic is a bioinert ceramic that is used in ossiculoplasty.[9] Its advantage is that it stays mobile in the middle ear chain, and there is no resorption or reaction of the body. Because of its bioinertness, however, integration is less favorable.

The bioactive ceramics glass ceramics and calcium phosphate ceramics are used in otology. There are different types of glass ceramics, and every glass ceramic has its own distinct composition and reactivity with the surrounding tissue. They are mainly used for the reconstruction of the middle ear chain in the form of columella prostheses.[10] They can be difficult to shape, and long-term studies have shown that resorption occurs. Therefore, we studied calcium phosphate ceramics. Their composition resembles that of bone tissue. There are different types of calcium phosphates, and we have focused our interest on hydroxyapatite, which is the mineral matrix of living bone tissue. It has proved to be a bioactive material that achieves a real integration with bone tissue without encapsulation. Hydroxapatite can be made in porous as well as in dense forms, depending on the surgical requirements. The continuation of the remodeling of the porous forms is also controlled in infected surroundings. The interaction with epithelium and connective tissue is excellent, with a direct bond between the material and the tissue. The attachment of epithelium to the apatite surfaces has been shown to take place by means of hemidesmosomes, and the implants are not encapsulated by fibrous tissue. The disadvantages of hydroxyapatite are its brittleness and its insufficient tensile strength; therefore, only non–load-bearing defects in the bone can be repaired with it. The use of this ceramic in long-term clinical studies in middle ear surgery has validated its biocompatibility and usefulness.[11–18] Otologous and homologous materials are often considered ideal for the reconstruction of defects in the middle ear. However, after preservation, the remodeling of the body with these implant materials takes place in the same way as with the biomaterials, which we have chosen for our reconstructive procedures.

The advantage of the hydroxyapatite implant for bony reconstruction is that the material is readily available. Because of standard manufacturing procedures, resorption and remodeling are controlled. There is no possibility of transmission of diseases, and this material can be shaped ac-

cording to individual demands. If these implants are used in combination with good surgical criteria, the body will remodel these implants as appropriate or integrate them biologically where needed, which will finally lead to a good, lasting result. The usefulness of these materials is also demonstrated with retrieved implants that were removed in patients because of problems that are discussed later. The histology of these implants proved their utility in reconstruction of the middle ear, and the results in the human body are comparable to those studied in vitro and in long-term animal experiments.[19–23]

Hydroxyapatite cement[23] has been developed, but data on its otologic clinical application in long-term studies are not available. Another cement is ionomer cement, a polymaleinate ionomer, introduced in otology as bone replacement and ossicles. It is easy to shape and therefore attractive for reconstructive surgery, but with resorption, aluminum comes free, and in contact with the brain has given rise to lethal storage in cerebro. Therefore, it is not approved for use.[24–26]

Since the introduction of hydroxyapatite, composite ossicles, mostly of Plastipore and hydroxyapatite, have become available. The Plastipore shaft is easy to trim, and the interface with the tympanic membrane hydroxyapatite is ideal.[27, 28] The use of a combination of biomaterials is mostly based on surgical needs. However, the biologic integration of these implants in long-term studies has yet to be determined.

SURGICAL TECHNIQUE

The development of new implant materials for a reliable and lasting reconstruction of defects in the middle ear makes it possible to separate eradication and reconstruction. This separation has the advantage that during the eradication, all the diseased tissue and adjacent bone can be removed. Only in cases in which the cholesteatoma is lateral of the ossicular chain, without ingrowth in the facial recess of sinus tympani, can the eradication and the reconstruction be done in the same stage. In more extensive cholesteatomas, an eradication is done first with an open technique, and reconstruction is done in a second stage, if indicated.

Eradication

The skin incision is made retroauricularly, and a cranial-based periosteal flap is mobilized. A lateral flap in the posterior skin of the ear canal is made, and after retraction of the flaps, the middle ear is inspected by mobilization of the tympanomeatal flap anteriorly. The remnants of the ossicular chain and the extent of the cholesteatoma in the middle ear are inspected. The ear canal is widened, and via an endaural approach, the cholesteatoma is now exposed. The first landmark is the tegmen tympani, exposed by drilling away the remnants of the scutum and opening up the epitympanic area until the tegmen tympani is seen. The cholesteatoma is followed and exposed posteriorly. The next landmark is the sinodural angle. The posterior border is found by widening of the bony ear canal and exposure of the cholesteatoma. The facial recess is not opened in this stage. Along the tegmen tympani, the supratubal cells are opened anteriorly, and the cog is drilled away.

The surgical landmarks of the anterior epitympanum are superior to the tegmen tympani, anterior to the zygoma root, medial to the bone plate covering the geniculate ganglion, and inferior to the canal of the tensor tympani (Fig. 14–1). The eustachian tube is found via the anterior epitympanum. From there, the cholesteatoma can be mobilized posteriorly, and the landmark of the canal of the tensor tympani leads to the cochleariform process.

The head of the malleus and, if present, the incus are removed, and superior to the cochleariform process, the horizontal part of the facial nerve is found. The cholesteatoma matrix is mobilized in continuity with the perimatrix, and the facial recess is now opened. The oval window is identified via the hypotympanum and via posterior so as not to luxate remnants of the stapes superstructure. The cholesteatoma is further exposed by drilling away the cortex of the mastoid. The facial ridge is lowered, and in this way the total cholesteatoma is exposed and can be removed. A meatoplasty is performed, and the cranial-based periosteal flap covers the skin of the meatoplasty, forming a lateral lining of the cavity. With use of the endaural approach for eradication, the patient has the smallest cavity possible. This is an advantage in sclerotic mastoids. If the stapes is present, a modified radical resection is done using a type III tympanoplasty. If the footplate is empty but mobile, plastic sheeting is put in the middle ear, and myringoplasty is performed without trying to reconstruct the sound-transforming mechanism in this stage. This approach ensures that the patient has a cholesteatoma-free ear without problems, especially in patients with a sclerotic mastoid. If necessary, a reconstruction of the middle ear can be done in a second stage. Residual cholesteatoma will be seen in cavities within 1 year postoperatively. To be sure that the reconstruction can be done in a cholesteatoma-free ear, it is therefore wise to delay the reconstruction for at least 1 year.

Reconstruction

The indications for reconstruction of a cavity are as follows:

1. The patient wishes to hear better.
2. The patient has recurrent infections of the cavity and wants a dry ear.
3. The patient wants to be able to swim.
4. The patient needs better canal conformation for fitting of a hearing aid.
5. The patient becomes dizzy if the ear is exposed to wind.
6. The patient has any combination of the above.

Patient Selection

In general, I do not advise reconstruction in children if they still have frequent upper respiratory infections; I wait until the child is 7 to 10 years old. In cases of a cavity in both ears, the ear in which the cavity is worse is always operated on first. If the main indication for operation is hearing improvement, the goal of a better hearing ear is taken into account.

The better ear is never operated on, and the contralateral ear must be kept safe and dry. There is no use in gaining 20 dB in the "worse" ear if the combination of both ears does not lead to better hearing. For the reconstruction, the ear must be as dry as possible, or it can be made dry during the operation by excision of the diseased tissue.

Preoperative Care

It is important that the cavity be free of cholesteatoma. For a successful reconstruction, enough healthy epithelium for the covering of the new canal is necessary. Although in many cases of large infected cavities the only way to get a dry ear is to reoperate, it is still advisable to have the cavity as dry as possible with regular preoperative cleaning and local and sometimes systemic antibiotics prescribed based on a proper culture. Upper respiratory infections must be cured before reconstruction.

Canal Wall Reconstruction

For the reconstruction of the canal wall, a prosthesis made of porous hydroxyapatite ceramic, chemical composition $Ca_{10}(PO_4)_6(OH)_2$, is used. The material has a macroporosity of 30 per cent, a pore size of approximately 100 μm, and a microporosity of less than 5 per cent (pore size, approximately 3 μm). With this porosity, bone ingrowth will take place in about 9 months, and it serves as the mineral matrix of bone.

A postauricular incision is made, the skin is elevated up to the concha, and the lateral lining of the cavity is kept intact. Posterior to the cavity, an incision is made in the periosteum, parallel to the skin incision. The periosteum is mobilized in the right plane, up to the border of the cavity without opening the cavity. Then, with a sharp knife, the periosteal flap is mobilized from the lining of the cavity, from inferior to superior. By mobilizing this periosteal flap and cutting it from the concha, a cranial-based periosteal flap is formed. This cranial-based flap is needed for the covering of the canal wall prosthesis at the end of the operation. Therefore, a cranial-based periosteal flap is mobilized because the undersurface of the periosteum is the bone-inducing surface, and the contact between this periosteal flap and the canal wall will stimulate new bone formation. If the epithelial lining of the cavity is not expected to be sufficient, a larger periosteal flap is needed. The soft tissue covering of the new canal wall prosthesis is very important.

Now, the lateral epithelial lining of the cavity is incised with a knife pointing anteriorly and not downward, especially in old cavities, because of the danger of cutting into an exposed sinus or an exposed dura. The lateral skin lining of the cavity is mobilized, and incisions are made at 12 and 6 o'clock in the meatal skin. In this way, the lateral epithelium of the former ear canal is mobilized. In this stage, it is important to control whether a good meatoplasty is made. If not, part of the conchal cartilage has to be removed. The new ear canal will be wider, and therefore this epithelial flap must be in direct contact with the new ear canal. The cranial-based periosteal flap and the epithelial flap are very important for a successful integration of the canal wall of hydroxyapatite. With a large diamond burr, the lining of the mastoid cavity is mobilized, and with an elevator, this lining is further mobilized from posterior to anterior.

In case of a very thin epithelium in the cavity, the epithelial lining is mobilized carefully. In case of disruption of the continuity, the adjacent bone is drilled away. In this way, the tegmen tympani is identified, and the skin lining is mobilized along the tegmen tympani to the anterior epitympanic area and the zygoma root. In many old cavities, the anterior epitympanic area is not opened sufficiently, and the remnant of the cog has to be removed, as well as the anterior buttress, so that there is a complete overview of the anterior epitympanic area. Often in old cavities, residual cholesteatoma is present in this area. Reconstruction will not be performed in these cases, and an operation with a modified radical is done.

With the overview of the anterior epitympanic area the patient is turned away from the surgeon. The entrance of the eustachian tube can be found with identification of the canal of the tensor tympani. From there, often granulation tissue or scar tissue can be present in the protympanum; suprisingly, in most cavities the eustachian tube itself has no disease. Now the epithelial lining is mobilized posteriorly along the canal of the tensor tympani. The cochleariform process is identified, and from there the horizontal part of the facial nerve is found, and the skin is mobilized along the facial nerve, even if it is denuded. Care is taken that the epithelial lining is mobilized in continuity. The middle ear is not opened at the area of the oval window niche so as not to luxate the stapes, if present.

Once the level of the facial nerve is identified, the mastoid epithelium is mobilized out of the mastoid tip, taking care to preserve much of the cortex in this place because this area will later provide stability for the canal wall prosthesis. Now, the whole lining of the cavity is put forward and outward. Via the hypotympanum, the middle ear cleft is entered, and from inferior and posterior, the oval window niche area is inspected. The epithelium and the remnants of the tympanic membrane are lifted from the remnants of the stapes superstructure or, if the structure is not present, from the footplate. In this way, the whole tympanomeatal flap, including a large piece of skin lining of the cavity, is mobilized outward. If the tensor tympani is still present, it is cut to lateralize the tympanic membrane completely. Now a good inspection of the eustachian tube and the protympanum can be performed, and the mobility of the footplate and/or the stapes superstructure is tested with the round window reflex. Also in this stage of the operation, the skin of the tympanomeatal flap can be trimmed, taking care that there is enough skin lining for the canal wall and that the skin lining will fit exactly on the new ear canal wall prosthesis (Fig. 14–2). Also, the edges of a tympanic membrane perforation are freshened.

Two grooves for the canal wall prosthesis are drilled. Anteriorly, the groove is made in the zygomatic root, just underneath the tegmen tympani, superior of the former location of the ear canal. Therefore, the tegmen tympani is drilled as flat as possible, and a groove is made in the zygomatic root. The reason for placing this anterior groove directly adjacent to the tegmen is that with a new ear canal no epitympanic area will be left, so in cases of retraction of the tympanic membrane, recurrent cholesteatoma will not occur. The level of the new annulus can be chosen as far lateral as possible.

The posterior groove is drilled in the facial ridge, lateral of the facial nerve. The stability of the groove is especially important in the cortex of the mastoid. If there is no mastoid cortex left, the groove has to be drilled in the floor of the former ear canal, anterior of the facial ridge, to get a stable position for the canal wall prosthesis (Fig. 14–3). This action, of course, yields a smaller ear canal, and it is preferable to have a wide, round ear canal for self-cleaning. With a width-measurement instrument, the width between the two grooves is measured, and with a depth-measurement instrument, the depth of the posterior groove is measured (Figs. 14–4 and 14–5). The canal wall prosthesis is drilled with a large diamond drill with water or with a diamond drill blade without water. The porous canal wall prosthesis is as brittle as bone but can be shaped easily. In the anteromedial part of the canal wall prosthesis, the annulus goes up and can therefore be drilled before the canal wall is placed. The canal wall prosthesis is placed into the two grooves with stability, especially at the cortex of the mastoid tip and in the facial ridge (Fig. 14–6). The new annulus is far more lateral than the original and leaves a wide posterior tympanotomy opening, but there is no epitympanic area. Therefore, the retraction of the tympanic membrane can be done anteriorly, but the membrane will then be part of the ear canal, or it can be done posteriorly through the wide posterior tympanotomy. Because of this wide opening, such a retraction is self-cleaning.

Obliteration of the mastoid cavity is not advisable. Even with good biomaterials, such as granules of hydroxyapatite, complete ossification of the mastoid cavity is not certain, and holes will stay under the obliteration. In addition, there is also a possibility of leaving epithelium or perhaps residual disease, which in the case of obliteration is not advisable.

In reconstruction of the canal wall, without obliteration, residual disease in the mastoid cavity can become evident and be noticed via the middle ear. In addition, the middle ear cleft will be smaller. There is no air reserve, which is a disadvantage for a well-functioning middle ear. With the canal wall prosthesis in place, a strip of absorbable gelatin film (Gelfilm) is placed from mastoid through the posterior tympanotomy to the eustachian tube orifice, and in the case of denuded promontory, a piece is also placed in the middle ear. A fascia graft is used as an underlay in case of a tympanic membrane perforation, with the support of some absorbable gelatin sponge (Gelfoam) anteriorly in the middle ear.

The ossiculoplasty is now performed (as described later), and the tympanomeatal flap is placed in contact with the canal wall prosthesis. It is important that the canal wall prosthesis have a good contact anteriorly with the anterior canal wall. Then the cranial-based periosteal flap is turned into the new ear canal underneath the tympanomeatal flap. A skin defect will be present laterally, but the new ear canal is covered by soft tissue. The lateral skin defect is

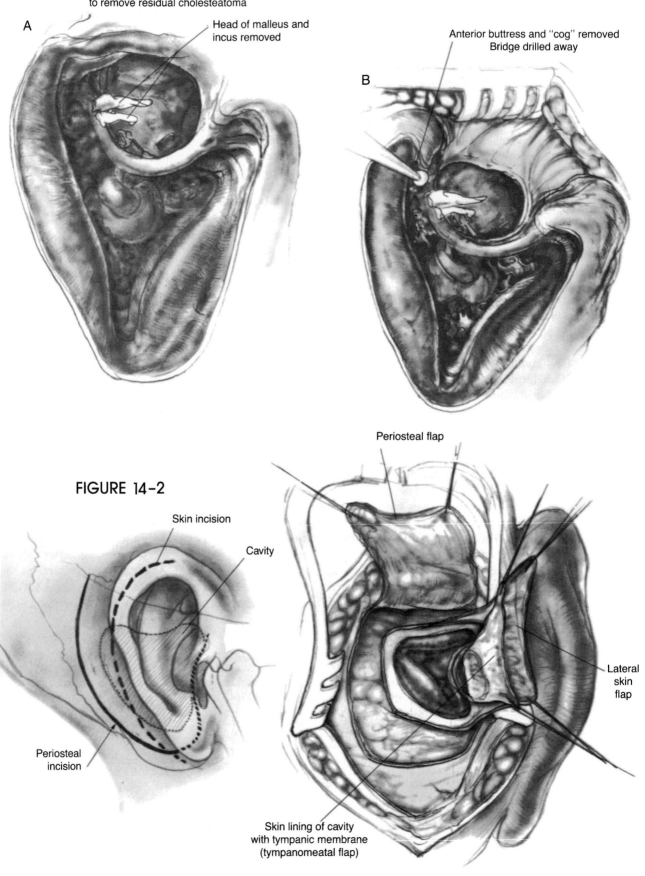

FIGURE 14-1

A

Remove old cavity and open anterior epitympanum to remove residual cholesteatoma

Head of malleus and incus removed

B

Anterior buttress and "cog" removed
Bridge drilled away

FIGURE 14-2

Periosteal flap

Skin incision

Cavity

Periosteal incision

Lateral skin flap

Skin lining of cavity with tympanic membrane (tympanomeatal flap)

FIGURES 14–1 and 14–2. *See legends on opposite page*

covered with the concha-based epithelium flap, which was the lateral skin lining of the cavity. When the pinna is turned backward, this skin flap falls in place (Fig. 14–7). It is important that the ear canal wall prosthesis be at the same level as the former cortex of the mastoid, so that this epithelial flap will not fall behind the new ear canal. Now, the tympanomeatal flap and the lateral skin flap are kept in place with gelatin sponge in the new ear canal, and loose oxytetracycline-soaked cotton wool is used the first week. The incision is stitched in one layer. The cotton wool is removed after 7 days, and in only a few cases, depending on the state of the skin lining of the new ear canal, is it replaced for another week.

If necessary, local antibiotic eardrops can be administered. The need for total covering of the canal wall prosthesis is also demonstrated by others.[29, 30] Black[30] uses a large periosteal flap underneath the temporalis muscle to cover the hydroxyapatite and also promotes the use of perichondrium and cartilage to support the posterosuperior part of the tympanic membrane.

Postoperative Problems

More than 1200 reconstructions have been performed since 1980, and although most of the patients have a nondraining ear and can swim, over the years some problems have been encountered.

Defects in the Skin Lining. A skin defect can be present, mostly in the medial part of the canal wall, especially in cases of insufficient skin lining in the cavity or insufficient covering of a large, cranial-based periosteal flap. With high magnification, there is clearly a one-layer epithelium, but the borders of this skin defect can be vulnerable, and therefore the patients are not allowed to swim. In most cases, this skin defect heals gradually in several months. In cases of a persistent defect, the skin is mobilized after the total integration of the canal wall prosthesis, which is in about 9 months, and then this defect can be closed with a skin graft.

Denuded Medial Part of the Ear Canal Prosthesis. In some cases, the tympanomeatal flap is not of adequate size and grows underneath the annulus of the new ear canal, leaving a denuded medial part of the canal wall prosthesis. These patients are not allowed to swim, and with local eardrops, the ear canal can be kept dry. After total integration in 9 months, this medial part of the denuded canal wall prosthesis can be drilled away with a diamond drill. The skin lining comes into view and leaves a small cavity, although the mastoid tip is covered. In cases of continuous ear drainage postoperatively, there are different possibilities.

Infected Lateral Pocket. If the meatoplasty was not wide enough, the lateral skin lining may not be in good contact with the canal wall prosthesis, and a pocket behind the lateral skin lining may be formed. This lateral pocket can then become infected, and although the medial part of the ear canal is normalized and integrated and the tympanic membrane can be completely normal without signs of infection of the middle ear and mastoid, this lateral pocket can have granulation and purulent discharge, which in most cases necessitates reoperation. Reintervention must be done, preferably as late as possible so as not to interfere with the integration of the canal wall prosthesis after 9 months.

Retraction and Atelectasis of the Middle Ear. Retraction and even atelectasis of the middle ear are possible. This problem results from the original disease, mostly the scar tissue. The retraction can take place anteriorly but will then be controlled and cleaned via the wide new ear canal. There is no epitympanic area. Retraction of the tympanic membrane may also occur posteriorly, through the posterior tympanotomy, but this is a very wide opening, and so far this problem has led to recurrent cholesteatoma in only a few patients over long postoperative periods. Patients with retractions are not allowed to swim so as to avoid infection of this pocket.

Residual Cholesteatoma. In cases of a residual cholesteatoma behind the lining of the former cavity, I advise not to reconstruct in the same stage. In cases in which I did reconstruct in the same stage, residual cholesteatoma recurred in half. This problem, however, will be readily apparent because of the wide posterior tympanotomy and the wide new ear canal.

Fracture of the New Ear Canal. In some cases in which trauma resulted from manipulation in the new ear canal, fracture of the brittle new ear canal prosthesis occurs. It takes 9 months before this ear canal is completely integrated; therefore, such trauma has to be avoided.

Infection of the Middle Ear and Mastoid. In cases of upper respiratory infections, some patients tend to develop middle ear infections again. These infections are treated in the usual way, with antibiotics, and the ear drains only temporarily. However, in some cases, a massive granulation develops in the middle ear as well as in the mastoid. When reoperation is necessary, the canal wall prosthesis is removed. The retrieved canal wall prostheses have been examined histologically over the years and have revealed that hydroxyapatite is resistant to infection and that new bone formation has taken place, indicating the capacity of the material. If ossiculoplasty is not done in the same stage as the canal wall reconstruction, transcanal ossiculoplasty can be performed after 1 year. Via incision in the skin of the posterior canal wall, the tympanomeatal flap can be elevated in the usual way, as in the normal middle ear.

Results

Two hundred patients with a cavity had reconstruction surgery and were followed up for at least 10 years. For the reconstruction of the posterior canal wall, a canal wall prosthesis of porous hydroxyapatite was used. The indication for operation was in most cases a combination of

---

FIGURE 14–1. Landmarks of the attic.

FIGURE 14–2. Soft tissue flaps: cranial-based periosteal flap, lateral skin flap, and tympanomeatal flap.

FIGURE 14-3

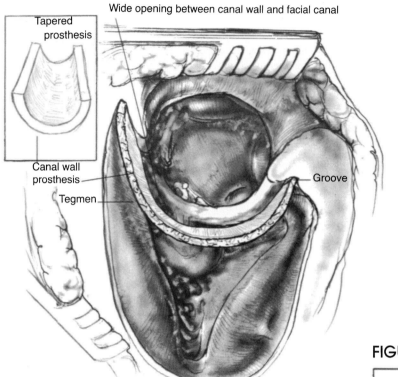

Wide opening between canal wall and facial canal

Tapered prosthesis

Canal wall prosthesis

Tegmen

Groove

FIGURE 14-6

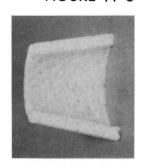

FIGURE 14-7

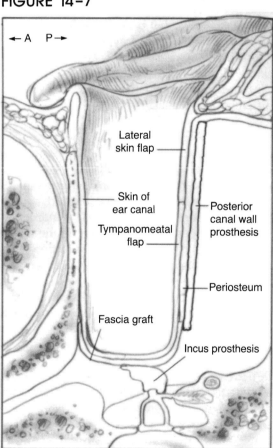

← A   P →

Lateral skin flap

Skin of ear canal

Tympanomeatal flap

Posterior canal wall prosthesis

Periosteum

Fascia graft

Incus prosthesis

FIGURE 14-4

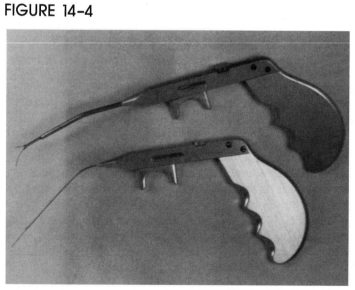

FIGURE 14-5

FIGURES 14–3 to 14–7. *See legends on opposite page*

hearing loss and draining ear. Persistent drainage of the cavity was present in 77 patients (38.5 per cent), and after the reconstruction only 8 patients (4 per cent) had persistent otorrhea. Recurrent otorrhea was present in 53 patients (26.5 per cent), and postoperatively, 33 (16.5 per cent) of these patients had a draining ear after one or two episodes of upper respiratory infection. The tympanic membrane was perforated preoperatively in 154 patients (77 per cent), and in 24 patients (12 per cent) there was a perforation postoperatively. Of the 200 patients, 25 (12.5 per cent) had a retraction pocket, but this pocket had such a large opening via the wide posterior tympanotomy that it was self-cleaning.

In 4 patients (2 per cent), reintervention was necessary because of a laterally infected new ear canal because the lateral skin of the new ear canal was not in contact with the canal wall prosthesis. Therefore, a meatoplasty had to be done to get a good alignment of the lateral skin of the new ear canal. The pocket between the skin and the new ear canal was infected and continued to drain.

Another problem was the denuded medial part of the canal wall prosthesis. In 5 patients, this problem resulted from the tympanomeatal flap being located behind the new ear canal; in these cases, reintervention was necessary. In the 200 patients, a residual cholesteatoma was found in 12 patients (6 per cent), and these were all cases in which I had done a reconstruction in a cavity with cholesteatoma. In this series, only one recurrent cholesteatoma (0.5 per cent) occurred, and the canal wall had to be removed. In all the cases of reintervention, the canal wall had to be removed, and histology showed living bone tissue.

After 15 years 75 per cent of the patients had a normal ear canal. In 25 per cent the ear canal had to be removed because of recurrent suppurative otitis media and collapse of the middle ear. The significant preoperative indication for failure was a history of more than three ear operations necessitated by recurrent infection before the reconstruction.[31]

The conclusion from the long-term follow-up studies is that it is possible to reconstruct a cavity with a new ear canal. The ear canal is ossified within 9 months, and there is no resorption. The patients are allowed to swim if there is a closed tympanic membrane and no retraction pocket.

Ossiculoplasty

The most reliable way to perform an ossiculoplasty is to reconstruct the defect in the ossicular chain in such a way that the ossicular chain is moved via the tympanic membrane by its contact with the handle of the malleus and that the lever mechanism of the ossicular chain is part of the transmission, making a proper piston-like function possible.

Different possibilities for a defect in the ossicular chain can be encountered:

1. Malleus present, stapes superstructure present, incus absent
2. Malleus present, stapes superstructure absent, incus absent
3. Malleus absent, superstructure present
4. Malleus absent, incus absent, stapes superstructure absent but a mobile footplate present

To overcome the defects in the ossicular chain, there are two approaches for the reconstruction: using a columella or bridging the defect in the ossicular chain.

For the columella there are two possible approaches. When the stapes superstructure is present, a short columella from the stapes head to tympanic membrane can be used in the form of a partial ossicular replacement prosthesis, When the stapes superstructure is missing but a mobile footplate is present, a long columella connecting the mobile footplate with the tympanic membrane can be used. This is a total ossicular replacement prosthesis.

Using a columella in the reconstruction of the ossicular chain has several disadvantages. Even with the use of a good biomaterial, the postoperative results are uncertain. The function of a columella depends on a good contact with the footplate or stapes superstructure, as well as over a larger surface area with the tympanic membrane. The healing process of the tympanic membrane is not predictable and can lateralize. There is also a possibility that the columella may integrate with the tympanic membrane but lateralizes with no contact with the footplate or stapes. Another possibility is that the tympanic membrane will fold over the columella in time. This result is often blamed on a eustachian tube dysfunction or the implant material itself, but from animal experiments it is clear that a mobile tympanic membrane always tends to fold over something that is placed against it, and even without effusion can eventually extrude the columella, even if it is made of homologous ossicles.

Bridging defects in the ossicular chain, therefore, yield more predictable results with implanted ossicles that bridge such that the handle of the malleus, which is integrated in the tympanic membrane, drives the ossicular chain. Another advantage of this assembly technique is the restoration of the lever mechanism of the ossicular chain. With this technique, the function of the ossicular chain is independent of the level of the tympanic membrane, and because of good integration with the remnants of the ossicular chain, extrusion will not occur.

A set of dense hydroxyapatite prostheses is used for tympanoplasty. The dense hydroxyapatite is integrated in

---

FIGURE 14–3. Anterior and posterior groove and the canal wall prosthesis.

FIGURE 14–4. Width measurement instrument.

FIGURE 14–5. Depth measurement instrument.

FIGURE 14–6. Porous hydroxyapatite canal wall prosthesis.

FIGURE 14–7. The different layers on top of the reconstruction.

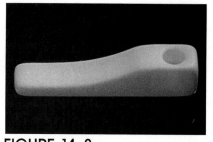

FIGURE 14-8

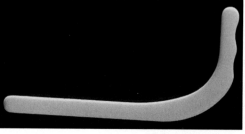

FIGURE 14-10

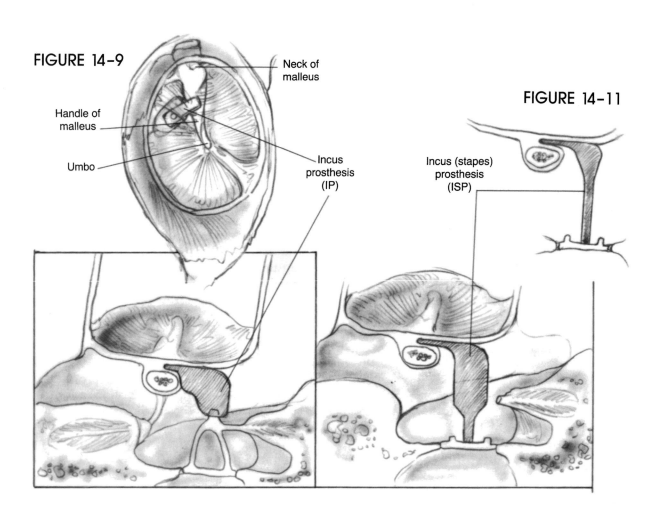

FIGURE 14-9

Neck of malleus

Handle of malleus

Umbo

Incus prosthesis (IP)

FIGURE 14-11

Incus (stapes) prosthesis (ISP)

FIGURE 14–8. Incus prosthesis of dense hydroxyapatite.

FIGURE 14–9. Incus prosthesis between the stapes head and malleus.

FIGURE 14–10. Incus-stapes prosthesis.

FIGURE 14–11. Incus-stapes prosthesis between the footplate and malleus.

the ossicular chain and it is covered by mucosa in a few days. The dense hydroxyapatite is not resorbed and resists infections of the middle ear.

Incus Prosthesis

In cases of a missing incus, a dense hydroxyapatite incus prosthesis is used to bridge the gap between the handle of the malleus and the mobile stapes (Fig. 14–8). The incus prosthesis has a corpus with a depression that fits on the stapes head. It overcomes the height difference between the stapes head and the handle of the malleus with a handle which connects the stapes head with the handle of the malleus. The longest distance between the stapes head and the handle of the malleus is chosen, necessitating removal of half of the handle in most cases. The incus prosthesis can be shaped with a diamond drill, but the handle of the incus prosthesis can also be cut with a small chisel. At the neck of the malleus, there is a loose connective tissue connection between the tympanic membrane and the handle of the malleus; therefore, it is easy to make a natural pocket between the tympanic membrane and the handle of the malleus, just inferior to the lateral process of the malleus.

The distance between the stapes head and the handle of the malleus is measured with the width-measurement instrument, and the incus prosthesis is cut to an individual length. The corpus of the incus prosthesis is placed with the niche on top of the head of the stapes, and the handle is placed on top of the handle of the malleus in the pocket, underneath the tympanic membrane (Fig. 14–9). The new incus integrates in the ossicular chain via the contact at the malleus and stapes head. The incus prosthesis can also be placed underneath the handle of the malleus, but this is a less stable position, and if there is a long distance between the stapes head and the malleus handle, the prosthesis can fall onto the promontory. The dimensions of the incus prosthesis are such that no contact exists between the annulus or facial ridge, thereby avoiding bony contact and fixation.

Problems with the Incus Prosthesis. It is important to establish the right distance between the stapes head and the handle of the malleus. If the handle of the incus prosthesis is too long, it may perforate the tympanic membrane. In such cases, there is a good integration of the incus prosthesis, but crusts can occur around the perforated tympanic membrane. If the handle of the incus is just on top of the malleus in the pocket, there is good integration and no problem with the interface of the tympanic membrane and the new incus prosthesis. Another problem can be the contact of the stapes head with the incus prosthesis: When a tendon of the stapedial muscle inserts at the top of the head of the stapes, the contact between the corpus of the incus prosthesis and the stapes head can be insufficient. Therefore, a groove must be drilled in the corpus of the incus prosthesis, or the tendon of the stapedial muscle has to be cut. A piece of gelatin sponge is placed underneath the bony annulus on top of the incus prosthesis to keep the incus prosthesis in close contact for the first few days, to secure good integration. There is a fibrous layer on top of the stapes head and mostly also a periosteum on the mal-

leus; therefore, the contact between the incus prosthesis and the malleus and stapes head is fibrous.

To get predictable postoperative results, the stapes superstructure and the footplate must be inspected carefully. In cases of a missing anterior or posterior crus, which in many instances can be fibrous, it is advisable not to use an incus prosthesis but to use an incus-stapes prosthesis between the remnants of the stapes on the footplate, in connection with the handle of the malleus. This is described later.

In cases in which the stapes superstructure is bent to the promontory by scar tissue, the results with an incus prosthesis are also poor, because the transfer mechanism in this case is not piston-like. In these cases, the use of an incus-stapes prosthesis is advised.

In cases of a missing lenticular process, the remnant of the long process of the incus is cut off, whereas the corpus of the incus, if mobile, is left in place. This prevents scar tissue formation in the epitympanic area. The incus prosthesis is used as a bridge between the stapes head and the handle of the malleus. The function and mobility of the reconstruction are tested via the round window reflex.

Results. In 200 patients with an incus prosthesis who have been followed for at least 10 years, the air-borne gap closure was within 20 dB in 80 per cent. Two patients required reoperation because the incus prosthesis was too long and perforated the tympanic membrane. These patients were not allowed to swim, and the incus prosthesis was well integrated. The connection between the handle of the malleus and the stapes superstructure was fibrous. A shorter incus prosthesis was implanted. In 10 cases of no improvement, incus prostheses were reinspected. In these cases, a problem occurred with the stapes superstructure being partly fibrous or bending to the promontory, resulting in poor function. In these cases, an incus-stapes prosthesis was used. There were no extrusions, and good results remained constant. There were no signs of resorption or fixation.

Incus-Stapes Prosthesis

In cases of a present malleus, an absent incus and stapes superstructure, and a present mobile footplate, an incus-stapes prosthesis of dense hydroxyapatite is used as a connection between the handle of the malleus and the mobile footplate (Fig. 14–10). The incus-stapes prosthesis consists of a shaft, with a dimension of 0.6 mm of dense hydroxyapatite, and a handle. The handle is placed in the pocket, as described earlier. It is a natural pocket in the loose connective tissue between the tympanic membrane and the handle of the malleus, just inferior to the lateral process. The shaft of the incus-stapes prosthesis is placed in the middle of the mobile footplate. To secure the shaft in the middle of the footplate, gelatin sponge can be used. It is also possible to cut a small strip of gelatin film. The strip of gelatin film around the incus-stapes prosthesis is pushed in the oval window niche, keeping the incus-stapes prosthesis in the center of the footplate. There is no need for an interface between the prosthesis and the footplate, and only in cases of a hypermobile or fractured footplate is a vein graft placed on top of the footplate. The handle is cut to an individual length, and the incus-stapes prosthesis stands stable between the handle of the malleus and the footplate (Fig. 14–11) The mucosa on the footplate is not removed, resulting in a fibrous contact between the hydroxyapatite shaft and the footplate. A piece of gelatin sponge is put underneath the bony annulus to secure a good adaptation for the first days. The bioactive material induces a good integration within a few weeks. The mobility of the new ossicular chain is tested via the round window reflex. In cases of a remnant of a mobile stapes superstructure, an incus-stapes prosthesis with a 0.6-mm shaft can be easily placed between the anterior and the posterior crura, securing the place of the incus-stapes prosthesis. In cases of overhang of the facial nerve, the shaft can also be drilled in a smaller dimension. A piece of gelatin film is placed between the incus-stapes prosthesis and the facial nerve.

Results. Two hundred patients with an incus-stapes prosthesis have been followed for at least 10 years. In 118 patients, this prosthesis was used as an assembly that connected the malleus and the footplate. The air-bone gap closure was within 20 dB in 74 per cent, and no improvement was found in 16 per cent. There was no extrusion in this long follow-up period. Once a good result was estab-

lished, it remained constant during the entire 10-year observation period; no resorption or fixation took place.

Since 1982, the incus-stapes prosthesis has also been used as a columella in 82 cases of a missing handle of the malleus. In these cases, the results were not as good: airbone gap closure within 20 dB in 34 per cent, and no improvement in 74.7 per cent. Extrusion was observed in 4.7 per cent. The extrusion took place via the following mechanism: The tympanic membrane gradually folded over the columella. There was no erosion or granulation of the tympanic membrane, but finally the incus-stapes prosthesis was extruded. The experience with this incus-stapes prosthesis as a columella indicated that either the design of the prosthesis was not ideal for the columella technique or the columella gave less favorable results. Therefore, a tympanic membrane–malleus prosthesis is preferred in cases of an absent malleus.

Total Alloplastic Middle Ear

In cases of a missing handle of the malleus, an incus or incus-stapes prosthesis, which can bridge the gap in the ossicular chain, cannot be used. Therefore, the concept of

FIGURE 14–12

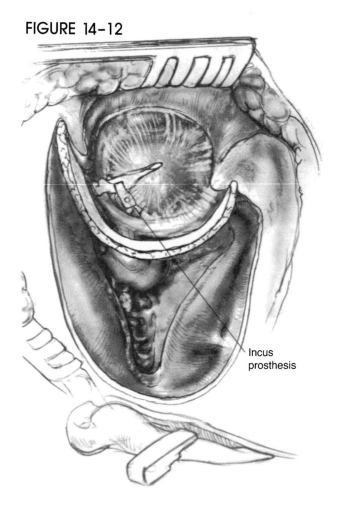

Incus
prosthesis

FIGURE 14–12. Total alloplastic middle ear.

the total homologous implant, including tympanic membrane, malleus, incus, and stapes, was used to make a total alloplastic middle ear (Fig. 14–12). It was shown that a tympanic membrane–malleus prosthesis was necessary to obtain a complete equivalent of the normal-functioning middle ear. Therefore, in vitro and in vivo studies were performed to find a degradable bioactive polymer to serve as a substitute for the middle layer of the tympanic membrane and for the integration of the handle of the malleus. Myringoplasty yielded good results with fascia, but for the development of the tympanic membrane–malleus prosthesis, a soft tissue replacement biomaterial was necessary.

In vivo studies and long-term animal studies resulted in the selection of a new biomaterial for this purpose: a degradable copolymer (Polyactive).[32] Polyactive is the first bioactive polymer showing a direct bond with the surrounding tissue. Exposed to bone, it enhances new bone formation, and in soft tissue, for instance in the tympanic membrane, it serves as a scaffold for the ingrowth of collagen and elastic fibers, forming a good middle layer. Polyactive has been used as an underlay, and a tympanic membrane–malleus prosthesis was developed to use in a total artificial middle ear, which includes the use of a canal wall prosthesis, a tympanic membrane–malleus prosthesis as an underlay under the remnants of the tympanic membrane, and an incus or incus-stapes prosthesis connecting the stapes superstructure or the mobile footplate with the handle of the malleus in the artificial tympanic membrane.

This technique makes total reconstruction of an empty middle ear possible. There are several advantages to the combination of these prostheses. The eradication can be done in the first stage without any concessions to the reconstruction. All diseased tissue can be removed, and in a second stage even an empty middle ear cavity can be reconstructed. The tympanic membrane–malleus prosthesis is placed underneath the remnants of the tympanic membrane in such a way that the pocket between the artificial tympanic membrane and the malleus is formed superiorly and in the same anatomic relation with the cochleariform process. The advantage of the canal wall prosthesis is that the level of the annulus can be chosen as far lateral as possible, thereby permitting the formation of a wide middle ear mastoid cleft. Then the incus or incus-stapes prosthesis is placed on the stapes or the footplate, as described before. It connects the new artificial handle of the malleus with stapes superstructure or footplate. With gelatin sponge, the prosthesis is stabilized for the first few days, and gelatin film secures the drainage from the mastoid–middle ear cleft to the eustachian tube. It will take several weeks before the epithelium has completely covered the tympanic membrane material; degradation of the new tympanic membrane scaffold takes place in 6 months, and remodeling in collagen and elastic fibers continues in that period. The main problem with the new tympanic membrane material is infection. If a purulent middle ear infection occurs in the first month, this material will degrade even faster, and, being a polymer, it will have more reaction.

Results. In 20 patients in whom an empty cavity was reconstructed with a total artificial middle ear, tympanic membrane closure occurred in 80 per cent of the patients with sufficient epithelium and an air-bone gap closure within 20 dB occurred in 45 per cent. Long-term results,

however, showed that the new middle ear collapsed and suppurative otitis media recurred. This is probably due to more extensive scar tissue in the totally empty middle ears, and as with the 15-year results of the cavity reconstructions, it shows that healthy mucosa is necessary to obtain a lasting result in the reconstructions.[33] The problems with the absence of the malleus are therefore not solved.

SUMMARY

I introduced hydroxyapatite for the reconstruction of the bony defects in the middle ear, and for 15 years it has proved its usefulness. It is the mineral matrix of bone, and it can be used in different forms, depending on the defect to be bridged and the demands of remodeling and resorption. This flexibility makes different prosthetic designs possible. It is my practice to stage eradication and reconstruction if cholesteatoma is present. With the new prostheses, we are no longer depending on the former anatomy. On the contrary, a new wide middle ear cleft can be made with a new round ear canal in which the epitympanic area is taken into the new ear canal, thereby avoiding future problems. Obliteration is not ideal, because of the possibility of burying diseased tissue that induces uncontrollable problems. For new middle ear function, it is also good to have a wide middle ear–mastoid cleft. For the reconstruction of the ossicular chain, the assembly technique gives the most predictable results. The hydroxyapatite ossicles bridge the gap in the ossicular chain, so that the tympanic membrane drives the ossicular chain via the handle of the malleus. The ossicular chain is moved with a lever mechanism and a piston-like function on the footplate.

If the principles we learned from the homologous implants are used, more predictable and uniform ways of reconstruction are possible. The development of new materials in otology gives new possibilities for the future.

References

1. Jansen C: The combined approach for tympanoplasty (report of 10 years' experience). J Laryngol 82: 776–793, 1968.
2. Grote JJ: Tympanoplasty with calcium phosphate. Am J Otol 6: 269–271, 1985.
3. Smyth GDL: Chronic Ear Disease. New York, Churchill Livingstone, 1985.
4. Homsy CA: Biocompatibility in selection of materials for implantation. J Biomed Mater Res 4: 341–356, 1970.
5. Gjuric M, Schagerl S: Gold prostheses for ossiculoplasty. Am J Otol 19: 273–6, 1998.
6. Austin DF: Ossicular reconstruction. Arch Otolaryngol Head Neck Surg 94: 525–535, 1971.
7. Brackmann DE, Sheehy JL: Tympanoplasty with TORPs and PORPs. Laryngoscope 89: 108–114, 1979.
8. Emmett JR: Plastipore implants in middle ear surgery. Otolaryngol Clin North Am 28: 265–72, 1995.
9. Jahnke K, Schmidt C: Histological studies on the suitability of Macor ceramic implants. *In* Grote JJ (ed): Biomaterials in Otology. Boston, Martinus Nijhoff, 1984, pp 74–79.
10. Reck R: Bioactive glass-ceramics in ear surgery: Animal studies and clinical results. Laryngoscope 94(Suppl 33): 1–54, 1984.
11. van Blitterswijk CA, Koerten HK, Bakker D, et al: Biodegradation-dependent trace element accumulation: A study on calcium phosphate ceramics and polymers. *In* Williams KR, Lesser THJ (eds): Interface Medicine Mechanics. Trowbridge, England, Dotesios Printers, 1990, pp 110–119.

12. van Blittersswijk CA, Grote JJ: Biological performance of ceramics during infection and inflammation. Crit Rev Biocompatibil 5: 23–43, 1989.

13. van Blitterswijk CA, Grote JJ, Koerten HK, et al: The biological performance of calcium phosphate ceramics in an infected implantation site: III. Biological performance of B-whitlockite in the non-infected rat middle ear. J Biomed Mater Res 20: 1197–1218, 1986.

14. van Blitterswijk CA, de Groot K, Daems WT, et al: The biological performance of calcium phosphate ceramics in an infected implantation site: I. Biological performance of hydroxyapatite during *Staphylococcus aureus* infection. J Biomed Mater Res 20: 989–1002, 1986.

15. van Blitterswijk CA, Bakker D, Grote JJ, Daems WT: The biological performance of calcium phosphate ceramics in an infected implantation site: II. Biological performance of hydroxyapatite during short-term infection. J Biomed Mater Res 20: 1003–1006, 1986.

16. van Blitterswijk CA, Grote JJ, Kuijpers W, et al: Macropore tissue ingrowth: A quantitative and qualitative study on hydroxyapatite ceramic. Biomaterials 7: 137–143, 1986.

17. van Blitterswijk CA, Kuijpers W, Daems WT, Grote JJ: Epithelial reactions to hydroxyapatite: An in vivo and in vitro study. Acta Otolaryngol (Stockh) 101: 231–241, 1986.

18. Grote JJ, van Blitterswijk CA: Reconstruction of the posterior auditory canal wall with a hydroxyapatite prosthesis. Ann Otol Rhinol Laryngol 95(Suppl 123): 6–9, 1986.

19. Grote JJ, Kuijpers W, de Groot K: use of sintered hydroxyapatite in middle ear surgery. ORL J Otorhinolaryngol Relat Spec 43: 248–254, 1981.

20. Grote JJ, van Blitterswijk CA, Kuijpers W: Reconstruction of the middle ear with hydroxyapatite implants. Ann Otol Rhinol Laryngol 95(Suppl 123): 1–12, 1986.

21. Grote JJ: Tympanoplasty with calcium phosphate. Am J Otol 6: 269–271, 1985.

22. Grote JJ: Reconstruction of the ossicular chain with hydroxyapatite prostheses. Am J Otol 8: 396–401, 1987.

23. Kveton JF: Obliteration of the eustachian tube using hydroxyapatite cement: A permanent technique. Laryngoscope 106: 1241–1243, 1996.

24. Geyer G, Dazert S, Helms J: Performance of ionomeric cement (Ionocem) in the reconstruction of the posterior meatal wall after curative middle ear surgery. J Laryngol Otol 111: 1130–1136, 1997.

25. Geyer G, Helms J: Ionomer cement prostheses in reconstructive middle ear surgery. HNO 45: 442–447, 1997.

26. McElveen JT Jr, Feghali JG, Barrs DM, et al: Ossiculoplasty with polymaleinate ionomeric prosthesis. Otolaryngol Head Neck Surg 113: 420–426, 1995.

27. Black B: Spanner malleus-stapes/footplate assembly. Laryngoscope 104: 775–777, 1994.

28. Goldenberg RA: Ossiculoplasty with composite prostheses: PORP and TORP. Otolaryngol Clin North Am 27: 727–745, 1994.

29. Lenis A: Middle ear reconstruction with modifed hydroxyapatite prosthesis. Laryngoscope 100: 1020–1021, 1990.

30. Black B: Prevention of recurrent cholesteatoma: Use of hydroxyapatite plates and composite grafts. Am J Otol 13: 273–278, 1992.

31. Grote JJ: Results of cavity reconstruction with hydroxyapatite implants after 15 years. Am J Otol 19: 565–568, 1998.

32. Grote JJ, Bakker D, Hessling SC, van Blitterswijk CA: New alloplastic tympanic membrane material. Am J Otol 12: 329–335, 1991.

33. Grote JJ: Total artificial middle ear: Preliminary report. Am J Otol 6: 797–800, 1995.

15

Surgery of Acute Infections and Their Complications

J. Gail Neely, M.D., F.A.C.S. ▪ Mark S. Wallace, M.D., F.A.C.S.

DEFINITION AND CLINICAL SIGNIFICANCE

Complications of suppurative ear disease, acute or chronic, manifest acutely and are medical and surgical emergencies. They are defined as a spread of infection beyond the confines of the pneumatized spaces and the attendant mucosa.

Complications are classified into two groups: aural (intratemporal) and intracranial. Aural complications include (1) mastoiditis, (2) petrositis, (3) labyrinthitis, and (4) facial paralysis. Intracranial complications are (1) extradural abscess or granulation tissue, (2) dural venous sinus thrombophlebitis, (3) brain abscess, (4) otitic hydrocephalus, (5) subdural abscess, and (6) meningitis (Fig. 15–1).[1, 2]

Because of the significant reduction in absolute numbers of complications, individual clinicians do not have extensive experience in treating patients with complications of suppurative ear disease. This contributes to decreased familiarity and recognition of otogenic complications.[3, 4] The combination of lack of awareness and masking of early signs and symptoms leads to delay in diagnosis and subsequent treatment. Physician delay has been noted to be the most significant factor in late diagnosis and treatment of otogenic complications. Delay in diagnosis and treatment of complications of suppurative ear disease is associated with worsening morbidity and mortality.[3, 5]

ETIOLOGY AND PATHOGENESIS

The organisms responsible for otogenic complications in the acute setting are *Streptococcus pneumoniae* and *Haemophilus influenzae*. Organisms that cause complications in chronic otitis media are frequently gram-negative and/or anaerobic.[6] The presence of anaerobes is significantly associated with complications.[7–9]

In patients with intratemporal complications, isolates from cultures of middle ear effusions, otorrhea, and mastoid have demonstrated *S. pneumoniae* to be the most common organism,[10] followed by *Pseudomonas aeruginosa* and *Streptococcus pyogenes*,[11] *Staphylococcus aureus*, and *H. influenzae*.[12, 13] However, *P. aeruginosa* was the most common organism found in a recent review of 134 patients with acute mastoiditis.[14]

S. pneumoniae[15] and *H. influenzae* type B are the most common cause of bacterial meningitis.[16] *Proteus mirabilis*, *P. aeruginosa*, and staphylococcal organisms are common

pathogens isolated in patients with intracranial complications.[17] Gram-negative isolates have been major organisms in other series.[18, 19] Polymicrobial cultures are common in brain abscess.[8]

Obstruction of the aditus ad antrum, congenitally preformed pathways through the oval or round window, or acquired pathways from fractures or chronic erosive infection, granulation tissue, or cholesteatoma, especially virulent organisms such as type B *H. influenzae*, and synergistic pathogenicity resulting from anaerobic organism microenvironmental changes all may play a role in the pathogenesis of complications (Fig. 15–2).[20–22]

Clinically, several important observations can be made that help alert the physician to the possible occurrence of a complication and may reflect some of the pathobiology. Signs and symptoms of possible impending complications are (1) persistent acute infection for 2 weeks; (2) recurrent symptoms of infection within 2 weeks; (3) acute, fetid exacerbation of chronic infection; (4) fetid discharge during treatment; (5) *H. influenzae*, type B, or anaerobes cultured from the ear; or (6) fever in the presence of a chronically perforated tympanic membrane, with or without cholesteatoma.

CLINICAL PRESENTATION

When the possibility exists that the patient has a complication from suppurative ear disease, the complete list of the 10 complications and the fact that more than one complication is likely can be somewhat overwhelming. Fortunately, the complications tend to manifest in some obvious or predictable clinical patterns.[22]

The three most obvious complications are facial paralysis, labyrinthitis, and meningitis. Facial paralysis is obvious, and if it occurs as a result of acute infection, it is usually the only complication. If it occurs as a result of cholesteatoma, a horizontal canal fistula may also exist.

Labyrinthitis presents in an obvious manner, manifesting as ipsilateral sensorineural hearing loss, nystagmus toward the contralateral side, and vertigo. It is classified according to what enters the perilymphatic space: serous labyrinthitis (toxins), suppurative labyrinthitis (bacteria), or chronic labyrinthitis (soft tissue, such as cholesteatoma). Suppurative labyrinthitis destroys all the hearing and may rapidly progress to meningitis. Labyrinthitis with some hearing, resulting from acute infection, is usually serous and isolated without other complications. Labyrinthitis with hearing,

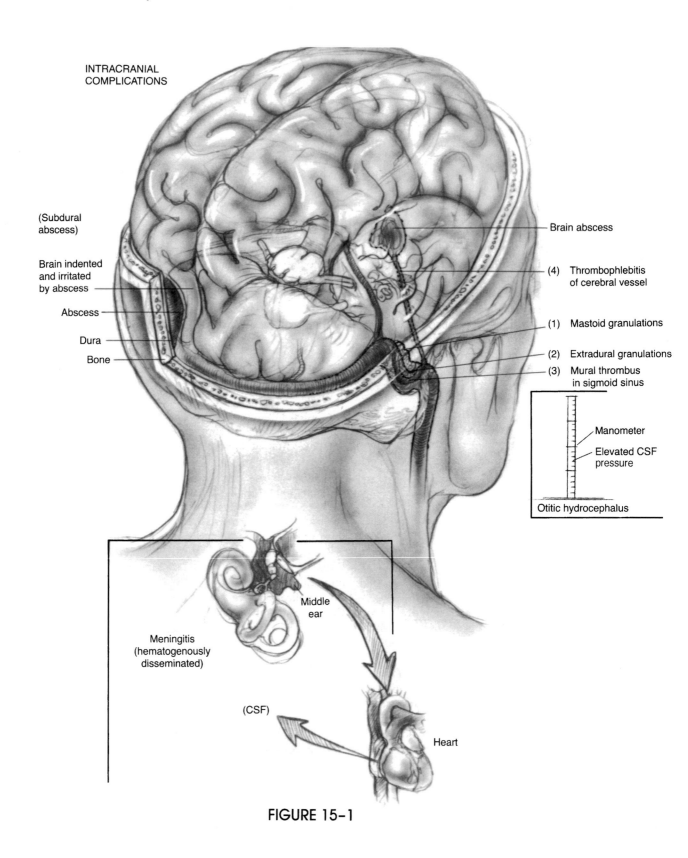

FIGURE 15-1. Artist's illustration of intracranial complications. The predictable pattern of associated complications is numbered in order of progression with the ultimate outcome being brain abscess and/or otitic hydrocephalus.

resulting from a cholesteatoma, may well be associated with a labyrinthine fistula of the horizontal canal and a dehiscence of the fallopian canal, with or without facial paralysis.

Meningitis also presents in an obvious manner. Meningitis associated with acute otitis media almost always is the result of hematogenous dissemination, and other complications are rare. Meningitis associated with chronic suppurative otitis media is usually the result of a dehiscence in the dura that allows continuity between an extradural abscess and the cerebrospinal fluid.

Mastoiditis may be rather obvious if a subperiosteal abscess is present; however, without such a recognizable sign, "masked mastoiditis" may present as mild discomfort in the ear, with or without mastoid tenderness. If the mastoid infection spreads along the vessels laterally through the outer cortex of the mastoid at McEwen's triangle and purulent debris accumulates under the periosteum, a subperiosteal abscess results. Patients have mastoid tenderness, pain, swelling, and an anteroinferior displacement of the ear. Rarer subperiosteal or soft tissue abscesses can occur in the deep neck or zygoma. If purulent debris escapes through eroded bone and along vessels from the medial tip cells and diploic bone medial to the digastric muscle and enters the neck through the incisura digastrica, a Bezold's abscess is formed. Purulent debris deep to the fascial planes of the sternocleidomastoid and trapezius muscles is difficult to localize by palpation.[23] If pus tracks along the external auditory canal and accumulates under the temporalis muscle, the rare Luc's abscess is formed.[24]

Less obvious complications follow. Subdural abscesses are extremely rare, usually devastatingly obvious by coma and focal neurologic signs and easily seen by magnetic resonance imaging (MRI). If there is any doubt that a catastrophic intracranial lesion exists, the chance of a subdural abscess being present is remote. Otitic hydrocephalus characteristically presents with headache, some degree of lethargy, and severe papilledema. Almost without exception, otitic hydrocephalus is associated with occlusive sigmoid sinus thrombophlebitis and extradural abscess. Petrositis presents with retro-orbital pain; however, the patient may not volunteer this symptom. It is crucial to ask about retro-orbital pain to be assured of its absence. Petrositis is rarely, if ever, present without mastoiditis. Intracranial complications are more frequent with petrositis. The full classic triad of Gradenigo—ear infection, ipsilateral retro-orbital pain, and abducens palsy—often thought to be pathognomonic of petrositis, is rarely present in petrositis unless an extradural medial petrous abscess is present.

The remaining four complications of suppurative ear disease are masked mastoiditis, extradural abscess or granulation tissue, dural venous sinus thrombophlebitis, and brain abscess. Unfortunately, these can be silent but extremely serious. Fortunately, they occur together in predictable patterns. Mastoiditis may occur alone but often results in a silent accumulation of extradural abscess or granulation tissue. The extradural infection may occur, in the case of cholesteatoma, in the middle fossa at the tegmen, but it characteristically occurs along the extraluminal surface of the lateral wall of the sigmoid sinus, creating an often

FIGURE 15-2

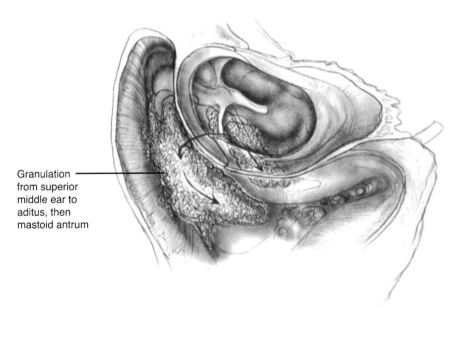

Granulation from superior middle ear to aditus, then mastoid antrum

FIGURE 15–2. Artist's illustration of obstruction of the aditus ad antrum, a principal key to the development of complications.

silent, nonoccluding phlebitis of the sinus wall and an induced mural thrombus, sigmoid sinus thrombophlebitis. In every case of suspected or operated mastoiditis, extradural granulation tissue and sigmoid sinus thrombophlebitis should be sought, preoperatively and intraoperatively. Brain abscess occurs as a result of retrograde thrombophlebitis of cerebral or cerebellar veins that are tributary to the inflamed sigmoid sinus or other adjacent dural sinuses. Brain abscesses have four stages, as follows:

1. *Invasion,* the initial onset of cerebritis. This stage creates vague symptoms of mild headache, lethargy, and malaise that last several days and then resolve.
2. *Localization,* the stage of quiescence and latency. This stage is totally silent for weeks.
3. *Enlargement,* in which most abscesses manifest with seizures or focal neurologic signs.
4. *Termination,* in which the abscess catastrophically ruptures into the ventricle or subarachnoid space.

Brain abscesses are silent, take weeks from onset to be detectable, even with imaging, and can be devastating. It is prudent to look for brain abscesses in cases of mastoiditis initially and again 3 to 4 weeks later (Fig. 15–3).

The pathophysiologic and diagnostic key to occult complications is mastoiditis. Without careful medical care, the classic presentation of acute coalescent mastoiditis with an associated subperiosteal abscess characterizes the clinical presentation of mastoiditis.[25] Masked mastoiditis, in patients with seemingly adequate care, however, is much harder to diagnose, can be much more devastating, and is more often associated with intracranial complications.[26, 27] Patients with any of the signs and symptoms of impending complication, particularly with a recurrence of deep, not necessarily severe, pain, may have masked mastoiditis. If bone destruction is present, the diagnosis is made. However, masked mastoiditis may exist without early bone destruction. If pain persists despite adequate culture-guided antibiotic administration, surgical exploration and aggressive medical treatment are indicated.

DIAGNOSIS

The most powerful, rapid, efficient, and useful diagnostic tools are the expertly performed history and physical examination. In the history, look for the following:

1. Symptoms suggesting impending complications
2. Symptoms of retro-orbital or deep, boring head pain
3. Symptoms of lethargy, headache, or both, currently and within the past 2 months

In the physical examination, look for the following:

1. Signs suggesting impending complications
2. Signs diagnostic of obvious complications
3. Signs of catastrophic neurologic disease
4. Funduscopic examination for papilledema

Investigators reporting recent series have found the following early findings to be associated with impending or established intratemporal or intracranial complications:

1. Pain and fever lasting more than 4 days despite appropriate treatment for acute otitis media[10]

2. Persisting fever and headache[3]
3. Radiographic evidence of a lytic lesion, presence of anaerobes, or excessive granulation tissue at surgery associated with chronic suppurative otitis media[7]
4. Chronic suppurative ear disease with fever, headache, ear pain, or vertigo[28]
5. Increasing otorrhea, meningeal signs, or impairment of consciousness[17, 29]
6. Headache with vomiting in patients with chronic otitis media[8]

The most important error in diagnosis is a poor or nonexpert history with little attention paid to the details of previous symptoms and the associated time courses. Another error is to assume that the organisms cultured from the ear canal drainage accurately reflect the organism causing the complication; aspiration and intraoperative cultures from the complication and the involved tissues of the ear best reflect the responsible pathogens.

When a complication is suspected, high-resolution computed tomography (CT) of the temporal bone and associated brain, with and without contrast infusion, is indicated. CT allows a good look at the bone and a reasonable look at the intracranial structures.[9, 17, 23, 24, 30–32] If bone is eroded over the sigmoid sinus or at the tegmen, MRI is indicated to get a better appreciation of possible extradural, intradural, subdural, and intracerebral granulation, edema, or abscess.[8] MRI is more sensitive than CT in detecting early cerebritis and cerebral edema.[9] MRI may be useful in imaging lesions at the petrous apex in Gradenigo's syndrome.[33] MRI is the most sensitive diagnostic tool in identifying the site and size of epidural, subdural, and brain abscess and is more sensitive than CT in detecting extraparenchymal spread to the subarachnoid space or ventricle.[34]

If mastoiditis, and particularly sigmoid sinus phlebitis, is surgically proven, repeat MRI is indicated 3 to 4 weeks postoperatively to detect the subsequent development of an occult brain abscess.

In cases of suspected meningitis or otitic hydrocephalus, a thorough funduscopic examination and CT scan should precede lumbar puncture to determine the presence of simultaneous intracranial abscess.[9, 17] Typical findings on lumbar puncture for meningitis are high protein and low glucose levels and the presence of microorganisms on Gram's stain. In otitic hydrocephalus typical findings on lumbar puncture are normal protein and glucose levels, negative Gram's stain, and elevated opening pressure.

Careful surgical observations, through thin bone, of the dura at the tegmen, the sigmoid sinus, and the facial nerve are crucial for complete diagnosis (Fig. 15–4).

Diagnoses are made from the history, physical examination, and surgical exploration. Imaging is crucial to observe brain and subdural abscesses, but reliance on imaging modalities at the expense of these three elements, carefully done, will lead to serious errors.

TREATMENT

The treatment of all complications is admission to the hospital, use of antibiotics that are culture guided from the ear and the complication, and surgical intervention as outlined in this section.

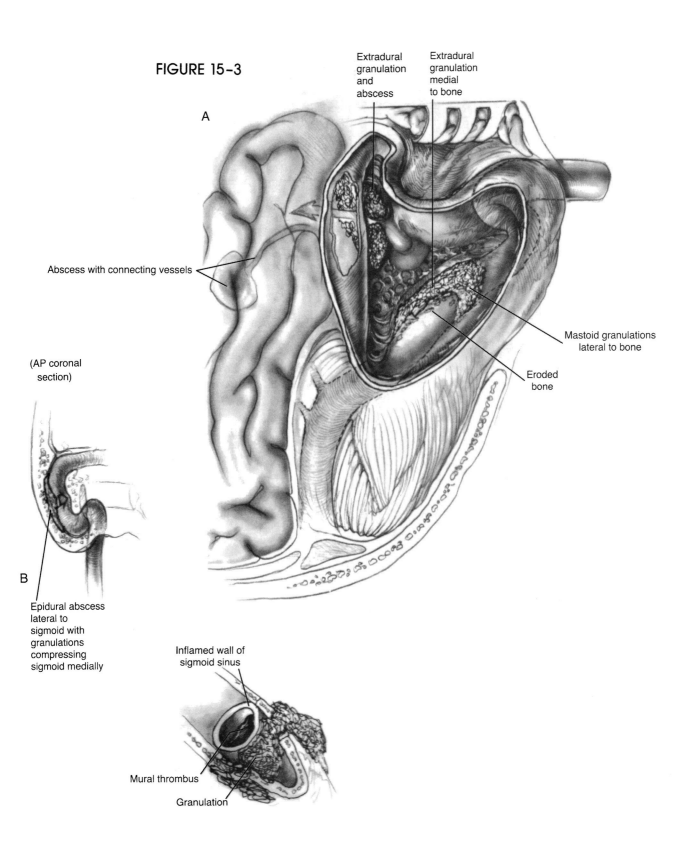

FIGURE 15-3

A

Extradural granulation and abscess

Extradural granulation medial to bone

Abscess with connecting vessels

Mastoid granulations lateral to bone

Eroded bone

(AP coronal section)

B

Epidural abscess lateral to sigmoid with granulations compressing sigmoid medially

Inflamed wall of sigmoid sinus

Mural thrombus

Granulation

FIGURE 15–3. Artist's depiction of mechanism of development of brain abscess by retrograde thrombophlebitis of cerebral vessels, usually above the tentorium, from inflamed sigmoid and transverse sinus secondary to mastoid and extradural granulations.

FIGURE 15-4

RADICAL MASTOIDECTOMY WITH INTACT OSSICLES

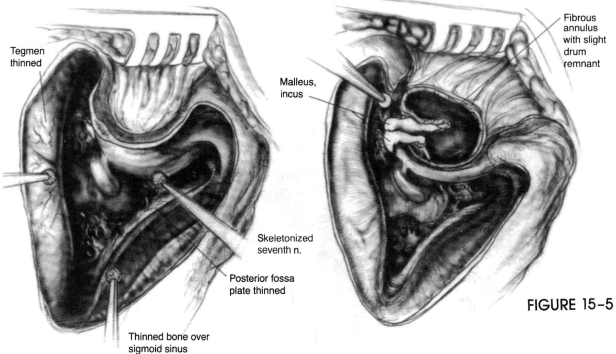

Tegmen thinned

Malleus, incus

Fibrous annulus with slight drum remnant

Skeletonized seventh n.

Posterior fossa plate thinned

Thinned bone over sigmoid sinus

FIGURE 15-5

A PETROSITIS—Lateral approach—Tracts to petrous apex
First stage

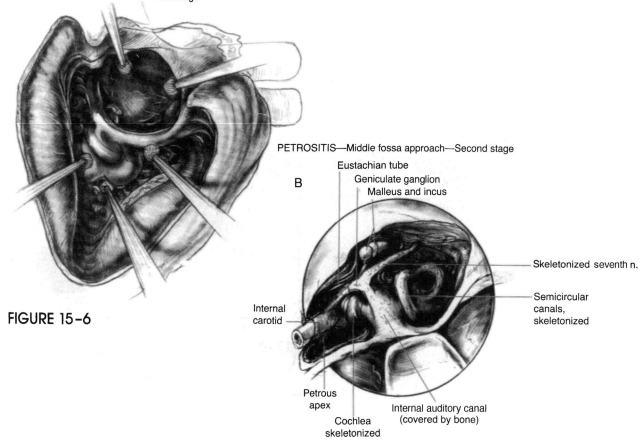

PETROSITIS—Middle fossa approach—Second stage

B

Eustachian tube
Geniculate ganglion
Malleus and incus

Skeletonized seventh n.

Semicircular canals, skeletonized

Internal carotid

FIGURE 15-6

Petrous apex

Cochlea skeletonized

Internal auditory canal (covered by bone)

FIGURES 15-4 to 15-6. *See legends on opposite page*

The treatment of acute coalescent mastoiditis and masked mastoiditis, with or without subperiosteal abscess, is wide myringotomy, complete canal wall up mastoidectomy, and wide facial recess approach from the mastoid into the middle ear. The aditus ad antrum obstruction cannot be adequately maintained patent without the additional facial recess window. Sometimes the granulation tissue is severe in the middle ear and mastoid, and symptoms suggest petrositis; in these cases, total resection of the tympanic membrane with careful maintenance of the ossicles in situ and resection of the posterosuperior canal wall allows adequate drainage. Reconstruction of the tympanic membrane can be done later in a healed ear (Fig. 15–5).

Chronic mastoiditis is a diagnostic dilemma; the primary way to establish the diagnosis is to intraoperatively identify granulation tissue–induced erosion of bone, usually over the sigmoid sinus. The treatment of most chronic mastoiditis is the same as for cases of chronic suppurative otitis media, with or without cholesteatoma. Most of these cases improve with removal of disease and reconstruction of the middle ear at the same setting, with canal wall up or canal wall down procedures.

In all patients undergoing mastoidectomy for suppurative disease, inspection of the dura of the tegmen, the sigmoid sinus, and the facial nerve through thin bone is crucial. Otherwise, granulation tissue in the middle and posterior fossa and along the facial nerve may go unrecognized and untreated.

The treatment of petrositis may require two stages, but the second stage is usually not necessary. The first stage is a radical mastoidectomy, or the modification of the radical procedure mentioned earlier in which the ossicular chain is left intact, the drum is removed, and the five tracts to the petrous apex are opened as far as possible.[35] The second stage, if the first does not resolve the infection, is a middle fossa approach for the total exenteration of disease in the petrous apex and in the perilabyrinthine cells. This dissection is combined with the previous lateral approach, and all pneumatized spaces in the temporal bone are removed, sparing the vital structures of the inner ear, facial nerve, carotid artery, jugular bulb, and sigmoid and the contents of the internal auditory canal. The cavity is left open (Fig. 15–6).

The surgical treatment of labyrinthitis in acute infection is confined to myringotomy. The treatment of labyrinthitis in chronic otitis media, with or without cholesteatoma, is tympanoplasty and mastoidectomy following the surgeon's usual preference. If a fistula is identified in the cochlea, it is usually better to leave the cholesteatoma matrix on the fistula, close the ear, and return to remove it when the ear is well healed and sterile. This is a good technique for wide, deep fistulas in the vestibular labyrinth as well. For narrow, shallow fistulas in the semicircular canals, the cholesteatoma matrix may be carefully removed and the fascia placed over the fistula; if the matrix appears to be attached to the membranous labyrinth, dissection should cease and the matrix left to be removed later. An important point to re-emphasize is that one cannot be sure prospectively if the labyrinthitis is toxic (serous) or suppurative; nor can one be comfortable that a serous labyrinthitis may not become suppurative. Suppurative labyrinthitis may be soon associated with meningitis. Thus, hospitalization and intravenous antibiotics need to be continued until the infection has been eradicated.

The surgical treatment of facial paralysis from acute infection is myringotomy. If subacute or chronic infections are present, mastoidectomy to eradicate disease and to explore the fallopian canal for invasive granulation tissue is indicated; this exploration can be done by thinning the bone of the canal to allow observation of the contents. Decompression may not be worthwhile. Opening the sheath and exposing the nerve in the face of infection are probably contraindicated. If invasive granulation tissue is found within the osseous canal, the canal should be opened for at least the length of the extent of the granulation. External epineurial sheath granulations may be removed, but no attempt should be made to remove granulations from within the sheath; granulation tissue tends to infiltrate between fibers, and attempts to remove it will result in fiber destruction.

The treatment of preoperatively or intraoperatively discovered extradural granulation tissue or abscess is the wide exposure of the abnormal dura. Careful attempts to bluntly remove excess granulation tissues are appropriate; it is not necessary to remove all granulations. Abscesses should be completely drained into the mastoid. If an abscess is encountered, the canal wall should be taken down so that complete drainage is ensured (Fig. 15–7).

Dural venous thrombophlebitis rarely requires additional surgical treatment beyond a complete mastoidectomy and management of the extradural granulations or abscess; opening the sinus is not usually required.[36] Medical therapy includes antibiotic therapy and measures to reduce any intracranial pressure using hyperventilation, therapeutic lumbar puncture, mannitol, and dexamethasone.[37] In the rare case in which classic preoperative spiking fever and chills precede the discovery of a completely solidified sinus, careful opening of the sinus to explore for an intra-

FIGURE 15–4. Illustration of the very important exploration of dura of the sigmoid sinus, middle fossa, posterior fossa, and sheath of the facial nerve as inspected through thin bone intraoperatively. It is not necessary to thin all the bone and certainly not necessary to transverse the bone to the structure, unless granulations or pus is found.

FIGURE 15–5. Artist's illustration of Neely's modification of a radical mastoidectomy in which the drum and the posterior and superior canal wall are removed, but the ossicles are left intact. Tympanoplasty may later be performed.

FIGURE 15–6. Artist's illustration of the two phases of management of petrositis. The first phase (A) requires a radical mastoidectomy and following the five cellular tracts to the petrous apex. The second phase (B), if the first fails to resolve the infection, is the middle fossa approach to the complete petrosectomy.

FIGURE 15-7

FIGURE 15-8

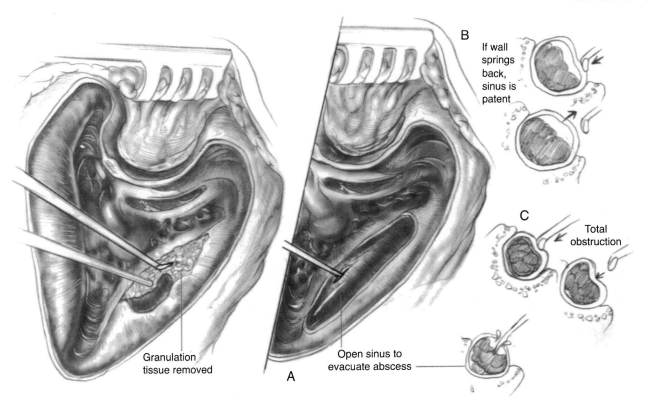

Granulation tissue removed

If wall springs back, sinus is patent

Total obstruction

Open sinus to evacuate abscess

A

B

C

REMOVAL OF DEEP BRAIN ABSCESS

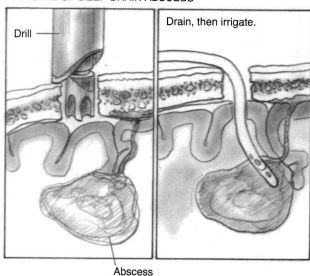

Drill

Drain, then irrigate.

Abscess

FIGURE 15-9

FIGURE 15–7. Artist's illustration of the management of granulations on the sigmoid sinus thrombo-phlebitis. A conservative approach is advisable.

FIGURE 15–8. Artist's illustration of exploration of the sigmoid sinus in search of an intraluminal abscess. This is very unusual and should not be performed without complete capability and familiarity with neurotologic surgery.

FIGURE 15–9. Artist's illustration of a burr hole over a brain abscess through a separate sterile approach and the aspiration, with or without irrigation with antibiotics. Aspiration, irrigation, or resection of brain abscesses may not be required.

luminal abscess may be indicated. Usually, a fibrotic, non-abscessing mural thrombus is found, for which no further intraluminal work should be done.[34, 38, 39] If an easily identifiable intraluminal abscess is found, it should be drained into the mastoid.[6, 34, 39]

If bleeding occurs with sinus opening, it can be controlled with an extraluminal piece of Surgicel, which is left in place at the conclusion of the procedure; a piece of fascia may be additionally placed lateral to this patch. Ligation of the internal jugular vein or use of anticoagulants and thrombolytics is not usually required; their use is still controversial.[34, 36, 39, 40] Some investigators avoid anticoagulants for fear of creating septic emboli and causing hemorrhagic complications.[17, 40] However, continuing sepsis, extension of thrombus, or pulmonary complication with continuous spiking fevers may be an indication for internal jugular vein ligation.[6, 17, 34, 40, 41] Anticoagulation is considered in cases of thrombosis spreading to the cavernous sinus.[6] If anticoagulants and thrombolytics have a role, it is in cases associated with otitic hydrocephalus (Fig. 15–8). In cases with progressive neurologic deterioration with evolution of thrombus, transvenous, direct intrasinus thrombolytic treatment with urokinase[42, 43] and streptokinase has been successful.[44]

The treatment of brain abscess is under the guidance of neurosurgery. Empiric treatment usually includes penicillin or β-lactam antibiotic, chloramphenicol, and metronidazole[9] and intravenous dexamethasone.[34] Additionally, increases in intracranial pressure may require mannitol, hyperventilation, or dexamethasone preoperatively.[9] In the past, the goal of traditional treatment was to surgically remove the intact, unruptured abscess capsule. However, burr hole aspiration and stereotactic drainage have been performed.[8, 15] Serial stereotactic aspiration may soon become the procedure of choice.[6] Many authors advocate delay of mastoid surgery until after neurologic stabilization.[8, 17] However, in a prospective study of 36 patients with otogenic intracranial abscess, Kurien and associates found that concurrent craniotomy and mastoidectomy avoids reinfection while the patient is waiting for definitive surgery, removes the source of infection at the same time complications are being treated, and results in a single, shorter hospital stay.[19]

CT-guided needle aspiration may be useful for aspiration for culture through a sterile field.[9] Aspiration for culture through a sterile field distant to the ear with or without intra-abscess instillation of antibiotics is not always done; systemic antibiotics may be the only treatment required to resolve the brain abscess, particularly in those patients with multiple brain abscesses (Fig. 15–9). Except for aspiration, these abscesses are usually not openly drained or resected, unless they fail to resolve. In cases with multiple abscesses, in a deep or dominant location, with concomitant meningitis, with early response to antibiotics, or in cases with abscesses less than 3 cm, repeated aspirations are preferred to complete excision.[9]

Mastoidectomy can be done prior to or under the same anesthetic[19] and after neurosurgical drainage of the abscess.[40] Rarely is the brain abscess in direct continuity with the ear[45]; if it is and it spontaneously drains into the mastoid, it can be drained through the ear (see Fig. 15–9).

The surgical treatment of otitic hydrocephalus is the management of mastoiditis, extradural granulations, and sigmoid sinus thrombophlebitis.[36, 38] Care must be taken to have an ophthalmologist follow the patient's vision. Long-term care of the intracranial hypertension by a neurologist may be necessary. Most cases of otitic hydrocephalus resolve spontaneously in months, and neurosurgical intervention (lumboperitoneal shunt) should be reserved for patients with deterioration of vision[34, 38] or disabling pulsatile tinnitus. Many cases can be effectively treated with acetazolamide and furosemide or systemic steroids.[17, 34, 38] Techniques of management of intracranial thrombophlebitis and chronic intracranial hypertension are controversial and rapidly evolutionary; optimal treatment is provided by a local team of expert consultants involved with the case. Ventricular shunting and optic nerve decompression may be required.[46] The main point of treatment is careful management of the ear and chronic intracranial hypertension. Blindness or brain herniation are serious concerns.[47]

The treatment of subdural abscess occurs under the guidance of neurosurgery. The medical treatment includes parenteral antibiotics, anticonvulsants, and corticosteroids.[34] The surgical control of the mastoiditis, extradural granulations or abscess, and sigmoid sinus thrombophlebitis is crucial for recovery. Usually myringotomy for acute otitis media and complete mastoidectomy for coalescent mastoiditis or nonresolving otitis media are involved, as well as diagnostic subdural tap. If the subdural space contains purulent material, the empyema must be removed by craniotomy or burr holes and the subdural space must be irrigated.[9, 34, 36] Craniotomy with abscess excision is sometimes the neurosurgical treatment of choice.[6] Depending on the stability of the patient, the two surgical procedures (neurosurgical drainage with mastoidectomy) may be done together[19] or sequentially. Subdural abscesses are extremely rare from suppurative ear disease, tend to be quite severe, and may have direct connections through the infected dura. Experience with these lesions has led this primary author and neurosurgical colleagues to favor an aggressive approach.

The treatment of meningitis from acute ear infection is predominantly medical, except for myringotomy. With aggressive use of appropriate intravenous antibiotics, dexamethasone has been shown to reduce the incidence of neurologic sequelae, including deafness,[6] and should be considered. If severe Mondini's deformity with dehiscence of the medial wall of the vestibule is present on the infected side, intralabyrinthine obliteration is required after recovery of the meningitis (Fig. 15–10).[20]

Meningitis from chronic ear infection is a surgical and medical emergency because of the probability of a dehiscence in the dura and an ever-increasing flow of pus directly from the ear into the subarachnoid space. Radical mastoidectomy with exploration of all dural surfaces directly or through thin bone is necessary. When the extradural abscess is evacuated, care should be taken to identify the dural defect. When the defect is found, it may be repaired with fascia placed intradurally and extradurally. Wedging or suturing the graft is usually possible. Postoperative cerebrospinal fluid leak may occur but tends to close as the meningitis and excessive production of cerebrospinal fluid resolve.

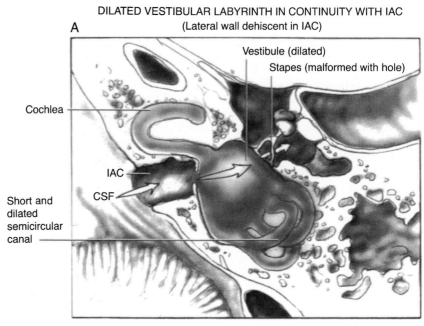

DILATED VESTIBULAR LABYRINTH IN CONTINUITY WITH IAC
(Lateral wall dehiscent in IAC)

A

Vestibule (dilated)

Stapes (malformed with hole)

Cochlea

IAC

CSF

Short and
dilated
semicircular
canal

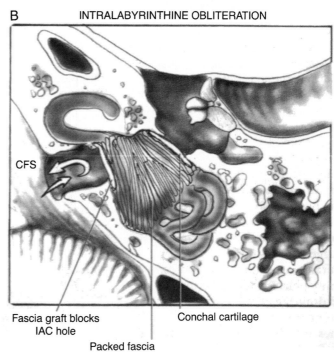

B   INTRALABYRINTHINE OBLITERATION

CFS

Fascia graft blocks
IAC hole

Conchal cartilage

Packed fascia

FIGURE 15–10

FIGURE 15–10. (A) Artist's illustration of severe Mondini malformation with CSF entering the vestibule through a dehiscence in the lateral wall of the internal auditory canal and then entering the middle ear through dehiscences in congenitally malformed stapes footplate and/or round window. (B) Treatment for this is fascia obliteration of the vestibule, taking care not to compress the facial nerve; a piece of cartilage is wedged through the oval window to create a self-retaining seal.

SUMMARY

Expertly performed, detailed, and time-specific history and physical examination are the most powerful tools of diagnosis. Imaging is the only way to detect brain abscess and subdural abscess. The complete diagnosis depends on carefully done intraoperative observations.

Complications of suppurative ear disease manifest in obvious or predictable patterns that help guide preoperative diagnosis and intraoperative discovery and treatment. Treatment of complications requires hospitalization, culture-specific intravenous antibiotics, expedient surgical exenteration of the ear disease, and a specific tailored approach to the complication.

References

1. Neely J: Complications of Suppurative Otitis Media: I. Aural Complications: A Self-Instructional Package from the Committee on Continuing Education in Otolaryngology. Washington, DC, American Academy of Otolaryngology, a Division of American Academy of Ophthalmology and Otolaryngology, 1978.
2. Neely J: Complications of Suppurative Otitis Media: II. Intracranial Complications: A Self-Instructional Package from the Committee on Continuing Education in Otolaryngology. Washington, DC, American Academy of Otolaryngology—Head and Neck Surgery, 1983.
3. Albers F: Complications of otitis media: The importance of early recognition. Am J Otol 20: 9–12, 1999.
4. Friedberg J, Gordon D: Acute otitis media: The evolution of surgical management. J Otolaryngol 27: 2–8, 1998.
5. Wang N, Burg J: Mastoiditis: A case-based review. Pediatr Emerg Care 14: 290–292, 1998.
6. Youngs R: Complications of suppurative otitis media. In Ludman H, Wright T (eds): Diseases of the Ear. London, Arnold, 1998, pp 398–415.
7. Panda N, Sreedharan S, Mann S, Sharma S: Prognostic factors in complicated and uncomplicated chronic otitis media. Am J Otolaryngol 17: 391–396, 1995.
8. Yen P, Chan S, Huang T: Brain abscess: With special reference to otolaryngologic sources of infection. Otolaryngol Head Neck Surg 113: 15–22, 1995.
9. Brook I: Brain abscess in children: Microbiology and management. J Child Neurol 10: 283–288, 1995.
10. Harley E, Sdralis T, Berkowitz R: Acute mastoiditis in children: A 12-year retrospective study. Otolaryngol Head Neck Surg 116: 26–30, 1997.
11. Goldstein N, Casselbrant M, Bluestone C, Kurs-Lasky M: Intratemporal complications of acute otitis media in infants and children. Otolaryngol Head Neck Surg 119: 444–454, 1998.
12. Gliklich R, Eavey R, Iannuzzi R, Camacho A: A contemporary analysis of acute mastoiditis. Arch Otolaryngol Head Neck Surg 122: 135–139, 1996.
13. Rosen A, Ophir D, Marshak G: Acute mastoiditis: A review of 69 cases. Ann Otol Rhinol Laryngol 95: 222–224, 1986.
14. Khafif A, Halperin D, Hochman I, et al: Acute mastoiditis: A 10-year review. Am J Otolaryngol 19: 170–173, 1998.
15. Grigoriadis E, Gold W: Pyogenic brain abscess caused by *Streptococcus pneumoniae*: Case report and review. Clin Infect Dis 25: 1108–1112, 1997.
16. Haddad J: Treatment of acute otitis media and its complications. Otolaryngol Clin North Am 27: 431–441, 1994.
17. Kangsanarak J, Navacharoen N, Fooanant S, Ruckphaopunt K: Intracranial complications of suppurative otitis media: Thirteen years' experience. Am J Otol 16: 104–109, 1995.
18. Hlavin M, Kaminski H, Fenstermaker R, White R: Intracranial suppuration: A modern decade of postoperative subdural empyema and epidural abscess. Neurosurgery 34: 974–981, 1994.
19. Kurien M, Job A, Mathew J, Chandy M: Otogenic intracranial abscess. Arch Otolaryngol Head Neck Surg 124: 1353–1356, 1998.
20. Neely J: Classification of spontaneous cerebrospinal fluid middle ear effusion: Review of 49 cases. Otolaryngol Head Neck Surg 93: 625–634, 1985.
21. Neely J: Complications of temporal bone infections. In Cummings CW, Fredrickson J, Harker L, et al (eds): Otolaryngology—Head and Neck Surgery, Vol 4, 2nd ed. St. Louis, Mosby, 1993, pp 2840–2864.
22. Neely J: Intratemporal and intracranial complications of otitis media. In Bailey B, Johnson J, Kohut R, et al (eds): Head and Neck Surgery—Otolaryngology. Philadelphia, JB Lippincott, 1993, pp 1607–1622.
23. Castillo M, Albernaz V, Mukherji S, et al: Imaging of Bezold's abscess. AJR Am J Roentgenol 171: 1491–1495, 1998.
24. Spiegel J, Lustig L, Lee K, et al: Contemporary presentation and management of a spectrum of mastoid abscesses. Laryngoscope 108: 822–828, 1998.
25. Hawkins D, Dru D: Mastoid subperiosteal abscess. Arch Otolaryngology 109: 369, 1983.
26. Holt R, Gates G: Masked mastoiditis. Laryngoscope 93: 1034–1037, 1983.
27. Bluestone C, Klein J: Intratemporal complications and sequelae of otitis media. In Bluestone C, Stool S (eds): Pediatric Otolaryngology, Vol 1. Philadelphia, WB Saunders, 1983, pp 513–564.
28. Schwaber M, Pensak M, Bartels L: The early signs and symptoms of neurotologic complications of chronic suppurative otitis media. Laryngoscope 99: 373–375, 1989.
29. Kangsanarak J, Fooanant S, Ruckphaopunt K: Extracranial and intracranial complications of suppurative otitis media: Report of 102 cases. J Laryngol Otol 107: 999–1004, 1993.
30. Shanley D, Murphy T: Intracranial and extracranial complications of acute mastoiditis: Evaluation with computed tomography. J Am Osteopath Assoc 92: 131–134, 1992.
31. Scott T, Jackler R: Acute mastoiditis in infancy: A sequela of unrecognized acute otitis media. Otolaryngol Head Neck Surg 110: 683–687, 1989.
32. Bizakis J, Velegrakis G, Papadakis C, et al: The silent epidural abscess as a complication of acute otitis media in children. Int J Pediatr Otorhinolaryngol 45: 163–166, 1998.
33. Murakami T, Tsubaki J, Tahara Y, Nagashima T: Gradenigo's syndrome: CT and MRI findings. Pediatr Radiol 26: 684–685, 1996.
34. Nissen A, Bui H: Complications of chronic otitis media. Ear Nose Throat J 75: 284–292, 1996.
35. Mawson S: Diseases of the Ear. Baltimore, Williams & Wilkins, 1974.
36. Gower D, McGuirt W: Intracranial complications of acute and chronic infectious ear disease: A problem still with us. Laryngoscope 93: 1028–1033, 1983.
37. Gettelfinger D, Kokmen E: Superior sagittal sinus thrombosis. Arch Neurol 34: 2–6, 1977.
38. Commins D, Koay B, Milford C, Renowden S: Otitic hydrocephalus. J Otolaryngol 26: 210–212, 1997.
39. Garcia R, Baker A, Cunningham M, Weber A: Lateral sinus thrombosis associated with otitis media and mastoiditis in children. Pediatr Infect Dis J 14: 615–623, 1995.
40. Samuel J, Fernandez C, Steinberg J: Intracranial otogenic complications: A persisting problem. Laryngoscope 1986: 272–278, 1986.
41. Leiberman A, Lupu L, Landsberg R, Fliss D: Unusual complications of otitis media. Am J Otolaryngol 15: 444–448, 1994.
42. Tsai F, Higahida R, Matovich V, Alfieri K: Acute thrombosis of the intracranial dural sinus: Direct thrombolytic treatment. AJNR Am J Neuroradiol 13: 1137–1142, 1992.
43. Barnwell S, Higashida R, Halbach V, et al: Direct endovascular thrombolytic therapy for dural sinus thrombosis. Neurosurgery 28: 135–142, 1991.
44. Kermode A, Ives F, Taylor B, et al: Progressive dural venous sinus thrombosis treated with local streptokinase infusion. J Neurol Neurosurg Psychiatry 58: 107–108, 1995.
45. Kumar R, Sharma R, Tyagi I: Spontaneous evacuation of cerebellar abscess through the middle ear: A case report. Neurosurg Rev 21: 66–68, 1998.
46. Horton J, Seiff S, Pitts L: Decompression of the optic nerve sheath for vision-threatening papilledema caused by dural sinus occlusion. Neurosurgery 31: 203–211, 1992.
47. Gower D, Baker A, Bell W, Ball M: Contraindications to lumbar puncture as defined by computed cranial tomography. J Neurol Neurosurg Psychiatry 50: 1071–1074, 1987.

16

Mastoidectomy: The Intact Canal Wall Procedure

James L. Sheehy, M.D.

There are two ways of handling mastoidectomy in cases of cholesteatoma. The canal wall down (CWD) technique will be discussed by Arriaga in Chapter 17. The canal wall up (CWU) technique is dealt with here.

This chapter covers not only the technique for CWU but also the evolution of the technique, controversies in regard to CWU versus CWD, indications for CWD procedures, a discussion of the facial nerve in surgery for chronic ear disease, and management of the labyrinthine fistula.

DEFINITIONS

The common mastoid operations performed for chronic ear infections are listed in the following sections. Technical surgical variations peculiar to each surgeon do not alter the fundamental classification.[1]

Radical Mastoidectomy

Radical mastoidectomy is an operation performed to eradicate middle ear and mastoid disease in which the mastoid antrum, tympanum, and external auditory canal are converted into a common cavity exteriorized through the external meatus. This operation involves removal of the tympanic membrane and ossicular remnants, with exception of the stapes, and does not involve any reconstructive or grafting procedure. Frequently, the surgeon places a plug of soft tissue in the tubotympanum or may even lay soft tissue over the middle ear to assist in healing, but this does not alter the name of the procedure.

Modified Radical Mastoidectomy

Modified radical mastoidectomy is an operation performed to eradicate mastoid disease, in which the epitympanum, mastoid antrum, and external auditory canal are converted into a common cavity exteriorized through the external meatus. This technique differs from the radical operation in that the tympanic membrane, or remnants thereof, and ossicular remnants are retained to preserve hearing. (This operation does *not* involve any reconstructive procedure.)

Tympanoplasty with Mastoidectomy

Tympanoplasty with mastoidectomy is an operation performed to eradicate disease in the middle ear and mastoid and to reconstruct the hearing mechanism, with or without tympanic membrane grafting.

There are essentially three variations of this operation; the classic type of procedure involves permanent exteriorization of the epitympanum and mastoid, a CWD procedure. A different approach is to perform a CWD procedure and then obliterate the cavity or reconstruct the external auditory canal. Finally, there is the CWU procedure, the intact canal wall tympanoplasty with mastoidectomy, which is the subject of this chapter.

EVOLUTION OF TECHNIQUE

Prior to the mid 1950s there were essentially two operations for chronic otitis media with cholesteatoma: radical mastoidectomy and modified radical mastoidectomy. These are classic operations that are still indicated at times. Their object is to create a safe ear by exteriorizing the disease, and preserve hearing, if possible.

When tympanoplasty was first introduced by Wullstein[2] and Zollner,[3] exenteration of the mastoid was the rule. Two problems eventually became apparent. Moisture in the cavity had a deleterious effect on the full-thickness skin used to graft the tympanic membrane, and the narrowed middle ear space created in the classic types III and IV tympanoplasty was prone to collapse, nullifying any hearing improvement (see Chapter 13).

It became apparent that if satisfactory hearing results were to be obtained, some method of avoiding a narrow middle ear space would be necessary. Many thought that the best way of solving this problem was by not creating an exteriorized cavity but by reconstructing the tympanic membrane in a normal position and then inserting some type of tissue or prosthetic device to re-establish the sound pressure transfer mechanism (see Chapter 13). Although this concept led to better hearing results, many problems developed over the course of the years, some of which are still being seen.

It was learned that the harder one tried to obtain a good functional result, the more problems (and failures) one had. To avoid these problems, some surgeons still advocate the classic modified radical and radical mastoidectomy, nonreconstructive procedures.

The physicians at the House Ear Clinic (HEC) began performing the intact canal wall tympanoplasty with mastoidectomy in 1958, under the direction of William House.[4] By 1961, over half of all cholesteatoma cases were so managed at the HEC, but many revision operations were required for correction of recurrence of cholesteatoma due to retraction pockets. As a result, many at the HEC reverted to taking the CWD and then obliterating the cavity with muscle, based on a procedure suggested by Rambo.[5] In 1963, 50 per cent of cholesteatoma cases were so managed.

By 1964, it was realized that the technique of obliteration did not eliminate the cavity and the problems involved. In addition, the routine use of plastic sheeting through the facial recess in the intact canal wall procedure was reducing the number of cases that had to be revised because of retraction pockets (recurrent cholesteatoma). From that point on, the percentage of cases managed by a CWD technique gradually decreased to 10 per cent in 1970. Since then, there have been yearly fluctuations: 15 to 25 per cent CWD procedures over the last 16 years.

THE CONTROVERSY

The controversy over CWU versus CWD centers mostly on safety: safety of the operation procedure and safety over the ensuing years.[6] The consideration should—but rarely does—include the technical ability of the surgeon. In the surgery of aural cholesteatoma, be it CWU or CWD, judgment and technical ability are major factors in the outcome.[7]

Let us assume that the technical ability and judgment are superior in the two groups. Why is there a difference in opinion as to what is best for the patient?

Are hearing results a factor? Not really. The HEC physicians do not find much difference. Of course, they are very careful not to narrow the middle ear space (see Chapter 13) and stage the operation almost as frequently as in CWU (see Chapter 18).

Is there a difference in the healing? Yes—CWU procedures, with lateral surface grafting (see Chapter 9), may well take 6 to 8 weeks to heal. Open cavities frequently require 3 to 4 months and occasionally 6 to 8 months, and there is a small percentage that are never free of minor moisture problems.

What about residual and recurrent disease? Most surgeons who use both CWU and CWD procedures find little difference in the incidence of middle ear residual disease, or disease left behind. They also find little difference in the incidence of staging the operation (see Chapter 18).

Recurrent cholesteatoma is a different matter. Recurrent cholesteatoma characteristically results from a posterosuperior retraction pocket,[8, 9] which occurs only in CWU procedures. Those who have reported a 20 to 40 per cent incidence of recurrent cholesteatoma have failed, with rare exceptions, to stage the operation when indicated (75 per cent of the time) and have failed to use plastic sheeting through the facial recess, even when the operation was being performed in one stage. Advocates of the CWU procedure, those who have had extensive experience, have less than a 5 per cent incidence of recurrent cholesteatoma.

Everyone knows that when a cavity is created it is usually necessary to clean (remove dead skin) every 6 to 12 months for the rest of the patient's life. One must see the CWU patient only every 1 to 2 years for about 10 years.

Precautions relative to not getting water in the ear are necessary 50 per cent or more of the time in CWD cases, depending on whether the cavity is healed, how large it is, whether an adequately sized meatus was created, and whether the cavity is round, rather than bean shaped.

Finally, the adequate-sized meatus is relevant. If one creates a meatus large enough to have a trouble-free ear and allow water in the ear, the size can pose a problem with fitting a hearing aid, if and when there is a need for the aid in the future. The problem consists of getting a secure fit and preventing feedback. Fortunately, the behind-the-ear aid usually solves this problem and is the best aid anyway for use in an ear that may have some drainage from a cavity.

INDICATIONS FOR MASTOIDECTOMY

Mastoidectomy may be indicated in tympanoplasty surgery to eliminate disease, to explore the mastoid to ensure that there is no disease, to enlarge the air-containing middle ear–antral space, or on occasion, to create temporary post-auricular drainage (with a catheter) in patients with compromised eustachian tube problems or uncontrolled mucosal infection.[10] By far the most common indication, however, is the treatment of cholesteatoma and the associated infection.

What about those who recommend at least a cortical ("simple") mastoidectomy in all tympanoplasties? The rationale appears to be that it is "good practice" and that "it's better to be safe than sorry." There are also arguments, mentioned earlier, that this practice can increase the middle ear cleft space and that this is a good idea if there is compromised eustachian tube function.

In fact, the indication for mastoidectomy is made on the basis of the clinical history and the appearance of the ear in the physician's office. The final decision is made during the surgery. There are some patients for whom a mastoidectomy is not done when it was thought necessary or when the decision had not been realized preoperatively.

Radiographs and imaging studies play little part in making the diagnosis, the decision to do the surgery, or management of the mastoid at surgery.

INDICATIONS FOR AN EXTERIORIZED MASTOID CAVITY

The HEC physicians prefer not to create a cavity, but they may do so at times. That decision may be made preoperatively, but more often than not, the operation is begun as a CWU procedure, and the decision to exteriorize the mastoid is made intraoperatively.[11]

Preoperative Decisions

The decision to perform a CWD procedure is made preoperatively in some cases. This decision is based on the consideration of the hearing in the involved ear, the status of the opposite ear, the preoperative complications, the degree of posterior canal wall destruction by disease, and the age and health of the patient.

With rare exceptions, a cholesteatoma requiring mastoid surgery in an only hearing ear is managed with a CWD technique. Usually, the procedure is a classic modified radical mastoidectomy, leaving the middle ear and hearing the way they are. A classic modified radical mastoidectomy may be used in cases in which the affected ear has serviceable hearing and the opposite ear has a severe uncorrectable impairment. One does not wish to jeopardize the only serviceable ear.

In labyrinthine fistula cases, one may decide preoperatively to use a CWD operation if the mastoid is small or if the opposite ear has a cholesteatoma that will require surgery. If the hearing is serviceable, one will probably perform just a classic modified radical procedure, particularly for patients in poor health or in the elderly.[11-13]

A CWD operation may be decided on preoperatively if it can be seen that the cholesteatoma has destroyed a significant portion of the posterior canal wall. If the opposite ear already has a cavity, one may elect to create a cavity on the other ear at the time of surgery. In elderly patients or those in poor health, we are more likely to use a classic modified radical mastoidectomy—the less done, the better.

Intraoperative Decisions

Advocates of the CWU procedure generally start the operation in this manner unless the decision has been made preoperatively. When one encounters a very contracted mastoid, particularly with an ear canal slanting up and forward, or if one encounters an unsuspected canal wall destruction, one would not hesitate to take the canal wall. Intraoperative decisions normally (at HEC) account for two thirds of the decisions for CWD.

PREOPERATIVE EVALUATION AND TREATMENT

How does one make the diagnosis of cholesteatoma? What tests are necessary? How vigorously does one treat the chronically draining ear preoperatively?

The diagnosis of cholesteatoma is based on a well-taken history by the physician and a careful examination of the ear under an operating microscope to confirm ingrowth of skin into the middle ear, at the epitympanum, or both.

The only routine testing is the hearing test. This test is not related to making the diagnosis but is to allow proper counseling. Occasionally, the hearing test will result in a change of approach to the surgery, as noted in the preceding section.

Radiographs or imaging studies play little part in making the diagnosis or directing the surgical approach. These tests are usually obtained if there is a complication or if one is considered likely, for example, semicircular canal fistula, facial paralysis, meningitis, or other intracranial complications.[13] Under these circumstances, imaging studies rarely make a difference in the overall surgical approach but should allow the surgeon to predict any complications or

sequelae. The patient and family can be counseled properly and forewarned of problems.

Treatment of the Chronically Draining Ear

How much, if any, treatment of the draining ear is indicated prior to surgery? Must the ear be dry before the surgery? If so, for how long? How vigorous should treatment be? Are cultures of the drainage indicated?

The HEC physicians rarely take cultures of draining ears unless there appears to be a subacute mastoiditis or a suspected complication. Then a culture may be indicated.

In the noncholesteatomatous ear (the benign central perforation), local treatment is indicated to obtain a dry ear prior to surgery (see Chapter 8). One would like to have the ear dry for 3 or 4 weeks prior to tympanic membrane grafting. If the ear is draining at the time of surgery, it is probably best to perform at least an antrotomy through the mastoid cortex and place a catheter drain (to ensure drainage while the tympanic membrane graft is healing).[10] Furthermore, it is more likely that a mucosal problem could dictate staging the operation if the ear is still draining at the time of surgery (see Chapter 18).

Many ears with cholesteatoma have only intermittant discharge, if any. These ears usually respond quickly to various local medications. If the cholesteatomatous ear has a history of almost continual drainage and there are no associated symptoms requiring treatment, it may be best to leave the ear alone. Certainly, if local treatment is started, it should be effective quickly, if it is going to help at all. The exception to this course is the actively draining ear with polyps; these should be treated with local medication. Resolution of discharge despite the history is common.

PREOPERATIVE COUNSELING

Using a Chronic Ear Patient Discussion Booklet, I explain to the patient how a normal ear functions. I then show on a second drawing of the ear how skin grows into the ear and forms a cholesteatoma. The following extract is a summary of my description of the procedure at the HEC that I then offer to the patient:

Cholesteatoma is an ingrowth of skin into the mastoid. This forms a skin-lined cyst that we call a cholesteatoma. It is not a tumor or truly a growth. But it does tend to get larger as time goes on if the ear continues to drain.

There are three reasons why the ear should have surgery at some time. In the first place, it is potentially dangerous. If the drainage continues, we know that about 20 per cent of these patients will eventually develop severe dizziness because the cholesteatoma breaks into the balance canal. There is about a 1 per cent chance that it may break into the nerve to the face or break into the covering of the brain.

Secondly, the longer the problem goes on, the more damage may be done to the hearing. If the cholesteatoma should break into a balance canal, the patient might then lose all hearing permanently.

Thirdly, there is the matter of the drainage.

The objectives of surgery are to get a safe, dry, and hearing ear. Getting a safe, dry, healed ear is almost certain. Unfortunately, to obtain a good hearing ear it is frequently necessary to do the operation in two stages. There is a 60 to 70 per cent chance of helping the hearing with the second operation.

There is nothing urgent about having the surgery. You certainly can have it done in a month or 3 months, but I would not put it off indefinitely. It is like sitting on a keg of dynamite. It is not a very good place to sit; you are not quite sure whether the dynamite will ever explode and cause a serious problem.

I have made notations of all of this in the booklet. In the back of the booklet there is an area called Risks and Complications of Surgery. The only serious complication that happens with any degree of regularity, and it is serious, is a total, 100 per cent loss of hearing in the ear operated on. The likelihood of this happening is no more then a 1 to 2 per cent chance; all of the other things listed here are either very remote or are temporary. (The Risk and Complications sheet appears as Appendix 1 in Chapter 9).

If the patient has a labryinthine fistula, as between 5 and 10 per cent of our patients with cholesteatoma do, the patient is then told that there is a 10 per cent chance of a total loss of hearing and prolonged dizziness, which would eventually clear up.

PREOPERATIVE PREPARATION OF THE PATIENT

Preoperative preparation of the patient differs little from what was described for tympanic membrane grafting (see Chapter 9). The operation is done under general anesthesia unless the patient requests otherwise.

SURGICAL TECHNIQUE

Just as the preparation before and in surgery is the same as that described for tympanic membrane grafting (see Chapter 9), the initial steps are also identical: making canal incisions, elevating the vascular strip, turning the ear foreward, removing and dehydrating the temporalis fascia, removing canal skin, enlarging the ear canal by removing the overhanging bone anteriorly and inferiorly, and assuring that the remnant is de-epithelized.[14]

Removal of Middle Ear Disease

Cholesteatoma should be dissected in continuity to ensure total removal. All diseased tissue is dissected from the bone or mucosa, beginning in the anterosuperior quadrant, proceeding inferiorly, then posteriorly, and superiorly until the superior edge of the promontory, the lower edge of the oval window, is reached. Normal mucosa should not be sacrificed.

No attempt should be made at this time to remove cholesteatoma that surrounds the stapes or is in the oval window. Manipulations in this area should be postponed until the mastoidectomy has been completed and the facial recess is open. Removal of oval window disease should always be deferred until the end of the procedure, so that if a fistula develops inadvertently, the operation may be terminated expeditiously.

Before proceeding with the mastoidectomy, one must determine the status of the incudostapedial joint. If there is an intact chain, the incudostapedial joint should be separated at this time. This facilitates removal of the incus after the facial recess is opened and prevents possible trauma to the inner ear, which could occur should the drill inadvertently touch the incus when the epitympanum or facial recess is being opened.

Mastoid Exenteration

The mastoid is exenterated, under the microscope, using a drill with various-sized round cutting burrs. Continuous suction-irrigation during drilling is used to cool the bone, to keep the field clean at all times, and to prevent clogging of the burr by bone dust.

The initial burr cut is made along the linea temporalis. This marks the lowest point of the middle fossa dura in most cases. The second burr cut is along a line perpendicular to the one just described and tangent to the posterior margin of the ear canal (Fig. 16–1). These two burr cuts outline a triangular area, the apex of which is at the spine of Henle. Projected into the mastoid, parallel to the direction of the ear canal, the apex of this triangle is directly over the lateral semicircular canal. The only structure of importance lying within this triangle as one proceeds with the exenteration is the lateral (sigmoid) sinus.

The deepest mastoid penetration is always at the apex of this triangle. This ensures that the antrum is entered and the lateral canal identified before deeper penetration in other areas. The dural plate is skeletonized superiorly and the lateral sinus skeletonized posteroinferiorly as the dissection proceeds. Uncovering the middle fossa or sigmoid sinus dura is not necessary but should not result in any problem. It is not considered a complication.

After the lateral semicircular canal has been identified and the cortical mastoidectomy has been completed, the zygomatic root is exenterated to allow access to epitympanum. The posterior bony canal wall is thinned at this time (Fig. 16–2).

I have certain "rules of thumb" that I use in teaching in regard to the initial approach to the mastoid. Let me comment on each of these.

Always keep the deepest area of penetration into the mastoid at the apex of the two initial burr cuts. The direction in which one proceeds is not necessarily perpendicular to the bone; it should be parallel to the ear canal. Following parallel to the ear canal will lead to the mastoid antrum.

Do not dig a "deep dark hole." One must remember to saucerize the margins, to open the exposure as one proceeds deeper. In this way, it is possible to see what one is doing and also to use the suction-irrigation with the drill.

Always use the largest burr possible. If one should inadvertently uncover the middle fossa dura or the facial nerve or the sigmoid sinus, one is less likely to do serious damage with a large burr as opposed to a very small burr. Furthermore, if there is a problem, one will be able to see what was done.

Finally, "if lost on the way to the antrum, go high and forward." This is exactly what I say to students taking our temporal bone surgical dissection course. And this is in fact what I do when I sit down with one of them who has

FIGURE 16–1

FIGURE 16–2

FIGURE 16–3

FIGURE 16–4

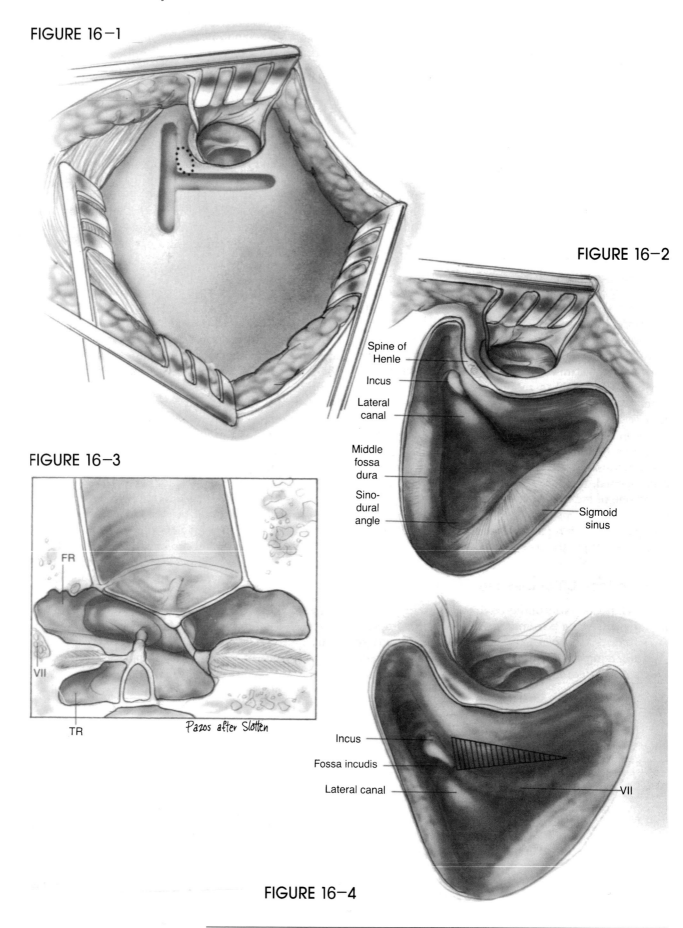

Spine of
Henle

Incus

Lateral
canal

Middle
fossa
dura

Sino-
dural
angle

Sigmoid
sinus

FR

VII

TR

Pazos after Slotten

Incus

Fossa incudis

Lateral canal

VII

FIGURES 16–1 to 16–4. *See legends on opposite page*

gotten halfway through the dissection and is lost. By going high, one identifies the middle fossa dural plate. By going forward, one then squeezes into the angle between the dural plate and the ear canal. Going medial in that direction leads to the epitympanum and avoids the matter of fenestrating the lateral semicircular canal or getting into other troubles should the mastoid antrum be filled with bone.

Opening the Facial Recess

The facial recess is one of the posterior recesses of the middle ear. It is bordered laterally by the chorda tympani, medially by the upper mastoid segment of the facial nerve, and superiorly by bone of the fossa incudis (Fig. 16–3). This recess is frequently the seat of cholesteatoma, particularly when cholesteatoma is associated with a perforation below the posterior malleal fold. Bone in this area may be cellular even in poorly developed mastoid.

The landmark for opening into the facial recess is the fossa incudis. One visualizes the triangular area that is inferior to the fossa and is bordered by bone of the fossa incudis superiorly, the upper mastoid segment of the facial nerve medially, and the chorda tympani laterally (Fig. 16–4). The bone is saucerized in this area with a large cutting burr. When the bony canal wall lateral to the recess has been thinned satisfactorily (care being taken not to perforate into the external canal), bone removal is continued with a smaller cutting burr. One should always stroke with a burr parallel to the direction of the nerve, never allowing the burr to pass the bone of the fossa incudis superiorly (Fig. 16–5).

The facial recess is opened from the mastoid to remove disease in the area, to gain additional access to the posterior middle ear (oval and round windows), to gain a better view of tympanic segment of the facial nerve, and to facilitate postoperative aeration of the mastoid. Opening into the middle ear through the facial recess is a key step in performing an intact canal wall tympanoplasty with mastoidectomy; with rare exceptions, it should not be omitted (Fig. 16–6).

There are two things one may notice when approaching the facial nerve in this area. Frequently, bleeding is encountered from one of the vessels intimately associated with, but lying outside, the bony canal of the nerve. Before actually uncovering the nerve, one may note its white sheath showing through the thin bone. Often this sheath is highlighted by the sight through the bone of one of the vessels on the sheath.

Identification of the facial nerve provides an additional landmark for opening into the facial recess. A small cutting burr is used to enter into the middle ear, just lateral to the nerve, and then the opening is enlarged to the extent possible with diamond stones. It is usually possible to obtain at least a 2-mm opening.

It is not necessary to expose the nerve with this approach, but there is no harm in doing so. Fortunately, the facial nerve is quite resistant to gentle trauma.[15] One can use the cutting burrs when approaching the nerve in the region of the facial recess. Bone removal is quicker than with the diamond stone, and it is easier to determine when the nerve is exposed. To make this differentiation, the exposed area can be probed with a mobilizing needle. If the exposed area is nerve sheath, it rebounds immediately after release of the probe; it "bounces back." If what has been uncovered is mucosa or cholesteatoma, one may note that it will "come back at you" but that it does not bounce back or rebound. After the recess has been opened, the incus, if present, is removed along with bone of the fossa incudis. It is possible to see the pyramidal eminence, the oval and round windows, and that part of the tympanic portion of the facial nerve lying posterior to the cochleariform process.

Elimination of Disease

As disease is encountered in the mastoid it is removed by dissecting it *from behind forward*. It is important to remove all cholesteatoma matrix in continuity so that no remnant of epithelium remains. The mastoid is exenterated to the extent indicated by the disease process and to the extent necessary to obtain adequate exposure. It is not necessary to remove normal-appearing cells, to exenterate all cells, as one would do in a CWD procedure.

From the mastoid approach, all mastoid and facial recess disease may be removed by elevating it and dissecting it toward the epitympanum and middle ear. Unless there is an unusually narrow angle between the tegmen and the superior wall of the ear canal, it should be possible to remove all epitympanic disease. When the cholesteatoma has contacted the malleus head, as it frequently has, the entire malleus should be removed. This exposes the opening into the supratubal recess and facilitates dissection of disease from behind and through the ear canal simultaneously.

Posterosuperior middle ear disease is removed at this time through both the ear canal and mastoid (via the facial recess). The cholesteatoma matrix is dissected in continuity, if possible.

The areas that are most difficult to see with this or any other approach, even radical mastoidectomy, are the posterior middle ear recesses: infrapyramidal and tympanic.[16] These are the areas posterior to and between the

---

FIGURE 16–1. Burr cuts to begin mastoidectomy. Note lateral semicircular canal ghosted in.

FIGURE 16–2. Exenteration of the mastoid is completed.

FIGURE 16–3. Horizontal cross section of temporal bone, looking at the upper segment from below. Note facial recess (FR) and tympanic recess (TR).

FIGURE 16–4. Facial recess area outlined by triangle: borders are the bone of the fossa incudis, upper mastoid segment of the facial nerve, and chorda tympani.

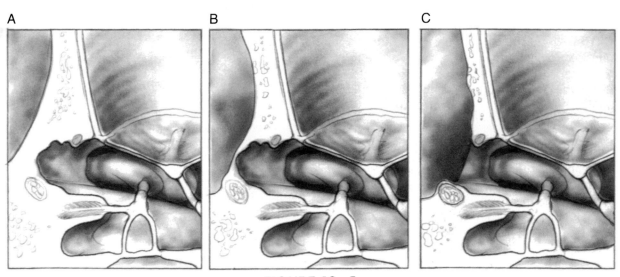

FIGURE 16-5

FIGURE 16-6

FIGURE 16-7

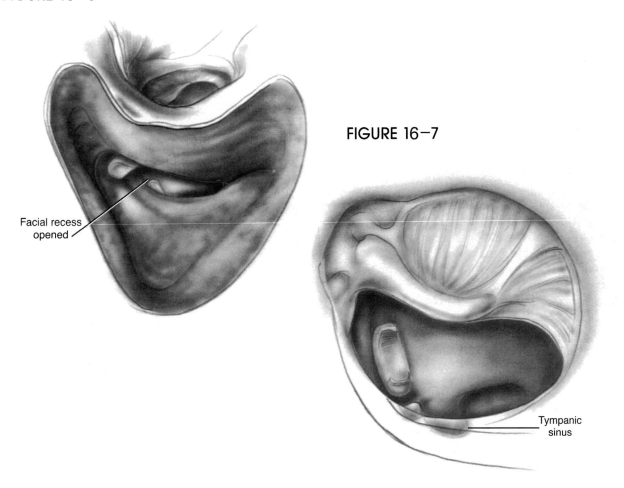

Facial recess opened

Tympanic sinus

FIGURE 16-5. *A* to *C*, Horizontal cross section showing progressive saucerization and opening into the facial recess; compare with Fig. 10–13.

FIGURE 16-6. Facial recess is open and incus is removed.

FIGURE 16-7. View through the ear canal showing location of tympanic sinus, medial to the facial nerve.

oval and round windows (Fig. 16–7). They extend for a variable distance medial to the pyramidal process and facial nerve (and lateral to the posterior semicircular canal). They are often the seat of cholesteatoma, particularly in cases associated with perforations below the posterior malleal ligament. The area must be cleaned with a right-angle dissector. Removal of the pyramidal process and adjacent bone with a diamond burr may be necessary at times to facilitate the cleaning but can be done safely only in a case where the stapes superstructure and tendon are missing. If the tympanic recess is deep and there is disease in it, it can be approached in a well-developed mastoid from the mastoid side, medial to the facial nerve and lateral to the posterior semicircular canal. This approach is not usually feasible, or necessary, but is to be kept in mind. It is an approach commonly used in connection with glomus tumor surgery.

Use of Plastic Sheeting

Plastic sheeting is used routinely in the intact canal wall procedure, regardless of the status of the middle ear mucosa, to prevent adhesions between the raw undersurface of the tympanic membrane graft and the denuded bone of the epitympanum and facial recess area. (Other uses of plastic sheeting are discussed in Chapter 18.)

Before it was realized that plastic sheeting should be used through the facial recess, there were many cases of recurrence of cholesteatoma due to retraction of the tympanic membrane into the facial recess and epitympanum (Fig. 16–8). If the operation is not being staged, thin silicone sheeting is used through the recess. An opening can be created in the plastic to allow for reconstruction to the stapes capitulum (Fig. 16–9). When staging of the operation is indicated, as it usually is in cholesteatoma cases, either thick silicone sheeting or Supramid is used (see Chapter 18) (Fig. 16–10).

Completion of the Operation

The tympanic membrane remnant is grafted with rehydrated fascia, the ear canal skin is replaced on the denuded bone, packing is inserted, the vascular strip is replaced, and closure postauricularly is with subcutaneous suture, all as described for tympanic membrane grafting (see Chapter 9).

In the occasional case in which the mastoid is badly infected and this infection has broken out of the confines of the cholesteatoma, it is wise to irrigate the mastoid with antibiotic solution. In this situation, it is also wise to place a catheter drain to the antrum, bringing it out to a separate incision. The drain may be left until the first postoperative visit. The purpose of this procedure is to make sure that anything that can drain out will and does not interfere with the tympanic membrane graft take.

A superficial Penrose drain is occasionally indicated when oozing has been a problem. The drain extends from the area of the fascia removal and exits at the lower part of the incision. This drain may be removed on the first postoperative day.

Dressing and Postoperative Care

There is no difference between the dressing or postoperative care for this procedure and that for tympanic membrane grafting (see Chapter 9) except that it is much more common to keep the patient overnight with this procedure. The schedule and plan for office visits are the same.

THE FACIAL NERVE IN SURGERY OF CHRONIC OTITIS MEDIA

One of the greatest fears of the inexperienced surgeon is that damage to the facial nerve may occur during a mastoidectomy.[15] This fear may result in avoidance of the nerve rather than positive identification. This can result in inadvertent damage to the nerve that has not been identified. In CWD surgery, this fear certainly results in the inadequacy of some of the surgical procedures, leaving the posterior bony canal wall high, creating a bean-shaped cavity.

Familiarity with the facial nerve results in respect: respect for helping to guide one throughout the temporal bone and respect for its ability to withstand manipulations and minor trauma.

There are three segments to the facial nerve: labyrinthine, tympanic, and mastoid. In surgery of chronic otitis media, concern is with the tympanic and mastoid segments.

Tympanic Segment

The tympanic segment is that portion of the nerve extending from the geniculate ganglion to the second genu (adjacent to the pyramidal process). Landmarks for identification of the nerve in its tympanic course are the cochleariform process, the oval window, and the pyramidal process. From the mastoid approach, the lateral semicircular canal and the cog are useful. These are discussed later.

The upper edge of the oval window is bordered by the facial nerve (Fig. 16–11). If this is not apparent, the cochleariform process may be identified. The facial nerve lies both posterior and superior to the cochleariform. One may also identify the pyramidal process and note that the facial nerve lies both above and behind this structure.

When none of these landmarks are apparent, the semicanal for the tensor tympani may be identified in the anterior middle ear and followed posteriorly. Its inferior border is continuous with the upper margin of the oval window, the facial nerve.

On rare occasions, one may need to identify the vertical groove on the promontory for the tympanic nerve. This groove is then followed superiorly to the cochleariform process or its remnants. The facial nerve is both posterior and superior to the cochleariform process.

From the mastoid approach, there are two landmarks to the tympanic course of the facial nerve: the lateral semicircular canal and the cog. The posterior half of the tympanic segment is immediately inferior to the lateral canal. The nerve course is anteriorly, passing superior to the cochleariform process and anterior to the cog.

The cog is a ridge of bone that extends inferiorly from

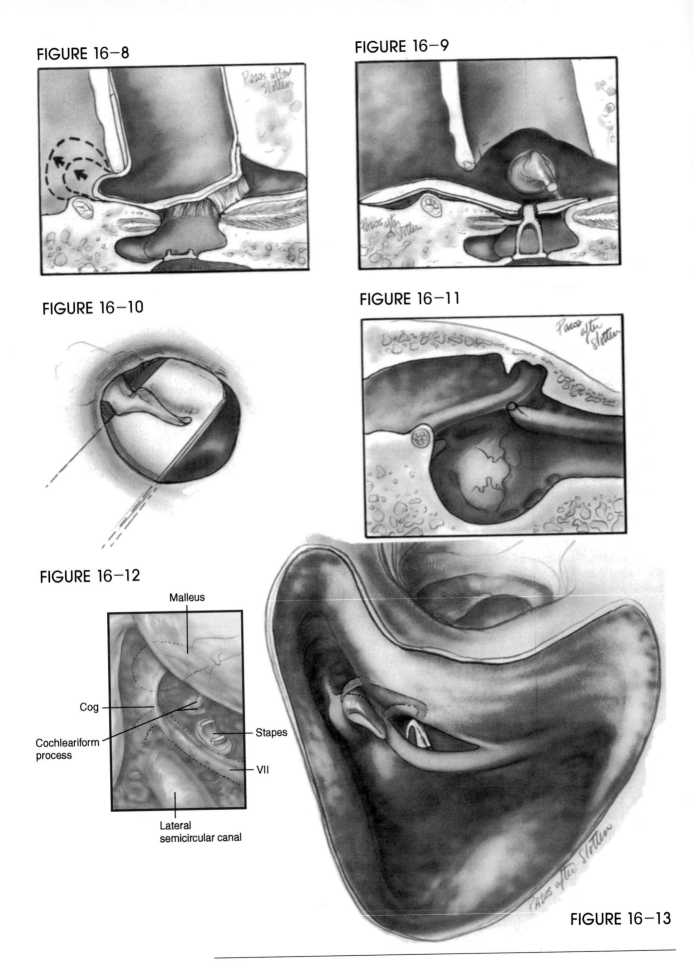

FIGURE 16-8

FIGURE 16-9

FIGURE 16-10

FIGURE 16-11

FIGURE 16-12

Malleus

Cog

Cochleariform process

Stapes

VII

Lateral semicircular canal

FIGURE 16-13

FIGURES 16-8 to 16-13. *See legend on opposite page*

the tegmen epitympani and partially separates the anterior tympanic compartment (supratubal recess) from the meso-epitympanum. The cog lies immediately superior to, and just slightly posterior to, the cochleariform process and anterior to the head of the malleus (Fig. 16–12). As the facial nerve runs between the cochleariform process and the geniculate ganglion, it courses under the base of the cog and anterior to it in the floor of the supratubal recess.

Mastoid Segment

In mastoidectomy, the initial landmarks within the temporal bone are the mastoid antrum and the lateral semicircular canal. Once the lateral canal is identified, the surgeon knows where the facial nerve is and is prepared to remove all the diseased tissue from the mastoid (Fig. 16–13).

The short crus of the incus is located inferior, and slightly lateral, to the anterior portion of the lateral canal bulge. The fossa incudis is at the tip of the short crus. The facial nerve lies medial to the fossa incudis and inferior to the lateral canal. As the nerve travels inferiorly in its course to the stylomastoid foramen, it travels in a slightly posterior direction, in most instances, and also travels laterally. (The reader would be well served by reading the article by Litton and associates on the relationship of the facial canal to the tympanic sulcus.[17]

Two further landmarks to the mastoid segment of the facial nerve are the digastric groove and the posterior semicircular canal. Neither are usually involved (in facial nerve identification) in surgery of chronic otitis media because of the lack of cellular development in most cases of this type. The digastric groove leads to the stylomastoid foramen. The inferior portion of the posterior semicircular canal travels medial to the facial nerve.

MANAGEMENT OF THE LABYRINTHINE FISTULA

There is no way of knowing for certain preoperatively that a patient with cholesteatoma does not have a labyrinthine fistula; as many as 10 per cent do.[12]

Each mastoid must be approached as if a fistula existed. When the cholesteatomal sac is encountered in the mastoid, it should be opened, and the medial wall of the sac lying on the lateral semicircular canal should be palpated to detect any bony dehiscence. Bony erosion may be obvious by flattening of the usual prominence of the lateral canal.

If there appears to be a fistula, a decision has to be reached as to management of the mastoid: continue as an intact canal wall procedure, or create an open cavity? If an open cavity is to be created, the matrix may be left on the fistula permanently.[11]

If the operation is to continue as an intact canal wall procedure, carefully incise the matrix around the fistula. The rest of the matrix may be removed without removing the segment covering the fistula. If a decision has been reached that the operation is to be performed in two stages (see Chapter 18), leave the matrix over the fistula. It will be removed at the planned second stage when the ear is healed. If the operation is to be performed in one stage, complete the operation, including grafting, ossicular chain reconstruction, and packing of the ear canal. If you suspect that the fistula is small, it is reasonable to remove the matrix at this time and cover the fistula immediately with fascia. If on the other hand the fistula appears to be large or the ear is infected, it is probably best to leave the matrix and come back into the mastoid in 6 months to remove it.

REPAIR OF CANAL WALL DEFECTS

Defects in the posterior or superior bony canal wall need to be repaired to prevent recurrence of cholesteatoma from retraction pockets. Defects may be the result of the disease or the surgery.

Defects due to Disease

It is not unusual for cholesteatoma to erode some of the lateral epitympanic wall, but it may at times destroy a larger portion of the posterior canal wall. If the canal wall

---

FIGURE 16–8. Retraction of new tympanic membrane into the facial recess, caused by scar tissue; plastic sheeting was not used. *Arrows* indicate development of recurrent cholesteatoma.

FIGURE 16–9. Thin plastic through the facial recess; capitulum is protruding through the opening to allow reconstruction.

FIGURE 16–10. Thick plastic sheeting extending from the mastoid into the middle ear through the facial recess.

FIGURE 16–11. Parasagittal section through the middle ear of the right temporal bone to show landmarks. Facial nerve lies superior to the oval window and posterior (also superior) to the cochleariform process. The nerve lies superior, and also posterior, to the pyramidal process and anterior to the cog in the floor of the supratubal recess. The cog is a ridge of bone extending inferiorly from the tegmen epitympani, above the cochleariform process (refer to Fig. 16–12). Note the relationship of semicanal for the tensor tympani and a groove in the promontory for the tympanic nerve of Jacobson.

FIGURE 16–12. View from the mastoid into the epitympanum (facial recess has been opened). Malleus head has been ghosted in to show the relationship to the cog (compare with Fig. 16–11). The cog is a ridge of bone extending inferiorly from the tegmen epitympani, anterior to the malleus head, above the cochleariform process.

FIGURE 16–13. Facial nerve (labyrinthine, tympanic, and mastoid segments) has been ghosted in to show the relationship to the ossicles, facial recess opening, and lateral semicircular canal.

destruction is extensive, it is probably wise not to repair the defect but to change to a CWD procedure.

In most cases, canal wall destruction is limited to the lateral epitympanic wall (Fig. 16–14). If a second-stage procedure is planned (see Chapter 18), it is wise not to reconstruct the defect; the Supramid or thick silicone sheeting will prevent a retraction pocket between stages 1 and 2. At stage 2, after removing the plastic, one may see through the defect to detect any residual disease. The defect may be repaired at that time with bone pate or cartilage.

If a second-stage operation is not indicated, then the defect may be repaired in similar way after the graft has been tucked under the bony defect (Fig. 16–15).

Defects due to Surgery

If one is using an intact canal wall technique, it is unwise to perform atticotomy. At times, however, it is necessary to do so, particularly anteriorly, if the middle fossa dural plate is low or the ear canal is angled in such a way that one cannot obtain adequate vision into the supratubal recess. The repair of these problems is the same as mentioned earlier.

At times, there will be an inadvertent opening made in the canal wall when the mastoid is drilled. To avoid this, the ear canal bone should be thinned as the final step in the procedure before the facial recess is opened. This procedure prevents inadvertently knocking a hole in the wall while drilling in the mastoid. Should such a defect occur, it may be repaired with a shaving of cartilage over the hole on the canal side prior to replacement of the ear canal skin.

ACKNOWLEDGMENT

Many of the illustrations are modified from *Otolaryngology*, Vol. 1, published by J. B. Lippincott Company.

References

1. Committee on Conservation of Hearing of the American Academy of Ophthalmology and Otolaryngology: Standard classification for surgery of chronic ear infection. Arch Otolaryngol Head Neck Surg 81: 204–205, 1965.
2. Wullstein H: Theory and practice of tympanoplasty. Laryngoscope 66: 1076–1093, 1956.
3. Zollner F: Principles of plastic surgery of the sound-conducting apparatus. J Laryngol Otol 69: 637–652, 1955.
4. Sheehy JL, Patterson ME: Intact canal wall tympanoplasty with mastoidectomy. Laryngoscope 77: 1502–1542, 1967.
5. Rambo JHT: Further experience with musculoplasty. Arch Otolaryngol Head Neck Surg 71: 428–436, 1960.
6. Sheehy JL: Intact canal wall tympanoplasty with mastoidectomy. *In* Snow JB (ed): Controversies in Otolaryngology. Philadelphia, WB Saunders, 1980.
7. Sheehy JL, Brackmann DE: Surgery of Chronic Ear Disease: What We Do and Why We Do It. Instructional Courses, Vol 6. St. Louis, CV Mosby, 1993.
8. Sheehy JL: Cholesteatoma surgery: Residual and recurrent disease. Ann Otol Rhinol Laryngol 86: 451–462, 1977.
9. Sheehy JL, Robinson JV: Cholesteatoma surgery at the Otologic Medical Group: Residual and recurrent disease. A report on 307 revision operations. Am J Otol 3: 209–215, 1982.

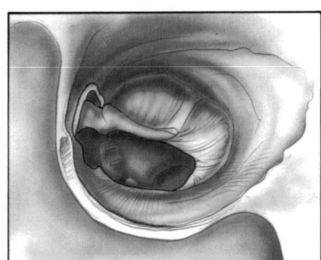

FIGURE 16-14

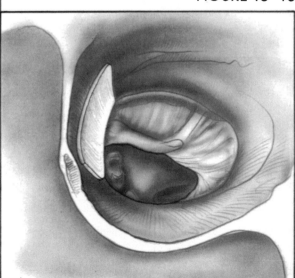

FIGURE 16-15

FIGURE 16–14. Defect in lateral epitympanic wall.

FIGURE 16–15. Repair of lateral wall defect with cartilage.

10. Sheehy JL: Chronic tympanomastoiditis. *In* Gates GA (ed): Current Therapy in Otolaryngology—Head and Neck Surgery, Vol 4. Philadelphia, BC Decker, 1990, pp 19–22.
11. Sheehy JL: Cholesteatoma surgery: Canal wall down procedures. Ann Otol Rhinol Laryngol 97: 30–35, 1988.
12. Sheehy JL, Brackmann DE: Cholesteatoma surgery: Management of the labyrinthine fistula. Laryngoscope 89: 78–87, 1979.
13. Sheehy JL, Brackmann DE, Graham MD: Complications of cholesteatoma: A report on 1024 cases. *In* McCabe B, Sade J, Abramson M (eds): Cholesteatoma, First International Conference. Birmingham, AL, Aesculapius, 1977.
14. Sheehy JL, Brackmann DE: Surgery of chronic otitis media. English GM (ed): *In* Otolaryngology. Philadelphia, JB Lippincott, 1994, Chapter 20.
15. Sheehy JL: Facial nerve in surgery of chronic otitis media. Otolaryngol Clin North Am 7: 493–503, 1974.
16. Donaldson JA, Anson BJ, Warpeha RL, et al: The surgical anatomy of the sinus tympani. Arch Otolaryngol Head Neck Surg 91: 219–227, 1970.
17. Litton WB, Krause CJ, Anson BA, et al.: The relationship of the facial canal to the annular sulcus. Laryngoscope 79: 1584–1604, 1969.

Additional Reading

Sheehy JL: Management of cholesteatoma. *In* Controversies in Otolaryngology. New York, Thieme, In press.

17

Mastoidectomy: The Canal Wall Down Procedure

Moisés A. Arriaga, M.D.

There are two ways of handling a mastoidectomy in patients with cholesteatoma and chronic otitis media. The canal wall up (CWU) technique has already been discussed in detail in Chapter 16. This chapter describes the technique for canal wall down (CWD) surgery. Related topics included in this chapter are the role of atticotomy, mastoid obliteration procedures, reconstruction of CWD cavities that have not been previously reconstructed, management of dural venous sinus injury during chronic ear surgery, and a discussion of facial nerve monitoring in chronic ear surgery.

DEFINITIONS

The surgeon may perform a series of mastoidectomy procedures that involve sacrificing a portion or all of the ear canal in continuity with the mastoidectomy.

Modified Radical Mastoidectomy (Bondy). This is the classic modified radical mastoidectomy. The epitympanum and CWD mastoidectomy and external auditory canal are converted into a common cavity. The tympanic membrane and middle ear are left undisturbed.

Radical Mastoidectomy. This is an operation that eradicates middle ear and mastoid disease by converting the mastoid antrum, middle ear, and external auditory canal into a common cavity. The tympanic membrane and ossicular chain are sacrificed. No effort is made at reconstructing a middle ear space; however, a tissue plug or graft is usually placed to seal the orifice of the eustachian tube.

Tympanoplasty with CWD Mastoidectomy. In this procedure, the mastoid air cells are exteriorized and form a common cavity with the external auditory canal. The middle ear is reconstructed by grafting the tympanic membrane and possibly reconstructing the ossicular chain. The terminology can sometimes be confusing. Some authors refer to this procedure as a *modified radical mastoidectomy.* To be accurate, that terminology should be applied to the Bondy modified radical mastoidectomy.

Atticotomy. In this mastoid procedure only a limited portion of the wall of the external auditory canal is sacrificed. A small attic cholesteatoma is exteriorized by drilling the scutum to the limits of the cholesteatoma sac. The defect is reconstructed with a cartilage graft or autologous bone.

Mastoid Obliteration Procedure. This refers to a possible modification of the just-discussed mastoid procedures in which soft tissue, bone pate, or even biocompatible materials are used to fill the space of the mastoid cavity in an effort to limit postoperative mastoid cavity problems.

Mastoid Reconstruction Procedure. This two-stage procedure involves creating an air-containing space with tympanoplasty and Silastic sheeting in a previous radical mastoidectomy. A subsequent procedure is then performed for ossicular reconstruction.

INDICATIONS FOR CWD MASTOIDECTOMY

Mastoidectomy in chronic ear surgery is designed to eliminate mastoid disease in the face of suppurative otitis media and, more commonly, cholesteatoma of the middle ear or mastoid. In general, CWU surgery is preferred to maintain the normal anatomic contours of the mastoid. Certain factors are strong indications for CWD surgery, including (1) extensive damage by disease to the posterior canal wall, (2) severely contracted mastoid with low-lying tegmen and far forward sigmoid sinus preventing adequate visualization through a standard CWU approach, (3) cholesteatoma in an only-hearing ear, and (4) labyrinthine fistula in an ear with extensive cholesteatoma. Some authors have argued that CWD surgery permits excision of cholesteatoma in the sinus tympani region.[1] Anatomically this is not full visualization because the depths of the sinus tympani are medial to the facial nerve. Nonetheless, Hulka and McElveen recently demonstrated that CWD procedures do permit additional visualization in the anterior epitympanum and sinus tympani region.[2] The latter is not fully visualized with any technique. Another relative indication for CWD mastoidectomy is failure of previous CWU procedures with recurrent cholesteatoma from epitympanic retraction pockets. The anatomy of a CWD mastoidectomy with full exteriorization of the epitympanum makes retraction pocket recurrences of cholesteatoma unlikely because the whole epitympanum has been exteriorized. Although the use of Silastic in CWU facial recess surgery and staging has been significant in reducing the incidence of recurrent cholesteatoma with CWU surgery, the presence of a scutal edge and a distinct epitympanum in cases with persistent eustachian tube dysfunction can produce recurrent cholesteatoma.

DECISION MAKING

With the exception of the preoperative identification of an attic cholesteatoma in an only-hearing ear, usually the decision to perform a CWD technique is made intraoperatively. Such characteristics as extensive canal wall destruction by cholesteatoma, a large labyrinthine fistula with an extensive cholesteatoma, and a severely contracted mastoid all are features identified intraoperatively. Furthermore, as the operation proceeds, the surgeon may discover that certain areas of the mastoid such as the epitympanum are poorly visualized and may elect to perform a CWD procedure for purposes of exposure. Similarly, as the operation is proceeding in a patient with multiple previous recurrences in the epitympanum through retraction pockets, the surgeon may elect to convert the mastoid into a CWD cavity, especially if no clear technical reason for failure of the previous procedures has been identified other than chronic eustachian tube dysfunction.

PREOPERATIVE EVALUATION

A detailed microscopic examination of the ear is necessary preoperatively. Attic retraction pockets should be viewed with suspicion if the surgeon is unable to see the depths of the pocket. Using a right-angle pick to feel the depths of such a retraction is often helpful. The use of otoendoscopes has been quite helpful to permit a "fish-eye" view of these pockets. This technique permits wider visualization of the pocket. In these cases, computed tomographic (CT) scan can be helpful to define whether what seems to be a small retraction represents the neck of a cholesteatoma or is merely a small retraction. Although the CT scan may underestimate the extent of disease in this area, a large cyst extending into the antrum would certainly be identified with CT scan. An attic pocket, in which the depths cannot be palpated, that is beginning to retain debris is an indication for surgery. If the scan does not show a large cyst in the antrum, an atticotomy may be considered.

Similarly, a distinct attic cholesteatoma with a positive fistula test and the subjective symptom of dizziness is also an indication for imaging. The possibility of a labyrinthine fistula must be considered. Especially if there is a large cholesteatoma, a CWD procedure should be considered.

In a pre-existing CWD cavity that is draining or is retaining significant debris, the surgeon must evaluate four specific characteristics of the cavity: (1) adequacy of saucerization of the mastoid cortex margins, (2) adequate lowering of the facial ridge, (3) adequate management of the mastoid tip, and (4) adequacy of the meatus. Problems with any of these characteristics can contribute to cavity failures. In chronic drainage situations, areas of persistent mucosalization should be identified so that these are dealt with appropriately in the revision procedure.

Audiometric studies are routinely obtained preoperatively. In general, we repeat audiometric studies done elsewhere before the patient undergoes surgery. This is particularly emphasized if the "outside" audiograms do not coincide with tuning fork tests. Special attention must be given to the adequacy of masking with the audiometric studies performed.

PREOPERATIVE COUNSELING

As with any otologic procedure, we counsel patients that there are three principal risks: (1) hearing loss that may

even be total in the operated ear (< 1 per cent), (2) dizziness that is usually temporary but rarely can become permanent, and (3) facial nerve paralysis, which is quite rare but an obvious and distressing complication for the patient. In general, patients who undergo CWD surgery will also have facial nerve monitoring. Our indications and rationale for this are discussed later.

Patients undergoing CWD surgery should be specifically advised that the ear canal will be larger postoperatively. Healing following a CWD procedure takes longer than in a CWU procedure. Even at the preoperative visit, patients are counseled that they should begin applying otologic antibiotic drops immediately following surgery to begin dissolving the packing. After the initial postoperative visit at 2 weeks, half-strength vinegar irrigations are used to remove residual packing and limit granulation tissue formation. These cavities are usually healed between 2 and 3 months postoperatively.

SURGICAL TECHNIQUES

Patient Preparation

The patient is placed supine on the operating table with the head turned away. Hair is shaved approximately 2 to 3 fingerbreadths behind the pinna. Adhesive plastic drapes are applied surrounding the edges of the shaved hair. Approximately 3 to 4 ml of lidocaine (Xylocaine) 1 per cent with epinephrine 1:100,000 is injected in the postauricular region and also in the posterosuperior aspect of the ear canal. Sterile preparation is then accomplished with povidone-iodine solution, allowing solution to enter the ear canal as well.

In cases in which facial nerve monitoring is used, electromyographic needle electrodes are placed in the orbicularis oculi and orbicularis oris muscles as well as in the forehead and ipsilateral shoulder to act as ground for monitoring and for stimulating, respectively.

Sterile towels are then placed around the prepared area. The area is dried with a sterile towel and a large sterile adhesive drape is applied that overlies the sterile prepared area and holds the sterile towels in position.

As mentioned previously, the decision to convert a mastoid operation from CWU to CWD is usually made intraoperatively. Accordingly, the usual steps for tympanoplasty with mastoidectomy surgery would have been accomplished, including canal incisions, as described in the previous two chapters on tympanoplasty (undersurface and lateral graft). The ear has been reflected forward, the middle ear work has been completed, the tympanic membrane remnant has been prepared for grafting, and the mastoidectomy has begun.

Basic Techniques

The basic principle of CWD mastoidectomy surgery is to eliminate all of the disease and exteriorize the mastoid antrum in continuity with the external auditory canal. In addition to removing all diseased air cells, the following four steps are basic to creating a trouble-free mastoid cavity:

1. ADEQUATE SAUCERIZATION. (Fig. 17–1)
   Removal of bone from the edges of the mastoid defect saucerizes or bevels the edges of the defect so that there is no overhanging bone obstructing the wider cavity below. This ensures that there is no disease tissue laterally. Also, this permits soft tissue surrounding the mastoid to slide into the defect. Paradoxically, removing additional bone around the margins of the mastoid cortex in this saucerization step actually makes a smaller cavity rather than a larger cavity.

2. ADEQUATE LOWERING OF THE FACIAL RIDGE. (Fig. 17–2)
   The boundary between the external auditory canal and the mastoid cavity is defined by the height of the facial nerve. Leaving excessive bone overlying the facial nerve (facial ridge) between the external auditory canal and the mastoid cavity creates a situation in which there is a deep trough on the mastoid side. This high ridge is sometimes referred to as a "beginner's hump." Occasionally novice mastoid surgeons leave a large ridge of bone overlying the facial nerve for fear of injuring it. This creates a difficult situation postoperatively with trapped mastoid spaces that are hard to clean in the office, and it also prevents natural cleaning. The surgeon should lower the ridge of bone overlying the facial nerve so that the fallopian canal is barely visible with a thin amount of bone overlying the vertical segment of the facial nerve.

   Inferiorly, toward the stylomastoid foramen, the nerve takes a medial-to-lateral trajectory. In this area, it is helpful to bevel the bone of the external auditory canal to parallel this more lateral track of the facial nerve inferiorly. Three adjuncts are used for appropriately identifying the level of the facial nerve. First, the nerve itself can be identified at the second genu where the short process of the incus points directly to the facial nerve. If a facial recess has already been accomplished, this level can be followed from superiorly toward inferiorly. The second adjunct is the periosteum and tendon of the digastric muscle in the digastric ridge inferiorly in the region of the mastoid tip. This also leads directly to the facial nerve. This periosteum surrounds the nerve as it exits the stylomastoid foramen. Finally, if facial nerve monitoring is employed, soft tissue structures that parallel the course of the nerve can be stimulated directly with the facial nerve stimulator to confirm the anatomic position of the nerve. The latter is more often useful in revision cases in which scar tissue may obscure the anatomy. The objective in adequately lowering the facial ridge is to make the cavity more rounded rather than kidney shaped, which will facilitate postoperative hygiene.

3. MANAGEMENT OF THE MASTOID TIP. (Fig. 17–3)
   If the mastoid tip is not pneumatized, it is incapable of retaining debris and suppurative mucosal air cells—accordingly, no specific management is necessary. Often in chronic draining situations, a pneumatized tip is encountered. This must be removed. There are two basic techniques. The mastoid air cells lateral to the digastric muscle can simply be drilled away, in this manner allowing the soft tissue of the skull base to obliterate the space. Alternatively, the digastric ridge can be followed from posterior to anterior. A Kocher clamp can be placed on the mastoid tip and a curved Mayo scissors can be used to remove the muscular attachments from the mastoid tip to permit complete

FIGURE 17-1

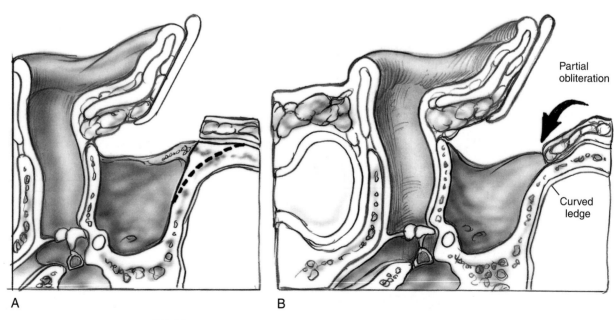

A   B

FIGURE 17–1. A and B, Saucerization. Removal of ledges and overhanging bone facilitates visualization and permits adjacent soft tissue to "obliterate" part of the cavity.

FIGURE 17-2

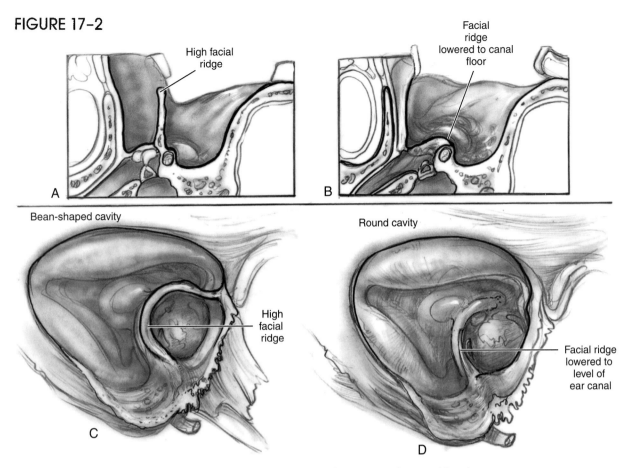

FIGURE 17-2. Facial ridge. *A* and *B,* Lowering the ridge permits easier access to the mastoid cavity. Bean-shaped *(C)* and round *(D)* cavities are created by lowering the facial ridge to the level of the floor of the ear canal.

amputation of this structure. Once again, this eliminates the tip and allows the soft tissue of the skull base to prolapse into the defect.

4. ADEQUATE MEATOPLASTY. (Fig. 17–4)

An adequate meatus is essential to allow aeration, epithelialization, and adequate drainage of the cavity. Of the four steps for a trouble-free cavity, small errors in the first three can be compensated by an adequate meatus. The converse is usually not true. An adequate meatoplasty involves extending the vascular strip incisions laterally through the conchal cartilage. The conchal cartilage is then removed to permit this extended vascular strip complete mobility so that it can even be everted through the ear canal. The cartilage can be removed posteriorly by first freeing the soft tissue from the conchal cartilage. This soft tissue can remain pedicled medially and be used to partially obliterate a large mastoid cavity. In general, we simply discard this tissue. At this point, the cartilage can be incised carefully to not transect the skin on the ear canal side. The wedge of cartilage can be removed. Alternatively, the vascular strip can be grasped from the ear canal side and the level of the cartilage can be identified and peeled from the medial side. Additional conchal cartilage adjacent to the edges of the vascular strip should also be removed to allow this whole posterior aspect of the incision complete mobility to overlie the bony mar-

gins. Once the posterior meatoplasty has been accomplished, attention is focused anteriorly. At the superior edges of the tragal cartilage there is usually a significant amount of soft tissue. By undermining the skin overlying the anterior canal and tragal cartilage, a portion of the tragal cartilage can be trimmed along with the adjacent soft tissue to permit the soft tissue mass from obliterating the meatus with either scar or contracture. Once the soft tissue meatoplasty has been accomplished anteriorly and posteriorly, we have found that placement of sutures near the edge of cartilage removal is useful in the early postoperative period to maintain the patency of the meatus. In this manner, stenting is not necessary to keep the meatus open during the initial healing phases.

The four steps just described are the basic building blocks for an adequate CWD mastoidectomy procedure.[3] These techniques as they apply to specific CWD procedures are described in the following sections.

MODIFIED RADICAL MASTOIDECTOMY—BONDY
(Fig. 17–5)

The Bondy modified radical mastoidectomy is the original modified radical mastoid operation. Before this procedure

FIGURE 17-3

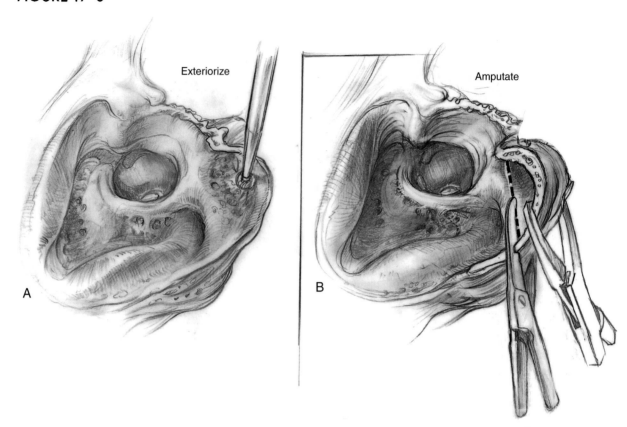

FIGURE 17–3. Mastoid Tip. *A,* The mastoid tip is exteriorized with a burr. *B,* The tip is grasped with a Kocher clamp and amputated by cutting with curved Mayo scissors along the digastric ridge.

FIGURE 17-4

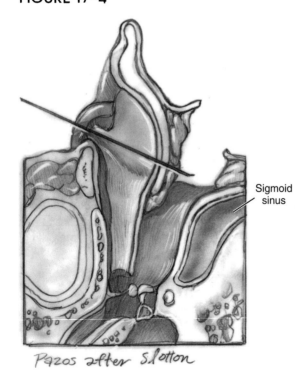

FIGURE 17–4. Meatoplasty. Rosen needle marks the area of conchal carti-lage removal.

FIGURE 17-5

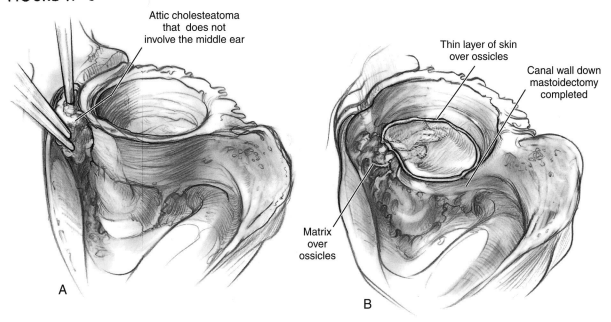

Attic cholesteatoma
that does not
involve the middle ear

Thin layer of skin
over ossicles

Canal wall down
mastoidectomy
completed

Matrix
over
ossicles

A

B

FIGURE 17–5. *A* and *B,* Modified radical mastoidectomy. An attic cholesteatoma is exteriorized without entering the middle ear. The canal wall down mastoidectomy is completed and the matrix covers the ossicle in the epitympanum.

was developed, mastoid surgery entailed complete exenteration of the middle ear–transducing mechanism, including the tympanic membrane and ossicular chain. Despite its historical development, at this time this procedure is indicated for cholesteatoma that has spared the middle ear. An attic cholesteatoma that has extended through the attic into the epitympanum and mastoid antrum can be managed by this technique, which spares the tympanic membrane and middle ear. This is particularly useful in cholesteatoma in an only-hearing ear, in elderly patients in whom staging and multiple surgeries would not be advised, and even in cases of lateral canal fistulas from extensive atticoantral cholesteatoma that has spared the middle ear.

After the ear is reflected forward with standard vascular strip incisions, the CWD mastoidectomy is created in the usual manner as described in the techniques section. The edges of the cavity are saucerized. The facial ridge is brought down to the level of the nerve with management of the mastoid tip if it is pneumatized, as well as adequate meatoplasty. The hallmark is that the tympanic membrane is left in position. Middle ear work such as ossicular reconstruction is not performed. Cholesteatoma matrix that is lining the epitympanum or overlying a semicircular canal fistula can be left in place as this begins the epithelialization process.

CWD MASTOIDECTOMY WITH TYMPANOPLASTY (Fig. 17–6)

CWD mastoidectomy with tympanoplasty is the procedure that has been renamed by some authors as a *modified radical mastoidectomy*. The difference between this procedure and the procedure described in the previous section is

that tympanic membrane grafting, staging, and ossicular reconstruction are performed with this procedure. In general, it is preferable to accomplish the middle ear work first. We adhere to the strategy described in the previous chapter for addressing middle ear pathology prior to the mastoid pathology. Middle ear disease in the anteroinferior, anterosuperior, and posteroinferior quadrants is managed first. The posterosuperior quadrant is saved for the final manipulation in the event that an oval window fistula is encountered to permit expeditious termination of the procedure.

The mastoidectomy procedure is then performed. Initially, the strategy would be to perform a CWU mastoidectomy; however, if any of the characteristics described earlier are encountered, which require changing over to a CWD procedure, the technical steps of saucerization, managing the facial ridge, managing the tip, and performing adequate meatoplasty are accomplished. Once the technical maneuvers for the CWD procedure have been completed, the decision is made whether primary reconstruction can be performed. In the case of extensive cholesteatoma, the usual area for residual disease is not the mastoid but the mesotympanum. Accordingly, if the cholesteatoma has not been removed in continuity or if there is a question of complete cholesteatoma removal or there is extensive mucosal disease, staging is performed with Silastic in the middle ear prior to tympanic membrane grafting. If ossicular reconstruction can be accomplished at the same stage, this is performed. We prefer porous polyethylene partial and total ossicular prosthesis. These prostheses are covered with large cartilage grafts. In cases with a mobile stapes suprastructure, ossicular reconstruction in CWD surgery often requires only covering the capitulum with autologous cartilage because the middle ear space is narrow. The

FIGURE 17-6

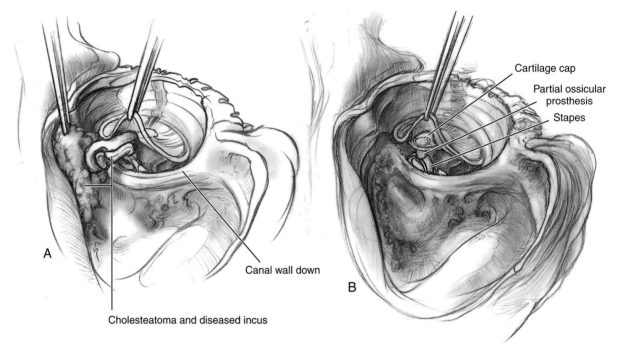

Cartilage cap

Partial ossicular prosthesis

Stapes

Canal wall down

Cholesteatoma and diseased incus

A

B

FIGURE 17–6. *A and B, Canal wall down (CWD) mastoidectomy with tympanoplasty. In addition to the CWD cavity, disease is removed from the middle ear and ossiculoplasty can be accomplished.*

cartilage is usually left with an attached tail of perichondrium that serves to anchor the prosthesis-cartilage complex in position. Preservation of the canal wall has not been a prognostic factor for hearing results in our cases or in those of others.[4] If primary ossicular reconstruction is planned without staging in CWD surgery, medial grafting is performed if possible when a substantial anterior tympanic membrane remnant is present and the annulus is intact anteriorly. This technique has less risk of lateralization that would affect the ossicular reconstruction in a primarily reconstructed case.

ATTICOTOMY (Fig. 17–7)

In cases of limited attic cholesteatomas, drilling the scutum around the epitympanic margins of the cholesteatoma can preserve a near-normal contour for the ear. This procedure is limited to patients with cholesteatoma confined to the central epitympanic area. The surgeon must be prepared to convert to a complete CWD mastoidectomy if necessary. Preoperative CT has been useful to ascertain that a cyst is limited to the attic. Clinically, the clue that an attic pocket is transitioning into a cholesteatoma is when it is no longer self-cleaning and debris begins to accumulate. Even in a CWU procedure with staging and facial recess, this region of the scutum would require reconstruction with either cartilage or bone pate.

The procedure is approached such that conversion to a full CWD mastoidectomy with tympanoplasty is straightforward. Standard vascular strip incisions are performed followed by a postauricular incision and reflecting the ear anteriorly. The edge of the scutal defect is drilled with a small diamond burr and gradually widened. The bone of the superior ear canal is thinned and saucerized to permit adequate visualization. Once the margins of the cholesteatoma sac are identified, this is exteriorized. Often the cholesteatoma debris itself is excised and the matrix can be reflected inferiorly and a small cartilage graft or bone chip can be placed in the scutal defect and the inferiorly based tympanomeatal flap can be returned. The vascular strip is returned to position and the ear is packed with Gelfoam.

If the disease has been underestimated and the cholesteatoma extends significantly toward the antrum, the surgeon at this point is usually committed to a full mastoidectomy with tympanoplasty.

RADICAL MASTOIDECTOMY
(Fig. 17–8)

In this procedure, extensive disease does not permit ossicular reconstruction; instead, the middle ear and mastoid cavity are exteriorized. Middle ear mucous membrane must be excised along with all deceased mastoid air cells. The eustachian tube must be addressed specifically. If it is left open, nasopharyngeal reflux can create a moist cavity. Although the tube may be packed with pledgets of temporalis muscle, a small temporalis fascia graft over the eustachian tube orifice works effectively.

MASTOID OBLITERATION PROCEDURE

Patients with particularly large mastoid cavities occasionally have difficulty with drainage from retained moisture

FIGURE 17–7

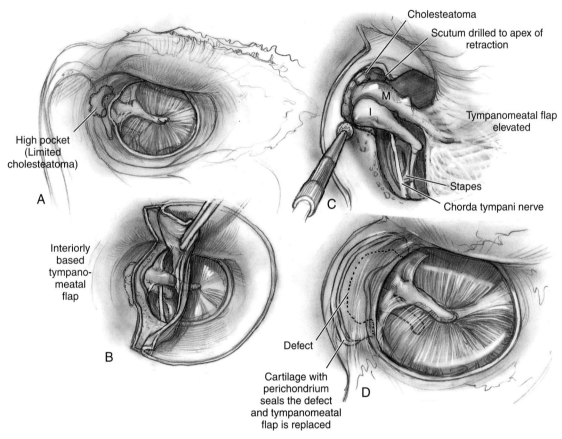

FIGURE 17–7. Atticotomy. *A,* Atticotomy is limited to small pockets in the epitympanum without extension into the antrum. *B* and *C,* An inferiorly based tympanomeatal flap is gradually elevated as the scutum is drilled to the apex of the retraction. *D,* Cartilage with attached perichondrium seals the defect.

FIGURE 17-8

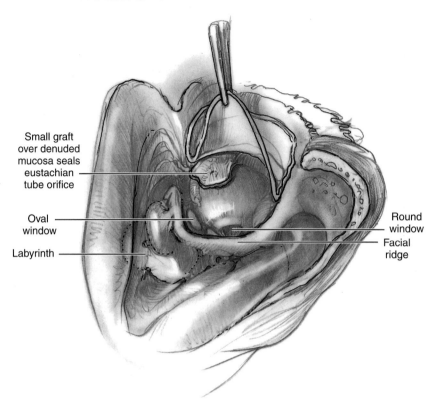

Small graft over denuded mucosa seals eustachian tube orifice

Oval window

Labyrinth

Round window

Facial ridge

FIGURE 17–8. Radical mastoidectomy. Fascia is used to seal the eustachian tube orifice after completing the canal wall down cavity and removing middle ear mucous membrane. No effort is made at tympanic membrane or ossicular reconstruction.

or difficulty being fitted with the hearing aid because of the volume of the cavity. In an attempt to eliminate this problem, soft tissue flaps, bone pate, and biocompatible materials may be placed to obliterate the volume of the cavity. Rambo[5] and Palva[6] described a series of muscular flaps for mastoid obliteration. The former used inferior flaps and the latter used more posteriorly fashioned flaps. Recent studies indicate that the long-term effect of mastoid obliteration is negligible because the obliterated and non-obliterated cavities ultimately heal with essentially the same mastoid volume.[7] In portions of the cavity that are difficult to exteriorize, such as deep retrofacial air cells, fascia or muscle grafts can be used to seal these air cells to encourage their drainage into the eustachian tube through the air cell system. If the surgeon wishes to seal off a portion of the cavity, the soft tissue that is freed from the posterior aspect of the vascular strip prior to freeing the cartilage during meatoplasty can be left pedicled to the vascular strip and used as a vascularized flap to obliterate a portion of the cavity. Mastoid obliteration to reduce the volume of the cavity is an infrequently used technique in our practice. Instead, wide saucerization to permit prolapse of adjacent soft tissue is a preferred method.

RECONSTRUCTION OF A RADICAL CAVITY

In some patients who have undergone previous radical mastoidectomy, the ear itself becomes quiescent. Despite obliteration of the eustachian tube, recanalization occurs and an air-containing space can be identified. This air space is usually limited to the protympanum directly over the eustachian tube area. In the absence of weeping mucous membrane or disease in the rest of the cavity, these patients are candidates for reconstruction of the middle ear sound transforming mechanism. The patient must understand that this will require a two-stage procedure.

Any form of revision surgery must be done with great caution, particularly in elevating the tympanomeatal flap over the level of the facial ridge. The initial surgeon may have lowered the ridge to the level of the nerve itself and not left bony cover. Alternatively, chronic osteitis may have dissolved the remaining thin bone over the facial nerve. Furthermore, any previous labyrinthine fistula is in jeopardy. The tympanomeatal flap tends to shrink following elevation. Accordingly, the incisions are usually made along the superior aspect of the lateral semicircular canal and on the posterior aspect of the facial ridge, leaving adequate room in the event of flap shrinkage so that the mesotympanum itself will be covered (Fig. 17–9). In these cases, we encourage the anesthesiologist to use nitrous oxide to further inflate whatever air-containing space exists within the middle ear. Facial nerve monitoring is useful in these cases to confirm the position and the adequacy of bony cover of the facial nerve.

The tympanomeatal flap is elevated along with the epithelialized layer covering the promontory. Often this will elevate most of the mucosa over the promontory as well.

FIGURE 17-9

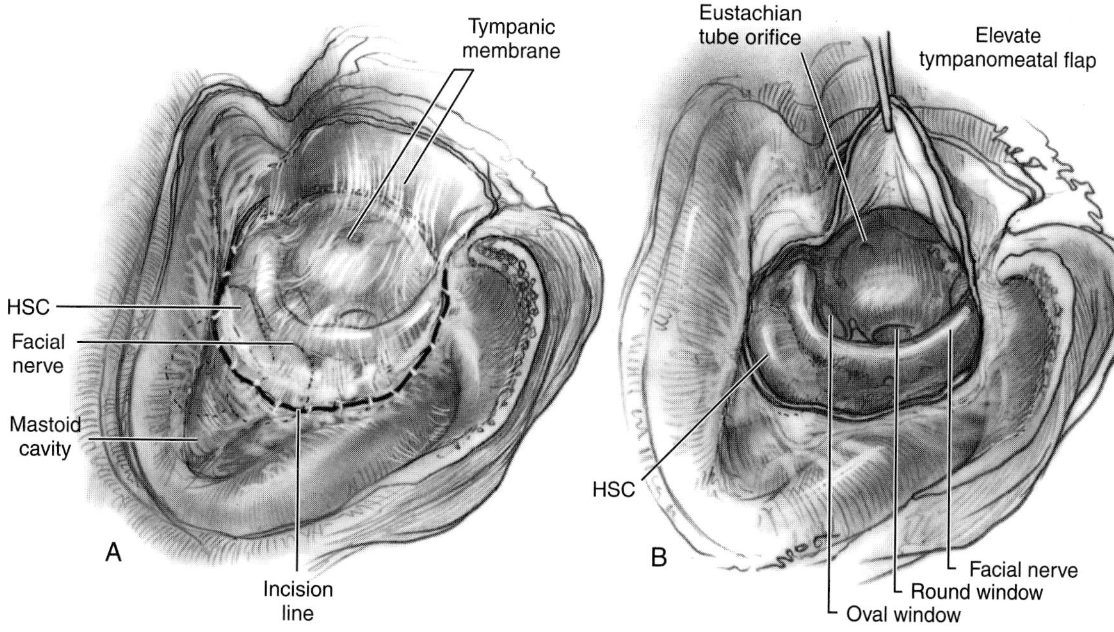

FIGURE 17–9. *A* and *B*, Incisions for tympanomeatal flap. The tympanomeatal flap incisions are made along the superior edge of the horizontal semicircular canal (HSC).

Once this is accomplished, the eustachian tube itself is examined carefully. We have encountered a number of patients whose eustachian tubes have been obliterated by previous surgeons using an ossicular remnant. This should be removed with care because the petrous carotid artery is just medial to the eustachian tube in this area. Once the eustachian tube patency is confirmed, Silastic is placed in the middle ear, the drum is regrafted if necessary with a medial technique with the fascia extending over the level of the facial ridge, and the tympanomeatal flap is returned. Six months later, this Silastic is removed and the ossicular reconstruction can be accomplished. We have found the argon laser (similar to the method used for laser stapedotomy) to be a useful adjunct for excising fibrous tissue and defining the anatomy of the oval window and stapes footplate itself. Reconstruction is usually accomplished with a total ossicular prosthesis and a cartilage graft that brings the level of the reconstruction barely above the level of the tympanic and vertical segments of the facial nerve.

REVISION CWD SURGERY

Revision CWD surgery requires certain technical modifications. Specifically, it is difficult to accomplish vascular strip incision because the bone of the canal is missing. Furthermore, if the tegmen has been thinned, blindly cutting toward the tegmen could injure the dura or underlying structures. Accordingly, the principal technical modification in revision canal wall surgery is that no canal incisions are made at the outset. Instead, a postauricular incision is made and the epithelialized covering of the contours of the mastoid is elevated in continuity. This tissue usually cannot be elevated to the level of the facial nerve, and once the cavity is entered medially, vertical incisions (the equivalent

of 6 and 12 o'clock incisions) can be fashioned from medial to lateral to permit reflection of the ear anteriorly. At this point, the tympanomeatal flap is elevated in a similar manner to that described earlier for reconstruction of a radical cavity. Care must be taken with regard to the facial nerve and possible labyrinthine fistulas. The middle ear pathology can be dealt with as described previously, and the specific problem with the cavity can be corrected, with the surgeon being methodical in performing each of the four steps described previously (saucerization, facial ridge, mastoid tip, and adequate meatoplasty). If areas of retained air cells with mucosal discharge have been identified preoperatively, these are drilled. Areas that cannot be fully exteriorized, such as deep retrofacial air cells or perilabyrinthine cells extending toward the apex, are covered with a graft to encourage drainage toward the eustachian tube.

POSTOPERATIVE CARE

We pack CWD cavities with moistened Gelfoam. Antibiotics containing potentially ototoxic medications are specifically avoided. Neomycin-containing otologic preparations are not used. Instead, cefazolin is usually placed in the irrigation fluid for drilling and for irrigating bone dust at the completion of drilling. The Gelfoam itself is moistened in saline and packed over the tympanic membrane and in the cavity. As described in the section on meatoplasty, the meatus is held open with two absorbable sutures (3-0 Vicryl) placed from the posterior aspect just at the edge of cartilage removal from the concha. The periosteum and subcutaneous tissue are reapproximated with interrupted 3-0 absorbable sutures. Steri-Strips are applied, and the remainder of the cavity is packed with large pieces of Gelfoam.

The patient is instructed to begin otologic drops (usually a sulfa and steroid preparation) the day following surgery; this is continued until the 2-week postoperative visit. At that point, most of the packing is removed in the office from the cavity. The patient is then instructed in using a dilute vinegar solution (acetic acid) to wash out the remainder of the packing and minimize granulation formation. The patient irrigates twice a day and uses the antibiotic drops at bedtime. The second postoperative visit is 6 weeks following the surgery. At that time any residual packing is cleaned. Significant granulations are managed with judicious application of silver nitrate, vinegar irrigations at home, and antibiotic-steroid drops.

POTENTIAL PITFALLS

Dural Venous Sinuses

Although management of the dural venous sinus is not usually considered a component of chronic ear disease, these structures are intimately related to the surgical field, and the surgeon must be comfortable in managing any injuries to these structures because cholesteatoma itself can affect them. The principle outlined in Chapter 16 of using the largest possible burr is necessary for preserving the safety of the dural venous sinuses. A large cutting burr essentially will bounce off the wall of the sigmoid sinus,

whereas a small cutting burr with the same amount of force applied will lacerate the sinus, necessitating management. If the sigmoid sinus is entered, the immediate management is to remove the suction aspirator from the field and place a finger over the opening. This is venous bleeding, and usually pressure is adequate for its control. A large piece of Gelfoam over the *surface* of the opening with gentle pressure such as with a cottonoid is usually adequate for coagulation and termination of the venous bleeding. If there is a surrounding bony cover, bone wax can be used effectively. Care must be exercised if any material is placed intraluminally to maintain a tail of the packing material extraluminally. Packing material that is placed within the lumen of the sinus continues through the jugular bulb into the central venous circulation and produces pulmonary emboli. An injury to the superior petrosal sinus can usually be repaired with bipolar cautery of the sinus or placement of bone wax. Injury of the jugular bulb is usually more problematic. Again, temporary occlusion with the surgeon's finger or a cottonoid is necessary. In the meantime, a patch can be prepared combining Surgicel or Gelfoam with a large piece of bone wax to cover the injured area and apply pressure for coagulation to occur. If conservative methods are unsuccessful, the surgeon must be prepared to ligate the jugular vein in the neck and proceed with intraluminal packing.

FACIAL NERVE (Fig. 17–10)

The floor of the epitympanum must be approached cautiously because the facial nerve labyrinthine segment is

FIGURE 17-10

(Canal wall down)

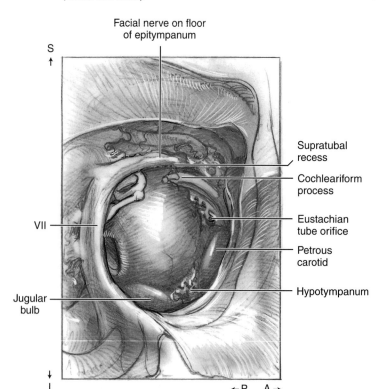

FIGURE 17–10. Facial nerve on floor of epitympanum. Schematic view of labyrinthine segment of the facial nerve just medial to the epitympanum. S, superior; I, inferior; P, posterior; A, anterior.

just medial to the geniculate ganglion, and aggressive dissection in this region can injure the nerve.

FACIAL NERVE MONITORING

Facial nerve monitoring in ear surgery has become a contentious topic. We do *not* believe that facial nerve monitoring is the current standard of care in surgery for chronic ear disease. Nonetheless, because our team is involved in a significant number of neurotologic cases as well, we monitor most otologic cases done under general anesthesia. Therefore, the surgical team is comfortable with the use of a facial monitor; the anesthesiologist knows muscle relaxants are not used in otologic cases, and the quality of monitoring improves. With regard to monitoring in CWD surgery, revision CWD surgery (because of the risk to the facial nerve in the previously lowered facial ridge as well as in a large cholesteatoma) is a definite indication for facial nerve monitoring. Although the monitoring is not a substitute for anatomic knowledge, chronic ear disease can distort the anatomy, making monitoring useful. We have even encountered cases in which edematous changes to the dehiscent tympanic segment of the nerve have increased its diameter threefold so that the nerve itself appeared to be a mound of granulation tissue. Furthermore, in large cholesteatomas when the fallopian canal has been eroded, monitoring permits separation of the cholesteatoma from the nerve with auditory feedback from the monitor in a similar manner to removal of an acoustic tumor from a facial nerve in cerebellopontine angle surgery. The advantages of facial monitoring include identification of unexpected anatomic variations; identification of anatomic distortions from chronic ear disease; assistance with lowering the facial ridge to an appropriate level; and in cases of dehiscent nerves or significant dissection of granulation from the nerve, anatomic integrity of the facial nerve can be confirmed by stimulating proximal to the questionable area prior to the conclusion of the procedure.

OUTCOMES

Adherence to the principles of CWD surgery outlined earlier results in more than 90 per cent of cavities requiring yearly or biannual cleaning without drainage or infection. The anatomy of the ear has been changed by CWD surgery. Failure to débride desquamated epithelium can produce infections, cholesteatomas, and serious complications. We counsel patients that cholesteatoma is a lifelong disease that is either active or inactive. Periodic follow-up is necessary to prevent reactivity.

We prefer patients to have otologic drops available at home in the event of cavity drainage. Three drops, three times a day for 3 days at the onset of drainage will prevent development of a severe infection. If drainage persists, office follow-up is advised.

References

1. Edelstein DR, Parisier SC: Surgical technique and results in cholesteatoma. Otolaryngol Clin North Am 22: 1029–1040, 1989.
2. Hulka GF, McElveen JT Jr: A randomized blinded study of canal wall up versus canal wall down mastoidectomy determining the differences in viewing middle ear anatomy and pathology. Am J Otol 19: 574–578, 1998.
3. Sheehy JL: Surgery in chronic otitis media. *In* English GM (ed): Otolaryngology, Vol 1, Philadephia, JB Lippincott, 1984.
4. Sheehy JL, Beneche JE: Middle ear reconstruction: Current status, Adv Otolaryngol Head Neck Surg. 1: 143–170, 1987.
5. Rambo JHT: Musculoplasty. Ann Otol Rhinol Laryngol 74: 535, 1965.
6. Palva T: Meatally based musculoperiosteal flap in cavity obliteration. *In* Sade J (ed): Cholesteatoma and Mastoid Surgery: Proceedings, Second International Conference. Amsterdam, Kugler, 1982.
7. Toner JL, Smyth GD, Kerr AG: Realities in ossiculoplasty. J Laryngol Otol 105: 529–533, 1991.

18

Tympanoplasty: Staging and Use of Plastic

James L. Sheehy, M.D.

Elimination of disease and restoration of function are the two aims of tympanoplasty. In most teaching situations, one can separate the two aims, limiting the discussion to one or the other. The staging of the operation and the use of plastic in the middle ear, however, require that the discussion consider both objectives.

Staging the operation involves both disease and function, and it is not technique oriented; that is, staging does not vary significantly with the technique of tympanic membrane grafting or of restoring the sound pressure–transfer mechanism, or even the management of the mastoid.

This chapter discusses the history of, and indications for, tympanoplasty, as well as techniques used in performing tympanoplasty in two stages. The controversies surrounding the procedure are discussed at the end of the chapter.

HISTORICAL ASPECTS

In the mid 1950s, a persistent problem in obtaining satisfactory hearing results in tympanoplasty was the maintenance of an aerated middle ear space. When the space collapsed, eustachian tube malfunction was blamed.[1]

By the late 1950s, many recognized that although eustachian tube malfunction played a part in this collapse, a major contributing factor was surgical technique. Creating an open cavity and adapting the graft to whatever ossicular remnants remained resulted in narrowing of the middle ear space. As a result of this realization, many otologists stopped creating open cavities routinely, leaving the bony annulus and epitympanic plate intact (see Chapter 16). This procedure required that a prosthesis be used between the more normally positioned tympanic membrane and the stapes or stapes footplate (see Chapter 13). Although these efforts often led to successful results, collapse of the space continued to be a problem. This problem, however, was compounded by prosthesis extrusion and, at times, formation of a cholesteatoma resulting from retraction pockets into the epitympanum (recurrent cholesteatoma). Many investigators continued to blame collapse of the middle ear space on eustachian tube malfunction.

Rambo[2] recognized that much of the problem was caused by the formation of adhesions between the graft and the denuded medial wall of the middle ear. He recommended a two-stage procedure, the first stage of which involved filling the middle ear with paraffin. Paraffin maintained the space quite nicely, preventing adhesions and allowing normal mucous membrane to cover the denuded areas. For many reasons, Rambo's principle of staging the operation to obtain this mucous membrane–lined, air-containing middle ear space was not appreciated at the time.

The principle of staging the operation was refined by Tabb[3] in 1963, but he described a three-stage procedure. This seemed excessive to many otologists, who were still blaming eustachian tube malfunction for most of the problem. Nonetheless, from then on, staging the operation attracted more attention.

Various thin plastic sheetings (polyethylene, polytetrafluoroethylene [Teflon], silicone rubber) were used, but it was soon learned that this thin sheeting was ineffective in many of the worst ears.[4] The sheeting was pushed aside by fibrous tissue and extruded when pushed against the tympanic membrane.

By the late 1960s, some surgeons began using stiffer plastic in planned, two-stage procedures. Stiffer plastic maintained its position, accomplishing what Rambo had earlier accomplished with paraffin.[5–8]

INDICATIONS FOR STAGING

There are two reasons for staging the operation in tympanoplasty: obtaining a permanently disease-free ear and obtaining permanent restoration of hearing.[7–9] Whether one finds any indication for staging depends on how vigorously a good functional result is pursued in badly diseased ears.

The decision to stage or not to stage is made at the time of surgery. With experience, one usually can make this judgment preoperatively and thereby alert the patient to the possible necessity of a two-stage procedure. The decision is based on three factors: the extent of the mucous membrane problem, the certainty (or lack thereof) of removal of cholesteatoma, and the status of the ossicular chain. Taking these three factors into account, about 40 per cent of tympanoplasty operations are staged by House Ear Clinic (HEC) physicians: 10 to 15 per cent of ears without cholesteatoma and 75 per cent or more of ears with cholesteatoma.

Mucosal Disease Factors

There are frequently large areas of diseased or absent mucosa in the chronically infected middle ear. Groundwork is necessary to promote regrowth of normal mucosa. The first step is elimination of infection prior to surgery, if possible. The second step is removal of all squamous epithelium, granulations, and irreversibly diseased mucosa at the time of surgery. The middle ear is then sealed with a graft to prevent squamous epithelium from migrating back into the middle ear. This sealed middle ear space will fill with a blood clot, and this clot supports fibroblastic invasion with eventual formation of scar tissue or adhesions between the denuded surfaces. To prevent these adhesions from forming, and to allow mucosa to migrate in, plastic sheeting is used over the denuded areas.

A two-stage operation is indicated to obtain the best hearing results and to prevent recurrence of cholesteatoma (retraction pocket) in patients with extensive mucous membrane destruction. The object of the two-stage procedure is to obtain a well-healed ear with a mucosa-lined pneumatized middle ear cleft so that ossicular reconstruction may be performed later under ideal circumstances.

Ossicular Chain Factors

There has been an increase in the incidence of sensorineural hearing impairment in patients in whom the inner ear has been opened in the presence of actual or potential infection. Because of this result, a fixed stapes should not be removed at the time of tympanic membrane grafting. In cases of otosclerosis, a two-stage procedure is almost always indicated. When the fixation is due to tympanosclerosis, it may be possible to mobilize the stapes, depending on the area of fixation. If the oval window is *diffusely* involved, the procedure should be staged.

Residual Cholesteatoma Factor

It may seem quite illogical to leave behind epithelial disease, removing it at a planned second-stage procedure, but this is exactly what is done under certain circumstances.

Removal of cholesteatoma in the middle ear may be questionable, at times, in an acutely inflamed ear in which differentiating between granulation tissue and matrix is difficult. Differentiating becomes a particular problem when granulations fill the oval and round windows. Excessive manipulation in these areas could result in an inner ear complication.

The surgeon may have torn the matrix when removing it from the tympanic recess and may not be certain of complete removal, which presents a considerable problem under the pyramidal process, an area hidden from view regardless of the technique of surgery, whether it is an open- or closed-cavity technique. Removal of the pyramidal process with a diamond burr may or may not resolve the problem.

It is much easier to be certain of cholesteatoma removal from the mastoid, especially in a small apneumatic one. Extensive cholesteatoma in a pneumatized mastoid poses a problem. In using the intact canal wall procedure, one should usually revise the mastoid in such cases within 1 to 2 years to be certain not to leave disease behind.

The mastoid and epitympanum are often re-explored in patients in whom excessive bleeding occurred at surgery.

Unexpected residual disease in the epitympanum has been noted in some cases of this type in the past.

Timing the Second Stage

The second-stage operation may be performed in 6 to 9 months if the primary indication for staging was an ossicular or a mucous membrane problem. The middle ear should be well healed by that time.

If the primary reason for staging is reinspection of the mastoid and epitympanum for possible residual cholesteatoma, it is best to wait 9 to 18 months. The delay allows time for any residual disease to have grown to a 1- or 2-mm cyst so that it may be identified with greater ease. The only exception to this rule is if this disorder occurs in a child or if serous otitis media develops; a residuum may grow faster under these circumstances.

PREOPERATIVE EVALUATION AND COUNSELING

The ability to predict the need for staging the operation depends on one's experience and philosophy regarding the badly diseased ear.

At HEC, the physicians have a section in the *Patient Discussion Booklet* dealing with a planned second-stage procedure. Furthermore, the second-stage operation is mentioned as a possibility under the section on tympanoplasty without mastoidectomy and a probability under that on tympanoplasty with mastoidectomy.

If the patient has dry central perforations with normal mucosa, then the possibility of a second-stage operation need not be mentioned unless there is reason to believe that the stapes is fixed (otosclerosis or tympanosclerosis). When fixation is suspected or there is a major mucous membrane problem, staging is likely. As the HEC booklet states,

I think the outlook for obtaining a healed, dry ear is excellent—90 to 95 per cent chance. But it may be necessary to perform a second operation for hearing improvement. That depends on whether it is necessary to replace the third ear bone; it is not safe to do that at the same time as I graft the ear drum. [Or I say "that depends on how badly diseased the middle ear is."]

If it is necessary to do the operation in two stages, the hearing will probably be worse between step 1 and step 2, for a period of 6 to 12 months.

In cases of cholesteatoma in the middle ear, and in any case requiring mastoid surgery, the patient should be told that a two-stage operation is probable. Again, the HEC booklet states,

The outlook for obtaining a healed, dry, safe ear is excellent—90 per cent or better chance. Unfortunately, it is usually necessary to do a second operation to improve the hearing and to make sure that all the skin growth is out. Your hearing will be worse for 9 to 12 months, until I perform the second surgery.

There is no need to further elaborate on this preoperatively unless the patient asks for more information. If details are necessary, be frank. There is nothing to hide. Elaborate.

When the decision is made at surgery that a second stage is needed, one should explain at the time of the first postoperative visit exactly why this was done. Use a diagram, explain in simple terms, and record a note in the chart that this counseling has been done.

PLASTIC IN THE MIDDLE EAR

The most common middle ear indication for staging the operation is a mucous membrane problem. To avoid confusion, the following discussion is limited to that problem. The techniques are the same when there are other indications.[10]

Plastic Sheeting

Polyethylene film was used initially, then Teflon film. Since 1964, various thicknesses of silicone sheeting have been used and, at times, Supramid.

Silicone sheeting will be referred to here as "thin" and "thick." The thin sheeting is 0.005 inch; the thick sheeting is 0.040 inch. Silicone sheeting is distributed by Invotec International, Inc., Jacksonville, Florida.

Thin silicone sheeting is malleable. It adapts easily to the middle ear space and does not tend to curl when exposed to body temperature. Thick silicone sheeting is stiff and is not deformed by fibrous tissue that may develop in the middle ear. Although stiff, it is malleable enough to be withdrawn from the mastoid and middle ear through a tympanotomy exposure.

Supramid Extra is the trade name for a medical-grade nylon 6. The sheeting thickness of Supramid Extra Foil is 0.3 mm. Because it is thinner than thick silicone sheeting, it is easier to insert. It is not malleable, however, and this quality prevents it from being extracted from the mastoid without a mastoid re-exploration.

Mucous Membrane Indications

When the mucous membrane problem is limited, there is no need for staging (Fig. 18–1). Adhesions form between denuded bone of the middle ear and the tympanic membrane graft but usually do not pose a long-term problem. Nonetheless, thin silicone sheeting is frequently placed over the denuded areas to prevent adhesions (Fig. 18–2). The silicone sheeting may be left in place indefinitely. Alternatively, one may use absorbable gelatin film (Gelfilm), if desired.

In more diseased ears one may find that normal mucosa remains only in the tubotympanum, facial recess, and epitympanum (Fig. 18–3). Reconstruction of this ear without regard to the mucous membrane problem usually results in a fibrosed middle ear.

When thin silicone sheeting was used in such cases in the early 1960s, the results were frequently disappointing. The silicone sheeting was rolled up or deformed by advancing fibrous tissue. If the silicone sheeting contacted the

tympanic membrane, extrusion often occurred. To obtain the best hearing results in such cases, it was necessary to perform the reconstruction in two stages. At the initial operation, the tympanic membrane was grafted over a piece of thick silicone sheeting that filled the middle ear (Fig. 18–4). Six months later, the thick silicone sheeting was removed, and a suitable prosthesis was inserted.

In badly infected ears, there may be no mucosa remaining in the middle ear cleft except for the tubotympanum (Fig. 18–5). Some believe that nothing can be done to reconstruct such an ear; radical mastoidectomy has been advised. Ears of this type can be reconstructed by staging the tympanoplasty, as long as some mucosa remains in the tubotympanum and the plastic sheeting can reach the area to prevent eustachian tube closure.

In cases of extensive or total mucous membrane destruction, it may be wise to perform an intact canal wall mastoidectomy even though there may not be other indications for a mastoid exploration. The mastoid is opened into the middle ear through the facial recess for insertion of a sheet of Supramid or thick silicone sheeting (Fig. 18–6). This process ensures that the plastic will not roll up, hence, no fibrous tissue. During revision, the plastic is removed, and a suitable prosthesis may be placed between the stapes capitulum or footplate and the mobile tympanic membrane in a well-healed normal middle ear.

Canal Wall Down Procedures

The principles and indications involved in staging the operation in canal wall down procedures are the same as in canal wall up procedures, but the technique is different. Many who use both techniques in tympanoplasty have stated that their hearing results are less satisfactory in canal wall down cases. The probable reason for these results is the narrowing of the middle ear space, which should not be allowed to occur in canal wall down procedures (see Chapter 13).

In staging the operation in canal wall down procedures, a wide middle ear space is obtained by extending the thick silicone sheeting onto the fallopian canal. It is important to bevel the superior edge of the plastic to help delay extrusion; the graft rests on that edge.

Plastic Extrusion

There is no question that plastic material placed in the middle ear may extrude if an edge of the plastic comes in contact with the tympanic membrane. At HEC, where surgeons have used the techniques described herein over the past 32 years, extrusion has occurred in less than 0.5 per cent of the cases. Those who have reported a major problem with extrusion are probably using thin silicone sheeting in situations in which they should have used thick plastic and staged the operation.

It might be of interest for me to mention two patients, each of whom had plastic in the ear for more than 20 years between stage 1 and stage 2. I performed a canal wall down operation on a 6-year-old child and staged the operation, leaving in thick silicone sheeting. The patient returned

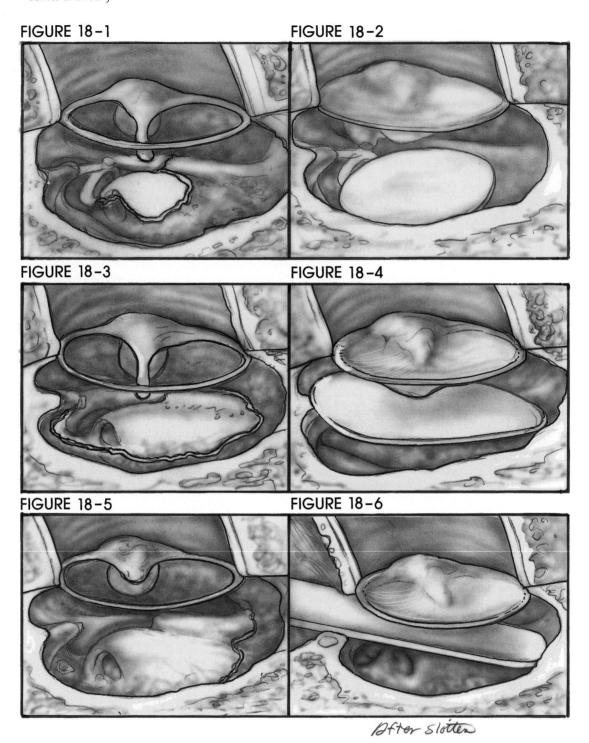

FIGURE 18–1

FIGURE 18–2

FIGURE 18–3

FIGURE 18–4

FIGURE 18–5

FIGURE 18–6

After slotten

FIGURE 18–1. Absence of mucosa over promontory.

FIGURE 18–2. Silicone sheeting has prevented adhesions between tympanic membrane graft and denuded promontory.

FIGURE 18–3. More extensive mucous membrane destruction and absence of the stapes. Good mucosa remains in the recesses and the epitympanum.

FIGURE 18–4. Stiff plastic sheeting holds its position and prevents adhesions between the tympanic membrane graft and the raw areas of bone.

FIGURE 18–5. Mucous membrane destruction is extensive. Note a few islands, here and there, of mucosa and some in the tubotympanum.

FIGURE 18–6. Thick silicone or Supramid sheeting will not be displaced by fibrous tissue. Mucosa should regrow over all denuded bone and the undersurface of the graft.

at age 26, having had no further problem, and decided that it was time to have the second stage. There had been no ill effect from the thick silicone sheeting.

A second example is a patient in his mid-40s in whom cholesteatoma matrix was left over the lateral semicircular canal fistula. An intact canal wall procedure was performed, and a 1.2-cm sheet of Supramid was placed through the facial recess. The patient came in for initial follow-up and made it clear that he was going to do nothing further and was lost to follow-up. He returned 21 years later and said that he wanted his second-stage procedure. Not only was the Supramid in good condition, as was the rest of the ear, but the matrix that had been left over the fistula had disappeared, and the fistula was closed by bone.

THE CONTROVERSY

There is considerable difference of opinion among experienced otologists in regard to staging the operation. The major difference occurs over the more diseased ears, usually with cholesteatoma, and is related not to the management of the mastoid (canal wall up or down) but instead to the surgeon's philosophy.[11]

The following quotation is taken from the article "Tympanoplasty: To Stage or Not to Stage."[9] The quotation is from a well-known otologist who stages "sometimes":

My hunch is that there might be a slight edge to those with a planned second stage, as you describe. However, this advantage, I think, would be overshadowed by the significant number that initially look like they needed a second stage, but heal amazingly well and end up with an excellent result in spite of the massive pathology in the tympanic cavity. With a philosophy of a planned second stage procedure, these patients might be denied the opportunity to have had success with the first operation, thus requiring a needless second procedure. My inability to predict the frequent, excellent healing response makes me go all out in attempting to reconstruct the conductive mechanism the first time, hoping for a good healing and a good initial result.[9]

Quoted here, from the same article, is the opinion from another highly regarded otologist who feels that there is essentially no indication to stage the operation:

I do not believe that staging should be a routine procedure.

Every effort should be made to eliminate disease and maximize hearing results at the first operation. Should the hearing results be unsatisfactory, and if the postoperative status regarding pneumatization of the middle ear, etc., is satisfactory, a revision operation can be done. In most cases revisions are not necessary and, therefore, the staging procedure is avoided.[9]

The HEC physicians believe that the great divergence of opinion on staging that one encounters is related to two factors. How hard does the individual pursue a good functional result in the most severely diseased ear? What does one accept as a satisfactory functional result? Certainly, in the ear with no remaining mucosa except in the tubotympanum, the HEC physicians have seen that unless the operation is staged, one cannot usually obtain a satisfactory functional result. Staging the operation has resulted in a satisfactory functional result in 50 to 60 per cent of cases—not perfect, but nonetheless good.

ACKNOWLEDGMENT

Many of the illustrations are modified from *Otolaryngology*, Vol. 1, published by J. B. Lippincott Company.

References

1. Sheehy JL: Testing eustachian tube function. Ann Otol 90: 562–564, 1981.
2. Rambo JHT: Use of paraffin to create a middle ear space in musculoplasty. Laryngoscope 71: 612–619, 1961.
3. Tabb HG: Surgical management of chronic ear disease with special reference to staged surgery. Laryngoscope 73: 363–383, 1963.
4. House HP: Polyethylene in middle ear surgery. Arch Otolaryngol Head Neck Surg 71: 926–931, 1960.
5. Austin DF: Types and indications of staging. Arch Otolaryngol Head Neck Surg 89: 235–242, 1969.
6. Smyth GDL: Staged tympanoplasty. J Laryngol 84: 757–764, 1970.
7. Sheehy JL: Plastic sheeting in tympanoplasty. Laryngoscope 83: 1144–1159, 1973.
8. Sheehy JL, Crabtree JA: Tympanoplasty: Staging the operation. Laryngoscope 83: 1594–1621, 1973.
9. Sheehy JL, Shelton C: Tympanoplasty: To stage or not to stage. Otolaryngol Head Neck Surg 104: 399–407, 1991.
10. Sheehy JL, Brackmann DE: Surgery of chronic otitis media. *In* English GM (ed): Otolaryngology. Philadelphia, JB Lippincott, 1994.
11. Sheehy JL, Brackmann DE: Surgery of Chronic Ear Disease: What We Do and Why We Do It. Instructional Courses, Vol. 6. St. Louis, CV Mosby, 1993.

19

Management of Complications of Chronic Otitis Media

Richard J. Wiet, M.D. ▪ Steven A. Harvey, M.D.
George P. Bauer, M.D.

Chronic otitis media can present a formidable challenge to the otologic surgeon. Competent operative management requires a thorough knowledge of the anatomy of the temporal bone as well as the pathologic subtleties of the disease. Because avoidance of complications is a major goal, steps toward prevention should begin with a thorough history and physical examination. In addition to the benefits of surgery, specific complications and their possible outcome must be discussed with the patient. Even the most experienced surgeon, however, will at some point in his or her career confront an intraoperative complication. When this does happen, the surgeon first must recognize that a complication has indeed occurred. Second, he or she must be capable of handling the complication in a way that minimizes subsequent morbidity. This ability to properly manage such complications requires a careful blend of knowledge and judgment.

This chapter emphasizes the management of complications from surgery for chronic otitis media, including otic capsule fistulas due both to the disease process and to the surgical treatment. Fistulas due to disease are discussed because improper management can lead to further morbidity. Other topics are sensorineural hearing loss from various causes, iatrogenic facial nerve trauma, ossiculoplasty complications, and dural and vascular injury. Specific surgical techniques to prevent or deal with these problems are mentioned as appropriate.

PREOPERATIVE COUNSELING

It is essential that the patient understand the goal of the surgery. The principal goal of ear surgery for chronic otitis media is elimination of infection. Correction of hearing loss is the secondary goal, often accomplished in a second procedure.

Preoperative counseling depends on a complete history and thorough examination. A history of vertigo or sensorineural hearing loss would be an important finding with respect to counseling. The location of the tympanic membrane perforation may help in counseling the patient and in planning treatment. Central perforations are usually not associated with cholesteatoma, whereas marginal perforations are often more problematic. Those located in the attic are most often associated with secondary acquired cholesteatoma. Usually, hearing loss of greater than 30 to 35 dB implies erosion of the ossicular chain. Many times,

in the presence of cholesteatoma in the posterior superior quadrant, hearing is normal. The patient must be forewarned that sound transmission is occurring *through* the cholesteatoma, and hearing will probably decrease after surgery. Hearing improvement often requires a second-stage procedure. Management of the patient with an only-hearing ear often necessitates a more conservative approach than of the patient with bilateral hearing. Management of the diseased better-hearing ear may require immediate postoperative aural rehabilitation with a bone conduction aid.

We not only explain the procedure to the patient in simple layman's terms but also describe to the patient his or her medical diagnosis. The probability of surgical success is often explained in simple ratios, such as "eight or nine times out of ten we succeed in closing the perforation with a subsequent gain in hearing." The risks and the benefits of the procedure are discussed in detail. Our group follows the example outlined by Sheehy.[1] We then explain the potential risk of partial or total sensorineural hearing loss, dizziness, facial weakness, and other complications related to mastoid surgery.

An appropriate discussion of postoperative care and follow-up is outlined to the patient before discharge from the outpatient or inpatient setting. This discussion includes proper aural hygiene, water precautions, activity limitations, and the use of antibiotics, when deemed necessary.

If a complication requiring management occurs, the surgeon who is involved should freely consult with other experts for advice. This is especially true if the surgeon has managed very few complications resulting from disease or an iatrogenic cause. An example may be unexpected immediate onset of facial paralysis following surgery for cholesteatoma. It is considered good practice to consult with another physician when in doubt about a management decision.

LABYRINTHINE FISTULA SECONDARY TO CHRONIC OTITIS MEDIA

Labyrinthine fistulas are well-known complications of chronic otitis media. They are an unusual, but by no means rare, clinical entity and present a significant risk. The inexperienced surgeon may not be prepared for the possibility of a fistula, and some cases of postoperative dead ear may result from the opening of an undiagnosed fistula. The incidence of labyrinthine fistulas secondary to chronic otitis media in the modern literature varies from a low of 3.6 per cent, reported by Palva and colleagues,[2] to a high of 12.9 per cent, reported by Sanna and coworkers.[3] Although the incidence of other complications due to chronic otitis media such as meningitis, sigmoid sinus thrombosis, and intracranial abscess have greatly decreased over the years, labyrinthine fistulas have had a remarkably stable rate of occurrence of about 10 per cent.[4]

The most common location for labyrinthine fistulas is the lateral semicircular canal in all reported series (see Fig. 19–1). Most authors have reported the incidence of isolated lateral canal fistulas to be about 80 per cent, but this figure ranges from 57[5] to 90 per cent[6] and is indicative of the fact that the lateral semicircular canal is the most exposed (to cholesteatoma) of the three canals. The remainder of fistulas in most series generally involved the lateral canal along with one or several other sites.

Distinction should be made also between a bony erosion and a fistula. Erosion is present when the endosteal layer of bone remains intact and may appear as a blue or gray line under the operating microscope; it does not represent a true fistula.[5] When the endosteal bone layer is eroded, only the endosteal membrane separates the cholesteatoma matrix from the perilymphatic space. In this manner, direct pressure can be transmitted to the membranous labyrinth and is seen in most instances of described fistulas.

Many authors describe fistulas as small or large without quantifying the terms. Sanna and coworkers,[3] however, have classified fistulas as small (0.5 to 1 mm), medium (1 to 2 mm), and large (>2 mm) according to intraoperative findings. They found that large fistulas made up the majority (74 per cent), followed by medium (18.4 per cent) and small (7.6 per cent) ones. Gacek also has classified fistulas as either small or large and uses 2 mm in greatest dimension as the cutoff point.[5] Although he states that 2 mm was chosen as an arbitrary dividing point, he points out that in fistulas smaller than 2 mm, the bony margin of the opening is able to support the cholesteatoma matrix and separate it from the underlying endosteal membrane by a layer of connective tissue. This allows for safe removal of the matrix from the fistula.

Although the surgeon should be prepared to deal with a possible fistula in any ear with chronic otitis media, the length of symptoms may heighten suspicion. Sheehy and Brackmann, reporting on 97 cases of labyrinthine fistulas, noted that over 50 per cent had a history of chronic otitis media for 20 years or longer.[7] Ritter also noted that many of his patients had suffered from lifelong otorrhea, often dating back to childhood.[8]

Vestibular symptoms also increase the possibility of a labyrinthine fistula. Sheehy and Brackmann noted that almost two thirds of patients experienced dizziness, and it was of a constant nature in 12 per cent.[7] Ritter noted that 76 per cent of patients complained of vertigo, which was usually of a brief nature, lasting several seconds to minutes.[8] Ostri and Bak-Pedersen,[9] reporting on 20 fistula cases, and Gormley,[10] on 35 cases, both noted frank vertigo in 65 per cent of patients. In cases of chronic otitis media without a fistula, dizziness has been noted much less com-

monly. One review found this figure to be 15 per cent in such cases and more related to age rather than duration of disease.[11] McCabe noted the highest incidence of vestibular symptoms (90 per cent) of any larger series, reporting on 79 cases of fistula.[4] In addition, a higher incidence of positive results on fistula tests (72 per cent) was noted.[4] McCabe has given an excellent detailed description of the test along with the expected eye movements based on the location of the fistula (Table 19–1).

A positive result on a fistula test in the case of a postampullary lateral canal fistula (the most common site) is denoted by conjugate deviation (*not* nystagmus) of the eyes to the opposite ear with compression of air in the external canal. In this instance, endolymph and therefore the cupula are deviated anteriorly. If the positive pressure is sustained, nystagmus then results toward the diseased (test) ear. Subsequently, if the air pressure is pulsed, deviation to the opposite ear initially occurs, and as the pressure is released, the eyes drift back toward the midline. If the fistula is located at the junction of the lateral canal ampulla and vestibule (preampullary region), positive pressure will lead to posterior displacement of the cupula and subsequent conjugate deviation of the eyes toward the diseased ear. Positive pressure on a fistula of the vestibule will lead to deviation of the horizontal and superior canal ampullas and the associated rotary-horizontal eye movements noted in Table 19–1.

Dizziness may result from several factors. Extension of infection into the perilymph from the middle ear would be expected to lead to purulent labyrinthitis and complete loss of vestibular function. Serious labyrinthitis would be expected when only toxic byproducts and inflammatory cells gain entrance to the labyrinth, with subsequent vertiginous attacks.[8] Also, pressure changes transmitted from the middle ear into the perilymphatic space, the basis of the fistula test, may lead to cupular displacement and subsequent vestibular symptoms.

The level of preoperative hearing may serve as a clue to a possible labyrinthine fistula. Sheehy and Brackmann found a sensorineural impairment in over half of their fistula cases, compared with only 20 per cent of nonfistula cases.[7, 11] Sensorineural levels were more commonly diminished in patients with extensive fistulas at sites other than the lateral canal. Preoperative anacusis was found in 12 per cent of such cases.[7] Ritter also found decreased sensorineural levels in his series—70 per cent of patients had a loss of bone conduction, which averaged 26 dB.[8] A

TABLE 19–1. Site of Labyrinthine Fistula and Associated Eye Movements

SITE OF FISTULA	EYE MOVEMENTS
Lateral canal, postampulla	Horizontal, toward normal ear
Lateral canal, preampulla	Horizontal, toward fistulous ear
Vestibule	Rotary, horizontal, toward fistulous ear
Superior canal	Rotary, toward fistulous ear
Posterior canal	Vertical, with an arc

Adapted from McCabe BF: Labyrinthine fistula in chronic mastoiditis. Ann Otol Rhinol Laryngol 93(Suppl 112): 138–141, 1983.

discrimination score below 80 per cent was seen in 20 per cent of patients, and 30 per cent were deaf. Farrior has reported nonserviceable hearing preoperatively in 13 per cent of 31 fistula cases.[12] Ostri and Bak-Pedersen found anacusis in 15 per cent of their patients.[9]

Preoperative facial nerve weakness, although rare in fistula cases, is more common than in nonfistula cases: 4 per cent versus 1 per cent.[7] All series, however, report a high incidence of facial nerve dehiscence in fistula cases, including Gormley[10] (27 per cent), Ritter[8] (36 per cent), Sheehy and Brackmann[7] (50 per cent), and Ostri and Bak-Pedersen[9] (55 per cent). Thus, intraoperative facial nerve trauma, dealt with in another section of this chapter, represents a significant potential risk in these patients.

INTRAOPERATIVE MANAGEMENT OF LABYRINTHINE FISTULAS

Removing cholesteatoma matrix versus leaving it in situ and performing intact canal wall versus canal wall down mastoidectomy is a long-standing controversy in the management of labyrinthine fistulas that has not been resolved to this day. This controversy was first brought into sharp focus by Walsh and Baron in 1953. In a symposium regarding management of cholesteatoma matrix, Walsh advocated removing the matrix in all cases, feeling that this tissue had a chemical osteolytic effect on underlying bone.[13] Baron presented his views that bone erosion from cholesteatoma resulted mainly from a pressure effect and that exteriorization of the sac was sufficient.[14] Since that time, various techniques have been advocated.

Several general comments regarding the management of labyrinthine fistulas secondary to cholesteatoma are universally advocated by all authors. First, when a cholesteatoma sac is found in the mastoid, it should be opened and the contents evacuated (Fig. 19–1). The medial wall of the sac should be carefully palpated to detect any bony erosion, especially on the dome of the lateral canal. Once a fistula is identified, matrix should be left over the site to protect it (even if eventual removal is planned) while the remainder of the ear is cleared of disease. This protects the area from subsequent bone dust and irrigation solution. If removal of matrix is planned at that operative setting, it should be the last maneuver performed prior to completing the operation and closing the ear. When the fistula is exposed, it should be quickly covered with a tissue seal (e.g., fascia, vein, or perichondrium) (Fig. 19–2). The possibility of "tisscal"—a blood product to seal the fistula—seems promising in this regard. Most authors advocate leaving matrix over extensive fistulas involving other semicircular canals, the vestibule, or cochlea (Fig. 19–3) because of the high incidence of postoperative sensorineural impairment. Sheehy and Brackmann reported a postoperative severe or total sensorineural hearing loss of 56 per cent in their cases of extensive fistulas when the matrix was removed.[7] Gacek reported a partial or profound hearing loss in all three cases in which matrix was removed from a cochlear fistula.[5] He states that the membranous semicircular canals and ampullas have thicker, more rigid walls than Reissner's or the basilar membrane of the cochlea and thus are less likely to rupture with removal of cholesteatoma matrix. Also, the cochlear

duct occupies the outermost portion of the bony cochlea, thus allowing it to more readily come in contact with overlying matrix. Other authors who normally advocate matrix removal also feel that it should be left in situ in cases of multiple fistulas or those involving the vestibule or cochlea.[3, 10] A promontory cochlear fistula is considered one of the few absolute indications for radical mastoidectomy.[15]

With regard to the isolated lateral canal fistula, some authors think that matrix always should be left undisturbed because of risk to the inner ear.[8, 16, 17] Ritter recommends performing a canal wall down mastoidectomy and leaving the matrix intact over the fistula site.[8] He reported that a decrease in hearing was noted in 47 per cent of cases in which the matrix was removed as opposed to 22 per cent in which matrix was left undisturbed. However, in his series of the cases in which matrix was removed, 80 per cent were not covered over with a tissue seal, which could lead to a significant increased risk of inner ear damage. The first author (RJW) agrees with Ritter and Gacek regarding this opinion, especially when the fistula appears to be greater than 2 mm on computed tomographic (CT) scan.

Other surgeons advocate performing a canal wall down tympanomastoidectomy along with removal of the fistula matrix in cases of isolated lateral canal fistula. Farrior prefers this method in a single-stage operation but cautions against matrix removal from an acutely inflamed or better-hearing ear.[12] He recommends a classic modified radical mastoidectomy in many cases of better-hearing ears with fistulas. Palva and associates likewise prefer a canal wall down tympanomastoidectomy with matrix removal at a single operation.[2] They base this preference on the finding of periodic otorrhea and continued vertigo on fistula manipulation postoperatively in cases in which matrix was left intact. All cases in which matrix was removed from the fistula and the area sealed with tissue subsequently healed with no further otorrhea or symptoms of vestibular upset.

Gacek believes that the decision to remove matrix should be based on the following factors:[5]

1. Ability and experience of the surgeon—If the surgeon does not feel confident in his or her ability to remove the matrix over the fistula atraumatically, then it is wise to leave it undisturbed.

2. Location and size of fistula—In lateral canal fistulas less than 2 mm in diameter, Gacek states that removal of matrix can be undertaken safely, because there is minimal risk to the inner ear. In canal fistulas larger than 2 mm, only an experienced surgeon should attempt removal, and if the matrix appears to be adherent to the underlying membranous labyrinth, it is better left alone.

3. Function of the fistulous ear and relationship to the contralateral ear—In a fistulous ear with profoundly depressed function, the risk of underlying disease in the labyrinth takes precedence, because there is no risk to further hearing loss. Thus, the matrix should be removed and a labyrinthectomy considered. In the significantly better- or only-hearing ear with a fistula, no attempt should be made to remove matrix if the opening is over 2 mm. Only in the case of a very-small-canal fistula should an experienced surgeon attempt removal in this situation.

FIGURE 19-1

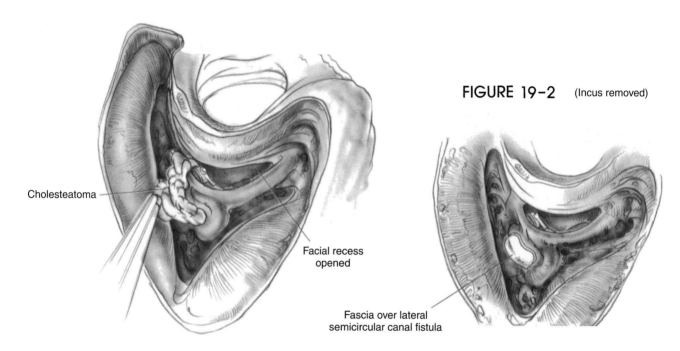

Cholesteatoma

Facial recess
opened

FIGURE 19-2 (Incus removed)

Fascia over lateral
semicircular canal fistula

FIGURE 19-3

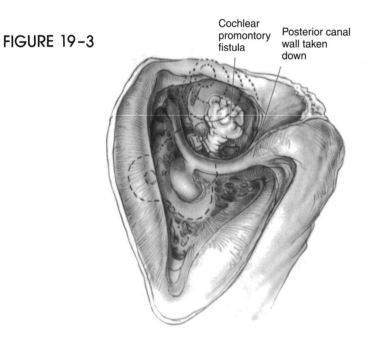

Cochlear
promontory
fistula

Posterior canal
wall taken
down

FIGURE 19–1. Cholesteatomatous fistula of the lateral semicircular canal. Facial recess has been opened.

FIGURE 19–2. Fascia placed over lateral semicircular canal fistula after removal of cholesteatoma matrix.

FIGURE 19–3. Cochlear promontory fistula secondary to cholesteatoma. Posterior canal wall is taken down in this dissection.

4. Mechanism of bone erosion by the cholesteatoma—In cases in which the osteolysis appears to be secondary to pressure from an expanding cholesteatoma sac, one may elect only to exteriorize the disease, allowing for decompression, and leave the matrix intact over the fistula. This situation may be seen with noninfected or "dry" cholesteatomas, in which the keratin debris does not liquefy but remains impacted within the sac. On the other hand, if the bone destruction appears to be secondary to a biochemical effect of the matrix, it may be more beneficial to remove this source of osteolysis. This situation may occur when granulation tissue is present in conjunction with cholesteatoma. The enzyme collagenase, which can lead to bone resorption, is present in cholesteatoma matrix and granulation tissue. When these two are present together, the activity of this enzyme is considerably increased.[18–20]

Sheehy and Brackmann take an eclectic approach to the problem of lateral canal fistulas also. They consider all of the factors mentioned by Gacek, except for the fourth one, in the decision-making process.[7] They do not feel that the mechanism of bone erosion by cholesteatoma plays an important part in the decision regarding fistula management. They prefer the intact canal wall tympanomastoidectomy approach with removal of the matrix over the fistula at a second-stage operation 4 to 6 months later once the infection is cleared and the ear is well healed. Only in the case of a small lateral canal fistula (they do not define "small") in a noninfected ear with normal bone conduction do they feel it is reasonable to remove the matrix at the first stage.

When a fistula is found in a much better-hearing or only-hearing ear, Sheehy and Brackmann,[7] like Farrior,[12] advocate a classic modified radical mastoidectomy to avoid further risk to the ear or a second-stage operation. They do feel that when the mastoid is exteriorized, matrix should be left over the fistula rather than removed.

Sanna and associates[3] and Gormley[10] (reporting on Smyth's series of labyrinthine fistulas) both take a similar approach to that of Sheehy and Brackmann.[7] They prefer a staged intact canal wall tympanomastoidectomy with matrix removal from the fistula at the second-stage operation when the opposite ear is normal. In the presence of an only-hearing ear, a large posterior canal wall defect, multiple fistulas, or an elderly patient, Sanna and associates recommend exteriorizing the mastoid and leaving matrix over the fistula.[3]

Ostri and Bak-Pedersen advocate removal of the matrix over a fistula (even large fistulas) in conjunction with an intact canal wall mastoidectomy in a single-stage procedure.[9] They cite improvement in hearing in the majority of cases and a low incidence of postoperative anacusis as justification for this approach.

A wide variety of surgical procedures have been advocated for the management of labyrinthine fistulas, including at one extreme always exteriorizing the mastoid and leaving matrix over the fistula to removing the matrix over even large fistulas in a closed mastoid at one operation.[8, 9] Other authors take an approach between these diametrically opposed viewpoints.[3, 5, 7, 10, 12, 21]

Several technical points deserve mention for removal of cholesteatoma matrix from a fistula. As already stated, this procedure should be the last part of the operation prior to closing the ear. On elevating matrix, a determination should be made about whether the underlying membranous labyrinth is attached, and if so, attempts at further elevation should be aborted.[5] However, Bellucci thinks that matrix does not become attached to the underlying endosteal membrane or membranous labyrinth and, therefore, can always be elevated under high magnification.[22] He states that damage to the labyrinth is secondary to suction or instrumentation. Farrior supports this concept and believes that instrumentation or suction should not be applied directly to the fistula site.[12] He recommends using strips of cellulose sponge applied to the matrix to help with dissection in a blunt manner. This material has a slightly abrasive quality and helps scrub the bony surface, ensuring complete removal of matrix. Irrigation should be gentle and is important for preventing contamination of the fistula by infected debris.

Preservation of sensorineural hearing levels is certainly a desirable goal in the management of labyrinthine fistulas. Postoperative hearing results vary among authors. However, direct comparison is impossible, because each series was managed by differing surgical approaches and the extent of disease varied. Gormley[10] reported a 3.3 per cent incidence of anacusis postoperatively in ears that were functioning preoperatively. Ostri and Bak-Pedersen[9] reported a 5 per cent incidence of anacusis, whereas Sanna and associates[3] divided their results based on whether an open (9.5 per cent) or closed (2.6 per cent) mastoidectomy was performed. Gacek had a 14 per cent incidence of anacusis, all in ears in which matrix removal from a cochlear fistula was attempted.[5] Sheehy and Brackmann noted severe or total loss of hearing in 8 per cent of lateral canal fistulas and in 56 per cent of fistulas involving other sites (predominantly cochlear fistulas).[7] Law and colleagues noted postoperative anacusis in 22 per cent of patients.[21]

A decrease in sensorineural levels or discrimination scores without total hearing loss postoperatively has been reported as follows: Sanna and associates[3] (4 per cent—closed mastoidectomy, 6.4 per cent—open mastoidectomy), Gacek[5] (7 per cent), Ostri and Bak-Pedersen[9] (17 per cent), and Ritter[8] (37 per cent). Thus, the potential for postoperative sensorineural hearing loss is very real, and this possibility must be discussed preoperatively with any patient suspected of harboring a fistula.

Extensive destruction of the labyrinth does *not* invariably lead to loss of hearing, however. Phelps discussed a patient with an extensive cholesteatoma involving the vestibule along with the basal and middle turns of the cochlea who retained hearing preoperatively (destroyed after surgery).[23] We have also observed this phenomenon in four patients who had slowly progressing cholesteatomas. Bumstead and coworkers reported on four cases of extensive labyrinthine destruction in which vestibular function was destroyed but hearing preserved (both preoperatively and postoperatively).[24] They theorized that the inflammatory response walled off the cochlea on an acute basis, allowing for preservation of hearing. They proposed four anatomic sites where this walling off may have occurred: (1) ductus reuniens, (2) saccular duct, (3) utricular duct, and (4) utriculoendolymphatic valve. At least one other report documents a case of labyrinthine fistula with preoperative anacusis and a significant gain in hearing postoperatively.[25]

The preoperative hearing loss was thought to result from serous labyrinthitis that resolved after surgery.

An additional reconstructive technique that has recently been employed for fistula repair involves use of hydroxyapatite cement (BoneSource, Leibinger Corp., Dallas, TX). The cholesteatoma matrix is gently elevated off the fistula, observing the technical points noted earlier. A tissue seal is immediately placed over the site, followed by the hydroxyapatite cement. The powder is mixed with either water or sodium phosphate as the catalyst to form a semidry paste that is contoured over the fistula, forming a solid protective layer. Solidification time is reduced with the sodium phosphate compared with water. Care must be taken not to hydrate the paste too much (or form a "slurry") because the time to solidification can be quite prolonged. Placing cotton pledgets around the material to prevent contact with surrounding blood or middle ear effusion also hastens the hardening process. As the paste hardens, there is no exothermic response.

Additional soft tissue (i.e., fascia) can then be layered over the hardened hydroxyapatite to promote mucosalization (if used in an intact canal wall mastoidectomy) or epithelialization (in a canal wall down setting) of the site. The technique may be employed at the time of initial surgery (noninfected cholesteatoma) or at the time of a second-stage procedure. We have found that hydroxyapatite reconstruction seems to render the vestibular apparatus less susceptible to the effects of barometric changes (such as in sneezing and the Valsalva maneuver).

IATROGENIC LABYRINTHINE FISTULA

It has classically been taught that the accidentally opened labyrinth will necessarily lead to a dead ear. Although the labyrinth is at risk during surgery for chronic otitis media, this is, thankfully, a relatively infrequent complication. The three sites that are most at risk for injury during surgery for chronic otitis media are the lateral semicircular canal, the promontory, and the oval window.[26] Injury to the membranous labyrinth does not always lead to loss of hearing, as evidenced by the number of case reports during the fenestration era describing accidental tearing of this structure with preserved sensorineural levels.[27–30]

Palva and associates reported iatrogenic injury to the lateral canal in the absence of a cholesteatomatous fistula in 0.1 per cent of chronic otitis media cases (2 of 2192).[31] One of these had approximately a 20-dB loss in bone conduction for the speech frequencies, and the other had no change in hearing thresholds. Jahrsdoerfer and colleagues described two cases of accidental drilling into the lateral canal with no subsequent postoperative loss of cochlear function.[32] A more recent review by Canalis and coworkers[33] reported a 0.08 per cent incidence of this mishap, similar to the figure given by Palva and associates.[31] They made several interesting observations regarding this injury.[33] Noted in cases with an ultimately favorable outcome was a moderately severe sensorineural loss that occurred acutely; however, it returned to near preoperative levels over a period of 3 to 6 weeks. Permanent high-frequency losses of a mild nature were common, but speech discrimi-

nation scores returned to normal, and tinnitus was a rare complaint. Acute vertiginous symptoms and nystagmus were expected; however, these symptoms commonly continued well beyond the usual period of central compensation. Patients may demonstrate unsteadiness and positional vertigo along with spontaneous nystagmus 1 to 2 years following surgery, which is in keeping with a partial labyrinthine injury in which continued active impulses are generated.

Canalis and coworkers believed that opening the lateral canal at its posterior limb away from the ampullary end in a previously normal inner ear was associated with a better outcome.[33] In this situation, symptoms may result from hemorrhage and serous labyrinthitis rather than from the chemical injury of endolymph contamination of the perilymphatic space. The latter effect may be more common with injury near the ampullary end and may lead to permanent cochlear damage. They postulated that the cochlear protection seen in their cases was due to local changes at the site of the fistula. The walls of the membranous labyrinth possibly collapse due to loss of fibrovascular support from the periotic tissue within the perilymphatic space. This, along with a sudden loss of endolymph and decreased pressure, may lead to collapse of the membranous walls and sealing off of the endolymphatic space from the surrounding perilymph.

Jahrsdoerfer and colleagues present a somewhat different theory on cochlear preservation.[32] They postulate a sealing off of the pars superior from the pars inferior at the level of the utriculoendolymphatic valve. With an acute loss of endolymph from the vestibular labyrinth, the utricular wall collapses, sealing off the valve area and protecting the cochlea from fluid decompression. They advocated sealing iatrogenic fistulas with a fascia plug. Bone wax[34] and muscle plugs[33] have also been suggested for sealing off iatrogenic fistulas.

Accidental fistulization of the inner ear appears to occur more commonly at the oval window than the lateral canal. Palva and associates reported a 1.4 per cent incidence of accidentally opening the labyrinth, and of their 12 cases, 11 occurred at the oval window.[2] Even though infection was present at the time of surgery, none of the ears developed total sensorineural hearing loss in the immediate postoperative period. However, three did subsequently exhibit depressed bone conduction thresholds several months after surgery. The loss was assumed to result from serous labyrinthitis with subsequent fibrosis. Of their 11 cases, two had complete avulsion of the footplate, three had dislocation, and the remaining six suffered fracture without dislocation. In a follow-up report 5 years later, they added a single case of oval window fistulization in an additional 1362 cases of chronic otitis media, for an overall incidence of 0.5 per cent.[31] This is still higher than the reported rates of lateral canal fistulization mentioned earlier.

This relative retention of sensorineural hearing in the majority of patients supports the findings of an earlier report by Weichselbaumer.[35] He described 27 cases of accidental fistulization at the oval window but no postoperative dead ears. Only two patients developed a postoperative decrease in bone conduction (each by 20 dB). Of his cases, complete footplate avulsion occurred in 11, partial avulsion in 12, and footplate perforation in the remaining five cases.

Likewise, Sheehy and Brackmann, in their report on labyrinthine fistula secondary to cholesteatoma, noted inadvertent fistulization of the oval window from surgical manipulation (not cholesteatoma) in 11 cases—none of which resulted in a sensorineural impairment.[7]

Several guidelines can be offered to minimize the possibility of oval window fistulization secondary to surgical manipulation. Cholesteatoma should be removed from the oval window—stapes region by dissecting parallel to the stapedius tendon, which stabilizes the stapes and prevents inadvertent mobilization (Fig. 19–4).[12] Manipulation in a superinferior direction, along with depression of the stapes, must be strictly avoided to prevent disruption of the annular ligament (Fig. 19–5). In situations in which remnants of cholesteatoma cannot be safely dissected from the stapes, one may try laser with a mildly defocused beam. Otherwise, it is safer to reconstruct the tympanic membrane, seal the ear, and perform a second-stage operation 6 to 9 months later. At that time, surrounding inflammation has subsided, and an epithelial pearl is usually found that can be easily removed, followed by ossicular reconstruction. If fistulization occurs at the second stage, there is less risk of contamination to the inner ear and subsequent sensorineural depression.[12] Should opening into the oval window occur, it should immediately be sealed with fascia that has already been prepared. Palva and associates recommend delaying ossicular reconstruction until a stable tissue seal has formed over the area.[31] Absolute avoidance of suction is also necessary.

If granulation tissue and thickened mucosa surround the stapes, the surgeon should be very conservative in their removal, because this will quickly resolve once the remainder of the middle ear cleft is cleared of disease and sealed with tympanic membrane reconstruction.[36] The laser has proved useful in atraumatically clearing disease from the stapes and oval window region.[37, 38]

SENSORINEURAL HEARING LOSS

Postoperative sensorineural hearing loss in patients with chronic otitis media may obviously result from either cholesteatomatous or iatrogenic fistulization of the labyrinth, as already discussed. However, it may also occur from excessive manipulation of the ossicular chain (without fistulization) or other unidentifiable factors. Smyth reviewed his personal series of 3000 chronic ear disorder operations and found the overall incidence of cochlear damage to be 2.5 per cent from all causes.[39] He defined significant sensorineural depression as a 10-dB drop from 500 to 4000 Hz or a 10 per cent reduction in speech discrimination.

In reviewing his tympanoplasty procedures (without mastoidectomy), he found the incidence of cochlear injury to be twice as high when the ossicular chain was disarticulated (2.6 per cent) compared with when it was left intact (1.3 per cent). This difference was attributed to intentional disarticulation during the process of removing tympanosclerotic plaques. In cases of intact canal wall tympanomastoidectomy with a facial recess approach (combined approach tympanoplasty), the incidence of sensorineural impairment was reversed: higher for intact-chain

cases (5.6 per cent) than for disarticulated chain cases (2.5 per cent). Loss of hearing in the intact-chain situations resulted equally from contact of the drill with the incus and excessive manipulation of the malleus in removing cholesteatoma from its medial surface (Fig. 19–6). In the case involving a disarticulated ossicular chain due to either disease or intentional sectioning, the majority of losses are theorized to develop after excessive manipulation of the stapes during disease removal or reconstruction of the ossicular chain. When a canal wall down procedure with cavity obliteration was performed, there was a higher incidence of sensorineural loss when the ossicular chain was left intact (50 per cent) but no losses when it was disarticulated.

Palva and associates reported their incidence of sensorineural hearing loss following chronic ear surgery to be 4.5 per cent in 1680 cases.[36] They noted that the majority of hearing losses were high frequency, in the range of 4000 to 8000 Hz (57 per cent). Only 8 per cent occurred across all test frequencies, and all ears demonstrated some recovery during the first 3 months postoperatively. Following that time, there was no appreciable change for better or worse in hearing thresholds. Discrimination scores remained above 80 per cent if the hearing loss occurred at 2000 Hz or greater. If low frequencies were affected, discrimination varied between 50 and 80 per cent. They found that the majority of losses occurred in ears with an intact ossicular chain (81 per cent) and when considerable disease was cleaned from the epitympanum.

These studies allow one to make several generalizations about minimizing the incidence of postoperative sensorineural impairment. When squamous epithelium is removed from the malleus handle, dissection should be parallel, not perpendicular, to this structure and performed in a slow, deliberate manner, which allows the stapes to move across its longitudinal diameter, disturbing inner ear fluid movements the least.[31] Slow dissection allows time for the perilymph to pass through the helicotrema toward the round window without damaging the organ of Corti.[39] Cholesteatoma should be dissected off the lateral surface of the incus in a posterior-to-anterior direction and parallel to the long process. This process allows for partial stabilization of the incus by its posterior and lateral suspensory ligaments and by the malleus head.[12] If dissection in the epitympanum is required, it is safest to disarticulate the incudostapedial joint first (working parallel to the stapedius tendon) and remove the incus.[36] Careful drilling in the region of the antrum and aditus along with raising and lowering the irrigant level to allow early identification of the incus (the so-called water sign) help prevent vibratory transmission to this ossicle or its dislocation.[2]

Management of disease in the stapes and oval window region is as detailed in the previous section. Additionally, caution in attempts to remove significant tympanosclerotic plaques must be advised. Although delaying stapedectomy until a second stage decreases cochlear risk from acute inflammation, many patients may be better served with a hearing aid in this situation.[39]

Using many of these guidelines, Palva and associates, in a 3-year follow-up report on an additional 512 procedures for chronic otitis media, noted no further cases of high-frequency sensorineural hearing loss.[31] They did report

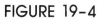

FIGURE 19-4

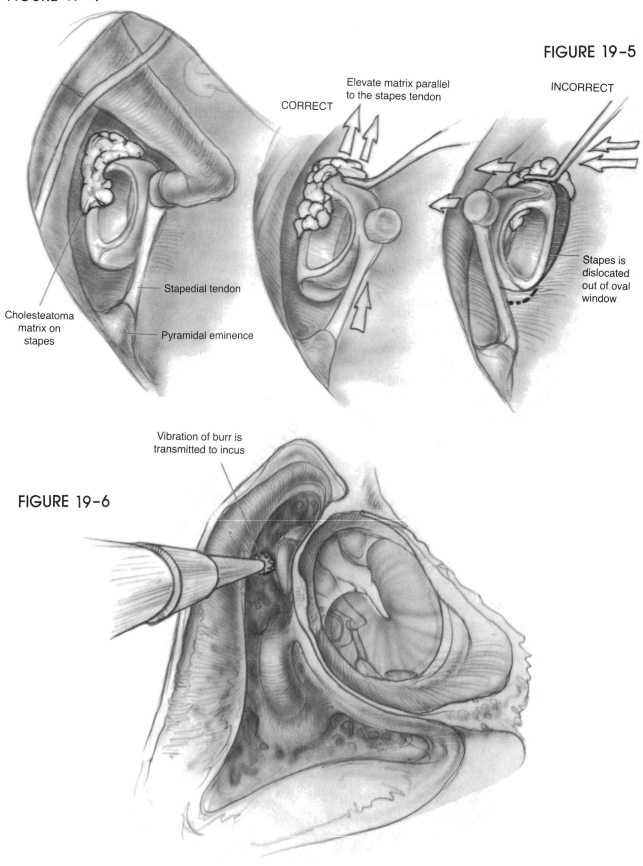

FIGURE 19-5

Elevate matrix parallel
to the stapes tendon

CORRECT

INCORRECT

Cholesteatoma
matrix on
stapes

Stapedial tendon

Pyramidal eminence

Stapes is
dislocated
out of oval
window

Vibration of burr is
transmitted to incus

FIGURE 19-6

a 0.2 per cent incidence of unexplained deafness in the postoperative period that could not be attributed to a specific factor. Noise from the drill and suction-irrigation may play a role. Even low-intensity noise can lead to spasm of the vessels in the zona arcuata of the basilar membrane in laboratory animals.[40] The greater metabolic needs of hair cells in the presence of noise may lead to ischemia and subsequent damage.[39]

FACIAL NERVE INJURY

The literature[22, 41–44] supports the precept that the best precaution for preventing facial nerve injury is a thorough knowledge of temporal bone anatomy, specifically, the landmarks used for identification of the facial nerve. This knowledge is acquired only by repeated, meticulous dissection in the temporal bone laboratory combined with careful, attentive dissection in surgery and years of clinical experience. The useful landmarks to accurately identify the facial nerve are the mastoid antrum and the prominence of the lateral semicircular canal. Once the lateral canal is identified, the fossa incudis is located at the tip of the short process of the incus. The facial nerve lies medial to the fossa incudis and immediately inferior to the horizontal semicircular canal.[43]

The incidence of iatrogenic facial paralysis from otologic surgery has been reported to range from 0.6 to 3.6 per cent, and is as high as 4 to 10 per cent in revision cases.[26, 43] In one large series of 958 operations for chronic otitis media, only two patients had a transient postoperative facial palsy after radical mastoidectomy.[42] In one case, a dehiscent tympanic segment was present. There was no apparent dehiscence in the other case. Both of these nerves recovered to full function several weeks following surgery. The authors reemphasized the need for thorough knowledge of temporal bone anatomy combined with careful surgical dissection when operating for chronic otitis media, because normal facial nerve landmarks may be destroyed.[42]

Transection of the mastoid segment of the facial nerve with the cutting burr is the most frequently encountered injury (Figs. 19–7 and 19–9).[41] Special care is needed in revision cases because of altered anatomy. Drilling under continuous suction-irrigation to prevent thermal injury to the nerve is necessary.[43] Furthermore, cool irrigation has a hemostatic effect on the bleeding encountered from the inflammatory response of chronic mastoiditis and cholesteatoma and allows for better visualization.

If facial nerve injury is recognized during surgery, the facial canal should be opened proximally and distally to ensure continuity of the nerve. Paparella and colleagues[44] recommend preserving the nerve sheath unless discontinuity of the nerve is suspected because this condition will invite fibrous proliferation and reduction of nerve regeneration. Other authors[22, 43] recommend decompression of the edematous segment (if there is no nerve substance loss) by opening the nerve sheath until normal-appearing nerve is found proximal and distal to the site of injury.

If the surgeon is unaware of a facial nerve injury and the patient awakens with a facial paralysis, several reasons should be considered. If intramastoid ear packing has been used, it could be in direct contact with the facial nerve, producing the paralysis from pressure. The surgeon should loosen the packing.[43] Also, the use of a local anesthetic could lead to a temporary facial nerve paralysis.[43] The effects of the local anesthetic must be allowed to wear off. If enough time has elapsed, the packing has been loosened, and the patient still has facial paralysis, the decision concerning re-exploration must be entertained.

FACIAL NERVE GRAFTING

Because results of early repair of facial nerve transection are more favorable, the clinician must carefully consider the clinical situation, using objective studies and historical information provided by any previous surgeon. If a first surgeon identified the nerve and is confident that it was not transected, neuropraxia is likely the problem. An expectant course based on electrical study can be maintained. If, however, electrical silence is observed beyond 3 days after the event and doubt exists regarding the degree of trauma, inspection is warranted. Most authors believe that if the diameter of the nerve is disrupted by one third or greater, ultimately better return of facial function can be obtained with resection of the segment and grafting (Figs. 19–8 and 19–10).[45–49]

If resection and reanastomosis or grafting are required, several factors affect the timing of repair, including (1) connective tissue proliferation, (2) proximal neuroma formation, (3) distal glioma formation, and (4) axoplasmic flow.[48] Connective or fibrous tissue formation is evident within several days of neural injury and is capable of infiltrating distal endoneural tubules to the exclusion of regenerating axons. The main source of this fibrosis is not surrounding connective tissue but rather the epineurium itself.[41, 50, 51] Approximately 10 to 14 days following injury, Schwann cells proliferate, which in the proximal nerve stump intermingle with connective tissue and axonal filaments, leading to neuroma formation. Distally, the Schwann cells and connective tissue lead to glioma formation at the nerve stump.[48] Multiple studies have shown that maximal axonal regenerative ability is present 21 days following injury.[52–54]

Previous studies have advocated delaying repair for several weeks to allow maximal axonal regeneration and sub-

---

FIGURE 19–4. Correct method for removal of cholesteatoma from stapes. Dissection should be from posterior to anterior, allowing stapedius tendon to stabilize stapes.

FIGURE 19–5. Incorrect method for removal of cholesteatoma from stapes. Stapes is not stabilized by stapedius tendon and is thus at risk for inadvertent dislocation or subluxation.

FIGURE 19–6. Inadvertent contact between mastoid burr and intact incus. This situation could lead to dislocation of the incus or vibratory transmission to stapes if incudostapedial joint is intact.

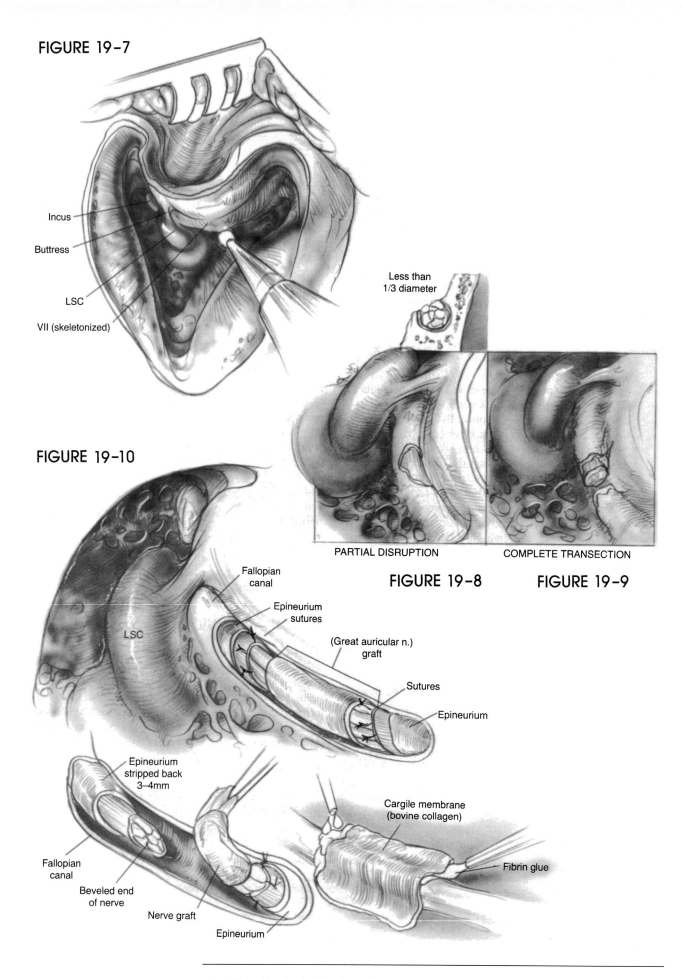

FIGURE 19-7

Incus

Buttress

LSC

VII (skeletonized)

Less than
1/3 diameter

PARTIAL DISRUPTION

COMPLETE TRANSECTION

FIGURE 19-8

FIGURE 19-9

FIGURE 19-10

Fallopian
canal

Epineurium
sutures

LSC

(Great auricular n.)
graft

Sutures

Epineurium

Epineurium
stripped back
3–4mm

Fallopian
canal

Cargile membrane
(bovine collagen)

Beveled end
of nerve

Fibrin glue

Nerve graft

Epineurium

FIGURES 19–7 to 19–10. *See legends on opposite page*

sequently push the axons across the anastomotic site.[55, 56] However, more recent literature supports *early repair* within several days of injury and certainly within 30 days.[57–59]

Once the decision has been made to resect the injured portion of the facial nerve, it must be determined whether end-to-end anastomosis or interposition cable grafting is better suited for reconstruction. Rerouting of the labyrinthine and tympanic segments (in a nonhearing ear) to gain additional length can be performed by sectioning the greater superficial petrosal nerve. A gap width of up to 1 cm has been proposed as the cutoff point for attempted rerouting and primary anastomosis.[45] The first author (RJW) has not found this method of repair to be successful. Some authors feel that if tensionless end-to-end anastomosis can be obtained, the results are ultimately better than those of interposition grafting. However, in rerouting procedures, the blood supply is necessarily disrupted, and this fact must be taken into consideration.[45, 60, 61] Others think that interposition grafts yield results equal to those of end-to-end anastomosis.[62] This has been our experience also.

For interposition cable grafting, the ipsilateral greater auricular nerve is the donor site of choice.[43, 45] This nerve can be used for grafting segments up to 10 cm in length. The proximal-distal orientation of the graft is reversed to prevent regenerating facial nerve axons from growing into endoneural tubes that leave the donor nerve trunk prior to the end of the graft.[63] The graft length should exceed that of the gap to be repaired by 3 to 5 mm both proximally and distally to allow for tensionless reapproximation.[64]

The use of epineural versus perineural coaptation in grafting is controversial.[65] Fisch and Lanser, however, advocate removal of 3 to 4 mm of epineurium from the end of the graft and nerve stump site.[63] This recommendation is based partly on the work of Millesi and Berger[50, 51] and also on the ability to better assess the true anastomotic cross section of the graft end. The greater auricular nerve has a fascicular pattern of axonal location, whereas the facial nerve changes from a monofascicular to multifascicular pattern as it is followed from the geniculate region to the stylomastoid foramen.[63]

A clean, oblique cut should be made on both the nerve stumps and the cable graft. This allows for increased contact surface area and permits a greater number of regenerating axons to cross the anastomotic site.[45, 66, 67] Determination of the site for freshening the proximal nerve stump can be difficult, and no adequate guidelines are available. Axonal sprouting by the proximal facial nerve stump can take place up to at least 10 mm proximal to the site of injury in experimental animals.[57]

Sutureless reapproximation is the preferred anastomotic technique, because no motion is present within the temporal bone, in contrast to the situation with extratemporal nerve grafting.[45, 48] Also, the fallopian canal provides an excellent cradle for the interposition graft.[47] The use of fibrin glue has been advocated to stabilize the anastomosis, as has the placement of bovine collagen membrane (Cargile) over the site (Fig. 19–10).[45, 63] This material is reabsorbed within 4 to 6 weeks and helps protect the repair site from fibrous tissue infiltration during this period. The material has increased the number of regenerating neurofibrils across the anastomosis in animal experiments.[63] Other materials that have been used to cover the anastomotic site include topical thrombin, absorbable gelatin sponge (Gelfoam), gold foil, and skin grafts.[44, 47] Brackmann recommends splinting the anastomosis with clotted blood without the use of any other supporting material.[46] Other authors also rely on natural tissue adhesiveness for intratemporal facial nerve grafting.[45, 48]

In conjunction with interposition grafting, another proposed technique is peripheral ligation of the zygomatic and buccal branches of the facial nerve so that selective rerouting of regenerating neurofibrils can be directed to the more important fronto-orbital and marginal mandibular branches.[63] This effect has occurred in experimental studies.[68]

In spite of careful, tensionless approximation, epineural stripping, and wrapping with absorbable collagen, only 20 to 50 per cent of the original facial nerve fibers will traverse the graft site to innervate motor endplates.[63, 69] Fisch and Lanser state that maximal restoration of facial movement following grafting does not exceed 75 per cent of normal, which corresponds to a grade III on the House-Brackmann scale.[63] Farrior also states that 60 to 80 per cent recovery of facial function can be expected with meticulous repair.[12] Synkinesis is always a problem because of sprouting of the regenerating fibers and intermixing secondary to disruption of endoneural tubes in the graft and peripheral nerve stump.[64] One may expect some return of facial nerve function within 5 to 7 months following repair of the tympanic or mastoid segment of the nerve.[61]

OSSICULOPLASTY COMPLICATIONS

The issue of ossicular reconstruction is covered extensively in other chapters and the discussion here is limited to the topic of prosthesis extrusion. A variety of materials have been advocated for ossicular reconstruction, including autologous tissue (bone or cartilage), polyethylene, polymaleinate ionomer, and hydroxyapatite.[70–73] Multiple variables

---

FIGURE 19–7. Injury to mastoid segment of facial nerve with drill. Complete transection of the nerve occurs most commonly at this location. LSC, lateral semicircular canal.

FIGURE 19–8. Partial disruption of facial nerve involving less than one third of total diameter.

FIGURE 19–9. Complete transection of facial nerve.

FIGURE 19–10. Greater auricular interposition graft. Ends of graft and facial nerve are beveled to increase available surface area for coaptation. Epineurium is stripped back 3 to 5 mm to prevent fibrous proliferation at anastomotic site. Area is sealed with bovine collagen membrane and fibrin glue. LSC, lateral semicircular canal.

exist in the setting of chronic otitis media that may play a role in prosthesis extrusion. These include underlying eustachian tube dysfunction (and its ability to aerate the middle ear postoperatively), the extent and severity of mucosal inflammation or granulation tissue, the status of the native tympanic membrane, and the method of grafting employed. Many of these factors are not under the control of the surgeon.

Multiple techniques to inhibit extrusion have been proposed. This includes engaging the prosthesis beneath an intact malleus manubrium and the use of a cartilage platform placed over the head of the device, especially when using polyethylene.[74] Hydroxyapatite is probably the material of choice today with most surgeons, with its excellent biocompatibility and lack of need for cartilage protection from the tympanic membrane. However, the extrusion rate of this material is still 4 to 7 per cent even in short-term follow-up.[73, 75]

Under certain circumstances, an extruding prosthesis can be carefully observed. This would include the dry, noninfected ear without evidence of progressive sensorineural hearing loss or dizziness as long as water precautions are observed. The presence of infection that does not promptly resolve with oral and/or topical antibiotics, formation of granulation around the prosthesis, or residual/recurrent cholesteatoma leading to the extrusion usually mandate active intervention. This should be managed in the operating room under controlled conditions, and an extruding prosthesis should *never* be extracted in the office setting due to the potential for injury to the oval window.

The use of autologous tissue is certainly not a novel concept for ossicular reconstruction but may be the preferred choice in a severely diseased ear to minimize the risk of extrusion. In the setting of advanced disease (usually requiring a canal wall down mastoidectomy), we may use cartilage blocks in various configurations. Good hearing results with essentially absent extrusion rates have been reported.[70, 76] The double-cartilage block (DCB) ossiculoplasty as originally described by Luetje and Denninghoff[76] is often used.

A rectangular block of cartilage (conchal or tragal) measuring approximately 3 × 6 mm is harvested. Perichondrium is stripped off one surface only, and the cartilage is cut in half (avoiding transection of the perichondrium on the opposite surface) (Fig. 19–11). The cartilage is folded over on itself, and a shallow acetabulum is created in one leaf of the cartilage to accept the stapes capitulum. Tympanoplasty is performed in the usual fashion, draping the fascia over the DCB. Short-term results have been favorable with no extrusions to date.[77]

DURAL INJURY

Inadvertent exposure of the dura usually presents no serious problems.[44] Normal dura composed of two layers—an inner thin (meningeal) layer that covers the brain and an outer thick layer composed of collagen bundles serving as the endosteum for the skull—is quite capable of supporting the cerebrum without bony support. In most cases, simple dural exposure without injury requires no therapy.

With the use of the otologic microscope and general

improvements in operative techniques, the incidence of dural injury has decreased.[78] Dural injury is often caused by indiscriminate cauterization of bleeding dural vessels and can usually be prevented with either the use of bipolar cautery or lower-power settings with unipolar cautery. Another mechanism of injury is direct trauma caused by the rotating burr or the curette.[22] Once the dura is injured, cerebrospinal fluid can be seen leaking from the site of dural penetration (Fig. 19–12).

If dural injury with cerebrospinal fluid leakage is noted at the time of surgery, repair should be undertaken immediately. Small leaks from the middle cranial fossa dura may close spontaneously because of the presence of abundant arachnoid tissue at this location.

With middle cranial fossa dural injury, Paparella and colleagues recommend removal of surrounding bone to expose normal dura 5 mm circumferentially.[44] A fascial graft can then be placed between the normal dura and surrounding bone to ensure repair (Fig. 19–13). We have found that macerated muscle gently placed in the defect will stop most leaks. If the dural defect is more in the form of a slit, it may be repaired by suture. The other option may be a long, inferiorly based Palva flap.

Posterior fossa dural injury is more problematic because of the decreased arachnoid tissue available to aid in spontaneous repair. More profuse cerebrospinal fluid leaks are likely. Repair involves again exposing normal dura for approximately 1 cm in each direction by removing bone.[44] A fascia graft can then be applied. Postoperatively, the patient may require a few days of bed rest with the head elevated to help reduce the intracranial cerebrospinal fluid pressure and to facilitate healing. If the cerebrospinal fluid leak persists, serial lumbar punctures or the placement of an indwelling lumbar drain may be needed to reduce the cerebrospinal fluid pressure.[22, 44]

Materials other than temporalis fascia can be used to repair large middle fossa defects (Fig. 19–14). Bellucci recommends using fascia, skin, or bone and emphasizes the use of tight intramastoid packing to secure the tissue graft in firm contact with the dura.[22] Neely and Kuhn described the use of a cartilage-perichondrial graft to repair the defect.[79] Silicone sheeting can be used to repair a defect of middle cranial fossa dura but should not be used in the presence of infection. Larger defects may require rotational flaps, fat obliteration, or pedicled or free muscle flaps to support the fascia during healing.[80] Kamerer and Caparosa further recommend the use of surgical packing in the mastoid cavity to support the repair.[80] Packing should remain in place postoperatively for up to 3 weeks. They also recommend intraoperative and postoperative antibiotic coverage.[80]

VASCULAR INJURY

The three major vascular structures at risk during surgery for chronic otitis media are the sigmoid sinus, jugular bulb, and internal carotid artery. Iatrogenic injury to these structures is more likely in cases of anatomic variation, in poorly pneumatized mastoids, and in revision surgery. Venous injury is relatively more common than arterial injury.[22]

Sigmoid Sinus

The sigmoid sinus is commonly encountered during mastoidectomy. It may be identified by a bluish coloration beneath an intact bony plate or by a change in pitch of the rotating drill bit to a higher frequency on contacting the compact bone overlying the sinus. The most common anatomic anomaly of the sigmoid sinus is anterior displacement into the mastoid cavity.[26] The sinus is intradural, as are all of the intracranial sinuses, enclosed by two layers that split to envelop this structure. The outer layer (toward the mastoid cavity) is the thinner of the two layers, being approximately half the thickness of the inner or intracranial portions.[81] The wall of the sinus has no contractile muscular elements and cannot collapse unless overlying bone is removed. Laceration of the sigmoid sinus may be prevented by initially identifying this structure in the sinodural angle superiorly and then following it down from

there to the mid- and inferior portions of the sinus.[26] When the sinus is displaced far anteriorly, obscuring more medial structures, such as the labyrinth, it can be collapsed with a self-retaining retractor once all of the overlying bony plate is removed.

The mastoid emissary vein enters the sigmoid sinus in its upper third and on the posterolateral aspect. Multiple veins may occasionally be found. This structure may be lacerated or avulsed during mastoidectomy. To prevent or control bleeding, the vein should be skeletonized first with a cutting burr and then completely exposed with a diamond burr. It can then be coagulated with bipolar cautery and divided. The distal bony foramina are then obliterated with bone wax.[82, 83]

Bleeding from the sigmoid sinus may be either minimal or profuse (Fig. 19–15), depending on the nature of the injury. Oozing may occur from small dural veins overlying the sinus, and small lacerations of the sinus wall itself may

FIGURE 19-11

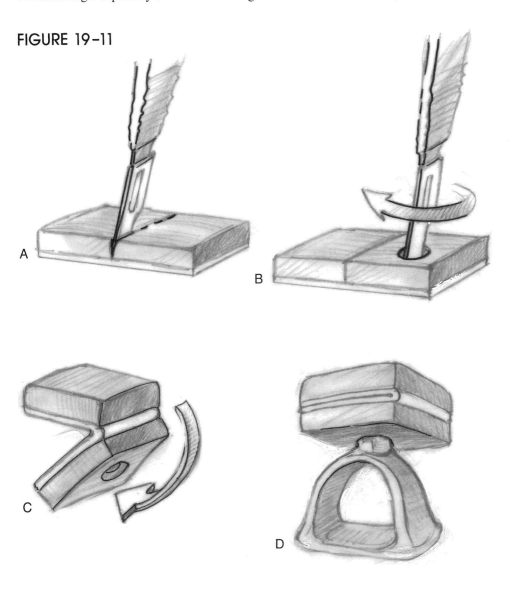

FIGURE 19–11. *A* to *D*, Steps in creating the double-cartilage block. Care must be taken not to transect the perichondrium on the contralateral side.

FIGURE 19-12

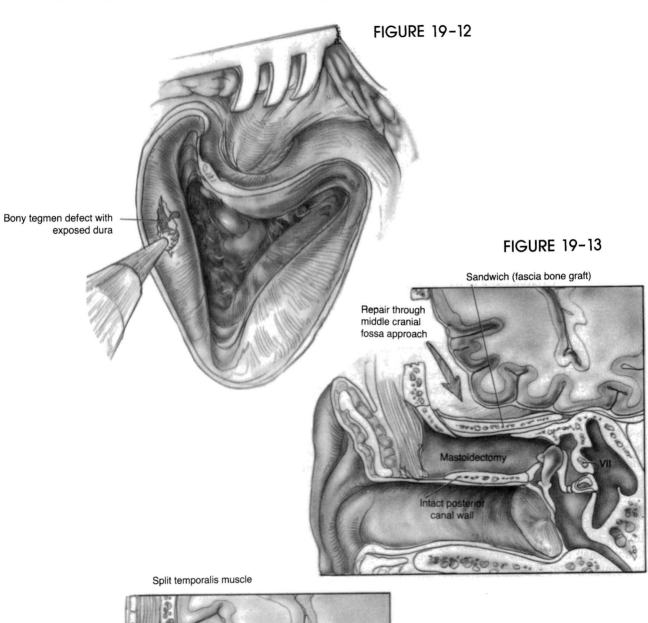

Bony tegmen defect with exposed dura

FIGURE 19-13

Sandwich (fascia bone graft)

Repair through middle cranial fossa approach

Mastoidectomy

VII

Intact posterior canal wall

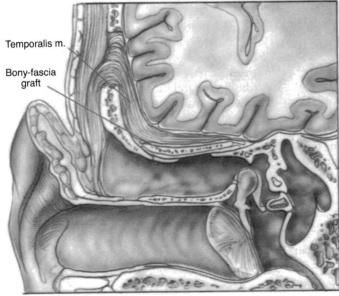

Split temporalis muscle

Temporalis m.

Bony-fascia graft

FIGURE 19-14

FIGURES 19–12 to 19–14. *See legends on opposite page*

be produced by the edge of a bone fragment. These can often be controlled with gelatin sponge soaked in thrombin or with bipolar cauterization. Long segments of the sinus should be coagulated in a stripping fashion rather than a spotting one.[83]

Larger lacerations require either extraluminal or intraluminal packing. Prior to packing, however, bone must be completely removed circumferentially around the site of hemorrhage. The simplest method of packing is to obliterate the sinus extraluminally by placing a large sheet of Surgicel between the bone and wall of the sinus distal to the laceration. The sinus can also be obliterated intraluminally distal to the site of hemorrhage. In either case, a large sheet of Surgicel (4 × 4 cm) should be used to prevent embolization (Fig. 19–16).[83]

Another method is to place a bolus of Surgicel directly over the laceration and then cover it with bone wax to secure it in place. This packing can also be held in place with through-and-through dural sutures on both sides of the sinus.[83] The advantage of packing over the sinus is that it prevents total obstruction of the lumen.

In severe hemorrhage, the sinus must be obliterated both above and below the laceration. First, the internal jugular vein must be ligated in the neck to prevent embolization. Then, inferior to the laceration, the sinus is occluded intraluminally while bleeding above is controlled with extraluminal compression by packing Surgicel between bone and the sinus wall. Another method of control requires exposure of dura in front of and behind the sinus both above and below the laceration. The dura is punctured, and large hemoclips are placed to obliterate the sinus lumen (Fig. 19–17).[84]

Superior Petrosal Sinus

The superior petrosal sinus may occasionally be lacerated when the posterosuperior cell tract is drilled out in a well-pneumatized mastoid. Usually, this problem can be managed with biopolar cautery. If not, control must be gained by isolating the sinus both medial and lateral to the laceration. Medially, the lumen can be obliterated by an intraluminal or extraluminal technique.[83]

Jugular Bulb

The jugular bulb may show great anatomic variation. The average dimensions of the bulb are 15 mm wide × 20 mm high; however, the latter figure may vary as much as 10 mm.[81, 85] In most individuals, the right jugular bulb is slightly larger than on the left side. The dome of the bulb is generally covered by bone and resides in the hypotympa-

num. However, the more anteriorly placed the sigmoid sinus, the higher the dome of the bulb lies.[81] One study[86] has shown a 6 per cent incidence of the jugular bulb lying above the level of the inferior tympanic annulus, and another, quoted by Graham,[81] has shown a 7 per cent incidence of dehiscent bone over the bulb. Injury to an exposed jugular bulb may occur during dissection of cholesteatoma from either the hypotympanic or retrofacial air cells. Also, elevation of a tympanomeatal flap has been reported to cause massive hemorrhage due to entering an exposed bulb.[81, 87, 88] An exposed bulb is especially prone to injury, because the vessel wall is extremely thin in this area. The sigmoid sinus wall superiorly gains support from the dura that ends as the sinus leaves the posterior fossa. Inferiorly, once the jugular vein leaves its foramen, a heavy adventitial layer surrounds the vessel. These extra layers of support are missing in the region of the jugular dome.[81] High-resolution CT is the most sensitive means of diagnosing a high or dehiscent jugular bulb.[89]

Bleeding from the bulb can be managed in several ways. Small openings may be occluded with bone wax or gelatin sponge that is pressed into place with a cotton applicator or neurosurgical cottonoid.[82] Larger lacerations may be controlled by packing Surgicel between the bony defect and the bulb.[83] This material may be held in place with bone wax if further dissection in the area is required. Care should be taken not to overpack the area, because unwanted pressure on cranial nerves IX, X, and XI could result. If this procedure does not control the hemorrhage, the jugular vein should be ligated in the neck to prevent embolization, then the bulb and proximal sigmoid sinus lumen should be obliterated with packing.

Should hemorrhage from a high bulb occur with elevation of a tympanomeatal flap, the flap should be replaced and the external auditory canal packed firmly with petrolatum gauze,[81] which should be left in place for 1 week, then slowly advanced over several days to a week.

Carotid Artery

Carotid artery injury is rarely encountered in chronic ear surgery. However, it is closely related to several anatomic structures within the middle ear and may be exposed either congenitally or secondary to disease. The vertical portion of the petrous carotid normally lies slightly medial and anterior to the basal turn of the cochlea. At the genu where the artery turns into the horizontal segment, it lies anteroinferior to the cochleariform process, medial to the eustachian tube orifice, and anterior to the cochlea.[90] Usually, the petrous carotid artery is well covered by bone; however, the bone may be less than 0.5 mm thick in the area of the eustachian tube orifice and in 1 per cent of cases is dehiscent.[49, 91]

FIGURE 19–12. Laceration of exposed middle cranial fossa dura by mastoid drill with subsequent cerebrospinal fluid leak.

FIGURE 19–13. Repair of dural and tegmental defect with bone graft–fascia sandwich placed via middle cranial fossa approach.

FIGURE 19–14. Repair of dural and tegmental defect with bone graft–rotation temporalis muscle flap placed via middle cranial fossa approach.

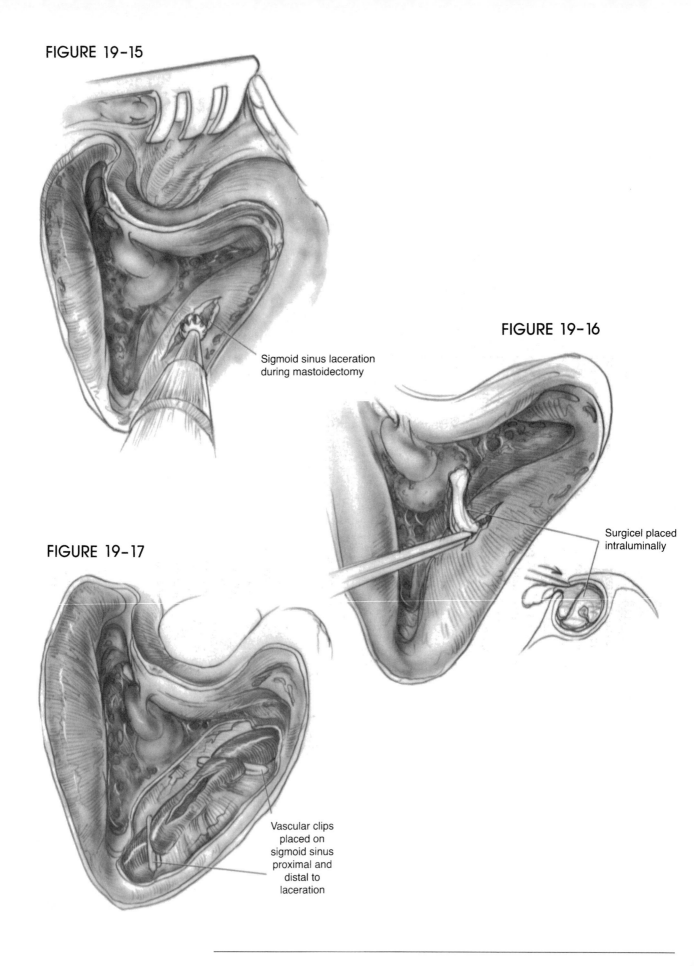

FIGURE 19-15

Sigmoid sinus laceration
during mastoidectomy

FIGURE 19-16

Surgicel placed
intraluminally

FIGURE 19-17

Vascular clips
placed on
sigmoid sinus
proximal and
distal to
laceration

FIGURES 19–15 to 19–17. *See legends on opposite page*

Quite rarely, the petrous carotid artery may take an anomalous course through the temporal bone. Normally, the artery is found medial to the vestibular line, which is a vertical plane that runs through the lateral aspect of the vestibule and approximates the level of the promontory.[78, 92] The anomalous vessel can be lateral to this line, and the carotid foramen may be seen opening into the posterior hypotympanum.[92, 93]

An exposed artery must be kept in mind, whenever dissection in the anterior mesotympanum and eustachian tube is undertaken. The lack of pulsations in the petrous carotid artery makes positive identification more difficult.[22] Often, bleeding from this area is from the vasa vasorum within the wall of the artery, rather than the artery itself. A true rupture of the carotid wall is exceedingly difficult to manage through the limited exposure afforded by the usual approaches for chronic otitis media. Small lacerations can repaired with No. 7 to No. 10 Prolene suture if temporary proximal and distal vessel occlusion can be obtained in time.[82] Larger lacerations can be controlled with temporary balloon occlusion until the damaged area is resected and grafted, or if adequate collateral circulation via the circle of Willis is present, simple ligation can be performed.[94, 95] However, these maneuvers first require greater exposure of the carotid artery within the temporal bone.

SUMMARY

Specific surgical complications in the management of chronic otitis media have been discussed. Thankfully, these problems do not arise commonly. Largely because of this, however, an added element of difficulty is present when complications do occur, because the surgeon may be unfamiliar with subsequent proper management. Varied manifestations of chronic otitis media and the subtle differences found in temporal bone anatomy from patient to patient also must be considered. This combination of factors leads to the creation of a unique situation in every operative case that requires thoughtful judgment. Thorough knowledge and careful technique guide the surgeon in his or her quest for that most important goal first stated by Hippocrates, "Above all, do no harm."

ACKNOWLEDGMENT

The authors gratefully acknowledge the work of Ann Hileman in the manuscript preparation.

References

1. Sheehy JL: Surgery of chronic otitis media. In English GM (ed): Otolaryngology, Vol 1. Philadelphia, Harper & Row, 1985, pp 1–86.
2. Palva T, Kårjå J, Palva A: Opening of the labyrinth during chronic ear surgery. Arch Otolaryngol Head Neck Surg 93: 75–78, 1971.
3. Sanna M, Zinni C, Gamoletti R, et al: Closed versus open technique in the management of labyrinthine fistula. Am J Otol 9: 470–475, 1988.
4. McCabe BF: Labyrinthine fistula in chronic mastoiditis. Ann Otol Rhinol Laryngol 93(Suppl 112): 138–141, 1983.
5. Gacek RR: The surgical management of labyrinthine fistulae in chronic otitis media with cholesteatoma. Ann Otol Rhinol Laryngol 83(Suppl 10): 3–19, 1974.
6. Wayoff MR, Friot JM: Analysis of one hundred cases of fistulas of the external semicircular canal. In McCabe BF, Sadé J, Abramson M (eds): First International Conference on Cholesteatoma. Birmingham, AL, Aesculapius Press, 1977, pp 463–464.
7. Sheehy JL, Brackmann DE: Cholesteatoma surgery: Management of the labyrinthine fistula—a report of 97 cases. Laryngoscope 89: 78–87, 1979.
8. Ritter FN: Chronic suppurative otitis media and the pathologic labyrinthine fistula. Laryngoscope 80: 1025–1035, 1970.
9. Ostri B, Bak-Pedersen K: Surgical management of labyrinthine fistulae in chronic otitis media with cholesteatoma by a one-stage closed technique. ORL J Otorhinolaryngol Relat Spec 51: 295–299, 1989.
10. Gormley PK: Surgical management of labyrinthine fistula with cholesteatoma. J Laryngol Otol 100: 1115–1123, 1986.
11. Sheehy JL, Brackmann DE, Graham MD: Complications of cholesteatoma: A report of 1024 cases. In McCabe BF, Sadé J, Abramson M (eds): First International Conference on Cholesteatoma. Birmingham, AL, Aesculapius Press, 1977, pp. 420–429.
12. Farrior JB: Surgery for cholesteatoma. In Wiet RJ, Causse JB (eds): Complications in Otolaryngology—Head and Neck Surgery, Vol 1. Philadelphia, BC Decker, 1986, pp 69–76.
13. Walsh TE: Why I remove the matrix. Symposium on the Surgical Management of Aural Cholesteatoma. Trans Am Acad Ophthalmol Otolaryngol 57: 687–693, 1953.
14. Baron SH: Why and when I do not remove the matrix. Symposium on the Surgical Management of Aural Cholesteatoma. Trans Am Acad Ophthalmol Otolaryngol 57: 694–706, 1953.
15. Glasscock ME: The open cavity mastoid operations. In Glasscock ME, Shambaugh GE Jr (eds): Surgery of the Ear. Philadelphia, WB Saunders, 1990, pp 228–247.
16. Freeman P: Fistula of the lateral semicircular canal. Clin Otolaryngol 3: 315–321, 1978.
17. Ruedi L: Acquired cholesteatoma. Arch Otolaryngol Head Neck Surg 78: 252–261, 1963.
18. Abramson M: Collagenolytic activity in middle ear cholesteatoma. Ann Otol Rhinol Laryngol 78: 112–125, 1969.
19. Abramson M, Gross J: Further studies on a collagenase in middle ear cholesteatoma. Ann Otol Rhinol Laryngol 80: 177–185, 1971.
20. Abramson M, Huang CC: Localization of collagenase in middle ear cholesteatoma. Laryngoscope 87: 771–791, 1977.
21. Law KP, Smyth GDL, Kerr AG: Fistulae of the labyrinth treated by staged combined-approach tympanoplasty. J Laryngol Otol 89: 471–478, 1975.
22. Bellucci R: Iatrogenic surgical trauma in otology. J Laryngol Otol 8(Suppl): 13–17, 1983.
23. Phelps P: Preservation of hearing in the labyrinth invaded by cholesteatoma. J Laryngol Otol 83: 1111–1114, 1969.
24. Bumstead RM, Sadé J, Dolan KD, McCabe BF: Preservation of cochlear function after extensive labyrinthine destruction. Ann Otol Rhinol Laryngol 86: 131–137, 1977.
25. Sheehy JL: Dead ear? Not necessarily: A report of three cases of chronic otitis media. Am J Otol 4: 238–239, 1983.
26. Wiet RJ, Herzon GD: Surgery of the mastoid. In Wiet RJ, Causse JB (eds): Complications in Otolaryngology—Head and Neck Surgery, Vol 1. Philadelphia, BC Decker, 1986, pp 25–31.
27. Cawthorne T: The effect on hearing in man of removal of the membranous lateral semicircular canal. Acta Otolaryngol 78(Suppl): 145–149, 1948.

FIGURE 19–15. Large laceration of sigmoid sinus during mastoidectomy.

FIGURE 19–16. Large sheets of Surgicel placed intralumenally for sigmoid sinus obliteration.

FIGURE 19–17. Vascular clips placed proximal and distal to large sigmoid sinus laceration. Dural exposure is required anterior and posterior to sinus for intradural placement of clip.

28. Jonkees LBW: On the function of the labyrinth after destruction of the horizontal canal. Acta Otolaryngol (Stockh) 38: 505–510, 1950.

29. Sadé-Sadowsky N: The damage to the membranous labyrinth during fenestration and its influence upon hearing. J Laryngol Otol 69: 753–756, 1955.

30. Thomas R: Fenestration operation: Experience of first ninety-six (consecutive) cases. J Laryngol Otol 65: 259–274, 1951.

31. Palva T, Kårjå J, Palva A: Immediate and short-term complications of chronic ear surgery. Arch Otolaryngol Head Neck Surg 102: 137–139, 1976.

32. Jahrsdoerfer RA, Johns ME, Cantrell RW: Labyrinthine trauma during ear surgery. Laryngoscope 88: 1589–1595, 1978.

33. Canalis RF, Gussen R, Abemayor E, Andrews J: Surgical trauma to the lateral semicircular canal with preservation of hearing. Laryngoscope 97: 575–581, 1987.

34. Cullen JR, Kerr AG: "How I do it." Iatrogenic fenestration of a semicircular canal: A method of closure. Laryngoscope 96: 1168–1169, 1986.

35. Weichselbaumer W: The opening of the vestibule during tympanoplasty. Z Laryngol Rhinol Otol 44: 457–464, 1965.

36. Palva T, Kårjå J, Palva A: High-tone sensorineural losses following chronic ear surgery. Arch Otolaryngol Head Neck Surg 98: 176–178, 1973.

37. McGee TM: Argon laser in chronic ear and otosclerotic surgery. Laryngoscope 93: 1177–1182, 1983.

38. Parkin JL: Lasers in tympanomastoid surgery. Otolaryngol Clin North Am 23: 1–5, 1990.

39. Smyth GD: Sensorineural hearing loss in chronic ear surgery. Ann Otol Rhinol Laryngol 86: 3–8, 1977.

40. Lawrence M: In vivo studies of the microcirculation. Adv Otorhinolaryngol 20: 244–255, 1973.

41. May M, Wiet RJ: Iatrogenic injury—prevention and management. In May M (ed): The Facial Nerve. New York, Thieme, 1986, pp 549–560.

42. Vartiainen E, Kårjå J: Immediate complications of chronic ear surgery. Am J Otol 7: 417–419, 1986.

43. Wiet RJ: Iatrogenic facial paralysis. Otolaryngol Clin North Am 15: 773–780, 1982.

44. Paparella MM, Meyerhoff WL, Morris MS, DaCosta SS: Mastoidectomy and tympanoplasty. In Paparella MM, Shumrick DA, Gluckman JL, Meyerhoff WL (eds): Otolaryngology, Vol 2, 3rd ed. Philadelphia, WB Saunders, 1991, pp 1405–1439.

45. Adkins WY, Osguthorpe JD: Management of trauma of the facial nerve. Otolaryngol Clin North Am 24: 587–611, 1991.

46. Brackmann D: Otoneurosurgical procedures. In May M (ed): The Facial Nerve. New York, Thieme, 1986, pp 589–618.

47. Kamerer DB: Intratemporal facial nerve injuries. Otolaryngol Head Neck Surg 90: 612–616, 1982.

48. McCabe BF: Symposium on trauma in otolaryngology: I. Injuries to the facial nerve. Laryngoscope 82: 1891–1896, 1972.

49. Myerson MD, Ruben H, Gilbert JG: Anatomic studies of the petrous portion of the temporal bone. Arch Otolaryngol Head Neck Surg 20: 195–210, 1934.

50. Berger A, Millesi H: Nerve grafting. Clin Orthop 133: 49–55, 1978.

51. Millesi H: Healing of nerves. Clin Plast Surg 4: 459–473, 1977.

52. Grafstein B: The nerve cell body response to axotomy. Exp Neurol 48(Part II): 32–51, 1975.

53. McCabe BF: Facial nerve grafting. Plast Reconstr Surg 45: 70–75, 1970.

54. Sunderland S: Some anatomical and pathophysiological data relevant to facial nerve injury and repair. In Fisch U (ed): Facial Nerve Surgery. Birmingham, AL, Aesculapius Press, 1977, pp 47–61.

55. Ducker TB, Kauffman FC: Metabolic factors in surgery of the peripheral nerves. Clin Neurosurg 1: 406–424, 1977.

56. McQuarrie IG, Grafstein B: Axon outgrowth enhanced by previous nerve injury. Arch Neurol 29: 53–55, 1973.

57. Barrs DM: Facial nerve trauma: Optimal timing for repair. Laryngoscope 101: 835–848, 1991.

58. May M: Facial reanimation after skull base trauma. In May M (ed): The Facial Nerve. New York, Thieme, 1986, pp 421–440.

59. May M: Management of cranial nerves I through VII following skull base surgery. Otolaryngol Head Neck Surg 88: 560–575, 1980.

60. Harker L, McCabe BF: Temporal bone fractures and facial nerve injury. Otolaryngol Clin North Am 7: 425–431, 1974.

61. Johns M, Crumley R: Facial Nerve Injury: Repair and Rehabilitation (SIPac), 2nd ed. Alexandria, VA, American Academy of Otolaryngology, 1977, p 9.

62. Fisch U, Rouleau M: Facial nerve reconstruction. J Otolaryngol 9: 478–492, 1980.

63. Fisch U, Lanser MJ: Facial nerve grafting. Otolaryngol Clin North Am 24: 691–708, 1991.

64. Fisch U: Facial nerve grafting. Otolaryngol Clin North Am 7: 517–529, 1974.

65. Orgel MG: Epineurial versus perineurial repair of peripheral nerves. Clin Plast Surg 11: 101–104, 1984.

66. Yamamoto E, Fisch U: Experiments on facial nerve suturing. ORL J Otorhinolaryngol Relat Spec 36: 193–204, 1974.

67. Yasargil MG, Fisch U: Unsere Ertahrungen in der mikrochirurgischen exstirpation der akustikusneurinome. Arch Ohrenheilk 194: 243, 1969.

68. Mattox DE, Felix H, Fisch U, Lyles CA: Effect of ligating peripheral branches on facial nerve regeneration. Otolaryngol Head Neck Surg 6: 558–563, 1988.

69. Ashur H, Vilner Y, Finsterbush A, et al: Extent of fiber regeneration after peripheral nerve repair: Silicone splint vs. suture, gap repair vs. graft. Exp Neurol 97: 365–374, 1987.

70. Altenau MM, Sheehy JL: Tympanoplasty: Cartilage prosthesis—a report of 564 cases. Laryngoscope 88: 895–904, 1978.

71. Slater PW, Rizer FM, Schuring AG, Lippy WH: Practical use of total and partial ossicular replacement prostheses in ossiculoplasty. Laryngoscope 107: 1193–1198, 1997.

72. McElveen JT, Feghali JG, Barrs DM, et al: Ossiculoplasty with polymaleinate ionomeric prosthesis. Otolaryngol Head Neck Surg 113: 420–426, 1995.

73. Goldenberg RA: Hydroxylapatite ossicular replacement prosthesis: A four-year experience. Otolaryngol Head Neck Surg 106: 261–269, 1992.

74. Brackmann DE, Sheehy JL, Luxford WM: TORPs and PORPs in tympanoplasty: A review of 1042 operations. Otolaryngol Head Neck Surg 92: 32–37, 1984.

75. Black B: A universal ossicular replacement prosthesis: Clinical trials of 152 cases. Otolaryngol Head Neck Surg 104: 210–218, 1991.

76. Luetje CM, Denninghoff JS: Perichondrial attached double-cartilage block: A better alternative to the PORP. Laryngoscope 97: 1106–1108, 1987.

77. Harvey SA, Lin SY: Double-cartilage block (DCB) ossiculoplasty in chronic ear surgery. Laryngoscope 109: 911–914, 1999.

78. Glasscock ME, Dickins JR, Jackson CG, et al: Surgical management of brain tissue herniation into the middle ear and mastoid. Laryngoscope 89: 1743–1764, 1979.

79. Neely JG, Kuhn JR: Diagnosis and treatment of iatrogenic cerebrospinal fluid leak and brain herniation during or following mastoidectomy. Laryngoscope 95: 1299–1300, 1985.

80. Kamerer DB, Caparosa RJ: Temporal bone encephalocele—diagnosis and treatment. Laryngoscope 92: 878–881, 1982.

81. Graham MD: The jugular bulb: Its anatomic and clinical considerations in contemporary otology. Laryngoscope 87: 105–125, 1977.

82. Leonetti JP, Smith PG, Grubb RL: Control of bleeding in extended skull base surgery. Am J Otol 11: 254–259, 1990.

83. Moloy PJ, Brackmann DE: "How I do it." Control of venous bleeding in otologic surgery. Laryngoscope 96: 580–582, 1986.

84. Hotaling AJ, Rejowski JE, Kazan RF, Wiet RJ: Control of sigmoid sinus in glomus jugulare tumor resection. Laryngoscope 95: 481–482, 1985.

85. Glasscock ME, Dickins JR, Jackson CG, Wiet RJ: Vascular anomalies of the middle ear. Laryngoscope 90: 77–88, 1980.

86. Overton SB, Ritter FN: A high-placed jugular bulb in the middle ear: A clinical and temporal bone study. Laryngoscope 83: 1986–1991, 1973.

87. Hough JVD: Congenital malformations of the middle ear. Arch Otolaryngol Head Neck Surg 78: 335–343, 1963.

88. West JM, Bandy BC, Jafek VW: Aberrant jugular bulb in the middle ear cavity. Arch Otolaryngol Head Neck Surg 100: 370–372, 1974.

89. Lo WWM, Solti-Bohman LG: High-resolution CT of the jugular foramen: Anatomy and vascular variants and anomalies. Radiology 150: 743–747, 1984.

90. Leonetti JP, Smith PG, Linthicum FH: The petrous carotid artery: Anatomic relationships in skull base surgery. Otolaryngol Head Neck Surg 102: 3–12, 1990.

91. Goldman NC, Singleton GT, Holly EH: Aberrant internal carotid artery. Arch Otolaryngol Head Neck Surg 94: 269–273, 1971.
92. Valvassori GE, Buckingham RA: Middle ear masses mimicking glomus tumors: Radiographic and otoscopic recognition. Trans Am Otol Soc 62: 85–91, 1974.
93. Lapayowker MS: Presentation of the internal carotid artery as a tumor of the middle ear. Radiology 98: 293–297, 1971.
94. Andrews JC, Valavanis A, Fisch U: Management of the internal carotid artery in surgery of the skull base. Laryngoscope 99: 1224–1229, 1989.
95. De Vries EJ, Sekhar LN, Janecka IP, et al: Elective resection of the internal carotid artery without reconstruction. Laryngoscope 98: 960–966, 1988.

20

Dural Herniation and Cerebrospinal Fluid Leaks

Malcolm D. Graham, M.D. ▪ Larry B. Lundy, M.D.

The otologic surgeon may have occasion to manage dural defects in the temporal bone that manifest as brain herniation into the middle ear or mastoid or as cerebrospinal fluid escaping from a temporal bone defect. Appropriate management depends on proper diagnosis, which can range from the obvious to the very difficult, and the application of a few fundamental principles for surgical repair. There are several different causes of dural herniation and cerebrospinal fluid leakage (Table 20–1).

Two major categories of defects—dural herniation and spontaneous cerebrospinal fluid leaks—are covered in this chapter. Dural or brain herniation associated with chronic otitis media can result directly from the disease process or from a postsurgical defect. Spontaneous cerebrospinal fluid leaks arising from the temporal bone may have a childhood or adult onset. This chapter describes the characteristics, diagnostic techniques, and surgical management of the two major categories. Post-traumatic, neoplastic, congenital, and miscellaneous causes are well recognized but are beyond the scope of this chapter. However, surgical repair of these defects still follows the basic principles that are elaborated herein.

CHRONIC OTITIS MEDIA–RELATED ENCEPHALOCELE

The successful management of dural and brain herniation and cerebrospinal fluid leakage via the temporal bone depends on a fundamental understanding of the pathophysiology, accurate preoperative diagnosis, and appropriate surgical techniques for repair of the lesion.

Protrusion of brain and dura out of the cranial cavity into the mastoid and middle ear has been variously called *brain hernia, brain prolapse, cerebral hernia, brain fungus, endaural encephalocele, fungus cerebri, encephalocele,* and *meningoencephalocele.* The clinical spectrum of presentations include herniation associated with a space-occupying lesion (brain abscess or tumor),[1, 2] temporal lobe seizures,[3–10] recurrent meningitis,[11–16] spontaneous cerebrospinal fluid otorrhea,[13, 17, 18] and rhinorrhea.[13, 19] The circumstances under which these occur, and their character, have changed with the evolution of otology.[20]

Around the turn of the century, brain herniation was frequently related to otitis media and brain abscess.[21] Acute or chronic otitis media was a primary source of brain abscess, and the only treatment was surgical drainage. Not surprisingly, in this preantibiotic, preimaging, and premicrosurgical technique era, the mortality under such dire circumstances was extremely high, primarily because of purulent meningitis and the brain abscess itself.[21] Faced with a patient who has a possible brain abscess and a draining ear, surgeons would trephine through the infected mastoid and dura and then use their finger to probe into the brain in an attempt to locate and drain the abscess.[22, 23] Frequently, a delayed, secondary brain hernia would develop that was infected from the abscess or was prolapsing through the infected mastoid. In 1910, Dean[22] significantly altered this standard management of brain abscess by advocating exploratory trephination through a clean field unless there was an actively discharging sinus. Rand, as quoted by Hall,[1] concurred with this change of basic principle, and both noted a dramatic drop in brain hernia as well as mortality. In 1939, Hall[1] noted that "the important clinical point is that this complication of abscess surgery, which was common many years ago, has become very rare during the past 25 years." He also noted that "brain hernia is a rare complication in mastoid surgery . . . and in the majority of cases, an avoidable complication."

Although the incidence of brain hernia into the mastoid is a rare complication of mastoid surgery (Fig. 20–1), it still exists,[1, 4, 9, 12, 24–32] and has been well recognized in the 1990s.[33–39] In 1961, Alberti and Dawes[24] clearly documented the relationship of chronic otitis media with cerebrospinal fluid leak and meningitis. They reported on six patients: two had meningitis, two had prior ear surgery, and five had cholesteatoma. Brain hernia can also occur in chronic ear disease without prior surgery.[5, 24, 35, 38, 40–42] In 1963, Blatt[43] noted one case of cerebrospinal fluid leakage and brain hernia 11 weeks after a radical mastoidectomy as well as two cases of exposed brain found at the time of surgery for active chronic otitis media. In 1960, Schurr[9] reviewed three cases of postmastoidectomy endaural cerebral hernia, two of which had known dural penetration at the time of initial surgery, and the third had dural exposure.

TABLE 20–1. Causes of Dural Herniation and Cerebrospinal Fluid Leak

Related to chronic otitis media	Neoplastic
Direct inflammation	Congenital neural tube defects
Postoperative	Miscellaneous
Spontaneous	Postradiation therapy
Adult onset	Infectious
Childhood onset	Degenerative
Post-traumatic	

FIGURE 20-1

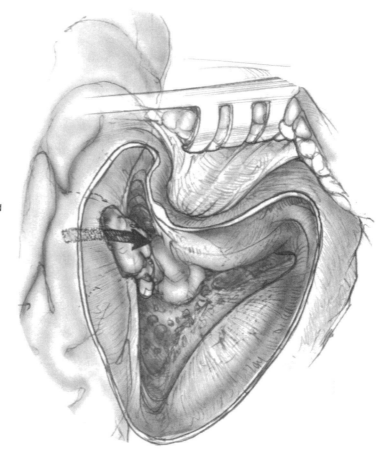

FIGURE 20–1. Temporal lobe herniation into the mastoid cavity through tegmen defect.

In 1969, Stout and associates[32] reported a case of postmastoidectomy dural herniation, which recurred after repair with Silastic sheeting. In 1969, Baron[25] reported on three patients with brain herniation into the mastoid cavity. Baron noted that none of the three had cerebrospinal fluid leakage and that brain hernia can easily be mistaken for a blue dome or chocolate cyst.

In 1970, Dedo and Sooy[20] added 11 cases to the 30 cases published from 1934 to 1970 (i.e., after the antibiotic era had begun). Only three of these cases were associated with brain abscess, and in those, drainage of the abscess occurred through the mastoid. Twenty-six of these 41 cases resulted from known dural perforation at the time of surgery, with the most common site being the tegmen antri or the tegmen tympani. They mentioned that if dural defects are noted during surgery, herniation can be prevented by covering the defect with temporalis fascia or temporalis muscle, or both, and supporting it with packing in the mastoid bowl with iodoform gauze for 10 days in closed mastoid bowls, then 6 to 12 weeks in open mastoid bowls. In 1971, Levy and colleagues[44] described a case of what they believed to be spontaneous herniation of dura and cerebral tissue into the middle ear with a 30-year history of conductive hearing loss and no prior history of significant ear disease. In 1977, Fernandez-Blasini and Longo[28] reported on four cases of postmastoidectomy dural herniation into the mastoid cavity.

Although rare, dural exposure with resultant herniation and cerebrospinal fluid leakage can occur as a result of chronic otitis media with or without cholesteatoma.[24, 27, 35, 42, 45] Paparella and coworkers[42] in 1978 and Glasscock and associates[5] in 1979 added 10 cases and 11 cases, respectively, to this number. Paparella and coworkers[42] reported on 10 cases of patients with brain hernia, all of whom had chronic otitis media, and 6 of whom had not had prior surgery. Dural prolapse is typically found incidentally at the time of surgery and can be mistaken for granulation tissue. Paparella and coworkers[42] speculated that in the present era of antibiotics, brain herniation could be an abortive attempt at brain abscess formation when mastoiditis is present. They noted the chronic low-grade infection involving the mastoid and middle ear likely led to destruction of tegmen with extension to dura, followed by involvement of adjacent brain and herniation. In their cases, only 2 patients had cholesteatoma, whereas all had granulation tissue.

Eight of the 11 cases presented by Glasscock and colleagues[5] were associated with chronic otitis media and prior surgery. They noted that granulations from infection on exposed dura compromised the integrity of dura. Therefore, the dura was no longer a protective barrier and allowed local cerebritis to occur.

Glasscock and colleagues[5] noted that one contributing factor to the decreased incidence of brain herniation was

FIGURE 20-2

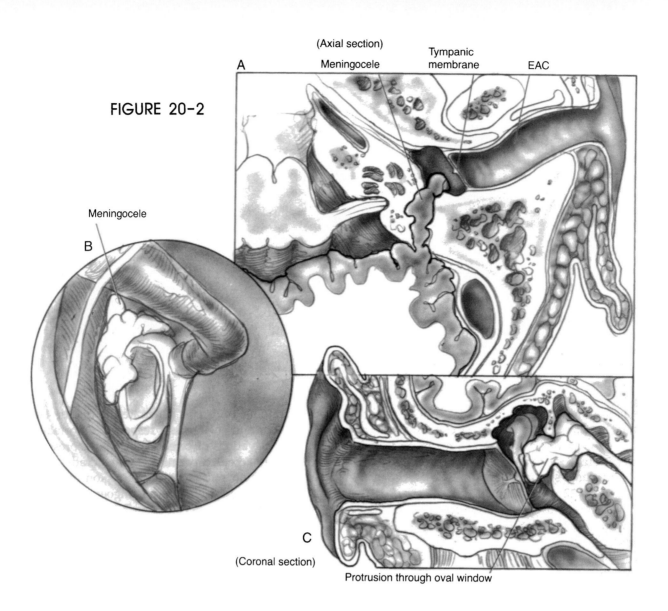

A (Axial section)

Meningocele

Tympanic membrane

EAC

B Meningocele

C (Coronal section)

Protrusion through oval window

FIGURE 20-3

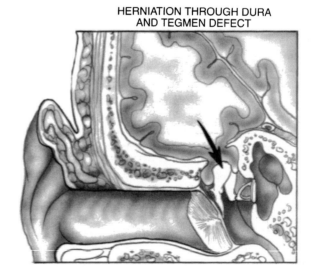

HERNIATION THROUGH DURA AND TEGMEN DEFECT

FIGURES 20–2 and 20–3. *See legends on opposite page*

the progression of surgical techniques to include the operating microscope and high-speed drills rather than chisels, gouges, and curettes. Glasscock's data were updated by Jackson and colleagues[38] to a total of 35 cases and it was reported that 27 of 35 had prior surgery. All groups note, as others have, that herniated tissue is functionless and should be excised.[4, 5, 7, 10, 13, 27, 28, 31, 42, 45–48] Several authors stress the importance of sending supposed granulation tissue for histologic confirmation.[5, 8, 10, 42, 44, 49]

In the 1980s and 1990s, 165 cases of brain herniation and cerebrospinal leaks secondary to chronic otitis media were identified, 114 (69 per cent) of which occurred postoperatively.[3, 4, 6–8, 10, 26, 29, 31, 33–39, 45, 46, 48, 50–60]

SPONTANEOUS CEREBROSPINAL FLUID LEAKAGE

Spontaneous cerebrospinal fluid otorrhea is a rare but potentially life-threatening condition with two different subtypes: (1) children with otic capsule defects and sensorineural hearing loss, and (2) adults with meningoencephaloceles. The two subtypes have distinctly different manifestations.

The concept of spontaneous cerebrospinal fluid leakage was first positively established by Thomson[19] in 1899. He quoted Escat (1897) as reporting the first case of spontaneous cerebrospinal fluid otorrhea in a 10-year-old girl. The source was identified as a fine white line in the inner one third of the external auditory canal. Escat reported that this flow ceased after galvanocautery was applied to it; however, follow-up lasted only 2 months. In 1933, Kline[18] reported on a 54-year-old man with spontaneous cerebrospinal fluid otorrhea that occurred after stooping. The patient subsequently died 8 days later from fulminant meningitis. An autopsy revealed a 2.5-mm defect in the floor of the middle cranial fossa and dural herniation in a fistulous tract, which was considered the duct of a congenital cyst.

In 1987, Wetmore and coworkers[59] reviewed the literature on spontaneous cerebrospinal fluid otorrhea and added four cases of their own to total 87 cases. Of these 87 cases, 63 (72 per cent) were of the childhood type, with the median age of onset of 4 years. Seven of these 63 were diagnosed as adults. Subsequently, three authors[61–63] have added 10 additional cases to the literature, one of which had bilateral oval window fistulas. By combining these data for the childhood-onset type, a high incidence of certain features is noted. Meningitis occurred in 93 per cent, profound sensorineural hearing loss in 82 per cent, and Mondini's defect in 83 per cent. These numbers are likely higher for sensorineural hearing loss and Mondini's defects because audiograms and accurate imaging were not always reported in some of the earlier literature. The most common site of the cerebrospinal fluid leakage was the otic capsule (92 per cent).[14, 59, 63–66] The stapes footplate and oval window area account for approximately 75 per cent

FIGURE 20-4

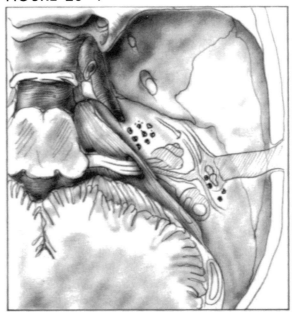

FIGURE 20–4. View of middle cranial fossa floor demonstrating frequent sites of bony defects.

of the fistulas[58, 61–67] frequently associated with a Mondini-type defect (Fig. 20–2).[58, 63, 65, 68] Other miscellaneous sites include the round window,[68, 69] the eustachian tube area,[68] the promontory,[14] Hyrtl's fissure,[70] the hypotympanum,[59] and the fallopian canal.[71]

The second major subtype of spontaneous cerebrospinal fluid leakage from the temporal bone occurs in adults[17] and has distinctly different characteristics and presentations. The site of the defect and leak is usually (88 per cent) in the floor of the middle cranial fossa (Fig. 20–3), occasionally in the posterior fossa wall.[51, 52, 59, 72] Leakage occurs in two primary areas in the floor of the middle cranial fossa[17, 55] anteromedially or the tegmen tympani or mastoideum (Fig. 20–4). Of the 57 cases reported in the literature,[34–36, 73–75] 40 per cent had two or more defects when reported. A common presentation is that of serous otitis media.[17, 35, 49–52, 55, 76, 77] In this disorder, clear, watery, thin fluid escapes and continues to drain on myringotomy. Alternatively, cerebrospinal fluid can drain through a patent eustachian tube and present as cerebrospinal fluid rhinorrhea, and the source is commonly mistaken for the anterior cranial fossa and cribriform plate area.[60]

Meningitis occurs in up to 36 per cent of adult-onset patients.[52] Profound sensorineural hearing loss, Mondini's malformation, and otic capsule fistulas are not associated with adult-onset spontaneous cerebrospinal fluid leaks (Table 20–2).

The pathophysiologic mechanism for adult-onset cerebrospinal fluid leaks is not completely understood. In 94

FIGURE 20–2. Meningocele filling a Mondini defect and protruding through the oval window.

FIGURE 20–3. Spontaneous encephalocele through tegmen.

consecutive autopsies, Ahren and Thulen[78] noted a 6 per cent incidence of multiple (5 to 10) bone defects in the tegmen tympani. In 15 per cent of their autopsy specimens, there were fewer than 5 perforations. Therefore, 21 per cent of their temporal bones had tegmen defects. An additional 16 per cent had only a thin, transparent cortical bone covering the pneumatic air cells of the tegmen tympani and, "when demonstrated, the bone defects were mainly found bilaterally and similarly distributed."[78] Lang[79] found 20 per cent of 70 temporal bones had bony tegmen defects, and Kapur and Bangash[80] found 34 per cent of 50 bones had these defects. Ferguson and associates[52] found a 22 per cent incidence of tegmen defects in 27 preserved, dried temporal bones examined, usually with 4 to 10 defects, 0.5 to 2.0 mm in diameter. These four temporal bone studies indicate the range of bony tegmen defects is 20 to 34 per cent, and when all are averaged, it is 25 per cent (60/241).

The high incidence of middle cranial fossa floor bony defects accompanied by the rarity of spontaneous cerebrospinal fluid leaks is difficult to reconcile. Congenital bony defects have also been implicated in cerebrospinal fluid rhinorrhea. In addition to congenital defects of the cribriform plate, numerous small "pit holes" have been noted in the anterior medial portion of the middle cranial fossa, independent of any history of spontaneous cerebrospinal fluid rhinorrhea.[81] If these pits appear juxtaposed to sphenoid or ethmoid air cells, cerebrospinal fluid rhinorrhea may occur.[60, 81–83] Kaufman and colleagues[81] speculate that these defects result from normally occurring arachnoid villi and draining veins that penetrate the middle cranial fossa floor and enlarge as a response to normally occurring elevations of cerebrospinal fluid pressure. A commonly accepted premise is that decades of cerebrospinal fluid pulsations in the region of the bony defect are necessary before meningoencephalocele or meningeal dehiscence can occur.[84] Increased intracranial pressure is a possible contributing factor, but four cases in which a computed tomographic (CT) scan was obtained preoperatively showed normal-sized ventricles, a finding that questions the concept of increased intracranial pressure playing a significant role.[50, 59]

Gacek[71] further elaborated on adult-onset cerebrospinal fluid leaks. He reported on a case of aberrant arachnoid granulation tissue on the posterior mastoid dural surface of the temporal bone responsible for cerebrospinal fluid leakage. A subsequent examination of 188 temporal bones revealed that 9 per cent had posterior fossa mastoid plate dural arachnoid granulations.[71]

Arachnoid granulations are macroscopic enlargements or distentions of minute projections of arachnoidea mater, termed *arachnoid villi*. Arachnoid granulations project into the intradural venous sinuses, and the centers of the arachnoid granulations are filled with cerebrospinal fluid. Cerebrospinal fluid passes from the center of the arachnoid granulations into the intradural venous sinuses, providing for resorption of cerebrospinal fluid into the blood stream.[85]

The concept of bony pits associated with arachnoid tissue is not new. In 1870, Von Recklinghausen reported on the first case of multiple cerebral herniations, and in 1898, Beneke reported on two others.[2] In 1908, Wolbach[2] reported on nine autopsy cases of increased intracranial pressure: six resulted from tumors, two from acquired internal

TABLE 20–2. Conditions Associated with Spontaneous Cerebrospinal Fluid Leak

	CHILDHOOD TYPE (%)	ADULT TYPE (%)
Meningitis	93	36
Profound sensorineural hearing loss	82	—
Otic capsule defect	83	—
Cerebrospinal fluid otorrhea or rhinorrhea	—	Very common
Dural defect	—	Always

hydrocephalus, and one from massive cerebral hemorrhage. Wolbach noted numerous pits in the skull bone and gave Beneke credit for the concept that these pits were partly preformed by arachnoid villi. Wolbach also noted that "the most striking anatomical relationship is that to the vessels of the dura. This was particularly marked about the middle meningeal vessels and their branches in the middle fossa. It is probable that the distribution of minute arachnoid villi is far more widespread than has been believed."[2]

Arachnoid granulations are not limited to the intradural venous sinuses but are "disseminated over a considerable area; they increase in number and size as age advances. They cause absorption of bone and so produce the pits or depressions"[86]

Schuknecht and Gulya[87] called attention to the structures on the middle fossa and posterior fossa surfaces of the temporal bone. The size and location of arachnoid granulations, as well as the degree of pneumatization of the mastoid air cell system, could create an opportunity for communication between cerebrospinal fluid and the mastoid air cell system. The same scenario could apply to the sphenoid and ethmoid sinuses, thereby producing cerebrospinal fluid rhinorrhea. Infection from suppurative otitis media can also ascend into the subarachnoid space, producing meningitis. As support for the clinically relevant role of temporal bone arachnoid granulations, Gacek[76] reported on seven patients with temporal bone arachnoid granulations, one of whom had meningitis. Arachnoid granulations can be suggested by CT scans and magnetic resonance imaging (MRI), depending on their size and location.

DIAGNOSIS

The diagnosis of dural herniation and cerebrospinal fluid otorrhea is primarily clinical, with supplemental information provided by various imaging tests. History and physical examination quite often provide all the necessary information for a diagnosis. As discussed previously, brain herniation related to chronic otitis media can occur alone or with cerebrospinal fluid leak.

In an ear with chronic otitis media without prior surgery, typical presentations can range from clear watery discharge,[17, 29, 50–52, 55, 76, 77] conductive hearing loss,[29, 44, 76, 88] seizures,[3–7, 9, 10, 55] or meningitis,[5, 6, 9, 18, 21, 40, 41, 43, 46, 53, 55, 89] in addition to the characteristic signs and symptoms associated with chronic otitis media. The same applies for a prior intact canal wall mastoid procedure. In these circumstances, if suspicion is aroused, high-resolution CT scan with bone windows may provide additional information, although it is seldom conclusive.[52, 55] In a radical or modified radical mastoid cavity, the same symptoms can manifest, as can the presence of a mass.[6] Baron[25] noted that these encephaloceles can mimic a blue dome cyst.

A key point in differentiation between the two is that the encephalocele will pulsate and enlarge with the Valsalva maneuver, whereas the blue dome cyst will not.[25, 27] CT scans can assess bony integrity, and recently, MRI has proved to be of benefit in differentiating brain versus cholesteatoma.[3, 90] Jackson and colleagues[38] noted in their series that CT is 64 per cent accurate, MRI is 80 per cent accurate, and the combination of the two is 89 per cent accurate in identifying the lesion preoperatively.

Spontaneous cerebrospinal fluid leakage from the temporal bone is primarily a clinical diagnosis, but it can be quite difficult to make if the quantity of the fluid is limited. Also, if cerebrospinal fluid presents as rhinorrhea, the diagnosis and preoperative localization become more difficult. Cerebrospinal fluid in sufficient quantities has a clear, watery, thin appearance. Cerebrospinal fluid leakage in children can be assessed by the history of meningitis (especially recurrent), severe-to-profound sensorineural hearing loss, and CT evidence of otic capsule abnormality. Middle ear exploration may be ultimately required as a diagnostic measure. In adults, cerebrospinal fluid flow will increase with Valsalva maneuvers, pressure occlusion of the jugular vein, and a dependent head position.

Glucose testing with commercially available test papers has been of little clinical value, especially if the result is negative. Immunoelectrophoretic identification of β_2-transferrin is pathognomonic for cerebrospinal fluid.[91] This test can be of great value if the quantity of suspected fluid is small and contaminated. However, this sophisticated test is not always readily available in most clinical laboratories.

CT scan with metrizamide contrast[56, 68, 92] can demonstrate extracranial extravasation of cerebrospinal fluid for diagnosis and location. The main limitation is with very small sites of leakage or intermittent leakage, both of which can make the tests falsely negative. Other techniques used to demonstrate cerebrospinal fluid leakage include injection of colored dyes into the subarachnoid space (fluorescein, methylene blue, indigo carmine, and toluidine blue) or radioactive isotopes[16, 23, 47, 52, 93–97] (radioactive sodium, ^{111}In-DTPA, ^{99m}Tc-DTPA, [99m]TcHSA). With these techniques (dye or tracer), pledgets are placed at the suspected site to absorb with the dye or tracer, then visually inspected or submitted for radiation counting techniques. Methylene blue (methylthionine chloride) has been abandoned as an intrathecal injection technique to detect cerebrospinal fluid leaks because of severe reactions, including transverse myelitis.[27] Fluorescein is usually safe[27, 50, 51, 77, 93, 98–100] to use intrathecally, although transient paraplegia and seizures were reported once[101] when it was used in high concentration. Suspected ear fluid is examined 2 hours later visually or with the aid of a Wood's lamp.

SURGICAL MANAGEMENT

As expected, surgical management techniques depend on the type of defect as well as the location. Substances used

for repair need only be strong enough to withstand normal intracranial pressure (<200 mm H_2O) and be compliant enough to form a seal. For a temporal lobe herniation through the floor of the middle cranial fossa into a radical or modified radical cavity, the herniation is usually broad based. The favored technique (Fig. 20–5) consists of a combined mastoid-temporal craniotomy with fascia-bone-fascia support.[6, 35, 55] Lundy and associates,[35] using this basic approach philosophy in 18 of 19 cases, had no recurrent or persistent cerebrospinal fluid leaks and no complications (seizures, brain abscess, hemorrhage, postoperative meningitis, wound infection, or death). In addition to being safe and effective, the inclusion of the middle fossa craniotomy portion of the procedure allows for identification of multiple defect sites and their direct repair, which could easily be missed with a transmastoid-only approach, especially for spontaneous cerebrospinal fluid leaks.[35]

A wide mastoidectomy is performed and the extent of dural and temporal lobe herniation determined. Fibrous adhesions between the dura and adjacent soft tissues are separated; however, reduction of the temporal lobe is not attempted. A middle cranial fossa temporal skin incision is then made, and a large piece of temporalis fascia is acquired and dried for future use. A temporal craniotomy is then fashioned with the cutting drill and suction-irrigation. Dura is elevated off the floor of the middle cranial fossa, and the herniated temporal lobe is elevated and supported by the House-Urban middle fossa retractor. A portion of the squamous temporal bone removed at craniotomy is then fashioned to lie on the floor of the middle cranial fossa, bridging the tegmen defect. Two layers of dry temporalis fascia are then placed over and under the bony plate. The dural defect should be closed with sutures, if possible. If the defect is too large to close primarily, it should be covered by fascia to prevent cerebrospinal fluid leak. The dura middle fossa retractor is removed and the temporal lobe allowed to re-expand slowly. The wound is then closed in layers without drainage. Recently, Jackson[38] and Aristegui[37] and their colleagues advocated intradural placement of temporalis fascia in a large defect.

There are alternative approaches for this repair. Canfield[21] in 1913 and Dandy[11] in 1944 corrected dural defects with prolapse of the temporal lobe following mastoidectomy by suturing dura and fascia into the dural defect. In 1963, Blatt[43] described dural defect repair with fascia and bone graft and amputation of the herniated dura. In 1970, Dedo and Sooy[20] reviewed nine cases and described the surgical method of correction by temporalis muscle flap rotation to the mastoid cavity to seal the defect after the brain herniation had been excised, the flap being held in place by packing. In 1977, Fernandez-Blasini and Longo[28] described four cases of temporal lobe herniation through the radical mastoid defect and the successful correction by middle fossa temporal parietal osteoplastic craniotomy. They also described dural hernia and bony defect repair by pedicled temporalis muscle and fascia graft. In 1977, Bhatnager[102] described an instance of temporal lobe herniation following intact canal wall tympanoplasty with mastoidectomy. The prolapse eroded through the posterior bony canal wall postoperatively; the defect was successfully closed by temporalis fascia. In 1978, Iliades[30] described a case occurring 19 months after radical mastoidectomy that

FIGURE 20-5

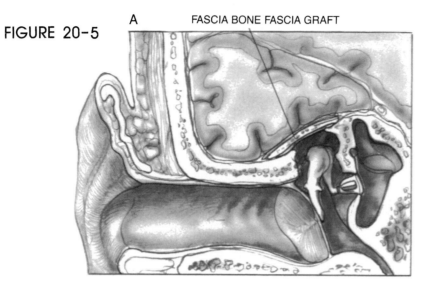

A

FASCIA BONE FASCIA GRAFT

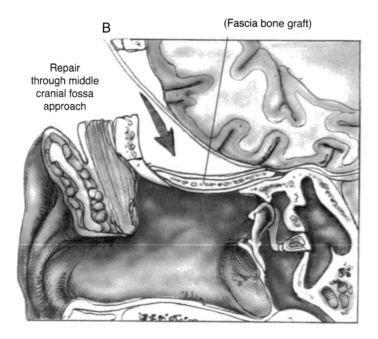

B

(Fascia bone graft)

Repair
through middle
cranial fossa
approach

FIGURE 20–5. A, Tegmen defect covered by fascia-bone-fascia technique via a temporal craniotomy approach. B, Temporal lobe herniation reduced and supported by fascia-bone-fascia technique.

FIGURE 20–6. Fascia "dumbbelled" through small dural defect.

FIGURE 20-6

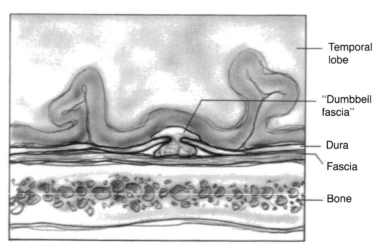

Temporal
lobe

"Dumbbell
fascia"

Dura

Fascia

Bone

was followed by *Pseudomonas* infection. This defect was not repaired. In 1978, Paparella and associates[42] used a temporalis fascia graft to cover a defect on the mastoid side and a split-thickness skin graft carefully placed to line the remaining cavity. A firm pack held the graft in place for 2 weeks. In 1979, Glasscock and coworkers[5] discussed in depth the problem of brain tissue herniation into the middle ear and mastoid cavity and reviewed methods of repair, that is, from below via mastoidectomy and by a combined intracranial and mastoid approach.

The surgeon should be prepared to deal with an encephalocele encountered incidentally during surgery for chronic otitis media. Typically, the mass is pedunculated through a small opening. This herniated tissue is functionless and should be amputated.[4, 5, 7, 13, 27, 28, 31, 35, 37, 38, 42, 45–48] The surgeon must decide whether this problem can be repaired from below (mastoid approach) or above (middle cranial fossa approach).

Various options for transmastoid repair include temporalis fascia or fascia lata[3, 11, 24, 48] inserted intracranially but extradurally with or without firm support, such as conchal cartilage graft[4, 31, 45, 46] or cortical bone.[4, 6, 26, 55] Another option includes rotating pedicled temporalis muscle flap[3, 17, 24, 25, 27, 28, 32, 41, 46, 47, 49–52, 54, 70, 103] for additional support or abdominal fat graft[59, 77, 100] in the mastoid cavity. Some authors[3, 5, 27, 32, 47, 53, 57] have used synthetic material (silicone sheeting, Marlex, stainless steel mesh, Vivosil, acrylic, methyl methacrylate) for bony defect closure, but there is a higher incidence of infection, recurrence, and extrusion with these materials.[3, 5, 32] Others[3, 5, 12, 14, 24, 27, 28, 43, 45] have advocated packing the cavity (open or closed) until healing is well under way, then removing the packing. With a temporal craniotomy, an intradural temporalis fascia or fascia lata graft can be placed and provides a better anatomic seal for large defects.[37, 38] A combined mastoidectomy-minicraniotomy approach has been successfully used.[4, 8, 45]

For children with otic capsule defects, the oval window is by far the most common site because there is almost always no functional hearing; therefore, a total stapedectomy is performed, with soft tissue obliteration of the vestibule.[14, 58, 61–67, 93, 104, 105] For the rare miscellaneous sites of otic capsule defects, a radical mastoidectomy with obliteration of the eustachian tube, middle ear, and mastoid, and blind sac closure of the external auditory canal are recommended.[14, 59, 77, 106, 107] This procedure provides the best chance of permanent closure of cerebrospinal fluid fistula and control over recurrent meningitis, while maintaining cochlear function.

Probably the most challenging issue is the adult onset of spontaneous cerebrospinal fluid leakage. As noted earlier, the source can be posterior fossa mastoid dural surface, middle fossa dural surface, or, very rarely, the middle ear. Multiple sources of cerebrospinal fluid leaks are frequently encountered.[8, 11, 17, 25, 35, 43, 50, 52, 55, 59, 60, 69, 81–83] Therefore, a combined mastoid-subtemporal craniotomy approach is recommended.[6, 35, 55] The dural surfaces of the mastoid and posterior fossa should be thoroughly explored, as should the middle ear. The final portion of the procedure is the subtemporal craniotomy with wide exposure of the entire middle cranial fossa floor, especially the anteromedial portion. Experience has shown that the multiple small sites

would easily be missed from a mastoid-alone approach. If the dural defects are small, an oversized piece of fascia can be "dumbbelled" into the opening, and then an extradural fascia graft can be done[35] (Fig. 20–6).

SUMMARY

Dural or brain herniation and cerebrospinal fluid leakage from the temporal bone are a widely recognized, but infrequently encountered, challenge for the otologic surgeon. Two major categories are reviewed in this chapter: dural herniation secondary to chronic otitis media and spontaneous cerebrospinal fluid leaks. Dural herniation secondary to chronic otitis media can result from the chronic otitis media itself or from surgery for chronic otitis media. Spontaneous cerebrospinal fluid leakage from the temporal bone has two recognized subtypes: childhood onset and adult onset. Each has distinctly different characteristics and presentations.

Regardless of the underlying cause, a break in the integrity of the intracranial-extracranial barrier poses significant risk of complications, such as meningitis[5–7, 9, 12, 14–16, 18, 21, 40, 41, 43, 46, 49, 53, 59, 62–67, 88, 89, 93, 94, 104, 105, 107, 108] and seizures.[3–10]

References

1. Hall C: Brain hernia: A postoperative complication in otology. Ann Otol Rhinol Laryngol 48: 291–309, 1939.
2. Wolbach SB: Multiple hernias of the cerebrum and cerebellum due to intracranial pressure. J Med Res 19: 153–173, 1908.
3. Bowes AK, Wiet RJ, Monsell EM, et al: Brain herniation and space-occupying lesions eroding the tegmen tympani. Laryngoscope 97: 1172–1175, 1987.
4. Feenstra L, Sanna M, Zini C, et al: Surgical treatment of brain herniation into the middle ear and mastoid. Am J Otol 6: 311–315, 1985.
5. Glasscock ME, Dickins JRE, Jackson CG, et al: Surgical management of brain tissue herniation into the middle ear and mastoid. Laryngoscope 89: 1743–1754, 1979.
6. Graham MD: Surgical managment of dural and temporal lobe herniation into the radical mastoid cavity. Laryngoscope 92: 329–331, 1982.
7. Hyson M, Andermann F, Olivier A, Melenson D: Occult encephaloceles and temporal lobe epilepsy: Developmental and acquired lesions in the middle fossa. Neurology 34: 363–366, 1984.
8. Iurato S, Ettorre GC, Selvini C: Brain herniation into the middle ear: Two idiopathic cases treated by a combined intracranial mastoid approach. Laryngoscope 99: 950–954, 1989.
9. Schurr PH: Endaural cerebral hernia. Br J Surg 47: 414–417, 1960.
10. Williams DC: Encephalocele of the middle ear. J Laryngol Otol 100: 471–473, 1986.
11. Dandy WE: Treatment of rhinorrhea and otorrhea. Arch Surg 49: 75–85, 1944.
12. Lillie HI, Spar AA: Escape of cerebrospinal fluid into the wounds of operations on the temporal bone. Arch Otolaryngol Head Neck Surg 46: 779–788, 1947.
13. Mosberg WH: Spontaneous cerebrospinal fluid rhinorrhea and otorrhea. Md Med J 8: 62–65, 1959.
14. Nenzelius C: Spontaneous cerebrospinal otorrhea due to congenital malformations. Acta Otolaryngol (Stockh) 39: 314–328, 1951.
15. Precechtel A: The problem of recurrent meningitis in ORL. Acta Otolaryngol 45: 427–430, 1954.
16. Spitz EB, Wagner S, Sataloff J, et al: Cerebrospinal fluid otorrhea and recurrent meningitis. J Pediatr 59: 397–400, 1961.
17. Dysart BR: Spontaneous cerebrospinal fluid otorrhea—a report on a case with successful surgical repair. Trans Am Laryngol Rhinol Otol Soc 62: 381–387, 1959.
18. Kline OR: Spontaneous cerebrospinal otorrhea. Arch Otolaryngol Head Neck Surg, 18: 34–39, 1933.

19. Thomson St C: The Cerebro-spinal Fluid: Its Spontaneous Escape from the Nose. New York, William Wood & Company, 1899.

20. Dedo HH, Sooy FA: Endaural brain hernia (encephalocele): Diagnosis and treatment. Laryngoscope 80: 1090–1099, 1970.

21. Canfield RB: Some conditions associated with the loss of cerebrospinal fluid. Ann Otol Rhinol Laryngol 22: 604–622, 1913.

22. Dean LW: Operative procedure for brain abscess of otitic origin. Ann Otol Rhinol Laryngol 19: 541–556, 1910.

23. DiChiro G, Ommaya AK, Ashburn WL, Briner WH: Isotope cisternography in the diagnosis and followup of cerebrospinal fluid rhinorrhea. J Neurosurg 28: 522–529, 1968.

24. Alberti PWRM, Dawes JDK: Cerebrospinal otorrhea and chronic ear disease. J Laryngol Otol 75: 123–135, 1961.

25. Baron SH: Herniation of the brain into the mastoid cavity: Postsurgical, postinfectional, or congenital. Arch Otolaryngol Head Neck Surg 90: 127–133, 1969.

26. Bartels L, Luk LJ, Balis G, Bald C: Endaural brain hernia: Repair using mastoid cortical bone. Am J Otol (Suppl): 121–125, 1985.

27. Dedo HH, Sooy FA: Endaural encephalocele and cerebrospinal fluid otorrhea: A review. Ann Otol Rhinol Laryngol 79: 168–177, 1970.

28. Fernandez-Blasini N, Longo R: Surgical correction of dural herniation into the mastoid cavity. Laryngoscope 87: 1841–1846, 1977.

29. Gavilan J, Trujillo M, Gavilan C: Spontaneous encephalocele of the middle ear. Arch Otolaryngol Head Neck Surg 110: 206–207, 1984.

30. Iliades CE: Brain hernia: A postoperative complication in otology. Ear Nose Throat J 57: 39–43, 1978.

31. Neely JG, Kuhn JR: Diagnosis and treatment of iatrogenic cerebrospinal fluid leak and brain herniation during or following mastoidectomy. Laryngoscope 95: 1299–1300, 1985.

32. Stout JJ Jr, Trowbridge WV, Ruggles RL: Surgical repair of dural herniation into the mastoid bowl. Arch Otolaryngol Head Neck Surg 89: 72–77, 1969.

33. Gottlieb MB, Blaugrund JE, Niparko JK: Imaging quiz case: Tegmental encephalocele. Arch Otolaryngol Head Neck Surg 124: 1274–1277, 1998.

34. Golding-Wood DG, Williams HO, Brookes GB: Tegmental dehiscence and brain herniation into the middle ear cleft. J Laryngol Otol 105: 477–480, 1991.

35. Lundy LB, Graham MG, Kartush JK, et al: Temporal bone encephalocele and cerebrospinal fluid leaks. Am J Otol 17: 461–469, 1996.

36. Ramanikanth TV, Smith MC, Ramamoorthy R, et al: Postauricular cerebellar encephalocele secondary to chronic suppurative otitis media and mastoid surgery. J Laryngol Otol 104: 982–985, 1990.

37. Aristegui M, Falcioni M, Saleh E, et al: Meningoencephalic herniation into the middle ear: A report of 27 cases. Laryngoscope 105: 513–518, 1995.

38. Jackson GC, Pappas DG, Manolidis S, et al: Brain herniation into the middle ear and mastoid: Concepts in diagnosis and surgical management. Am J Otol 18: 198–206, 1997.

39. Souliere CR, Langman AW: Combined mastoid/middle cranial fossa repair of temporal bone encephalocele. Skull Base Surgery 8: 185–189, 1998.

40. Mealey J Jr: Chronic cerebrospinal fluid otorrhea—report of a case associated with chronic infection of the ear. Neurology 11: 996–998, 1961.

41. Moore GF, Nissen AJ, Yonkers AJ: Potential complications of unrecognized cerebrospinal fluid leaks secondary to mastoid surgery. Am J Otol 5: 317–323, 1984.

42. Paparella MM, Meyerhoff WL, Oliviera CA: Mastoiditis and brain hernia (mastoiditis cerebri). Laryngoscope 88: 1097–1106, 1978.

43. Blatt IM: Surgical repair for cerebrospinal otorrhea due to middle ear and mastoid disease—a report of six cases. Laryngoscope 73: 446–460, 1963.

44. Levy RA, Platt N, Aftalion B: Encephalocele of the middle ear. Laryngoscope 81: 126–130, 1971.

45. Adkins WY, Osguthorpe JD: Mini-craniotomy for management of CSF otorrhea from tegmen defects. Laryngoscope 93: 1038–1039, 1983.

46. Jahn AF: Endaural brain hernia: Repair using conchal cartilage. J Otolaryngol 10: 471–475, 1981.

47. Jahrsdoerfer RA, Richtsmeier WJ, Cantrell RW: Spontaneous CSF otorrhea. Arch Otolaryngol Head Neck Surg 107: 257–262, 1981.

48. Ramsden RT, Latif A, Lye RH, Dutton JEM: Endaural cerebral hernia. J Laryngol Otol 99: 643–651, 1985.

49. Kramer SA, Yanagisawa E, Smith HW: Spontaneous cerebrospinal fluid otorrhea simulating serous otitis media. Laryngoscope 81: 1083–1089, 1971.

50. Adams GL, McCoid G, Weisbeski D: Cerebrospinal fluid otorrhea presenting as serous otitis media. Minn Med 65: 410–415, 1982.

51. Briant TD, Bird R: Extracranial repair of cerebrospinal fluid fistula. J Otolaryngol 11: 191–197, 1982.

52. Ferguson BJ, Wilkins RH, Hudson W, Farmer J Jr: Spontaneous CSF otorrhea from tegmen and posterior fossa defects. Laryngoscope 96: 635–644, 1986.

53. Hicks GW, Wright JW Jr, Wright JW III: Cerebrospinal fluid otorrhea. Laryngoscope 80(Suppl 25): 1–25, 1980.

54. Kamerer DB, Caparosa RJ: Temporal bone encephalocele: Diagnosis and treatment. Laryngoscope 92: 878–882, 1982.

55. Kemink JL, Graham MD, Kartush JM: Spontaneous encephalocele of the temporal bone. Arch Otolaryngol Head Neck Surg 112: 558–561, 1986.

56. Myer CM, Miller GW, Ball JB: Spontaneous cerebrospinal fluid otorrhea. Ann Otol Rhinol Laryngol 94: 96–97, 1985.

57. Richardson GS: Brain herniation into the mastoid antrum. Am J Otol 2: 39, 1980.

58. Weider DJ, Geurkink NA, Saunders RL: Spontaneous cerebrospinal fluid otorhinorrhea. Am J Otol 6: 416–422, 1985.

59. Wetmore SJ, Herrmann P, Fisch U: Spontaneous cerebrospinal fluid otorrhea. Am J Otol 8: 96–102, 1987.

60. Yeates AE, Blumenkopf B, Drayer BP, et al: Spontaneous CSF rhinorrhea arising from the middle cranial fossa: CT demonstration. AJNR Am J Neuroradiol 5: 820–821, 1984.

61. MacRae DL, Ruby RRF: Recurrent meningitis secondary to perilymph fistula in young children. J Otolaryngol 19: 222–225, 1990.

62. Phillipps JJ: Bilateral oval window fistulae with recurrent meningitis. J Laryngol Otol 100: 329–331, 1986.

63. Quiney RE, Mitchell DB, Djazeri B, Evans JNG: Recurrent meningitis in children due to inner ear abnormalities. J Laryngol Otol 103: 473–480, 1989.

64. Barr B, Warsall J: Cerebrospinal otorrhea with meningitis and congenital deafness. Arch Otolaryngol Head Neck Surg 81: 26–28, 1965.

65. Bennett RJ: On subarachnoid tympanic fistula—a report of two cases of the rare indirect type. J Laryngol Otol 80: 1242–1252, 1966.

66. Biggers WP, Howell NN, Fisher ND, Himadi GM: Congenital ear anomalies associated with otic meningitis. Arch Otolaryngol Head Neck Surg 97: 399–401, 1973.

67. Tschiang HH, Harrison MS, Ozsahinaglu CAN: Cerebrospinal otorrhea. J Laryngol Otol 87: 475–483, 1973.

68. Park TS: Spontaneous cerebrospinal fluid otorrhea in association with a congenital defect of the cochlear aqueduct and Mondini dysplasia. Neurosurgery 11: 356, 1982.

69. Brodsky L: Spontaneous cerebrospinal fluid otorrhea and rhinorrhea co-existing in a patient with meningitis. Laryngoscope 94: 1351–1354, 1984.

70. Gacek RR, Leipzig B: Congenital cerebrospinal otorrhea. Ann Otol 88: 358–365, 1979.

71. Gacek RR: Arachnoid granulation cerebrospinal otorrhea. Ann Otol Rhinol Laryngol 99: 854–862, 1990.

72. Finsnes KA: Lethal intracranial complication following insufflation with a pneumatic otoscope. Acta Otolaryngol 75: 436–438, 1973.

73. Wilkins SA, Radtke RA, Burger PC: Spontaneous temporal encephalocele: A case report. J Neurosurg 78: 492–498, 1993.

74. Mostafa BE: Spontaneous CSF leak from the temporal bone. Skull Base Surg 7: 139–144, 1997.

75. Pappas DG, Pappas DG, Hoffman RA, et al: Spontaneous cerebrospinal fluid leaks originating from multiple skull base defects. Skull Base Surg 6: 227–230, 1996.

76. Gacek RR: Evaluation and management of temporal bone arachnoid granulations. Arch Otolaryngol Head Neck Surg 118: 327–332, 1992.

77. Schuknecht HF, Zaytoun GM, Moon CN: Adult onset of fluid in the tympanomastoid compartment. Arch Otolaryngol Head Neck Surg 108: 759–765, 1982.

78. Ahren C, Thulin CA: Lethal intracranial complications following inflation in the external auditory canal in treatment of serous otitis media and due to defects in the petrous bone. Acta Otolaryngol 60: 407–421, 1965.

79. Lang DV: Macroscopic bony deficiency of the tegmen tympani in adult temporal bones. J Laryngol Otol 97: 685–688, 1983.

80. Kapur TR, Bangash W: Tegmental and petromastoid defects in the temporal bone. J Laryngol Otol 100: 1129–1132, 1986.
81. Kaufman B, Yonas H, White RJ, Miller CF: Acquired middle cranial fossa fistulas, normal pressure, and non-traumatic in origin. Neurosurgery 5: 466–472, 1979.
82. Brisman R, Hughes JEO, Mount LA: Cerebrospinal fluid rhinorrhea. Neurolology 22: 245–252, 1970.
83. Kaufman B, Nulsen FE, Weiss MH, et al: Acquired spontaneous non-traumatic normal pressure cerebrospinal fistulas originating from the middle fossa. Radiology 122: 379–387, 1977.
84. Ommaya AK: Cerebrospinal fluid rhinorrhea. Neurology 15: 106–113, 1964.
85. Weed LH: The absorption of cerebrospinal fluid in the venous system. Am J Anat 31: 191–221, 1923.
86. Warwick R, Williams PL (eds): Gray's Anatomy, 35th British ed. London, WB Saunders, 1973, p 991.
87. Schuknecht HF, Gulya AJ: Anatomy of the Temporal Bone with Surgical Implications. Philadelphia, Lea & Febiger, 1986, pp 125–126.
88. Koch H: Meningocele of the temporal bone. Acta Otolaryngol (Stockh) 38: 59–61, 1950.
89. Feenstra L, Blom ER: Mastoid approach for brain herniation into the middle ear. Clin Otolaryngol 8: 187–190, 1983.
90. Kaseff LG, Seidenwurm DJ, Neiberding PH, et al: Magnetic resonance imaging of brain herniation into the middle ear. Am J Otol 13: 74–77, 1992.
91. Irjala K, Suompaa J, Laurent B: Identification of CSF leakage by immunofixation. Arch Otolaryngol Head Neck Surg 105: 447–448, 1979.
92. Loew F: Traumatic spontaneous and postoperative CSF rhinorrhea. Adv Tech Stand Neurosurg 11: 169, 1984.
93. Harris HH: Cerebrospinal otorrhea and recurring meningitis: Report of three cases. Laryngoscope 88: 1577–1585, 1978.
94. Kaseff LG, Neiberding PH, Shorago GW, Huertas G: Fistula between the middle ear and subarachnoid space as a cause of recurrent meningitis: Detection by means of thin-section, complex motion tomography. Radiology 135: 105–108, 1980.
95. Ommaya AK, DiChiro G, Baldwin M, Pennybacker JB: Non-traumatic cerebrospinal fluid rhinorrhea. J Neurol Neurosurg Psychiatry 31: 214–225, 1968.
96. Ray BS, Bergland RM: Cerebrospinal fluid fistula: Clinical aspects, techniques of localization, and methods of closure. J Neurosurg 30: 399–405, 1969.
97. Rotillio A, Andrioli GC, Scanarini M, et al: Concurrent spontaneous CSF otorrhea and rhinorrhea. Eur Neurol 21: 77–83, 1982.
98. Kirchner FR: Use of fluorescein for the diagnosis and localization of cerebrospinal fluid fistulas. Surg Forum 12: 406–408, 1961.
99. Kirchner FR, Proud GO: Method for identification and localization of cerebrospinal fluid, rhinorrhea, and otorrhea. Trans Am Laryngol Rhinol Otol Soc 70: 786–796, 1960.
100. Montgomery WW: Surgery for cerebrospinal fluid rhinorrhea and otorrhea. Arch Otolaryngol Head Neck Surg 84: 92–104, 1966.
101. Mahaley MS Jr, Odom GL: Complications following intrathecal injection of fluorescein. J Neurosurg 25: 298–299, 1966.
102. Bhatnager HN: Meningoencephalocele of the mastoid. Ear Nose Throat J 56: 20–28, 1977.
103. Andrew WF: Temporal lobe herniation through traumatic defect in tegmen of temporal bone with cerebrospinal fluid otorrhea. Ann Otol Rhinol Laryngol 60: 622–626, 1951.
104. Gundersen T, Haye R: Cerebrospinal otorrhea. Arch Otolaryngol Head Neck Surg 91: 19–23, 1970.
105. Herther C, Schindler RA: Mondini's dysplasia with recurrent meningitis. Laryngoscope 95: 655–658, 1985.
106. Neely J, Neblett CR, Rose JE: Diagnosis and treatment of spontaneous cerebrospinal fluid otorrhea. Laryngoscope 92: 609–612, 1982.
107. Schindler RA: Congenital deafness, recurrent meningitis, and neural tube defects. Transpac Coast Oto Ophthalmol Soc 82: 275–282, 1976.
108. Hall GM, Pulec JL, Hallberg OE: Persistent cerebrospinal fluid otorrhea. Arch Otolaryngol Head Neck Surg 86: 43–47, 1967.

21

Total Stapedectomy

Howard P. House, M.D. ▪ Jed A. Kwartler, M.D.

The goal of stapes surgery is to re-establish sound transmission through an ossicular chain stiffened due to otosclerosis. Various techniques have been used to accomplish this goal, including stapes mobilization, fragmentation, small fenestration, and partial as well as total stapes footplate removal.

The history of surgery for otosclerosis is a fascinating story that began to unfold in the latter part of the nineteenth century. A group of pioneering surgeons, including Kessel,[1] Boucheron,[2] Miot,[3] Faraci,[4] and Passow,[5] began to mobilize the stapes. At about this time, Jack[6] reported on a series of cases in which he removed the stapes entirely.

The unacceptably high rate of inner ear injury and infection led to the abandonment of stapes surgery. As stated by Goodhill,[7] "it was probably Siebenmann[8] along with Moure[9] who closed the door on further stapes surgery at the turn of the century."

Surgery for otosclerosis was reactivated in 1923, when Holmgren[10] bypassed the stapes area by creating a fenestra in the horizontal canal to stimulate inner ear fluids in response to sound, and the fenestration operation was reborn. In 1937, Sourdille[11] presented a series of fenestration cases before the New York Academy of Medicine. It was Lempert,[12] however, who in 1938 introduced his unique one-stage fenestration technique using his endaural approach and a dental drill to create the fenestra. Surgeons throughout the world beat a path to his door to learn his technique, which became the standard. He will forever be known as the father of otosclerosis surgery.

In 1952, Rosen[13] reintroduced stapes mobilization for otosclerosis. For a brief time, this technique was widely used and threatened to replace the Lempert procedure. It was soon realized that refixation of the footplate often occurred. Fortunately, Shea[14] introduced his technique of total stapedectomy. After removing the total stapes, he covered the oval window with a vein graft and introduced an artificial stapes made of polytetrafluoroethylene (Teflon) by Harry Treace to make the connection with the incus. This reactivation of stapedectomy by Shea replaced both Lempert's fenestration procedure and Rosen's mobilization operation and, with modification, is now used universally throughout the world. We indeed are greatly indebted to Shea for his tremendous contribution to otosclerosis surgery.

PATIENT COUNSELING

All patients should be told that even though their hearing loss is hereditary, their children or grandchildren will not necessarily have a similar problem. They should be assured that they are not going to become totally deaf. The mechanics of the hearing loss should also be explained in detail, preferably by use of a suitable illustration.

Patients who are suitable for stapes surgery should be told that they have the option of wearing hearing aids, and if there is any doubt about the decision to have surgery, they should be encouraged to have a trial period with hearing aids unless they are already wearing them.

The expected hearing result as well as all possible risks, such as further or even total hearing loss, taste disturbance, dizziness, the effect on tinnitus (if present), and the very remote possibility of a partial or total facial paralysis, should be clearly understood.

Hearing improvement is in direct proportion to the preoperative bone conduction level, and the patient must understand the degree of improvement to be expected.

SELECTION OF PATIENTS FOR STAPES SURGERY

All patients who are suitable for stapes surgery should be thoroughly informed of both the advantages and the possible complications of the operation. For some, serviceable hearing will be restored with no need for a hearing aid. In others, the hearing will be improved so they may need a hearing aid only for distant conversation. In still others, the hearing will be improved, and they may be able to convert their postauricular aid to an all-in-the-ear aid or from an all-in-the-ear aid to an intracanal aid.

Occasionally, patients will have a totally blank audiogram and still be suitable for stapes surgery. This situation occurs when the bone conduction level exceeds the capability of the audiometer. There may be a 75 or 80 dB bone conduction level but a 40 to 50 dB air-bone gap. Typically, when the patient is initially evaluated, he or she is hearing surprisingly well with a powerful hearing aid and possesses excellent speech quality. On examination, one may note a positive Schwartze's sign, but the 512 tuning fork is not helpful. Following surgery, these patients are most grateful because they can now wear the less powerful hearing aids with fewer feedback problems.

Indications for Stapes Surgery

The patient should understand the details of the operation, including the operative procedure itself, and all admission and discharge procedures. The following principles also apply:

1. The patient should be in reasonably good health, especially if general anesthesia is contemplated.

2. The age of the patient is not a factor in the decision to perform surgery. The youngest in our series was 7 years of age, and the oldest was 98.

3. The poorer-hearing ear, based on the patient's statement and not necessarily on the audiogram, should be chosen for surgery. In children, the poorer-hearing ear should be operated on so that the hearing aid can be eliminated before they enter school. Surgery for the second ear should be delayed until they are old enough to make their own decision.

4. Tuning forks should be used to confirm the audiometric findings. If bone conduction is heard louder than air conduction with a 512 or a 1024 tuning fork, with proper masking of the better ear, the individual is a suitable candidate for surgery. If one reverses the 2048 fork, he or she is an excellent candidate. The minimum air-bone gap should be 15 dB, as averaged in speech frequencies.

5. Speech discrimination is not a great factor in determining stapes suitability. If the patient understands sentences and answers questions correctly using a speaking tube while masking the opposite ear with a Bárány apparatus, he or she is suitable, providing the earlier criteria are met. The improvement the patient receives with a cochlear implant substantiates the value of any sound that helps patients hear and react better to their environment.

6. Indications for stapes surgery are essentially the same whether the hearing loss is unilateral or bilateral. Surgery in the opposite ear can occur 6 months later, provided it is then the poorer-hearing ear.

Contraindications of Stapes Surgery

Stapes surgery is contraindicated in patients

1. In poor physical health
2. With a current balance problem, such as active Ménière's disease or a fluctuating type of hearing loss
3. With pre-existing tympanic membrane perforation
4. With active external or middle ear infection
5. With an inadequate air-bone gap confirmed by an audiogram and the 512 tuning fork

SURGICAL TECHNIQUE

Step 1. Stapes surgery may be performed either with a local or a general anesthetic. Our preference is local anesthesia with adequate sedation that may be supplemented during the procedure with intravenous midazolam (Versed) or diazepam (Valium), if necessary. We prefer local anesthesia because there is less bleeding, and the surgeon is alerted if any vertigo occurs while working on the footplate, inserting the prosthesis, or removing the prosthesis, in a revision case.

Step 2. During surgery, the patient's vital signs are monitored by electrocardiography, blood pressure, and oxygen saturation. The auricle and the surrounding area are cleaned with povidone-iodine (Betadine) solution and plastic drapes and folded towels are applied. A final head drape

with an opening exposing the ear is placed over the head and rested on a metal support to help prevent the feeling of claustrophobia.

Step 3. The operating table is placed slightly in Trendelenburg's position and rotated toward the surgeon so he or she can see directly down the ear canal from the sitting position.

Step 4. The ear canal is washed with warm saline solution to remove the povidone-iodine, and local anesthesia containing 2 per cent lidocaine fortified by 1:100,000 of epinephrine is infiltrated. The initial injections are made with a 30-gauge needle around the periphery of the entrance to the ear canal. Approximately 2.5 to 3 ml of this solution is injected, and 1 or 2 drops is placed in the vascular strip just external to the tympanic membrane. This helps reduce the bleeding at the time of the incision. The tissue to be used, whether vein, fascia, perichondrium, or fat, may be obtained before or after the canal surgery is started.

Several sizes of speculums, both oval and round, should be on the tray, and the largest one that can be seated into the canal is used. The shaft of the instruments entering the speculum are in firm contact with the middle finger, which in turn is stabilized against the speculum and the speculum stabilized by the other fingers against the head. A fixed speculum holder is not used. The advantage of not using a fixed speculum holder is flexibility of the speculum for viewing purposes and for allowing the patient to move his or her head, if desired. The speculums as well as all instruments should be plain metal, because black speculums and instruments absorb much-needed light. The shafts of the needles and hooks should be malleable so that they can be bent slightly to reach difficult areas.

The inferior and superior vertical incisions are made at 6:30 and 11:30 o'clock positions (Fig. 21–1). The point of the sickle knife is started 1 mm from the edge of the tympanic membrane to prevent a possible tear. It is extended externally approximately 8 mm, and this distance can be confirmed when the curve of the incision knife strikes the edge of the properly inserted speculum. If one extends the incisions further externally, the skin becomes thicker, and more bleeding occurs. Several sweeps are made to be certain that one cuts through the periosteum.

The horizontal incision begins by elevation of the skin from the depth of the suture indentation and then continues inferiorly in short increments toward the inferior vertical incision to avoid tearing of the skin toward the eardrum. Several clean sweeps of the knife are again made to ensure that the periosteum that connects to the inferior vertical incision has been cut through. A similar superior incision is made in increments halfway to the superior vertical incision. Again, several sweeps are made on this partially completed incision. The knife is inserted beneath the remaining skin to elevate it. Scissors are then used to connect with the end of the superior vertical incision. Scissors crush the vessels in the vascular strip and help reduce the bleeding.

Following these incisions, a broad separator is used to elevate the skin flap in a uniform manner toward the eardrum. Considerable pressure is applied on the instrument, especially inferiorly, to stay under the periosteum until it enters the middle ear area posterior to the ligament.

FIGURE 21-1

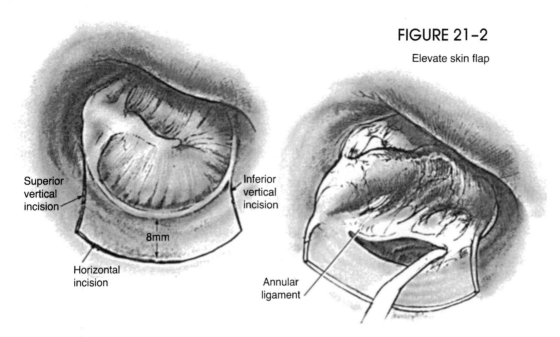

FIGURE 21-2

Elevate skin flap

Superior vertical incision

Inferior vertical incision

8mm

Horizontal incision

Annular ligament

FIGURE 21-4

FIGURE 21-3

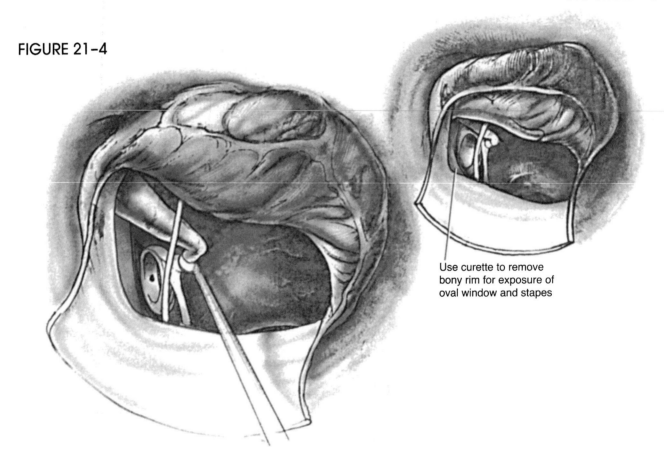

Use curette to remove bony rim for exposure of oval window and stapes

FIGURE 21-1. The inferior and superior vertical incisions.

FIGURE 21-2. Elevating the skin flap.

FIGURE 21-3. Middle ear exposure.

FIGURE 21-4. Separating the incudostapedial joint.

228

A curved Rosen needle is used superiorly to elevate the eardrum and identify the position of the chorda tympani nerve (Fig. 21–2). Once the nerve is identified, the needle is inserted superiorly to the nerve and carried forward to contact the malleus. This action provides the superior exposure. The needle is then used inferior to the chorda tympani to identify the beginning of the tympanic membrane ligament. An elevator is used to lift the ligament inferiorly and to identify the round window. At this point, a cotton ball soaked in the lidocaine-epinephrine solution is placed on the raw surface of the skin flap to lessen the bleeding for a moment. The entire skin flap is then elevated anteriorly, and a few drops of lidocaine-epinephrine are dropped onto the mucosa of the middle ear for anesthesia and to control any mucosal bleeding later as work is done in the stapes area.

To visualize the footplate, bone of the posterior scutum is removed. At the upper limit of exposure superiorly, one should observe the lower half of the transverse portion of the fallopian canal (Fig. 21–3). If one can see the beginning of the curve of the body of the incus, a subsequent retraction pocket may develop. The posterior exposure is limited to observation of the stapedial tendon and the attachment of the posterior crus of the stapes to the footplate. If more bone is removed, a posterior retraction pocket may develop. This exposure is usually done with curettes, but a diamond burr may be necessary to expose the posterior portion of the chorda tympani. On completion of this exposure, a square area is created posterosuperiorly. When the curette or the burr is used, the patient under local anesthesia should be forewarned of the noise that will be created so there will be no surprise to the patient.

If the footplate area appears to be thin, a sharp needle is used to make a small perforating hole in the thinnest area. This small hole will later provide an opening in which an obtuse hook can be inserted if the footplate is inadvertently mobilized at the time the crura are fractured toward the promontory.

A small, round, right-angle knife is used now to separate the incudostapedial joint (Fig. 21–4). The intact stapedial tendon helps prevent an inadvertent mobilization from occurring. In this manipulation, a mild pressure and "jiggling" of the knife blade back and forth is used because if strong direct pressure is applied, dislocation of the incus may occur when the joint is suddenly separated.

The necessary limits of exposure are the round window inferiorly, the lower half of the fallopian canal superiorly, the stapedial tendon pyramidal eminence and posterior crus posteriorly, and the malleus anteriorly (Fig. 21–5).

The malleus is now checked to determine its mobility. One in 200 patients has a fixed malleus. If fixed, alternative techniques must be used (described later).

The stapedial tendon is cut; then the patient is forewarned that a loud sound is forthcoming. The Rosen mobilizing needle is placed on the superior side of the stapes arch near the neck, and the superstructure is sharply fractured toward the promontory and removed (Fig. 21–6).

The distance from the top of the incus to the thin, fixed footplate is measured (Fig. 21–7). Some surgeons measure from the inferior surface of the incus, and the prosthesis length is made accordingly. The prosthesis length should be checked before it is inserted. The measurement from the outer portion of the incus to the footplate is usually 4.5 mm but may vary from 3.5 to as much as 5.5 mm.

The membrane is left intact over the footplate because it helps prevent bony chips from dropping into the vestibule. Obtuse, right-angle hooks and finally the Hough hoe is used to remove the posterior and then the anterior portion of the footplate, thereby effecting a total removal (Fig. 21–8).

Great caution must be used to avoid suction of the perilymph when blood is suctioned from around the oval window. During footplate removal, bone chips or blood entering into the vestibule are left undisturbed.

The previously prepared tissue of choice, measuring about 5×5 mm, is grasped with a nonserrated alligator forceps and slipped over the oval window so that it covers all the edges and is positioned superiorly over a portion of the fallopian canal (Fig. 21–9). The prosthesis is then inserted with a nonserrated forceps into the center area of the oval window and over the incus (Fig. 21–10). A crimper is used to close the loop on the incus, and the wire is moved toward the lenticular process.

The skin flap is then placed back in its normal position, and a small gauze wick is inserted into the hypotympanic area. A cotton pledget is placed over the opening of the external ear canal, and a Band-Aid or two holds the cotton in position, thereby completing the procedure.

In our experience, whether one totally or partially removes the footplate or uses the small fenestra technique or whether one uses the diamond burr or the laser to create the small fenestra, the end result is quite similar. More surgeons are using the small fenestra technique, and the postsurgery imbalance is less noticeable because perilymph disturbance is minimal.

It is not the technique, the instruments, or a particular prosthesis that leads to a successful result but rather the hands and mind behind the instruments. If one is closing the air-bone gap in 90 per cent of the cases and encountering no more than a 1 per cent severe sensorineural loss, one should stay with that technique.

POSTOPERATIVE CARE

Some patients may have dizziness for a few hours following surgery. They are cautioned not to blow their nose hard. If patients sneeze, they should do so with their mouth open, and they should avoid excessive straining for 2 weeks. If operated on in the morning, the patient usually can go home that night and remove the Band-Aid, cotton, and gauze wick the following morning. Patients are allowed to travel by air 3 days after surgery and are instructed to use a nose spray and swallow frequently on descent.

Most patients hear immediately after surgery, but their hearing level may drop back somewhat a few hours later. Barring complications, patients should have their first hearing test 3 weeks after surgery, at which time most have recovered their hearing. In others, the hearing will improve over the next 3 months. The hearing they have at this time is what they will keep. We do not do revision surgery on any patient until 4 months have passed. All patients are routinely placed on a sodium fluoride and calcium carbon-

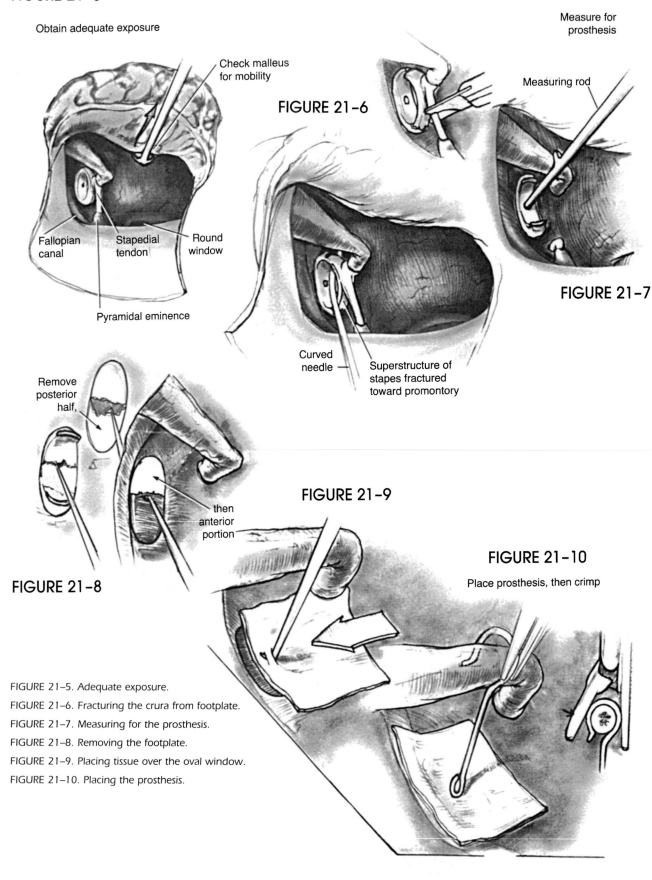

FIGURE 21–5

Obtain adequate exposure

Check malleus for mobility

FIGURE 21–6

Measure for prosthesis

Measuring rod

FIGURE 21–7

Fallopian canal

Stapedial tendon

Round window

Pyramidal eminence

Curved needle

Superstructure of stapes fractured toward promontory

Remove posterior half,

then anterior portion

FIGURE 21–9

FIGURE 21–10

Place prosthesis, then crimp

FIGURE 21–8

FIGURE 21–5. Adequate exposure.
FIGURE 21–6. Fracturing the crura from footplate.
FIGURE 21–7. Measuring for the prosthesis.
FIGURE 21–8. Removing the footplate.
FIGURE 21–9. Placing tissue over the oval window.
FIGURE 21–10. Placing the prosthesis.

ate supplement (Florical), 8 mg three times a day, and are followed up routinely on an annual basis.

INTRAOPERATIVE PITFALLS

Chorda Tympani Nerve

During the procedure, the chorda tympani nerve may be enlarged or may be in a position to interfere with proper visualization of the stapes area (Fig. 21–11). The chorda tympani may be gently moved superiorly and inferiorly. If it is stretched to the point of a partial tear, it should be severed rather than left partially functioning—the patient has less taste disturbance than when a partially functioning chorda is left intact. One should not sever the chorda if the opposite ear is operated on, because a dry mouth and a severe taste disturbance may result.

Eardrum Perforation

If a small perforation of the tympanic membrane occurs during surgery, it will often heal if the edges are placed together. If a larger tear occurs, tissue is used with an underlay technique.

Malleus Fixation

If the malleus is fixed and the stapes is mobile, further stapes surgery is abandoned (Fig. 21–12). The incudostapedial joint is carefully separated, and the incus is removed. The head and neck of the malleus are further exposed anteriorly, and the Lempert snipper is used to sever the neck. Fixation usually results from tendon ossification, and tapping with a small chisel on the head of the malleus will free it, thereby enabling removal. Continuity between the mobile stapes and the eardrum then may be re-established by reconstruction.

If the stapes is also fixed, an incus replacement prosthesis is used. Incisions are made to separate the periosteum from the middle one third of the malleus, and an incus replacement wire prosthesis is inserted through the opening. A right-angle hook is used to rotate the loop portion and placed on the surface of the footplate to determine if the length is proper. The usual length is 5.5 mm. Following this step, the loop is elevated away from the footplate, and the head and neck of the malleus are removed. The footplate is removed, and the loop of the prosthesis is placed into the oval window. The shaft of the prosthesis is grasped with a nonserrated alligator forceps to stabilize it, and with the right hand, it is tightened on the malleus by use of a right-angle hook. Fat or absorbable gelatin sponge (Gelfoam) centers the loop in the oval window.

Other types of prostheses, such as clamp-on plastic pistons, are available, and for some surgeons, these are more easily attached and inserted into the oval window. Another option is to use a total ossicular replacement prosthesis.

Facial Nerve Abnormalities

The facial nerve is often dehiscent in its tympanic segment, but the dehiscence is rarely seen because it often occurs on its undersurface. If the dehiscence is extensive, a prolapse covering half of the footplate area may occur. In this case, the facial nerve may be carefully elevated superiorly, and an opening may be made in the footplate for insertion of the prosthesis. If the shaft of the prosthesis needs to be bent, it usually does not provide a satisfactory hearing result. If the prosthesis rubs on the prolapsed facial nerve, it will not disturb facial nerve function.

A marked prolapse covering the entire oval window requires a prosthesis from the malleus. In these cases, the incus is removed, and the facial nerve is moved slightly so the inferior part of the footplate can be visualized and then fragmented for insertion of the incus replacement prosthesis with the loop into the fragmented area.

Floating Footplate

The most difficult complication in otosclerosis surgery is the solid floating footplate. When one encounters either this or the large prolapsed facial nerve, it is best to terminate the case and send it to your worst enemy! This requires the most complicated and difficult procedure encountered in stapes surgery and should be managed only by highly experienced surgeons.

In this problem, a small cutting burr is used posteroinferiorly on the promontory "side" of the oval window to gain room. The drilling stops 1 mm from the floating footplate. Straight and obtuse needles are used to enter the vestibule along the side of, but at no time touching even the edge of, the floating footplate.

A right-angle hook is inserted into the opening and then rotated to the undersurface of the footplate. It is elevated outward and anteriorly toward the fallopian canal. Blood adhesiveness allows the plate to remain there after the hook is removed and reinserted under the edge of the footplate to then slip it up and over the fallopian canal, where it can be grasped. Only then can the surgeon take his or her first breath with a sigh of relief!

Solid or Obliterated Footplate

By observation, the surgeon cannot determine whether the footplate is minimally fixed at the edges or is obliterated (Fig. 21–13). In each instance, it is necessary to use a cutting burr with a gentle paintbrush-type stroking motion anteroposteriorly. If the slightest give is felt with the drill, minimal fixation and a floating footplate exist. Perilymph escape is noted around the edges. The technique to be used is the same as for the solid floating plate.

Obliterated Footplate

With an obliterated footplate, a cutting burr is used anteroposteriorly and around the edges to develop a thin blue area. The burr is then used to enlarge the opening sufficiently to cover the area with a graft and to insert the prosthesis of choice. The edges are always jagged because there is no demarcation between the attachment of the footplate to the surrounding bone as there is in the solid

FIGURE 21-11

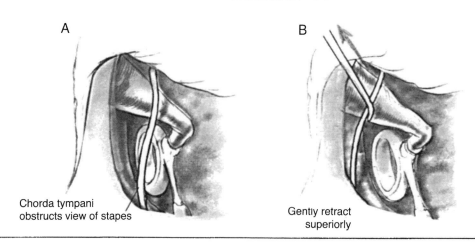

A

Chorda tympani
obstructs view of stapes

B

Gently retract
superiorly

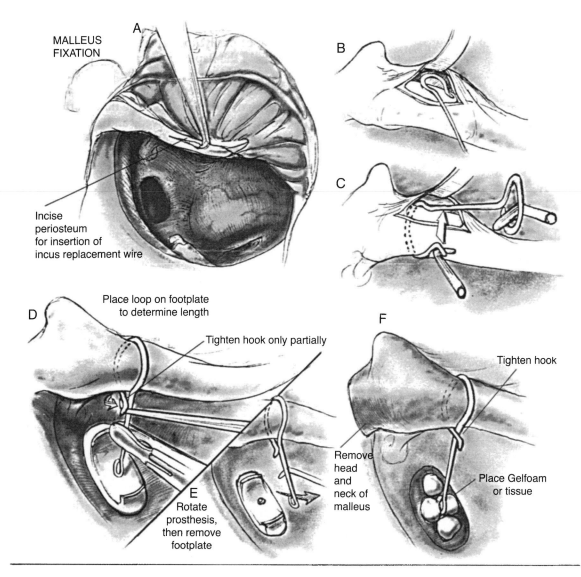

A

MALLEUS
FIXATION

Incise
periosteum
for insertion of
incus replacement wire

B

C

D

Place loop on footplate
to determine length

Tighten hook only partially

E

Rotate
prosthesis,
then remove
footplate

F

Tighten hook

Remove
head
and
neck of
malleus

Place Gelfoam
or tissue

FIGURE 21-12

FIGURES 21–11 and 21–12. *See legends on opposite page*

FIGURE 21-13

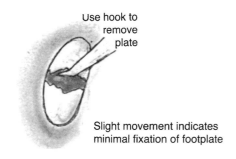

Use hook to remove plate

Slight movement indicates minimal fixation of footplate

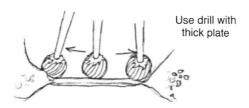

Use drill with thick plate

FIGURE 21–13. A minimally fixed solid footplate.

footplate. These patients respond well either to the small fenestra, the subtotal footplate, or the total removal technique. The floating footplate does not occur in obliterated cases.

Round Window Closure Due to Otosclerosis

A round window closure due to otosclerosis is a rare occurrence that is best left undisturbed. In these cases there is always a fibrous band leading to the round window that is apparently sufficient to produce the necessary relationship between the oval window and the round window. Complete drilling out of the round window has not given the desired result and may make the hearing worse.

Perilymph Gusher

When the cochlear aqueduct is widely patent, it may result in an excessive perilymph flow after the surgeon perforates the footplate. If it is a massive gusher, like a broken fireplug, one should not proceed with the removal of the stapes. It would be best to scrape the membrane of the footplate and the surrounding oval window area with suction in one hand, followed by the placement of small pieces of fascia or perichondrium in the arch of the stapes that will help hold them in place. On one such occasion, we proceeded to remove the stapes and its footplate. The tissue

placed over the oval window floated away, and it needed to be held in place with a suction tip in one hand until the prosthesis was inserted onto the incus. We packed the middle ear solid with gelatin sponge and replaced the flap, only to note the flap being elevated by the flow of perilymph. The ear canal was tightly packed to hold the flap in place, and the patient was elevated to a sitting position. The mastoid dressing was changed repeatedly until the flow stopped.

Intraoperative Vertigo

When patients are under local anesthesia, their response to sudden vertigo is immediately noted by the operating surgeon. This may occur more often in revisions if the covering tissue membrane is inserted too deeply into the vestibule or if the prosthesis is too long. If the cause is tissue, it should be carefully removed and replaced. If the prosthesis is too long, it should likewise be removed and replaced with a shorter one. In revision, the incidence of further sensorineural loss is slightly more common than in a primary case.

Deep Oval Window

In some cases, the oval window niche is very narrow and very deep. If this condition results from otosclerotic encroachment on the sides of the oval window, it can be enlarged by use of a cutting burr. If there is another cause, a broad posterior crus located in the deep narrow niche may be difficult to fracture from the footplate. In this instance, after a small perforating hole has been made in the footplate, a tiny cutting burr or a laser may be used to cut through the posterior crus, thereby making removal of the superstructure of the stapes possible.

SUMMARY

Training surgeons is difficult because of the scarcity of suitable otosclerotic patients, and it is most difficult for residents to obtain sufficient experience to ensure good hearing results in their patients.

We again emphasize that if a surgeon is obtaining the results being reported in the literature, namely, 90 per cent closure of the air-bone gap within 10 dB and no more than 1 per cent further sensorineural loss, there is no need to change technique. We stress again—it is not the instruments or technique that ensure success, but rather the minds and the hands in control of the instruments.

FIGURE 21–11. A and B, Superior retraction of chorda tympani for visualization.

FIGURE 21–12. A to F, Incus replacement prosthesis.

References

1. Kessel J: Uber das Mobilisieren des Steigbugels durch Ausschneiden des Trommelfelles, Hammers und Amboss bei undurchgagikeit der Tuba. Arch Ohrenheilkd, 13: 69–88, 1878.
2. Boucheron E: La mobilisation de l'etrier et son procede operatoire. Union Med Can 46: 412–416, 1888.
3. Miot C: De la mobilisation de l'etrier. Rev Laryngol Otol Rhinol (Bord) 10: 49–54, 1890.
4. Faraci G: Importanza acustica e funzionale della mobilizzazione della staffa: Risultati di una nuova serie di operazioni. Arch Ital Otol Rinol Laringol 9: 209–221, 1899.
5. Passow KA: Operative anlegung einer offnung in die mediale pauken-hohlenwand bei stapesankylose. Ver Dtsch Otol Ges Versamml 6: 141, 1897.
6. Jack FL: Remarkable improvement of the hearing by removal of the stapes. Trans Am Otol Soc 284: 474–489, 1893.
7. Goodhill V: Stapes Surgery for Otosclerosis. New York, Paul B. Hoeber, 1961.
8. Siebenmann F: Traitement chirurgical de la sclerose otique. Cong Int Med Sec Otol 13: 170, 1900.
9. Moure EJ: De la mobilisation de l'etrier. Rev Laryngol Otol Rhinol (Bord) 7: 225, 1880.
10. Holmgren G: Some experiences in surgery of otosclerosis. Acta Otolaryngol (Stockh) 5: 460, 1923.
11. Sourdille M: New technique in the surgical treatment of severe and progressive deafness from otosclerosis. Bull NY Acad Med 13: 673, 1937.
12. Lempert J: Improvement in hearing in cases of otosclerosis: A new, one-stage surgical technic. Arch Otolaryngol Head Neck Surg 28: 42, 1938.
13. Rosen S: Restoration of hearing in otosclerosis by mobilization of the fixed stapedial footplate: An analysis of results. Laryngoscope 65: 224–269, 1955.
14. Shea J Jr: Fenestration of the oval window. Ann Otol Rhinol Laryngol 67: 932–951, 1958.

22

Stapedectomy: Use of Natural Material

J. V. D. Hough, M.D. ▪ Michael McGee, M.D.
R. Stanley Baker, M.D. ▪ Graham Bryce, M.D.

Despite 40 years of ever-improving technology and new techniques, there is still no universally accepted surgical technique for restoration of hearing in patients with stapedial otosclerosis. In view of the amazing, even perplexing, anatomic and pathologic differences the surgeon encounters in and around the oval window, it is perhaps best that we not adopt a single strategy. Fortunately, today's popular techniques, properly done, give similar excellent results. The total stapedectomy, partial stapedectomy, and stapedotomy techniques are at the forefront of today's surgical armamentarium. These three accomplish the essential requirements for long-term success; that is, they first open the oval window by removing enough of the footplate for unimpeded sound entry into the inner ear, and they provide effective sound conduction from the incus to the labyrinth by using an artificial prosthesis or by preserving the stapedial crura in a functional state. Each of these techniques seems to have unique and distinctive advantages applicable in certain circumstances, and under diverse anatomic and pathologic conditions.

We use all three of these techniques but predominantly perform a stapedectomy with preservation of the posterior crus while using a tragal perichondrial graft to seal the opening of the oval window. This method eliminates the need for an artificial prosthesis and the resultant complications caused by a foreign body.

The first stapedectomy with preservation of the posterior crus was done by the senior author (JVDH) quite by accident in 1956 while doing a stapes mobilization using the improved Fowler anterior crurotomy procedure.[1]

In this patient, as prescribed by the technique, the footplate had been transected and the anterior crus cut, thus liberating the posterior footplate, bypassing the anterior otosclerotic focus. But while a portion of the stump of the anterior crus was being removed, the entire anterior half of the footplate came out. Because there was no trauma to the labyrinth, the hearing result was excellent and remained so. From a surgical perspective, these results seemed good: the involved anterior portion of the footplate had been removed and the normal portion of the stapes preserved.

Total stapedectomy was also introduced during that year, but it required routine removal of the crural arch, necessitating the use of a prosthesis between the incus and the oval window. Since that time, much effort and frequent changes have been made by many surgeons trying to find the proper prosthesis to insert between the incus and the oval window. The proper choice of prosthesis to rebuild the ossicular chain is still debated.

Also during this time, we and others had been trying to find better techniques and instrumentation that allowed more frequent preservation and use of the posterior crus. We are now able to avoid using an artificial prosthesis by preserving the posterior crus in over 70 per cent of ears. We also believe that a diverse-technique approach is preferable to make use of the advantages of other methods in ears for which the posterior crus cannot be preserved.

The second most common technique we use is total stapedectomy with restoration of hearing using a homograft prosthesis. The process of microlathing the prothesis in the bone laboratory prior to surgery has reduced both time and expense. The end result is a precise, nonartificial homograft bone that looks like a factory-produced prosthesis, yet contains all the characteristics inherent in other homograft ossicles. It is well tolerated, does not cause incus erosion, is invaded by host osteocytes, and basically lasts for a lifetime. The results are very good. The technique is described later.

PATIENT SELECTION

The object of stapedial surgery is to improve the patient's hearing. This simple statement has important implications and, if applied, broadens the indications for stapedectomy. A surgeon should not withhold a chance for the patient to obtain improvement in hearing, provided that improvement is beneficial, and the procedure is not deleterious to the patient's well-being. The following conditions would *not* be exclusions or contraindications unless other medical, psychologic, or physical constraints make it impractical or unreasonable to do the surgical procedure.

1. Unilateral conductive impairment. (Binaural hearing is important!)
2. Age.
3. Profound hearing loss (i.e., speech reception threshold > 90 dB or discrimination < 10 per cent) with a significant detectable air-bone gap. (Many of these patients' hearing can be restored to acceptable levels with a hearing aid.)
4. Mild-to-moderate hearing loss. (e.g., a 30- to 35-dB speech reception threshold with a 12- to 15-dB air-bone gap in a patient requiring better hearing for job performance.)
5. Moderately severe hearing impairment with a good air-bone gap, but bone conduction indicating that the patient will still require hearing aids for good socially adequate hearing. (Functionally, many of these patients can be improved dramatically.)

SURGICAL TECHNIQUE

Surgical Preparation Room

Preoperative Medications (Use Routine Orders)

Sedation should be given 30 minutes prior to the surgical intervention. We use an analgesic, barbiturate, and atropine combination.

Surgical Preparation

The ear is not instrumented or cleaned before surgery. A hearing aid mold should not be used in the ear for 1 week prior to surgery. The ear is prepared with a povidone-iodine solution, or its equivalent, 20 minutes before surgery. The ear canal should be filled and the scalp scrubbed along with the face and neck in an area 3 inches in diameter around the ear canal. The ear is allowed to soak until draped and is irrigated later in the operating room.

During this time, an intravenous line is started with 5 per cent dextrose and Ringer's lactated solution. The hair is not shaved but is retracted to expose the ear and surrounding area for sterilization. The patient's clinic chart, as well as the hospital record, is with the patient and is carefully checked to verify the identifying information, such as correct ear for surgery, name, and allergies.

Operating Room Procedures

The patient is moved to the operating room and properly placed on the surgical table. It is important that the surgical table be an adjustable, motor-driven table. The controls should be on a panel at the head of the table, with control buttons easily palpable by the surgeon's fingers through the drapes. The table should be movable in three dimensions:

1. Up and down
2. Head up or down
3. Rotated from side to side (away from or toward the surgeon)

The latter direction is extremely important in allowing good visualization of the tympanic cavity anteriorly and posteriorly to accommodate the large variety of ear canal configurations encountered.

The patient's head is placed on a small, 2-inch-thick flat foam pillow with a 3-inch neck roll edge, which provides stability and comfort. Electrodes are attached, and cardiovascular and respiratory monitoring is established. Properly trained personnel are in constant attendance to observe the vital signs throughout the procedure. During this time, if the patient is observed to be unusually anxious, 5 mg of diazepam (Valium) is given intravenously at least 5 minutes before the first injection of the local anesthetic. Later, during the procedure, the dose may be repeated in 2.5 mg increments, up to a total of 10 mg for an adult. Ondansetron (Zofran), 4 mg intravenously, is given at the beginning of the procedure.

Draping

The patient is draped in the usual fashion with a complete body drape followed by a regional ear drape, leaving only the external ear exposed. The face of the patient should remain exposed under a canopy provided by a semicircular adjustable gooseneck arch, which is placed lateral to, and in front of, the head. This allows an attendant seated in front of the patient and opposite the surgical side of the table to see the patient's face, monitoring their reactions and reassuring them by verbal communication.

The patient's head should be almost flush with the end of the table, and the arm on the side toward the surgeon should be stretched slightly toward the knee to bring the shoulder down, thus increasing access to the ear.

Suction tubing is provided from a constant central vacuum source and passes through a surgeon-controlled foot pedal valve system (Hough-Cadogan foot pedal control) placed conveniently on the floor under the surgeon's foot. This allows the suction to be immediately stopped and the line exhausted. It also allows various degrees of intensity of the suction to be controlled by the foot pedal.

Preference in microscope design, flexibility, and lens distance is variable. We prefer a light, highly maneuverable microscope with a 200mm lens for stapes surgery and a 225mm lens for all other temporal bone surgery. When the microscope is brought into the field, it should be finally set so that the surgeon is in a comfortable position. The table, the microscope, and the rest of the materials should be brought to the surgeon so that he or she is not in an awkward position or stretching or reaching for the patient.

Anesthetic

Local anesthetic is preferred for all patients except children and unusually tense adults. In these, a general anesthetic is used.

The solution of local anesthetic is composed of 2 per cent lidocaine hydrochloride (Xylocaine) with 1:30,000 epinephrine with hyaluronidase (Wydase) added for perfusion. This mixture is administered through a 1 ml Luer-Lok syringe firmly attached to a 1½-inch, 25-gauge needle.

The first injection is introduced into the soft tissue just inside the superior canal area between the helix and the tragus, depositing approximately 0.2 ml of local anesthetic solution. Another injection is made in the inferior area of the canal just medial to the conchal cartilage.

The ear is then irrigated copiously to remove all antiseptic solution and debris. By the time this step is accomplished, the discomfort of the next two injections is much less noticeable. The next injection is more medial in the ear canal, superiorly in the vascular strip. This area is infiltrated with approximately 0.1 ml of local anesthetic solution. The infiltration should be seen lifting and slightly blanching the soft tissue to near the tympanic membrane. The last canal injection is inferiorly in the external canal just exterior to the junction of the thicker skin at the external orifice and the very thin skin over the bony external canal. This juncture is always clearly visible. The needle should penetrate the thicker skin near the juncture and be inserted to the bone so that blanching caused by subperiosteal infiltration can be clearly seen advancing deep toward the tympanic membrane. The placement of these last two injections is extremely important if good anesthesia and homostasis are to be obtained for successful surgery. Lastly, the dome of the tragus is injected subcutaneously with approximately 0.1 ml of local anesthetic solution.

The total anesthetic solution used ranges from 0.6 to 0.9 ml. The remainder of the solution in the syringe can be used later for topical anesthesia of the mucous membranes of the tympanic cavity.

A spatula can then be used to mold the flexible canal to facilitate insertion of the speculum. After the incision and flap elevation, the canal tissues will frequently be dilated enough by the speculum to allow the use of a larger speculum for more complete exposure of the tympanic cavity.

Incision and Elevation of the Tympanomeatal Flap

The incision is made with a Hough modification of the Rosen knife. The modification is simply a rounding off of the very acute–angle tip of the original Rosen knife. The incision is made by the sharp sides or leading edge of the knife and is done in a sweeping motion or occasionally in a guillotine-like cutting fashion. Because of the angle of the knife, the semilunar incision line is made with the limbs of the incision closer to the tympanic membrane both superiorly and inferiorly. The arch of the incision is made just medial to the area where there is a clear distinction between the thick lateral canal skin and the thin skin nearer the tympanic membrane. It is important to make the incisions completely through the skin, subcutaneous tissue, and periosteum.

Elevation of the tympanomeatal flap is usually made by carefully dissecting the periosteum off the bone, which is successfully done by using the same knife to scrape the periosteum off the bone down to the annular rim. A commercially prepared No. 3 preformed dental cotton ball rested against the elevated flap is helpful in protecting the flap and in maintaining a dry, clean field. If the tympanomeatal flap is dissected hard against the bone, the annulus of the tympanic membrane is not in danger of being overrun. Once it is identified, it should be elevated out of the sulcus tympanicus (at about the 9 o'clock position in the right ear and the 3 o'clock position in the left ear). The mucous membrane of the tympanic cavity usually separates at this point, but if not, it is incised with a pick in a sweeping motion, staying hard against the bone of the annulus. The tympanomeatal flap and tympanic membrane are elevated inferiorly to the 6 o'clock position and superiorly all the way to the notch of Rivinus (12 o'clock position).

Removal of the Posterosuperior Canal Bone to Expose the Oval Window

Usually, it is necessary to remove bone from the posterosuperior bony canal wall to properly visualize the oval window. The No. 3 dental cotton ball is again helpful and is placed inferiorly, holding the tympanomeatal flap anteriorly, and being in position to catch bone chips. With a serrated Hough curette, the edge of the curette is engaged along the bony margin. The notch of Rivinus usually makes an easy beginning point. With care taken to stay well above and away from the chorda, the bone is curetted by twisting motions counterclockwise, and the cutting pressure is directed posteriorly. If the bone is thick and dense, it is prudent to gradually thin it superiorly before finally cracking it off just superior to the chorda tympani. Contrary to initial perception, the chorda tympani is best preserved by curetting the bone with counterclockwise twists to crack the fragments against the nerve rather than elevating the nerve and curetting upward. Enough bone should be removed to visualize the stapedius tendon at its entry into the pyramidal eminence. In approximately 5 per cent of cases, the nerve must be sacrificed for exposure.

All bone chips are now removed, and the cotton ball previously placed inferiorly is removed. The tympanic cavity is now properly exposed. A drop or two of lidocaine is now applied to the mucosa of the oval window and provides instant topical anesthesia.

Examination of the structures of the middle ear is now done in a systematic fashion. Vascular structures, nerve elements, and ossicular variations, as well as the pathology producing the hearing impairment, must be carefully evaluated to allow proper choice of surgical techniques and possible variations.

The mobility of the ossicular chain should be tested, beginning with the malleus. Experience provides assurance in determining mobility or fixation. The lack of mobility of the incus may be misleading if the stapes is firmly fixed. Careful observation of the movements of the mucous membrane at the incudostapedial joint is helpful.

Evaluation of the Oval Window

The oval window is examined. Commonly seen primitive mesenchymal strands and cicatricial bands need to be removed. Frequently, mucosal vessels cross the footplate. These need to be severed so that adequate time for natural hemostasis can occur early in the procedure. However, mucous membrane should not be stripped from the footplate, because it later provides a natural holding blanket to keep the footplate fragments from falling into the labyrinth. More profuse bleeding can occur from larger blood vessels in the mucous membrane anterior to the oval window, and it is sometimes advantageous also to cut these vessels early.

A dehiscent facial nerve is commonly present superior to the oval window. Other than being careful not to penetrate or scrape it with sharp picks, it may be ignored. More rarely, the nerve bulges over the oval window to obscure portions of the field. Usually, it can be partially retracted or worked around for successful completion of the task.

Choice of Stapedial Procedures

Pathology and Anatomy of the Oval Window and Stapes

In approximately 80 per cent of ears, the otosclerotic pathology will be confined to the anterior footplate. In approximately 18 per cent, circumscribed otosclerosis will involve most of the footplate (biscuit-type otosclerosis with areas of the annular ligament still identifiable). In approximately 2 per cent, there will be diffuse obliterative otosclerosis (the oval window will be covered, and no identifiable annular ligament margins exist).

In our hands, all of the first group and most of the second are candidates for stapedectomy with preservation of the posterior crus. The diffuse obliterative otosclerosis group and some of the circumscribed, biscuit-type otosclerosis group may be primary candidates for a stapedectomy with a piston technique or the use of a nonossicle homograft stapes replacement technique.[5]

Before the oval window is opened or the superstructure of the stapes is cut or removed, the distance between the footplate and the incus is measured. This step prepares for any variation in the usual technique that might necessitate employing a prosthesis or a homograft bone transplant.

Certain anatomic restrictions or operative conditions may also make preservation of the posterior crus unwise, such as

1. An extremely narrow oval window niche. Frequently, on first observation this condition may seem to be an impossible barrier. The picture may change dramatically, however, once the stapedial arch is out of the oval window and the footplate is removed. Regardless of how narrow the oval window niche is, attempting to preserve the posterior crus does no harm. It can always be removed later during the procedure if it cannot be used. We *always* try to preserve the posterior crus until it is determined to be useless.

2. A stapes that lies at an acute angle against the promontory, making it difficult to reposition the posterior crus so that it will not be too adherent to the oval window margins or the promontory.

3. Surgical conditions described later.

Stapedial Surgery for Preservation of the Posterior Crus

Opening the Footplate

Usually, a thin portion of the footplate can be visualized. This area is opened by barely thrusting a fine pick through the bone in several places, preferably joining them with a fracture line (Fig. 22–1).

Note. This step should be done *before* cutting the tendon, cutting the crus, or otherwise manipulating the superstructure because any of these maneuvers may cause complete mobilization of the stapes, producing a floating footplate, whereupon further attempts to open the footplate with any downward pressure with instruments could be dangerous. Although rare, a floating footplate requires a surgical decision. One can (1) abandon further attempts and terminate the operation as a completed stapes mobilization; (2) attempt to remove the superstructure and drill out a pothole entry into the labyrinth on the promontory side of the oval window for removal of the footplate; or (3) use the laser to safely open the oval window.

If the footplate has circumscribed, biscuit-type otosclerosis (annular ligament can be identified), and it is palpated to be impenetrable by the pick, the superstructure

can be lifted out of the oval window and the entire footplate visualized for safer instrumentation. Usually, however, even when the footplate is thick, enough of it is visualized around the arch to allow the use of a small burr in one or more places even before removal of the superstructure.

Cutting the Anterior Crus

The anterior crus is sectioned high, preferably about one third of the distance from the stapedial head to the footplate. This is done with specially designed angulated bone-cutting forceps (crural nippers). In the past, sectioning had been done with scissors, whirlybirds, and motor-driven saws, but all of these are not nearly as uniformly successful or as safe as the nippers (Fig. 22–2).

Note. When the crural nippers are used, after the cut has been made, the tendency is to bring the forceps out laterally and inferiorly, which may fracture the remaining stapedial arch. Remember to move the instrument medially, anteriorly, and then inferiorly before bringing it out, which will fracture the anterior stump attached to the footplate but will not disturb the remaining arch.

Inadvertent fracture of the neck, arch, or posterior crus seems to occur most often as the anterior crus is being manipulated while being transected. One of the authors has found that this problem can be managed by using the HGM Argon Laser–otoprobe to cut the crus. The 0.2-mm laser fiber can be custom shaped to blindly palpate the anterior crus while it is transected with laser energy.

Cutting the Stapedial Tendon

Cutting the stapedial tendon may also be done with the laser but is usually done with Bellucci's scissors. The scissor blades should not reach downward and engage the posterior crus—often, the tendon is resting on the posterior crus (Fig. 22–3).

The primitive mesenchymal strands, heavy sheets of mucous membrane, and scar bands should now be removed with the laser or with curved and right-angle picks in a gentle, sweeping motion parallel to the posterior crus. This tissue may, if left alone, later cause fracture of the posterior crus or joint separation during manipulation.

Occasionally, a portion of the posterior crus may be hidden by the overhang of the pyramidal eminence. The pyramidal eminence may be easily shaved away with fenestration excavators for better exposure.

Cutting the Posterior Crus at the Footplate

The earlier steps all have been taken in systematic order for specific reasons. Until now, it has been important that the arch remain attached to the footplate to prevent floating, and that it not be twisted so that the posterior crus could be prematurely fractured in the wrong place, making it too short.

Now the posterior crus is to be separated from the footplate. The whirlybird instrument is placed under the crural arch in the obturator foramen. According to the patient's anatomy, it may be inserted either on the facial nerve side or on the promontory side of the arch. The blade of the instrument is passed inside the arch and onto the

FIGURE 22–1

FIGURE 22–2

FIGURE 22–3

FIGURE 22–4

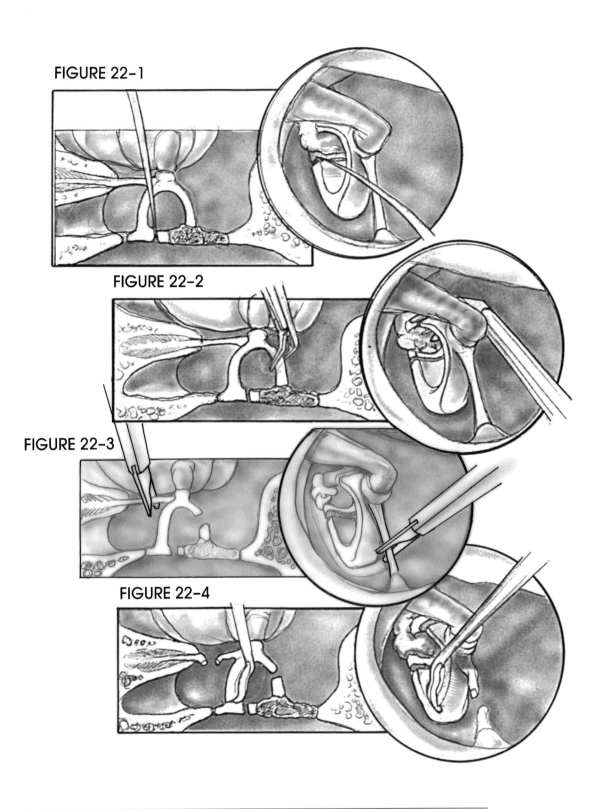

FIGURE 22–1. Opening the footplate.

FIGURE 22–2. Anterior crurotomy.

FIGURE 22–3. Cutting the stapedial tendon.

FIGURE 22–4. Cutting the posterior crus with a whirlybird.

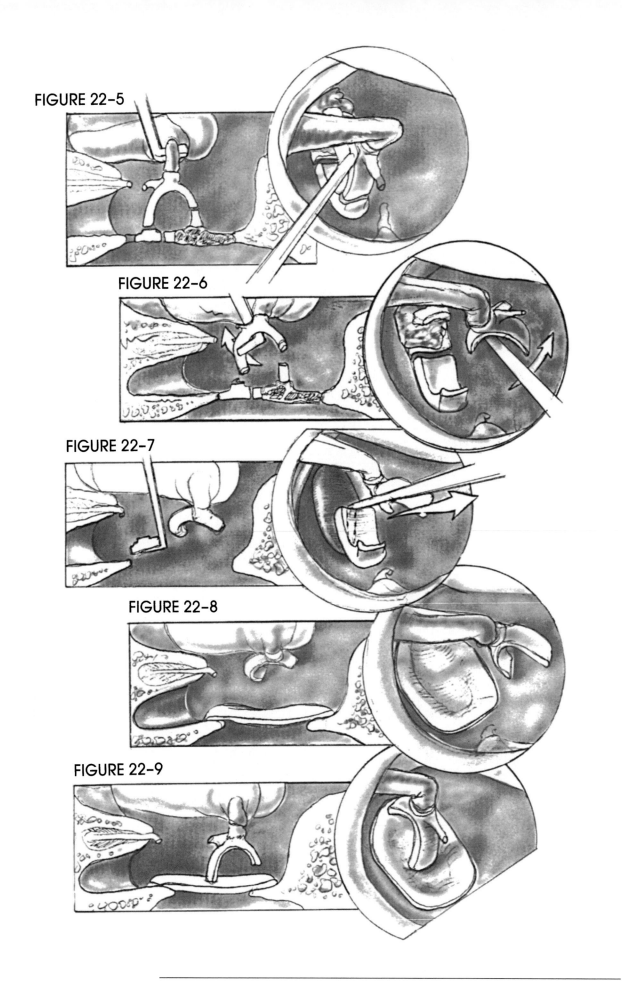

FIGURE 22–5

FIGURE 22–6

FIGURE 22–7

FIGURE 22–8

FIGURE 22–9

FIGURES 22–5 to 22–9. *See legends on opposite page*

footplate. It is moved along the footplate posteriorly until it encounters the posterior crus (Fig. 22–4). This portion may or may not be visualized. With the blade of the whirlybird flush against the footplate and pushing firmly in a posterior direction against the posterior crus, a twisting motion is made, which will fracture the posterior crus at the footplate. The posterior crus can be easily palpated and cut, even blindly, by this maneuver. Fortunately, the posterior crus has its weakest, most cancellous bone at the footplate and is therefore most likely to fracture at the desired point. Even if it should fracture so that the posterior crus is only three fourths its normal length, it can still be used successfully. Long-term results with a shortened crus are still highly successful, as discussed later.

Lifting the Posterior Crus and Resting It on the Inferoposterior Promontory

Lifting the posterior crus and resting it on the inferoposterior promontory is the most delicate maneuver of the technique and is perhaps the reason most surgeons do not attempt the procedure. Once mastered, however, it quickly becomes a worthwhile routine.

Before attempting to lift the crus out of the oval window, it is important that all adhesions and binding mucous membrane be removed from the posterior crus. A right-angle excavator (Hough's hoe) is now placed under the incus and lifted laterally to test the stiffness of the incudal joints and ligaments (Fig. 22–5). Watching the posterior crus, the surgeon lifts the incus slightly laterally to cause some flexibility in joints that have been chronically out of use. Be careful that binding mucous membrane does not hold the stapedial arch down, causing a separation of the incudostapedial joint during this maneuver. The right-angle excavator is then placed in the obturator foramen under the neck of the stapes. Depending on the anatomy, it may be engaged under the arch, either on the superior or inferior surface of the arch. With firm, steady, continuous pressure, the arch is then lifted out gently and rotated so that the posterior stapedial crus clears the promontory and rests on its posterior slope (Fig. 22–6).

The exposure of the oval window is now excellent. Because the incus has been retracted slightly laterally and the arch is completely out of the oval window, the exposure of the oval window and footplate is definitely more complete than with any other stapedectomy or stapedotomy technique.

The two advantages to preserving the arch in this manner are that it provides

1. Better visualization of the entire oval window
2. Possible use of the posterior crus rather than a prosthesis

Obtaining the Perichondrial Graft

Rationale

The use of tragal perichondrium to seal the oval window has been an excellent contribution to stapedial surgery since Goodhill described it in 1961.[3] We have used it in thousands of ears, and its record of successful results has been repeated by many other otologists. Of significance is the fact that we have not encountered a single incident of long- or short-term postoperative fistulas when it has been used. Some of the advantages of its use in stapedial surgery are

1. It is already in the field. One does not need to change to another body site to obtain a graft. Therefore, the procedure saves time and reduces the chances of contamination.
2. It is histologically akin to the normal inhabitants of the oval window.
3. It forms a natural little "boat" that nestles down in the oval window for an excellent fit.
4. Because of its boat or "tray" edges in the oval window, it naturally centers the posterior crus so that it will not drift or adhere to the bony margins of the oval window, thus preventing refixation.
5. It can be made extremely thin for ears with a very narrow oval window niche. The graft can easily be thinned with scissors and placed in an absorbable gelatin sponge (Gelfoam) press. Also, it can be left thick for ears in which the preserved posterior crus fractures high and is short (not quite full length).

Surgical Technique for Removal of Perichondrium

If the tragus is pushed forward with the thumb, the dome of the tragus is outlined through the skin. With a scalpel, an incision is made over the dome of the tragal cartilage. The edge of the incision is grasped with thumb forceps and retracted forward. With curved scissors, the soft tissue is dissected to the dome of the tragal cartilage. If the scissors are used in a penetrating, spreading manner, soft tissue is dissected away from the perichondrium on both sides of the tragus, approximately 1 cm. The tragus is then grasped in the thumb forceps while the dome of the tragal cartilage with its perichondrium is removed with curved iris scissors. To prevent hematoma, the external wound is closed with only one silk suture.

The cartilage and perichondrial tissue are placed on a polytetrafluoroethylene (Teflon) disk. With the whirlybird, the cartilage is broken away in pieces and cleanly removed from the perichondrium. With curved scissors, the graft is cleared of all useless soft tissue, thinned, and cut for the size of the oval window. If the niche is narrow, the graft

---

FIGURE 22–5. Lifting the incus.

FIGURE 22–6. Lifting the posterior crus out of the oval window arch to the promontory.

FIGURE 22–7. Removing the footplate.

FIGURE 22–8. Sealing the oval window with perichondrial graft.

FIGURE 22–9. Replacing the posterior crus in the oval window.

may be pressed in a House gelatin sponge press, which will facilitate the use of the posterior crus or a prosthesis in a narrow space.

The graft is usually placed on the promontory at this time, to be ready for closing the oval window once the procedures in the oval window have been accomplished.

Removal of the Footplate of the Stapes

A small, right-angle 0.3-mm pick is inserted through the fracture line of the footplate. It should be inserted only deep enough to engage the medial surface of the footplate. Usually, the pick can be visualized through the bone. The point of the pick is usually turned to point posteriorly. A fragment of bone is then lifted out. If only a small segment of bone is removed, a right-angle excavator (Hough's hoe) is then used to remove the remainder of the footplate. This instrument has a flat surface and is not sharp on the tip or along its edges, thus making it the safest instrument to use below the footplate.

Occasionally, the entire half of the posterior footplate is removed cleanly from the oval window in one piece (Fig. 22–7). Even though the entire posterior edge of the oval window may not be visible, the rim of the footplate is identifiable as it is removed, and one is assured of clean and complete removal. Removal of as much of the footplate as can be easily extracted is accomplished using this instrument. Remember not to insert the instrument deeper than is necessary to engage the medial surface of the footplate. Also, do not pick at the edges of the footplate, because this may cause it to loosen en masse and to tumble into the labyrinth. Rather, try to remove as much as will easily lift out of the window by engaging the full right-angle surface of the excavator. On occasion, a very hard, trapped anterior portion of the footplate may be left in place so that the labyrinth is not traumatized by attempted forceful removal. Fragments of the footplate that have been lifted out of the oval window are then extracted by the use of forceps or suction. The variable on/off control of suction is extremely important in removing fluid, blood, and footplate fragments in the oval window niche. This can be done safely only by using suction that is controlled by the surgeon's foot, that is, the foot-pedal suction control (i.e., Hough-Cadogan foot-pedal suction).

Sealing the Oval Window with the Perichondrial Graft

After the oval window has been cleared of footplate fragments, the perichondrial graft is moved into the niche from its anterior end. This perichondrial dome of the tragus makes a perfect boat that nestles down to seal the oval window. Fortunately, its tray edges also center the posterior crus in the window, preventing refixation (Fig. 22–8).

Replacing the Posterior Crus in the Oval Window

With a right-angle excavator, the posterior crus is carefully lifted back into the oval window niche and placed in the center, or the widest portion, of the oval window. It is lifted back just as it was lifted out with the excavator under

the arch (Fig. 22–9). The crus can then be moved toward the center by placing the excavator under the bony projection provided by the insertion of the stapedius tendon on the posterior rim of the crus.

Occasionally, the graft may be tucked behind the crus to prevent it from drifting posteriorly. The incudostapedial joint may become somewhat loose during the various proceeding manipulations, and occasionally it is necessary to lift the incus and the stapedial arch simultaneously in a two-handed maneuver.

The techniques we use when the posterior crus fractures too high or the incudostapedial joint is completely disrupted are discussed later.

Replacement of the Tympanic Membrane and Canal Packing

The tympanic membrane and tympanomeatal flap are replaced so that the incision lines are reapproximated. Gelatin sponge strips soaked with physiologic solution (Physiosol) are placed over the incision lines, and an expandable cellulose wick (a Pope wick) is placed in the ear canal. A cotton ball covered with cortisone ointment is then used to occlude the ear canal, and another cotton ball is placed in the concha. No other head dressing need be used.

Conditions in Which the Posterior Crus Cannot Be Preserved

1. FRACTURE OF THE POSTERIOR CRUS CAUSING A SHORT CRUS.
   In this event, the posterior crus is anatomically not reasonable to use or is fractured too high to remain useful. However, if it is two thirds to three fourths its normal length, it is not always considered useless. When the arch is rotated forward toward the center of the oval window, it gains length by its rotation and can usually be used. Furthermore, the perichondrial graft can be left somewhat thicker so that the membranous oval window is higher postoperatively. Our statistical results among these patients indicate that there is no sacrifice of benefit and that hearing perception is equal to that of patients with normal-length crura.[4, 5]

2. INCUDOSTAPEDIAL JOINT SEPARATION OR PROBLEMS CAUSING DELIBERATE REMOVAL OF THE STAPEDIAL SUPERSTRUCTURE.
   Unfortunately, incudostapedial joint separation from manipulation of the arch or anatomic conditions causing removal of the arch can occur, necessitating treatment alternatives. These conditions occur in approximately 4 per cent of ears.

For years, the senior author (JVDH) resorted to artificial prostheses of various types in these cases, but only if the loose stapes and the joint could not be replaced. However, once the incudostapedial joint was dislocated, it was difficult to manipulate the posterior crus and the head of the stapes back into position.

Use of Homograft Transplants in Stapedial Surgery

Both the problems of joint separation and fracture of the stapedial arch have now been solved by the use of a sculptured homograft bone transplant. During the past several years, when irreparable joint separation or undesirable crural fracture occurs, a sculptured bone implant has been used. Since the technique of sculpturing homograft bone was developed by McGee[5] and refined by Bryce, this transplant is now used more often. The convenience and usefulness of this sculptured homograft has accelerated the use of natural materials in recent years.[5]

Initially, dense perilabyrinthine bone or nonpneumatized mastoid and petrous apex bone were used as transplant material.[5] These protheses were totally sculptured by hand. The shape was similar to a Robinson prosthesis without the bucket handle. This sculptured bone graft, without the handle, provided an ossicular replacement more easily used, with less trauma, than any artificial stapedial prosthesis in the surgical armamentarium. It required no crimping or other manipulation to attach it to the incus. It simply fit underneath the lenticular process. The use of perilabyrinthine or nonpneumatized temporal bone provided approximately 20 or more protheses per temporal bone.

In August 1992, two important changes were made that increased efficiency as well as decreased expenses. We began using cortical bone (femur) obtained from the American Red Cross, which reduced expenses drastically by allowing hundreds of prostheses to be made from each bone. Also, the discovery of the microlathing process reduced manufacturing time.

The homograft ossicle stapes prosthesis we use today still looks like a Robinson prosthesis without the bucket handle (Fig. 22–10). From a tiny section of homograft femur, the piston-shaped implant is microscopically sculptured using a lathe (Dremel drill), which holds and rotates the bone, and a conventional mastoid drill with a diamond burr. This sculpturing produces a precisely designed and measured natural tissue implant to be kept in the operating room bone bank ready for use.

These precision-shaped, carefully measured transplants are easily inserted after the oval window has been covered

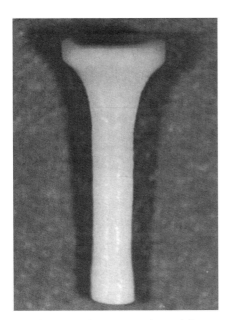

FIGURE 22–10. Stapes replacement sculptured from nonossicular homograft cortical bone.

with the perichondrial graft. The tip of the implant shaft is placed in the center of the oval window, and the implant is rotated so that the cup rests under the proximal portion of the long process of the incus (near the body of the incus). With a pick, the cup end of the homograft transplant is then depressed slightly into the oval window as the cup is moved inferiorly. Finally, it is fitted into place with the cup securely under the lenticular process of the incus. Gelatin sponge is not required to hold it in place.

This use of homograft bone has allowed us to use almost no artificial foreign material in stapedial surgery, except in diffuse obliterative otosclerosis (in approximately 2 per cent of ears). In these, a stainless-steel piston is used.

Management of Extensive Stapedial Otosclerosis

Circumscribed Otosclerosis (Biscuit-Type)

Circumscribed biscuit-type otosclerosis is distinguished by very thick, sometimes soft, biscuit-like otosclerosis confined to the footplate and involving the oval window margin only in a restricted area. The annular ligament area is usually clearly identifiable around the bulging footplate. We have found that the footplate can be transected with a pick or a fine drill in most of these ears. The biscuit footplate frequently rolls out completely in two large pieces, and the technique of posterior crus preservation can usually be carried out as routinely planned, or the sculptured homograft procedure discussed earlier is used. Regrowth and refixation are rare in patients with this pathology.[2, 4, 6]

Diffuse Obliterative Otosclerosis

Diffuse obliterative otosclerosis occurs in approximately 2 per cent of ears in North America. This pathologic process produces massive involvement of the entire footplate, annular ligament, and surrounding labyrinthine capsule. In contradistinction to circumscribed biscuit-type otosclerosis, diffuse obliterative otosclerosis leaves no annular ligament visible, even when the bone in the area is drilled away.

In the early history of stapedectomy, most surgeons recreated the oval window with a massive drill-out procedure, followed by the use of a prosthesis. Due to excessive labyrinthine trauma and bone regrowth, results were unsatisfactory.

The use of a metal piston prosthesis is now the procedure of choice. In our view, this condition is the only one for which the use of an artificial prosthesis in performing primary stapedectomy procedures is preferred.

The procedure begins the same as described earlier. After laying aside the crural arch with the crus on the promontory, the incus is held slightly laterally. When diffuse obliterative otosclerosis is identified, a shaft of 0.7 mm in diameter is slowly drilled into the labyrinth. The drill must be a microdrill designed for work in the tympanic cavity (e.g., Skeeter or Kerr drill). A diamond burr measuring 0.7 mm in diameter is used. The shaft or the hole into the labyrinth should be placed slightly inferior and posterior to the center of the footplate. If the bone is thicker than 1 to

1.5 mm, the operation should be terminated because the anatomic position of the labyrinthine structures may be obscure. We commonly use a 0.6-mm stainless-steel piston long enough to extend 0.25 mm into the labyrinth. Soft tissue is used to surround the shaft in the oval window.[2, 4, 6]

Postoperative Care

The inner cellulose wick and gelatin sponge are removed from the canal 5 days to 1 week postoperatively. Usually, the blood clot and gelatin sponge adhere to the wick, and the extraction is easily done. Suction may be used along the anterior canal wall to remove excessive fluids, but it is unnecessary to remove all the gelatin sponge. The hearing is then tested, and the patient is instructed to return for evaluation at 6 weeks, 6 months, and then every 2 years thereafter.

Results Using the Posterior Crus Preservation Technique

Over the past 40 years, results using the posterior crus preservation technique in several large series have been reported by the senior author (JVDH).[1, 2, 4, 5, 7] Good results with few complications have been the consistent findings. Results at 6 months or longer postoperatively show that

1. Approximately 90 to 95 per cent of patients closed the air-bone gap to within 10 dB of the preoperative bone conduction threshold in the three speech frequencies.

2. Eighty per cent overclosed or totally closed the air-bone gap. Overclosure simply represents recapture of the Carhart notch and probably does not represent actual improvement in inner ear cochlear function. Nevertheless, overclosure is important. In our opinion, this represents an added physiologic advantage in the preservation of normal tissues, which allows

    a. Maintenance of the normal incudostapedial joint.

    b. Firm normal tissue attachment of the stapedial crus to the soft tissues over the oval window.

3. The hearing was made worse from a slight 10-dB loss to profound loss of hearing in all the series in fewer than 1 per cent of cases. The total loss of useful hearing (loss of discrimination of ≥50 per cent) occurred an average of less than 0.25 per cent. These results are unsurpassed by any other stapedectomy or stapedotomy technique reported.

Use of Homograft Replacements

When the posterior crus cannot be used, we believe that the use of natural human materials is still the best option.

The results from the use of refined sculptured homograft bone transplants have been equally gratifying. Closure of the air-bone gap to within 10 dB of the preoperative bone conduction still occurs in over 90 per cent of cases, and overclosure of the air-bone gap is approximately 5 to 10 per cent less, but still equal to or better than that of other procedures using artificial materials.[2, 6]

SUMMARY

Depending on the dexterity, effort, and experience of the surgeon, human material can be used to reconstruct the ossicular chain in over 95 per cent of ears requiring stapedectomy. The benefits are the following:

1. No foreign body reaction, thus preventing soft tissue reaction in the oval window and bone erosion of the incus caused by artificial materials.

2. Better exposure. Excellent surgical exposure of the oval window is obtained without removal of the normal stapedial arch.

3. Better healing. More physiologic healing occurs at the oval window, and the normal incudostapedial joint is maintained.

4. Good results. In thousands of ears and in repeated series of cases reported, the short-term and long-term results with this technique are not excelled, and usually not equalled, by other techniques reported in the scientific literature.

5. We find that this technique, once mastered, can be accomplished more rapidly and with less effort.

6. Cost effectiveness. Because this technique seldom requires expensive adjunct equipment, such as drills and lasers, and seldom uses an artificial prosthesis, it is always more cost-effective.

References

1. Hough JVD: Partial stapedectomy. Ann Otol Rhinol Laryngol 69: 571, 1960.
2. Hough JVD: A critique of stapedectomy. J Laryngol Otol 90: 15, 1976.
3. Goodhill V: Tragal perichondrium as oval window graft. Laryngoscope 71: 975, 1961.
4. Hough JVD: Otosclerosis: The method of JVD Hough, MD. *In* Gates GA (ed): Current Therapy in Otolaryngology—Head and Neck Surgery, 1982–83. BC Decker, 1982, pp 24–30.
5. McGee M: Non-ossicle homograft bone prosthesis in the middle ear: II. Laryngoscope 100: 10 (Pt 2) (Suppl 51), 1990.
6. Hough JVD: Operative treatment for otosclerosis: Stapedectomy with preservation of the posterior crus and the use of perichondrial graft over the oval window. *In* Snow JB (ed): Controversy in Otolaryngology. Philadelphia, WB Saunders, 1980, pp 266–280.
7. Hough JVD: Ten-year results with stapedectomy. Panel presentation, Annual Meeting of the American College of Surgeons, San Francisco, CA, October 9, 1969.

23

Laser Stapedotomy

Rodney Perkins, M.D.

A new era in the treatment of otosclerosis began in 1956 when the stapedectomy procedure was introduced by John Shea.[1] Since then, variation from the original technique has occurred in three major areas: the design of the prosthesis, the nature of the oval window seal, and the small-fenestra technique. One only need look in an otologic prosthesis catalog to see the wide variation in design and materials used in prostheses for connecting the incus with the peri-lymphatic fluids of the vestibule. The literature from the past three decades is replete with reports of various bioma-terials (e.g., vein, perichondrium, fascia, absorbable gelatin sponge, and fat) that have been used to seal the oval window area. Although these variations in prosthesis de-sign and seal material have contributed to improvement of the original procedure, the development of the small-fenestration concept has probably been the most important variant of the stapedectomy procedure for otosclerosis.

The small-fenestra technique was primarily championed by European otologists during the 1970s. This technique involved careful manual dissection of a small hole in the footplate and the subsequent placement of a piston-type prosthesis in the created fenestra. The primary advantage of this procedure was that it minimized iatrogenic trauma to the inner ear and reduced the incidence of the prosthesis becoming malpositioned as a result of postoperative heal-ing dynamics or of being engulfed by scar tissue, which commonly fills the oval window niche after manual stape-dectomy. However, the technique had problems: it required an excellent technician to effect the procedure successfully, and it was not always possible to create a uniform circular fenestra because of the tendency of the footplate to crack, a circumstance that would, in some cases, force removal of the entire footplate.

As a result of observing the small-fenestra technique performed by skilled European otologists (Fisch, Marquet, and Smyth), I began to develop a technique to facilitate making a fenestra atraumatically and, in September 1978, performed the first laser stapedotomy.[2] This procedure has proved to be exceptionally safe and efficacious; although it has been refined, it is performed similarly today.

PREOPERATIVE PREPARATION

The laser stapedotomy procedure is done under local anes-thesia on an outpatient basis. To perform otologic surgery successfully with the patient under local anesthesia, the surgeon, the patient, and the operating room must be prop-erly prepared.

Surgeon Preparation

In addition to being familiar with the classic techniques of otosclerosis surgery, the surgeon must become familiar with the laser, its biologic characteristics, beam manipula-tion to achieve various surgical effects, and safety measures that protect the patient and operating room personnel. Otol-ogists planning to use the laser in otosclerosis surgery and other otologic surgery should take an appropriate training course and practice using the laser on temporal bone speci-mens prior to clinical application.

Microscope Preparation

It is crucial to set up the operating microscope and the laser in the following manner before laser stapedotomy when a microscope-mounted beam delivery system, such as the Microbeam device from Laserscope, is used. The following procedure makes the microscope parfocal, allowing the focus of the optical plane to remain the same when magnification is changed. When this procedure is followed by the laser preparation described later, the focus of the laser beam and that of the optical plane remain the same through changes in magnification. Otherwise, the laser spot will not be in focus at the optical plane, and the energy will not be appropriately delivered. In addition, these procedures ensure that the laser beam will have diminished energy density after the focal point, giving increased safety to the procedure.

Parfocal Procedure

- Position the microscope above a flat, stationary surface.
- Using a pen or pencil, make a dot on a piece of white paper to serve as a focus target and place it in the center of the illuminated field of the microscope.
- After adjusting both eyepiece diopter settings to "0," set the microscope fine-focus controls so that they are at the approximate midpoint of the fine-focus range.
- Advance the microscope to its highest magnification setting and focus, using the fine-focus control until a sharp image of the dot is obtained.
- Being careful not to shift microscope position, change the magnification setting to its lowest position, focus left and right eyepieces, *one at a time*, with the opposite eye closed, by turning the diopter rings. When these settings can be repeated to within one-quarter diopter, you may wish to record these settings for future use with this microscope.

Laser Preparation

- Identify the spot-size adjustment knob on the right side of the Laserscope Microbeam microscope adapter. Turn it fully counterclockwise (toward the user) to the minimum spot setting.
- Check that the system status on the video display screen is "ready" and that power and duration are at the minimum setting.
- Press the foot switch halfway down to activate the aiming beam.
- Identify the focus adjustment knob on the back of the adapter. Look through the microscope, and turn the focus adjustment knob either clockwise or counterclockwise until the aiming beam spot is as small as possible.
- The microscope and the laser are now parfocal together.

Patient Preparation

There are two components of patient preparation for otologic surgery performed under local anesthesia: psychologic and pharmacologic.

Psychologic

To reduce anxiety and create rapport, the surgeon should give the patient a full explanation of the procedure and its objectives, benefits, and risks. In addition, a surgical nurse or medical assistant should explain what will happen to the patient in the operating room by describing such elements as the operating room environment, use of an intravenous line for medication delivery, placement of monitor electrodes, and draping. By informing the patient and making him or her part of the process, the physician and nurse will reduce anxiety and ensure cooperation and less bleeding. Beyond the technical advantages achieved by such preparation, there is an ethical responsibility to inform the patient. In addition, the likelihood of the patient becoming litigious as a result of a poor outcome is markedly reduced if he or she has been informed of the procedure and the risks and benefits and has had an opportunity to discuss them with the surgeon before surgery.

Pharmacologic

The chemical preparation of the patient can be achieved in many ways. The pharmaceutic agents that I have employed have worked for me, but many premedication regimens will achieve a similar result.

In the average adult, I give pentobarbital (Nembutal), 150 mg, orally 1 hour prior to surgery. One half hour prior to surgery, meperidine (Demerol), 75 mg, and diazepam (Valium), 10 mg, are given by intramuscular injection. An intravenous catheter is started in the arm opposite the operative ear before the patient arrives in the operating room, and dextrose 5% in Ringer's solution is started with a Volutrol. Unless the patient appears very sedated, an additional 25 mg of meperidine is placed in the Volutrol and infused slowly over 30 to 45 minutes. In addition, patients receive penicillin VK, 250 mg, or another appropriate antibiotic 1 hour before surgery.

General anesthesia is contraindicated in otosclerosis surgery in mentally competent adult patients for four primary reasons. First, the surgeon should avoid unnecessary exposure of the patient to the risks of anesthesia. Second, in the fully anesthetized patient, there is no indication of cochleovestibular trauma occurring during the procedure, whereas in the sedated but awake patient, stimulation of the vestibular system during the procedure evokes nausea or subjective dizziness, which is usually reported by the patient immediately. This is a valuable early warning to desist from whatever manipulation is evoking the response. Third, vomiting in the postoperative period is more likely after general anesthesia. Although vomiting may have no effect on the ultimate outcome of the procedure, the increased cerebrospinal fluid and intracochlear pressures that would likely accompany vomiting may force development of a perilymphatic fistula. However, this concern is higher in conventional manual stapedectomy than in the laser stapedotomy procedure described here because there is an extremely good fit of the prosthesis of the fenestra and an excellent biologic seal. A fourth consideration is the cost of general anesthesia. In this procedure, general anesthesia is unnecessary and hence an additional financial burden on an already expensive health care system.

Site Preparation

The auricle and periauricular area are scrubbed with povidone-iodine (Betadine) solution. A plastic drape is placed over the area, with the auricle exteriorized through the opening in the drape. This drape is placed over an L-shaped bar that is fixed in the rail attachment of the operating table (Fig. 23–1). Attached to the bar is a small, low-volume office fan that provides a gentle cooling breeze to the patient's face during the procedure. The plastic drape forms a canopy, allowing the patient to see from under the drape and reducing the feeling of claustrophobia. In addition, a foam ear piece from a speaker is inserted into the opposite ear. This ear piece is connected to a compact disk

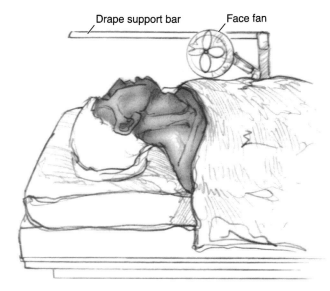

FIGURE 23–1. The drape support bar and face fan.

player and input microphone that allows the patient to listen to relaxing music and provides a pathway to converse with the patient if this is necessary. The dorsum of the ipsilateral hand is scrubbed with povidone-iodine solution and draped in preparation for the harvest of a vein graft later in the procedure.

Analgesia

It is important not only to achieve analgesia but also to maximize canal hemostasis with injections into the external auditory meatus. By using 2 per cent lidocaine (Xylocaine) with 1:20,000 epinephrine solution in a ringed syringe with a 27-gauge needle, a classic four-quadrant approach is used such that each injection falls within the wheal of the previous injection. I have also found an anterior canal injection useful; this is done with the bevel of the needle parallel to the bony wall of the external meatus (Fig. 23–2). After the needle is inserted, it is advanced a few millimeters, and 1 or 2 drops of the solution is injected extremely slowly. The solution infiltrates medially along the anterior canal wall and adds to the hemostasis in the anterior extent of the tympanomeatal incision.

OPERATIVE TECHNIQUE

The ear canal is cleansed of wax and epithelial debris and irrigated with povidone-iodine solution. Through as large an oval-beveled speculum as possible, incisions for a tympanomeatal flap are created. The initial incision is made with a sickle knife just lateral to the inferior annulus of the tympanic membrane at the 6 o'clock location and brought laterally along the floor of the canal approximately 4 mm. A second incision is made with a 2-mm round canal knife beginning at the lateral extent of the initial incision and extending in a curvilinear manner, first posteriorly and then anterosuperiorly until it terminates about 2 mm above the pars flaccida. This second incision is made in multiple small segments. Each segment is composed of an initial crushing application of the knife into the canal skin and a subsequent cutting action that connects that small segment with the previously cut segment. The crushing portion of this action seems to impart additional hemostasis. An additional advantage of making this incision in multiple small segments is that it eliminates the tendency of the tissue to tear, especially in patients in whom the superior medial canal skin is thick.

Through the use of a small round or lancet knife, the described skin flap is elevated progressively and equally toward the annulus. While the knife edge is kept tight to the bone, the fibrocartilaginous annulus is elevated from the bony sulcus. The investing tympanic cavity mucosa is torn with a blunted curved needle, and care is taken to identify and preserve the chorda tympani nerve. The tympanomeatal flap is then folded anteriorly, revealing the posterior tympanic cavity (Fig. 23–3). The superior portion of the manubrium of the malleus should be visible.

The malleus is palpated with a blunt, curved needle to assess the mobility of the malleus and incus and to rule out fixation of these ossicles as a cause for the conductive

impairment. The stapes is palpated as a preliminary confirmation of the diagnosis. The middle ear is inspected, with particular attention to the round window area, which may be obliterated in cases of extensive otosclerosis. A small amount of 2 per cent lidocaine with 1:20,000 epinephrine is infused into the middle ear and then immediately aspirated. This infusion provides analgesia to the sensory distribution in the middle ear space, and the rapid aspiration of the excess mitigates its potential absorption through the round window membrane, which might cause a temporary paresis of vestibular function and vertigo.

A sharp double-ended curette is used to remove an adequate amount of the posterosuperior medial canal wall bone (scutum) to give a satisfactory view of the stapes and the pyramidal process. In laser stapedotomy, it is sometimes advisable to curette slightly more bone than in conventional stapedectomy to provide an unobstructed pathway for the laser beam. The initial curettage should be lateral to the edge of the scutum (Fig. 23–4). Creating a furrow lateral to the edge of the scutum allows the surgeon to protect the incus from inadvertent disarticulation during the portion of the curettage when more pressure is applied to the curette (Fig. 23–5). Adequate scutum removal has been attained when the pyramidal process can be seen.

The stapes is inspected and palpated, and the diagnosis of otosclerosis is confirmed. The chorda tympani nerve is separated from the medial surface of the manubrium of the malleus with a curved needle or joint knife (Fig. 23–6). This maneuver allows any stretching of the chorda tympani nerve that might be necessary to be distributed along the full course of the intratympanic chorda tympani rather than only between the manubrial attachment and the iter chordae posterius, through which it emerges into the tympanic cavity. Any dehiscence in the bony covering of the facial nerve immediately above the stapes is noted. If mucosal adhesions are present between the promontory or facial nerve and the stapes, they are vaporized by slightly defocusing the minimally focused beam, using 100-msec bursts of about 2 W of the potassium titanyl phosphate crystal (KTP)/532 laser. Although these adhesions could be interrupted with a small pick, the laser is less likely to cause bleeding because of its coagulating characteristics.

A measurement is made of the distance between the footplate and the medial surface of the lower portion of the long process of the incus to select a prosthesis of appropriate length (Fig. 23–7). Although some surgeons make this measurement after the superstructure of the stapes has been removed, it is more accurately made before disarticulating the incudostapedial joint because this is the undisturbed natural position of the incus. To accommodate the entrance of the prosthesis slightly into the vestibule, 0.25 to 0.5 mm should be added to this measured distance for prosthesis length. If there appears to be reasonable access to the footplate, a stainless-steel bucket-handle prosthesis with a piston diameter of 0.8 mm is selected (Fig. 23–8). However, if a large facial nerve overhang or a narrow niche or other anatomic variation exists that compromises the surgeon's ability to see a large amount of footplate, selecting a 0.6-mm-diameter prosthesis may be advisable.

The tympanomeatal flap is placed back into position loosely to decrease mucosal drying and to prevent blood

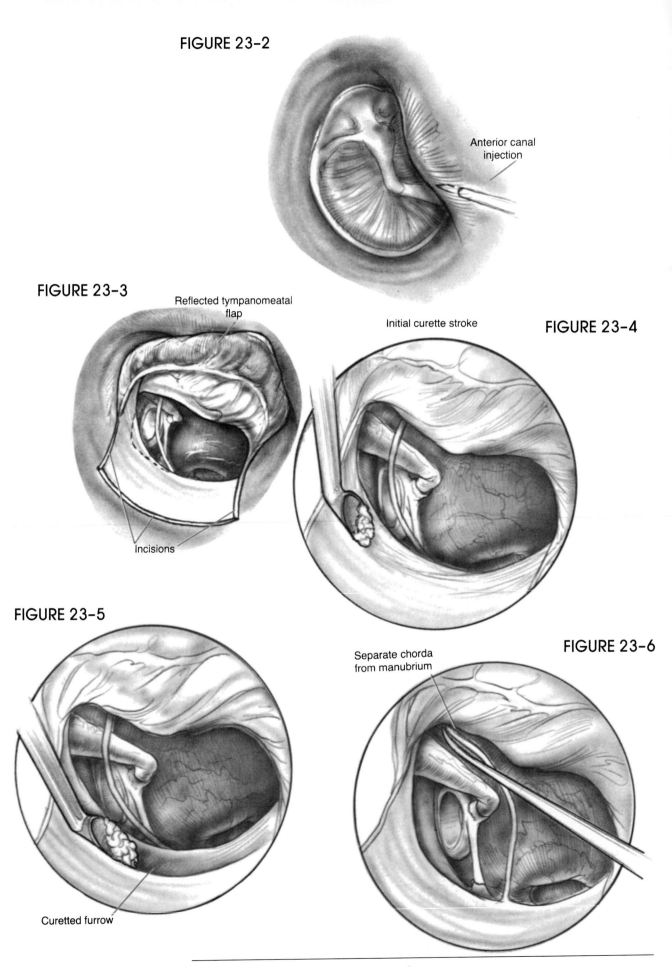

FIGURE 23-2

Anterior canal injection

FIGURE 23-3

Reflected tympanomeatal flap

Incisions

FIGURE 23-4

Initial curette stroke

FIGURE 23-5

Curetted furrow

FIGURE 23-6

Separate chorda from manubrium

FIGURES 23-2 to 23-6. *See legends on opposite page*

from entering the middle ear while a segment of vein is harvested from the hand. Attention is turned to the prepared dorsum of the ipsilateral hand, and the povidone-iodine residue is removed with a moist sponge. If the superficial venous structure is not readily visible, the surgeon may bring these into view by tightly grasping the patient's wrist to obstruct venous return. A venous segment is identified within 2 cm of the knuckles. Care is taken to avoid an incision too close to the knuckle fold because slower healing may occur in that dynamically moving area. The larger veins found more superiorly on the hand may be too thick for this application. The flat bevel of a 27-gauge needle is placed immediately over the desired vein, and a 1-cm intradermal wheal of 2 per cent lidocaine with 1:20,000 epinephrine is created. While this wheal is still elevated, a No. 15 scalpel is used to make a 0.75-cm incision through the dermis and subcutaneous tissues. Through the use of two mosquito clamps that have been honed to have narrow sharpened tines, tissues adjacent to the vein are separated by expansion of the tines parallel to the vein. The closed mosquito clamp is then passed beneath the vein and brought to the surface. The desired segment of the vein is then clamped at both ends with mosquito clamps, and the vein is grasped with a fine hand forceps and cut at the clamp site with a clean No. 15 blade that has not been used on the skin. The delivered vein segment is placed in a moist sponge, and the ends of the vein are tied with 4.0 polyglactin 910 (Vicryl) suture and the wound closed with 6.0 Dermalon. An adhesive bandage is applied parallel to the incision.

On a separate side table, the vein is prepared. Small, sharp-pointed scissors are inserted into the venous lumen, and the vein is stretched slightly by opening the tines. Excess adventitial tissue is removed by grasping this tissue with small sharp jeweler's forceps and tearing it from the vein. With a No. 15 scalpel, the stretched vein is incised longitudinally, and the adventitial side is placed over a hole (0.8 to 1.0 mm in diameter, depending on the thickness of the vein) in a polytetrafluoroethylene (Teflon) block (Fig. 23–9). Excess venous tissue is cut away with the scalpel, leaving a disk of vein that is approximately 2.5 to 3.0 mm in diameter. The previously selected stainless-steel bucket-handle prosthesis is then placed into the hole in the block, dragging the wet vein in with it (see Fig. 23–9). Any flange of vein remaining on the block is smoothed onto the piston shaft. This prosthesis-vein assembly is then left to air dry until needed.

The tympanomeatal flap is then reopened and the stapes area is brought into view. Through use of the incudostapedial joint knife, the joint is sectioned (Fig. 23–10). Because it is sometimes difficult to be sure of the exact location of the joint, it is advisable to shift the incus slightly in an anteroposterior direction while observing for the light reflex of the joint capsular ligament. The joint knife is first used to incise this ligament superiorly and inferiorly prior to insinuating it into the joint capsule with a slight rotating motion. After separation of this joint, the laser phase of the procedure is begun. Prior to using the laser, the speculum should be fixed in place with an articulated speculum holder. Usually, a larger speculum that increases visibility and enhances canal hemostasis can be used at this point. The smallest spot size, 100-msec pulses (2 to 2.5 W) of the KTP/532 laser are used to vaporize the stapedial tendon, and the smoke and vapor plume is aspirated with a 24-gauge suction tip (Fig. 23–11). Initial vaporization is enhanced by the placement of the aiming beam on a vessel on the tendon. The tendon removal should be adequate to allow a good view of the posterior crus (Fig. 23–12). Continuing with the same laser parameters, the surgeon vaporizes the posterior crus (Fig. 23–13). The char created is picked away with a 30-degree stapes pick (Fig. 23–14). Sometimes, portions of the crus remain unvaporized, and it is necessary to continue with additional pulses into these intact bone remnants. The posterior crus must be vaporized to as near the footplate as possible to allow a clear beam pathway to the footplate (Fig. 23–15).

Attention is then turned to vaporization of the anterior crus of the stapes, which is accomplished by use of a small mirror that has special optical coating to reflect the laser wavelength. First, the focused beam is placed on the anterior oval window niche area between the incus and the stapes. Then, with a No. 24 suction tip in the left hand and the mirror in the right hand (opposite if the surgeon is left-handed), the beam is directed into the anterior crus (Fig. 23–16). Should the previously warmed mirror fog with condensate, placing the suction tip near it will usually clear the surface. The anterior crus is vaporized just below the neck of the stapes (Fig. 23–17). Multiple pulses are placed into the anterior crus until char is created along 1 or 2 mm of the crus. The superstructure of the stapes is removed by a blunt right-angle hook (Fig. 23–18).

The topography of the footplate surface is now studied (Fig. 23–19). Bony ridges, thick areas of otosclerosis, and blood vessels are noted. By use of a 0.6- or 0.8-mm (preferable)-diameter measuring instrument, the target zone for the laser fenestra is identified (Fig. 23–20). The KTP/532 laser is set at the smallest spot size, 100-msec pulse, and 2 W. Ridges or areas of thickened bone are vaporized first. The rationale is to lower these areas to the same thickness as the thinner areas before perilymph comes onto the surface. The presence of perilymph makes vaporization slightly more difficult because it reflects some of the beam and becomes a surface heat sink. For the first pulse, it is frequently advantageous to start on a small blood vessel. The hemoglobin provides excellent absorption of the KTP/532 beam. The aim beam should be overlapped onto the

---

FIGURE 23–2. The anterior canal injection.

FIGURE 23–3. The tympanomeatal flap is reflected.

FIGURE 23–4. Curettage begins away from scutum edge.

FIGURE 23–5. A groove is created, facilitating removal of the thinned scutum edge.

FIGURE 23–6. The chorda tympani nerve is separated from the malleus.

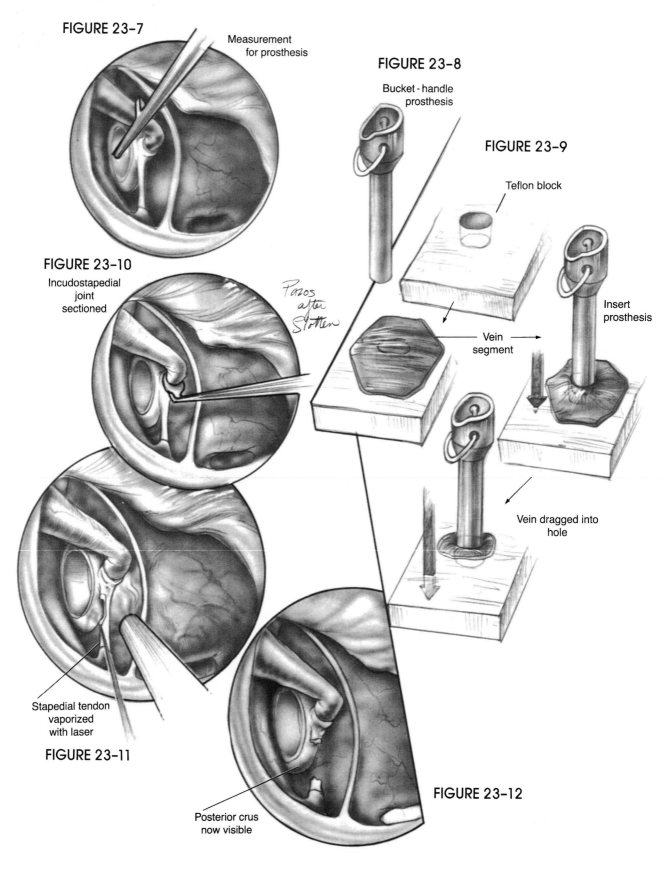

FIGURE 23-7

Measurement for prosthesis

FIGURE 23-8

Bucket - handle prosthesis

FIGURE 23-9

Teflon block

Insert prosthesis

Vein segment

Vein dragged into hole

FIGURE 23-10

Incudostapedial joint sectioned

Pazos after Stotten

FIGURE 23-11

Stapedial tendon vaporized with laser

Posterior crus now visible

FIGURE 23-12

FIGURES 23–7 to 23–12. *See legends on opposite page*

char of the previous hole as the progressive rosette pattern of holes is being made (Fig. 23–21). The dark char is a chromophore that absorbs the wavelength very well and optically "catalyzes" the next hole. Once the first hole is made, a small amount of perilymph will come onto the surface of the footplate. Small Nos. 26 and 28 suction tips placed away from the holes, but on the footplate surface, are used to safely remove this perilymph, facilitating the vaporization process (Fig. 23–22). After the rosette is completed, a central segment of bone may be unvaporized and can be vaporized in a similar manner. This process is continued until a completed rosette pattern of holes has been created that results in a fenestra of appropriate diameter (Fig. 23–23). The adequacy of the size of the fenestra is assessed with the measuring instrument (Fig. 23–24). It is not necessary to remove the charred bone lattice within the fenestra prior to placement of the prosthesis.

The prosthetic piston-vein assembly is then carefully removed from the Teflon block to keep the vein clad on the piston (Fig. 23–25). With the bucket-handle wire resting opposite the notch in the cup for the long process of the incus, the prosthesis is carried into the field and placed on the footplate. A 30-degree pick and a No. 24 suction tip help insert the prosthesis assembly into the stapedial fenestra, and the bucket-cup portion is manipulated onto the lenticular process of the incus. Slight lateral displacement of the long process of the incus with the pick while guiding the piston into position with the suction tip facilitates this maneuver. The bucket-handle wire is then brought over the lateral surface of the inferior long process (Fig. 23–26). Optionally, autogenous fibrin glue or a small piece of vein may be placed over it to improve stability of the bucket-handle position.

The footplate area should be inspected at this time to confirm that the vein has now hydrated and its flange lies on the footplate (see Fig. 23–26). If it does not surround the piston or looks as though an edge has been carried into the vestibule, consideration should be given to removing the piston, repositioning the vein over the fenestra, and reinserting the prosthesis. Palpation of the incus should confirm an easy motion of the prosthesis. If motion is difficult, the prosthesis may not be in the fenestra. This can be checked by gently pushing the shaft of the prosthesis anteriorly. If the piston is in the fenestra, it will not displace anteriorly, but if it is residing on the surface of the footplate, it will slip anteriorly when the pressure is applied. Gently checking for a round window reflex is desirable. However, if a good round window reflex is not seen, the prosthesis may still be in good position. Persistent move-

ment of the prosthesis to elicit a round window reflex should be avoided because the increased iatrogenic trauma is undesirable.

The tympanomeatal flap is placed back into anatomic position, and one or two small pledgets of absorbable gelatin sponge are placed over the incision. Alternatively, if available, a small amount of autogenous fibrin glue can be placed on the bony canal wall under the flap.

It is worthwhile to give a whisper test to the patient by having him or her repeat numbers spoken by the surgeon with decreasing intensity. The results may give some credence to good placement of the prosthesis in the absence of a round window reflex. However, variation in the alertness of the patient and the lack of control of the test make it difficult to ascribe any accurate objectivity to it.

After the drapes are removed, the patient can be evaluated for dizziness and nystagmus. The lack of nystagmus is a good sign, but the presence of slight nystagmus does not mean that a good result will not be obtained. A mastoid-type dressing is applied by the nurse, and the patient is taken to his or her room. Patients are routinely discharged the afternoon of the surgery. However, should they have significant vertigo, they should not be allowed to drive.

Conservation of the Stapedial Tendon

I have developed a variation of the classic laser stapedotomy technique that allows conservation of the stapedial tendon. Although it cannot be employed in every patient, it should be considered in all procedures for otosclerosis. The technique is similar to that just described; however, it necessitates the use of a piston prosthesis that crimps on the long process of the incus rather than the bucket-handle prosthesis that couples to the lenticular process of the incus.

The procedure is the same until the prosthesis is selected prior to vaporization of the stapedial tendon. Before the tendon is vaporized, the oval window niche anatomy is carefully inspected. Particular attention is paid to the ability to directly view the posterior crus looking both superior to and inferior to the stapedial tendon. By depressing the stapedial tendon inferiorly and elevating it superiorly with a No. 26 suction tip, one can decide if it is feasible to project the laser beam into the posterior crus sufficiently to vaporize it without vaporizing the stapedial tendon. Other mitigating factors such as an overhanging facial nerve or significant otosclerosis on the inferior oval win-

FIGURE 23–7. A measuring instrument is used to determine the length of the prosthesis.

FIGURE 23–8. Stainless-steel bucket-handle prosthesis.

FIGURE 23–9. A vein segment is placed over a hole in the Teflon block. The prosthesis is inserted into the hole, dragging the vein with it.

FIGURE 23–10. The incudostapedial joint is sectioned with the joint knife.

FIGURE 23–11. The stapedial tendon is vaporized with the KTP/532 laser, and the smoke and vapor plume is aspirated.

FIGURE 23–12. Adequate stapedial tendon vaporization brings into view the posterior crus of the stapes.

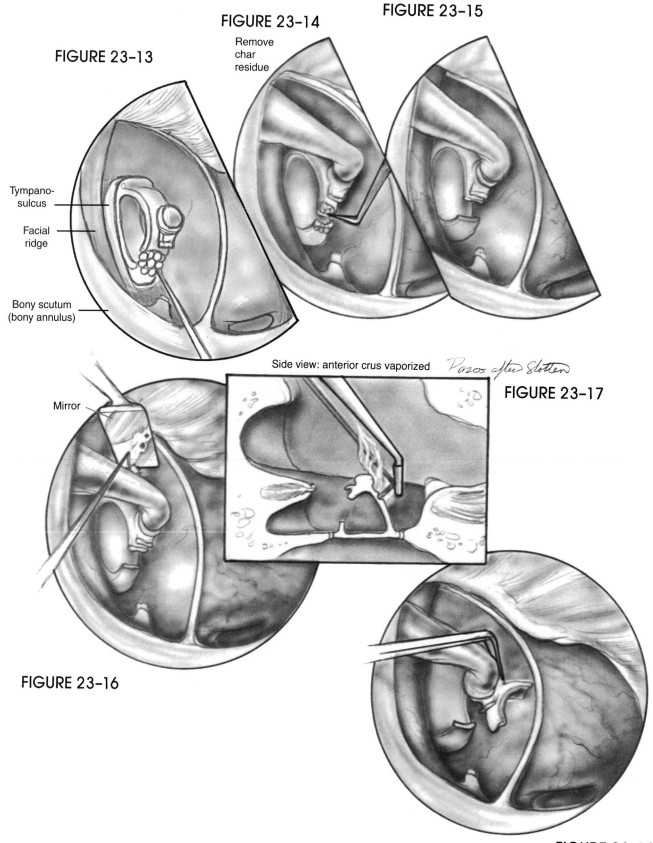

FIGURE 23-13

Tympano-sulcus

Facial ridge

Bony scutum (bony annulus)

FIGURE 23-14

Remove char residue

FIGURE 23-15

Mirror

FIGURE 23-16

Side view: anterior crus vaporized

Pazos after Slotten

FIGURE 23-17

FIGURE 23-18

FIGURES 23–13 to 23–18. *See legends on opposite page*

dow niche wall may make this technique more complicated and therefore inadvisable. Should the posterior crus not appear to be accessible or other mitigating factors be present, then proceeding with vaporization of the stapedial tendon and the technique described earlier is recommended.

If this does appear feasible, then the following technique resulting in maintenance of the stapedial tendon can be employed. Instead of selecting a bucket-handle piston prosthesis at this point, a wire Teflon piston prosthesis is chosen by adding 0.5 mm to the measured distance to the undersurface of the incus. The vein segment is trimmed as described earlier, then clad on the piston in the same manner as for the bucket-handle prosthesis.

Attention is then turned to the oval window niche. Using a relatively high-power magnification, the tendon is depressed inferiorly with the No. 26 suction tip, gaining a view of the superior portion of the posterior crus. This portion of the posterior crus is vaporized with the KTP/532 laser using the smallest spot size, 4 W, and 100-msec pulses (Fig. 23–27). In a similar manner the tendon is displaced superiorly and the same laser parameters are used to vaporize the inferior portion of the posterior crus (Fig. 23–28).

The anterior crus is vaporized in the same manner described for the more classic laser stapedotomy (Fig. 23–29). Using a blunt right-angle pick, the superstructure is displaced inferiorly, bringing into view the vaporized ends of the crura (Fig. 23–30). Care must be taken to not disengage the stapes superstructure from the lenticular process. With the superstructure displaced inferiorly and using the same beam parameters, both crura are shortened if possible (Fig. 23–31). This is done to decrease the possibility that they may impinge on the inferior oval window niche wall and diminish the hearing result.

Attention is then turned to the footplate and the laser fenestration of the opening for the prosthesis is done in the manner already described (Fig. 23–32). The piston prosthesis with the vein clad on it is removed from the block and introduced into the middle ear, being careful to avoid touching the ear canal skin with the prosthesis. The prosthesis is placed on the footplate and released from the carrying forceps. With a No. 24 suction tip and a 30-degree pick, the prosthesis is guided into the fenestra and onto the long process of the incus. The prosthesis is then crimped on the long process of the incus (Fig. 23–33).

This stapedial tendon conservation method has the advantage of keeping intact the normal protective function of the stapedial reflex, which may result in less acoustic trauma to the inner ear and perhaps better high-frequency performance in the decades following the procedure. However, this supposition has not been proved and would require a carefully done long-term study to corroborate it. Although this variation may not be advisable in every case, it should be considered in each patient.

SPECIAL CONDITIONS

The previous description depicts the technique employed in most cases. However, certain conditions call for special techniques to surmount unusual anatomic or pathologic problems.

Overhanging Facial Nerve

Usually, almost the entire width of the middle portion of the footplate is seen by the surgeon. This visibility allows access of the beam to create the fenestra and allows for the placement of the preferable larger-diameter prosthesis. However, one occasionally encounters a facial nerve whose bony covering is dehiscent in the area of the oval window, and the protruding nerve prevents direct observation of all but the inferior portion of the footplate. Two techniques that are helpful in these circumstances are the facial nerve displacement technique and the partial-promontory fenestra technique.

Facial Nerve Displacement Technique

The overhanging facial nerve is a problem for both conventional manual stapedectomy and for laser stapedotomy techniques. Although facial nerve displacement technique may be used in both, it is more satisfactory in laser stapedotomy because of the lower incidence of bleeding in the oval window area with laser stapedotomy compared with conventional manual stapedectomy. This technique can be used with both the dehiscent and nondehiscent overhanging facial nerve. Most overhanging facial nerves are dehiscent, but if a bony covering is present, it can be picked off and thus converted to a situation similar to a dehiscent facial nerve.

Facial nerve displacement is first employed during the assessment of the footplate stage of the operation and then during the creation of the laser fenestra. It involves displacement of the nerve for short periods, which can be done without causing damage. The side of a No. 24 suction tip is placed on the inferior edge of the dehiscent facial nerve adjacent to the midpoint of the stapes. With the application of slight pressure superiorly, the facial nerve compresses and provides an improved view of the footplate. This pressure is applied for short durations of up to

FIGURE 23–13. The posterior crus is vaporized.

FIGURE 23–14. Char residue is removed with a 30-degree stapes pick.

FIGURE 23–15. Further vaporization of the posterior crus base allows a beam pathway to the footplate.

FIGURE 23–16. The anterior crus is vaporized using a special optically coated miniature mirror.

FIGURE 23–17. The anterior crus is vaporized just below the neck of the stapes.

FIGURE 23–18. The head, neck, and upper crura are removed with a blunt pick.

FIGURE 23-19

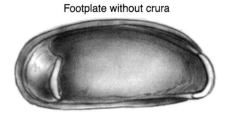

Footplate without crura

FIGURE 23-20

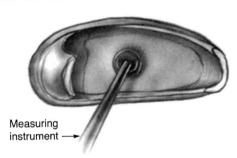

Measuring instrument →

FIGURE 23-21

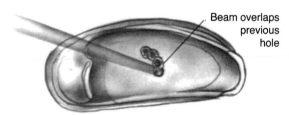

Beam overlaps previous hole

FIGURE 23-22

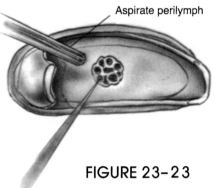

Aspirate perilymph

FIGURE 23-23

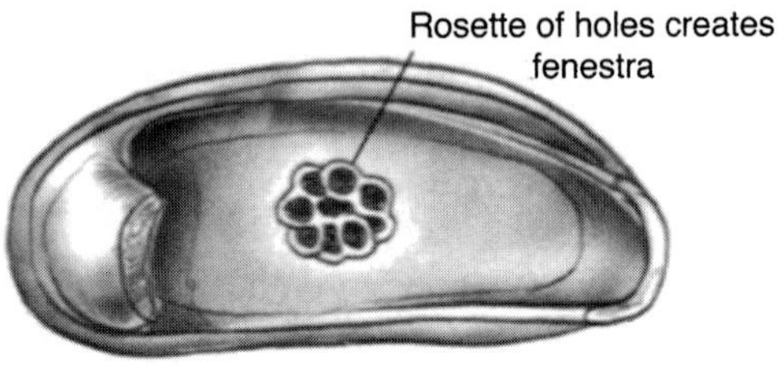

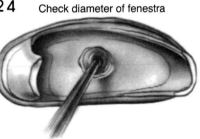

Rosette of holes creates fenestra

FIGURE 23-24

Check diameter of fenestra

FIGURE 23-25

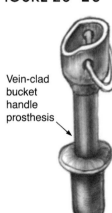

Vein-clad bucket handle prosthesis

FIGURE 23-26   Piston in place

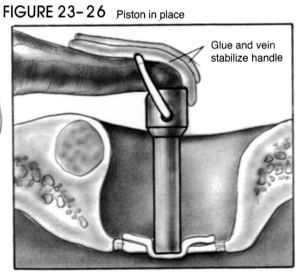

Glue and vein stabilize handle

A205 after Stotten

FIGURES 23–19 to 23–26. *See legends on opposite page*

5 seconds and released. After 10 to 15 seconds, the process is repeated until an assessment of the footplate and the target zone for the fenestra has been completed. During creation of the fenestra, the displacement process is repeated. While the nerve is displaced and the footplate is visible, the laser is pulsed. This is repeated until the rosette has been completed. In this situation, it is sometimes necessary to use a wire-type prosthesis that attaches to the long process of the incus. The wire may be bent to curve around the dehiscent nerve. When selecting such a prosthesis, it is advisable to add 0.50 to 0.75 mm to the selected length to accommodate the additional distance needed because of the bend around the nerve.

Partial-Promontory Fenestra Technique

When the facial nerve obstructs observation and obstructs the pathway of a prosthesis, the partial-promontory fenestra technique may be employed alone or in combination with the facial nerve displacement technique. The KTP/532 laser (4 W; 100-msec pulses) vaporizes the superior extent of the promontory, which forms the inferior wall of the oval window niche. The bone residue is removed with an oval window rasp, and this process is repeated until the removal is at the level of the footplate. In this situation, care should be taken not to pulse the laser too frequently because the higher energy level used here may cause rapid deposition, absorption of heat in the bone, and transient vertigo. Then, the rosette pattern is created such that the fenestra is partially in the inferior footplate and partially in the inferior wall of the oval window niche. The vein-clad prosthesis is placed as usual. Again, a wire prosthesis may be bent to accommodate the facial nerve obstruction, although with this technique, the prosthesis pathway is less likely to be obstructed.

Obliterated Footplate

Footplates that are thick or obliterated can be effectively managed with a variant of the laser technique described earlier. The laser is used to progressively vaporize several layers of the footplate until the perilymph is reached. This step is accomplished by starting with a rosette pattern that is a millimeter or so wide, removing the char that is created with a pick, and then vaporizing another rosette. The char is again removed and the process is continued until perilymph comes into the created hole by capillary action. Once this

occurs, it is more difficult to lase successfully, and a portion of the fenestra sometimes has to be removed with a small stapes pick. Alternatively, one could use a microdrill to thin the footplate and then make the entering fenestra with the laser. It is sometimes necessary to use a 0.6-mm-diameter prosthesis without the vein clad on it. If so, a small amount of venous blood should be infused into the oval window niche or minute pieces of gelatin sponge should be packed around the piston to provide a temporary seal. This blood may be obtained from an antecubital vein with a conventional syringe and infused with a blunted No. 22 spinal needle.

Floating Footplate

A floating footplate is not likely to be created when the laser stapedotomy technique is used. However, should it be created during the course of a conventional manual stapedectomy, the operation should be halted if no laser is available. After 4 months' healing, the patient should have reoperation using the laser. At this time, the rosette pattern is created, and a vein-clad prosthesis is installed, thereby avoiding the high risk of iatrogenic trauma that is attendant to manual management of the floating footplate.

POSTOPERATIVE CARE

Surgical Facility

The patient remains in the outpatient surgical facility for 2 or 3 hours after the procedure and is then driven home or to other appropriate accommodations. The marked reduction in iatrogenic vibratory trauma attendant to the laser procedure compared with manual procedures results in less postoperative dizziness and nausea and makes possible the management of otosclerosis as an outpatient procedure. Even with a smooth and uneventful procedure, an occasional patient will have nausea and vomiting and will be hospitalized overnight. Patients who have dysequilibrium, vertigo, or vomiting are given diazepam, 5 to 10 mg intramuscularly, every 4 hours as needed for vestibular suppression. It is also worthwhile to give patients diazepam, 10 mg orally, about 45 minutes before discharge to reduce the potential of vestibular disturbance initiated by an automobile ride to their destination.

FIGURE 23–19. The topography of the footplate is studied and a target zone is identified.

FIGURE 23–20. A measuring device is used to confirm the adequacy of the target zone.

FIGURE 23–21. The aimed beam slightly overlaps the previous hole.

FIGURE 23–22. Suctioning distal to rosette aspirates perilymph, facilitating vaporization.

FIGURE 23–23. The rosette of small vaporization holes creates a fenestra of appropriate diameter.

FIGURE 23–24. The measuring instrument is used to assess the adequacy of the fenestra.

FIGURE 23–25. The dried vein remains clad on the prosthesis after removal from the Teflon block.

FIGURE 23–26. The vein-clad piston in place with optional fibrin glue and vein stabilizing the bucket handle.

FIGURE 23–27

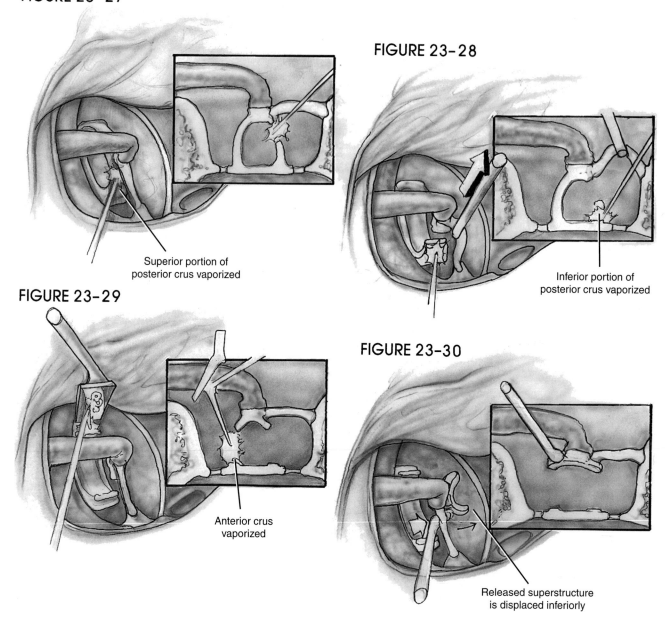

FIGURE 23–28

Superior portion of
posterior crus vaporized

Inferior portion of
posterior crus vaporized

FIGURE 23–29

Anterior crus
vaporized

FIGURE 23–30

Released superstructure
is displaced inferiorly

FIGURE 23–27. The superior portion of the posterior crus is vaporized.

FIGURE 23–28. The inferior portion of the posterior crus is vaporized while the tendon is deflected superiorly with a No. 26 suction tip.

FIGURE 23–29. The anterior crus is vaporized using the laser micromirror.

FIGURE 23–30. The released superstructure is displaced inferiorly.

Office

Patients from the local area are seen at 1 week, 1 month, 4 months, and 1 year after surgery. Patients from outside the area may travel by land or air the day following surgery. On the first visit, any gelatin sponge that has been placed in the canal is removed. Usually, no eardrops are prescribed unless there is evidence of a developing external otitis.

Medications

Patients are given a prescription for penicillin VK, 250 mg, three times a day, to be taken for 5 days after the surgery. An additional prescription for acetaminophen with codeine (30 mg) is given with the instructions to fill only if their pain is not alleviated by their usual over-the-counter pain remedy.

FIGURE 23-31

FIGURE 23-32

FIGURE 23-33

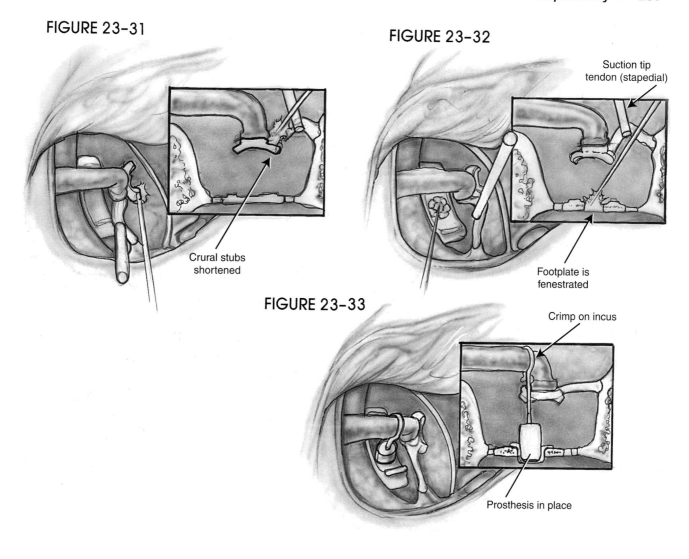

FIGURE 23-31. The inferiorly displaced crural stubs are shortened.

FIGURE 23-32. The footplate is fenestrated with a rosette pattern technique.

FIGURE 23-33. The prosthesis in place in the fenestra and crimped on the incus.

RESULTS

Patients who have laser stapedotomy experience far less labyrinthine disturbance in the postoperative period than do patients having manual stapedectomy. In fact, this is the primary reason that the procedure can be routinely performed on an outpatient basis.

In the most recent study of results, a comparative study of three prosthesis-seal combinations, a postoperative air-bone gap in speech frequencies of less than 10 dB was achieved in 90 per cent of patients who had laser stapedotomy with the vein-clad prosthesis.[3] The average postoperative air-bone gap in the speech frequencies was 4.5 dB. None of the patients in my series have had catastrophic hearing impairment in the operative or perioperative period in the years since the first laser stapedotomy.

In addition to the reduced morbidity and risk of adverse effect, laser stapedotomy will likely result in better high-frequency hearing compared with conventional manual sta-

pedectomy. In 1969, in a small unpublished study, I compared my last 15 manual stapedectomy patients with the first 15 laser stapedotomy patients and found better results at both 2000 and 4000 Hz in the latter group. This better efficacy has continued to be my clinical impression. I believe that the improvement derives from the reduction in iatrogenic vibratory trauma to the nearby hair cells in the high-frequency area of the basilar turn when laser stapedotomy is performed.

DISCUSSION

The Vein-Clad Bucket-Handle Prosthesis

In the first laser stapedotomy in 1978, I used a vein-clad stainless-steel wire piston in the first 15 or 20 cases.[2] Subsequently, the procedure was changed to employ an

FIGURE 23-34

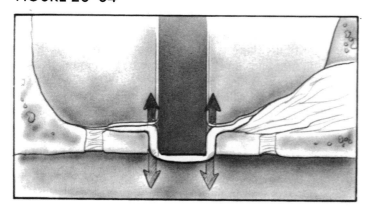

FIGURE 23-35

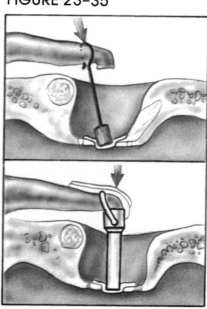

FIGURE 23-36

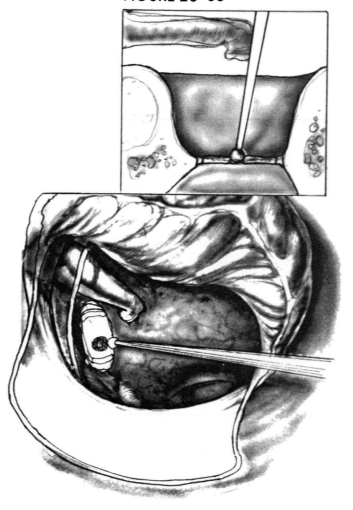

FIGURES 23–34 to 23–36. *See legends on opposite page*

autogenous blood seal in the oval window, along with a special platinum wire–Teflon piston. However, over time and in a larger number of cases, the wire prosthesis occasionally eroded the long process of the incus. Also, the hearing results with this platinum wire-Teflon piston blood seal combination did not seem to be quite as good as those in the initial small number of cases in which the vein-clad wire piston prosthesis was employed. Therefore, I have returned to the vein-clad prosthesis and am now using this concept with a bucket-handle piston prosthesis.

The vein-clad bucket-handle piston prosthesis appears to have numerous actual and theoretical advantages over other prostheses. By placing the vein on the end of the piston, one can easily, atraumatically, and simultaneously place the prosthesis and tissue seal into the fenestra. This is a much easier procedure than first manipulating the vein into position on the footplate and then searching for the location of the fenestra beneath a previously placed vein segment. When the dehydrated vein enters the footplate fenestra, it immediately hydrates and provides a moderate resistance to the entry of the piston into the vestibule. This action prevents the piston from dropping into the vestibule when it is displaced medially to manipulate the bucket receptacle up onto the lenticular process. Also, tissue material between the piston and the edge of the fenestra would be expected to form a superior seal. The normal annular ligament is an important part of the middle ear transducer function. The elastic nature of vein may provide a pseudoannular ligament or "biogasket" that could mimic the acoustic function of the annular ligament of the stapes (Fig. 23–34). This concept has been studied by Causse and associates, who believe them to be important.[4]

The bucket-handle prosthesis will likely evoke a lower frequency of erosion of the incus than metal wire prostheses attached to the incus long process. Also, theoretically, force transmission would be expected to be slightly better from the medial surface of the lenticular process than from the inferior portion of the long process of the incus, as is the case with wire or Teflon prostheses that attach to the inferior portion of the long process (Fig. 23–35).

KTP/532 Versus Argon Versus Carbon Dioxide Lasers

KTP/532, argon, and carbon dioxide lasers all have been used in performing laser stapedotomy. Visible-light lasers, such as KTP/532 and argon, have far greater target accuracy than does the carbon dioxide laser because their aiming beam is an attenuated version of the surgical beam. The spot size and the beam location of the aiming beam are exactly where the surgical beam will hit the target when released. This is not as important in gross applications of the laser, but in the oval window area, the accuracy and small beam size are important. The carbon dioxide laser,

being invisible, requires a separate second laser to act as an aiming beam. This is usually a red helium-neon beam, which has an ill-defined fuzzy perimeter, and its central axis may not be in alignment with the axis of the surgical beam. These factors make the actual spot size at tissue level difficult to determine. All of these factors tend to decrease precision and could increase the risk of damage to adjacent nontargeted structures.

KTP/532 and argon lasers are similar in their biosurgical effect. Although KTP/532 is somewhat better absorbed in hemoglobin, the observable clinical difference in these two lasers in stapedotomy application is negligible. Consideration should be given to the costs of operation and maintenance, which are higher in argon lasers because of tube degradation and tube replacement costs that are unnecessary in the solid-state KTP/532 laser.

Beam Versus Probe

A laser stapedotomy can be performed with a beam directed from a device mounted under the microscope or from a beam emitting from the end of a hand-held quartz fiber optic wave guide. I prefer the microscope-mounted delivery for stapedotomy, although I use the hand-held probe in all other otologic and neurotologic applications. By placing the finely focused aiming beam on the footplate, one can see exactly where the hole will occur, whereas with the microprobe, the instrument itself tends to obscure the field of vision. Also, unless the probe is touching the footplate, the size of the hole tends to vary, and the completeness of vaporization is erratic because of the varying spot size coming from the probe at differing attack distances. When contact vaporization is done with the probe, there is some risk of physical penetration of a thin footplate. The exquisite focus and the target accuracy of the focused spot coming from the KTP/532 Microbeam device mounted on the microscope result in extremely accurate spot placement and uniformity in the vaporization hole.

Vestibular Safety

When the laser stapedotomy procedure was developed, one of the obvious considerations was the potential effect that the laser might have on the vestibule. Would the thermal energy of the laser cause stimulation of the vestibular neural endings because of movement of vestibular fluids created by the thermal effect? Another consideration was the potential direct damage that laser energy might cause to the saccule or the macula of the utricle. This proposition was considered by Gantz and colleagues in a study in which cats were used as experimental animals.[5] They found that, with the beam parameters that were recommended

---

FIGURE 23–34. The pseudoannular ligament may mimic the acoustic function of the normal annular ligament.

FIGURE 23–35. A more normal force vector is present with a prosthesis driven by the lenticular process.

FIGURE 23–36. Stapedotomy performed using microdrill with diamond burr.

with an argon laser for laser stapedotomy, the cat saccule was damaged by beaming a laser pulse into the vestibule in some cases. This finding was of interest because I had tried to make an opening in the saccule in hopes of finding a means of treating Ménière's disease by creating a shunt from the endolymphatic system to the perilymphatic system. In fact, I found it difficult to do this because the saccular membrane is transparent and contains no chromophores to absorb the energy of the argon wavelength. In addition, the cat footplate is considerably thinner than that of the human, and the distance between the footplate and the saccule is much less. This laboratory finding was inconsistent with my experience in the laboratory in human temporal bones and completely insupportable by clinical results from hundreds of laser stapedotomies by myself and other clinicians. In a later study, Lesinski attempted to discredit visible-wavelength lasers in stapedotomy.[6] He reported the results of beaming a visible wavelength laser into the vestibule of temporal bones, measuring the heat, and drawing conclusions adverse to the use of visible wavelength lasers in stapedotomy. This experiment reflected a lack of understanding of the basic physics of laser absorption. It was flawed because the dark thermocouple used to measure the heat is itself a chromophore and absorbed the energy, whereas in the normal vestibule there is no such chromophore. In fact, and quite to the contrary, the lack of intraoperative vestibular effects resulting from the KTP/532 and argon lasers in stapedotomy has been extremely remarkable.

The lack of significant thermal effect seems to result from several factors. Probably most of the heat is dissipated in the vaporization of the bone and pulled off by the suction. The energy is delivered, not in one large pulse but in a series of pulses over time, allowing any heat build-up to be removed by the vasculature within the vestibule. In addition, the beam is in focus on the lateral surface of the footplate and immediately defocuses as it goes beyond the focal point. Engineering calculations suggest that the energy density of the defocusing beam is significantly decreased from its strength at the footplate by the time it arrives at the saccule some 1.8 mm medially.

Although these calculations are rough and may contain some error, they do underscore the fact that the beam below the footplate has less power density than the spot focused on the surface. However, even though the safety of the KTP/532 laser is well established, caution should be used to prevent beam penetration into an open vestibule when blood has entered the vestibule. In this situation, the hemoglobin of blood in the perilymph or perhaps lying on the saccule acts as a chromophore and will absorb the beam energy and create heat. This could cause thermal damage and perhaps a shunt between the endolymph and the perilymph.

Facial Nerve Safety

Concern often arises over damage to the facial nerve if a pulse hits the bone overlying it or the sheath of a dehiscent nerve. When the suggested laser parameters are used, pulses will not penetrate the bony covering over the nerve or the sheath in the case of a dehiscent nerve sufficiently to cause damage to the neural structures beneath. The bone of the fallopian canal is much thicker than the footplate, and the white neural sheath tends not to absorb much of the beam energy. However, one should always assess the location and status of the facial nerve before lasing in any case. An anatomic variant, such as a bifid facial nerve with a portion of it traveling inferior to the oval window niche, may be present. If this is not identified and the partial promontory technique described earlier is employed, the unidentified aberrant nerve could be damaged by the repeated laser pulses.

SUMMARY

The laser stapedotomy procedure has been proved to be safe and effective for the treatment of otosclerosis. It represents part of the continuum of development and refinement of the surgery for otosclerosis. The low level of iatrogenic vibratory trauma attendant to this procedure reduces the chances of catastrophic loss of hearing and vestibular disturbance postoperatively and provides the basis for the outpatient surgical treatment of otosclerosis on a routine basis. Experience with laser stapedotomy has proved it to be a safe and effective procedure of choice for otosclerosis.

EDITORIAL COMMENT

Microdrill Small Fenestra Stapedotomy

Although this editor preferentially uses a laser to perform small-fenestra stapedotomy, similar to the method described in this chapter, a laser is not required for this technique. A small fenestra can easily be created using one of the microdrills that are now available from several manufacturers. To make the footplate opening, a 0.7-mm diamond burr is used, which allows sufficient clearance for a 0.6-mm piston prosthesis. After the stapes superstructure has been removed, the burr is lightly placed on the footplate (Fig. 23–36). Pressure is not exerted against the footplate, and a light touch is used. The drill motor is activated, and when the fenestration is completed, the surgeon will sense a subtle resistance change. The appropriate prosthesis can then be placed. This technique results in quick and reliable fenestration of the footplate and yields results similar to those obtained with other techniques.

C.S.

References

1. Shea JJ: Fenestration of the oval window. Ann Otol Rhinol Laryngol 67: 932–951, 1958.
2. Perkins RC: Laser stapedotomy for otosclerosis. Laryngoscope 91: 228–241, 1980.
3. Perkins R, Curto FS Jr: Laser stapedotomy: A comparative study of prostheses and seals. Laryngoscope 102: 1321–1327, 1992.
4. Causse JB, Causse JR, et al: The Annular Ligament of the Stapes Footplate: Reconstitution of Its Function in Otosclerosis and Dysplasia Surgery. International Workshop on Otosclerosis, Rome, April 25–27, 1989.
5. Gantz BJ, Jenkins HA, Fisch U, Kishimoto S: Argon laser stapedotomy. Ann Otol Rhinol Laryngol 91: 25–26, 1982.
6. Lesinski SG: Lasers for otosclerosis: CO_2 versus argon and KTP-532. Laryngoscope 99(Suppl 46): 1–8, 1989.

24

Partial Stapedectomy

Mendell Robinson, M.D., F.A.C.S.

Many surgeons prefer a partial stapedectomy technique for the surgical treatment of otosclerosis. However, I can endorse a partial stapedectomy only when the surgeon follows certain basic principles in stapedial footplate surgery. This chapter covers those surgical principles and the manner in which they apply to the partial stapedectomy technique. Additionally, this chapter addresses the application of these principles to the total stapedectomy and the stapedotomy techniques.

HISTORY

In 1958, Shea advocated total stapes footplate removal when using the polyethylene strut prosthesis and a vein graft to seal the oval window.[1] Shortly thereafter, Schuknecht[2] advocated the use of a wire and fat prosthesis, and House and Greenfield[3] advocated the use of a wire with absorbable gelatin sponge (Gelfoam) prosthesis. The use of the wire-Gelfoam or wire-fat prosthesis necessitated a total footplate removal for the wire prosthesis to function satisfactorily. Other methods that could be considered a partial stapedectomy technique included the shattered footplate procedure with the use of a polyethylene strut and the subluxated footplate procedure, both of which necessitated removal of the superstructure of the stapes.[4] The two techniques quickly fell into disrepute because of the associated sensorineural hearing loss due to either surgical trauma or a perilymphatic fistula. In 1961, the piston concept was introduced in which a cup-piston prosthesis was used with a connective tissue graft of vein to seal the oval window.[5] The introduction of the piston prosthesis no longer required a total removal of the stapes footplate. Thus, the concept evolved of "removing only that part of the footplate which comes out easily."[6] As a result, this newly introduced surgical technique produced more successful hearing results and fewer inner ear complications. The same technique could be used for the thin blue footplate with minimal otosclerotic involvement, or for the obliterative footplate, in which only a stapedotomy opening ("drill-out") could be created. Measurement of the distance between the long process of the incus and stapes footplate was eliminated because a 4-mm prosthesis would protrude into the vestibule 0.2 to 0.3 mm in virtually every case. This slight protrusion would create its self-centering effect. By interposing a vein graft between the prosthesis and vestibule, there was rarely a regrowth of otosclerotic bone, including the obliterative type. Also, because of this protrusion, migration of the piston in subsequent years was virtually unknown.

Because of the unique design of the cup-piston, the surgeon was permitted a choice of a total stapedectomy or partial stapedectomy or stapedotomy. The classic cup-piston prosthesis was fabricated of 316L stainless steel, an alloy that is inert in living tissue and is also nonmagnetic. Its design enhanced the self-centering effect because of the cup attachment to the lenticular process of the incus (the true physiologic point of attachment), and also because of the axially placed stem protruding minimally through the footplate opening. The four holes in the cup and the hole on the distal end of the piston encouraged tissue and vascular ingrowth to secure the prosthesis and to allow capillaries to vascularize the lenticular process, thereby eliminating the avascular necrosis that so frequently occurred with the polyethylene strut. The 4-mm length is used in virtually every stapedectomy case whether it is a drill-out stapedotomy, a partial footplate removal, or a total footplate removal. Any connective tissue can be used with this prosthesis, but my preference is a vein graft that outlines the oval window opening and ensures a complete immediate seal of the oval window. Moon advocates the cup-piston with areolar tissue.[7] The cup-piston prosthesis is radiopaque and easy to localize and identify on routine mastoid radiographic views. Comparison of impedance studies of various stapes prostheses has shown the stainless-steel cup-piston to be the closest in compliance to that of a normal mobile stapes.[8] Hearing results reported by otologic surgeons who have used this technique have consistently confirmed a 96 per cent air-bone gap closure to within 10 dB.[9-11] Similarly, the complete closure (and overclosure) rate has been repeatedly confirmed at the 80 per cent level, which the wire-tissue prosthesis and wire-pistons have yet to attain.

Because the stapes does not increase in size with age, the 4-mm cup-piston prosthesis has been used in children as young as 5 years of age as well as in adults and the elderly.

All patients who demonstrate an air-bone gap and normal results on otologic examination are candidates for stapedectomy surgery if stapedial fixation is found at the time of the middle ear exploration. Approximately 22 per cent of otosclerotic patients have a diminished cochlear reserve with a Shambaugh preoperative bone conduction classification of D or E. These patients have very severe mixed hearing losses, and in many, only a partial footplate removal can be obtained. These also are the patients who most frequently show complete closure and overclosure of the air-bone gap. For these, the extra 10 dB of hearing gain is crucial because of their mixed hearing loss. Approximately 74 per cent of the patients undergoing surgery have a partial or total footplate removal that does not necessitate drilling. The remaining 26 per cent require drilling to create a fenestra 0.8 mm in diameter or larger to accept the vein graft and cup-piston prosthesis.[6]

In 1980, Austin[12] compared the results of total stapedectomy and partial stapedectomy, tissue seal and no tissue seal, and the small fenestra of Smyth. His statistical analysis, using chi-square tables for success or failure, sensorineural hearing loss, fistula, and complete air-bone gap closure, was computed. He concluded that a tissue seal provides a better success rate, a significantly lower risk of fistula, and a better hearing result in terms of complete closure or overclosure of the air-bone gap. He also noted that in addition to the increased risk of sensorineural complications and fistulas, the small-diameter pistons used in stapedotomies did not provide as good a hearing result.[12]

SURGICAL TECHNIQUE

Stapedectomy footplate surgery follows a very basic principle—*be as atraumatic as possible in removing the footplate of the stapes*. This principle is contingent on removal of "only that part of the footplate which comes out easily."[6]

The routine stapedectomy is divided into three stages. The first stage is exposure of the middle ear, incus, stapes, and footplate area. The second is removal of the stapes superstructure. The third is removal of the stapes footplate. If the opening is 0.8 mm or larger, the piston will function satisfactorily. The new fenestra must be sealed with a tissue graft, and a self-centering 4-mm cup-piston will then bridge the gap from the oval window membrane to the incus (Figs. 24–1 to 24–5).

Footplate surgery can be classified as follows:

1. Total footplate removal, in which a blue footplate with all oval window margins is visualized
2. Partial footplate removal, in which absent margins are in part of the circumference of the footplate, but where there is a blue area for perforating
3. Total footplate removal with drilling, in which a thick footplate with margins and without a blue center exists for perforating the footplate (biscuit footplate)
4. Partial footplate removal with drilling, in which absent margins are in part of the circumference of the footplate, and there is no blue area for perforating the footplate
5. The drill-out for obliterative otosclerosis, in which no margins of the oval window and thick-mounding otosclerotic bone exist.

The technique used in this method involves the use of the cup-piston stainless-steel stapes prosthesis and a vein graft to seal the re-created oval window. The vein graft is usually taken from the dorsum of the opposite hand by an assistant surgeon at the same time the ear is being operated on. After the vein is opened, it is thinned and as much of the adventitia is removed as possible. It is then trimmed to a final size of 4 × 8 mm. The graft is placed in a small bowl of intravenous saline until it is ready for insertion. The vein is folded over the tip of a smooth-jawed microalligator forceps, umbrella style, and it is inserted into the middle ear, avoiding contamination by not touching the ear speculum or the wall of the external auditory canal. The vein is placed over the oval window opening with its adventitial surface facing the vestibule. It is indented slightly into the vestibule with a fine, curved needle so that the exact location of the oval window is visualized. Measurement of the distance between the long process of the incus and the oval window is not necessary, as the 4-mm-long prosthesis is used in virtually every case. If there is a drill-out, a 4.5-mm prosthesis may optionally be used to ensure the self-centering effect by protruding 0.7 mm into the vestibule. This will also retard formation of new otosclerotic bone. The prosthesis is grasped at its cup end with a small, smooth alligator forceps and targeted into the dimpled portion of the vein graft. It is then engaged on the lenticular process of the incus by slightly depressing the socket with the curved needle and then allowing the prosthesis to rise up and lock onto the lenticular process. The wire loop is rotated over the long process of the incus. The wire is not crimped, because the fit is precise. Mucosa will grow over the wire loop and secure its position. Before the middle ear is closed, the malleus is gently palpated to be certain that there is mechanical transmission of vibration from the malleolar handle to the prosthesis. The vein graft is inspected to be certain that the edges of the graft overlap the entire oval window area and that there is no inversion of any of the edges toward the vestibule; otherwise this problem may predispose to a perilymphatic fistula. The tympanomeatal flap is replaced, and the ear canal is packed with a strip of silk and an expandable methyl cellulose otowick and saturated with Neosporin (neomycin and polymyxin B) solution. The canal packing is removed in 1 week. Prophylactic antibiotics are used preoperatively and postoperatively (tetracycline), and steroid-antibiotic eardrops (Cortisporin otic suspension) are used in the ear canal for 1 week to maintain sterility of the ear canal and to prevent the otowick from drying out.

This prosthesis, because of its unique design, is a "smart" prosthesis—it can be fitted to the incus under many circumstances. It can fit an angled lenticular process; an extra-large lenticular process; an extra-long long process; a short long process; or a fractured, atrophic, or necrotic long process. When a narrow oval window niche or a prolapsed facial nerve is present, the prosthesis easily self-centers into the vein graft. When there is only a partial footplate removal or a drill-out for obliterative otosclerosis, the vein graft and prosthesis align perfectly because of the self-centering feature.[9]

MODIFICATIONS OF THE CUP-PISTON STAPES PROSTHESIS

Infrequently, an anatomic variation in the middle ear may result in a prosthesis that performs less than optimally. For these infrequent situations, a cup-piston prosthesis with an offset shaft will compensate for a short long process of the incus, a prolapsed facial nerve, and an abnormally high rise of the promontory.

When the lenticular process of the incus is absent or there is erosion of the long process of the incus, the modified Robinson-Moon-Lippy stapes prosthesis will compensate for the absent lenticular process. A cutout is in the cup of the prosthesis to accept the eroded long process of the incus, and the shaft is offset in a way similar

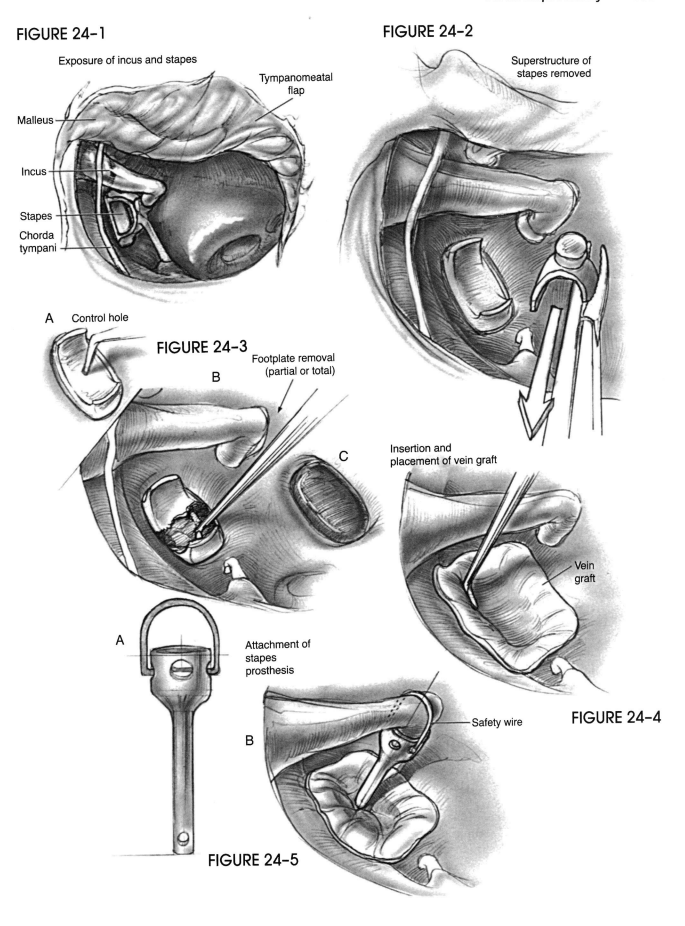

FIGURE 24-1

Exposure of incus and stapes

Tympanomeatal flap

Malleus

Incus

Stapes

Chorda tympani

FIGURE 24-2

Superstructure of stapes removed

A   Control hole

FIGURE 24-3

B   Footplate removal (partial or total)

C

Insertion and placement of vein graft

Vein graft

A   Attachment of stapes prosthesis

B   Safety wire

FIGURE 24-4

FIGURE 24-5

to the Moon modification. The length of this prosthesis should be 4.5 mm to compensate for the fact that the long process is in the socket rather than above it.

The standard dimension of the cup is 0.875 mm, inside diameter, and 0.6 mm, stem diameter, with a 4-mm length. The cup-piston prosthesis is available with a large well (1.0 mm) and a narrow stem (0.4 mm) for the large lenticular process or the narrow oval window niche.

INDICATIONS FOR THE CUP-PISTON PROSTHESIS

The partial or total stapedectomy technique described in this chapter is used for stapes fixation due to otosclerosis, tympanosclerosis, and osteogenesis imperfecta. It is also used for congenital stapes anomalies and stapedial injuries, including fracture or dislocation of the stapes.

POSTOPERATIVE RESULTS

The postoperative hearing results with this partial-total stapedectomy technique have been consistent and repeatable since first reported in 1961. Subsequent reports by myself and others have repeatedly shown a success rate of closure to within 10 dB of the air-bone gap to be 96 per cent. A partial success rate of 3 per cent exists in closure to within 20 dB, leaving only 1 per cent unsuccessful.

Delayed hearing losses have been infrequent. In a 21-year period, the incidence of delayed conductive losses was 1.6 per cent, and cochlear losses of more than 10 dB was 1.2 per cent. Thus, the total continued long-term success rate is 93 per cent. These data were derived from a 20-year study of 4815 stapedectomy cases.[13] The causes of a delayed conductive loss and their incidence are as follows: otosclerotic regrowth, 3/1000; tympanofibrosis, 2/1000; malleus fixation, 1/1000; postoperative tympanic membrane perforation, 1/1000; incus necrosis, 1/1000; prosthesis migration, 1/3000; prosthesis extrusion (preoperatively healed perforation), 3/1000; and perilymphatic fistula (first vein graft too small), 1/1000.

Delayed cochlear losses resulted primarily from perilymphatic fistula (vein graft too small), 1/2000; cochlear otosclerosis, 1/1000; presbycusis, 4/1000; and viral labyrinthitis, 2/1000.

DISCUSSION

Comparison with Wire-Stapes Prosthesis

With wire prostheses, design, fabrication, and measurement are not standardized. Wires attach to the incus on its long process and not at the physiologic site where the capitulum of the stapes is attached to the incus. Wires are at a disadvantage when there is a short incus, an eroded incus, or a prolapsed facial nerve. Over a long period, there is usually notching of the long process of the incus and occasionally a necrosis of the long process from the notching. Wire-tissue prostheses require a total footplate removal, which can be traumatic, and wires are not self-centering and frequently develop a delayed conductive hearing loss due to migration and impingement on the margin of the oval window.

Wire-piston prostheses also exhibit some of the same disadvantages, including the lack of standardization and the incus attachment problems mentioned earlier. The oval window opening must be precise, because an exact fit is mandatory for the stapedotomy technique. The length must be precise: the piston must protrude 0.2 mm into the vestibule. When a stapedotomy opening is created, microfractures of the footplate may occur, increasing the risk of a perilymphatic fistula.

Results with wire prostheses vary greatly: success rates range from 80 to 95 per cent. With wire-piston stapedotomy procedures, there frequently is a residual, small air-bone gap in the low frequencies. Complete closure reports are sparse, but the wire-fat complete closure rate has been reported at 15 to 20 per cent, and the wire-piston stapedotomy procedure complete closure rate has been reported at not more than 50 per cent. However, the cup-piston complete closure rate has consistently been at the 80 per cent level. Impedance studies have shown that wires have a very high compliance, whereas cup-piston prostheses have a compliance similar to that of a normal mobile stapes. This high compliance of wire prostheses reflects the less-than-perfect attachment to the incus because the wire is crimped over the long process and eventually loosens slightly when the notching of the incus occurs. Notching and loosening do not occur with the cup-piston prostheses.[8]

Stainless Steel Prostheses Versus Teflon Prostheses

Many materials have been used and advocated for the fabrication of stapes prostheses. Polytetrafluoroethylene (Teflon) has many advocates because of its inertness and lack of tissue reaction. The stainless steel cup-piston, which is fabricated of 316L stainless steel, has also shown lack of tissue reaction. The main difference between both materials is the weight. A Teflon cup-piston prosthesis weighs 3.3 mg, and a stainless-steel cup-piston weighs 12.5 mg. An intact stapes freshly removed from the ear weighs 6 mg. Bluestone first reported that by loading a polyethylene stapes prosthesis with a steel core, he would obtain a 10 dB increase in hearing at 4000 and 8000 Hz compared with that of the control group.[14] I reported a study comparing the hearing results in patients with a Robinson stainless-steel cup-piston prosthesis and vein graft in the first ear and a Robinson Teflon cup-piston prosthesis and vein graft in the second ear.[15] This study eliminated all variables except the difference in weight of the prosthesis. The preoperative hearing level in each ear was the same, as was the footplate pathology in both ears. The design of the prosthesis was exactly the same, and only the weight differed. The stainless-steel prosthesis weighed almost four times that of the Teflon prosthesis. The results demonstrated that the high-frequency gains in hearing were slightly better for the stainless-steel ear (14 dB) than for the Teflon ear (11 dB).

The rate of complete closure and overclosure of the air-bone gap was significantly greater in the stainless-steel ear (80 per cent) than in the Teflon ear (52 per cent), even though the overall closure of the air-bone gap to within 10 dB was 97 per cent in the stainless-steel ear and 96 per cent in the Teflon ear. Impedance studies of this group again showed that the compliance of the stainless-steel stapes prosthesis most resembled that of the normal mobile stapes, whereas the Teflon prosthesis showed a slightly reduced compliance (high impedance), but as a cup-piston, its compliance curves were more within the range of the mobile stapes than any of the wire prostheses.

This study proved that the heavier prosthesis resulted in a much greater complete closure and over-closure of the air-bone gap, and that there was a small but significant hearing advantage in postoperative results when a metallic prosthesis was used (6 dB). In the mixed-type hearing loss, this increased hearing can have a significant effect on the patient's reaching a serviceable postoperative hearing level.[15]

Juvenile Otosclerosis

Otosclerosis is usually considered to be a disease of young and middle-aged adults, but juvenile otosclerosis occurs in 15.1 per cent of stapedectomy cases before the age of 18. I presented an in-depth study of 610 patients out of a total of 4014 who developed clinical otosclerosis before the age of 18 and underwent stapedectomy.[16] Of these 610 patients, 35 underwent surgery before the age of 18, and 574 underwent surgery after the age of 18, but their hearing loss had developed during their juvenile years. The youngest patient was aged 5 years, and the average age of onset was 11.5 years.

The surgical technique performed on all 610 patients consisted of a partial or total footplate removal, as described in this chapter. All the patients younger than 18 received general anesthesia, whereas all the patients older than 18 had local anesthesia (lidocaine [Xylocaine] 2 per cent with 1:30,000 epinephrine). The surgical footplate pathology varied considerably between those younger than 18 and those older than 18. In the juvenile group, 66.7 per cent had a thin blue footplate, which was totally removed, whereas in those older than 18, only 45.1 per cent had similar pathology. Partial footplate removal was performed in 5.5 per cent of the juveniles and 9.7 per cent of the group older than 18. More significantly, drilling of the footplate because of diffuse otosclerosis involvement was necessary in 27.8 per cent of the juveniles and in 45.2 per cent of those who waited beyond the age of 18 years. Obliterative otosclerosis, which required drill-outs, was 5.6 per cent in the juvenile group and 12 per cent in their older counterparts. This result is in contrast to 3 per cent prevalence of obliterative otosclerosis for all stapedectomies.

The hearing results were more favorable in those who underwent surgery before the age of 18. One hundred per cent had an air-bone gap closure of 10 dB or less, and 77.6 per cent had complete closure or overclosure of the air-bone gap. Those who waited until after the age of 18 had a very successful closure rate, but only 93.6 per cent had their air-bone gap closed to within 10 dB. Similarly, 77.3 per cent had complete closure or overclosure. A postoperative delayed conductive hearing loss (20 dB) occurred in only one patient 5 years after the initial surgery in the juvenile group. The postoperative hearing level in all juveniles (4000 Hz) remained the same or improved.

This study also revealed a very high incidence of bilateral otosclerosis (92 per cent) when the hearing loss appeared before the age of 18. Eighty per cent of juvenile otosclerotics had excellent cochlear reserve and did not show a deterioration of sensorineural function following stapedectomy. The longer the hearing loss existed, the greater the degree of footplate pathology that occurred. The probability of requiring a drill-out for obliterative otosclerosis increased fourfold when surgery was deferred to over the age of 18. Deferring a stapedectomy procedure in a juvenile may not be in the best interest of the patient because of the progressive nature of the footplate pathology and the increased necessity of drilling the footplate.[16]

SUMMARY

Stapedectomy and stapedotomy for the correction of hearing loss due to otosclerotic bony fixation of the stapes are surgical procedures that have evolved almost entirely in the "golden era" of otologic surgery (1955 to 1985). This era has passed, and even the most popular of the nationally known stapedectomists have experienced a dramatic decrease in the caseload for stapedectomy. This, in addition to the dispersion of patients to a larger number of trained otolaryngologists, has to some degree compromised the position of the otologic surgeon not only in developing skills and judgment but also in maintaining the acquired skill necessary to perform the more complicated and precise techniques. General otolaryngologists as well as otologists should, therefore, adopt a technique that is uncomplicated, relatively easy to perform, predictable, and safe for the patient. This technique should be standardized so that it can be performed in the same way for all stapedectomies. Reducing the variables and making one technique work for all cases of stapes fixation will allow the general otolaryngologist to gradually develop the high degree of skill necessary for this procedure. The technique adopted should have minimal risks and complications, either immediate or delayed and, if at all possible, should have the lowest incidence of revision, because revisions demand more skill, judgment, and knowledge than do primary stapedectomies.

More than 200,000 stapedectomies have been performed in the United States with the technique and prostheses described in this chapter. Despite the overall drop in the number of stapedectomy procedures performed annually, the number of Robinson cup-piston stapes prostheses used each year continues to increase, indicating the popularity of this simpler and safer technique.

References

1. Shea JJ Jr: Fenestration of the oval window. Ann Otol Rhinol Laryngol 57: 932, 1958.
2. Schuknecht H: Stapedectomy and graft prosthesis operation. Acta Otolaryngol (Stockh) 51: 241–243, 1960.

3. House HP, Greenfield EC: Five-year study of wire-loop absorbable gelatin sponge technique. Arch Otolaryngol Head Neck Surg 89: 420–421, 1969.

4. Goodhill V: Stapes Surgery for Otosclerosis. St. Louis, Paul B Hoeber, 1961, p 136.

5. Robinson M: The stainless-steel stapedial prosthesis: One year's experience. Laryngoscope 73: 514, 1962.

6. Robinson M: A four-year study of the stainless-steel stapes. Arch Otolaryngol Head Neck Surg 82:217–235, 1965.

7. Moon C: Stapedectomy connective tissue graft and the stainless-steel prosthesis. Laryngoscope 78: 798–807, 1968.

8. Feldman A: Acoustic impedance measurement of post-stapedectomized ears. Laryngoscope 79: 6, 1132–1155, 1969.

9. Schondorf J, Pilorget J, Graber S: [The influence of the stapes prosthesis on the long-term results of stapedectomy.] HNO 28: 153–157, 1980.

10. Elonka D, Derlacki E, Harrison W: Stapes prosthesis comparison. Otolaryngol Head Neck Surg 90: 263–265, 1982.

11. Girgis T: Stapedectomy: Robinson Stapes Prosthesis Versus Wire Prosthesis. American Society of Otology, Rhinology, and Laryngology. Middle Section Meeting. Chicago, January 1985.

12. Austin DF: Stapedectomy with tissue seal. *In* Snow JB Jr (ed): Controversy in Otolaryngology. Philadelphia, WB Saunders, 1980.

13. Robinson M: Total footplate extraction in stapedectomy. Ann Otol Rhinol Laryngol 90: 630–632, 1981.

14. Bluestone CD: Polyethylene stainless-steel core in middle ear surgery. Arch Otolaryngol Head Neck Surg 76: 303, 1962.

15. Robinson M: Stapes prosthesis: Stainless steel versus Teflon. Laryngoscope 84: 1982–1995, 1974.

16. Robinson M: Juvenile otosclerosis. Ann Otol Rhinol Laryngol 92: 561–565, 1983.

25

Laser Revision Stapedectomy

Larry B. Lundy, M.D.

In recent years, the safety and efficacy of revision stapedectomy have come under scrutiny. Experienced surgeons report that the results of revision stapedectomy are often worse than results of primary stapedectomy and that the risks of sensorineural hearing loss, tinnitus, and vertigo are increased. With the application of laser technology to revision stapes surgery, less traumatic and more precise techniques can be applied, thereby allowing better results and diminished risks, as compared with those of revision stapedectomy without lasers. This chapter reviews the clinically relevant principles of laser technology, compares results of revision stapedectomy with and without laser application, defines candidates for surgery, and reviews surgical technique.

LASER PHYSICS AND PRINCIPLES

Laser energy is derived from the release of energy (photons) occurring when stimulated electrons return to their resting orbital. As proposed by Einstein in 1917, when photons of the appropriate wavelength strike excited atoms, a second additional photon is released as the electron returns to its ground state (Fig. 25–1). In this stimulated emission situation, both photons that are emitted from the excited atom have exactly the same frequency, direction, and phase as the incident photon, providing laser energy that is collimated, coherent, and monochromatic.

Lasers are typically named by the active medium, or the source of atoms that are excited and undergo stimulated emission of photons. The active medium can be either a liquid, solid, or gas. Common gas lasers include CO_2,

argon, and helium-neon. An example of solid state lasers are the neodymium:yttrium-aluminum-garnet (Nd:YAG) and the potassium titanyl phosphate crystal (KTP). The KTP laser is simply a Nd:YAG laser beam that passes through a KTP crystal, which halves the wavelength and doubles the frequency of the laser beam (Table 25–1).

The wavelength of the emitted photons, or laser beam, has important characteristics for tissue interaction. Lasers whose wavelengths fall into visible (380 to 700 nm) and infrared (700 nm to 1 mm) portions of the electromagnetic spectrum are considered thermal lasers. Interaction of these lasers with normal biologic materials is mediated by a photothermal process. On contact with tissue, the laser energy is converted to thermal energy, resulting in a rapid rise in tissue temperature. The laser-tissue interaction depends as much on the tissue type and its composition (e.g., bone, muscle, cartilage, or nerve) as it does on the laser energy.

Visible-spectrum laser (argon and KTP) energy absorption by tissue is partially dependent on tissue color. For soft tissue work, chromophores of hemoglobin and melanin absorb most of the energy. Lighter color tissues reflect most of the laser energy. Energy absorption from the invisible CO_2 laser is primarily by intracellular and extracellular water, which is instantaneously converted to steam.

For any laser, the magnitude of the laser-tissue interaction can be regulated by the laser's power output, the power density at the point of impact, and the energy fluence. Every surgeon who uses a laser should thoroughly understand these fundamental concepts. Power is the time rate at which energy is emitted and is expressed as watts. The power output is directly adjusted by the control panel

FIGURE 25–1. According to the Bohr atomic model, an electron can absorb a photon, and the electron makes a transition to a higher energy level from its normal ground state. The electron will eventually return to the ground state by the spontaneous emission of a photon. In the condition of stimulated emission, a photon of appropriate energy interacts with the electron already in its excited state, thereby causing the release of two photons. (From Weisberger EC: Lasers in Head and Neck Surgery. New York, Igaku-Shoin, 1991.)

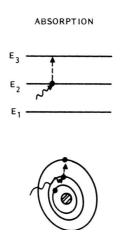
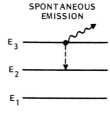
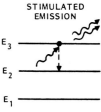
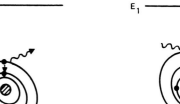

ABSORPTION

SPONTANEOUS EMISSION

STIMULATED EMISSION

TABLE 25–1. Characteristics of Laser Types

	LASER TYPE		
CHARACTERISTIC	**Argon**	**KTP-532**	**CO₂**
Medium	Gas	Crystal	Gas
Wavelength	488–514 nm	532 nm	10,600 nm
Color	Blue-green	Green	Invisible
Smallest spot size	0.150 mm	0.150 mm	0.150 mm
Delivery	Handpiece or micromanipulator	Handpiece or micromanipulator	Micromanipulator
Absorption	Pigment	Pigment	Water

on the laser console. Laser energy is delivered through a focusing lens. Power density is a measure of the intensity, or concentration, of the laser beam spot size (Fig. 25–2). It is the ratio of power to surface area of the spot size and is expressed in terms of watts per square centimeter:

$$\text{Power density} = \frac{\text{power (W)}}{\text{area of spot size (cm}^2)}$$

where area of spot size is πr^2 and where r = spot size radius in centimeters.

Power density is inversely proportional to the square of the radius of the spot size. Consequently, for any specific power output, changes in the spot size can have a tremendous effect on power density (Fig. 25–3).

The third fundamental, practical concept is that of fluence, which is simply the power density × time. This is the total amount of energy delivered to the tissues:

$$\text{Fluence (J)} = \frac{\text{power (W)} \times \text{exposure time (sec)}}{\text{area of spot size (cm}^2)}$$

As fluence increases, the volume of affected tissue also increases. The thermal energy having an impact on tissue rises dramatically as the time of exposure increases. If power density W/cm² is held constant and exposure time is doubled, the energy delivered is doubled. However, the thermal effect of the tissue increases significantly because

the rise in temperature is continuous. For example, assume the laser power is set at 2.0 W, the spot size is 0.2 mm², and exposure time is 0.2 seconds. Is this the same as delivering two separate impulses at 0.1 seconds each? Yes and no. Yes, it is the same in terms of energy delivered *from* the laser. But no, it is not the same in terms of thermal energy imparted *to* the tissue, because during the time between the two separate 0.1-second pulses, no matter how brief, the tissue is cooling (Fig. 25–4). Granted, other factors come into play, such as the absorption characteristics of the damaged tissue in the center of the laser spot as well as dissipation of heat, but the important concept is that of the rise and fall of the temperature.

HISTORY OF REVISION STAPEDECTOMY

Background

Following the introduction of the stapedectomy procedure by Shea[1] in 1958, the surgical treatment of otosclerosis was truly revolutionized. During the 1960s and 1970s, otologic surgeons performed hundreds of thousands of stapedectomies. It was not uncommon for a single otologic surgeon to perform literally thousands of stapes procedures during his or her peak professional years. The accepted success rate (as defined by closure of the air-bone gap to

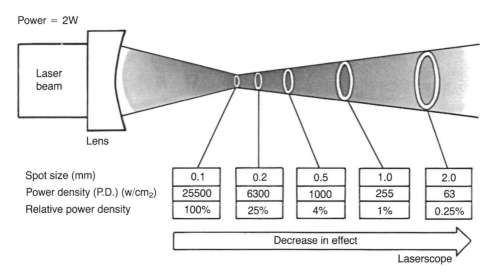

Power = 2W

Spot size (mm)	0.1	0.2	0.5	1.0	2.0
Power density (P.D.) (w/cm₂)	25500	6300	1000	255	63
Relative power density	100%	25%	4%	1%	0.25%

Decrease in effect

Laserscope

FIGURE 25–2. Illustration of planes of focus with spot size and power density.

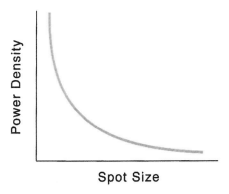

FIGURE 25–3. Schematic representation of relationship between spot size and power density.

≦10 dB) was 90 per cent or more, with a 1 per cent or less incidence of significant sensorineural hearing loss, including deafness. The most common technique by far during this time period was the total stapedectomy, with removal of the entire stapes footplate. The small fenestra technique began gaining some acceptance, although not universal, in the early 1980s.

As with any surgical procedure, the success rate of stapedectomy was not 100 per cent; therefore, with even a small percentage of failures (i.e., air-bone gap closure of >10 dB) in such a large pool of patients, there was a significant number of patients who were candidates for revision stapes procedures. Stapes surgeons soon discovered two important facts: The success rate of revision

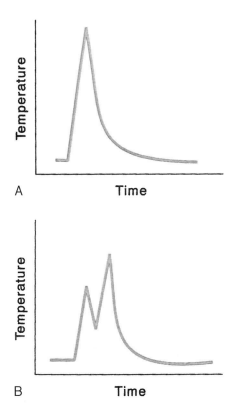

FIGURE 25–4. Schematic representation of temperature–time of exposure relationship for a single pulse (A) versus two separate pulses (B).

stapedectomy was not nearly as high as that of primary stapedectomy, and the incidence of significant sensorineural hearing loss, including dead ears, was significantly higher than the incidence for primary stapedectomy. Prominent otologists obtained air-bone gap closure within 10 dB in 50 per cent or less of revision cases.[2–7] The incidence of significant postoperative sensorineural hearing loss ranged from 3 to 20 per cent, with up to 14 per cent having profound loss.[2, 3, 6, 8] Glasscock[2] and Sheehy[3] and their associates and Lippy and Schuring[8, 9] advocate leaving the oval window neomembrane intact and undisturbed, if possible, in revision cases to reduce the risk of severe sensorineural hearing loss, even though it may result in fewer patients with postoperative hearing improvement. Feldman and Schuknecht,[4] Pearman and Dawes,[10] and Derlacki[5] reported opening the neomembrane to identify the vestibule and ensure correct prosthesis placement.

To diminish the risk of significant sensorineural heaing loss, the surgeon would often not open the oval window and vestibule, and then place a prosthesis on the existing oval window membrane. By doing so, the prosthesis would often rest on a thick fibrous oval window membrane or perhaps a residual bony footplate or new bone growth. Although this technique protected against sensorineural hearing loss, the lower incidence of closure of the air-bone gap to within 10 dB remained. The stark contrast of results of revision stapedecomy compared with primary stapedectomy, plus technologic advances in hearing aids, diminished the enthusiasm for revision stapes surgery in all but the most experienced hands.

The Laser

Concomitant with the realization that revision stapedectomy surgery was not as successful as primary stapedectomy was the introduction of lasers in temporal bone surgery. The use of the laser in temporal bone surgery was the object of experiments as early as 1967 by Sataloff[11] and 1972 by Stahle and colleagues.[12] The evolution of laser otologic surgery has been based on a mixture of clinical, experimental animal, and laboratory observations. In 1977, Wilpizeski and coworkers[13] examined argon and CO_2 lasers on monkeys by performing a myringotomy, ossicular amputation, stapes fenestrations, lysis of stapedial tendon, and crurotomy. They noted damage to the organ of Corti in monkeys after using "excessive power." Escudero and associates[14] were the first to use a laser in human otologic surgery in 1977. They used the argon laser with a fiberoptic handpiece to tack temporalis fascia to tympanic membrane perforations. Perkins,[15] in 1979, presented a preliminary report of argon laser stapedotomy with excellent initial results in 11 patients. In 1980, DiBartolomeo and Ellis[16] expanded argon laser applications in 30 patients for middle ear and external ear soft tissue and bony problems. In 10 patients, otosclerosis was corrected, including one revision case. In 1983, McGee[17] reported on the use of argon laser in more than 500 otologic cases, 100 of which were primary stapedectomies. There were no laser-related complications in his study. This has held true over time, because in 1989 McGee[18] reported an update on 2500 tympanomastoid procedures, of which 510 were primary stapedectomies. By comparing 100 consecutive laser stapedectomies with a previous 139 small fenestra stapedectomies using instruments, McGee found that the laser technique permitted much shorter hospital stay, less vertigo, and excellent hearing results (93 per cent air-bone gap closure within 10 dB at 6 months). This large study indicated the safety of argon laser use for stapedectomy and yielded comparable hearing results and less vertigo. This clinical evidence is not consistent with experimental animal studies, in which temporary changes of cochlear microphonics and saccular perforations were noted.[17, 19, 20] Clinical experience from several centers has illustrated the safe use of lasers in ear surgery; however, arguments and opinions persist regarding the best type of laser.[21–25]

Comparison of Lasers

The visible spectrum lasers were used initially because they were the only ones that were precise and accurate enough for stapes surgery. Like any tool or instrument, each type of laser has advantages and disadvantages. The visible-wavelength lasers (argon and KTP) have the practical advantage of precision because the aiming beam and the working beam are one and the same. The blue-green (argon) or green (KTP) aiming beam has clear, crisp margins, which allows extreme precision. The CO_2 laser beam is invisible; therefore, a separate aiming beam (helium-neon) is required. This aiming beam is coaxial and focuses in a different plane from the CO_2 laser beam because of the differences in wavelength of the helium-neon and CO_2 lasers. Therefore, with these lasers, there is more potential for misalignment and a greater margin of error than with the KTP. It is critical that the CO_2 laser and its helium-neon aiming beam be calibrated precisely and checked frequently during the procedure to ensure maximum accuracy.

The tissue absorption of the visible-laser energy is color dependent, and for the argon and KTP lasers, peak absorption is dark red. For lightly colored tissues, such as a neomembrane or bone, a significant amount of laser energy is reflected rather than absorbed. A practical solution involves placing a minute quantity of blood in the field, or applying several bursts (*not* in rapid succession) to get a dark char, thereby increasing the laser energy absorption. With the CO_2 laser, this absorption is not a problem, because the laser beam is invisible, and absorption by water and tissue is not color dependent.

The visible-wavelength laser beam can be carried by thin fiberoptic cables, which allow two modes of delivery: a micromanipulator attached to the microscope or a hand-held probe (Fig. 25–5). The hand-held probe provides greater angle of divergence of the laser beam (i.e., rapid deterioration of power density) and must be placed very close to the tissue. This instrument is directly in the operative field and can obstruct a portion of the visual operative field. With the micromanipulator, the angle of the laser beam is less divergent. It does not require an instrument in the field (except a suction for smoke plume removal) but does require the use of a "joystick" control mechanism to direct the beam. The CO_2 laser energy cannot be carried by a fiberoptic cable; therefore, use of a micromanipulator system is the only choice. Older CO_2 lasers have a system of articulated arms and mirrors that significantly reduces accuracy. However, newer models allow the optical chamber to be attached to the side of the microscope, a significant technologic advance.

In recent years, questions have arisen regarding the safety of visible-spectrum laser in stapedectomy and revision stapedectomy. The issue revolves around depth of penetration of laser energy into an open vestibule with potential injury to inner ear structures, such as the saccule or utricle. No laser surgeon advocates firing any type of laser beam into an open vestibule. These concerns have not been borne out, as experience with hundreds of patients and multiple authors have indicated.[15, 16, 21–23, 25, 26]

Serious theoretical safety issues related to visible spectrum lasers arose when Lesinski[23] pointed out that the shorter wavelength of the visible wavelength lasers (argon and KTP) penetrates tissue more deeply than the longer wavelength CO_2 lasers. By constructing a model of the

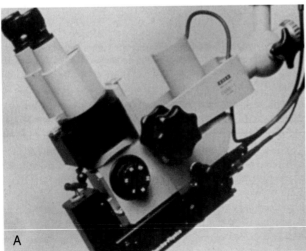
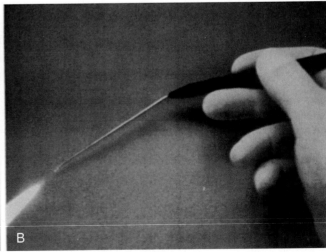

FIGURE 25–5. *A*, Micromanipulator delivery system. *B*, Hand-piece delivery system.

vestibule and placing a black painted thermocouple in it at a depth comparable to the saccule or utricle, he measured very high temperatures when the visible laser was allowed to strike the thermocouple directly. This effect was not noticeable with the CO_2 laser. He concluded there was the potential for the visible lasers to traumatize the saccule and/or the utricle, therefore risking sensorineural hearing loss.

However, years of clinical experience with visible lasers used for both primary and revision stapes surgery had failed to show clinical evidence to support this concept. This discrepancy between theoretical and clinical experience is probably best explained by the fact that visible laser energy is maximally absorbed by darkly colored or pigmented structures. A thermocouple painted black would therefore absorb most of the laser energy of the KTP (green) and the argon (blue-green) laser. However, in the human inner ear, there are no darkly colored structures. The saccule and the utricle are a light pink; therefore, the laser energy is much more likely to be reflected rather than absorbed. A second possible reason that clinical experience fails to support the theoretical concern is the possibility that microperforations of the saccule and/or utricle do occur but may have no clinical significance or measurable effect on hearing.

The 1990s

The renewed interest in laser use for revision stapes surgery combined with the theoretical issues of "best" type of laser (visible vs. invisible) sparked a series of self-appraisals by stapes surgeons. The two major concerns of revision stapes surgery—successful outcome (air-bone gap ≦ 10 dB) versus sensorineural hearing loss—continue their importance, regardless of use of the laser or not. In essence, revision stapes surgery has improved as surgeons have employed better selection criteria. A recurring theme throughout the literature is that patient selection for revision stapes certainly affects the outcome. For example, if a patient never had a good result to begin with, the chances are less that a good result will be obtained by revision. Likewise, patients with vertigo and reaccumulation of the air-bone gap do not fare as well. The results of revision stapes surgery without the laser are better than historical controls of the 1970s and 1980s (Table 25–2).[27–32] The results of revision stapes surgery using the laser are also better than the historical controls and show a lesser incidence of sensorineural hearing loss (Table 25–3).[23, 26, 33–37]

Analysis of Failed Stapes Surgery

The analysis of the long-term success and failure rate of primary stapes surgery is difficult for several reasons. The original surgeon seldom has the opportunity to follow all of the patients long term: therefore, the surgeon would be unaware of some of the failures. Most of the revision stapes surgery performed is often done by another surgeon other than the original. In our mobile society, patients often move to other locations. If their original successful result deteriorates, they may simply seek a hearing aid. Younger and middle-aged patients may outlive the older experienced surgeon, or at least live longer than the surgeon's active practicing years. Finally, it is not uncommon that the original operative reports and audiograms are unavailable years later when the revision stapes is being considered. Although these circumstances are not unique to otosclerosis and otology, it certainly increases the difficulty of establishing the long-term outcome of stapes surgery and of comparing different techniques, prostheses, and surgeons' outcomes.

Nonetheless, several factors responsible for the reaccumulation of the air-bone gap have been repeatedly identified in almost all studies. Findings at the time of revision stapes surgery can be generally classified as common or uncommon:

Common	Uncommon
Displaced prosthesis	Dislocated incus
Incus erosion	Prosthesis too long
Fibrosis of oval window	Fixation of malleus/incus
New bone growth	Depressed footplate fragment
Prosthesis too short	Reparative granuloma
	Perilymph fistula

Although there are no excellent long-term follow-up data to support or implicate any one technique due to the previously mentioned social factors, certain conclusions can still be reached. Recall that most of the primary stapes surgery involved total or near-total removal of the footplate during the years of frequent stapes surgery. Regardless of the prosthesis used, the oval window tissue seal is much larger than the prosthesis. All of the soft tissue seals (lobule fat, areolar fascia, temporalis fascia, vein, tragal perichondrium) have to occlude the oval window to prevent peri-

TABLE 25–2. Revision Stapes Without Laser, 1990s

STUDY	NO. OF CASES	NO. (%) WITH ≤10 dB AIR-BONE GAP	NO. (%) WITH SNHL	NO. (%) WITH DEAD EAR
Hammerschlag et al[27]	250	200 (80)	13 (5.2)	0
Han et al[28]	74	34 (46)	3 (4.1)	1 (1.4)
Prasad and Kamerer[29]	66	30 (46)	5 (7.6)	0
Langman and Lindeman[30]	66	40 (61)	2 (3)	0
Cokkesser et al[31]	49	8 (16)	0	2 (4)
Farrior and Sutherland[32]	99	58 (59)	0	0
Total	**604**	**370 (61)**	**23 (3.8)**	**3 (0.5)**

SNHL, sensorineural hearing loss.

TABLE 25–3. Revision Stapes With Laser, 1990s

STUDY	NO. OF CASES	NO. (%) WITH ≤10 dB AIR-BONE GAP	NO. (%) WITH SNHL	NO. (%) WITH DEAD EAR
Lesinski[23]	59	39 (66)	0	0
McGee et al[26]	77	62 (80.5)	1 (1.3)	0
Wiet et al[33]	23	12 (52)	0	0
Nissen[34]	21	9 (43)	1 (5)	0
Horn et al[35]	32	24 (75)	0	0
Haberkamp et al[36]	25	16 (65)	2 (8)	0
Silverstein et al[37]	38	19 (50)	0	2.6 1 (2.6)
Total	**275**	**187 (66)**	**4 (1.5)**	**1 (0.4)**

SNHL, sensorineural hearing loss.

lymph leak. Subsequently, a snug fit of this tissue results in either prolapse of the tissue into the vestibule to some degree, or a relative heaping up of the tissue in the oval window niche, or both. As this tissue heals, portions within the vestibule could easily band to the saccule or utricle,[38, 39] since the vestibule is only a few millimeters deep. When this tissue in the oval window is removed mechanically during revision surgery, tears and avulsions of the saccule and/or utricle could easily occur, thereby resulting in vertigo and/or significant sensorineural hearing loss. Obviously, this potential for inner ear damage can only be estimated, since there is no good way to assess this possible condition preoperatively or intraoperatively.

Accurate centering of the prosthesis in the oval window with these tissue grafts and total footplate removal is difficult, since the margins of the oval window are obscured by the tissue grafts. As healing occurs, this tissue fibroses and matures, presumably resulting in scar contracture, which causes the distal end of the prosthesis to migrate to the margin of the oval window where it adheres to the bony margin of the oval window. Subsequently, the combination of this adhesion/fixation and the inefficient angle of vibration of the prosthesis results in a conductive hearing loss.

With total or near-total footplate removal using mechanical techniques, footplate fragments can be left in the oval window or depressed into the vestibule. This may well be under-recognized, since the purpose of revision stapes surgery is to re-establish an efficient conductive mechanism, not the total exploration of the oval window. These bone fragments, if contacting the prosthesis, will impede the motion of the prosthesis, thereby resulting in a conductive hearing loss. Bone fragments can be embedded in the soft tissue scar as well as being in contact with the saccule and/or the utricle. The removal of the scar tissue with mechanical techniques can concomitantly remove the embedded bone fragment and tear the membranous structures in the vestibule. Again, there is no certain way to assess this possible condition preoperatively or intraoperatively.

Incus erosion at the lenticular process at the attachment of the prosthesis is another common finding in revision cases.[40] One theory of causation holds that a tightly crimped shepherd's crook results in ischemia and subsequent necrosis of the lenticular process.[7, 41, 42] Another theory holds that a loose-fitting shepherd's crook, either from a poorly performed crimping initially, or due to the "spring-back" nature of stainless steel used in the shepherd's crook, results in a loose-fitting shepherd's crook.[43] This laxity results in differential vibration of the incus and wire, ultimately eroding a notch in the lenticular process. The appearance of the lenticular process is that it has been "sawn" through from repeated vibration. Several prostheses are available with platinum ribbons for the shepherd's crook, supposedly for easier and better fitting crimping.

Uncommon findings such as a subluxated incus, previously unrecognized malleus/incus fixation, and improper prosthesis length are avoidable causes of failure with proper training and clinical experience. Bony regrowth in the oval window due to otosclerosis is a condition without a proven prevention strategy.

The Case for Use of Lasers in Revision Stapes Surgery

During the 1990s, several studies analyzed the success and complication rates of laser revision stapes surgery (see Table 25–3). The results are fairly consistent regardless of the type of laser used or the method of delivery of the laser energy. The average success rate in closing the air-bone gap to within 10 dB is 66 per cent, with the incidence of significant sensorineural hearing loss at 1.5 per cent and dead ears at 0.4 per cent. While these results do not equal those of primary stapes surgery, they do represent an improvement of the historical controls.

How could the laser account for some of this improvement, particularly when there has also been an improvement in the results of revision stapes surgery without the use of lasers? The answer lies in the management of the underlying cause of the original failure. Lasers give the surgeon an additional resource with which to deal with unforeseen or difficult circumstances.

Proponents of the laser use in revision stapes surgery maintain it is less traumatic and more precise than mechanical instruments. Laser energy in the soft tissue of the oval window clearly results in less bleeding than with instrumentation, which improves visualization. Laser "hits" vaporize soft tissue, allowing for precise delineation of the margin of the oval window, prosthesis—soft tissue interface, regrowth of bone, existing bone fragments, and precise sizing of the fenestra. For example, if a bony fragment is identified within the fibrous tissue of the oval window in the ideal site of planned prosthesis placement, it can be vaporized without having to manipulate it with instruments. Even with otosclerotic bony regrowth in the oval window, the laser can be used to create the fenestra and avoid the microdrill or pick. This ability to better manage the oval window partly accounts for the improved success rates and the decreased rate of sensorineural hearing loss.

Limitations of Laser

One of the primary limitations of the laser is the learning curve associated with the micromanipulator or the fiberoptic handpiece. The visible lasers have both options, whereas the CO_2 laser utilizes the micromanipulator only, due to the physics of the long wavelength of CO_2 and fiberoptic cables.

The potential for build-up of thermal energy in the oval window tissue is real; therefore, the rapid-fire sequence of laser hits should be avoided. Experienced laser surgeons recommend a 2-second pause between hits to allow for adequate tissue cooling. Evacuation of the smoke plume with a small suction also dissipates heat from this area by providing regional airflow around the oval window. No laser surgeon advocates allowing laser energy delivery directly into an open vestibule, regardless of the laser type. The precision of contemporary lasers permits avoiding this event.

Lastly, the laser imparts no advantage outside of the oval window area. It obviously has no benefit in managing the necrotic incus, reattaching a prosthesis, or stabilizing a subluxed incus. These conditions make a successful closure of the air-bone gap quite difficult, laser or no laser.

TECHNIQUE

Stapedectomies, either primary or revision, can be performed with the patient under local anesthesia with intravenous sedation, or under a general anesthetic. For intravenous sedation anesthesia, typically 50 to 100 μg of fentanyl citrate plus 1 to 2 mg of midazolam are administered intravenously before the ear is prepared and draped. A short-acting barbiturate (50 to 100 mg of thiopental) is administered intravenously just prior to infiltration of the ear canal. This agent allows a brief somnolence, thereby allowing painless infiltration of the local anesthetic. One per cent lidocaine (Xylocaine) with 1:15,000 dilution of epinephrine is used to infiltrate the ear canal skin with a 27-gauge needle. Typically, only 0.3 to 0.5 ml of this solution is used. The relatively high concentration of epinephrine is not necessary for adequacy of vasoconstriction but is used for a more rapid onset of vasoconstriction. During the surgical procedure, if the patient is restless and appears inadequately sedated, additional medication can be given. Caution must be exercised because an impatient surgeon or an inexperienced anesthetist can overmedicate, which paradoxically increases restlessness and movement.

Over the last several years, general anesthesia has become preferred. With general anesthesia, the patient is absolutely motionless. Local infiltration of the canal skin is with the same mixture noted earlier. With the use of laryngeal mask anesthesia, the "extubation" is smooth, without the patient coughing and bucking, because there is no tracheal stimulation.

A transcanal tympanomeatal-stapedectomy flap is raised with the patient under local anesthesia with vasoconstriction and intravenous sedation. On entry into the middle ear, the cause of the conductive hearing loss is assessed (Fig. 25–6). The malleus and incus are inspected and gently palpated to rule out fixation. Any obstructing middle ear fibrous adhesions are lysed with the laser. The chorda tympani nerve, if present, is frequently adhered to the tympanomeatal flap and can be sharply dissected with the laser. At the appropriate setting, the obliterating tissue of the oval window surrounding the prosthesis is vaporized until the exact oval window margins and depth are identified. For the KTP laser, the spot size is 0.15 mm, the power setting is 1.2 to 1.4 W, and the pulse duration is 0.1 second. For the CO_2 laser on the superpulse mode, the spot size is also 0.15 mm, the power setting is 0.8 to 1.0 W, and the pulse duration is 0.1 second. The attachment of the prosthesis at the incus is freed or loosened with a right-angle hook. The prosthesis may be removed at this point or may require further lysis at its base (Fig. 25–7). A series of laser hits are applied to the oval window neomembrane in a nonoverlapping rosette pattern (Fig. 25–8). A minimum of 2-second intervals between bursts is necessary to minimize heat build-up of the neomembrane and perilymph. A 0.6-mm stapedotomy is created and is incomplete until the vestibule and clear perilymph are identified. The stapedotomy size is confirmed by use of a 0.5-mm McGee-Farrior rasp. If the incus long process is satisfactory, a McGee 0.5-mm stainless-steel piston with a platinum ribbon is used. A length of 4.25 mm is used in 90 to 95 per cent of cases. If the lenticular process is unsatisfactory, a McGee 0.6-mm stainless-steel piston with a large hook is used from the malleus to the fenestra. The most commonly used length for this instrument is 4.50 to 4.75 mm. After crimping, the ossicular chain is gently palpated to ensure freedom of movement and appropriateness of prosthesis length. The oval window is sealed with areolar fascia. The tympanomeatal flap is returned to its anatomic position and secured with saline-moistened absorbable gelatin sponges or antibiotic ointment.

SUMMARY

The use of lasers for revision stapedectomy represents a significant advantage over standard instrument techniques. Not only has the clinical safety of properly used lasers for revision stapedectomy been demonstrated, but this technology has also yielded superior audiologic results. Any laser is simply a tool, and as such, has benefits and limitations. The appropriate use of lasers for revision stapedectomy requires a thorough comprehension of the principles of laser energy and technology, proper training, and hands-on experience in the laboratory as well as in clinical settings.

ACKNOWLEDGMENT

I would like to acknowledge Roger Vail, C.R.N.A., B.S., for consultation and advice concerning the anesthetic technique.

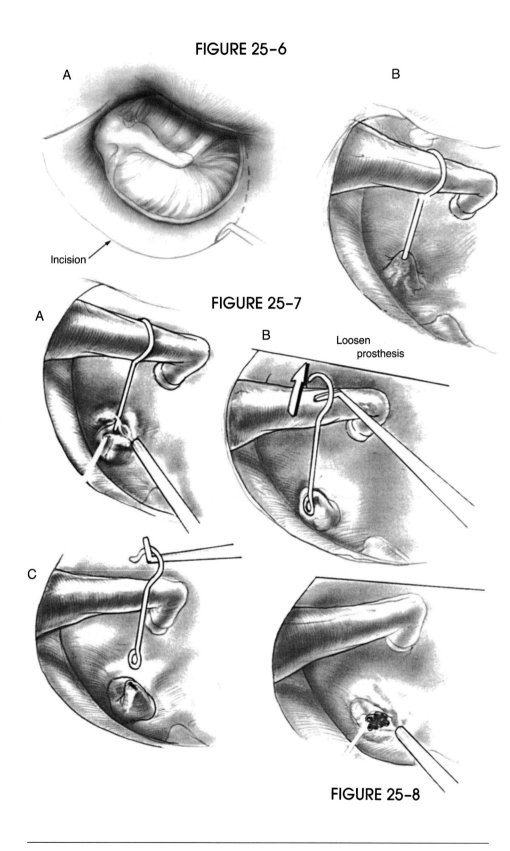

FIGURE 25–6

A

B

Incision

FIGURE 25–7

A

B

Loosen
prosthesis

C

FIGURE 25–8

FIGURE 25–6. *A,* Elevation of tympanomeatal flap. *B,* Migrated prosthesis with oval window obliteration.

FIGURE 25–7. *A,* Dissection of distal stapes prosthesis. *B,* Loosening of prosthesis at the incus. *C,* Removal of prosthesis.

FIGURE 25–8. Opening of vestibule.

References

1. Shea JJ: Fenestration of the oval window. Ann Otol Rhinol Laryngol 67: 932–951, 1958.
2. Glasscock ME III, McKennan KX, Levine SC: Revision stapedectomy surgery. Otolaryngol Head Neck Surg 96: 141–148, 1987.
3. Sheehy JL, Nelson RA, House HP: Revision stapedectomy: A review of 258 cases. Laryngoscope 91: 43–51, 1981.
4. Feldman BA, Schuknecht HF: Experiences with revision stapedectomy procedures. Laryngoscope 80: 1281–1291, 1970.
5. Derlacki EL: Revision stapes surgery: Problems with some solutions. Laryngoscope 95: 1047–1053, 1985.
6. Crabtree J: An evaluation of revision stapes surgery. Laryngoscope 90: 224–227, 1980.
7. Lippy WH: Stapedectomy revision. Am J Otol 2: 15–21, 1980.
8. Lippy WH, Schuring AG: Stapedectomy revision of the wire-Gelfoam prosthesis. Otolaryngol Head Neck Surg 91: 9–13, 1983.
9. Lippy WH, Schuring AG: Stapedectomy revision following sensorineural hearing loss. Otolaryngol Head Neck Surg 92: 580–582, 1984.
10. Pearman K, Dawes JDK: Post-stapedectomy conductive deafness and results of revision surgery. J Laryngol Otol 96: 405–410, 1982.
11. Sataloff J: Experimental use of the laser in otosclerotic stapes. Arch Otolaryngol Head Neck Surg 85: 58–60, 1967.
12. Stahle J, Hoegberg L, Engstrom B: The laser as a tool in inner ear surgery. Acta Otolaryngol (Stockh) 73: 27–37, 1972.
13. Wilpizeski CR: Otological applications of laser. In Wolbarsht MK (ed): Laser Applications in Medicine and Biology, Vol 3. New York, Plenum, 1977, pp 289–328.
14. Escudero LH, Castro AO, Drummond M, et al: Argon laser in human tympanoplasty. Arch Otolaryngol Head Neck Surg 105: 252–253, 1979.
15. Perkins RC: Laser stapedotomy for otosclerosis. Laryngoscope 90: 228–241, 1980.
16. DiBartolomeo JR, Ellis M: The argon laser in otology. Laryngoscope 90: 1786–1796, 1980.
17. McGee TM: Argon laser in chronic ear and otosclerosis. Laryngoscope 93: 1177–1182, 1983.
18. McGee TM: Lasers in otology. Otolaryngol Clin North Am 22: 233–238, 1989.
19. Gantz BJ, Kischimoto S, Jenkins HA, et al: Argon laser stapedotomy. Ann Otol Rhinol Laryngol 91: 25–26, 1982.
20. Vollrath M, Schreiner C: Influence of argon laser stapedotomy on cochlear potentials. Acta Otolaryngol (Stockh) 385(Suppl): 1–31, 1982.
21. Bartels L: KTP laser stapedotomy: Is it safe? Otolaryngol Head Neck Surg 103: 685–692, 1990.
22. Horn K, Gherini S, Griffin G: Argon laser stapedotomy using an endo-otoprobe system. Otolaryngol Head Neck Surg 102: 193–198, 1990.
23. Lesinski S: Lasers for otosclerosis. Laryngoscope 99(Suppl): 1–24, 1989.
24. McGee TM, Kartush JM: Laser-stapes surgery. Laryngoscope 100: 106–108, 1990.
25. Vernick DM: CO_2 laser safety. Laryngoscope 100: 108–109, 1990.
26. McGee TM, Diaz-Ordaz EA, Kartush JM: The role of KTP laser in revision stapedectomy. Otolaryngol Head Neck Surg 109: 839–843, 1993.
27. Hammerschlag PE, Fishman A, Scheer AA: A review of 308 cases of revision stapedectomy. Laryngoscope 108: 1794–1800, 1998.
28. Han WW, Incesulu A, McKenna MJ, et al: Revision stapedectomy: Intraoperative findings, results, and review of the literature. Laryngoscope 107: 1185–1192, 1997.
29. Prasad S, Kamerer DB: Results of revision stapedectomy for conductive hearing loss. Otolaryngol Head Neck Surg 109: 742–747, 1993.
30. Langman AW, Lindeman RC: Revision stapedectomy. Laryngoscope 103: 954–958, 1993.
31. Cokesser Y, Naguib M, Aristegui M: Revision stapes surgery: A critical evaluation. Otolaryngol Head Neck Surg 111: 473–477, 1994.
32. Farrior J, Sutherland A: Revision stapes surgery. Laryngoscope 101: 1155–1161, 1991.
33. Wiet RJ, Kubek DC, Lemberg P, Byskosh AT: A meta-analysis review of revision stapes surgery with argon laser: Effectiveness and safety. Am J Otol 18: 166–171, 1997.
34. Nissen RL: Argon laser in difficult stapedotomy cases. Laryngoscope 108: 1669–1673, 1998.
35. Horn KL, Gherini SG, Franz DC: Argon laser revision stapedectomy. Am J Otol 15: 383–388, 1994.
36. Haberkamp TJ, Harvey SA, Khafagy Y: Revision stapedectomy with and without CO_2 laser: Analysis of results. Am J Otol 17: 225–229, 1996.
37. Silverstein H, Bendet E, Rosenberg S, Nichols M: Revision stapes surgery with and without laser: A comparison. Laryngoscope 104: 1431–1434, 1994.
38. Hohmann A: Inner ear reaction to stapes surgery (animal experiments). In Schuknecht HF (ed): Otosclerosis. Boston, Little Brown, 1982, pp 305–317.
39. Linthicum F: Histologic evidence of the cause of failure in stapes surgery. Ann Otol Rhinol Laryngol 80: 67–68, 1971.
40. Krieger LW, Lippy WH, Schuring AG, Rizer FM: Revision stapedectomy for incus erosion: Long-term hearing. Otolaryngol Head Neck Surg 119: 370–373, 1998.
41. Morganstein KM, Manace ED: Incus necrosis following stapedectomy. Laryngoscope 78: 600–619, 1968.
42. Alberti PW: The blood supply of the incus long process and the head and neck of the malleus. J Laryngol Otol 79: 966–970, 1965.
43. McGee TM: The loose wire syndrome. Laryngoscope 91: 1478–1483, 1981.

26

Special Problems of Otosclerosis Surgery

William H. Lippy, M.D. ▪ Leonard P. Berenholz, M.D.

As the incidence of otosclerosis declines, fewer surgeons acquire adequate experience in stapes surgery, and even fewer surgeons treat the problems of either complicated or unsuccessful stapedectomy. This chapter presents a comprehensive approach and diagnostic criteria for selection of these unusual patients. It then defines and illustrates intraoperative problems and solutions. The solutions are presented in a logical, safe, stepwise manner to avoid irreversible results.

Before the technical aspects of the chapter, a few practical and philosophical points should be presented. When surgery is scheduled, a significant family member or friend should accompany the patient so that another person fully understands the goals and risks of the proposed surgery. During surgery, the surgeon should terminate the procedure if he or she encounters a problem that might further jeopardize the patient's hearing. Both patient and surgeon can more easily accept termination than a bad result. Do not lose focus just to be compulsively neat during stapedectomy. For example, do not search for the superstructure should it fall into the hypotympanum; do not remove pieces of footplate floating in the perilymph; do not force on a prosthesis or a wire keeper that is excessively tight. Remember that second-stage procedures can be done.

This chapter reviews the technique of stapedectomy and the principles that prevent misadventures and discusses solutions to unusual problems. In addition, revision techniques for failed stapedectomy are detailed. Finally, experience is presented in specific areas such as far-advanced otosclerosis with little or no testable hearing, and stapedectomy in children, in elderly patients with small air-bone gaps, and in fighter pilots.

INTRAOPERATIVE AUDIOMETRY

In the past, surgeons demonstrated the success of stapedectomy when the patient, under local anesthesia, heard sound ranging from a soft whisper to a loud voice. More sophisticated methods are now applied with great success. By using a portable audiometer in the operating room, the surgeon can precisely measure a patient's hearing before and after surgery. Such improved assessment benefits both surgeon and patient.

Any portable audiometer can be used. One of the earphones is removed from the headset and inserted into a sterile plastic sleeve, which is available as a disposable orthopedic drill sleeve. The surgeon holds the sterile earphone to the patient's ear or speculum. (Fig. 26–1). Testing begins at an easily heard threshold for the patient. Threshold progressively descends until the patient cannot hear most tones. The frequency with the greatest air-bone gap is usually used for single-frequency testing. Circulating nurses can easily learn to operate the audiometer. Hearing is tested at the beginning and the end of the operation to measure the hearing gain. In spite of the disturbed eardrum and blood in the middle ear and in the perilymph, the hearing will usually be within 15 dB and often as close as 5 dB of the final hearing result. The result is qualitative, not quantitative, so you are testing for a hearing gain.

Testing by an audiometer in the operating room offers several advantages. First, the surgeon and the patient have instant and accurate feedback on the success of the operation. Second, the improvement of hearing defines the end point of surgery. Third, in revision cases, the surgeon can explore the footplate area without opening the oval window by repositioning the prosthesis in various locations in the oval window. Finally, in difficult cases, different techniques can be attempted to determine the best prosthesis and best placement for optimum hearing.[1]

ROUTINE STAPEDECTOMY

The basic technique of our routine stapedectomy, which has remained largely unchanged for 37 years, illustrates the principle of a safe approach. Use of this technique and the application of the principles described earlier have

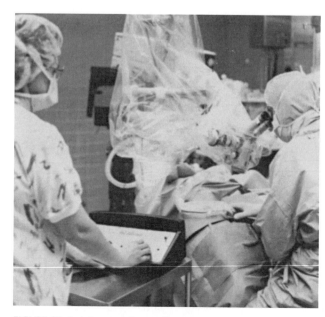

FIGURE 26–1. Intraoperative audiometer set-up.

closed the air-bone gap in 96 per cent of 15,500 cases. More importantly, overclosure of the air-bone gap occurs in 75 per cent of the cases. Worse hearing ears developed in only 0.5 per cent.

Before surgery, our own surgical nurse carefully explains the procedure to each patient. This knowledge helps an otherwise anxious patient to be calm and cooperative. The anesthesiologist or nurse anesthetist begins an intravenous infusion and monitors the patient during the stapedectomy.

The operation begins with the injection in four quadrants of the ear canal with a mixture of 0.5 ml of epinephrine 1:1000 solution and 4.5 ml of 2 per cent lidocaine. This solution results in maximal control of bleeding and minimal cardiovascular changes or symptoms. If the patient remains anxious, intravenous medication is administered in a dose that keeps the patient comfortable but awake enough to permit intraoperative audiometry.

Each step of the operation should be completed carefully and exactly. Precision in one step makes the next step easier and results in perfection.

The speculum holder, which is always used, is positioned to see each portion of the tympanomeatal flap incision as it is made. The flap should be elevated carefully to prevent damage to the skin and tympanic membrane. As the middle ear is entered, an absorbable gelatin sponge (Gelfoam) pledget soaked in the previously mixed anesthetic solution is placed into the middle ear to anesthetize the middle ear mucosa. As the drum is pushed back, the manubrium of the malleus and incus can be seen and palpated. Any fixation should not preclude completion of the operation but should be noted so that the patient can later be advised if the hearing result is suboptimal.[2]

A sharp, strong curette simplifies the task of curetting the ear canal. Enough of the scutum should be removed to see the origin of the stapedius tendon, the facial nerve, and the entire footplate area.

A control hole is placed in the footplate at the junction of the anterior one third and the posterior two thirds of the footplate. The hole may facilitate later removal of the footplate. It also permits early detection of a rare perilymph gusher, when it can be more easily controlled. In addition, should the footplate come out with the superstructure, the hole will reduce the sudden change of pressure in the vestibule. If the footplate is too thick for a needle, the argon laser is used to make the control hole.

After the incudostapedial joint is severed and the tendon cut, the superstructure is fractured toward the promontory and removed to expose the footplate. The control hole can now be extended across the footplate, and then the footplate posterior to the hole is removed. A stapedotomy or partial stapedectomy is then done. We have found no significant difference in outcome when comparing stapedotomy, partial stapedectomy, or total stapedectomy, except for the lower rate of overclosure in stapedotomies.[3] A vein from the forearm, previously harvested, pressed, and prepared, is immediately placed across the oval window with the adventitial side down to seal and protect the vestibule.

The Robinson stainless-steel stapes prosthesis is used in all cases. This prosthesis comes with either a standard or large well, 0.4- or 0.6-mm stem width, and in various lengths. We have found that a prosthesis with a large well,

narrow stem, and length of 4 mm is suitable in 99 per cent of cases, thus eliminating the need to measure.

The prosthesis is then placed by use of a two-handed technique. One hand lifts the incus with an incus hook while the other gently directs the prosthesis with a strut guide. A controlled study evaluating hearing results with various prostheses widths revealed similar hearing results in 0.4- and 0.6-mm prostheses. The narrow stem prosthesis is used because the 0.6 mm occasionally can be too wide for a narrow oval window niche.[4] Because this prosthesis centers itself in the oval window opening, middle ear packing is not used. The patient's hearing can be tested immediately after the tympanic membrane is replaced. If the wire keeper does not easily swing over the lenticular process, it is not necessary to employ it. Forcing it may displace the prosthesis from the center of the oval window (Fig. 26–2).

Intraoperative Problems

Tympanomeatal Flap Tears. To avoid tearing the flap as it is lifted, the speculum is repositioned frequently for better vision, especially when dissection is near the annulus, where most tears occur. A torn flap need not stop the operation: it can be repaired by approximation or with tissue, such as vein, fascia, or perichondrium, whatever tissue is used to seal the oval window. In our surgery, it is placement of the vein tissue underneath the tear that gives the best result. Enough tissue should have been previously harvested both to cover the oval window and to repair any tears or perforations.

Tympanic Membrane Perforation. Tears that involve the tympanic membrane are repaired in the same manner as are tympanomeatal flap tears. When a perforation develops centrally as a result of manipulation, a piece of tissue is placed under the perforation and packed against the tympanic membrane with absorbable gelatin sponge. The edges of the perforation are not freshened.

Atrophic Tympanic Membrane. An atrophic tympanic membrane may signal a poor blood supply to the incus. This has been observed on exploration in revision stapedectomy with erosion of the lenticular process being one of the more common findings.[5] As in treatment of a perforation, the intact tympanic membrane is reinforced from the underside of the tympanic membrane with tissue. This procedure should thicken the tympanic membrane and protect the incus by providing a better blood supply.

Ossicular Dislocation. During stapedectomy, the incus may be inadvertently loosened in several situations. Loosening may occur when the scutum is curetted away, when a wire is placed on the incus, or when an instrument strikes the incus. The practical solution is to attach a piston stapes prosthesis to the lenticular process that will help hold the incus in place. Surprisingly, two thirds of these cases will be successful; only a small number of unsuccessful cases will need a revision with a different technique.

Fixed Malleus. The malleus must always be routinely palpated with the same instrument under the surgeon's direct vision from the underside of the tympanic membrane. The malleus may be slightly fixed, moderately fixed, or totally fixed. If slight or moderate, the final result of

FIGURE 26-2

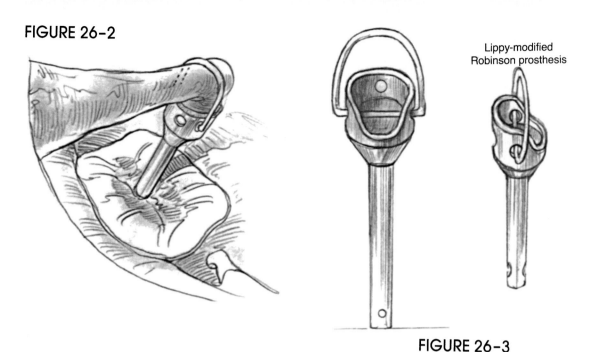

Lippy-modified
Robinson prosthesis

FIGURE 26-3

FIGURE 26-4

Modified 4.5mm
Robinson prosthesis

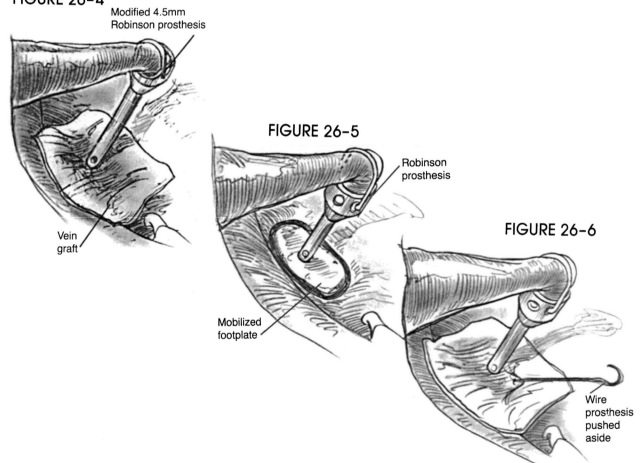

Vein
graft

FIGURE 26-5

Robinson
prosthesis

FIGURE 26-6

Mobilized
footplate

Wire
prosthesis
pushed
aside

FIGURE 26–2. Routine stapedectomy.

FIGURE 26–3. The Lippy modified Robinson prosthesis.

FIGURE 26–4. Modified 4.5-mm Robinson prosthesis in place on vein graft covering oval window.

FIGURE 26–5. Robinson prosthesis in place on mobilized footplate.

FIGURE 26–6. Revision stapedectomy wire prosthesis is pushed aside.

stapedectomy will be as if the malleus were not fixed at all. The success rate will be the same (96 to 97 per cent), but the overclosure rate will be substantially reduced.[2, 6] Thus, partial malleus fixation should be ignored. When the malleus (and probably the incus) is totally fixed, a stapedectomy should be completed, if the patient also has a fixed footplate. Most of the footplate should be removed to create a large enough oval window opening for a second future procedure (malleus or tympanic membrane to oval window technique). Sixty-eight per cent of the totally fixed malleus cases will be successful to within 10 dB, and the air-bone gap will be closed to within 10 to 20 dB in an additional 15 per cent. Cases with an air-bone gap of 25 dB or more should be considered for a second-stage procedure. Applying this simple solution over the past 20 years, we have enjoyed surprisingly good hearing results, and no patient with otosclerosis and a fixed malleus has had a further sensorineural hearing loss (Table 26–1). A more complex or possibly traumatic procedure can be postponed until an oval window tissue seal is present. Procedures to free the head of a fixed malleus are usually nonrewarding on a permanent basis.

Fused Incudostapedial Joint. If the joint cannot be separated with a joint knife, the laser can be used instead.

Partial Absence of the Incus. When a partial absence of the long process of the incus is found in a patient with otosclerosis, a stapedectomy is still done. Incus erosion is the second most common finding in revision stapes surgery with a crimped wire prosthesis causing the erosion twice as often as does the Robinson prosthesis. In place of the standard prosthesis, the Lippy modified Robinson prosthesis is used. The fenestra should be somewhat larger than usual because the prosthesis will not self-center.[6, 7] The technique of prosthesis placement is important to success. The lower stem end of the prosthesis is placed on the vein graft, the upper end with the open well, toward the eroded incus. The prosthesis is then guided onto the remaining incus from the direction of the promontory. A significant foreshortening of the eroded incus or overhang of the facial nerve will necessitate use of an offset Lippy modified prosthesis yielding more length to avoid the facial nerve.[5] In long-term follow-up using the Lippy modified prosthesis in nonrevision cases, initial success (<10 dB air-bone gap) was 90 per cent with long-term hearing (<10 dB air-bone gap) maintained in 86 per cent of patients.[5] If the lenticular process comes to a pointed rather than a blunted end, the laser is used to square the end. The laser can also be used to thin or sculpture an incus that is too thick to accept the Lippy modified prosthesis (Figs. 26–3 and 26–4).

Dehiscent Facial Nerve. In otosclerosis surgery, the facial nerve rarely interferes with a stapedectomy except in a congenitally deformed middle ear or when the facial nerve canal is completely dehiscent. If any part of the footplate is visible, a stapedectomy usually can be accomplished. A hole should first be made in the visible part of the footplate. Often, a large portion of the footplate can be removed from underneath the dehiscent nerve by retraction of the facial nerve with the shaft of the same instrument used to extract the footplate. If the footplate cannot be removed, the technique is to shatter the footplate with a pointed pick—even blindly, if necessary. After a vein graft is placed across the open oval window, the prosthesis is inserted by compressing the facial nerve with the prosthesis. In our experience, this technique of compressing the facial nerve has never caused permanent facial nerve paralysis. However, the success rate is slightly lower for these cases, probably because the nerve pushes the prosthesis out of optimal position.

Obliterative Otosclerosis. An obliterative footplate is saucerized with a 0.5-mm-diameter carbide burr. As large an area as possible is drilled to saucerize the footplate. A small opening of the footplate should be avoided until a wide area is saucerized because enlargement of a small footplate opening surrounded by thick, hard footplate may be impossible. The aim is to develop a blue eggshell appearance over as large an area of the footplate as possible, without penetrating the footplate. Occasionally, only the membrane under the footplate remains after drilling. It is helpful to drill off a small portion of the promontory adjacent to the footplate when the oval window niche is too narrow. The bit rests on the footplate, and several gentle outward strokes from the footplate are made. The footplate is then opened with a needle and removed with picks. Generally, more footplate is removed in this procedure than in routine stapedectomy in an attempt to prevent otosclerosis regrowth. If mobilization of the footplate occurs, the drilling is terminated and a prosthesis placed (see under Floating Footplate). In the moderately thick footplate, a laser may be used.

In the 1960s 30 per cent of the footplates were drilled, in the 1970s 9 per cent, in the 1980s 4 per cent, and in the 1990s 6 per cent. Fifty-five per cent of the cases overclosed, 80 per cent were successful, and 0.2 per cent were worse. Although the results of drill-out cases are certainly acceptable, they are not as good as routine cases. Preoperatively, the surgeon should be more suspicious of a possible drill-out in an obliterated footplate if the patient presents with a more than 30 dB air-bone gap and/or has had otosclerosis for many years. Suspicion should also be high in patients whose hearing loss begins early in life.[8]

Floating Footplate. The footplate can mobilize when the surgeon is drilling a hole in the fixed footplate, fracturing the stapes superstructure, or extracting the fixed footplate. The most common cause of a floating footplate from the 1960s to the early 1980s was drilling on a solid footplate. From the early 1980s through the 1990s the most common cause was fracturing the superstructure.[9] Once the footplate is mobilized, regardless of whether it is solid (white) or diffuse (blue), a vein graft is placed on top of the mobilized footplate, followed by placement of a Robinson prosthesis attached to the lenticular process (Fig. 26–5).[6, 10] This conservative method gives excellent long-term results.

TABLE 26–1. Malleus-Incus Fixation and Otosclerosis Hearing Results (n = 102)

| DEGREE OF FIXATION | AIR-BONE GAP (%) | | | |
	Overclosed	Within 10 dB	Worsened Conduction	Sensorineural Loss
Slightly (n = 40)	70	96	0	0
Moderately (n = 28)	29	97	0	0
Totally (n = 34)	24	68	9	0

If the mobilized footplate is mostly blue with diffuse otosclerosis, the hearing success rate is 97 per cent. Long-term hearing results at 3 years remained the same for the mobilized blue footplate with no refixation. If the footplate is thick, white, or biscuit shaped, the hearing success rate is 52 per cent. If the thick, white footplate later refixes, it can be revised during a revised stapedectomy. Refixation occurred in 30 per cent of mobilized thick, white, obliterative footplates. If we add the results of the unsuccessful cases that required revisions to the initially successful cases, the final success rate is 76 per cent. If the footplate again mobilizes during the revision procedure, no future surgery should be planned. Following this protocol, none of 147 cases of a floating footplate in a series of 8000 cases developed a further sensorineural loss (Table 26–2). In recent years the laser has been employed in the moderately thick footplate, preferably before it mobilizes.

REVISION STAPEDECTOMY

Our experience is based on over 1500 cases.[13, 14] Cases are divided into two major categories: sensorineural hearing loss and conductive hearing loss. These cases are further divided by the type of prosthesis and oval window covering used in the primary surgery.

We do not revise our cases (Robinson-vein) during the first 6 weeks after surgery. Previously, when we attempted early revision, tissue reaction was found throughout the middle ear, hindering our effort to analyze the problem. Furthermore, no patient gained improved hearing and many lost further hearing.

Patients with a negative attitude might not be candidates for revision. Because the risks are slightly higher in revision than in primary surgery, the patient must be prepared to accept a potentially poor result.

Sensorineural Hearing Loss. In patients with delayed sensorineural hearing loss after stapedectomy with a piston and an oval window tissue seal, revision is indicated only for a history of trauma or dizziness. Prior to this directive, in 27 cases, 79 per cent had negative surgical findings with no evidence of a surgical problem or oval window fistula. Only one case had a fistula.[11] We now revise only an occasional case with unexplained persistent dizziness or cases in which a rare fistula is highly suspected. Twenty per cent of patients who are dizzy before revision gain at least some relief after revision. Parenthetically, we have never been able to improve a sensorineural hearing loss.

In cases with a delayed or immediate sensorineural hearing loss and without an oval window tissue seal, the find-

TABLE 26–2. Prosthesis on Mobilized Footplate

HEARING	FOOTPLATE	
	Thick White (n = 56) (%)	Thin Blue-Mixed (n = 92) (%)
Successful	52	95
Conduction worse	7	2
Sensorineural loss worse	0	0
Successful after revision	76	—

TABLE 26–3. Surgical Findings in Revision of Sensorineural Cases

SURGICAL FINDINGS	TISSUE SEAL (n = 29) (%)	NO TISSUE (n = 42) (%)
Negative findings	79	24
Fistula	4	50
Long prosthesis	0	21
Tissue reaction	10	5
Lateral vein	7	0

ings at revision surgery are more dramatic. Most cases had a wire prosthesis with either absorbable gelatin sponge or a blood clot as an oval window seal. Fifty per cent of the cases had oval window fistulas. These cases were revised with an oval window tissue seal and a Robinson prosthesis. Hearing improved in a few cases, and dizziness improved in 75 per cent. The next most common findings were cases with negative surgical findings and prostheses that were too long when placed. Table 26–3 illustrates findings in the cases with sensorineural hearing loss by comparing those with and without a tissue graft.

In summary, the surgeon should seriously consider a revision stapedectomy in patients with a sensorineural hearing loss without an oval window tissue seal. If a tissue graft was used to seal the oval window, the surgeon should be reluctant to do a revision.

Conductive Hearing Loss. The deciding factor for revision of conductive hearing loss is the hearing history after the primary procedure.[11, 12] The most appropriate surgical candidates have hearing improvement postoperatively and then development of another conductive hearing loss. Patients with the same or worse hearing postoperatively have a low revision-surgery success rate (Table 26–4).

The operative experience of the previous surgeon is another factor. The greater the surgical experience, the less likely a reversible problem will be solved. Patients whose first surgeon was an experienced stapes surgeon and whose hearing did not improve are usually poor candidates for revision.[13, 14]

The type of prosthesis used and whether an oval window tissue graft was used are also important. Conductive hearing loss with a Robinson prosthesis and vein is most frequently due to incus erosion, prosthesis malfunction, or negative findings. In the eroded incus cases, many tympanic membranes were atrophic. In these cases the tympanic membrane is reinforced with fascia or vein. To decrease prosthesis malfunction, a large well with a narrow shaft is used in all stapedectomies, allowing the prosthesis more freedom of movement to center in the oval window.[5] Incus erosion is common with a wire prosthesis and can

TABLE 26–4. Audiologic Patterns and Hearing Results

AIR-BONE GAP	SUCCESSFUL HEARING (%)
Delayed conduction	70
No change in hearing	35
Increased conduction	25

be revised with good hearing results. Partial stapedectomy, in which the crus is mobilized into an opened covered oval window, is a procedure that is usually revised with a good result. Another successful revision occurs with or without conductive loss with distorted hearing or vibrations because of a prosthesis that is too short. The symptoms may be eliminated by the addition of a second vein graft and the placement of a new prosthesis 4 mm in length whether the original prosthesis was a piston or a wire.

Surgical Technique

Intraoperative testing is an important tool in revision surgery, allowing surgeons to obtain the most information with the least amount of trauma to the labyrinth. The patient must be under local anesthesia and should be instructed to inform the surgeon of any dizziness.

The surgical technique includes removing the previously placed prosthesis without disturbing the oval window seal and then placing a vein graft and a Robinson prosthesis. In cases with a wire prosthesis in which the patient experiences dizziness on manipulation, the end of the wire that is attached to the incus is detached and pushed aside, leaving the distal end of the wire in the oval window seal (Fig. 26–6). A vein graft is then placed over the oval window area with a slit cut in the graft to accommodate the wire. A Robinson prosthesis is then placed.

The Argon laser otoprobe is often used in revision stapedectomy. It is particularly useful in slowly removing tissue around the distal end of a wire prosthesis in the oval window. The prosthesis may be removed less traumatically using the laser at low wattage (1 W) and using brief bursts to avoid excessive vestibular stimulation. Once perilymph is identified a vein graft may be placed on the oval window followed by a Robinson prosthesis. At this point, the tympanomeatal flap is replaced, and the hearing is tested. If the hearing improves, the surgical procedure is finished.

If the hearing is not improved, the surgeon should consider other causes, such as previously inadequate footplate removal, otosclerosis regrowth, or a misdirected stapes prosthesis. The bottom of the prosthesis should first be moved slightly to search for an opening into the oval window. In the routine stapedectomy technique, the prosthesis is always self-centering. However, in a revision, because the tissue graft is healed and therefore less compliant, adjustment may be necessary. Should repositioning of the prosthesis not improve hearing, further exposure of the oval window covering with the laser may be necessary.

Surgical Findings

Incus Erosion. This is the most common finding with wire prostheses. The pressure of the wire around the long process of the incus causes necrosis and erosion. If the only problem is a loose wire, the prosthesis can be crimped again. With prostheses that attach to the lenticular process of the incus, such as the Robinson, incus erosion most often results from a previous infection, manifested by a healed perforation or an atrophic tympanic membrane and incus. For both wires and pistons, the success rate of

revision with the Lippy modified Robinson prosthesis is 80 per cent.[12]

Prosthesis Malfunction. Prosthesis malfunction in cases with a Robinson prosthesis on an oval window tissue seal is uncommon because of the self-centering ability of the prosthesis. A lenticular process that is too large can misdirect the piston from self-centering. This unusual problem can be avoided in the original procedure by using a 4-mm polytetrafluoroethylene (Teflon) prosthesis with a large well. This well is 0.2 mm larger than that of the Robinson prosthesis with a large well. This prosthesis accommodates the occasional extra-large lenticular process without causing misdirection. Malfunction is likely to occur in cases in which the stapes prosthesis becomes fused to the incus lenticular process and directed out of its self-centering position. If the fused prosthesis cannot be easily removed from the lenticular process, it may be removed with the laser. A prosthesis that is too short and used with a tissue graft may give a good result at first. However, a conductive loss will develop as the tissue graft thins out. These problems can be corrected by revision. Wire prostheses, which lack rigidity, are more likely to migrate. The distal looped end of the wire commonly rests on the promontory or is fixed to a margin of the oval window. In addition, a loose attachment of the wire prosthesis on the long process of the incus may occur with incomplete crimping or gradual erosion of the incus. Lastly, short wire prostheses are frequently found, resulting from either improper measurement or inadvertent shortening when the prosthesis is crimped to the incus. Revision stapedectomy will correct these problems.

Negative Findings. An interesting situation occurs when no problem can be recognized, the so-called negative surgical finding category. In cases with an oval window tissue seal and a piston prosthesis, a revision stapedectomy did not improve hearing. However, hearing improved in 60 per cent of cases in which a wire prosthesis without a tissue seal was replaced by a Robinson prosthesis on a vein (Table 26–5). The reason for this disparity appears to be the efficiency of the Robinson prostheses. The heavier and more rigid piston prosthesis more closely resembles the stapes mass than does the wire prosthesis and is, therefore, more efficient. With the use of laser there are fewer cases that we call "negative findings" patients.

Malleus Fixation. Malleus and incus fixations are discussed under intraoperative problems. Malleus fixation may have been present but ignored at the initial surgery, or it may have progressed in the interim. The totally fixed cases can be revised with a footplate-to-drum prosthesis or a malleus-to-footplate prosthesis when an oval window tissue seal is present.

Other Findings. Adhesions that are dense enough to impede the prosthesis are extremely rare. Adhesions are

TABLE 26–5. Hearing Results in Negative-Findings Cases

PROSTHESIS	HEARING RESULTS (%)	
	Successful Hearing	Worse Hearing
Wire–no tissue	60	0
Robinson–tissue	0	9

often found during revision, but the hearing rarely changes when they are removed. Intraoperative audiometry allows the surgeon to evaluate the affect of such adhesions when they are removed.

Tissue graft lateralization, which is uncommon, can be revised by placing a new tissue graft on top of the old one, followed by a rigid piston prosthesis. Aggressive, mounded up regrowth should not be removed, because the chances of further regrowth or further sensorineural loss are high. In cases where the previous drilling was well described and limited, a new area may be drilled. However, otosclerosis regrowth is rare.

Fistula. We have found only six fistulas in our cases with a Robinson prosthesis and a tissue seal. All six were women with smaller-than-usual vein grafts in whom fistulas occurred years after the original procedure. Each patient had a sudden hearing loss following descent either in a car or an airplane. The fistulas were found at the margin where the facial nerve canal adjoins the oval window. We now take a larger vein in women and attempt to remove some of the mucosa from the facial nerve canal or the facial nerve to create a surface to which the tissue seal will adhere and not slide toward the promontory. Fistulas were fairly common in conductive cases without tissue grafts.

Small Fenestra. In revision stapedectomy of cases that have had a small fenestra technique, the most common surgical finding is displacement of the prosthesis from the small fenestra. The revision technique is to ignore the previous small fenestra to avoid manipulating adhesions that may have formed in the vestibule. Often, a larger fenestra can be placed in the remaining portion of the footplate with picks or the laser. Both fenestrae are covered by a tissue graft and a Robinson prosthesis placed in the new larger opening.

Recommendations

In cases of revision stapedectomy, the following measures are recommended:

1. Local anesthesia should be used both to monitor any dizziness and to permit intraoperative audiometry.

2. Intraoperative audiometry should be performed. A hearing gain is evidence of a successful technical solution. The surgeon then need not further explore the oval window area. If hearing is not improved, the prosthesis should be moved. If the hearing is still not improved, then more of the oval window covering is exposed with the laser, to search for an intact otosclerotic footplate or otosclerosis regrowth.

3. A tissue seal should be used over the oval window, whether or not it was opened, for three reasons. First, tissue provides a seal of the oval window and therefore prevents fistulas. Second, fistulas of the oval window are not always evident, because they can be minute or temporarily closed. Third, the seal produced by absorbable gelatin sponge or mucosa will not safely support a rigid-piston prosthesis.

4. The oval window should not be routinely reopened. When the oval window is reopened, the incidence of hearing loss increases for the following reasons. First, routine stapedectomy can cause vestibular adhesions from indenta-

tion of the oval window seal by the prosthesis. Therefore, reopening the oval window can cause vestibular trauma because manipulation of the adhesions damages the membranous labyrinth. Second, the most critical part of stapedectomy is removing the footplate. Reopening the oval window in the absence of the footplate as a landmark is more technically difficult and thus carries the risk of greater surgical trauma. Third, delayed sensorineural hearing loss, which occurs rarely and inexplicably after stapedectomy, is probably related to a labyrinthine tissue reaction. Thus, the less trauma to the labyrinth, the less chance of a delayed sensorineural hearing loss. Again, the oval window seal should not be opened routinely.

5. Aggressive otosclerosis regrowth should not be removed. When it is encountered, the surgical procedure should be terminated. The reasons for not reopening the oval window seal are further supported by the difficult task of drilling and removing the otosclerosis regrowth. Even when the otosclerosis regrowth is successfully removed, the hearing gain is temporary in most patients. The incidence of a greater hearing loss is more than 50 per cent in our experience.

6. The distal loop of the wire prosthesis should be left in place in many cases. If the distal loop appears deep within the oval window seal, or if the patient experiences dizziness, the loop in the oval window seal is not removed. Removal may reopen the oval window, which will increase the likelihood of a hearing loss or dizziness. However, if the patient's main problem is significant incapacitating dizziness, the wire must be removed even if hearing is possibly sacrificed.

7. If the problem cannot be identified (negative findings), the case with a tissue seal should not be revised unless a laser is used. On the other hand, cases without a tissue seal should be revised with good results.

FAR-ADVANCED OTOSCLEROSIS

Far-advanced otosclerosis is defined as no measurable air or bone conduction or, at best, air conduction no better than 95 dB and bone at 55 to 60 dB at one frequency only. The history may include a family member with otosclerosis, previous audiograms showing a conductive hearing loss, and progressive hearing loss. The patient may be wearing a hearing aid successfully or may have previously worn an aid. Findings would also include better-than-expected speech patterns and a softer voice than expected with such a severe sensorineural hearing loss.

Most important is the ability to hear, not just feel, the 512 Hz tuning fork on the upper teeth. This practical test gives up to 10 dB more gain than when the tuning fork is placed on the mastoid. Edentulous patients are tested on their dentures or on their gums if they have no dentures.[15] In some patients, this test is the only one to yield measurable hearing evidence of far-advanced otosclerosis. Patients with some of these findings should be considered for a stapedectomy.

Surgical Technique

In far-advanced otosclerosis, the surgical techniques are the same as in the routine stapedectomy, but the surgical findings are different. Fifty per cent of the patients will have obliterative otosclerosis; therefore, the surgeon must be prepared to drill the footplate extensively, as recommended previously.[16]

Results

Success is measured by improved air conduction, improved speech discrimination, and more benefit from a hearing aid. In our surgical experience with 72 far-advanced otosclerosis patients, the average hearing gain was 20 dB, and 70 per cent benefited more from a hearing aid.[17] Discrimination was improved by more than 15 per cent in 54 per cent of cases. In addition, there is a high correlation of success between ears: the patient who gained hearing after surgery in one ear also did well in the other; the patient who did not achieve a good result in the first ear did not do well in the second ear.

The results of stapedectomy for far-advanced otosclerosis are often dramatic. They will reinforce the surgeon's resolve to double-check patients with no measurable hearing.

STAPEDECTOMY FOR SMALL AIR-BONE GAPS

Although most otologic surgeons advocate at least a 20 dB pure tone average air-bone gap as an indication for stapedectomy, recent review by the senior author (WHL) reveals that even smaller air-bone gaps may be corrected. In reviewing 136 cases overclosure was achieved in more than 80 per cent of the patients with mean overclosure of 8.1 dB.[18] These patients had a 10 dB or slightly less preoperative air-bone gap with an average 16.7 dB improvement postoperatively. Five-year follow-up revealed that almost all patients maintained their initial gains.[18]

STAPEDECTOMY IN CHILDREN

Approach and management of juvenile otosclerotic patients differ from those of adults with the disorder. In our review of 47 children 7 to 17 years of age, footplate pathology was greater in children necessitating drill-outs in 27 per cent of cases for obliterative otosclerosis.[19] Where inner ear malformations were suspected, they were ruled out with computed tomography imaging and therefore there are no such cases identified in this study. Some of the older children can be operated with a local anesthetic. There is a greater than 90 per cent chance of closing the air-bone gap to within 10 dB. In 5-year follow-up the mean pure tone average deteriorated an average of 8.1 dB. Overclosure is not as great as in the adult population.

STAPEDECTOMY IN THE ELDERLY

Although otosclerosis usually presents in patients younger than 40 years of age, some will delay surgery until the patients are older than 70 years of age. In a review of 154 patients ranging in age from 70 to 92 years of age, 91 per cent closed the air-bone gap to within 10 dB.[20] Results were stable at 5 years with 2.5 dB deterioration at 5 years. There was no increase in complications in the elderly compared with a comparison younger group, with transient dizziness occurring in less than 2 per cent of the patients postoperatively.

STAPEDECTOMY IN PILOTS

High-performance pilots with otosclerosis are a special group that deserves attention. Six fighter pilots underwent stapedectomy, with three having bilateral stapedectomy.[21] All the pilots returned to their active flight duties with no vestibular symptoms. Full flight status may be resumed after an altitude pressure test and a waiting period of a few months.

References

1. Lippy WH, Schuring AG, Rizer FM: Intraoperative audiometry. Laryngoscope 105: 214–216, 1995.
2. Lippy WH, Schuring AG, Ziv M: Stapedectomy for otosclerosis with malleus fixation. Otolaryngol Head Neck Surg 104: 338–389, 1978.
3. Rizer FM, Lippy WH: Evolution of techniques from the total stapedectomy to the small fenestra stapedectomy. Otolaryngol Clin North Am 26: 443–451, 1993.
4. Fucci MJ, Lippy WH, Schuring AG, Rizer FM: Prosthesis size in stapedectomy. Otolaryngol Head Neck Surg 118: 1–5, 1998.
5. Krieger LW, Lippy WH, Schuring AG, Rizer FM: Revision stapedectomy for incus erosion: Long-term hearing. Otolaryngol Head Neck Surg 119: 370–373, 1998.
6. Lippy WH, Schuring AG: Solving ossicular problems in stapedectomy. Laryngoscope 93: 1147–1150, 1983.
7. Lippy WH, Schuring AG: Prosthesis for the problem incus in stapedectomy. Otolaryngol Head Neck Surg 100: 237–239, 1974.
8. Lippy WH, Berenholz LP, Burkey JM: Otosclerosis in the 1960s, 1970s, 1980s, and 1990s. Laryngoscope 109: 1307–1309, 1999.
9. Lippy WH, Fucci MJ, Schuring AG, Rizer FM: Prosthesis on a mobilized stapes footplate. Am J Otol 17: 713–716, 1996.
10. Lippy WH, Schuring AG: Treatment of the inadvertently mobilized footplate. Otolaryngol Head Neck Surg 98: 80–81, 1973.
11. Lippy WH, Schuring AG: Stapedectomy revision following sensorineural hearing loss. Otolaryngol Head Neck Surg 92: 580–582, 1984.
12. Lippy WH, Schuring AG: Stapedectomy revision of the wire-Gelfoam prosthesis. Otolaryngol Head Neck Surg 91: 9–13, 1983.
13. Lippy WH, Schuring AG, Ziv M: Stapedectomy revision. Am J Otol 2: 15–21, 1980.
14. Lippy WH: Revision stapedectomy. AAO-HNS Instructional Courses. St. Louis, Mosby–Year Book, 1994.
15. Lippy WH, Rotolo AL, Berger KW: Bone conduction measurement: Mastoid versus upper central incisor. Trans Am Acad Ophthalmol Otolaryngol 70: 1084–1088, 1966.
16. Lippy WH, Battista RA, Schuring AG, Rizer FM: Far-advanced otosclerosis. Am J Otol 15(5 Part 2): 225–228, 1994.
17. Lippy WH, Burkey JM, Schuring AG, Rizer FM: Word recognition score changes following stapedectomy for far-advanced otosclerosis. Am J Otol 19: 56–58, 1998.
18. Lippy WH, Burkey JM, Schuring AG, Rizer FM: Stapedectomy in patients with small air-bone gaps. Laryngoscope 107: 919–922, 1997.
19. Lippy WH, Burkey JM, Schuring AG, Rizer FM: Stapedectomy in children: Short- and long-term results. Laryngoscope 108: 569–572, 1998.
20. Lippy WH, Burkey JM, Fucci MJ, et al: Stapedectomy in the elderly. Am J Otol 17: 831–834, 1996.
21. Katzav J, Lippy WH, Shaniss A, Davidson BZ: Stapedectomy in combat pilots. Am J Otol 17: 847–849, 1996.

27

Avoidance and Management of Complications of Otosclerosis Surgery

Joseph B. Roberson, Jr., M.D.

Otosclerosis surgery is one of the most exciting and rewarding procedures that the otologic surgeon performs. The physical demands of the operation are among the most refined of the surgical disciplines. There is an extremely small tolerance for error even when the case goes along well with perfect equipment and perfect performance of support personnel. Small deviations from the surgical techniques so wonderfully illustrated in the remainder of this text regularly prove necessary to avoid complications with this procedure. The knowledge base and technical skills needed to handle these deviations add difficulty to an already challenging undertaking. With this difficulty, however, comes a large reward as patients experience improvement of their hearing with a successful outcome—frequently to the normal range!

As with other difficult procedures, the learning curve for otosclerosis surgery is not steep. Complete preparedness for each potential surgical obstacle or complication is necessary to achieve results approaching those of experienced surgeons in centers of excellence located throughout the world. The atmosphere in operating theatre is usually one of excitement and slight tension with this procedure—especially for those just beginning their careers. Thorough knowledge of and ability to deal with potential complications and surgical deviations help lower anxiety and allow the operating surgeon to focus on and complete the job at hand.

Reliable correction of otosclerotic conductive hearing impairment requires discipline, precision, knowledge, and judgment. Cognitive preparation can and should be complete before undertaking stapes surgery as the primary surgeon. Expert training and steady experience provide mastery of technical skill and development of operative judgment. Only then can the fullest potential as a stapes surgeon be reached.

This chapter is designed to serve as a source of knowledge based on my experience and of other contributors to the field who have courteously shared their experience as colleagues, professors, mentors, and authors. We focus on the preoperative, operative, postoperative, and reoperative situations a surgeon faces when he or she seeks to prevent or rectify complications.

PREOPERATIVE EVALUATION

Medical Conditions

A checklist, either mental or written, is useful to avoid overlooking an important medical feature during preoperative evaluation. It is helpful (and recommended) to have any and all family members in the office present in the examination room during the interview. A useful practice is to write the names of those persons present on the chart during the interview. In addition to a complete history and physical examination with attention to medical conditions germane to any surgical procedure, the prudent surgeon will attempt to identify the following conditions.

Fluctuating hearing loss, episodic vertigo, or low-frequency sensorineural hearing loss (SNHL) may indicate endolymphatic hydrops. Care must be taken to avoid confusing the early conductive hearing loss of prior audiograms (which may falsely appear as SNHL) with endolymphatic hydrops. Patients with endolymphatic hydrops who undergo stapes surgery have a higher rate of SNHL (presumably from dilation of the saccule that contacts the stapes footplate where it is at risk during stapedectomy or stapedotomy) and chronic dizziness. This condition may be a contraindication to surgery.[1]

A history of multiple fractures or blue sclera may allow the diagnosis of osteogenesis imperfecta to be made preoperatively[2] (see later for further management information).

Life-long hearing loss in one ear should alert the surgeon to the possibility of congenital footplate fixation. Congenital footplate fixation carries a higher-than-usual risk of gusher and SNHL.[3] A computed tomography scan should be performed preoperatively in those patients with suspected congenital footplate fixation to look for abnormal cerebrospinal fluid (CSF)-perilymph connections that predispose to gusher. Should a high risk of a gusher be found, amplification is recommended. A genetic pedigree focused on hearing loss is helpful in identifying patients with X-linked progressive mixed deafness. Patients with this disorder are rare and unique in that a conductive hearing loss is seen on the audiogram with intact stapedial reflexes.[4, 5] During surgery a stapes gusher is encountered with the attendant risk of SNHL. Although males are typically affected, heterozygous females may exhibit milder audiologic abnormalities.[6]

Imbalance may occur following otosclerosis surgery in spite of a well-done surgical procedure and an excellent hearing result. Patients with occupations such as professional athletes, high-rise steelworkers, and painters might be best advised to avoid surgery until the completion of their careers. In similar fashion, those patients who depend on their sense of taste for employment (such as wine tasters, coffee tasters, and professional chefs) may choose to avoid surgery. Changes in chorda tympani function felt too minor to most patients may be a source of disability in such professions. Commercial airline pilots usually are allowed to have stapes surgery without impacting their employability, but the operating surgeon or patient should secure written documentation of the patient's employer's policy prior to undertaking surgery.

A history of or exhibited characteristics of severe anxiety, neuropsychiatric disease, claustrophobia, restless leg syndrome and other conditions that would make the procedure difficult under sedation with an awake patient should be sought. When such patients have surgery, it should be performed under general anesthesia.

Physical Examination

A variety of findings impact upcoming surgery, including the following:

- Otitis externa must be completely treated for at least 1 month prior to undertaking surgery.
- Serous otitis media contains bacteria in approximately 50 per cent of patients. Entrance into the vestibule in this situation puts the patient at risk for bacterial labyrinthitis, SNHL, and meningitis.[7-9]
- Tympanic membrane perforation or chronic otitis media must be repaired with a separate procedure prior to stapes surgery to reduce the bacteria present within the operative field as much as possible. Six to 12 months should pass after the first-stage repair for eustachian tube function to declare itself and for the hyperemia attendant with the primary procedure to fade.
- Exostosis, common in cold water swimmers, should be corrected and allowed to heal before attempting stapes surgery.
- A small or unusually angled ear canal should be noted. In extreme circumstances, enlargement may be necessary. More commonly, the case is simply made more difficult.
- Limited neck rotation or obesity may require rotation of the surgical table to allow correct positioning of the ear for the procedure. If this rotation is more than about 15 degrees, patients having surgery under local anesthesia with sedation are concerned about sliding on the operating room table. Such situations are better handled with a general anesthesia where the patient can be positioned more securely on the table.
- Congenital auricular or periauricular anomalies may indicate congenital malformation of the middle ear structures.
- Abnormalities of the ossicles or of the chorda tympani nerve noted at otomicroscopy are markers for congenital abnormalities.
- Severe myringosclerosis or an area of bimeric tympanic membrane (where the fibrous layer of the eardrum is missing, leaving only a mucosal lining and an epithelial surface) increases the chance of tympanic membrane perforation occurring as a result of tympanomeatal flap elevation. Note should be made of the finding to the patient with an explanation of the procedure for correction intraoperatively or during a second procedure. Myringosclerosis may be an indicator of tympanosclerosis involving the stapes footplate (see later for tympanosclerosis management).
- Tuning forks should confirm a conductive hearing loss with Weber or Rinne consistent with the audiogram. Overestimation of the conductive hearing loss using some audiologic techniques occurs. Lack of a "flipped tuning fork" may not be a contraindication to surgery when bilateral disease is present.[10]
- Careful examination may reveal evidence of prior otologic surgery not mentioned by the patient.

Informed Consent

Medicolegal situations over complications that are expected to happen in a small percentage of patients are avoided by achieving written informed consent prior to the procedure. The reader is referred to other chapters within this text for more information on the subject.

OPERATING ROOM

Surgical Technique Prerequisites for Residents

While in training, much effort is put toward using proper methodology in the operating room. The technical difficulty associated with stapes surgery requires the surgeon to be facile with several key techniques. Residents and fellows should enter the operating room with previously demonstrated abilities in several areas. Preparation becomes more of an issue as the number of cases of surgically correctable otosclerosis decreases in most training programs.[11] Limitation of hospital privileges may become more of an issue in the future if case availability precludes ascent to an acceptable level on an individual's own learning curve. The following list is put forth for those in training to use as preparation for successful performance of stapes surgery while minimizing the risk of complication for the patient.

Parfocal Set-Up of the Operating Microscope. This allows the surgeon to change magnification without losing focus in the operative field. Safety, accuracy, and speed all are improved. Please see Chapter 23 for details on microscope adjustment to achieve a parfocal state.

Appropriate Microscope Triangulation Intraoperatively to Allow Depth of Field Perspective. To achieve depth of field information, the plane of view must be off-axis from the surgical instrument by several degrees. Movement of the microscope off-axis establishes a virtual triangle with its apex at the point of surgical interest (usually the tip of an instrument or an anatomic structure). The two points of the base of the triangle are formed by the microscope lens and the intersection of an imaginary line drawn perpendicular to the line of vision from the microscope where it intersects another imaginary line extending from the handle of the instrument (Fig. 27–1). Very small movements of the microscope can mean the difference between success and failure with delicate manipulations mandatory with stapedotomy.

Appropriate Use of Magnification Balancing Depth of Field with Surgical Detail. Increasing magnification

FIGURE 27-1

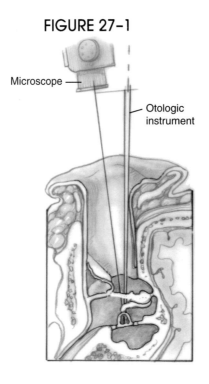

Microscope

Otologic
instrument

Tympanomeatal flap

FIGURE 27-2

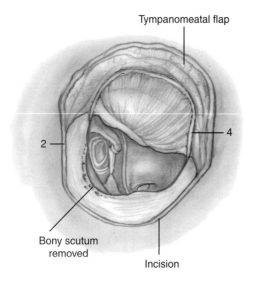

2

4

Bony scutum
removed

Incision

1. Bone of scutum (partially removed for exposure)
2. Tympanomeatal flap incision
3. Malleus
4. Fibrous annulus (elevated out of its sulcus)
5. Facial nerve ridge
6. Promontory
7. Round window niche
8. Stapes footplate
9. Saccule
10. Utricle
11. Chorda tympani nerve
12. Pyramidal eminence

FIGURE 27–1. Surgical technique of microscope triangulation.

FIGURE 27–2.

decreases depth of field and vice versa. The surgeon must balance the need for high magnification (such as is needed with footplate work) with the need for depth of field (such as is needed when securing the tympanomeatal flap with Gelfoam).

Laser Safety, Use, Beam Sizing, and Focus Coincident with Parfocal Microscope. Delivery of laser energy is a function of laser wavelength, generated power from the laser base unit, and power density as determined by the size of the working spot size in the operative field. If the laser is scope mounted, it should remain focused precisely with the vision at the working magnifications in which it will be needed. The surgeon should also be familiar with beam defocusing. This technique can be useful when taking measures such as stopping bleeding and shrinking tissue. Hand-held lasers diverge from the fiberoptic tip. In this instance, laser power can be manipulated by moving the probe tip to or away from the intended target.

Two-Handed Technique. It is critical that the operative surgeon be able to use two hands to perform surgical maneuvers. This skill is learned and starts with the use of two hands for otologic procedures beginning with tympanostomy tubes. Likewise, vision with two eyes is necessary to allow depth perception. Instruments must be grasped and used in a way that neither the right or left eye's visual pathway from the microscope is obstructed. Observer side arms are monocular, and the surgeon in training may not realize when binocular vision is missing when using the binocular microscope unless instructed. Professors of otologic surgery can ensure binocular vision while looking through the monocular side arm by watching the video monitor and the side arm in succession. Typically, the side arm is what the operating surgeon sees through one eye, while the video shows what is seen through the other eye.

Lack of Significant Tremor. Although many fine surgeons have rhythmic variation in fine muscle control, delicate otologic surgery and significant tremor are mutually exclusive. Nervousness and anxiety make tremor worse. Both the surgeon and professor of surgery should attempt to create and maintain an atmosphere of relaxed concentration and focus.

Canal Injection for Hemostasis. Local anesthetic provides anesthesia for the patient under sedation and is critical to procedure success. The mucosa of the middle ear receives innervation from deeper nerves and is not affected by the canal injection. A drop or two of local anesthesia instilled into the middle ear provides nearly instant relief. Anesthetic should be promptly removed from the middle ear to prevent absorption into the inner ear avoiding the coincident severe vertigo, nausea, and vomiting. A high percentage of epinephrine in the canal injection (such as 1:20,000) provides a maximal amount of vasoconstriction with a minimum of volume of injection. Turning the needle such that the bevel is against the bone allows delicate instillation of solution under thin skin. The majority of innervation proceeds down the canal, but small nerves traverse the fissures of Santorini in the anterior inferior canal adjacent to the annulus. These nerves are more of an issue when dissection is carried out in this area, but they may also need to be surrounded with local anesthetic to provide a comfortable patient under sedation. Use of identical syringes for each procedure will allow the surgeon to develop the feel necessary to perform excellent injections (we suggest a glass dental-type syringe holding 3 ml of solution). A perfect injection is an art that comes only with practice. Surgeons in training should perform and demonstrate proficiency with injections in cases where it is not as critical to the outcome of the procedure (such as tympanoplasty) before being allowed to inject for stapedotomy. Creation of large blebs cannot be rectified easily and markedly increases case difficulty.

Tympanomeatal Flap Design and Elevation. A recurring mistake of inexperienced surgeons occurs when the tympanomeatal flap is too short to reach anatomic position following curetting to expose the oval window niche (Fig. 27–2). One should avoid suctioning the elevated skin to prevent flap tears. Positioning the suction behind the round knife during flap elevation keeps the field dry and prevents inadvertent suctioning of the elevated skin. The vertical incisions of the flap should be kept 1 to 2 mm lateral to the annulus to reduce the likelihood of tearing the tympanic membrane.

Chorda Tympani Nerve Identification and Preservation. Surgeons should be able to identify and mobilize this nerve at the iter chordae posterius and also from the posterior surface of the malleus to maximize the chance of its preservation.

Curetting. Proficiency must be demonstrated in removing the posterosuperior canal wall to expose the facial nerve and pyramidal process while preserving the chorda tympani nerve.

Incudostapedial Joint Identification and Division. Correct identification of the joint is necessary to prevent removal of the lenticular process of the incus. This becomes more of an issue when a bucket handle prosthesis is used. Slight anterior pressure on the incus while focusing on the joint under high power allows correct identification of this plane.

Prosthesis Sizing. Understanding of the measurements used (Fig. 27–3) improves results. Measurement from the lateral surface of the footplate to the medial side of the incus is taken. To this figure is added 0.5 mm and an amount equal to the thickness of the stapes footplate. Footplate thickness may vary from 0.2 mm to several millimeters. The prosthesis should extend 0.5 mm beyond the medial surface of the footplate into the vestibule (Figs. 27–4 and 27–5).

Suction Sizing to Usage and Risk. Proper two-handed technique turns the suction into an instrument. Suction size must be scaled to use. Damage to middle and inner ear structures may occur with use of too large a suction or with improper use of any suction. Intraoperative electronystagmographic studies performed on stapedectomy patients in the prelaser era implicate suctioning over the vestibule (as well as drilling near the oval and round windows and manipulation of the stapes footplate) as the great offenders for vestibular and presumably for cochlear damage.[12]

Crus Division and Stapes Superstructure Removal. Fracture of the stapes superstructure with both crura intact and a fixed footplate is frequently possible. Division of the posterior crus prior to fracture decreases the chance of stapes footplate fracture, mobilization, and transmission of potentially damaging energy to the inner ear. A variety of methods are available for division of the posterior crus.

FIGURE 27-3

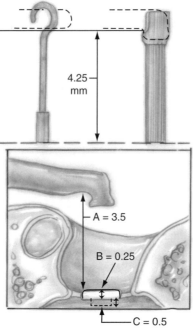

A = 3.5

B = 0.25

C = 0.5

(A = 3.5) + (B = 0.25) + (C = 0.5) = 4.25 mm

4.25 mm

FIGURE 27-4

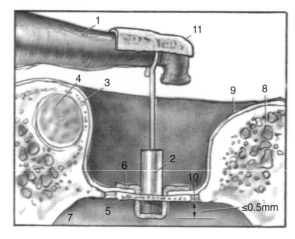

1. Incus
2. Piston
3. Bone of the facial nerve ridge
4. Facial nerve
5. Stapes footplate
6. Tissue seal
7. Vestibule
8. Promontory
9. Mesotympanum mucosa
10. Annular ligament
11. Tissue overlay

≤0.5mm

FIGURE 27-5

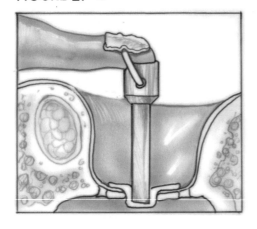

FIGURE 27-6

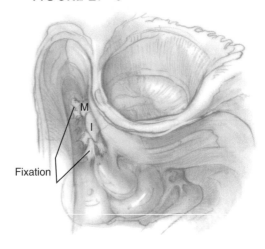

M

I

Fixation

FIGURES 27-3 and 27-6. *See legends on opposite page*

Our preferred method is laser vaporization, which carries with it a much-reduced risk for the inner ear. While some techniques advocate laser vaporization of the anterior crus, there is no indication that fracture of a single crus with a fixed footplate carries any risk of footplate mobilization.

Prosthesis Preparation and Loading. For those surgeons using a vein-clad technique, vein preparation, sizing, and vein-clad prosthesis preparation are steps in which small variations can produce postoperative conductive hearing loss. The stapedotomy, prosthesis, and attached vein should be approximately 0.9, 0.6, and 0.2 mm respectively. Variations in the thickness of the attached vein may cause the surgeon to vary the size of the stapedotomy. For this reason, the vein-clad prosthesis should be prepared before creation of the stapedotomy. In those situations where a vein is not attached to the prosthesis, the stapedotomy should exceed the size of the prosthesis by 0.2 to 0.3 mm. Bucket handle prostheses should be inserted with the bail inferior to the incus to allow it to be swung superiorly and secured with small pieces of tissue. Shepherd's crook pistons should be grasped with smooth forceps in a way that the open end of the wire hook can be placed directly over the incus.

Footplate Removal. The surgeon must be able to create a round and concentrically located stapedotomy by melding multiple round individual laser bursts. The tiny movements used to move the laser are more reliably produced by moving the microscope with pressure from a hand or nose than with the joystick, although both methods work. Vaporization of the footplate with a laser leaves a small meshwork of char. This need not be removed before prosthesis placement. Large fragments of footplate that enter the vestibule can give patients symptoms of positional vertigo. For this reason, all bony fragments within the stapedotomy that may mobilize with prosthesis placement should be vaporized. One should never attempt to "fish out" a fragment that has entered the vestibule. Use of a microdrill creates a round stapedotomy. Significant pressure on the footplate must be avoided to prevent drill overinsertion in the vestibule.

Prosthesis Placement. Resident surgeons should practice crimping techniques in the laboratory prior to undertaking the maneuver on a patient. Likewise, placement of a bucket handle prosthesis should be performed in the temporal bone laboratory setting first. Excess vein from operative procedures can be taken to the laboratory to create a realistic practice model.

Prosthesis Removal. Frequently, with revision surgery a prior prosthesis must be removed. It is also sometimes necessary, especially early in one's career, to remove a prosthesis that is the wrong size during primary surgery. This is best accomplished for a prosthesis attached to the incus with a wire by inserting a right-angle hook and rotating the hook to open the wire loop. In this way, traction forces on the incus are avoided. Laser ablation of the tissue surrounding the oval window segment of the prosthesis is a first step before removal to avoid traction damage of structures within the vestibule.

Those who have performed stapes surgery frequently understand that each individual step of the procedure itself must be performed to perfection or the ill effects become additive. (For example, a less than stellar injection makes every remaining portion of the procedure more difficult if blood continues to enter the operative field. Likewise, inadequate curetting limits exposure of the footplate, and so on.) A small amount of compromise in each step of the procedure quickly adds up to overall failure. This "law of additive inadequacy" has proven useful as a teaching concept. Viewing the procedure in this way emphasizes the need for perfection in each step before moving forward in the operation.

Similar to a preflight checklist, every skill must be checked off before allowing performance of a stapedotomy. Those that never master the listed techniques probably should not perform stapes surgery as part of their surgical practice—just as not every otolaryngologist is able to perform procedures such as blepharoplasty, partial laryngectomy, and laryngotracheal reconstruction.

Understandably, attending physicians are reticent to allow significant participation of residents and fellows if this means that several inadequacies have already summed to put the senior surgeon in a tough spot while completing the procedure. Residents and fellows gain the confidence of their attending surgeons as these skills are mastered allowing greater and greater participation. It is the duty of those of us who teach surgical technique to deliver to the next generation a cadre of well-trained individuals suited to stapes surgery without sacrificing success and safety for our current patients.

Surgical Equipment, Decisions, and Techniques

Prosthesis Type, Size, and Availability. Three general prosthesis types exist: piston/wire, bucket handle, and Teflon varieties. Little comparative data exist to compare the different types, but bucket handle prostheses may have a smaller incidence of incus necrosis in long-term follow-up. Piston/wire and Teflon varieties are probably easier to place.

Prostheses come in several different diameters, ranging from 0.3 to 0.8 mm most commonly. Experienced surgeons have indicated that 0.6 mm gives optimal results.[13] Several studies exist looking at alternative sizes, and there appears to be no degradation of results at 0.4 mm in the speech range.[14] Prostheses measuring 0.3 mm show worse hearing results when compared with those of 0.4 mm.[15] Data from our institute comparing 0.6 to 0.8 Robinson bucket handle prostheses reveal relatively equal function with a slight, but statistically insignificant, degradation in conductive hearing in the higher frequencies with larger prostheses—possibly due to weight.

FIGURE 27–3. Stapedotomy prosthesis measurement lengths.

FIGURE 27–6. Malleus and incus fixation.

Prosthesis length varies from patient to patient. Availability of the correct prosthesis is crucial to successful outcome. It is our preference to use a bucket handle prosthesis. Table 27–1 outlines those prostheses stocked in our operating suite. Note the inclusion of the incus replacement prosthesis (see the later discussion on incus necrosis).

Laser Stapedotomy Versus Drill Stapedotomy. It is generally agreed among most surgeons that use of the laser reduces the risk of mechanical transmission of vibratory energy to the inner ear, thereby making it a safer technique. Comparative data from primary stapedotomy question this tenet, viewing both techniques as effective and safe.[16] Use of a laser does improve results in revision cases.[17] In all cases, proper use of the laser reduces bleeding associated with tissue ablation, which is an advantage. Both techniques are accepted within the standard of care.

Stapedectomy Versus Stapedotomy. The procedure of choice for the majority of otologists for otosclerosis has become stapedotomy. When compared with stapedectomy, the limited fenestra improves results in the high frequencies, and most authors report a reduction in SNHL as a result of the procedure.[17–20] Stapedotomy carries a smaller rate of postoperative vestibular complaints. Stapedectomy remains a valuable alternative in the experience of some surgeons. Occasionally, a stapedotomy will need to be converted to a complete stapedectomy.

Stapedotomy Site. The stapedotomy should be placed posteroinferiorly in the central footplate region (see Fig. 27–2). This area does not overlay the saccule or utricle and gives the most margin for error. It is possible, and indeed frequently necessary, to move the stapedotomy to other areas of the footplate due to anatomic concerns of the incus or structures surrounding the oval window niche.

Footplate/Vestibular Relationships. Almost all patients

TABLE 27–1. Prosthesis Type and Size Stocked in Operating Suite

LENGTH	A	B	C	D	E	F
3.5		X	X	X	X	
3.75	X					
4.0	X	X	X	X	X	
4.25	X					
4.5	X	X	X	X	X	
4.75	X					
5.0	X	X	X	X	X	
5.75						X
6.0						X
6.25						X
6.5						X
6.75						X
7.0						X
7.25						X

A, Platinum-Teflon piston
B, Bucket handle piston 1.0 mm well × 0.6 mm piston
C, Bucket handle piston 0.875 mm well × 0.6 mm piston
D, Bucket handle piston 1.0 mm well × 0.8 mm piston
E, Bucket handle piston 0.875 mm well × 0.8 mm piston
F, Malleus piston prosthesis (incus replacement prosthesis)

have a minimum safe distance of 1.0 mm between the medial surface of the footplate and the utricle or saccule. Penetration of the vestibule by more than 1.0 mm with instruments or the prosthesis may impinge the structures of the membranous labyrinth, producing vertigo with prosthesis movement. Perforation of the saccule or utricle may induce SNHL, vertigo, or both.[21, 22]

Laser Type. Much controversy regarding laser type, efficacy, and safety has arisen since the first laser stapedotomy performed by Perkins.[23] Visible wavelength lasers have the added advantage of absorption by blood, thereby providing hemostasis. Appropriate adjustment of the CO_2 laser can provide hemostasis as well. Visible wavelength lasers have the technologic advantage of being able to use the laser light as the aiming beam. This avoids needing to produce a visible wavelength light that also serves as the aiming beam, which may not accurately reflect where the therapeutic beam is aimed (as can occur with the helium-neon aiming beam with CO_2 lasers). Theoretical concerns regarding absorption of energy from the KTP or argon laser by the inner ear have been voiced by several authors (visible wavelength lasers are transmitted through clear fluid). Several studies have proven equal safety of both visible wavelength and CO_2 lasers for laser stapedotomy.[24, 25]

Local Versus General Anesthesia. Local anesthesia for laser stapedotomy is cost effective, safe, and comfortable for patients. Under sedation a patient can supply feedback to the surgeon if any event that stimulates the vestibular system occurs. Such feedback may help to prevent damage to inner ear structures. Additionally, the patient's assessment of hearing ability after prosthesis placement and tympanomeatal flap replacement is helpful. Movement, which could be disastrous, is rarely experienced in the appropriately psychologically prepared and medicated patient. General anesthesia is used in those patients unable to comply with the demands of local anesthesia with sedation such as those with claustrophobia, young age, or who are non–English speaking. General anesthesia has appeal for teaching cases where operative time may be long.

Stapedotomy in Children. Stapedotomy can be performed safely in children with surgical results as least as good as those expected in adults.[26] Children should be beyond the age of otitis media, and surgery should be attempted only under general anesthesia. Congenital footplate fixation requires special considerations as mentioned later.

Prosthesis Ballottement. Following prosthesis placement, careful and gentle palpation of the incus reveals the degree of freedom of movement of the prosthesis. Prosthesis ballottement can be a useful measure for experienced surgeons to assess the function of the reconstruction on the operating table. If a prosthesis is too long and touching the membranous labyrinth (which could produce vestibular symptoms with loud sounds postoperatively), gentle motion of the reconstruction will induce vertigo in sedated patients allowing prosthesis replacement during the original procedure.

Prosthesis Displaceability at Stapedotomy. Following prosthesis placement, a gentle posterior to anterior force applied to the shaft of the prosthesis at the footplate helps identify a prosthesis of inappropriate length. A prosthesis well situated will not displace, whereas a too short prosthesis will be displaced from the stapedotomy. Because prosthesis displacement is the most common reason for failure of surgical success, proper sizing and positioning should receive special attention.

Oval Window Seal. A tissue seal at the oval window (our preference is vein taken from the dorsum of the hand) reduces, and in fact nearly eliminates, the risk of perilymphatic fistula.[27]

COMPLICATIONS ENCOUNTERED AT PRIMARY SURGERY: MANAGEMENT

Tympanic Membrane Perforation/Flap Tear. Skin or tympanic membrane tears can complicate elevation of the tympanomeatal flap. The case can be continued with an underlay graft of fascia or other collagen-containing tissue providing repair. With small tears, the defect heals if edges are approximated without an underlay graft. A similar repair can be used when the flap is made too short to cover the area of bone removal in the posterosuperior margin of the bony annulus. The flap incision should be at least 6 mm from the annular ligament to prevent inadequate flap length. The surgeon can estimate appropriate flap length to be twice the length of a large round knife.

Incus Dislocation. Dislocation of the incus precludes routine stapedotomy. The case should be halted and time given for the incus and malleus to reattach. In 4 to 6 months the patient is taken back to the operating room. If sufficient reattachment has occurred, stapedotomy is performed in the usual fashion. If not, the incus is removed and a malleus-to-footplate prosthesis is used.

Malleus/Incus Fixation. As a routine, every case should include a check of the mobility of the malleus and incus. This is best performed after division of the incudostapedial joint with gentle upward pressure on the undersurface of the handle of the malleus while watching for movement at the lenticular process of the incus. Documentation of the state of function of the first two ossicles is critical when evaluating and planning revision for those patients who do not enjoy adequate improvement of hearing with the primary procedure. In addition, in approximately 1 per cent of cases, fixation of the malleus and incus will be discovered, allowing rectification during the primary procedure. A small or moderate amount of limitation of motion of the malleus and incus will usually produce little in terms of conductive hearing loss, which is usually low frequency in nature. In cases where doubt exists as to the severity of malleus and incus fixation, performance of the stapedotomy with postoperative testing prior to work on the malleus and/or incus shows good judgment.

Operative repair of the situation is best addressed with a mastoidotomy with extension into the root of the zygoma to allow exposure of the body of the incus and head of the malleus in the epitympanum (Fig. 27–6). Usually, fixation occurs at the superior malleolar ligament from the tegmen. The posterior process of the incus may also be involved, as can any suspensory ligament of the ossicular chain.

Removal of offending bone and restoration of ossicular mobility can be performed with a laser. Larger wattages are necessary than those used on the stapes superstructure or footplate (we use the KTP laser with 5 to 8 W on continuous mode). A blood-soaked Gelfoam is placed as a "backstop" to protect the facial nerve with higher laser settings. Although a drill can remove bone as well, laser use minimizes the risk of transmission of damaging vibratory energy to the vestibule. If the stapes is also fixed, it is prudent to remove the stapes superstructure prior to mobilization of the malleus and incus. If the conductive hearing loss resides solely in the fixation of the malleus and incus, disarticulation of the incudostapedial joint to produce discontinuity is mandatory (sometimes interposition of Gelfoam is necessary to keep the lenticular process of the incus from touching the capitulum of the stapes). Removal of bone in the mastoid can be performed comfortably in most patients under sedation.

If a laser is not available, reconstruction can still be performed. Removal of the incus allows access to the head of the malleus through the mastoid. Removal of the head of the malleus superior to the lateral ligament is then performed with a malleus nipper or a tiny diamond drill. The chorda tympani nerve should be mobilized from the medial surface of the neck of the malleus and pushed inferiorly to prevent its injury with this maneuver. Reconstruction with a malleus to stapes footplate prosthesis completes the repair.

Persistent Stapedial Artery/Vascular Anomalies. Rarely, a persistent stapedial artery is encountered running from the facial nerve through the arch of the stapes to the carotid artery. Even less commonly, an aberrant carotid is seen. While the persistent stapedial artery is not seen with otoscopy, an aberrant carotid is visible and can be mistaken for a glomus tumor. The great majority of vascular anomalies occur in women patients.[28] If a persistent stapedial artery is small, fine bipolar cautery or laser coagulation may be used to remove the vessel from the field, thereby allowing completion of the procedure. With larger arteries, it may be prudent to stop the procedure and prescribe amplification.

Tympanosclerosis. One may discover ossicular fixation secondary to tympanosclerosis of the stapes footplate. Fixation of this type is not as vascular as otosclerosis and has a softer texture. Stapedotomy may be performed safely. Excellent early results may be achieved with some attrition over time.[29–31]

Osteogenesis Imperfecta. Osteogenesis imperfecta is a congenital disorder of bone inherited via autosomal dominant or autosomal recessive patterns. The triad of blue sclera, multiple fractures, and conductive hearing loss is known as Van der Hoeve's syndrome. The mean age of hearing impairment is in the early 20s.[32] Footplate fixation accounts for the conductive hearing loss. Footplates are typically thick and frequently very soft with increased vascularity, while crura may be atrophic.[33] Progressive SNHL can be seen in a small percentage of patients.[34] Despite a small increase in risk of SNHL in some series, stapedotomy remains a viable treatment for conductive hearing loss associated with this disorder.

Congenital Stapes Fixation. Complete absence of the

annular ligament of the stapes without evidence of otosclerotic bone growth may be congenital stapes fixation. Please refer to the discussion of this entity in the beginning of this chapter.

Round Window Obliteration. Severe otosclerotic overgrowth may completely obliterate the round window membrane. A remedy is not available for the excess bone and complete closure of the air-bone gap is unlikely postoperatively.

Overhanging Facial Nerve. The facial nerve can provide obstruction to completing successful stapes surgery and will be encountered regularly (Fig. 27–7). Recognition of an aberrant or dehiscent facial nerve will prevent injury. Twenty-five to 40 per cent of temporal bone specimens include dehiscence of the bony fallopian canal. Inconveniently located dehiscence may be sites of trauma due to surgical instrumentation. Local anesthetic agents may also penetrate these areas more readily, causing postoperative facial paralysis. The reader is referred to Chapter 23 for management options. In some situations, coupling the technique used for narrow oval window enlargement becomes necessary for prosthesis placement. Rarely will a dehiscent facial nerve prevent successful surgical repair.

Narrow Oval Window Niche. Anatomic abnormalities or impingement on the oval window area by the facial nerve can produce narrowing to the extent prosthesis placement is difficult or impossible. Enlargement of the inferior margin of the oval window niche at the mid point of the footplate just anterior to the junction of the subiculum and promontory can facilitate surgical success. Intermittent laser pulses produce char that is then removed with a rasp. Significant extra space can be gained with this technique, because the bone is quite thick in this area. Care must be taken to prevent caloric overstimulation of the vestibule. In addition, the stapedotomy can be shifted inferiorly to the margin of the oval window to facilitate prosthesis placement. Overlapping the margin of the oval window can be dangerous as Reissner's membrane and the basilar membrane occupy this area in the cochlear hook region.[35]

Congenitally Ectopic Facial Nerve. The facial nerve may be congenitally malpositioned entirely on the promontory side of the footplate split with a portion on either side of the footplate, or pass through the arch of the stapes.[36, 37] The stapes crura are not attached to the footplate a high percentage of the time with abnormalities in the course of the facial nerve. If prosthesis placement can proceed without iatrogenic injury to the nerve, the case can be completed with the prosthesis placed above, between, or around the aberrant nerve. Alternatively, few hearing devices produce facial paralysis!

Biscuit Footplate. Manipulation of a biscuit footplate puts the patient at increased risk for footplate mobilization and SNHL (Fig. 27–8). Use of the laser allows removal of bone and performance of a footplate fenestra without significant energy transfer to the tenuous footplate. Care should be used to prevent heat transfer to the vestibule that may put the inner ear at risk. Cases performed under local sedation allow the surgeon to sense when caloric stimulation begins for the patient as vertigo frequently begins. Cessation of laser use for several minutes allows cooling of the footplate and vestibule allowing resumption of the bone removal process. Patients operated under general anesthesia should have no more than 8 to 10 laser pulses in a row without allowing time for cooling. Excellent results are obtainable for the patient surgeon.

Obliterative Otosclerosis. Obliteration of the oval window niche occurs from otosclerotic bone growth in some cases (Fig. 27–9). The area should not be drilled out using a diamond burr because reactivation and reformation of the otosclerotic growth may be stimulated and a higher rate of SNHL realized. Bleeding is also frequently produced with such a technique.[38, 39, 40] Footplate fenestration may be accomplished as with a biscuit footplate outlined above.

Perilymphatic Gusher. The normal anatomic arrangement of the human ear allows flow of CSF into the perilymphatic space. Normally, extremely small connections between these two spaces exist. With enlarged connections (usually through the fundus of the internal auditory canal, the modiolus of the cochlea, and possibly through an enlarged cochlear aqueduct), a rapid outpouring of perilymph occurs when the stapes footplate is removed as a barrier in either a stapedectomy or stapedotomy. Known as a "gusher," such an event can be associated with SNHL.[41] Conditions known to increase the chance of this condition include enlarged vestibular aqueduct syndrome, X-linked progressive mixed deafness, congenital footplate fixation, and Mondini's dysplasia.

Successful repair is most easily accomplished with a bucket-type piston over a vein graft seal of the stapedotomy. The bucket-type prosthesis is recommended because of the possible CSF pressure extrusion of a piston-shepherd's crook–type prosthesis. If a watertight seal can be accomplished, no further treatment is necessary except restricted activity for 1 week.

Several authors recommend creation of a small control hole in the footplate prior to removal of the footplate if the technique of stapedectomy is used. It is much easier to handle this complication through a small footplate hole than with the entire footplate out. In the event a gusher is encountered that cannot be controlled with a vein and prosthesis, more extensive management becomes necessary. In this situation, management is similar to that of a CSF leak. Tissue is used to provide a seal for the oval window fenestra, preferably with a prosthesis providing tamponade (which is not always possible). A lumbar drain is placed to decrease the cerebrospinal and perilymph pressure. Postoperatively, the head of the bed is elevated at least 30 degrees and bed rest utilized. Fluids are restricted and oral acetazolamide may be prescribed. Prophylactic antibiotics are given.[42] Discharge is accomplished 24 hours after the lumbar drain is clamped with no further fluid leak as judged by CSF rhinorrhea. Bed rest at home is recommended for another week.

Fractured Footplate. Fragmentation occasionally occurs. Free-floating surface fragments should be removed and the surgery converted to a partial or complete stapedectomy. A tissue seal is mandatory in this setting.

Footplate Fragments in the Vestibule. No attempt should be made to remove any footplate fragments in the vestibule. Although positional vertigo is rarely a sequela of these fragments, most cause no harm. Attempted removal with an instrument in the vestibule carries a high rate of SNHL.

Sensorineural Hearing Loss. SNHL is perhaps the most

FIGURE 27-7

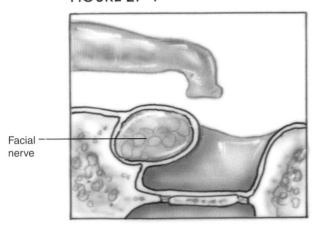

Facial nerve

1. Biscuit footplate

FIGURE 27-8

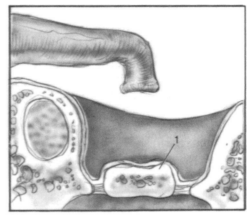

1. Posterior stapedial crura
2. Thickened footplate with obliterative otosclerosis
3. Incudostapedial joint

FIGURE 27-9

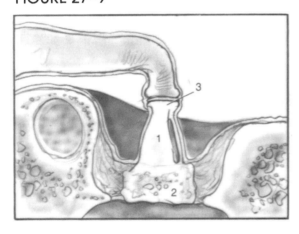

FIGURE 27-10

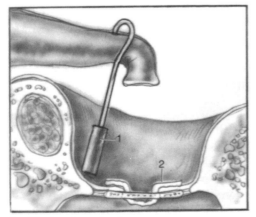
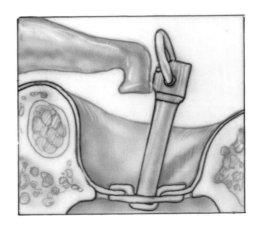

1. Displaced prosthesis
2. Tissue seal preventing perilymph fistula

disappointing and devastating complication for both the patient and surgeon. Complete or partial hearing loss can result from the most meticulously and appropriately performed stapes procedure. Most cases, however, probably are due to surgical trauma. Intraoperative electronystagmographic studies performed during stapedectomy in the pre-laser era implicate suctioning over the vestibule, drilling near the footplate, or oval window niche, and manipulation of the footplate as the great offenders for vestibular and presumably for cochlear damage.[43]

COMPLICATIONS FOLLOWING PRIMARY SURGERY: MEDICAL MANAGEMENT

Acute Otitis Media. Acute otitis media occurs in the postoperative period in patients who have had stapes surgery. The infection is usually successfully treated without sequelae. Entrance of pathogenic organisms into the perilymph can produce SNHL and vestibular damage. Progression into the CSF has been reported with meningitis.[44–47] Prophylactic antibiotics have not been shown to reduce the incidence of this complication and carry some risk and are, therefore, not recommended.

Barotrauma. Iatrogenic rearrangement of the normal anatomy may increase a patient's chance of suffering barotrauma of the inner ear following stapes surgery. It is our practice to allow patients to fly in pressurized aircraft 2 days following surgery. No restrictions are placed for snorkeling or scuba diving after healing has taken place, provided patients are able to self-insufflate through an open eustachian tube (as all patients should have for these activities even without previous ear surgery). A wide range of practices regarding postoperative restrictions exists among otologists. No significant differences have been demonstrated in the prevalence of barotrauma based on individual physician's recommendations for these activities.[48]

Dysgeusia. Approximately 20 per cent of patients note taste changes in the postoperative period when asked. Chorda tympani nerve dysfunction is usually transient, and fewer than 5 per cent of patients experience permanent deficits. "Second ears" and patients with a vocation involving taste deserve special consideration. Revision cases frequently involve a nerve adherent to the posterior surface of the tympanic membrane. Mobilization of an adherent nerve is best accomplished with a small sharp blade (such as a No. 5910 Beaver blade designed for corneal incisions).

Delayed Facial Nerve Paralysis. A small number of delayed facial nerve paralysis have occurred. Typically, the onset of paralysis occurs 7 to 10 days after surgery and is associated with pain. Treatment with a tapering dose of steroids (we use prednisone 30 mg bid tapering over 2 weeks) has brought about resolution in all cases.[49]

Hyperacusis. Almost all patients have some degree of phonophobia postoperatively. Reassurance is adequate treatment, with only a small number experiencing a persistent problem.[50]

Diplacusis Binauralis. The same tone will be perceived as different pitches in each ear in about one third of patients

following stapes surgery. By 6 weeks postoperatively, the condition fades without treatment.[51]

Otosclerotic Inner Ear Syndrome. Balance disturbance may result from ongoing growth of the otosclerotic focus postoperatively. Patients complain of brief episodes of motion not severe enough to be termed spinning or of diffuse, persistent unsteadiness. Such complaints are hard to distinguish from perilymphatic fistula and other causes of postoperative vestibular complaints. A high percentage of patients respond to the administration of fluoride when the complaint is due to ongoing otosclerosis.[52] We currently use calcium fluoride (MonoCal), two tablets twice daily. Sodium fluoride (FluroCal) has been associated with gastric intolerance in a higher percentage of patients.[53]

Sensorineural Hearing Loss Progression. Otosclerosis induces a progressive SNHL in a significant number of patients.[54–56] Otosclerosis can, in fact, be a cause of SNHL without a conductive component.[57] It can be extremely disappointing to see an excellent surgical result deteriorate due to progressive SNHL, leaving the patient with functionally significant hearing impairment. Convincing data exist that establish the role of fluoride in stabilizing SNHL associated with otosclerosis.[58–64] We place patients with SNHL present at the time of surgery on calcium fluoride (two tablets orally twice daily with meals) for 1 to 2 years following surgery. If hearing remains stable at that time, the treatment is stopped. Any further progression prompts further treatment. Patients who demonstrate new-onset SNHL in the postoperative period are treated similarly.

Serous Labyrinthitis. Patients who experience the onset of constant dysequilibrium several days following surgery are thought to have an inflammatory response in the inner ear. Frequently, a short course of steroids will improve symptoms and alleviate dizziness.

Vestibular Complaints. Vertigo with and following stapedotomy is less frequent than with stapedectomy. Approximately 1 or 2 in 10 patients will experience some balance complaint immediately following laser stapedotomy. Standard sedative vestibular suppressants provide relief allowing the problem to resolve on its own. Rarely does a patient suffer symptoms for more than 2 days postoperatively.

Wound Infection. Antibiotic-soaked absorbable gelatin sponges are placed against the tympanomeatal flap incision after return of the eardrum and skin to anatomic position. It is not necessary to fill the ear canal. The packing is removed 5 to 10 days following surgery. Antibiotic eardrops are prescribed once daily for 2 weeks. Water precautions are followed until 3 weeks postoperatively. With such a regimen, wound infections occur extremely rarely.

Upper Respiratory Infection. Infection in the postoperative period with influenza virus has been associated with an increase in SNHL.[65]

COMPLICATIONS FOLLOWING PRIMARY SURGERY: SURGICAL MANAGEMENT

Adhesions. Postoperative adhesions form in virtually every surgical case. Significant conductive hearing loss is rarely a result of adhesions for stapedotomy patients unless the healing process has displaced the prosthesis. When the middle ear is re-examined following primary surgery in these patients, a source of conductive hearing loss apart from adhesions must be sought. Stapedectomy patients have a higher tendency to form adhesions around the prosthesis foot in the oval window. Severe fibrosis in this area can displace or severely limit motion of the prosthesis producing conductive loss.

One of the most useful features of the laser for use in revision surgery is removal of adhesions with little to no bleeding. For insignificant adhesions, laser vaporization allows identification of the real cause of recurrent conductive hearing impairment without troublesome bleeding. In the case of oval window fibrosis, therapeutic removal of the adhesions with maintenance of a thin membrane separating the vestibule allowing prosthesis placement is possible.

Acute Facial Nerve Paralysis. As opposed to delayed facial nerve paralysis, which is a medically treated condition, acute paralysis may require surgical intervention. Adequate time (approximately 2 hours) should elapse following surgery to preclude a local anesthetic effect. Cases of persistent paralysis should be re-explored. Including a colleague for objectivity and future support and collaboration may be a prudent move.

Conductive Hearing Loss. Return of conductive hearing loss is by far the most commonly experienced postoperative complication of stapedotomy, accounting for 50 to 70 per cent of revision surgical procedures.[66-70] Although exact rates are difficult to determine, from 10 to 20 per cent of cases will require revision sometime during the patient's lifetime. With the decrease in primary surgery, many experienced stapes surgeons perform revision surgery a significant percentage of the time.

Prosthesis Displacement. Hearing deterioration may be acute, as the prosthesis becomes dislodged, or chronic, as it is gradually displaced out of position (Fig. 27–10). This complication may be encountered many years after stapes surgery. The diagnosis is definitively made at reoperation but may be suspected based on history and tuning fork and audiometric testing.

Incus Necrosis. Division of the incudostapedial joint reduces the blood supply to the distal incus. Vessels from the stapes superstructure provide a minority of perfusion while those coursing from the stapedial tendon bring most of the blood to the distal incus. Necrosis of this incus leads to prosthesis displacement (Figs. 27–11 and 27–12). Prostheses that crimp onto the incus may further reduce the only remaining blood supply coming from the direction of the body of the incus, increasing the chance of this complication. For this reason, some surgeons prefer a bucket handle prosthesis. Incus necrosis still occurs, no matter which prosthesis is used.

If an adequate amount of incus remains, a shepherd's crook prosthesis can be used by crimping the prosthesis more proximally on the incus during revision surgery. On occasion it will be necessary to bend the prosthesis around the facial nerve ridge to establish footplate contact. The amount of bend impacts the length of prosthesis needed. In the event the remnant incus cannot be used, the tympanic membrane is elevated from the lateral surface of the malleus and a malleus to stapes footplate prosthesis is placed.

Table 27–1 lists sizes of our preferred malleus-to-footplate prosthesis.

Prosthesis Extrusion. Prosthesis extrusion may occur in rare instances. Usually, contact of the prosthesis is first established by retraction of the eardrum. Over time, a perforation occurs and prosthesis extrusion becomes evident. A prosthesis that has partially extruded through the drum can be left in place as long as adequate function is maintained. In this event, the ear should be kept dry. Persistent tympanic membrane perforations should be repaired prior to replacing the stapes prosthesis to reduce the bacterial content of the middle ear prior to opening the vestibule. Placement of a tympanostomy tube or positioning of autologous tissue over the prosthesis helps discourage future extrusion.

Otosclerotic Regrowth. Otosclerosis continues to grow in some patients producing prosthesis fixation or displacement (Fig. 27–13). At revision surgery, the cause of the conductive hearing impairment is best handled with prosthesis removal, laser enlargement of the stapedotomy, and placement of a fresh prosthesis.

Wire Loop Prosthesis. The dominant prosthesis used for many years for stapes surgery was the wire loop prosthesis. The wire loop prosthesis was used only in the technique of total stapedectomy. Return of conductive hearing impairment prompting revision frequently shows displacement of the oval window portion of the prosthesis. As tissue was used to seal the stapedotomy in most instances, a large amount of scar usually exists in the oval window (Fig. 27–14). A properly adjusted laser allows removal of scar surrounding the oval window loop of the prosthesis and removal. The wire loop prosthesis should not be grasped and removed because it will frequently be attached to vital structures of the vestibule, producing a high chance of inner ear injury. It is necessary when revising these cases to leave a small membrane of tissue, if possible, over the vestibule or to insert autologous tissue with the new prosthesis.

Long Prosthesis Overinsertion. Overinsertion of the long prosthesis into the vestibule may cause a sensation of vertigo with loud sounds (Fig. 27–15). Should this occur, prosthesis removal and replacement with a shorter version usually fix the difficulty. Palpation of the freshly placed prosthesis by putting gentle pressure on the incus in those patients under sedation will identify too long of a prosthesis while still in the operating room. With too long a prosthesis, the patient will experience vertigo with this maneuver. Care should be used to avoid overstimulation of the vestibule, which could produce SNHL.

Loose Prosthesis Syndrome. Loose coupling of the prosthesis to the incus produces characteristic sensations of sound distortion[71] (see Fig. 27–11). A large conductive hearing loss may not exist on the audiogram; tuning forks may also be normal. Occasionally, severe symptoms of this type will prompt revision surgery. Tightening the crimp or changing to a different prosthesis can completely alleviate the difficulty.

Perilymphatic Fistula. Perilymphatic fistula is a cause of postoperative dysequilibrium and SNHL. The signs and symptoms of perilymphatic fistula may be indistinguishable from normal postoperative findings.[72, 73] In addition, a perilymphatic fistula may be discovered at revision surgery

FIGURE 27-11

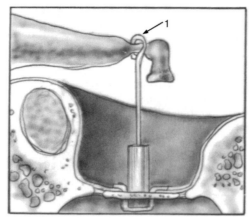

1. Incus erosion

FIGURE 27-12

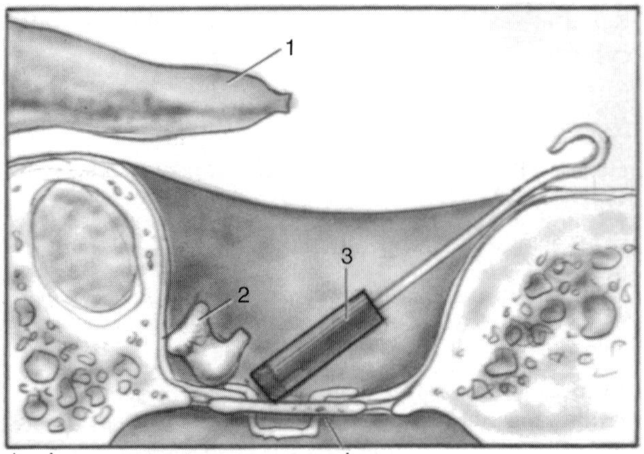

1. Incus remnant
2. Necrotic lenticular process
3. Displaced prosthesis
4. Tissue seal preventing perilymph fistula

FIGURE 27-13

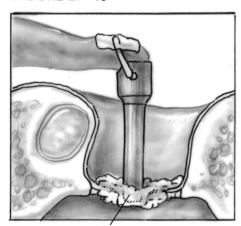

Regrowth of otosclerosis

FIGURE 27-14

Wire loop prosthesis

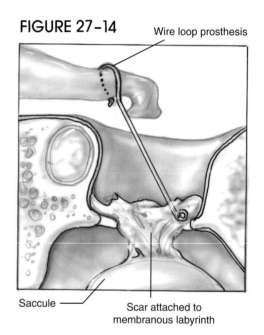

Saccule

Scar attached to membranous labyrinth

FIGURE 27-15

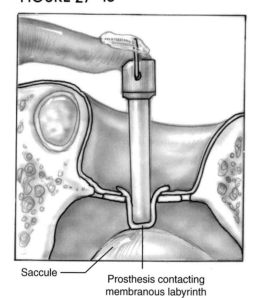

Saccule

Prosthesis contacting membranous labyrinth

FIGURE 27–13. Otosclerosis regrowth.

FIGURE 27–14. Adhesions from oval window to membranous labyrinth.

FIGURE 27–15. Excess prosthesis length, which contacts the membranous labyrinth.

with an asymptomatic patient. Fistulas appear to be much less common following stapedotomy as compared with stapedectomy. Progressive SNHL and/or unremitting vestibular complaints may prompt re-exploration. Repair of a symptomatic perilymphatic fistula relieves vestibular complaints in approximately half of patients.

Reparative Granuloma. Reparative granuloma is defined as a histologically confirmed formation of granulation tissue involving the prosthesis and oval window in a symptomatic patient following stapes surgery. The lesion does not involve granulomatous inflammation.[74] This unusual complication occurs in approximately 0.1 per cent of all cases. Presenting symptoms usually surface 1 to 6 weeks following surgery and most commonly involve vertigo but may include SNHL, progressive mixed hearing loss, sudden hearing loss, and tinnitus.[75] Management includes either immediate surgery with removal and replacement of prosthesis and grafting material or nonsurgical management comprising steroids and antibiotics. Surgical intervention appears to give a better outcome.

Introduced Ectopic Tissue. Occasionally, material introduced into the operative field brings about a return of conductive hearing loss. Introduced squamous epithelium can produce a cholesteatoma,[76] and perichondrium has been known to stimulate formation of cartilage.[77]

SURGICAL RISK REDUCTION IN REVISION SURGERY

Although variation occurs based on the adequacy and technique of primary surgery, revision stapes surgery is needed in a significant percentage of patients. Series from nations with centralized health care provide the best data due to controlled follow-up. A revision rate of 13 per cent in one series of 4000 cases amassed by several surgeons has been reported.[78] Revision may be necessary immediately following primary surgery or many years later, with an average time to revision of 8 to 12.5 years.[79, 80]

Success rates for revision surgery have improved significantly over the past 20 years. Early reports found postoperative conductive hearing loss of 10 dB or less in less than half of patients.[67, 81] Modern results more closely approach those of primary surgery with closure to 10 dB or less in 90 per cent of cases.

Use of a laser improves surgical outcome. Meta-analysis of revision stapes surgery comparing 11 studies without laser use (1147 patients) to four studies that employed laser technique (170 patients) showed a statistically significant ($P = 0.0002$) advantage in terms of safety and efficacy. Postoperative air-bone gaps of 10 dB or less were accomplished in 69 per cent of cases where a visible wavelength laser was used, whereas only 51 per cent of patients on whom standard techniques were used enjoyed the same results.[82]

The risk of SNHL is greater with revision surgery. Rates appear to be higher when revision of stapedectomy is undertaken when compared with those cases with stapedotomy as the primary technique. Oval window drill-out is associated with an unacceptably high rate of inner ear injury and hearing loss and should be avoided.[67] Reported rates of SNHL with revision surgery vary from 0 to 7.6

per cent.[40, 67, 79, 83] We currently quote patients a rate of SNHL twice that of primary surgery.

CONCLUSION

Successful performance of surgery for otosclerosis includes thorough mental and physical preparation. A solid knowledge base of potential complications and their management is vital to patient counseling, treatment, and outcome. Although complications are unavoidable and certain ones can be rectified, avoidance with proper surgical technique and planning is preferable for both patient and surgeon.

References

1. Smith MFW, Hopp ML: 1984 Santa Barbara State-of-the-Art Conference on Otosclerosis: Results, conclusions, consensus. Ann Otol Rhinol Laryngol 95: 1–4, 1986.
2. Garretsen TJTM, Cremers WRJ: Ear surgery in osteogenesis imperfecta. Arch Otolaryngol Head Neck Surg 116: 317–323, 1990.
3. Olson NR, Lehman RH: Cerebrospinal fluid otorrhea and the congenitally fixed stapes. Laryngoscope 78: 352–360, 1968.
4. Snik AF, Hombergen GC, Mylanus EA, et al: Air-bone gap in patients with X-linked stapes gusher syndrome. Am J Otol 16: 241–246, 1995.
5. Cremers CW: Audiologic features of X-linked progressive mixed deafness syndrome with perilymphatic gusher during stapes surgery. Am J Otol 6: 243–246, 1985.
6. Cremers CW, Huygen PL: Clinical features of female heterozygotes in the X-linked mixed deafness syndrome (with perilymphatic gusher during stapes surgery). Int J Pediatr Otorhinolaryngol 6: 179–185, 1983.
7. Brown JS: Meningitis following stapes surgery: The pathway of spread to the intracranial cavity. Laryngoscope 77: 1295–1303, 1967.
8. Clairmont AA, Nicholson WL, Turner JS: *Pseudomonas aeruginosa* meningitis following stapedectomy. Laryngoscope 85: 1076–1083, 1975.
9. Snyder BD: Delayed meningitis following stapes surgery. Arch Neurol 36: 174–175, 1979.
10. Gordon MA, Silverstein H, Willcox TO, et al: A re-evaluation of the 512-Hz Rinne tuning fork test as a patient selection criterion for laser stapedotomy. Am J Otol 6: 712–717, 1998.
11. Harris JP, Osborne E: A survey of otologic training in U.S. residency programs. Arch Otolaryngol Head Neck Surg 116: 342–345, 1990.
12. Majoras M: Electronystagmography during stapedectomy. Int Surg 47: 323–327, 1967.
13. Shea JJ: Thirty years of stapes surgery. J Laryngol Otol 102: 14–19, 1988.
14. Fisch U: Stapedectomy versus stapedotomy. Am J Otol 4:112–117, 1982.
15. Grolman W, Tange RA, de Bruijn AJ, et al: A retrospecive study of the hearing results obtained after stapedotomy by the implantation of two Teflon pistons with a different diameter. Eur Arch Otorhinolaryngol 254: 422–424, 1997.
16. Sedwick JD, Louden CL, Shelton C: Stapedectomy versus stapedotomy: Do you really need a laser? Arch Otolaryngol Head Neck Surg 123: 177–180, 1997.
17. Wiet RJ, Kubek DC, Lemberg P, et al: A meta-analysis review of revision stapes surgery with argon laser: Effectiveness and safety. Am J Otol 18:166–171, 1997.
18. Persson P, Harder H, Magnuson B: Hearing results in otosclerosis surgery after partial stapedectomy, total stapedectomy, and stapedotomy. Acta Otolaryngol 117: 94–99, 1997.
19. Kursten R, Schneider B, Zrunek M: Long-term results after stapedectomy versus stapedotomy. Am J Otol 15: 804–806, 1994.
20. Glasscock ME III, Storper IS, Haynes DS, et al: Twenty-five years of experience with stapedectomy. Laryngoscope 105: 899–904, 1995.
21. Anson BJ, Bast TH: Anatomical structure of the stapes and the relation of the stapedial footplate to vital parts of the labyrinth. Ann Otol Rhinol Laryngol 67: 389–399, 1958.
22. Pauw BKH, Pollack AM, Fisch U: Utricle and saccule and cochlear

duct in relation to stapedotomy: A histological human temporal bone study. Ann Otol Rhinol Laryngol 100: 966, 1991.

23. Perkins RC: Laser stapedotomy for otosclerosis. Laryngoscope 91: 228–241, 1980.
24. Vernick DM: A comparison of the results of KTP and CO_2 laser stapedotomy. Am J Otol 17: 221–224, 1996.
25. Antonelli PJ, Gianoli GJ, Lundy LB, et al: Early post-laser stapedotomy hearing thresholds. Am J Otol 19: 443–446, 1998.
26. Robinson M: Juvenile otosclerosis: A 20-year study. Ann Otol Rhinol Laryngol 92: 561–565, 1983.
27. Lippy WH, Schuring AG: Stapedectomy revision following sensorineural hearing loss. Otolaryngol Head Neck Surg 92: 580–582, 1994.
28. Pirodda A, Sorrenti G, Marliani AF, et al: Arterial anomalies of the middle ear associated with stapes ankylosis. J Laryngol Otol 108: 237–239, 1994.
29. Tos M, Lau T: Tynpanosclerosis of the middle ear: Late results of surgical treatment. J Laryngol Otol 104: 685–689, 1990.
30. Gormley PK: Stapedectomy in tympanosclerosis. Am J Otol 8: 123–130, 1987.
31. Giddings NA, House JW: Tympanosclerosis of the stapes—hearing results for various surgical treatments. Otolaryngol Head Neck Surg 107: 644–650, 1992.
32. Pedersen U, Elbrond O: Stapedectomy in osteogenesis imperfecta. ORL J Otorhinolaryngol Relat Spec 45: 330–337, 1983.
33. Garretsen TJTM, Cremers CWRJ: Stapes surgery in osteogenesis imperfecta: Analysis of postoperative hearing loss. Ann Otol Rhinol Laryngol 100: 120–130, 1991.
34. Garretsen TJTM, Cremers CWRJ: Ear surgery in osteogenesis imperfecta. Arch Otolaryngol Head Neck Surg 116: 317–323, 1990.
35. Stidham K, Roberson JB Jr: Cochlear hook anatomy: Evaluation of the spatial relationship of the basal cochlear duct to middle ear landmarks. Acta Otolaryngol 119: 773–777, 2000.
36. Leek JH: An anomalous facial nerve: The otologist's albatross. Laryngoscope 84: 1535–1544, 1974.
37. Willis R: Conductive deafness due to malplacement of the seventh nerve. J Otolaryngol 6: 1–4, 1977.
38. Gherini SG, Horn KL, Bowman CA, et al: Small fenestra stapedotomy using a fiberoptic hand-held argon laser in obliterative otosclerosis. Laryngoscope 100: 1276–1282, 1990.
39. Derlacki EL: Revision stapes surgery: Problems with some solutions. Laryngoscope 95: 1047–1053, 1985.
40. Farrior D: Abstruse complications of stapes surgery: Diagnosis and treatment. *In* Henry Ford Hospital International Symposium on Otosclerosis. Chicago, Little Brown, 1962, pp 509–521.
41. Glasscock ME: The stapes gusher. Arch Otolaryngol Head Neck Surg 98: 82–91, 1973.
42. Brodie HA: Prophylactic antibiotics for post-traumatic cerebrospinal fluid fistulae: A meta-analysis. Arch Otolaryngol Head Neck Surg 123: 749–752, 1997.
43. Majoras M: Electronystagmography during stapedectomy. Int Surg 47: 323–327, 1967.
44. Gristwood RE: Acute otitis media following the stapedectomy operation. J Laryngol Otol 80: 55–60, 1966.
45. Brown JS: Meningitis following stapes surgery: The pathway of spread to the intracranial cavity. Laryngoscope 77: 1295–1303, 1967.
46. Clairmont AA, Nicholson WL, Turner JS: *Pseudomonas aeruginosa* meningitis following stapedectomy. Laryngoscope 85: 1076–1083, 1975.
47. Snyder BD: Delayed meningitis following stapes surgery. Arch Neurol 36:174–175, 1979.
48. Harrill WC, Jenkins HA, Coker NJ: Barotrauma after stapes surgery: A survey of recommended restrictions and clinical experiences. Am J Otol 17:835–846, 1996.
49. Althaus SR, House HP: Delayed post-stapedectomy facial paralysis: A report of five cases. Laryngoscope 83:1234–1240, 1973.
50. Matthisen J: Phonophobia after stapedectomy. Acta Otolaryngol (Stockh) 68: 73–77, 1969.
51. Bracewell A: Diplacusis binauralis—a complication of stapedectomy. J Laryngol Otol 80: 55–60, 1966.
52. Cody T, Baker H: Otosclerosis: Vestibular symptoms and sensorineural hearing loss. Ann Otol Rhinol Laryngol 87: 778–796, 1978.
53. Das TK, Susheela AK, Gupto IP, et al: Toxic effects of chronic

fluoride ingestion on the upper gastrointestinal tract. J Clin Gastroenterol 18: 194–199, 1994.
54. Cole JM, Bartels LJ, Beresny GM: Long-term effect of otosclerosis on bone conduction. Laryngoscope 89: 1053–1060, 1979.
55. Vartiainen E, Virtaniemi J, Kemppainen M, et al: Hearing levels of patients with otosclerosis ten years after stapedectomy. Otolaryngol Head Neck Surg 108: 251–255, 1993.
56. Linthicum FH: Correlations of sensorineural hearing impairment and otosclerosis. Ann Otol Rhinol Laryngol 75: 512–524, 1966.
57. Balle V, Linthicum FH Jr: Proven cochlear otosclerosis: Sensorineural without conductive hearing loss. Ann Otol Rhinol Laryngol 93: 105–111, 1984.
58. Causse JR, Uriel J, Berges J, et al: The enzymatic mechanism of the otospongiotic disease and NaF action on the enzymatic balance. Am J Otol 3: 297–314, 1982.
59. Causse JR, Causse JB, Uriel J, et al: Sodium fluoride therapy. Am J Otol 14: 482–490, 1993.
60. Forquer BD, Linthicum FH, Bennett C: Sodium fluoride: Effectiveness of treatment for cochlear otosclerosis. Am J Otol 7: 121–125, 1986.
61. Bretlau P, Causse J, Causse JB, et al: Otospongiosis and sodium fluoride: A blind experimental and clinical evaluation of the effect of sodium fluoride treatment in patients with otospongiosis. Ann Otol Rhinol Laryngol 94: 103–107, 1985.
62. Bretlau P, Salomon G, Johnsen NJ, et al: Otospongiosis and sodium fluoride: A clinical double-blind, placebo-controlled study of sodium fluoride in otospongiosis. Am J Otol 10: 2–20, 1989.
63. Shambaugh GE Jr, Scott A: Sodium fluoride for arrest of otosclerosis. Arch Otolaryngol 80: 263–270, 1964.
64. Linthicum FH, House HP, Althaus SR: The effect of sodium fluoride on otosclerotic activity as determined by strontium 85. Ann Otol Rhinol Laryngol 82: 609–613, 1973.
65. Pedersen CB, Felding JU: Stapes surgery: Complications and airway infection. Ann Otol Rhinol Laryngol 100: 607–611, 1991.
66. Sheehy JL, Nelson RA, House HP: Revision stapedectomy: A review of 258 cases. Laryngoscope 91: 43–51, 1981.
67. Feldman BA, Schuknecht HF: Experiences with revision stapedectomy procedures. Laryngoscope 80: 1281–1291, 1970.
68. Glasscock ME, McKennan KX, Levine SC: Revision stapedectomy surgery. Otolaryngol Head Neck Surg 96: 141–148, 1987.
69. Pearman K, Dawes JDK: Post-stapedectomy conductive deafness and results of revision surgery. J Laryngol Otol 96: 405–410, 1982.
70. Farrior J, Sutherland A: Revision stapes surgery. Laryngoscope 101: 1155–1161, 1991.
71. McGee TM: The loose-wire syndrome. Laryngoscope 91: 1478–1483, 1981.
72. Moon CN: Perilymphatic fistulas complicating the stapedectomy operation: A review of 49 cases. Laryngoscope 80: 515–535, 1970.
73. Lippy WH, Schuring AG: Stapedectomy revision following sensorineural hearing loss. Otolaryngol Head Neck Surg 92: 580–582, 1984.
74. Fenton JE, Turner J, Shirazi A, et al: Post-stapedectomy reparative granuloma: A misnomer. J Laryngol Otol 110: 185–188, 1996.
75. Seicshnaydre MA, Sismanis A, Hughes GB: Update of reparative granuloma: Survey of the American Otological Society and the American Neurotology Society. Am J Otol 15: 155–160, 1994.
76. Von Haacke NP: Cholesteatoma following stapedectomy. J Laryngol Otol 101: 708–710, 1987.
77. Benecke JE, Gadre AK, Linthicum FH: Chondrogenic potential of tragal perichondrium: A cause of hearing loss following stapedectomy. Laryngoscope 100: 1292–1293, 1990.
78. Pedersen CB: Revision surgery in otosclerosis: Operative findings in 186 patients. Clin Otolaryngol 19: 446–450, 1994.
79. Pedersen CB: Revision surgery in otosclerosis—an investigation of the factors which influence the hearing result. Clin Otolaryngol 21: 385–388, 1996.
80. Prasad S, Kamerer DB: Results of revision stapedectomy for conductive hearing loss. Otolaryngol Head Neck Surg 109: 742–747, 1993.
81. Crabtree JA, Britton BH, Powers WH: An evaluation of revision stapes surgery. Laryngoscope 90: 224–229, 1980.
82. Wiet RJ, Kubek DC, Lemberg P, et al: A meta-analysis review of revision stapes surgery with argon laser: Effectiveness and safety. Am J Otol 18: 166–171, 1997.
83. Hammerschlag PE, Fishman A, Scheer AA: A review of 308 cases of revision stapedectomy. Laryngoscope 108: 1794–1800, 1998.

28

Perilymphatic Fistula

George T. Singleton, M.D. ▪ William H. Slattery, M.D.

Perilymphatic fistulas (PLFs) undoubtedly exist in association with stapedectomies and other invasive procedures of the cochlea. Likewise, severe head injury, abdominal blows, and rapid shifts in environmental pressure are accepted as causes of true PLF. Dissent remains, however, with regard to idiopathic PLF. Controversy stems from the interpretation of histopathologic findings of temporal bones in the region of the fissula ante fenestram and round window niche, the confusion of PLF with Ménière's disease, multiple tests that likely misidentify Ménière's disease as PLF, and the incidence of PLF in congenital forms of deafness. Some surgeons are doing large numbers of PLF operations based on these conjectural criteria; however, a national survey indicated that PLFs are uncommon.[1]

True PLF most commonly occurs as a result of external trauma to the head or abdomen or from rapid pressure shifts in the environment. Congenital defects of the middle ear space account for approximately 20 per cent of PLFs if abnormally placed round window membranes are included. Complications resulting from invasive procedures of the cochlea, including stapedectomy, the "tack" procedure, and cochleosacculotomy for the treatment of Ménière's disease, may result in persistent PLF.[2] Acute and chronic mastoiditis with erosion into the labyrinth as well as chronic granulomatous diseases, such as syphilis and tuberculosis, is of historical interest only in the development of PLF.

Homeostasis of the pressure differentials between endolymph and perilymph is maintained by the presence of both a patent endolymphatic duct and sac located in the dura of the posterior fossa and the cochlear aqueduct that leads from the scala tympani of the cochlea to the posterior fossa. In children and some young adults, this aqueduct is open. With maturity, the duct is normally criss-crossed with arachnoid strands; therefore, it functions as if sealed with a semipermeable membrane. Increased cerebrospinal fluid pressure in the normal adult results in equally increased pressures in the perilymphatic and endolymphatic space. Thus, damage to the endolymphatic membrane structure is unlikely.[3] The only outlet from increased intracochlear pressure is a tear of the round window membrane or annular ligament, which occurs most frequently anteroinferiorly, rarely superiorly, and never posteriorly around the stapes footplate. Congenital deformities of the stapes may occur and result in PLF. These deformities most commonly involve the posterior crus and posterior half of the footplate or occur as central perforations of the footplate. The round window membrane tears far less frequently; in the author's (GTS) series, only twice has a normal round window membrane torn.[26] In both instances, there was a severe blow to the head resulting in PLF at both the round and oval windows. The remaining tears to the round window membrane have occurred when its position was 45 degrees to the promontory and there was little or no overhanging promontory. In these cases, the round window membrane was directly visible when the middle ear was viewed transtympanically (Fig. 28–1A).[4, 5] This anomaly is probably associated with an abnormally patent cochlear aqueduct.[6] The cochlear aqueduct opens into the scala tympani adjacent to the round window.

The cribriform areas at the depths of the internal auditory canal are another source of potential transmission of increased cerebrospinal fluid pressure to the perilymphatic space. In rare instances, these areas are wide open with direct connections of cerebrospinal fluid to perilymph. This is particularly true in Mondini's deformities of the cochlea, which lead to gushers with any invasive operative procedure of the cochlea in these patients.

Goodhill coined the terms *implosive* and *explosive* pressure changes that result in PLF.[7] In reference to implosive, he states that increased pressure from the tubal tympanic region is directed via the ossicles to the perilymphatic space, resulting in a tear in the annular ligament or the round window membrane. This problem may occur with inadequate equalization of the middle ear or with blast injuries. The explosive route results from increased intracranial pressure due to a blow to the head or abdomen. Increased intra-abdominal pressure is transmitted via the vertebral veins to increase the cerebrospinal pressure, thus causing an increase of intracranial pressure. Pressure is placed on both the endolymphatic and perilymphatic systems, as outlined earlier, with rupture from inside out of either the annular ligament or the round window membrane.[7]

Early stapedectomy procedures were more likely to result in PLF than the methods practiced today. A pointed polyethylene strut prosthesis placed over absorbable gelatin sponge (Gelfoam) or a thin tissue seal was a common culprit when the patient was subjected to a change in barometric pressure, that is, ascent or descent in the mountains or in airplanes. Various wire procedures with a gelatin sponge seal had a similar plight. Piston procedures, when used without interposed tissue, commonly resulted in fistula development. The current small fenestra, small-piston, tissue seal techniques have dramatically lowered the incidence of PLF.[8–12]

Invasive procedures of the stapes footplate, including the Fick procedure and the tack procedure for Ménière's disease, were ultimately abandoned because of the relatively high incidence of sensorineural hearing loss. Later exploration of many of these ears revealed a persistent PLF. Likewise, the 20 per cent sensorineural hearing loss associ-

FIGURE 28-1

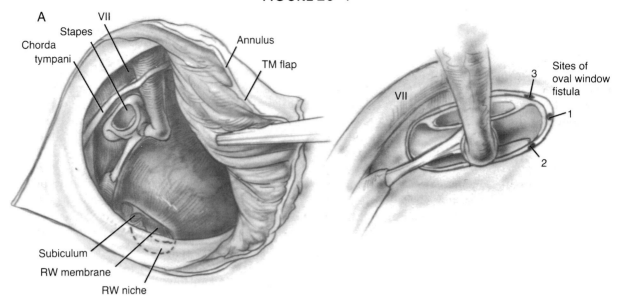

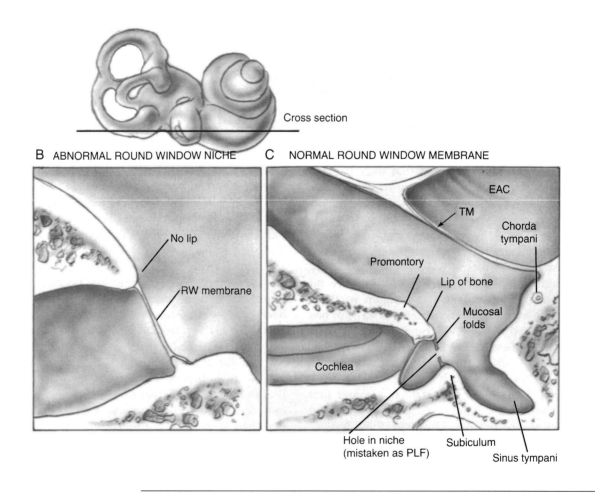

FIGURE 28–1. *A*, Right middle ear: surgeon's view with tympanomeatal, flap and drum folded forward. Sites of oval window fistula are numbered in order of occurrence (1 and 2 most common). *B*, Abnormal round window (RW) membrane at 45-degree right angle to promontory and no overhanging lip. *C*, Normal (RW) membrane hidden from view in depths of niche, with lip of bone overhang. Mucosal folds frequently appear to seal niche partially, with hole in center. EAC, external auditory canal; PLF, perilymphatic fistula.

ated with cochleostomy or cochleosacculotomy as it was originally described is probably related to a persistent round window PLF; surgeons did not remove the scutum, roughen the surface of the round window membrane, and seal the fistula they had made with the pick prior to closing the ear.[2]

Microfissures of the otic capsule may lead to PLF, although this hypothesis has never been confirmed in any patient or temporal bone.[13] Kohut and associates, in temporal bone studies, have suggested that microfissures around the round window niche may result in leaks if there is no dense collagen plug on the middle ear side.[14] This study also demonstrated an intact inner ear lining, endosteum, periosteum, and middle ear mucosa in the temporal bones with these fissures. These investigators also reported that leaks probably occur through the fissula ante fenestram where no bony or cartilaginous plug exists.[14] Again in these cases, multiple layers seal this area and no leak has been demonstrated. Hinojosa and associates reported seeing fluid in the area of the fissula ante fenestram after the mucosa in this area was destroyed with a pick or other instrument.[15] A follow-up study by Shazly and Linthicum[16] has shown that the fissures do occur and that the changes in the fissula ante fenestram as described by Kohut and associates are present. However, they demonstrated that there is absolutely no association between these findings and sudden sensorineural hearing loss and no evidence of a perilymphatic fluid leak.[16]

Numerous authors have added confusion to the issue of idiopathic PLF by describing the symptoms of PLF as exactly the same as those of Ménière's disease, that is, fluctuant sensorineural hearing loss, tinnitus, episodic vertigo, and pressure feeling in the involved ear. These authors use the same criteria to diagnose Ménière's disease and PLF. These criteria include the use of hyperosmolar solutions such as Renografin, urea, and glycerin to demonstrate an improvement in hearing exactly as would be expected in Ménière's cases (Weider and Johnson, unpublished data).[17] These same tests were used for predictive evaluation of Ménière's cases before endolymphatic shunt procedures were performed.

Some authors have touted electrocochleography as an effective technique for the differentiation of Ménière's disease from PLF,[18, 19] but results from another study suggest that electrocochleographic techniques are not valid for separating Ménière's patients from normal patients.[20] Meyerhoff and Yellin describe electrocochleographic changes after patching windows without PLF and attribute this phenomenon to a change in fluid dynamics.[19] One must question this interpretation; electrocochleographic changes most likely represent normal changes seen in Ménière's disease.

We have performed a surprising number of re-exploration procedures on patients who have had previous PLF surgery. These patients have an absolutely classic history of Ménière's disease. The initial surgeon's operative record describes a hole in the round window membrane. In every case explored, a perfectly normal round window membrane was found lying deep in the niche with no evidence that the round window had been touched. The first surgeon had simply sealed the mucosal folds that surround the round window niche (Fig. 28–1*B*).

For a time, patients with congenital deafness that exhibited fluctuating hearing loss were thought to have PLF. Studies by Reilly,[21] Parnes and McCabe,[22] Pappas and colleagues,[23] and Bluestone[24] have made it clear that PLF associated with congenital sensorineural hearing loss is quite uncommon. When a PLF is truly present and corrected, the associated dizziness is frequently improved, although the hearing is rarely improved, and only about half the time is it stabilized.[21–24] The Bluestone study[24] is fairly typical. In this group of 244 children with congenital hearing loss, only 6 per cent had a PLF; 36 per cent of the 44 ears selected for exploration had a fistula present. Only 23 per cent were improved by the operative intervention. Bluestone concluded that for a diagnosis of PLF in a case of congenital hearing loss to be correct, the patient had to have one of the following: labyrinthitis, meningitis, additional sensorineural hearing loss following acute otitis media, or hearing loss made worse by trauma. Our success in identifying PLF in congenital hearing loss cases has not occurred in those with fluctuating sensorineural hearing loss. However, in patients who have demonstrated positional nystagmus compatible with PLF, a positive eyes-closed-turning test result, a positive fistula test result, or a Tulleo response, a fistula has been identified without exception.[6]

PATIENT SELECTION

The typical patient with a PLF presents with a sudden onset of hearing loss or mild vertigo, or disequilibrium, or both, associated with a traumatic event. The onset is sudden in 94 per cent of proven PLF, and in 89 per cent of cases, trauma is related to the onset of symptoms. Trauma includes invasive inner ear surgical procedures, abdominal blows, head blows, blast injuries, or severe changes in environmental pressure, particularly in the presence of an upper respiratory infection or an acute allergic attack. Unsteadiness or dizziness is present in 90 per cent of cases, and the dizziness is usually positional in nature. Seventy-five per cent of patients will have a history of tinnitus, irrespective of whether a hearing loss is present.[6] Hearing loss is present in 53 per cent of patients and is not fluctuant in nature. PLF is *not* characterized by fluctuant hearing loss associated with episodic vertigo, tinnitus, and a full feeling in the ears, as some purport. That condition is Ménière's disease.

Significant physical findings in PLF include a characteristic positional nystagmus in 94 per cent of patients, a positive eyes-closed-turning test result to the side of the lesion in 89 per cent, a hearing loss in 53 per cent, a positive fistula test result in 25 per cent, and a positive Tulleo phenomenon in 4 per cent. The characteristic positional nystagmus may have a very short or no latency and a relatively long duration, and minimal or no fatigue is evident on repeated testing. Also, this nystagmus does not reverse direction on changing from the inducing position to the sitting position. It is not nearly as violent as that seen with benign paroxysmal postural vertigo. The nystagmus occurs with the involved ear undermost in 80 per cent of the cases, and it beats toward the involved ear in only 60 per cent. The nystagmus is rarely rotatory: from most to least frequent, it may be horizontal, diagonal, or vertical.[23, 24]

The hearing loss is usually sensorineural but may be predominantly conductive in the case of a slipped stapes prosthesis. When not associated with a slipped stapes prosthesis, the hearing loss is a sensorineural loss that may be flat, downsloping, or upsloping. The speech reception threshold is usually worse than one would anticipate from the pure tones and the discrimination score is usually lower than expected.[6]

Identification of the involved ear is sometimes quite difficult. If hearing loss is associated with the traumatic event that created the PLF, then the involved side is obvious. The side is also obvious in cases with a positive fistula test result or in the presence of a Tulleo phenomenon. As indicated earlier, positional nystagmus occurs with the involved ear undermost in only 80 per cent of cases. The direction of the nystagmus is of no diagnostic value in determining which ear is involved.

The eyes-closed-turning test result is positive in 90 per cent of patients with PLF and is highly specific to the side of involvement with only a 1 per cent error. The eyes-closed-turning test is performed by having the patient walk in a straight line with the eyes closed. The examiner taps the subject's shoulder, indicating to the patient to turn 180 degrees either right or left and stop in a position of attention with the eyes still closed (Fig. 28–2). A positive test result is readily recognized by the patient's swaying or having a tendency to lose balance when he or she has turned to the side of the lesion. Patients with significant central nervous system lesions are unable to perform the test; therefore, these patients are not at risk of misdiagnosis as PLF.[25, 26]

The Quix test has been recommended for identification of the involved side of the lesion; however, the result is positive only in about 20 per cent of cases.[27] This test involves having the patient stand erect with feet together, eyes closed, and arms outstretched. The examiner looks for a deviation of the arms to the side of the lesion.

No specialized audiometric or electronystagmography test has been of any value in identifying a PLF or the side of the lesion. Flood and coworkers recommended a test in which the involved ear is placed uppermost in an attempt

to get air into the vestibule and thus convert a neurosensory loss to a combined conductive neurosensory loss.[28] We have been unsuccessful in 25 cases of proven PLF in seeing this phenomenon develop.

Black and associates reported posturography as being highly specific and highly sensitive in detecting PLF.[29] This finding has not been corroborated by others, and a critical look at this study suggests that there is probably confusion with Ménière's disease in the study population. In this study, the identification of probable fistulas took place after mucosa of the middle ear had been significantly disturbed.[29]

Silverstein advocated the use of twin cruciate myringotomy incisions over the oval and round windows of the suspected ear and micropipette collection of fluid from the oval window recess and the round window niche.[30] This procedure has not gained much favor because of technical difficulties and the fact that false-negative results occasionally occur.

PREOPERATIVE EVALUATION AND PATIENT COUNSELING

Patients should have the usual preoperative evaluation required for local anesthesia with monitored anesthetic care in an ambulatory surgical setting. Healthy young adults receive only a hematocrit test preoperatively; older patients receive more extensive evaluation, as do those who have systemic diseases. Patients are advised to stop aspirin and nonsteroidal analgesic therapy 10 to 14 days before their surgical date. Patients are instructed to wash their hair the night before surgery and to put nothing on their hair. They are told that 3/4-inch of hair will be shaved from around the ear. Patients are advised that if PLF is found, a small incision will be made either over the tragus or above and behind the ear for obtaining a graft.

Patients are informed that if a leak is found, they will be on bed rest for 5 days with bathroom privileges only. They are advised that when they get up, they are to roll onto their side and push up with their arms so that they do not tighten their abdomen. They are advised that they will be placed on sedatives and that they will have stool softeners given to them so that they do not strain to have a bowel

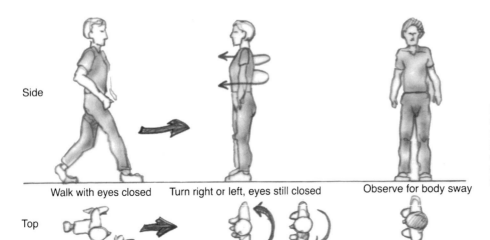

Side

Walk with eyes closed   Turn right or left, eyes still closed   Observe for body sway

Top

180°

FIGURE 28–2. Eyes-closed-turning test. Patient walks with eyes closed, turns quickly right or left, then stops in position of attention with eyes still closed. A positive test result consists of staggering or swaying on turn to the involved side.

movement. They are to sleep either in a recliner chair or in a bed that has the head elevated 4 to 6 inches. For 9 days after the 5 days of bed rest, they may get up and walk around the house but may do no heavy lifting and have no sexual activity. At 2 weeks, they may return to work if they have a sedentary job; if they are manual laborers, they are not allowed to work for 3 months. They are advised that they will be seen in the clinic 2 weeks postoperatively for follow-up.

SURGICAL PROCEDURE

Preoperative Preparation

Patients will have an intravenous line started in the preoperative holding area. They are asked to go to the bathroom immediately before coming back to the operative suite. If they are unusually nervous, they may receive a small amount of midazolam (Versed) before coming back to the operating room. Patients are placed backward on a standard operating table that is double-mattressed except at the head, thereby allowing room for the surgeon's legs. During surgical site preparation, the head is kept level on a folded towel or blanket. Approximately 3/4-inch of hair is shaved from around the ear, and all loose hair is removed with wide adhesive tape. The remaining hair is held back by brushing it with K-Y jelly so that it stays clear of the operative field. The anesthesiologist places the electrocardiographic monitors, chest stethoscope, and pulse oximeter on the patient. An automatic blood pressure cuff is placed on the arm opposite the operative ear. This action prevents accidental movement of the surgeon's arm during insufflation. The skin is prepared with povidone-iodine (Betadine) soap, wiped clean, then painted with povidone-iodine solution and dried, and the solution is wiped from around the ear. Skin around the ear is prepared with Mastisol adhesive. A 3M adhesive drape with a 2-inch hole is placed over the ear. The drape is folded so that it does not fall over the patient's mouth and nose. A disposable, lint-free, paper ear-draping pack is used to cover the patient and the remaining portion of the operating field. No towels or other lint-bearing materials are used. The front of the drape is held up on an intravenous line pole so that the patient can see the anesthesiologist, and, if the patient wishes, can watch the television monitor.

Surgical Instruments

A standard tympanostomy setup is used. Disposable, straight, and angled Beaver ear blades are used for flap incisions. A Skeeter Micro Drill with 1- to 1.4-mm diamond burrs is used for removing scutum. A sharp 0.5-mm, 90-degree pick is altered slightly by bending its shaft 20 degrees 2 inches from the end to allow better visualization of the tip. An angled-handle straight pick is used for work around the stapes footplate and to place grafts.

Surgical Technique

The folded blanket is removed from under the patient's head, and a single towel is placed between the patient's head and the table mattress. A four-quadrant injection of the ear canal with small amounts of 1 per cent lidocaine (Xylocaine) with 1:50,000 epinephrine is used to prevent the speculum from hurting the ear. The area of the tragus and the area above and behind the ear over the temporalis muscle are also injected for potential harvesting of graft tissue. The local anesthetic from the four quadrants is disbursed with a spreading speculum. The ear canal is then irrigated copiously with normal saline to remove the povidone-iodine, cerumen, and hairs. A 1.5-inch, 27-gauge needle is then used to inject the vascular strip area. Care is taken to produce no excessive injection or blisters. The inferior injection is placed posteroinferiorly at the bony cartilaginous junction, and care is taken to place the bevel of the needle against bone and under the periosteum. Administering the injection is a slow, deliberate process, with the surgeon watching carefully for blanching and making sure that it goes all the way to the annulus inferiorly. The surgeon now completes the removal of the desquamated epithelium from the ear canal with a small suction.

The inferior incision is made first by use of the No. 1 or straight Beaver blade. A cut is made from the 6 o'clock position and is angled to about 1-cm lateral to the annular ring on the posterior ear canal. The No. 2, or angled, Beaver blade is used to make an incision superiorly from 2 mm lateral to the short process of the malleus to join the tip of the other incision in the posterior ear canal. A duckbill elevator is used to elevate the skin of the posterior canal down to the annulus. If problems arise with fibers sticking in the suture line, a House No. 2 knife is used to separate these. Hemostasis is completed with the 20-gauge suction placed on the bleeder and touched with a Valley Lab cautery set between 5 and 7 o'clock. Hemostasis must be obtained before the middle ear is opened. The middle ear is opened at the notch of Rivinus by use of a Rosen needle. The chorda tympani nerve is then identified, and the beginning of the annular ring is raised with the Rosen needle. The entire posterior portion of the annular ring may be elevated with the Rosen needle, or a drum elevator may be used. The chorda tympani is gingerly dissected free of the tympanic membrane, and the posterior half of the tympanic membrane and the ear canal flap are folded forward so that the middle ear may be inspected (see Fig. 28–1).

Frequently, clear fluid is seen in the oval window recess and in the round window niche. This fluid is usually local anesthetic that has seeped into the middle ear space, and a 24-gauge suction is used to remove it. The patient is then asked to perform a Valsalva maneuver to observe if fluid reaccumulates. If fluid does reaccumulate and it is unclear whether a fistula is present, the fluid may be checked to determine if it is perilymph in two ways. A simple way is to put a small piece of absorbable gelatin sponge on an angled straight pick, soak up the solution, and then place it on a Clinistrip for glucose testing. If the glucose reading is approximately 100 mg/dl and if no blood has been allowed in the middle ear, the surgeon can be sure that the fluid is perilymph. Another technique is to use the Xomed Treace kit for measuring protein. This technique has been described by Silverstein: a micropipette is used to pick up the fluid, which is placed on indicator paper. The color change is compared with a standard. Again, the presence of protein in the absence of blood in the middle ear space identifies the fluid as perilymph.[30] Note that the scutum has not been removed and that the mucosa in the middle ear has not been touched except with the 24-gauge suction to remove the fluid that may have been present when the middle ear was opened. The round window niche has not been disturbed, nor has the lip of the promontory overlying it.

If the round window membrane is immediately visible when the middle ear is opened, that is, at about a 45-degree angle to the plane of the promontory, then the surgeon should become suspicious of a probable PLF in the round window membrane.[29–31] Only after checking for the recurrence of fluid in these recesses does the surgeon remove the scutum and get complete exposure of the oval window area. If fluid was not present earlier and fluid did not appear on Valsalva maneuver, the surgeon can place a straight pick on the lenticular process of the incus and press gently, looking for the accumulation of fluid around the annular ligament or in the round window niche. If no fluid accumulates in either place with both Valsalva maneuver and pressure on the stapes, no repair is performed. We believe that there is risk for creating some degree of conductive hearing loss and a possibility of injuring the inner ear by patching a round window or oval window with no PLF.

Most PLFs at the oval window are located directly anterior to the anterior crus or immediately below it; a few are superior to the anterior crus (Fig. 28–3). Generally the surgeon can see this area and can actually see the hole. Leaks in this area are best repaired by teasing away the surface mucosa either with the straight pick or with the tiny right-angle pick. A graft of adventitia is obtained from over the temporalis fascia. This graft is compressed and cut into the shape of a small set of trousers, about 3 mm long and 1.5 mm wide, and a 2-mm slit is made up the middle longways to form the pant's legs (Fig. 28–3A). The graft is then draped around the anterior crus and packed in place with gelatin sponge (Fig. 28–3B) soaked in Ringer's solution. This material is placed to the level of the tympanic membrane, and a sheet of absorbable gelatin film (Gelfilm) is placed over the gelatin sponge to prevent adhesions to the tympanic membrane.

If there is a congenital defect of the stapes footplate, the hole may be in the middle of the footplate or it may incorporate the entire posterior half of the footplate (Fig. 28–4). In these cases, the mucosa must be denuded all the way around the footplate. With larger perforations, we use perichondrium from the tragus because it is thicker and easier to handle to effect a seal. The area between the crura is packed full with gelatin sponge to hold the graft in place.

If the round window membrane has a fistula, the membrane will be in clear sight with no overhang of the round window niche. As a general rule, the tear will be readily visible somewhere around the annular ring of the membrane. Occasionally, it is in the center, particularly if it was made by a myringotomy knife or by a foreign body introduced into the ear. If the fistula is less than 2 weeks old, a fibrin clot or granulation tissue will be seen around the leak. The area around the perforation is roughened by use of the tiny right-angle pick. A thicker graft of perichondrium from the tragus is used. The graft is held in

place with absorbable gelatin sponge packed all the way to the level of the tympanic membrane, and then a sheet of absorbable gelatin film is placed to prevent adhesive bands from forming between the tympanic membrane and the round window seal. The tympanic membrane is replaced to its normal position, the skin flap in the canal is laid flat, and a 0.25 × 1.5-inch strip of Owen nonadherent surgical dressing is dampened in saline and laid over the tympanic membrane and the flap. The graft site is then closed with suitable sutures.

Dressing and Postoperative Care

A cotton ball is placed in the ear canal. The patient is returned to the recovery room in a semisitting position. If a PLF was found, the patient is sent home with instructions for absolute bed rest except for bathroom privileges for the first 5 days. The patient should sleep with the head of the bed elevated or in a reclining chair. The patient is advised to roll on his or her side and push up with the arms rather than sit up so that the abdominal muscles are not tightened, which would increase cerebrospinal fluid pressure and float the graft out. The patient is kept on small doses of diazepam (Valium), 5 mg, three times per day, and flurazepam (Dalmane), 30 mg, at bedtime. The sedatives are prescribed during the first 5 days of bed rest. A stool softener, such as bisacodyl (Dulcolax), is used for the first 2 weeks. The patient removes the cotton ball from the ear canal on the first postoperative day. This action also removes the rayon strip and any blood clot in the ear canal. The patient is advised to sneeze with the mouth open only and to not blow the nose for 2 weeks.

Pitfalls

There are two potential pitfalls of PLF surgery: The first is an inability to obtain adequate hemostasis and anesthesia, particularly in the lower portion of the flap. The second is obtaining adequate visualization of the oval window area without removing the scutum. Finally, some patients are quite uncomfortable when the surgeon begins to denude the area around the stapes or over the round window membrane in preparation for graft placement. We avoid putting 4 per cent lidocaine in the middle ear as is routinely done when the middle ear is opened for a stapedectomy, singular neuroectomy, or other middle ear procedures performed under local anesthesia. If lidocaine gets into the inner ear, the patient will become violently dizzy and lose all hearing in the ear for a short period.

Adhesive bands must not form between the tympanic membrane and a graft over the round window membrane. If the bands do form, the patient will have an apparent sensorineural hearing loss combined with a conductive loss, both of which will clear when the adhesion is lysed. Fat should be avoided as a graft material because the failure rate will exceed 50 per cent.[25]

Revision PLF Repair

If instability and mild vertigo persist after the repair has healed, and if the turning or fistula test results are still

FIGURE 28-3

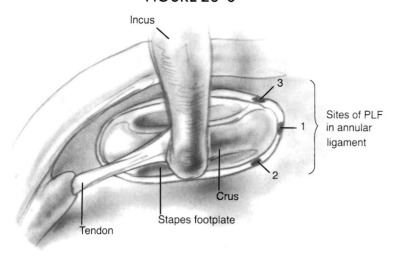

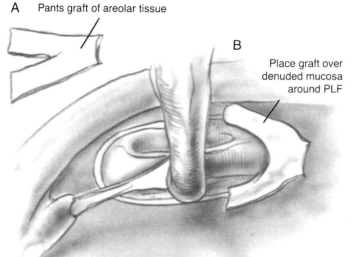

FIGURE 28-4

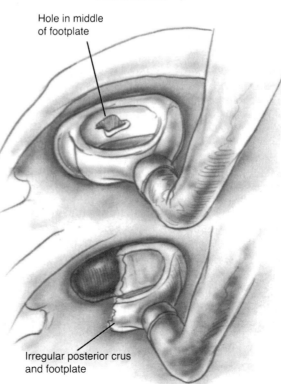

FIGURE 28–3. Details of oval window fistula sites in order of occurrence. Sites are in the annular ligament site. *A*, Pants graft of areolar tissue 3 × 1.5 mm with legs 2 mm long. *B*. Pants graft in place over denuded mucosa around perilymphatic fistula (PLF).

FIGURE 28–4. Congenital defects in posterior footplate.

positive, re-exploration should be considered. Failure occurs most frequently in cases with rather deep recesses of the oval window where one cannot get good access in front of the anterior crus to denude the bed and get the graft packed tightly enough into the area of the fistula tract. The procedure is identical to that used originally. Six weeks is allowed for the wound to completely heal before any revision is undertaken. The surgeon should attempt to re-repair a fistula at the oval window niche at least three times before considering doing a stapedectomy to close the fistula. For some reason, these PLF ears seem more sensitive than others to stapedectomy. In our hands, high-frequency sensorineural hearing loss has occurred every time a stapedectomy has been done for a PLF, whereas it rarely occurs with a small-window stapedotomy. If a stapedectomy is required to close a leak, one should use a perichondrial or fascial graft held in place with a 1-mm piston prosthesis.

RESULTS

There is a negative exploration rate of 40 to 50 per cent with our current diagnostic armamentarium. A better than 90 per cent first-time closure rate of round window membrane fistulas can be expected. The success rate with oval window fistulas, particularly if the recess is quite deep and narrow, is considerably lower—the first-time oval window failure rate is 20 to 30 per cent.

ALTERNATIVE TECHNIQUES

Patients seen in the first week after the development of a PLF should be treated with bed rest. The best recovery of hearing loss occurs with this group of patients. Only after bed rest for 5 to 7 days should surgical intervention be considered. If hearing loss is present, waiting more than 2 weeks from the onset of PLF significantly reduces the likelihood of improving the hearing with operative intervention. Therefore, these patients must be seen early and followed up carefully with audiometric testing. Positional testing should be avoided early in the convalescent period, because this may reopen the fistula.

Syms and associates have developed a new technique that involves injecting fluorescein intravenously in the patient approximately 20 minutes prior to the start of the operation.[31] By use of a special interference filter on the light source of the microscope to produce 490 nm of light, the surgeon is able to see fluorescence from a PLF.[31] It has been argued that all the surgeon is seeing is increased uptake of dye in the blood vessels on the promontory. If one looks at the clearance of the blood, particularly in experimental animals, most of the dye is gone very quickly: the dye seems to be concentrated in perilymph in experimental animals, reaching its peak in about 20 minutes. The animal study by Applebaum measured the dye through an intact round window membrane with blood vessels.[32] However, in the experimental animal groups, the dye is of such low concentration that it cannot be seen with the usual Wood's light techniques with the eye. Fluorescein does not accumulate in cerebrospinal fluid, so if one is dealing with a cerebrospinal fluid leak through a congenital defect, then the fluorescein is probably of little or no value.[32] The experience with this technique is somewhat limited and controversial. A repeat of the Syms study by Poe and colleagues, who carefully avoided blood loss, failed to demonstrate fluorescein in perilymph.[33]

References

1. House JW, Morris MS, Kramer SJ, et al: Perilymphatic fistula: Surgical experience in the United States. Otolaryngol Head Neck Surg 105: 51–61, 1991.
2. Singleton GT: Perilymph fistulas. Adv Otolaryngol Head Neck Surg 2: 25–38, 1988.
3. Allen GW: Endolymphatic sac and cochlear aqueduct. Arch Otolaryngol Head Neck Surg 79: 322–327, 1964.
4. Pullen FW: Round window membrane rupture: A cause of sudden deafness. Trans Am Acad Ophthalmol Otolaryngol 76: 1444–1450, 1972.
5. Rybak LP: "How I do it"—otology and neurotology. Laryngoscope 90: 2049–2050, 1980.
6. Singleton GT: Correlation of clinical symptoms of vertigo and/or hearing loss with anatomic site of surgically confirmed PLF. *In* Arenberg IK (ed). Inner Ear Surgery; Proceedings of the Third International Symposium and Workshops on Surgery of the Inner Ear. Snowmass-Aspen, CO, 1990. New York, Kugler, 1991, pp 395–397.
7. Goodhill V: Sudden deafness and round window rupture. Laryngoscope 81: 1462–1474, 1971.
8. Douek E: Perilymph fistula. J Laryngol Otol 89: 123–130, 1975.
9. Goodhill V: Stapedectomy revision commandments: Posterior arch stapedioplasty. Trans Pac Coast Oto-ophthalmol Soc 55:35–59, 1974.
10. Harrison WH, Shambaugh GE, Derlacki EL, et al: Perilymph fistula in stapes surgery. Laryngoscope 77: 736–849, 1967.
11. Hemenway WG, Hildyard VH, Black FO: Post stapedectomy perilymph fistulas in the rocky mountain area: The importance of nystagmography and audiometry in diagnosis and early tympanotomy in prognosis. Laryngoscope 78: 1687–1715, 1968.
12. House HP: The fistula problem in otosclerotic surgery. Laryngoscope 77: 1410–1426, 1967.
13. Kamerer DB, Sando I, Hirsch B, Takagi A: Perilymph fistula resulting from microfissures. Am J Otol 8: 489–494, 1987.
14. Kohut RI, Hinojosa R, Ryu J: Sudden-onset hearing loss in eleven consecutive cases: A temporal bone histopathologic study with identification of perilymphatic fistulae. Trans Am Otol Soc 77: 81–88, 1989.
15. Hinojosa R, Kohut RI, Lee JT, Ryu JH: Sudden hearing loss due to perilymphatic fistulae: II. Quantitative temporal bone histopathologic study. Trans Am Otol Soc 78: 121–127, 1990.
16. Shazly MA, Linthicum FH: Microfissures of the temporal bone: Do they have any clinical significance? Am J Otol 12: 169–171, 1991.
17. Lehrer JF, Poole DC, Sigal B: Use of the glycerin test in the diagnosis of post-traumatic perilymphatic fistulas. Am J Otolaryngol 1:207–210, 1980.
18. Arenberg IK, Ackley RS, Ferraro J, Muchnik C: ECoG results in perilymphatic fistula: Clinical and experimental studies. Otolaryngol Head Neck Surg 99: 435–443, 1988.
19. Meyerhoff WL, Yellin MW: Summating potential/action potential ratio in perilymph fistula. Otolaryngol Head Neck Surg 102: 678–682, 1990.
20. Campbell KCM, Karker LA, Abbas PJ: Interpretation of electrocochleography in Ménière's disease and normal subjects. Ann Otol Rhinol Laryngol 101: 496–500, 1992.
21. Reilly JS: Congenital perilymphatic fistula: A prospective study in infants and children. Laryngoscope 99: 393–397, 1989.
22. Parnes LS, McCabe BF: Perilymph fistula: An important cause of deafness and dizziness in children. Pediatrics 89: 524–528, 1987.
23. Pappas DG, Simpson LC, Godwin GH: Perilymphatic fistula in children with pre-existing sensorineural hearing loss. Laryngoscope 98: 507–510, 1988.
24. Bluestone CD: Otitis media and congenital perilymphatic fistula as a

cause of sensorineural hearing loss in children. Pediatr Infect Dis J 7: S141–S145, 1988.

25. Singleton GT, Karlan MS, Post KN, et al: Perilymph fistulas: Diagnostic criteria and therapy. Ann Otol Rhinol Laryngol 87: 797–803, 1978.

26. Singleton GT: Perilymph fistula. *In* Sharpe JA, Barber HO (eds): The Vestibulo-Ocular Reflex and Vertigo. New York, Raven Press, 1993.

27. Hart CW: The evaluation of vestibular function in healing and disease. *In* Otolaryngology. Hagerstown, MD, Harper & Row, 1972, pp 1–63.

28. Flood LM, Fraser JG, Hazell JWP, et al: Perilymph fistula: Four-year experience with a new audiometric test. J Laryngol Otol 99: 671–676, 1985.

29. Black FO, Lilly DJ, Nashner LM, et al: Quantitative diagnostic test for perilymph fistulas. Otolaryngol Head Neck Surg 96: 125–134, 1987.

30. Silverstein H: Rapid protein test for perilymph fistula. Otolaryngol Head Neck Surg 105: 422–426, 1991.

31. Syms CA III, Atkins JS Jr, Murphy TP: The use of fluorescein for intraoperative confirmation of perilymph fistula—a preliminary report. *In* Arenberg IK (ed). Inner Ear Surgery: Proceedings of the Third International Symposium and Workshops on Surgery of the Inner Ear, Snowmass-Aspen, CO, 1990. New York, Kugler, 1991, pp 379–381.

32. Applebaum EL: Fluorescein kinetics in perilymph and blood: A fluorophotometric study. Laryngoscope 92: 660–669, 1982.

33. Poe DS, Gadre AK, Rebeiz EE, Pankratov MM: Intravenous fluorescein for detection of perilymphatic fistulas. Am J Otol Am J Otol 14: 51–55, 1993.

29

Management of Bell's Palsy and Ramsay Hunt Syndrome

Bruce J. Gantz, M.D. ▪ Miriam I. Redleaf, M.D. ▪ Brian P. Perry, M.D.

Of the multitude of causes of facial paralysis, Bell's palsy and Ramsay Hunt syndrome are two of the most common. Although the diagnosis of Ramsay Hunt syndrome is generally quite obvious, Bell's palsy requires a thorough evaluation as well as close follow-up to establish a firm diagnosis. This chapter discusses the pathology, pathophysiology, evaluation, and management of these common disorders.

BELL'S PALSY

Sir Charles Bell (1774–1842) first described a patient with a facial paralysis in 1881[1]; subsequently, all patients with facial palsy of unknown etiology have come to bear his name. The etiology of this "idiopathic" disorder has become much clearer in recent years. Although first proposed in 1972 by McCormick,[2] herpes simplex virus (HSV) has only recently been identified as the disease vector,[3–5] and an animal model has been designed.[6] Murakami and associates identified HSV type 1 (HSV-1) DNA fragments in perineural fluid in 11 of 14 patients undergoing facial nerve decompression.[5] In this study, no control subjects had HSV-1 DNA in perineural fluid. Using polymerase chain reaction (PCR) to analyze the saliva of patients with Bell's palsy, Furuta and colleagues[3] identified HSV-1 DNA in 50 per cent of patients, which was significantly more often than controls. PCR has also been used to isolate HSV-1 genomic DNA from the geniculate ganglion of a temporal bone in a patient dying during the acute phase of Bell's palsy.[4] An animal model of Bell's palsy has been proposed by Sugita and coworkers.[6] Six days after inoculation of HSV-1 into either the auricle or tongue of mice, a temporary ipsilateral facial paralysis was identified that recovered spontaneously within 3 to 7 days. Histopathologically, neural edema, inflammatory cell infiltrate, and vacuolar degeneration were demonstrated in the affected facial nerve and nucleus. HSV-1 antigens were identified within the facial nerve, geniculate ganglion, and facial nucleus between 6 and 20 days after inoculation.[6] Similar pathologic findings have been demonstrated in rabbits after HSV-1 inoculation, but without the associated facial paralysis.[7]

In considering this evidence, the pathogenesis of Bell's palsy becomes more apparent: a virally induced, inflammatory response that produces edema within the nerve. Fisch and Felix first proposed that the facial nerve was entrapped at the meatal foramen as a result of neural edema.[8] Intraoperative conduction studies have shown an electrophysiologic blockage at this site.[9] The constriction imposed produces a conduction block at first; however, with prolonged or increased constriction, ischemia results. Subsequently, wallerian degeneration occurs, producing axonotmesis and/or neurotmesis. A spectrum of injury within the nerve from neuropraxia to neurotmesis may occur in Bell's palsy.[10, 11] The proportion of each of these determines the amount of facial function that returns when the acute phase of the disease subsides.

The clinical presentation of Bell's palsy is well known; however, the clinician must exclude other causes of facial paralysis based on history and physical examination findings. Patients describe an abrupt onset of unilateral paresis that occurs over a period of 24 to 48 hours. The paresis can progress over 1 to 7 days to complete paralysis. Occasionally, otalgia, dysgeusia, and a perception of some sensory change on the involved side will be present. Bilateral involvement, either simultaneously or consecutively, has been described.[12] A history of progression of weakness over weeks to months, repeated episodes of paralysis, and twitching of the facial muscles should not be considered symptoms of Bell's palsy. Other associated symptoms of hearing loss, vestibular symptoms, or other cranial nerve neuropathies also rule out the diagnosis of Bell's palsy.

On physical examination, the patient displays unilateral weakness or flaccid paralysis of all branches of the facial nerve. If forehead movement is normal, and there is strong eye closure and symmetric blinking, a central origin of paralysis should be suspected. The tympanic membrane should be of normal color and mobility. Careful bimanual palpation of the parotid gland may reveal a deep lobe parotid neoplasm. Oral cavity examination may demonstrate loss of papillae on the ipsilateral tongue. Cranial nerve testing is normal with the exception of the involved seventh nerve. Serial examinations are essential; if some evidence of recovery is not noted within 3 to 6 months, then an aggressive search for an underlying neoplasm should be undertaken.

Audiometric evaluation should reveal symmetric function except for an absent ipsilateral acoustic reflex. If unilateral hearing loss or acoustic reflex decay is present, further evaluation for retrocochlear pathology is necessary. If vestibular complaints are present, an electronystagmogram is performed and diagnosis of Bell's palsy should be questioned. If the history and clinical presentation are highly suggestive of Bell's palsy, magnetic resonance imaging (MRI) and computed tomographic (CT) scanning are not performed. High-resolution CT scans and MRI are obtained if patients have associated symptoms of otorrhea, vestibular complaints, and hearing loss. Planned surgical decompression and persistent dense paralysis after six months are also indications for imaging.

Electrodiagnostic testing is an important element of the diagnostic evaluation of facial paralysis. It can determine the extent of facial nerve injury and provide useful prognostic information for the development of management strategies. The technique of electroneuronography (ENoG), developed by Esslen, can distinguish the nerve fibers that have undergone wallerian degeneration from those that are temporarily blocked (neuropraxia).[13] ENoG testing is not performed until 3 to 4 days following the development of complete unilateral paralysis, because wallerian degeneration does not become apparent until 48 to 72 hours following an acute injury to the nerve. Electrodiagnostic testing is not performed when the patient exhibits paresis only. If the paresis progresses to total paralysis, electrodiagnostic testing is performed 3 days after the onset of total paralysis. Presence of voluntary movement 4 to 5 days following the onset of paresis indicates only minor injury, and complete recovery should be anticipated.

ENoG is most accurate when it is performed within 3 weeks of the acute injury. The test is performed using standard electromyographic (EMG) equipment but requires the use of special surface stimulating and recording electrodes.[14] The recording electrodes are in a hand-held carrier and are manipulated in the nasolabial fold with the Esslen technique. The recording electrodes are not taped to the skin, as has been described by others.[15]

An evoked electrical stimulus generates synchronous facial muscle movement that can be recorded from the skin surface (called the *compound muscle action potential* [CMAP]). The amplitude of the biphasic CMAP has been found to correlate with the number of blocked or neuropraxic nerve fibers. As the percentage of degenerated fibers within the nerve increases, the amplitude of the CMAP decreases compared with the normal side of the face. Fisch and Esslen have determined that if 90 per cent or more of the fibers within the facial nerve degenerate within the first 14 days of an acute paralysis, a severe injury has occurred, and the chances of complete recovery are less than 50 per cent.[16] Patients who do not reach the 90 per cent degeneration level by 3 weeks have a very good prognosis and will likely regain normal facial motion without synkinesis. The time course of degeneration is also important: the more rapid the degeneration, the more severe the injury.[17] A patient demonstrating greater than 90 per cent degeneration at 5 days will have a worse prognosis than someone with 90 per cent degeneration at 14 days.

Patients exhibiting 90 to 100 per cent degeneration or no response to electrical stimulation, in addition to ENoG, must undergo EMG testing. An EMG needle is placed in the orbicularis oris and oculi muscles, and the patient is asked to make a forceful contraction. Any voluntary motor unit activity indicates deblocking of the conduction block and a favorable prognosis. When deblocking occurs, fibers may not discharge at the same rate because of the previous injury and may fail to generate a surface CMAP, resulting in a false-positive test result on ENoG testing. As movement returns to the face, the surface CMAP may also be absent for the same reason. Voluntary evoked EMG testing is *mandatory* if a surgical decompression is planned. If a

facial paralysis has been slowly progressive over weeks to months, degeneration and regeneration of nerve fibers occur within the nerve, resulting is similar dis-synchronous discharge of evoked impulses and an inaccurate CMAP recording.

Topognostic testing is widely reported to be useful in determining the site of injury in acute facial paralysis; however, intraoperative studies have shown that the Schirmer test is not accurate in diagnosing Bell's palsy.[14] The Schirmer test may be used to determine the extent of lacrimation and the need for eye protection.

A review of the natural history of Bell's palsy shows that approximately 85 per cent of patients begin to display some return of facial movement within 3 weeks of the onset of paresis.[18] The remaining 15 per cent begin to improve 3 to 6 months after the onset of the disease. Most patients will display a complete return of facial function, but 10 to 15 per cent will have residual unilateral weakness and develop secondary deformities of synkinesis, tearing, or contracture. Some motion will return in almost all individuals with Bell's palsy by 6 months. If no movement returns, a vigorous search for another etiology should begin anew.

The management of patients with Bell's palsy is quite variable, depending on the type of specialist initially seeing the patient and on the training of the individual specialist. An overview of our management strategy is seen in Figure 29–1. Patients presenting within the first week of facial weakness with paresis are placed on steroid therapy (prednisone 60 to 80 mg per day for 7 days) and an antiviral agent (valcyclovir 500 mg three times per day for 10 days). If they are seen 7 to 10 days following onset and motor function is stable or improving, medical treatment is unnecessary. Patients are instructed to return in 1 week for re-evaluation to determine if neural degeneration has occurred. Electrodiagnostic testing is not necessary as long as voluntary facial movement is present. If total paralysis occurs in the interim, the total paralysis protocol of Figure 29–1 is followed. Stable or improving patients are seen in 1 month.

The use of steroids and antivirals in Bell's palsy is controversial; however, intrinsically it seems an appropriate management strategy for a viral syndrome. Three studies found much better outcomes in those treated with steroids,[19–21] whereas a fourth large series did not.[22] We use prednisone in a dose of 1 mg/kg daily for 7 days in all cases in which it is not medically contraindicated, in anticipation of speeding recovery, reducing the number of degenerating axons, and reducing the number of patients needing decompression. The combination of steroids and antivirals may be superior to either one alone. A double-blind, randomized, controlled trial of acyclovir and prednisone versus prednisone alone in the treatment of Bell's palsy demonstrated better results with the combination therapy.[23] This study documented poor facial function recovery in 23 per cent of the prednisone only group, compared with 7 per cent in the acyclovir plus prednisone group. Other studies have found no significant difference between this combination of drugs and the natural history of the disease.[24]

Patients presenting within 1 week of the onset of total unilateral paralysis undergo electrodiagnostic testing (if at

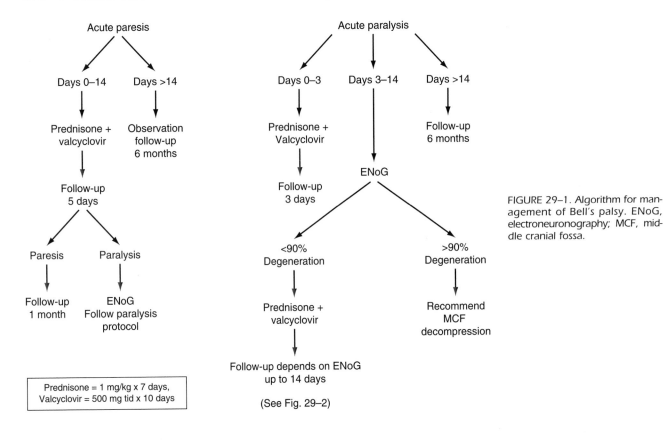

FIGURE 29–1. Algorithm for management of Bell's palsy. ENoG, electroneuronography; MCF, middle cranial fossa.

least 3 days have passed since the onset of paralysis) and are started on medical therapy. If the patient is seen in the first 3 days following the onset of paralysis, steroid and antiviral therapy are initiated and follow-up electrodiagnostic studies are arranged. The frequency of follow-up electrodiagnostic examinations is determined by the result of testing and the time interval following paralysis, as suggested by Fisch (Fig. 29–2).[25] Patients exhibiting nearly 90 per cent neural degeneration on ENoG examination, or who are degenerating quickly, undergo frequent electrodiagnostic testing (every 1 or 2 days). If greater than 90 per cent degeneration is reached, and there are no motor unit potentials on voluntary EMG testing, the patient is considered a candidate for middle cranial fossa decompression. When 90 per cent degeneration is not reached within 2 weeks (14 days) following the onset of paralysis, no further electrodiagnostic studies need be performed.

Patients seen for the first time more than 2 weeks follow-

ing the onset of paralysis undergo EMG evaluation to determine if regeneration has begun. They are scheduled for a six-month follow-up to make sure that some motor function has returned. If no movement is evident at 6 months, it must be assumed that Bell's palsy was an incorrect diagnosis, and a search for another disease process is begun.

RAMSAY HUNT SYNDROME

Ramsay Hunt syndrome (herpes zoster oticus) is the second most common cause of facial paralysis and is induced by the reactivation of the varicella zoster virus that remains latent in the geniculate ganglion after primary infection with chickenpox.[26] Classically, patients present with severe otalgia and unilateral facial paralysis. Vesicular eruptions may or may not be present initially but usually appear

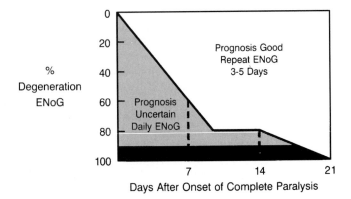

FIGURE 29–2. Recommended electroneuronographic (ENoG) testing schedule in acute facial paralysis.

within 3 to 5 days of the paralysis. The vesicular lesions can appear on the concha, ear canal, postauricular skin, and tympanic membrane. Occasionally the oral cavity, neck, and shoulder are also involved. Unlike Bell's palsy, the disease can affect other cranial nerves, including auditory, vestibular, trigeminal, glossopharyngeal, and the vagus, prompting the name *herpes zoster cephalicus*.[27] Also in contrast to Bell's palsy, the symptoms are more severe and the prognosis is worse in Ramsay Hunt syndrome. The frequency of complete neural degeneration of the facial nerve is substantially higher than with Bell's palsy, and complete recovery of facial motor function has varied from 10 to 31 per cent in several studies.[28–30] Patients with auditory and vestibular dysfunction in addition to facial paralysis generally have a worse prognosis.

The diagnosis of Ramsay Hunt syndrome is based on the history of otalgia, vesicular lesions or eschars, and facial paralysis. MRI demonstrates enhancement of a large portion of the facial nerve, often the vestibular and cochlear nerves, the labyrinth, and the dura lining the internal auditory canal as well.[31] Imaging as part of routine evaluation is unnecessary. Electrodiagnostic studies have not been reliable in herpes zoster oticus.

The management of this disease has changed with the development of antiviral agents. The natural history of the disease was evaluated by Devriese and Moesker, who identified only a 10 per cent rate of complete facial nerve recovery.[29] Many studies have identified a superior recovery rate using a combination of steroids and antiviral agents, as high as 75 per cent.[32–35] We have experienced similar successful results using either intravenous acyclovir (10 mg/kg tid) or oral valcyclovir (500 mg tid) for 10 days, in combination with 7 days of prednisone (60 to 80 mg/kg daily). Patients report rapid reduction in pain and occasionally experience return of facial movement during the medical therapy. The overall return of facial movement is better than with previous surgical decompressions; therefore, the surgical approach is no longer recommended.

FACIAL NERVE DECOMPRESSION FOR BELL'S PALSY

Decompression of the facial nerve for Bell's palsy has been reported since the 1930s[36] and is recommended in those patients who exhibit greater than 90 per cent degeneration on ENoG and no voluntary EMG activity within 14 days of the paralysis. Preliminary results suggested that early decompression of the labyrinthine, geniculate, and tympanic segments of the facial nerve through a middle cranial fossa approach improves recovery of severely degenerated cases,[13] whereas decompression of the mastoid segment alone did not alter the natural history of the disease.[37] Gantz and associates have shown a statistically significant difference in facial nerve outcome when decompression is performed within 2 weeks of onset of the paralysis.[38] The patients undergoing decompression exhibited House-Brackmann grade I ($N = 14$) or II ($N = 17$) in 91 per cent of cases; two patients had a grade III and 1 patient had a grade IV outcome. There were no grade V or VI results in the surgical group. Patients who met surgical criteria but elected not to undergo surgery had a 58 per cent chance of

a poor outcome. Within the nonsurgical group, 19 patients had a House-Brackmann score of either III or IV at 7-month follow-up.

Intraoperative evoked EMG is used to localize the region of the conduction block.[9] Intraoperative direct nerve stimulation is useful when the nerve is not completely degenerated, which includes most instances when preoperative ENoG reveals 100 per cent degeneration. This finding suggests that a small number of nerve fibers remain capable of stimulation even when ENoG demonstrates total nerve degeneration. In most cases, the nerve conduction block is localized between the geniculate ganglion and the internal auditory canal segments of the facial nerve. Failure to generate a motor unit potential when the tympanic segment of the nerve is stimulated indicates that the nerve is 100 per cent degenerated or that the conduction block is more distal. If the nerve appears normal in the tympanic portion while there is edema and erythema of the internal auditory canal segment, total degeneration should be suspected. If erythema and edema are apparent in the tympanic segment, a mastoid decompression is added.

Preoperative Preparation

The risks of middle fossa decompression of the facial nerve are discussed with the patient and include cerebrospinal fluid leak (4 to 6 per cent), infection (1 per cent), hearing loss (1 per cent), dizziness (1 per cent), intracranial hemorrhage (<1 per cent), and aphasia (<1 per cent). When the decision is made to proceed with surgical decompression, the procedure should be performed as soon as possible. Appropriate preoperative laboratory and imaging studies are obtained, along with a Stenvers projection plain radiograph of the temporal bone to identify the floor of the middle cranial fossa and superior semicircular canal. Cefazolin (Ancef) and dexamethasone (Decadron) are given prior to the skin incision and are continued for a total of six doses.

General anesthesia and transoral endotracheal intubation are accomplished; thereafter, the bed is rotated 180 degrees for access (Fig. 29–3). Paralytic agents must be reversed prior to the skin incision. A urinary catheter is placed to monitor fluids and diuresis. Hair is shaved approximately 10 cm above and 5 cm behind the ear. The entire side of the head and face are prepared, and EMG needles are placed in the orbicularis oculi and oris muscles (Fig. 29–4A) for facial nerve monitoring. A clear drape is placed over the prepared area to allow visualization of the entire side of the face in the case of monitoring equipment failure (Fig. 29–4B). Standard auditory brainstem evoked recording electrodes are placed in the right and left mastoid tips and the vertex and forehead (ground), and insert head phones are placed in both external auditory canals. The auditory brainstem response is monitored throughout the procedure.

Surgical Technique

The skin incision is marked as shown in Figure 29–5 and carried down to the level of the temporalis fascia. Mean-

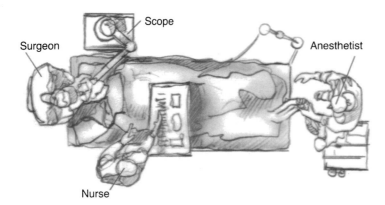

FIGURE 29–3. Operating room set-up for middle cranial fossa approach.

while, mannitol (0.5 g/kg body weight) and hyperventilation (P_{CO_2} of 25 mm Hg) are initiated by the anesthesiologist to relax the brain. After the posteriorly based skin flap is elevated, a 4 × 6 cm piece of temporalis fascia is harvested and set aside in a moist gauze for use at the time of closure. An anteriorly based, inferiorly staggered muscle flap is then elevated down to the level of the linea temporalis and reflected forward with an Adson cerebellar retractor. Staggering the incisions prevents dural exposure if wound dehiscence occurs. The zygomatic root identifies the floor of the middle cranial fossa and is the central landmark of the craniotomy. The skin and muscle flaps should be wrapped with moist sponges and secured with temporary retraction stitches.

The craniotomy should be approximately 4 cm in anteroposterior dimension and 5 cm cephalocaudal (Fig. 29–6A). The anteroposterior margins must be kept parallel for stability of the middle cranial fossa retractor. The craniotomy can be created with either cutting burrs or a craniotomy saw. The bone flap should be elevated with care by use of a blunt dural elevator. Occasionally, the middle meningeal artery will be imbedded within the bone, requiring bipolar coagulation to free it. The bone flap is wrapped in a moist gauze and set aside for use at closure.

Dural elevation from the floor of the middle cranial fossa is accomplished with a Freer or joker elevator, always in a posterior-to-anterior direction, which prevents injury to the greater superficial petrosal nerve and geniculate ganglion. The petrous ridge is identified at the posterior margin of the craniotomy, and the dura is slowly elevated over the arcuate eminence and meatal plane. Dural reflections are cauterized and sharply transected to allow elevation to the anterior petrous ridge. The hiatus of the facial canal with the greater superficial petrosal nerve and artery is the anterior margin of elevation. Further anterior elevation exposes the foramen spinosum and the pterygoid plexus of veins, which can cause troublesome oozing throughout the procedure. Following dural elevation, cottonoid sponges can be placed at the anterior and posterior margins of the elevation to help retract the dura during placement of the self-retaining middle cranial fossa retractor (Fig. 29–6B).

Prior to the bony exposure of the facial nerve, the Stenvers projection radiograph is re-examined to determine the depth of the superior semicircular canal in the temporal bone. The superior semicircular canal is the first structure to be located. Once its blue line is identified, the remaining intratemporal structures have consistent anatomic locations.

Landmarks of the middle cranial fossa floor can be quite subtle. The arcuate eminence may not be apparent and, in many instances, is not parallel with the superior semicircular canal. One consistent anatomic feature to remember is that the plane of the superior semicircular canal is almost always perpendicular to the petrous ridge (Fig. 29–7). If the arcuate eminence is not initially apparent, then drilling is begun posterior to the semicircular canal, slowly removing the tegmen mastoideum with a moderate-sized diamond burr. The whitish color of the membranous temporal bone can be distinguished from the yellow, dense otic capsule bone of the superior canal. Once the superior canal is identified, drilling in a parallel direction with the canal will gradually expose the blue line.

When the location of the superior canal is confirmed, an anterior line 60 degrees to the blue line locates the position of the internal auditory canal. The depth of the internal auditory canal is variable, but drilling medially near the petrous ridge provides a safe route to the canal. Drilling laterally near the anterior ampulla of the superior semicircular canal places the geniculate ganglion, labyrinthine segment of the facial nerve, and cochlea at risk. Once the blue line of the internal auditory canal is exposed, bone is removed in a lateral direction until the vertical crest is found (Fig. 29–8). Bone can now be removed over the geniculate ganglion and tegmen tympani.

The labyrinthine segment of the facial nerve is the narrowest portion of the fallopian canal and lies in an anterosuperior plane from the vertical crest to the geniculate ganglion. A 1-mm diamond burr is used to remove bone over the labyrinthine segment while the area directly anterior to the segment is closely observed for the blue line of the basal turn of the cochlea. The final layer of bone is removed with thin, angled hooks and blunt microelevators. At this point, marked swelling of the nerve in the internal auditory canal, labyrinthine segment, and geniculate ganglion is usually observed. Further swelling is apparent following neurolysis. A disposable microscalpel (Beaver No. 59–40) is used to slit the periosteum and epineural sheath.

Intraoperative EMG is used to localize the region of the nerve conduction block. Direct stimulation of the most distal exposed tympanic segment of the nerve is performed with monopolar or bipolar microforceps (Fig. 29–9). If the conduction block is medial to the point of stimulation and the nerve is not completely degenerated, a motor unit potential will be observed. Stimulating more medially to-

FIGURE 29-4

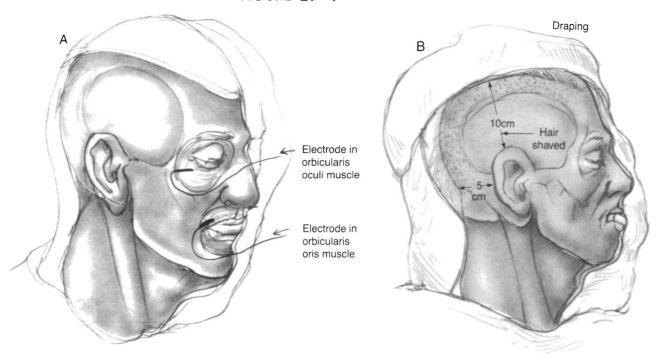

A

B

Draping

Electrode in orbicularis oculi muscle

Electrode in orbicularis oris muscle

10cm

Hair shaved

5 cm

FIGURE 29-5

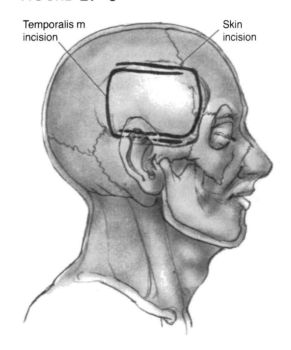

Temporalis m incision

Skin incision

FIGURE 29–4. *A*, Electrode placement for intraoperative electromyography. *B*, Draping with exposure of half the face for visual monitoring of facial movement.

FIGURE 29–5. *Skin incision for middle cranial fossa approach. Mastoid exposure can be obtained by extending the incision postauricularly. Incision of anteriorly based temporalis muscle flap is offset to keep suture lines from being directly in line.*

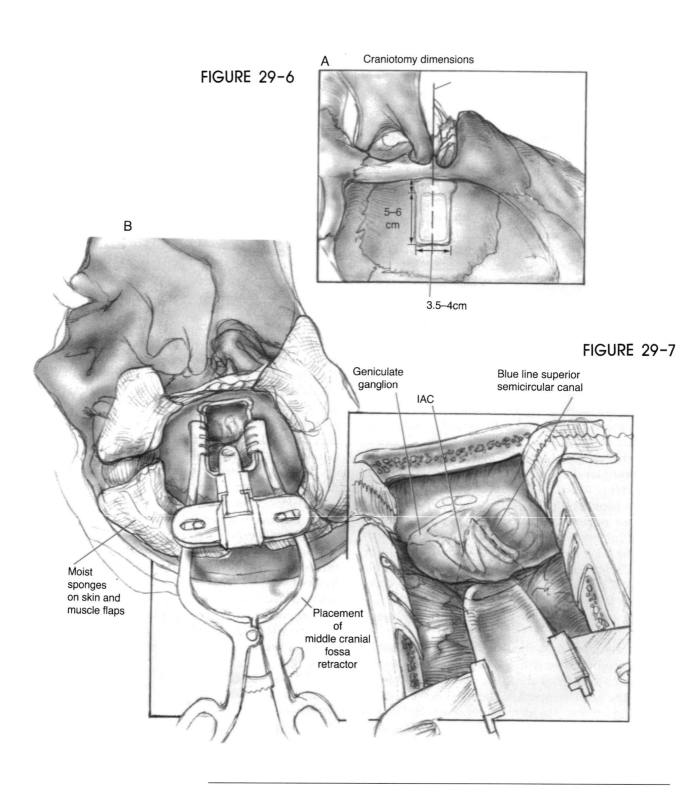

FIGURE 29-6

A Craniotomy dimensions

5–6 cm

3.5–4cm

B

Moist sponges on skin and muscle flaps

Placement of middle cranial fossa retractor

FIGURE 29-7

Geniculate ganglion

IAC

Blue line superior semicircular canal

FIGURE 29–6. *A,* Craniotomy for middle cranial fossa exposure. Inferior expansion of craniotomy allows more exposure during dural elevation. Vertical margins must be parallel for stability of retractor. Craniotomy should be centered on the temporal root of the zygoma *(dashed line). B,* Placement of House-Urban middle cranial fossa retractor.

FIGURE 29–7. Exposure of superior semicircular canal blue line and position of internal auditory canal 60 degrees anterior to a line through the blue line. Superior canal blue line almost always is perpendicular to petrous ridge. IAC, internal auditory canal.

FIGURE 29-8

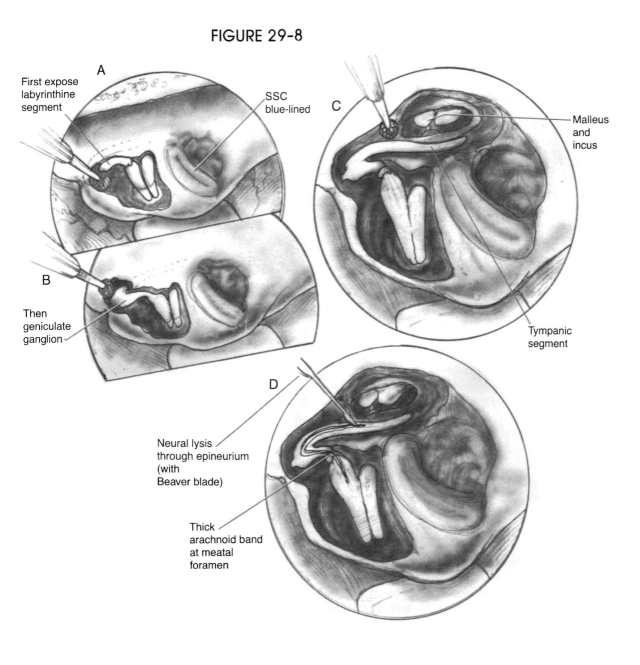

FIGURE 29–8. A to D, Middle cranial fossa exposure of cranial nerve (CN) VII and surrounding anatomy. Bone removed from tegmen tympani to expose tympanic segment of CN VII. Note edema of internal auditory canal segment CN VII, frequently found in Bell's palsy. SCC, semicircular canal.

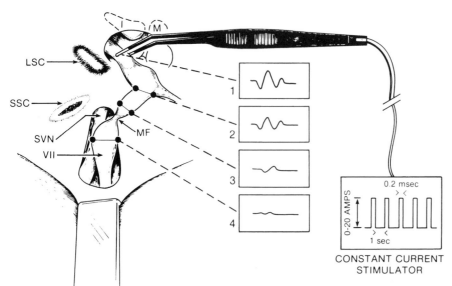

FIGURE 29–9. Intraoperative evoked electromyography to identify site of nerve conduction block. If conduction block is medial to geniculate ganglions, stimulation of tympanic segment results in motor unit potential (1); stimulation of internal canal segment (3) results in no response. Usually, conduction block is at meatal foramen (MF). LSC, lateral semicircular canal; SSC, superior semicircular canal; SVN, superior vestibular nerve.

ward the internal auditory canal will fail to elicit a motor unit potential if the conduction block is at the meatal foramen.

On completion of the decompression and confirmation of the site of the conduction block, the opened internal auditory canal is covered with a piece of temporalis muscle. The previously harvested temporalis fascia is placed over the opened floor of the middle fossa after bone waxing the opened mastoid air cells. The dural retractor is removed, and the anesthesiologist is asked to re-establish a normal P_{CO_2}.

A corner of the craniotomy bone flap is harvested and placed superior to the fascia to prevent herniation of the temporal lobe dura into the attic and internal auditory canal. The temporal lobe is allowed to re-expand into the middle cranial fossa floor. The remainder of the craniotomy flap is placed on the dura, and the temporalis is closed, creating a watertight seal with interrupted absorbable sutures. Skin is closed with a deep layer of interrupted absorbable sutures and an outer layer of nylon absorbable sutures. A mastoid-type dressing is applied. No drains are used.

Postoperative Care

Postoperative care includes intensive care observation overnight, limitation of fluids (1500 to 1800 ml per day), dexamethasone (6 mg every 6 hours for 36 hours), cefazolin (1 g every 8 hours for 36 hours), routine neural checks, and limitation of analgesia to codeine. There is little postoperative pain, and stronger narcotics may mask intracranial complications. The patient is transferred to a routine postoperative floor the next morning, encouraged to begin ambulation, and started on a diet as tolerated. On postoperative day 3, and daily thereafter, observations for cerebrospinal fluid rhinorrhea are made by asking the patient to lean forward with the head between the knees. If cerebrospinal fluid rhinorrhea occurs, a spinal drain must be placed for 4 to 5 days. Following this regimen, only

very rarely has a patient required surgical closure of the leak. Patients are usually discharged from the hospital on postoperative days 5 to 7. No intracranial complications, including intracranial hemorrhage, aphasia, or seizures, occurred in the Iowa series.[38]

Limitations and Special Considerations

The anatomy of the middle cranial fossa floor is quite variable and presents some difficulty in identification of landmarks. The surgeon must have a precise knowledge of the three-dimensional anatomy of the temporal bone. Many hours in the temporal bone dissection laboratory are required to attain the delicate microsurgical skills necessary for this type of surgery.

Dural elevation can be difficult, especially in patients older than 65 years of age. If a dural tear occurs, a temporalis fascia repair must be performed. Hearing loss can occur from contact of the rotating burr with an intact ossicular chain or by entrance into the cochlea or labyrinth. Vestibular dysfunction can occur in a similar fashion. If the membranous labyrinth is violated, immediate placement of a small amount of bone wax may preserve auditory and vestibular function.

Correct positioning of the craniotomy and maintaining parallel vertical margins are essential. Meticulous hemostasis must be maintained with bipolar cautery, oxidized cellulose, and pressure. A dry surgical field is critical for microscopic dissection of subtle landmarks and prevention of complications. If large apical air cells are opened, they must be plugged with temporalis muscle to prevent cerebrospinal fluid leaks.

References

1. Bell C: On the nerves, giving an account of some experiments on their structure and function, which led to a new arrangement of the system. Philos Trans 111: 398–424, 1821.

2. McCormick D: Herpes simplex virus as cause of Bell's palsy. Lancet 1: 937–939, 1972.
3. Furuta Y, Fukuda S, Chida E, et al: Reactivation of herpes simplex virus type 1 in patients with Bell's palsy. J Med Virol 54: 162–166, 1998.
4. Burgess RC, Michaels L, Bale JF Jr, Smith RJ: Polymerase chain reaction amplification of herpes simplex viral DNA from the geniculate ganglion of a patient with Bell's palsy. Ann Otol Rhinol Laryngol 103: 775–779, 1994.
5. Murakami S, Mizobuchi M, Nakashiro Y, et al: Bell palsy and herpes simplex virus: Identification of viral DNA in endoneurial fluid and muscle [see comments]. Ann Intern Med 124: 27–30, 1996.
6. Sugita T, Murakami S, Yanagihara N, et al: Facial nerve paralysis induced by herpes simplex virus in mice: An animal model of acute and transient facial paralysis. Ann Otol Rhinol Laryngol 104: 574–581, 1995.
7. Carreño M, Llorente J, Hidalgo F, et al: Aplicación de la reacción en cadeña de la polimerase a un modelo experimental de infección por el virus del herpes simplex tipo 1. Acta Otorrinolaryngol Española 49: 15, 1998.
8. Fisch U, Felix H: On the pathogenesis of Bell's palsy. Acta Otolaryngol 95: 532–538, 1983.
9. Gantz BJ, Gmuer A, Fisch U: Intraoperative evoked electromyography in Bell's palsy. Am J Otolaryngol 3: 273–278, 1982.
10. Proctor B, Corgill D, Proud G: The pathology of Bell's palsy. Trans Am Acad Ophthalmol Otolaryngol 82: 70–80, 1976.
11. Fowler E: The pathologic findings in a case of facial paralysis. Trans Am Acad Ophthalmol Otolaryngol 67: 187–197, 1963.
12. Cwach H, Landis J, Freeman J: Bilateral seventh nerve palsy: A report of two cases and a review. South Dakot Med J March: 99–101, 1997.
13. Esslen E: Electromyography and electroneuronography. In Fisch U (ed): Facial Nerve Surgery. Birmingham, AL, Aesculapius, 1977, pp 93–100.
14. Gantz BJ, Gmuer AA, Holliday M, Fisch U: Electroneurographic evaluation of the facial nerve: Method and technical problems. Ann Otol Rhinol Laryngol 93: 394–398, 1984.
15. Blumenthal F, May M: Electrodiagnosis. In May M ed: The Facial Nerve. New York, Thieme, 1986.
16. Fisch U, Esslen E: Total intratemporal exposure of the facial nerve: Pathologic findings in Bell's palsy. Arch Otolaryngol 95: 335–341, 1972.
17. Fisch U: Prognostic value of electrical tests in acute facial paralysis. Am J Otol 5: 494–498, 1984.
18. Peitersen E: Natural history of Bell's palsy. Acta Otolaryngol 492(Suppl): 122–124, 1992.
19. Katusic SK, Beard CM, Wiederholt WC, et al: Incidence, clinical features, and prognosis in Bell's palsy, Rochester, Minnesota, 1968–1982. Ann Neurol 20: 622–627, 1986.
20. Adour K, Wingerd J, Bell D: Prednisone treatment for idiopathic facial paralysis. N Engl J Med 287: 1276–1282, 1972.
21. Wolf S, Wagner J, Davidson S, Forsythe A: Treatment of Bell's palsy with prednisone: A prospective, randomized study. Neurology 28: 158–161, 1978.
22. May M, Wette R, Hardin W, Sullivan J: The use of steroids in Bell's palsy. Laryngoscope 86: 1111–1122, 1976.
23. Adour KK, Ruboyianes JM, Von Doersten PG, et al: Bell's palsy treatment with acyclovir and prednisone compared with prednisone alone: A double-blind, randomized, controlled trial. Ann Otol Rhinol Laryngol 105: 371–378, 1996.
24. Ramos Macías A, de Miguel Martínez I, Martin Sánchez AM, et al: Incorporación del aciclovir en el tratamiento de la parálisis periférica: Un estudío en 45 casos. Acta Otorrinolaringol Española 43: 117–120, 1992.
25. Fisch U: Surgery for Bell's palsy. Arch Otolaryngol 107: 1–11, 1981.
26. Ikeda M, Hiroshige K, Abiko Y, Onoda K: Impaired specific cellular immunity to the varicella-zoster virus in patients with herpes zoster oticus. J Laryngol Otol 110: 918–921, 1996.
27. Adour KK: Otological complications of herpes zoster. Ann Neurol 35(Suppl): S62–S64, 1994.
28. Peitersen E: Spontaneous course of Bell's Palsy. In Fisch U ed: Facial Nerve Surgery. Birmingham, AL, Aesculapias, 1977, pp 337–343.
29. Devriese P, Moesker W: The natural history of facial paralysis in herpes zoster. Clin Otolaryngol 13: 289–298, 1988.
30. Devriese P: Herpes zoster causing facial paralysis. In Fisch U ed: Facial Nerve Surgery. Birmingham, AL, Aesculapius, 1977, pp 419–420.
31. Brandle P, Satoretti-Schefer S, Bohmer A, et al: Correlation of MRI, clinical, and electroneuronographic findings in acute facial nerve palsy. Am J Otol 17: 154–161, 1996.
32. Stafford FW, Welch AR: The use of acyclovir in Ramsay Hunt syndrome. J Laryngol Otol 100: 337–340, 1986.
33. Murakami S, Hato N, Horiuchi J, et al: Treatment of Ramsay Hunt syndrome with acyclovir-prednisone: Significance of early diagnosis and treatment. Ann Neurol 41: 353–357, 1997.
34. Uri N, Greenberg E, Meyer W, Kitzes-Cohen R: Herpes zoster oticus: Treatment with acyclovir. Ann Otol Rhinol Laryngol 101: 161–162, 1992.
35. Dickens J, Smith J, Graham S: Herpes zoster oticus: Treatment with intravenous acyclovir. Laryngoscope 98: 776–779, 1988.
36. Balance C, Duel A: The operative treatment of facial palsy: By the introduction of nerve grafts into the fallopian canal and by other intratemporal methods. Arch Otolaryngol 15: 1–79, 1932.
37. May M, Klein SR, Taylor FH: Idiopathic (Bell's) facial palsy: Natural history defies steroid or surgical treatment. Laryngoscope 95: 406–409, 1985.
38. Gantz BJ, Rubinstein J, Gidley P, Woodworth GG: Surgical management of Bell's palsy. Laryngoscope 109: 1177–1188, 1999.

30

Traumatic Facial Paralysis

Herman A. Jenkins, M.D. ▪ Gregory A. Ator, M.D.

The facial nerve may be injured by many blunt and penetrating mechanisms. Common causes include motor vehicle accidents, stab or gunshot wounds to the face (frequently seen in urban areas), and iatrogenic injuries during head and neck surgical procedures. Primary mechanisms of injury include stretching, compression, and transection of the nerve.

The course of the nerve from the brainstem to the facial musculature can be divided into three segments: intracranial, intratemporal, and extratemporal or peripheral (Fig. 30–1). The pathophysiology of facial nerve disorders varies according to the segment of the nerve involved and is discussed individually.

INTRACRANIAL INJURY TO THE FACIAL NERVE

The intracranial facial nerve, extending from the brainstem to the fundus of the internal auditory canal, is rarely damaged by penetrating trauma because of the excellent protection afforded by the petrous bone and the cranial vault, but with severe trauma, stretch and shock wave–type injuries may still occur. Penetrating trauma to this region will likely be accompanied by extensive central nervous system pathology, which must first be evaluated and treated. Evaluation of the injured nerve begins with a careful examination of motor function as soon as possible after the injury is sustained. If the nerve is functional at presentation and becomes progressively paretic, a complete transection injury is unlikely. If the nerve manifests any motion, regular clinical observation can be used to follow up the status of the nerve. After the onset of complete paralysis, surgery is contemplated if the nerve shows electrical signs of near-total degeneration (see under *Timing of Surgery*).

INTRATEMPORAL INJURY TO THE FACIAL NERVE

The intratemporal facial nerve, extending from the internal auditory canal fundus to the stylomastoid foramen, is frequently damaged from blunt trauma to the skull that leads to a temporal bone fracture. Fractures produced by blunt trauma have been traditionally grouped into longitudinal and transverse varieties, although almost any type of fracture can be encountered. Two main groups of fractures are typically seen: longitudinal and transverse. Fractures with the main component parallel to the long axis of the petrous pyramid are classified as longitudinal (Fig. 30–2), whereas fractures perpendicular to the long axis (see Fig. 30–5) are considered to be transverse fractures. Longitudinal fractures are produced by trauma to the lateral aspects of the skull in the temporoparietal region and compose 80 per cent of fractures in most series.[1] Transverse fractures are produced by trauma to the occipital or frontal regions of the skull and compose about 20 per cent of fractures. Many fractures are oblique or combine elements of longitudinal and transverse fractures.[2] Severely comminuted and complex fractures of the temporal bone are commonly produced by penetrating gunshot wounds of the temporal bone.[3]

A longitudinal fracture (Fig. 30–2B and 30–3) is suspected when a step-off is present in the external auditory canal and is frequently accompanied by blood in the external auditory canal. A perforation or tear of the tympanic membrane may be present, and cerebrospinal fluid (CSF) otorrhea is occasionally seen. Sterile instruments should be used during the examination of the external auditory canal to avoid introducing contamination into the area and producing retrograde meningitis. A conductive hearing loss will usually be present and can have numerous causes. Perforation of the ear drum, hematoma in the middle ear cleft, disruption of ligaments supporting the ossicles in the attic region, and disruption of the ossicular joints all can lead to varying degrees of conductive hearing loss (see under *Ossicular Damage*). Facial paralysis is seen in only 20 per cent of longitudinal fractures but is the most common cause of facial paralysis in blunt trauma of the temporal bone because of the relative infrequency of transverse fractures. The facial nerve is involved in the perigeniculate region in 90 per cent of cases[4, 5] and less commonly in the mastoid segment by fractures of the posterior external auditory canal (Fig. 30–4). The pathology of the facial nerve injury in blunt temporal bone trauma, in decreasing order of occurrence, consists of intraneural hemorrhage, bony fragment impingement, and nerve transection.[6]

A transverse temporal bone fracture is suspected when a patient presents with sensorineural hearing loss and vertigo accompanied by facial paralysis. The external canal is frequently intact, and no evidence of canal wall discontinuity and hemotympanum may be present (Figs. 30–5B and 30–6). These patients have a 50 per cent incidence of facial paralysis, which occurs from damage to the geniculate ganglion region (Fig. 30–7).[7] The causes of injury are the same as for longitudinal fractures, and intraneural hemorrhage is the most common.

Gunshot wounds to the temporal bone region typically produce extensive damage, the degree of which is determined by the velocity of the projectile. Low-velocity civilian projectiles have relatively low energy and produce mainly locally destructive manifestations. On the other

FIGURE 30-1

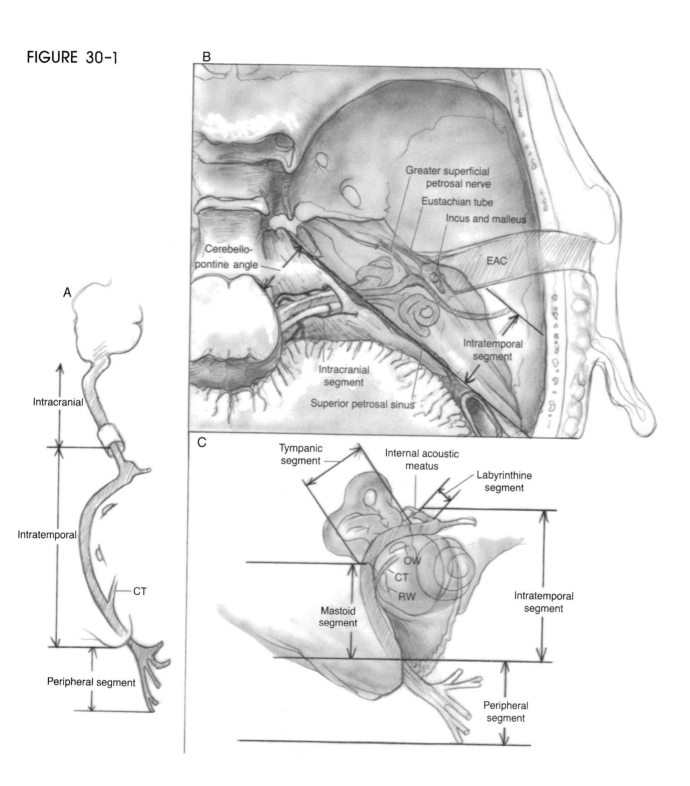

FIGURE 30–1. *A,* Schematic of facial nerve anatomy. *B,* Axial view. *C,* Lateral view. CT, chorda tympani nerve; EAC, external auditory canal; OW, oval window; RW, round window.

FIGURE 30-2

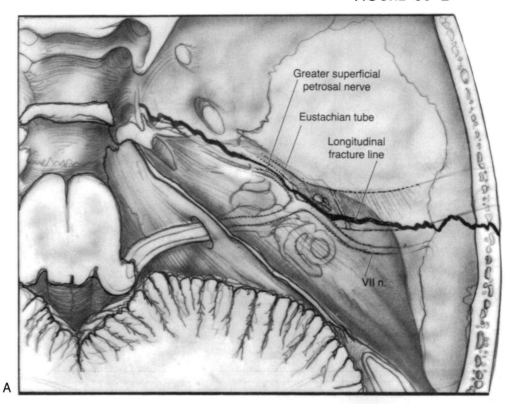

Greater superficial
petrosal nerve

Eustachian tube

Longitudinal
fracture line

VII n.

A

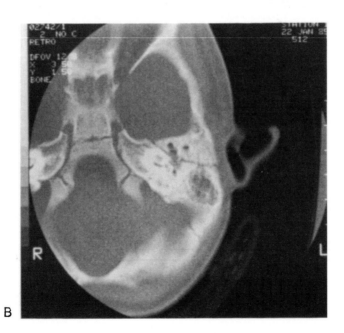

B

FIGURE 30–2. Longitudinal fracture of the temporal bone. *A,* Fracture line is parallel to the long axis. *B,* Computed tomographic scan of the fracture.

hand, high-velocity military weapons, which are increasingly being seen on city streets, are capable of widespread destruction, with extensive local and regional manifestations produced by the concomitant shock wave. People receiving low-velocity gunshot wounds to the intratemporal portion of the facial nerve have a 50 per cent incidence of facial nerve injury, with frequent injury to intracranial and extracranial structures. In a series of 22 cases of civilian gunshot wound injuries, Duncan and associates[3] found immediate onset of paralysis to be the most common presentation and violation of the facial nerve in vertical segment the most common site of injury. Other sites of injury were the tympanic portion in five cases; the stylomastoid foramen in two; and the labyrinthine segment in one. Treatment consisted of interposition grafts in five cases; transmastoid decompression in two; and rerouting with primary anastomosis in one. In summary, gunshot wounds of the temporal bone frequently result in loss of a segment of the nerve, usually in the tympanic portion, requiring interposition grafting for repair.[3] Associated central nervous system and vascular complications (32 per cent) are frequently present, and arteriography is recommended for evaluation of suspected damage to vascular structures of the temporal bone in these cases.[4]

EXTRATEMPORAL INJURY TO THE FACIAL NERVE

Facial paralysis after laceration or iatrogenic injury to the parotid region is best repaired primarily and as soon as the patient's condition permits. If no loss of nerve substance has occurred, the nerve should be repaired by direct anastomosis. When nerve substance loss has occurred, an interpositional graft should be used.

PATIENT EVALUATION

Electrical Prognostication

The presentation of facial nerve injuries greatly affects their management. The presence of a tightly enclosing fallopian canal around the intratemporal facial nerve makes

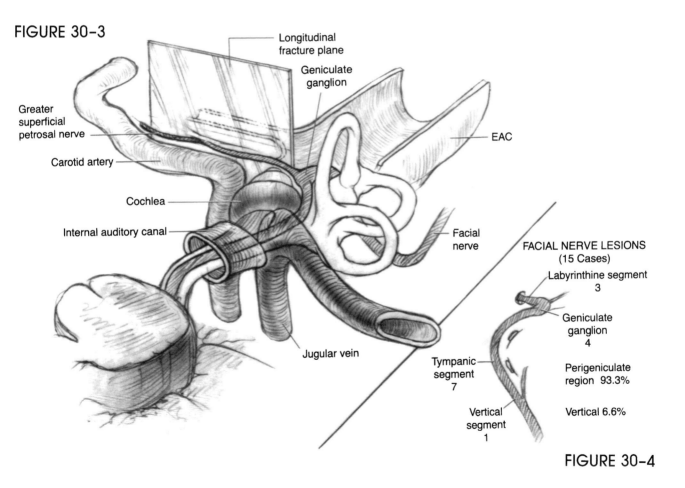

FIGURE 30–3

FACIAL NERVE LESIONS
(15 Cases)

FIGURE 30-4

FIGURE 30–3. Longitudinal fracture of the temporal bone. EAC, external auditory canal.

FIGURE 30–4. Location of lesion to facial nerve in 15 cases of longitudinal fractures. (From Coker NJ, Kendall KA, Jenkins HA, Alford BR: Traumatic intratemporal facial nerve injury: Management rationale for preservation of function. Otolaryngol Head Neck Surg 97: 262–269, 1987.)

FIGURE 30–5

A   TRANSVERSE FRACTURE

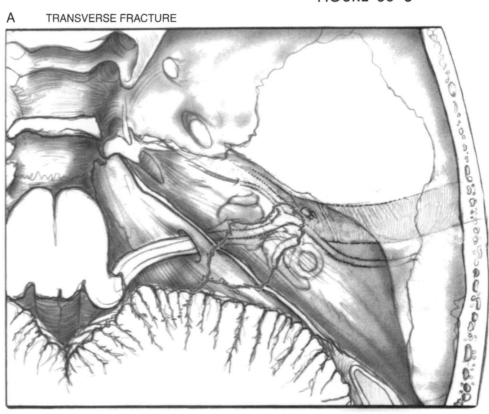

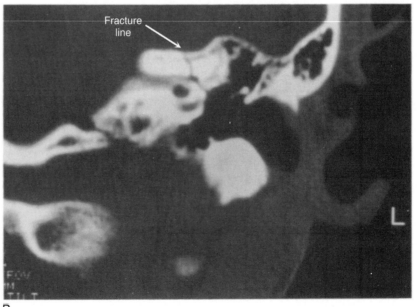

B

FIGURE 30–5. Transverse fracture of the temporal bone. *A,* Fracture line is perpendicular to the long axis. *B,* Radiography of transverse fracture *(arrow).*

the nerve much more susceptible to all types of trauma. Lack of any space to accommodate edema, which inevitably accompanies soft tissue trauma, leads to further neural injury. An injured nerve may not manifest significant clinical dysfunction initially, but later, once sufficient edema has occurred to prevent axoplasmic flow, the injury manifests. Fisch and others have shown that the area of the fallopian canal with the least expansion room for neural swelling is in the region of the meatal foramen.[6, 8–10] Because most injuries to the facial nerve occur in the perigeniculate area just distal to the meatal foramen, the edema produced in facial nerve injury is quite critical in the pathophysiology of this disorder. Precise analysis of facial nerve function must be made at the earliest opportunity after trauma has occurred, prior to the onset of edema. A nerve with diffuse weakness in all branches can be observed clinically, and if some function persists, expectant management can be employed. If this situation deteriorates to total paralysis, electrical testing should be used to follow up the nerve to ensure that total degeneration does not occur.

Fisch and Esslen have postulated that surgery can facili-tate return of facial nerve function if performed prior to complete degeneration. A level of 90 per cent degeneration, as determined by electroneuronography (ENoG), has been correlated with a uniformly good prognosis for return of function.[11] If the nerve is nonfunctional at the initial examination, the chance of a complete transection is high and will likely require surgery.

Patients with complete facial paralysis at the initial examination are screened daily with nerve excitability testing. This test uses direct transcutaneous stimulation of the nerve on each side of the face and determines a stimulation threshold that produces perceptible movement. The normal side is used as a control. If the threshold difference between the normal and dysfunctional sides exceeds 2.5 mA, ENoG is performed regularly thereafter. ENoG uses transcutaneous supramaximal stimulation of the facial nerve while simultaneously recording the evoked potential from antero-grade stimulation in the periphery of the face.[12] The maximal evoked response of the nerve is measured on each side by use of a nonfixed recording electrode technique. A side-to-side comparison is made, with the normal side serving as the control. The percentage of degeneration is calculated

FIGURE 30-6

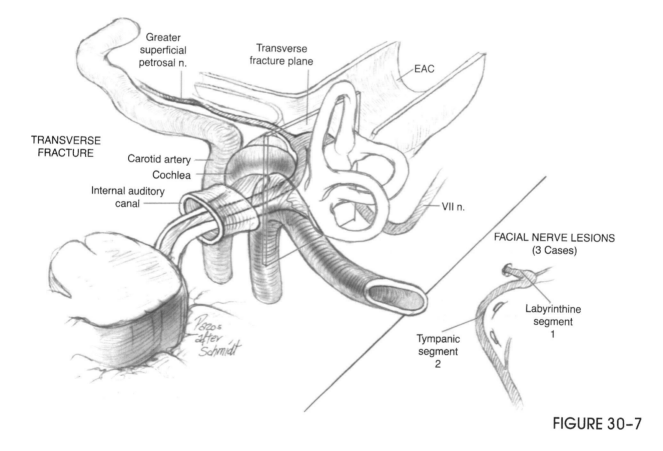

FIGURE 30–6. Transverse fracture of the temporal bone. EAC, external auditory canal.

FIGURE 30–7. Location of lesion in three cases of transverse temporal bone fracture. (From Coker NJ, Kendall KA, Jenkins HA, Alford BR: Traumatic intratemporal facial nerve injury: Management rationale for preservation of function. Otolaryngol Head Neck Surg 97: 262–269, 1987.)

as the difference between the two sides. Recent data have shown that a correlation exists between ENoG and nerve excitability testing: a 90 per cent degeneration score on ENoG correlates to about a 3.5 mA difference on nerve excitability testing.[13]

In a nonacute injury, ENoG can be relied on for up to 3 weeks, but after this period, a desynchronization (deblocking) of electrically evoked facial nerve discharge can occur, preventing a single unified discharge of all neurons in the trunk. This effect occurs because of the differing time courses over which recovering neurons re-establish electrical conductivity and the capability to conduct an action potential. At this stage, it is no longer possible to compare the diseased, asynchronously discharging side with the unaffected, synchronously discharging side, making accurate determination of the severity of degeneration by this technique alone impossible.

Electromyography (EMG) may be employed to establish whether recovering axons are present. Voluntary motor units and polyphasic potentials indicate that regeneration is in progress. Lack of the foregoing and fibrillation potentials indicate a fully degenerated nerve without evidence of ongoing recovery.

Radiologic Evaluation

Thin-cut computed tomographic (CT) examination of the temporal bone is routinely required for evaluation of trauma to the facial nerve. Evaluation of bone detail often establishes the anatomy of the fractures and allows prediction of neural segment damage. The geniculate ganglion region is most frequently involved in blunt trauma, and nondisplaced fractures across the tegmen may be difficult to recognize on CT scan. If facial nerve injury is suspected, special temporal bone views are necessary because the resolution in standard brain CT scans is not sufficient to delineate the intricate bony features of the fallopian canal.

Carotid arteriography is indicated if major vascular injury is suspected, particularly in gunshot injuries to the temporal bone. Traumatic pseudoaneurysms and arteriovenous fistulas are occasional sequelae and are readily identified by arteriography.

Timing of Surgery

Timing and even the necessity of surgery in some cases of facial nerve injury remains controversial. McCabe suggested that exploration and repair be accomplished at 21 days after injury based on studies of motor neuron proteosynthetic activity levels and maximal repair activity at a neural anastomosis.[14] Recent evidence does not support this theory but does show a trend toward lower regeneration rates with increasing time after onset of injury.[15]

Facial nerve paresis arising from blunt trauma to the peripheral portion of the facial nerve should be managed expectantly. If no recovery is evident at the end of 6 months, reconstitution of the dysfunctional portion of the nerve may be required. Facial paralysis ensuing after laceration or iatrogenic injury to the parotid region is likely a transection and is best repaired primarily and as soon as

the patient's condition permits. If a divided nerve cannot be repaired as soon as possible after the injury, then at least limited exploration of the wound should be performed to identify the severed ends of the nerve for subsequent repair. The use of an electrical nerve stimulator can be helpful for up to 48 hours after injury for stimulation of the distal ends of the severed nerve. The regional twitching of facial musculature then can be used as an aid to nerve identification.[4]

The role of surgery in delayed facial nerve injuries following blunt trauma remains controversial. However, significant sequelae from the injury exist in these patients. We managed these injuries similarly to those of patients with Bell's palsy. Surgery is performed once a significant level of degeneration of the facial nerve is evident, that is, 90 per cent on ENoG. The reasoning behind this strategy is to prevent conversion of the neural injury from a Sunderland class II to a class III. The latter has pronounced synkinesis in a large percentage of cases. The goal of surgery is to relieve the pressure on the nerve, thereby permitting the nerve to expand, and to decrease damage to the endoneural tubules from the external constriction.

ASSOCIATED TRAUMA

Other structures in the vicinity of the facial nerve may be injured from the trauma. These injuries may require either immediate or delayed management, depending on the circumstances.

Ossicular Damage

Trauma to the ossicular chain frequently occurs in concert with damage to the intratemporal facial nerve. The ossicles are most often damaged in longitudinal temporal bone fractures as the fracture line passes through the vicinity of the attic and posterosuperior external auditory canal wall. Ossicles may be damaged by dislocation brought about by relative movement of supporting structures or by inertial factors associated with sudden movements of the supporting structures.[16] Many different types of injury to the ossicles can occur, but the most frequent are dislocation of the incudostapedial joint, fractures of the stapes crura, and subluxation of the stapes footplate.[17] The malleus is rarely injured, but occasional fractures of the long process of the malleus are seen.

The treatment of ossicular trauma depends on the nature of the injury. Fractures of the distal long process of the malleus near the umbo are treated by excision of the fractured segment and reconstruction of the drum with temporalis fascia. More proximal fractures near the head of the malleus must be treated by removal of the malleus and incus and placement of a partial or total ossicular replacement prosthesis if the stapes is not normal.

Dislocation of the incus can be from incudostapedial disarticulation, incudomalleolar disarticulation, or both. Two approaches have been advanced for treatment of this condition: The traditional approach is an incus interposition, in which the incus is shaped into a strut with the former incudomalleolar joint area transformed into a notch for the malleus handle, engaging it near the region of the insertion of the tensor tympani. The tip of the former short process of the incus is fashioned into a cup to fit over the stapes capitulum. The overall length of the incus strut is determined by trial and error, and care is taken to ensure a slight amount of tension exists after placement between the malleus handle and stapes capitulum to enhance retention of the prosthesis and to promote good sound conduction. Bone dust from the shaping operation should be allowed to remain on the incus remnant to encourage fixation of the prosthesis in good position. An alternative approach is to reduce the dislocation at the malleus and stapes with careful packing of the incus in reduction from the mastoid and middle ear aspects. Good results are obtained by some authors using this approach, particularly when the joint is not completely separated. However, we favor incus interposition in most of these cases.

Fractures of the crura of the stapes render the ossicle ineffectual as a conductor of sound to the inner ear, and a stapes replacement procedure of some type must be undertaken to restore acoustic function. Stapedectomy or stapedotomy, at the surgeon's preference, can be performed in cases of a normal footplate, but if the footplate is fractured or subluxed, stapedectomy may be required. Fenestration of the footplate, or indeed most ossicular reconstruction, should not be performed in the presence of an infected middle ear cleft, and consideration should be given to using a staged reconstruction approach.

The choice between autograft versus prosthetic ossicular reconstruction methods is usually resolved in favor of autograft because of extrusion problems and the greater incidence of long-term tolerance problems with prosthetic materials. However, when the incus is not available, an incus-stapes replacement prosthesis can be used quite effectively to reconstruct the ossicular chain. In cases in which the entire long process of the malleus is missing, a total ossicular replacement prosthesis or partial ossicular replacement prosthesis made of hydroxyapatite with a platform is used. The incidence of extrusion is greatly reduced by cartilage reinforcement of the platform surface at the interface with the tympanic membrane.

Traumatic Otorrhea

The presence of CSF drainage from the ear or nose of a patient with head trauma is not unusual and represents a defect in the dural covering of the brain.[18] The incidence of meningitis in patients with CSF leaks lasting longer than 2 weeks is approximately 36 per cent,[19] and the mortality may be as high as 10 per cent in traumatic cases.[20] Only otologic sources will be considered in the chapter, but an anterior or middle cranial fossa defect in the sinus region should always be considered in the differential diagnosis of CSF rhinorrhea, especially in traumatic injuries. Fluid originating from a posterior or middle fossa fracture defect may enter the mastoid and middle ear and drain into the nose or the oropharynx. CSF otorrhea is frequently associated with longitudinal temporal bone fractures because the fracture defect may result in a dural tear, whereas a step-off in the external ear canal provides a direct channel for egress of the fluid from the middle ear.

Clear fluid in the ear should alert the examiner to the presence of CSF, and the diagnosis should be straightforward. The diagnosis of CSF rhinorrhea, however, is typically confounded by the appearance of clear nasal secretions frequently accompanying nasal trauma. An informal test to make this differentiation is the halo test, whereby the fluid is placed on filter paper and allowed to diffuse. Blood in the sample will be left behind, and a ring of clear fluid will surround the red ring of blood products. The glucose levels in nasal secretions have also been used to identify CSF; high levels (>50 mg/100 ml) are considered to be indicative of CSF. The most sensitive and specific method of differentiation appears to be protein electrophoresis of the sample: the β_2 fraction of transferring is specific to CSF.[21]

Potential help in localizing the source of the leak can be obtained from contrast-enhanced CT, radioisotope studies, and intrathecal dye instillation. Intrathecal dye methods are used infrequently because of potential adverse reactions, whereas radioisotope studies are more useful in studies of the anterior skull base. The metrizamide-enhanced CT scan provides the best localization for otorrhea because of the good detail of the bony defect usually accompanying the dural defect.

Pneumocephalus is a dreaded, potentially treacherous complication of a defect in the dural protective barrier of the brain.[22] It occurs when air is introduced into the cranial cavity via a fistula in the dura. Frequently, pneumocephalus is accompanied by CSF leakage, but it may occur in the absence of clinical evidence of fluid leakage. The major difficulty in this entity is the potential formation of a tension pneumocephalus from a ball-valve defect in the dura. Continued accumulation of air may induce intracranial hypertension, with resultant brain herniation. Aggressive management is required in CSF fistulas accompanied by persistent pneumocephalus.

The treatment of CSF otorrhea must take into account the natural history of the entity and, in particular, the incidence of meningitis. Conservative management is possible because of the high probability that the condition will heal spontaneously and because of the efficacy of present-generation antibiotics in meningitis. In a series of anterior cranial fossa CSF fistulas, 35 per cent resolved by 24 hours, and 85 per cent healed by 1 week.[23] The most common organisms isolated from post-traumatic meningitic cases are *Pneumococcus* species, and antibiotics are quite effective against them. Several measures may be implemented to aid spontaneous closure of CSF fistula. The most important treatment is bed rest and avoidance of activities that increase intracranial pressure, such as straining, lifting, or constipation. Placement of an indwelling lumbar subarachnoid drainage catheter may be useful in resistant cases. A closed-drainage system allows removal of fluid daily and permits regular monitoring of CSF cell counts to allow early identification of meningitis. Avoidance of the need for repeated lumbar punctures is also a major benefit with these systems.

The indications for operative management of CSF fistula include persistent leakage despite adequate conservative measures, recurrent meningitis, and persistent pneumocephalus.[24] These cases may be approached via the middle ear, mastoid, or middle fossa, depending on the extent and localization of the defect. In general, the defect should be identified and repaired with some form of soft tissue reinforced by bone, where possible. Discrete defects in the dura of less than 1 cm should be closed and the area reinforced with fascia. If a mastoid tegmen defect is identified, the dural defect is repaired, followed by soft tissue reinforcement, and finally bone graft support to stabilize the repair in the face of continuous CSF pulsation pressure and gravity.

SURGICAL TREATMENT

Preoperative Preparation

Patients with traumatic facial paralysis are often quite ill because of the multiple sequelae of severe head trauma. Trauma sufficient to produce fracture of the base of the skull and resulting facial nerve injury often damages intracranial contents as well as other structures throughout the body. Assessment of the entire patient must be made, with particular emphasis on the cervical spine, airway, and circulation. A thorough neurologic examination to rule out intracranial pathology, such as hematoma or parenchymal injury to the brain, must be performed and treatment rendered in a timely manner. Increased intracranial pressure is frequently seen as a result of head injury. High-dose steroids, hyperventilation, and head elevation are frequently required for pressure control, and intracranial pressure may be monitored by placement of an intraventricular catheter. Neurosurgical consultation should be obtained early in the treatment of these disorders. After stabilization of the overall neurologic status and treatment of any acute medical problems, the patient can be prepared for surgery to treat the facial nerve.

Patient Positioning

The patient is placed on the operating room table in the supine position with anesthesia located away from the head and neck region, down at the side. In addition to the standard postauricular access, the head of the table must be available in case a middle cranial fossa approach is required. The head is placed on a head holder with a recess that allows positioning of the opposite ear without compression. The entire table, and not the head, is moved during the course of the procedure to prevent flexion vascular compromise to the opposite auricle should the ear be folded when the patient's head alone is moved. Approximately half of the scalp is prepared and the hair shaved after the patient is asleep. The entire hemifacial area to the midline is included in the preparatory area, and the lower neck and face are included if vascular control will be required. Prophylactic antibiotics are given at this time, and 1:100,000 epinephrine solution is injected subcutaneously into the line of incision. If intraoperative EMG is to be used, the skin lateral to the angle of the mouth and the area inferior to the inner canthus is prepared with povidone-iodine (Betadine) swabs. Bipolar electrodes are placed in the muscles and the electrodes are gently tapped while recording to ensure that a discharge is elicited. A characteristic audio signal ("pop") is elicited by this maneuver, which is used as a check for proper electrode and recording system function. The electrodes are sutured in place using sterile technique, and the rest of the preparation and draping are performed. Care is taken to drape the entire half of the face out into the sterile field so that direct observation of the face can be used to confirm electrophysiologic events.

No special instruments are employed in these procedures.

Technique

Intratemporal Nerve Segment

The surgical technique for mastoid facial nerve exploration is discussed in Chapter 16. Details specific to post-traumatic treatment for paralysis are presented here. Surgery for intratemporal traumatic facial paralysis centers on exposure of the damaged segment of the fallopian canal, thereby facilitating surgical repair and providing the nerve room to expand. In treating damage to the nerve in the intratemporal segment, several factors must be taken into account: status of individual nerve fibers, percentage of nerve loss, and length of nerve trunk loss. The repair techniques used for the repair of common lesions are shown in Figure 30–8. In injuries to the fallopian canal, the bone fragments may be in good reduction, betraying the true extent of injury to the nerve. In these cases, an intraneural hematoma can be produced by free blood within the intact nerve epineurium. Blood staining is frequently observed, but in some cases, the nerve will appear diffusely enlarged without areas of visible sheath staining. The nerve sheath should be incised using sharp, atraumatic technique and taking special care to preserve all underlying nerve fascicles (Fig. 30–8A). The Ziegler ophthalmic knife (Storz) is useful for incising the nerve sheath.

After the nerve sheath has been opened, the degree of nerve loss is assessed. If a significant portion of the nerve fibers appears to be divided, clean division of the remaining trunk followed by an interposition graft should be considered. Bony fragments impinging on the nerve sheath should be atraumatically removed and the nerve assessed for intraneural hematoma and treated as discussed earlier (Fig. 30–8B). Complete transection situations can be repaired using nerve rerouting, when the anatomy permits, to avoid the need for an interposition graft (Fig. 30–8C and 30–9B). Gunshot wounds to the temporal bone with a tympanic or labyrinthine segment injury and a dead ear are the typical situation (Fig. 30–9).[6] The interposition graft should be performed with a donor nerve graft of the appropriate diameter. In many situations, creation of a bony channel can enhance nerve and graft alignment without the need for multiple stabilization sutures and attendant postoperative inflammation (Fig. 30–9A).[5] In all cases, the nerve should be widely decompressed until nonedematous nerve is encountered. In situations in which the loss of mastoid segment nerve tissue is minimal, the nerve can be dissected from the stylomastoid foramen region and the parotid facial nerve mobilized proximally to obviate an interposition graft.

FIGURE 30-8

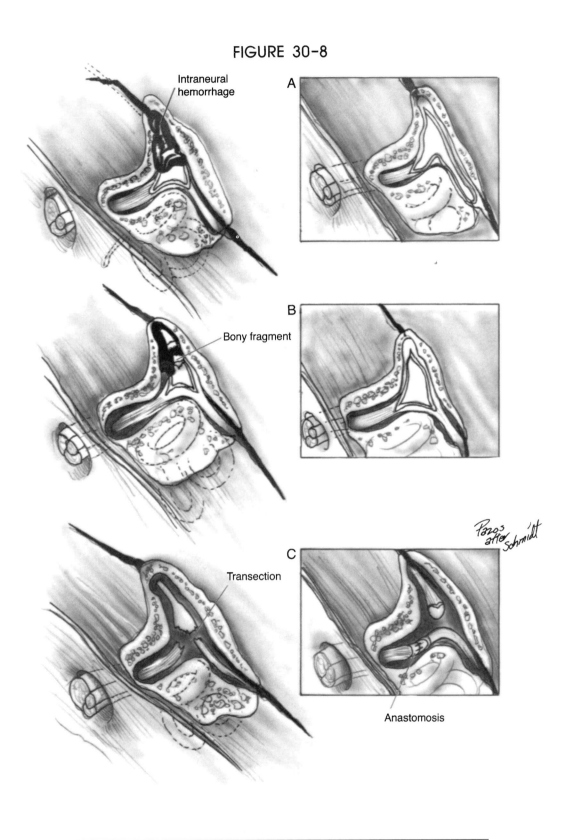

FIGURE 30–8. Surgical management of common facial nerve injuries in the perigeniculate region. *A,* intraneural hemorrhage. *Inset,* After opening nerve sheath. *B,* Bony fragment impingement. *Inset,* After fragment removal and opening of nerve sheath. *C,* Perigeniculate transection. *Inset,* Direct anastomosis after section of the superficial petrosal nerve.

FIGURE 30-9

A LOSS OF NERVE LENGTH IN VERTICAL SEGMENT

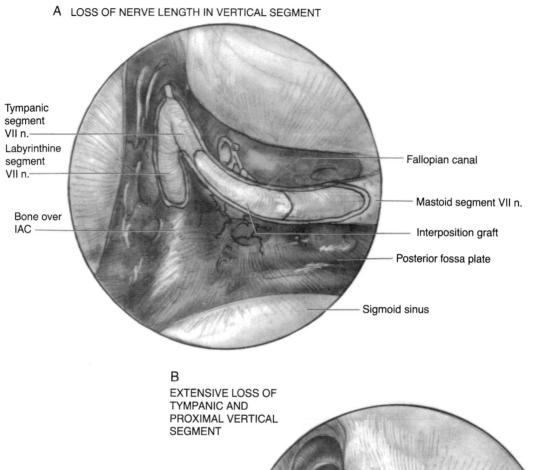

Tympanic segment VII n.

Labyrinthine segment VII n.

Bone over IAC

Fallopian canal

Mastoid segment VII n.

Interposition graft

Posterior fossa plate

Sigmoid sinus

B
EXTENSIVE LOSS OF TYMPANIC AND PROXIMAL VERTICAL SEGMENT

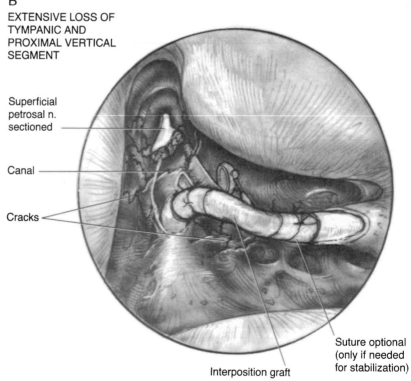

Superficial petrosal n. sectioned

Canal

Cracks

Interposition graft

Suture optional (only if needed for stabilization)

FIGURE 30–9. *A,* Loss of nerve length in the vertical segment in a nonhearing ear. A trough is created based on the fallopian canal, which helps maintain the graft and nerve in position and minimizes the need for suture fixation. *B,* Extensive loss of tympanic and proximal vertical segment of the facial nerve with rerouting from the internal auditory canal (IAC) to the vertical segment in a nonhearing ear. The superficial petrosal nerve is sectioned.

Electrical monitoring of the facial nerve is helpful in determining when surgical trauma is occurring to the nerve. Obviously, if the nerve is completely transected, this technique will be of no value, but if the injury has occurred within 3 days, use of intraoperative facial nerve EMG can be helpful because the nerve will remain electrically active distally even though complete transection has taken place. In general, if the results of ENoG do not reveal 100 per cent degeneration, facial nerve monitoring may have some value because a few neurons will be able to produce discharge in the facial musculature, although this activity is not detectable clinically. Facial nerve EMG monitoring is performed by placing a pair of transcutaneous needle electrodes in the orbicularis oculi and oris muscles. The electrodes are connected directly by a short length of wire to a preamplifier and sent to the main recording unit. Processing and display options vary among commercially available units, but all process the signal to provide audio output of the signal and perhaps a visual record of the actual action potential or at least a visual indication of the amplitude of the response. The output signal is usually filtered, and artifact rejection mechanisms may eliminate signals produced by electrocautery and other electrical noise sources in the operating room. We employ a Nicolet Compact Four (Nicolet Biomedical Instruments, Madison, WI) evoked potential unit, which requires a technician for operation and set-up as well as for monitoring and recording the waveforms during the operative case. Audio output is available to the surgeon throughout the procedure, and care is taken to ensure that the same filter settings are used at all times so that the sound of facial nerve discharge can be identified consistently. Occasional discharges of the nerve are not considered as significant as prolonged trains of discharge: the latter usually indicate a more severe, potentially nonreversible insult to the nerve. The face is always exposed via a clear plastic drape so that visual confirmation and correlation of electrophysiologic events can be obtained.

The most common area of damage to the intratemporal segment is in the perigeniculate region, but location of the precise area of damage should be ascertained on preoperative CT scans. The middle fossa approach to decompression is used when labyrinthine function must be preserved. If clinical suspicion is confirmed by preoperative CT scans and intraoperative findings warrant, decompression of the mastoid segment of the facial nerve can be performed via a mastoid approach (see Chapter 16). During middle fossa decompression of the proximal facial nerve, the condition of the distal nerve can be determined by examination of the tympanic portion as it is exposed. If the nerve appears to be in good condition with no hemorrhage or edema evident, and no other indications exist for exploration of the mastoid portion of the nerve, exploration need not be performed.[4]

In many cases of transverse fractures and gunshot wounds of the temporal bone, the patient will have minimal or no residual hearing on audiometric testing. In these cases, a translabyrinthine approach to expose the entire facial nerve is possible without resorting to middle cranial fossa surgery. The labyrinth is removed and the internal auditory canal is exposed. The nerve is identified in the tympanic segment adjacent to the lateral semicircular canal and in the labyrinthine segment distal to the internal auditory canal, and in this fashion, the entire intratemporal facial nerve is exposed.

During exposure of the nerve in the vertical and tympanic segments, surgical trauma to an already diseased nerve should be minimized. Minimal nerve trauma is produced because a thin shell of bone is left over the nerve throughout the decompression. At the conclusion of the gross exposure, a dissector is used to lift off the thin shell of bone as a large piece, thus avoiding contact of the diamond burr with the nerve sheath. At times, small fragments of the shell may be left in place without harm, and the goal of nerve decompression is still attained.

Repair should be performed at all anastomoses by use of neuroscopic technique, atraumatic handling of tissues, exact end-to-end anastomosis, tension-free closure, and the use of monofilament 9-0 or 10-0 suture.[5] Interposition grafts are employed when nerve tissue loss would produce tension in a direct anastomosis or when diseased nerve segments must be excised. The greater auricular nerve is adequate for defects less than 7 cm, and the sural nerve can bridge defects as long as 30 cm. The superiority of perineurial over epineurial repair has not been demonstrated, but meticulous techniques are clearly useful in reconstitution of the facial nerve.[25]

Extratemporal Nerve Segment

Establishing a functionally intact nerve in the frontal and marginal mandibular distribution of the face is important because of the limited anastomotic interconnection from adjacent branches of the facial nerve in these regions. Conversely, small branches in the midface region do not require extensive procedures to reestablish continuity, because of the rich anastomotic network that already exists. This quality leads to a much higher probability of a favorable outcome. Details of neural anastomosis techniques can be found in Chapter 31.

The technique for exposure of the peripheral nerve is based on techniques commonly used in parotid surgery. Penetrating trauma to the nerve at the stylomastoid foramen region may prevent identification of the nerve proximally, and the nerve will need to be found in the periphery and traced back proximally. Finding a branch of the marginal mandibular or frontal distribution is frequently useful.[26] If the exploration is performed within 2 days of the injury, the distal branches of the nerve will be able to be stimulated by electrical current, and observation of facial musculature twitching can help find the distal stump.

POSTOPERATIVE CARE

Postoperatively, a modified mastoid dressing is applied, extending superiorly to apply pressure over the midfossa incision if needed. The dressing is changed daily and the wound is examined for signs of infection or CSF collection in the wound. A dressing is left in place for 2 to 3 days in the case of midfossa surgery, and for 1 day for mastoid surgery in which the dura is not violated.

Intravenous antibiotics are continued for 24 hours postoperatively. The dressing is left in place for 24 hours and then removed and the wound is left exposed to allow easy observation. Any evidence of CSF collection in the wound is treated with pressure dressing and daily or twice daily observation to ensure that the fluid has not recurred. Needle aspiration is performed if indicated. Patients are asked to walk on the evening of surgery or the first day after surgery. Total hospital stay is 4 to 5 days.

PITFALLS OF SURGERY

The primary area of pathology in intratemporal injuries of the facial nerve is the labyrinthine segment. Frequently, the nerve must be exposed in this area if surgical intervention is required. If preservation of hearing is a goal, a middle fossa surgical approach will be required. Middle fossa surgery is a difficult technique because the anatomic approach is unfamiliar and the indications for its use are infrequent. These factors contribute to the difficulty in mastering this technique. However, the lack of good alternative procedures to address the anatomic region of greatest interest, the labyrinthine and meatal segment in the patient with intact hearing, makes maintenance of skills in middle fossa surgery a necessity for every active neurotologist.

RESULTS

The postoperative result depends largely on the severity of injury to the nerve and the timing of intervention to a lesser extent. Recovery is excellent for Sunderland's neurapraxic (1·) or axonotmetic (2·) lesions, which both involve intact endoneurial tubules. Primary anastomosis or interposition is required for neurotmesis (5·) injuries because complete separation of the nerve has occurred.[27] The best surgical result in this condition is a grade III or grade IV (AAO-HNS), with the latter being more typical. Crush and compression injuries are Sunderland 3· or 4· lesions, with varying degrees of endoneurial and perineurial disruption and no gross disruption of the nerve. These injuries present varying degrees of recovery, but grades III to V are usually attainable. The decision to resect and perform an anastomosis or to simply decompress is left to the surgeon; few physiologic data on which to base such a decision exist.[27] The best prognosis is obtained with early intervention in the acute phase of degeneration and prior to the onset of continuing endoneurial degeneration and fibrosis, which only impede the eventual re-establishment of competent axons.

COMPLICATIONS

CSF leakage is the most significant complication of surgical repair of traumatic facial nerve injuries. Leakage of CSF after middle fossa surgery is usually caused by access of the fluid to the air cell system of the mastoid. These cells can be exposed at the tegmen simply by lifting the dura over a natural dehiscence in the bone. Frequently,

cells will be opened as the dissection of the labyrinthine segment of the facial nerve is performed. Prevention is the best treatment, and careful attention must be given to blockage of any exposed air cell by the use of bone wax or fascia where needed.

Infection of a middle fossa wound has never occurred in the senior author's (HAJ) series.[28] Because of the low incidence of postoperative infection, it has not been necessary to modify our surgical approach to produce a staggered incision through the skin and temporalis muscles,[28] but rather, we use an incision straight through the skin down to bone.

A conductive hearing loss can occur after middle cranial fossa surgery if dura is allowed to contact the heads of the ossicles, thereby producing a reduction in motion. This reduction is generally minimal but may occasionally require revision surgery with interposition of a bone plate to prevent contact. Hearing loss and vestibular dysfunction are always possible with middle cranial fossa and mastoid surgery and can be prevented by extensive anatomic dissection in the laboratory and care in the operating room.

References

1. Cannon C, Jahrsdoerfer R: Temporal bone fractures. Arch Otolaryngol Head Neck Surg 109: 285–288, 1983.
2. Ghorayeb BY, Yeakley JW: Temporal bone fractures: Longitudinal or oblique? The case for oblique temporal bone fractures. Laryngoscope 102: 129–134, 1992.
3. Duncan NO, Coker NJ, Jenkins HA, Canalis RF: Gunshot injuries of the temporal bone. Otolaryngol Head Neck Surg 94: 47–55, 1986.
4. Coker NJ, Kendall KA, Jenkins HA, Alford BR: Traumatic intratemporal facial nerve injury: Management rationale for preservation of function. Otolaryngol Head Neck Surg 97: 262–269, 1987.
5. Coker NJ: Management of traumatic injuries to the facial nerve. Otolaryngol Clin North Am 24: 215–227, 1991.
6. Fisch U: Facial paralysis in fractures of the petrous bone. Laryngoscope 84: 2141–2154, 1974.
7. Lambert PR, Brackman DE: Facial paralysis in temporal bone fractures: A review of 26 cases. Laryngoscope 94: 1022–1026, 1984.
8. Esslen E: The Acute Facial Palsies: Investigations on the Localization and Pathogenesis of Meato-Labyrinthine Facial Palsies. Berlin, Springer-Verlag, 1977.
9. Lang J: Anatomy of the brainstem and lower cranial nerves, vessels, and surrounding structures. Am J Otol 6(Suppl): 1–19, 1985.
10. Xian-Xi G, Spector GJ: Labyrinthine segment and geniculate ganglion of facial nerve in fetal and adult human temporal bones. Ann Otol Rhinol Laryngol 90(Suppl 85): 1–12, 1981.
11. Fisch U: Prognostic value of electrical tests in acute facial paralysis. Am J Otol 5: 494–498, 1984.
12. Gantz BJ, Gmuer AA, Holliday M, Fisch U: Electroneurographic evaluation of the facial nerve: Method and technical problems. Ann Otol Rhinol Laryngol 93: 394–398, 1984.
13. Coker NJ, Fordice JO, Moore S: Correlation of the nerve excitability test and electroneurography in acute facial paralysis. Am J Otol 13: 127–133, 1992.
14. McCabe BF: Injuries to the facial nerve. Laryngoscope 82: 1891–1896, 1973.
15. Barrs DM: Facial nerve trauma: Optimal timing for repair. Laryngoscope 101: 835–848, 1991.
16. Hough J, Stuart W: Middle ear injuries in skull trauma. Laryngoscope 78: 899–937, 1968.
17. Belluci RJ: Traumatic injuries of the middle ear. Otolaryngol Clin North Am 16: 633–650, 1983.
18. Caniff JP: Otorrhea in head injuries. Br J Oral Surg 8: 203–210, 1971.
19. Westmore GA, Whittam DE: Cerebrospinal fluid rhinorrhea and its management. Br J Surg 69: 489–492, 1982.
20. Leech PJ, Paterson A: Conservative and operative management for

cerebrospinal fluid leakage after closed head injury. Lancet 1: 1013–1016, 1973.

21. Oberascher G: Cerebrospinal fluid otorrhea—new trends in diagnosis. Am J Otol 9: 102–108, 1988.
22. Andrews JC, Canalis RF: Otogenic pneumocephalus. Laryngoscope 96: 521–528, 1986.
23. Mincy JE: Post-traumatic cerebrospinal fluid fistula of the frontal fossa. Trauma 6: 618–622, 1966.
24. Marentette LJ, Valentino J: Traumatic anterior fossa cerebrospinal fluid fistulae and craniofacial considerations. Otolaryngol Clin North Am 24: 151–164, 1991.
25. Orgel MG, Terzis JK: Epineural vs. perineurial repair. Plast Reconstr Surg 60: 80–91, 1977.
26. Lore JM Jr: The parotid salivary gland. *In* Lore JM Jr (ed): An Atlas of Head and Neck Surgery. Philadelphia, WB Saunders, 1988, pp 708–713.
27. Coker NJ, Jenkins HA, Psifidis A: Electrophysiological prognostication of acute facial nerve trauma. *In* Fisch U, Valavanis A, Yasargil MG (eds): Neurological Surgery of the Ear and the Skull Base. Amsterdam, Kugler & Ghedini, 1989, pp 355–362.
28. House WF, Shelton C: Middle fossa approach for acoustic tumor removal. Otolaryngol Clin North Am 25: 347–359, 1992.

31

Facial Nerve Tumors

Clough Shelton, M.D.

Tumors of the facial nerve are rare causes of facial paralysis.[1-5] The two most common tumors are facial nerve neuromas, which are intrinsic to the nerve, and facial nerve hemangiomas, which are extraneural in origin. This chapter focuses on these two types of facial nerve tumors, although the techniques discussed can also be applied to other facial nerve neoplasms.

Because of their subtle presentation, facial nerve tumors may be difficult to diagnose and require a high degree of clinical suspicion.[6, 7] The presenting symptoms vary with the tumor location, size, and histology. Facial nerve neuromas that arise in the internal auditory canal and cerebellopontine angle may present with a progressive sensorineural hearing loss similar to that caused by an acoustic tumor,[8] and the true diagnosis may be established only at surgery.[9, 10] In a patient with a suspected acoustic tumor, the presence of coexisting facial nerve symptoms (rare with acoustic tumors) should warn the surgeon that a facial nerve tumor may be present.[11, 12]

Facial nerve neuromas usually do not cause symptoms until they are fairly large and may present initially with hearing symptoms.[12-14] Tumors arising in the middle ear may contact the ossicles and cause a conductive hearing loss.[15] In such cases, when a mass behind the tympanic membrane is not visible, the patient may be thought to have otosclerosis, and the correct diagnosis is made during tympanotomy for stapedectomy.[6] When a middle ear mass is encountered in such a situation, a biopsy must not be done because a facial nerve paralysis will likely develop postoperatively (see *Pitfalls of Surgery*).[1, 6, 13, 16, 17]

Should the tumor erode into the labyrinth (typically, the lateral semicircular canal at the external genu), the patient may present with dizziness.[3] On examination, the fistula test result may be positive.

Facial nerve hemangiomas characteristically cause severe symptoms when very small.[18, 19] Like facial nerve neuromas, hemangiomas can occur in the internal auditory canal and present as acoustic tumors.[20] They usually cause a relatively severe sensorineural hearing loss for the size of the tumor. Hemangiomas of the geniculate ganglion can cause profound facial nerve symptoms when of extremely small size.[21, 22] Hemangiomas are extraneural and cause paralysis by compression,[23] but the small size of the tumor can make diagnosis by imaging studies very difficult; therefore, a high degree of clinical awareness is required.[24]

Patients with either tumor type may present with facial nerve symptoms. Typically, these patients have recurrent Bell's palsy, although the facial nerve recovery is less complete with each episode.[14] Facial nerve twitching can be present in some patients, and others may suffer facial paralysis with no recovery or a slowly progressive facial

paralysis.[25, 26] When evaluating a patient with atypical facial nerve symptoms, one must always suspect facial nerve tumor.

Electrical testing can be helpful in establishing the diagnosis of a facial nerve tumor. Electroneuronographic results may be abnormal in patients with facial nerve tumors, even in the face of clinically normal function. Facial electromyography may show a pattern of simultaneous denervation and reinnervation in patients with tumors.[18] This pattern is seen in slowly progressive, pathologic processes and would not be expected with a rapid insult to the facial nerve, such as seen in Bell's palsy.

High-resolution magnetic resonance imaging (MRI) with gadolinium may sufficiently detect most facial nerve tumors (Fig. 31-1). Imaging of a facial nerve neuroma generally reveals a mass lesion and enlargement of the fallopian canal. However, small facial hemangiomas at the geniculate ganglion may require high-resolution computed tomographic (CT) scan (Fig. 31-2). These tumors exhibit characteristic bony changes termed *honeycomb bone*.[27] The medial extent of tumors arising at the geniculate ganglion can best be assessed with gadolinium-enhanced MRI. This medial extension has important ramifications regarding selection of surgical approach.

PATIENT SELECTION

The timing of surgery is perhaps the most difficult aspect of planning. Many patients with facial nerve tumors have normal or nearly normal facial function. The best anticipated facial function after a facial nerve graft is a House-Brackmann grade III to IV.[16] However, waiting too long to remove the tumor can adversely affect the ultimate facial nerve results. Patients with a long-standing facial nerve paralysis have worse results after facial nerve grafting than those who have grafting when they have normal facial function.[9, 13] Extraneural tumors, such as facial nerve hemangiomas, can be removed with preservation of facial nerve continuity; therefore, early surgery in such cases may offer the best hope for excellent facial nerve function. Labyrinthine fistula can develop from bony erosion by the tumor and can lead to deafness and dizziness if the tumor is neglected too long.[13, 28]

For an older patient in poor health who has a small tumor and good facial function, observation may be the best strategy. Younger patients with good facial function may also be followed up, but they must be aware of the possible risk to the ultimate facial nerve outcome and to their hearing if surgery is delayed.[12] In some cases, we follow patients until they show greater than 50 per cent

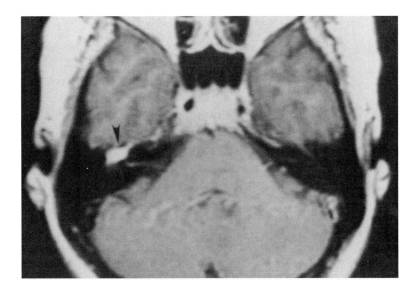

FIGURE 31–1. Magnetic resonance image of facial neuroma *(arrowhead)*.

denervation by electroneuronography. Once they reach this degree of denervation, we are concerned that facial nerve grafting after further loss of neural "firepower" will ultimately result in poor facial function.

Facial nerve neuromas in the internal auditory canal may be recognized during surgery for what was presumed to be an acoustic tumor.[29] (We counsel our acoustic tumor patients preoperatively about this unlikely possibility.) Usually, the tumor is resected and a nerve graft placed. In a few patients with a facial neuroma, tumor decompression is carried out, giving the patient several additional years of good facial function before definitive surgery is required.

Patient Counseling

The most important aspect of preoperative patient counseling is the expected postoperative facial function. Patients are told that a facial nerve graft will be needed, although patients with small hemangiomas are informed that it may be possible to preserve the continuity of the facial nerve. Patients should expect a postoperative facial paralysis lasting 6 to 12 months. Ultimate facial function after a facial nerve graft will not be "normal," and the consequences of synkinesis are discussed.

To describe a "good" result after facial nerve grafting, I tell my patients that they will look normal at rest and have active voluntary movement, but it will not be entirely symmetric motion. This asymmetry will be to the extent that family members will notice a difference, but a stranger on the street would not likely turn and stare (Fig. 31–3).

Patients with a preoperative facial nerve palsy are told to expect worse postoperative facial function after nerve grafting. The longer the duration or the greater the severity of the preoperative palsy, the worse the ultimate result. The other potential risks and complications of surgery are also discussed according to the surgical approach needed. For middle fossa and translabyrinthine cases, the risks are similar to those for acoustic tumor patients treated through these approaches (see Chapters 49 and 50).

Patients with tumor involvement of the ossicles may need ossicular reconstruction. In some cases, this procedure is best carried out at a second stage, and the patients are also informed of this possibility.

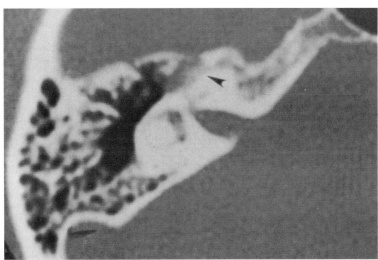

FIGURE 31–2. Computed tomographic scan showing hemangioma at geniculate ganglion with "honeycomb" bone *(arrowhead)*.

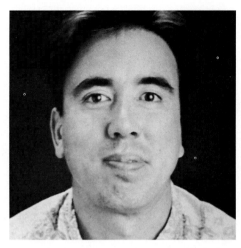

FIGURE 31–3. Patient postoperatively exhibiting a House-Brackmann facial function grade IV one year after facial nerve graft.

SURGICAL TECHNIQUES

Preoperative preparation, patient positioning, and instrumentation are described in Chapter 1. For patients needing a facial nerve graft, the upper neck is also prepared for harvesting of the greater auricular nerve.

The surgical approach is selected on the basis of tumor location, tumor size, and level of residual hearing. For small tumors around the geniculate ganglion in patients with good hearing, the middle fossa approach can be used. Besides providing access into the internal auditory canal, it can expose the horizontal facial nerve to approximately the midtympanic portion. However, because of the limited access, sewing a graft into the internal auditory canal can be difficult, and posterior fossa access is not provided. For patients with larger tumors or with poor hearing and involvement of the internal auditory canal, posterior fossa, or geniculate ganglion, the translabyrinthine approach can be used. This approach provides wide access for tumor removal and allows placement of a facial nerve graft.

Involvement of the horizontal and vertical facial nerve may also require a transmastoid facial recess approach. Erosion of the external auditory canal may necessitate a canal wall down procedure. The facial nerve can be followed into the parotid should tumor extension require the exposure. A staged procedure may be required in a chronically infected ear that requires an intracranial surgical approach for tumor removal.

Middle Fossa Approach

The initial middle fossa approach is carried out as described for acoustic tumors in Chapter 49. After the craniotomy window is made, the temporal lobe is supported by the House-Urban retractor, and the greater superficial petrosal nerve and the skeletonized superior semicircular canal are identified. The greater superficial petrosal nerve is followed posteriorly to the geniculate ganglion (Fig. 31–4). For patients with tumor involvement in this area, extreme care must be taken during the dissection because a tumor can distort the anatomy.

The internal auditory canal is dissected and the labyrinthine facial nerve identified. The amount of internal auditory canal exposure varies with the degree of tumor extension in that area and the need for access to place a graft (Fig. 31–5). The tegmen bone is also removed to expose the tympanic facial nerve (Fig. 31–6). Care is taken not to touch the ossicular heads with a burr during this removal because a sensorineural hearing loss will result.

Transmastoid Approach

Should additional distal exposure be needed, a transmastoid approach to the facial nerve can also be performed, as described in Chapter 16. The facial recess is opened and the nerve exposed to the stylomastoid foramen. Around the facial nerve, it is best to thin the bone over it with a diamond burr, to use copious irrigation, and then to remove the overlying "eggshell" of bone with an instrument such as a sickle or a whirlybird knife (Fig. 31–7). Because of tumor involvement or the need for additional room, the malleus head and incus can be removed and ossicular reconstruction performed at the end of the procedure.

Translabyrinthine Approach

The translabyrinthine approach is carried out as described in Chapter 50, and the facial nerve is skeletonized. The amount of medial bone removal varies with the tumor extent and the need for access for facial nerve grafting. The bone over the geniculate ganglion can be removed anteriorly to expose the greater superficial petrosal nerve (Fig. 31–8).

Tumor Removal

Tumor removal is accomplished with sharp and blunt dissection. Posterior fossa tumor removal is handled in a way

FIGURE 31–4. Exposure of the geniculate ganglion through the middle fossa approach. *A,* The greater superficial petrosal nerve and superior semicircular canal are skeletonized. *B,* Tumor is encountered at the geniculate ganglion.

FIGURE 31–5. The internal auditory canal and labyrinthine facial nerve are exposed medial to the geniculate ganglion.

FIGURE 31–6. After removal of tegmen bone, the facial nerve can be exposed to approximately the midtympanic portion.

FIGURE 31–7. Facial nerve neuroma is seen through a transmastoid approach. The facial recess is opened, and the thin eggshell of bone over the distal facial nerve is removed.

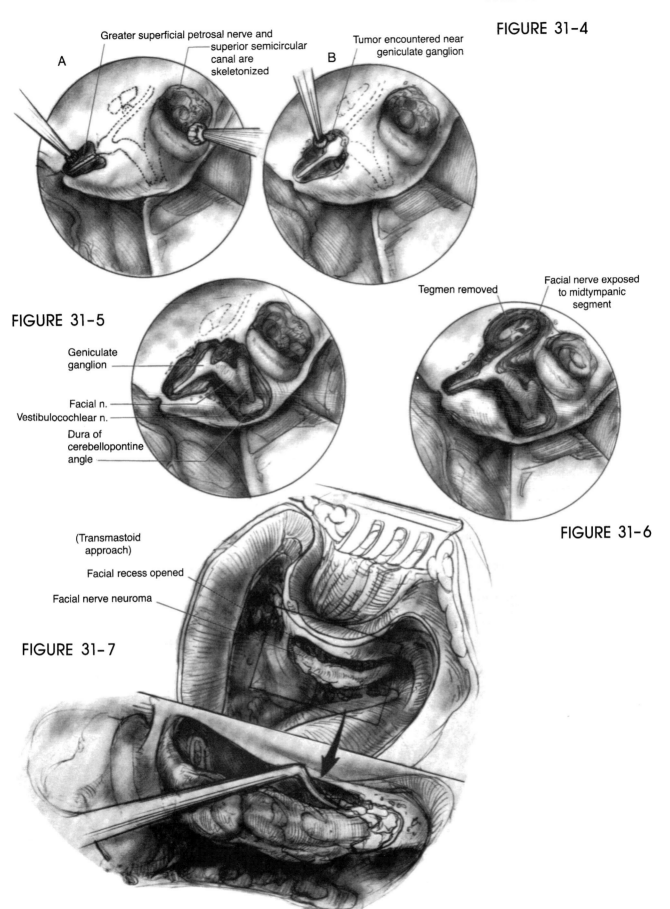

FIGURE 31–4

A — Greater superficial petrosal nerve and superior semicircular canal are skeletonized

B — Tumor encountered near geniculate ganglion

FIGURE 31–5

Geniculate ganglion

Facial n.

Vestibulocochlear n.

Dura of cerebellopontine angle

Tegmen removed

Facial nerve exposed to midtympanic segment

FIGURE 31–6

(Transmastoid approach)

Facial recess opened

Facial nerve neuroma

FIGURE 31–7

FIGURES 31–4 to 31–7 *See legends on opposite page*

similar to the technique used for acoustic tumors. After the tumor has been removed, frozen sections are taken from the remaining nerve ends to ensure total tumor removal.

In some extraneural tumors (hemangiomas), a plane can be developed between the tumor and nerve, allowing facial nerve preservation. In selected neuroma cases, it may also be possible to remove the tumor while maintaining partial continuity of the facial nerve.

Graft Material

The greater auricular nerve serves as an excellent donor nerve for grafting. The diameter match is good, and the donor deficit is minimal. Adequate length can be obtained to graft from the internal auditory canal to the stylomastoid foramen.

The greater auricular nerve can be found between the angle of the mandible and the tip of the mastoid process on the lateral surface of the sternocleidomastoid muscle,[30] posterosuperior to the external jugular vein (Fig. 31–9). The nerve can be harvested through an oblique skin incision placed in a skin crease. By dissecting the nerve from the posterior aspect of the sternocleidomastoid muscle, ample length is obtained. Another option for a donor graft is the sural nerve (Fig. 31–10), which has a larger diameter and length than the greater auricular nerve.

The ends of the graft are trimmed sharply, and excess fibrous tissue and epineurium are removed from the nerve stumps. Some surgeons advocate reversing the nerve direction to prevent axons from growing out branches of the graft.

Nerve Grafting

Within the temporal bone, if enough of the fallopian canal remains as a trough, placement of the graft in approximation to the nerve end is usually sufficient (Fig. 31–11). The anastomosis can be packed into place with Avitene, which forms a clot over the anastomosis.[31] When sutures are needed, two or three epineurial sutures of 9-0 Deklene II on a T-7 needle (Deknatel) work well (Fig. 31–12). The suture length is trimmed to 6 inches to make it easier to work under the microscope, and background material is cut, wetted, and placed beneath the anastomosis to give a smooth working surface. I prefer to cut the graft slightly longer than needed to ensure that no tension exists on the anastomosis. If possible, the graft is placed along the normal course of the facial nerve so that if further surgery is required, it can be easily identified. For patients requiring an ossicular reconstruction at a second stage, the graft of the horizontal facial nerve is placed in the epitympanum, superior to the oval window, so that it will not need to be manipulated during later ossicular reconstruction.

The placement of an anastomosis in the internal auditory canal or posterior fossa is much more difficult than that performed within the temporal bone because the intracranial facial nerve has no epineurium (Fig. 31–13). Usually, a single through-and-through suture of 9-0 Deklene is sufficient.[32] The suture is placed on the graft side first. When the suture is placed through the intracranial facial nerve stump, a fenestrated suction is used to support the facial nerve, and the needle is passed into a side hole of the suction (Fig. 31–14).[33]

Rerouting

Depending on the location and length of the facial nerve defect, it may be possible to remove the facial nerve from its canal and reroute it to gain extra length. This maneuver subjects the nerve to a great deal of manipulation and may interfere with its blood supply. However, for a defect in the cerebellopontine angle, rerouting (Fig. 31–15) gains additional nerve length and allows primary anastomosis.

The wounds are closed as described in Chapter 29, and abdominal fat packing is used when indicated. The standard mastoid dressing is used. The postoperative care for tumor removal from the translabyrinthine and middle fossa approaches is similar to that given to patients with acoustic tumors removed through these approaches (see Chapters 49 and 50).

An important aspect of postoperative care is attention to the paralyzed eye. This topic is detailed in Chapter 59. Depending on the anticipated time and quality of facial function recovery, some patients require the placement of an upper eyelid spring or gold weight.

PITFALLS OF SURGERY

Facial nerve tumors, particularly neuromas, tend to involve the nerve over long distances of its course. Underestimation of tumor extent is an important problem and can be overcome by high-resolution imaging studies. High-resolution

---

FIGURE 31–8. Translabyrinthine approach with exposure of the geniculate ganglion and greater superficial petrosal nerve. Tumor extends from the internal auditory canal (IAC) to the tympanic facial nerve.

FIGURE 31–9. The greater auricular nerve is located on the lateral surface of the sternocleidomastoid muscle, posterior to the external jugular vein. It lies between the tip of the mastoid and the angle of the jaw.

FIGURE 31–10. The sural nerve can be found on the lateral surface of the ankle posterior to the lateral malleolus.

FIGURE 31–11. Facial nerve graft is placed in apposition to the proximal facial nerve stump at the labyrinthine segment. Remaining fallopian canal holds graft in place, and sutures are not needed.

FIGURE 31–12. Nerve graft held in approximation to distal mastoid facial nerve stump with two epineurial sutures.

FIGURE 31-8

FIGURE 31-9

FIGURE 31-10

FIGURE 31-11

FIGURE 31-12

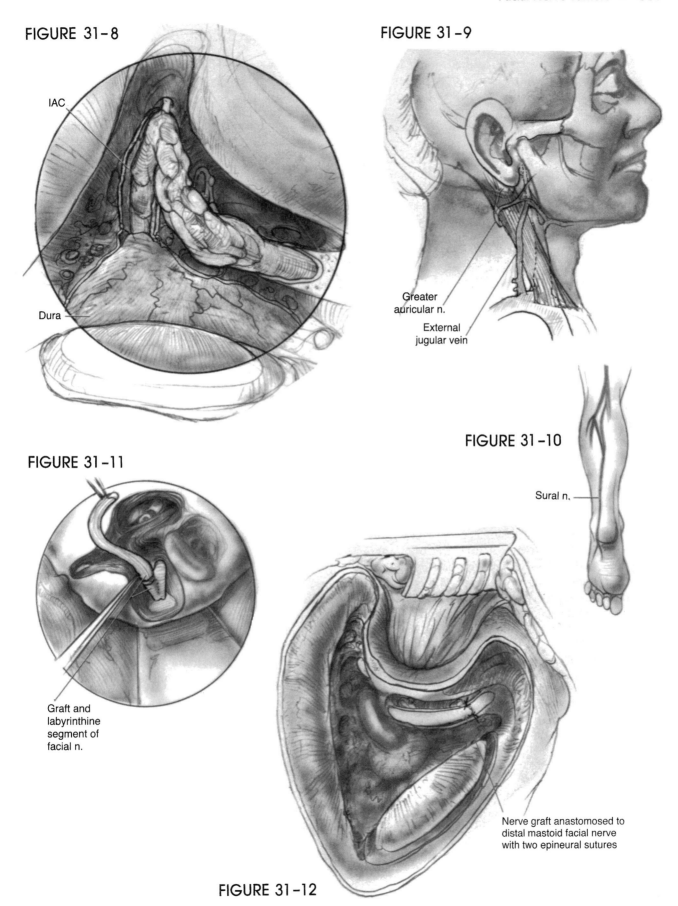

FIGURES 31–8 to 31–12 *See legends on opposite page*

FIGURE 31-13

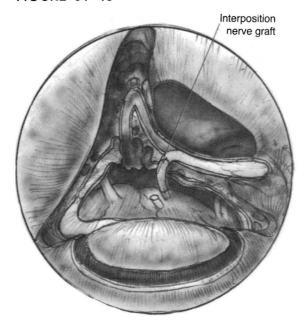

Interposition
nerve graft

FIGURE 31-14

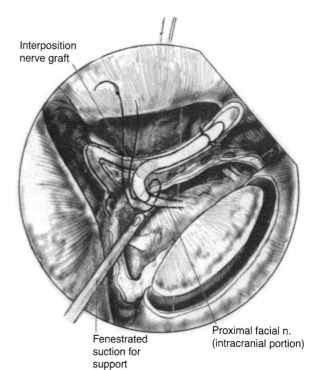

Interposition
nerve graft

Fenestrated
suction for
support

Proximal facial n.
(intracranial portion)

FIGURE 31-15

(Translabyrinthine approach)
Facial nerve rerouted gains
approx. 1.5 cm in length

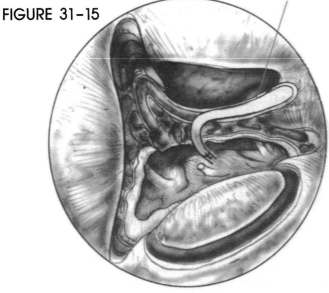

FIGURE 31–13. Facial nerve graft is placed into internal auditory canal through translabyrinthine approach. A single through-and-through suture holds the nerve ends together.

FIGURE 31–14. A fenestrated suction supports the intracranial facial nerve. The suture is passed through the nerve and into a side hole of the suction.

FIGURE 31–15. The facial nerve is rerouted in the translabyrinthine approach to gain approximately 1.5 cm of length.

CT of the temporal bone can show enlargement and erosion of the fallopian canal and indicate tumor involvement. When needed, gadolinium-enhanced MRI demonstrates extension of the tumor into the internal auditory canal and posterior fossa.

Some cases in our series were diagnosed elsewhere when a middle ear mass was encountered during tympanotomy to correct a conductive hearing loss. A biopsy must not be done on a middle ear mass in this situation. Of nine tumors for which biopsies were done by the referring surgeons in our series, 88 per cent suffered a postbiopsy facial paralysis.[34] For a patient going to surgery for a stapedectomy, the development of a postoperative facial paralysis from the biopsy can be extremely disturbing. When a middle ear mass is encountered, the ear should be closed, and a radiologic, not histologic, evaluation should be done. A high-resolution CT scan showing enlargement of the fallopian canal will yield a diagnosis of facial nerve tumor, and subsequent surgery can be planned based on the extent of the tumor.

The labyrinth is at risk for fistulization by bone erosion caused by tumor growth. Particularly vulnerable are the inferior surface of the lateral semicircular canal at the external genu and the cochlea near the geniculate ganglion. A patient with a facial nerve tumor (particularly one that does not involve the internal auditory canal) who exhibits dizziness or sensorineural hearing loss may have a labyrinthine fistula. Such fistulas can frequently be detected on high-resolution CT. However, the surgeon should always be alert to the possibility of encountering a fistula during surgery and must be prepared to repair it. In patients with a known fistula preoperatively, temporalis fascia can be harvested in anticipation of covering the fistula.

For a nerve graft to function, the anastomosis must be made to viable neural tissue at the nerve stump and not to residual tumor. Frozen section examination of the nerve stump is necessary not only to validate complete tumor removal but also to ensure that no tumor remains at the anastomotic site to impede axonal regrowth.

RESULTS

Facial Nerve Neuromas

A review of 64 facial nerve neuromas removed by members of the House Ear Clinic revealed that the facial nerve required repair (graft or primary anastomosis) in 72 per cent of these patients.[34] Of those with 1 year or more of follow-up, 83 per cent of the patients who had undergone repair had facial function graded as a House-Brackmann grade IV or better (Table 31–1). For those with preservation of facial nerve continuity, 70 per cent had postoperative facial function of House-Brackmann grade III or better at 1 year (see Table 31–1). Only one patient in long-term follow-up experienced no recovery of postoperative facial function.

Hearing was preserved near the preoperative level (within 10 dB pure tone average and 16 per cent speech discrimination score) in 53 per cent of patients, excluding those undergoing translabyrinthine tumor removal. Sixteen patients had fistulas of the inner ear, 11 involving a lateral semicircular canal, and 4 involving the cochlea. Hearing was lost in 4 patients, all with fistulas.

Facial Nerve Hemangiomas

Facial nerve hemangiomas tend to occur at the geniculate ganglion or in the internal auditory canal, with facial nerve repair most often required for tumors at the geniculate ganglion. Of the 34 facial nerve hemangiomas removed by the members of the House Ear Clinic, 47 per cent required facial nerve repair.[18] The vast majority of the repaired nerves achieved a House-Brackmann grade III or IV by 1 year or more after surgery (Table 31–2).

Hearing was maintained near the preoperative level in 64 per cent of patients. One patient had postoperative anacusis from a cochlear fistula caused by the tumor.

COMPLICATIONS AND MANAGEMENT

Postoperative cerebrospinal fluid leaks occurred in 6 per cent of the neuroma series, and postoperative meningitis developed in 3 per cent. Surprisingly, meningitis did not occur in patients who also experienced a cerebrospinal fluid leak. The management of these complications is similar to that after acoustic tumor removal by the translabyrinthine and middle fossa approaches, which are discussed in Chapters 49 and 50, respectively.

TABLE 31–1. Postoperative Facial Nerve Function for 34 Facial Nerve Neuroma Patients With More Than 1 Year Follow-Up

FACIAL NERVE FUNCTION*	FACIAL NERVE STATUS		
	Repaired (n = 24)	Intact (n = 10)	Total (n = 34)
I	—	3	3
II	—	1	1
III	9	3	12
IV	11	1	12
V	4	1	5
VI	0	1	1

*House-Brackmann classification.

TABLE 31–2. Postoperative Facial Nerve Results for 23 Facial Nerve Hemangioma Patients With More Than 1 Year Follow-Up

FACIAL NERVE GRADES*	FACIAL NERVE STATUS	
	Repaired	Intact
I	—	7
II	—	2
III	2	—
IV	8	1
V	1	—
VI	2	—

*House-Brackmann classification.
From Shelton C, Brackmann DE, Lo WW, Carberry JN: Intratemporal facial nerve hemangiomas. Otolaryngol Head Neck Surg 104: 116–121, 1991.

References

1. Pulec JL: Facial nerve neuroma. Laryngoscope 82: 1160–1176, 1972.
2. Rosenblum B, Davis R, Camins M: Middle fossa facial schwannoma removed via the intracranial extradural approach: Case report and review of the literature. Neurosurgery 21: 739–741, 1987.
3. Pearman K, Welch AR: Schwannoma of the intratemporal facial nerve: Case report. J Laryngol Otol 94: 779–784, 1980.
4. Liliequist B: Neurinomas of the labyrinthine portion of the facial nerve canal: A report of two cases. Adv Otorhinolaryngol 24: 58–67, 1978.
5. Pulec JL: Facial nerve tumors. Ann Otol Rhinol Laryngol 78: 962–983, 1969.
6. Jackson CG, Glasscock ME III, Hughes G, Sismanis A: Facial paralysis of neoplastic origin: Diagnosis and management. Laryngoscope 90: 1581–1595, 1980.
7. Wiet RJ, Pyle GM, Schramm DR: Middle fossa and intratemporal facial nerve neuromas. Otolaryngol Head Neck Surg 104: 141–142, 1991.
8. Lee KS, Britton BH, Kelly DL Jr.: Schwannoma of the facial nerve in the cerebellopontine angle presenting with hearing loss. Surg Neurol 32: 231–234, 1989.
9. King TT, Morrison AW: Primary facial nerve tumors within the skull. J Neurosurg 72: 1–8, 1990.
10. Dort JC, Fisch U: Facial nerve schwannomas. Skull Base Surg 1: 51–55, 1991.
11. Nelson RA, House WF: Facial nerve neuroma in the posterior fossa: Surgical considerations. In Graham MD, House WF (eds): Disorders of the Facial Nerve. New York, Raven Press, 1982, pp 403–406.
12. Bailey CM, Graham MD: Intratemporal facial nerve neuroma: A discussion of five cases. J Laryngol Otol 97: 65–72, 1983.
13. O'Donoghue GM, Brackmann DE, House JW, Jackler RK: Neuromas of the facial nerve. Am J Otol 10: 49–54, 1989.
14. Pillsbury HC, Price HC, Gardiner LJ: Primary tumors of the facial nerve: Diagnosis and management. Laryngoscope 93: 1045–1048, 1983.
15. Neely JG, Alford BR: Facial nerve neuromas. Arch Otolaryngol Head Neck Surg 100: 298–301, 1974.
16. Lipkin AF, Coker NJ, Jenkins HA, Alford BR: Intracranial and intratemporal facial neuroma. Otolaryngol Head Neck Surg 96: 71–79, 1987.
17. Wiet RS, Lohan AN, Brackmann DE: Neurilemmoma of the chorda tympani nerve. Otolaryngol Head Neck Surg 93: 119–121, 1985.
18. Shelton C, Brackmann DE, Lo WW, Carberry JN: Intratemporal facial nerve hemangiomas. Otolaryngol Head Neck Surg 104: 116–121, 1991.
19. Mangham CA, Carberry JN, Brackmann DE: Management of intratemporal vascular tumors. Laryngoscope 91: 867–876, 1981.
20. Pappas DG, Schneiderman TS, Brackmann DE, et al: Cavernous hemangiomas of the internal auditory canal. Otolaryngol Head Neck Surg 101: 27–32, 1989.
21. Fisch U, Ruttner J: Pathology of intratemporal tumors involving the facial nerve. In Fisch U (ed): Facial Nerve Surgery. Birmingham, AL, Aesculapius, 1977, pp 448–456.
22. Balkany T, Fradis M, Jafek BW, Rucker NC: Hemangioma of the facial nerve: Role of the geniculate capillary plexus. Skull Base Surg 1: 59–63, 1991.
23. Ylikoski J, Brackmann DE, Savolainen S: Pressure neuropathy of the facial nerve: A case report with light and electron microscopic findings. J Laryngol Otol 98: 909–914, 1984.
24. Glasscock ME, Smith PG, Schwaber MK, Nissen AJ: Clinical aspects of osseous hemangiomas of the skull base. Laryngoscope 94: 869–873, 1984.
25. Tew JM Jr, Yeh HS, Miller GW, Shahbabian S: Intratemporal schwannoma of the facial nerve. Neurosurgery 13: 186–188, 1983.
26. Valvassori GE: Neuromas of the facial nerve. Adv Otorhinolaryngol 24: 68–70, 1978.
27. Lo WW, Brackmann DE, Shelton C: Facial nerve hemangioma. Ann Otol Rhinol Laryngol 98: 160–161, 1989.
28. Sanna M, Zini C, Gamoletti R, Pasanisi E: Primary intratemporal tumours of the facial nerve: Diagnosis and treatment. J Laryngol Otol 104: 765–771, 1990.
29. Murata T, Hakuba A, Okumura T, Mori K: Intrapetrous neurinomas of the facial nerve: Report of three cases. Surg Neurol 23: 507–512, 1985.
30. Pulec JL: Facial nerve grafting. Laryngoscope 79: 1562–1583, 1969.
31. House JW: Facial nerve tumors and grafting. In Brackmann DE (ed): Neurological Surgery of the Ear and Skull Base. New York, Raven Press, 1982, pp 77–80.
32. Barrs DM, Brackmann DE, Hitselberger WE: Facial nerve anastomosis in the cerebellopontine angle: A review of 24 cases. Am J Otol 5: 269–272, 1984.
33. Arriaga MA, Brackmann DE: Facial nerve repair techniques in cerebellopontine angle tumor surgery. Am J Otol 13: 356–359, 1992.
34. Alavi S, Shelton C: Facial nerve neuromas: Comparison of results of facial nerve preservation versus facial nerve repair. Trans Pacific Coast Otoophthalmol Soc 74, 1993.

32

Surgery for Cochlear Implantation

William M. Luxford, M.D.

Although the first attempt to electrically stimulate the auditory system occurred nearly two centuries ago, the development of a cochlear prosthesis to restore hearing to patients with sensorineural hearing loss has happened only over the past four decades. The early pioneering work of Simmons, Michaelson, and House provided the stimulus to encourage others, including Bonfai, Chouard, Clark, Eddington, and the Hochmairs.[1] The initial acceptance of cochlear implants was slow; safety and efficacy were the concerns of the early investigators, and the greatest champions of the implant were the patients themselves. Time and technology increased the benefits gained by most patients from their cochlear implants. As a result, cochlear implants have become more widely accepted with each passing year. Of the more than 25,000 patients who have received cochlear implants worldwide, approximately 90 per cent have undergone implantation only since 1985.

Many centers throughout the world have investigated the cochlear implant, and many differences exist in the devices being investigated. In the United States, the Food and Drug Administration (FDA) has monitored these investigations. The FDA has approved the Nucleus 22-channel and the Nucleus 24-channel devices manufactured by the Cochlear Corporation for general use in adults and children.[2] The FDA has also approved the Clarion device manufactured by the Advanced Bionics Corporation for general use in adults and children.[3] The Combi 40+ device manufactured by Med EI Corporation is currently undergoing investigational FDA-controlled clinical trials in adults and children.[4] The criteria for these groups include age of 18 years or more in adults and age of 18 months to 17 years in children, bilateral profound-to-total sensorineural hearing loss, inability to benefit from conventional hearing aids, good physical and mental health, and the motivation and patience to complete a rehabilitation program.[5]

PATIENT SELECTION

Selection criteria of an appropriate implant candidate vary from center to center.

Audiologic Criteria

An audiologic assessment is the primary means of determining implant candidacy. A potential implant candidate has bilateral, profound-to-total sensorineural hearing loss, usually with a three-frequency average (500, 1000, and 2000 Hz), pure-tone unaided threshold in the better ear equal to or greater than 90 dB. Audiologic testing procedures differ between adults and children.

Adults

The prospective candidate is evaluated with appropriately powerful hearing aids. Factors regarding function with a hearing aid, such as recruitment and discomfort, are considered when the likelihood that the patient might perform better with an implant than with a hearing aid is evaluated.

If the patient cannot obtain an aided speech detection threshold of 70 dB sound pressure level or an approximate 53 dB hearing level or better, or performs very poorly on discrimination tests with conventional amplification, a cochlear implant is likely to provide greater benefit. Improvements in cochlear implant technology have provided more benefits to more recent implant patients; therefore, audiologic criteria for inclusion have been relaxed. Potential implant patients can now achieve as much as 40 per cent open-set sentence recognition testing in the better ear using taped presentation.

A full list of test procedures and criteria for patient selection recommended by the device manufacturers and principal investigators is typically specified in the product labeling or in the training manuals.

Children

Children evaluated for the cochlear implant undergo an extensive audiologic assessment. Tympanometry and otoscopy are performed to rule out middle ear pathology at the time of testing. Acoustic reflexes are measured. In children younger than 6 years of age, auditory brainstem response testing is required to confirm a profound hearing loss. Traditional behavioral audiometry or play audiometry with visual, social, or tangible reinforcers is used as needed. If there is no response to sound at maximal levels through the head phones, the child is conditioned to respond to a handheld bone oscillator to ensure that he or she understands the task.

Discrimination tests are performed with the aid that provides the best warble-tone threshold. With an appropriate hearing aid, the child's performance on the discrimination tests in the ear selected for implantation must be poorer than or equal to the average test results obtained from children using a cochlear implant.

Parent and teacher reports of the child's auditory ability must be consistent with the measured severity of the hearing loss. The child must also have a history of an appropriate hearing aid trial. If recently prescribed hearing aids or ear molds have not yielded optimal results, and if testing reveals that usable hearing may remain, a 3- to 6-month trial with appropriate aids and molds is required before a decision on the implant is made. In these cases, the parents and school are encouraged to provide intense auditory training during the trial period.

Medical Evaluation

The medical evaluation includes a complete history and physical examination to detect problems that might interfere with the patient's ability to complete either the surgical or rehabilitative measures of implantation. Appropriate laboratory studies should be ordered to eliminate any suspected medical disorder.

In adults and children receiving the cochlear implant, the etiology of deafness varies. From the variety of responses to cochlear implantation of patients with the same etiology, the etiology of hearing loss does not seem as important as the onset of loss. For cochlear implant candidates, the onset of profound hearing loss is best described as congenital (hearing loss present at birth) or acquired (hearing loss occurring after birth).

Adults deafened prior to acquisition of verbal language skills (congenital and early acquired) are considered prelingually deaf. Adults deafened after the acquisition of verbal language skills (late acquired) are considered postlingually deaf. Acquired deafness in children can be further defined by age of onset: prelingual ($\leq$1 year), perilingual (1 to 5 years), and postlingual ($\geq$5 years).

For adults, the postlingually deaf individual makes the best implant candidate; these are the majority of adults receiving implants. A smaller number of adult implant recipients have a congenital or very early onset of hearing loss. Prelingually deaf adults have a long period of auditory deprivation and may have had little experience with sound. Expectations for benefit from a cochlear implant must be adjusted accordingly. Although prelingually and postlingually deaf patients probably receive similar auditory information through a cochlear implant, prelingually deaf adults cannot use the information as effectively and have a higher rate of nonuse of the device.

For children, the later the onset of profound hearing loss, the greater the chance that the child will develop an auditory memory and realize the benefit of sound. Unlike adults, children with congenital, prelingual, or perilingual losses are usually able to effectively use the information provided by the implant and have a low rate of nonuse of the device when they receive the implant early.

Another important factor in patient selection is length of profound hearing loss. In a review of adult patients, Dowell and associates found no correlation between age and performance but a highly significant negative correlation between the length of profound deafness and performance.[6] For their patients, the performance was worse if hearing was lost more than 13 years before implantation. They found that patients with prolonged duration of deafness received similar information to that of the other implant patients but were unable to use the information as effectively in the recognition of running speech. Dowell and associates believed that this difference may have been caused by loss of central auditory processing resulting from the long period of sound deprivation.

Duration of profound deafness also seems to be an important factor in selection of an appropriate implant candidate in children, especially in those with onset of hearing loss prior to the acquisition of speech and language.

Even though a shorter duration between onset of hearing loss and implantation is beneficial, the interval must be long enough to be certain of the degree of hearing loss, to determine the full benefits of hearing aids, and to be sure that the profound loss has been accepted by both the patient and the family. The interval is 3–6 months for most adults and children.

For children, age does seem to be an important issue in patient selection. Teenagers are usually extremely poor candidates for cochlear implants. Although there are many reasons for this, peer pressure and cosmetic issues are the two factors cited most by teenagers who become nonusers. Counseling is an extremely important part of the patient selection with teenagers.

Physical Examination

It is important to identify preoperatively any external or middle ear diseases, including perforations of the tympanic membrane, that must be treated prior to cochlear implantation. For young children, the size of the implant in relation to the size of the child's skull must be evaluated, and issues involved with skull maturation must be considered. The distance between the cochlear promontory and the mastoid cortex, the approximate sites of the electrode array, and the receiver-stimulator increases about 1.7 cm from birth to adulthood, with one half of the increase occurring during the first 2 years of life.[7] The electrodes must be long enough to tolerate the increase in height and width of the skull that will occur with the child's growth. The accommodation occurs through the gradual straightening of the excess electrode length within the air-containing mastoid cavity.[8]

Radiologic Evaluation

High-resolution computed tomography (CT) of the temporal bone is performed in all cases to identify partial or complete ossification of the scala tympani, soft tissue obliteration of the scala, congenital malformation of the inner ear, and surgical landmarks.[9] Complete agenesis of the cochlea and an abnormal acoustic nerve, the result of either congenital malformation, trauma, or surgery, are contraindications for cochlear implant placement.[10]

Cochlear hypoplasia (Mondini's deformity) is not a contraindication for cochlear implantation. Adults and children with incomplete congenital cochlear malformations have received implants successfully.[11]

Ossification or fibrous occlusion of the cochlea or the round window does not exclude a patient from implantation, but it may influence outcome. Occlusion of the cochlea may lead to partial insertion of the electrode carrier. Magnetic resonance imaging has become more useful than CT in the evaluation of the membranous inner ear in detecting cochlear fibrosis.

Promontory Evaluation

Many implant teams perform an electrical stimulation test at either the promontory or the round window membrane.[12] A positive response is a perception of sound on stimulation. Some investigators do not feel that such testing is critical in the selection of candidates because patients with a negative response, particularly at the promontory, may respond to intracochlear stimulation with an implant.

Other Considerations

Although most implant programs no longer require a formal psychologic evaluation for implant candidates, numerous other factors are considered important in the final decision to perform the procedure. Counseling is often provided to families who have misconceptions or unrealistic expectations regarding the benefits and limitations of the cochlear implant. Support from family and friends is an important part in the rehabilitative process.

For children, the educational setting can play an important part in the selection process. Children in educational programs in which there is special emphasis on auditory training do better than those in settings with little or no auditory input.[13]

PREOPERATIVE EVALUATION

Once a candidate has been selected, the next decision is which side to place the implant. In the past, we always placed the implant in the worst-hearing ear. With experience, we have learned that the "hearing history" of each ear is important. In the potential candidate with a congenital onset of hearing loss in one ear and an acquired hearing loss in the opposite ear, better implant results would be attained if the latter ear received the implant. In the potential candidate with the different durations of profound hearing impairment in each ear, better results would be attained if the ear that had the shortest duration of deafness received the implant. In the potential candidate who has the same etiology for deafness and a similar duration of deafness in both ears but has used a hearing aid for sound awareness in only one ear with no benefit, as determined by the audiologic test procedures, placing the implant in the ear that used the hearing aid should be discussed with the patient. Potential candidates who have residual hearing in the ear to receive the implant must be told that, following implantation with the device's long electrodes, they will likely lose the residual hearing in the ear and be unable to use a hearing aid for sound awareness.

If there is no difference acoustically, then we place the implant in the better surgical ear, based on CT evaluation. The side with the least ossification or fibrosis within the scala tympani is chosen. Results from vestibular tests should be given the least weight in the selection of the side of cochlear implantation. The ear with the least caloric response should receive the implant.

In children, there are no absolute speech or language selection criteria; however, every child is given a full speech and language assessment, including speech production and expressive and receptive language testing. This information is important in helping the implant staff determine how to most effectively interact with the child. The results of these assessments may also influence the final decision regarding implantation by providing a more complete picture of the child's overall status. Reports from the child's educational setting are extremely helpful in completing the speech and language assessment.

The preimplant audiologic, psychologic, and speech and language evaluations provide baseline information against which improvements with the implant can be judged. These assessments are all repeated at regular follow-up intervals after the procedure.

SURGICAL TECHNIQUE

The details of implantation differ from prosthesis to prosthesis. The cochlear implant should be implanted only by qualified surgeons specifically trained to perform the procedure. Surgeons should avoid allowing any prosthetic material to have contact with the skin of the external ear canal. Therefore, the preferred procedure for placement of an implant in a patient with a normal external ear canal is via the transmastoid facial recess approach to the round window–scala tympani. In patients with mastoid cavities and an absent posterior external ear canal, the preferred procedure is total obliteration of the mastoid and closure of the external ear meatus.

The placement of a cochlear prosthesis in the child is essentially the same as in the adult because the key anatomic structures, including the cochlea, middle ear, ossicles, and tympanic membrane, are in place and in their adult configurations at birth. By age 18 months, the mastoid antrum and facial recess, which provide access to the middle ear for active electrode placement, are adequately developed. In fact, a few children younger than 18 months have had successful implantation.

A few modifications are required to accommodate these smaller dimensions of the mastoid process and the thinness of the scalp and temporal squama. The induction coil is firmly anchored to the squamous portion of the temporal bone, and the active electrode is sealed at the round window with connective tissue. Because the same electrode is used in children as in adults, the accommodation for skull growth occurs through gradual straightening of the excess electrode length that is left within the air-containing mastoid cavity. Fortunately, growth-related problems have not been identified in children with implants.

Preoperative Preparation

Implant patients are given the routine instructions that are provided to other patients undergoing mastoid surgery. The use of perioperative antibiotics varies among the implant groups. I do not routinely use perioperative antibiotics.

Preparation and Draping

As in routine chronic otitis media surgery, the patient is placed in the supine position with the surgeon and surgical nurse at the head of the bed and the anesthesiologist toward the foot. After induction of anesthesia and prior to preparation, the electrodes for monitoring the facial nerve are placed. This monitoring is used by many physicians. The position of the internal component of the implant is then determined and marked on the external skin surface. This position will vary among devices. Many different incisions have been designed to allow placement of the internal receiver stimulator. The amount of hair to be shaved depends on the design of the incision.

Operative Procedure

To prevent receiver-stimulator extrusion through the incision, the incision must be made at least 1 to 2 cm wider than the receiver-stimulator to be used (Fig. 32–1). Good vascular supply to the flap must also be maintained to decrease the chance of the wound not healing.

In adults and older children, the anterior postauricular flap is then elevated in the avascular plane between the scalp and temporalis muscle. Pieces of temporalis muscle are removed at and around the site of the receiver-stimulator. Postoperatively, the scalp heals against the bone around the receiver-stimulator, minimizing the thickness of the scalp over the internal device. As a result, the power required to transfer the stimulus from the external transmitter transcutaneously to the internal receiver is decreased. The decreased distance between the external transmitter and the internal receiver also improves the magnetic attraction between the two devices for those systems. In young children with thin scalps, the postauricular incision is carried down to bone. The temporalis muscle is elevated off the parietal portion of the skull with the skin as a single-layer flap forward to the spine of Henle.

The site for the internal receiver in the skull is created at the position previously determined so that there is a separation of at least 1 cm between the incision and the edge of the receiver-stimulator. Suture tunnel holes created on either side of the seat with a guarded burr will be used to help hold the receiver stimulator in place.

All implant systems use the transmastoid, facial recess approach to the round window and scala tympani. The mastoidectomy is done using conventional burrs and suction-irrigation techniques (Fig. 32–2). Unlike chronic otitis media surgery, the superior and posterior mastoid cortical margins are not saucerized. The margins can be undercut to create a bony overhang that will stabilize the coiled electrode within the matoid cavity. The bone removal extends back to the sigmoid, but retraction of the sigmoid is not required unless it is far forward. Enough of the bone in the attic is removed so that the top of the incus can be clearly seen. The incus should not be dislocated or removed because this method does not increase surgical exposure. The short process of the incus and its buttress are important landmarks in the development of the facial recess. The posterior bony ear canal wall is thinned without exposing the overlying vascular strip tissue. Thinning of the bony ear canal is necessary because in viewing the round window area, the direction of vision is parallel to the external auditory canal.

The facial recess is then opened (Fig. 32–3). The facial nerve is carefully skeletonized at the mastoid genu to avoid exposure of the nerve sheath. Once the facial recess is opened, the lip of the round window niche is usually visible just inferior to the stapedius tendon and oval window. To get a good look at the round window, one must open the facial recess more inferiorly and posteriorly. Usually, removing the chorda tympani is unnecessary to adequately visualize the round window niche area. If the facial recess is very restricted, the chorda can be removed, but because the chorda enters the middle ear at the level of the annulus, care must be taken not to damage the tympanic membrane.

With a small diamond stone and intermittent suction-irrigation, the lip of the niche is removed, and the round window membrane comes into clear view. To avoid possible damage to the facial nerve, the diamond stone is not rotated when it is passed through the facial recess to the round window area. In cases in which the round window niche is almost hidden under the pyramidal process, one must drill forward and thin the promontory until the scala tympani is entered.

In some cases, the round window niche and membrane are replaced with new bone growth.[14] This condition is more common in patients whose deafness is attributable to meningitis rather than to other diseases.[15] In these cases, the surgeon must drill forward along the basal coil for as much as 4 to 5 mm. Usually, the new bone is white and can be demarcated from the surrounding otic capsule. Following this white plug of bone with the drill will usually lead to the patent scala, allowing placement of the electrode array.[16] If new bone growth completely obliterates the scala tympani, the surgeon can drill superiorly and possibly enter a patent scala vestibuli.[17] In cases with complete ossifica-

FIGURE 32–1. Incision. The shape of the incision may vary from surgeon to surgeon, but it is important to maintain 1 to 2 cm from the edge of the implant to the incision. Good blood supply to the flap must be maintained both superiorly and inferiorly. An alternative incision to the classic wide C-shaped incision is an extension of a postauricular incision near the postauricular crease, extending superiorly over the temporal squama and middle fossa, curving slightly posteriorly at the most superior aspect of the incision. This incision allows a side-to-side closure.

FIGURE 32–2. Cortical mastoidectomy. Superior and posterior margins are not saucerized. Middle fossa plate, sigmoid sinus, antrum, lateral semicircular canal, and short process of the incus are identified.

FIGURE 32–3. Developing a facial recess. The facial nerve in its vertical portion is identified. Care should be taken not to expose the nerve sheath.

FIGURE 32–4. Opening into the scala tympani. The anteroinferior area of the true round window membrane is removed to allow entry into the scala tympani beyond the hook region of the cochlea.

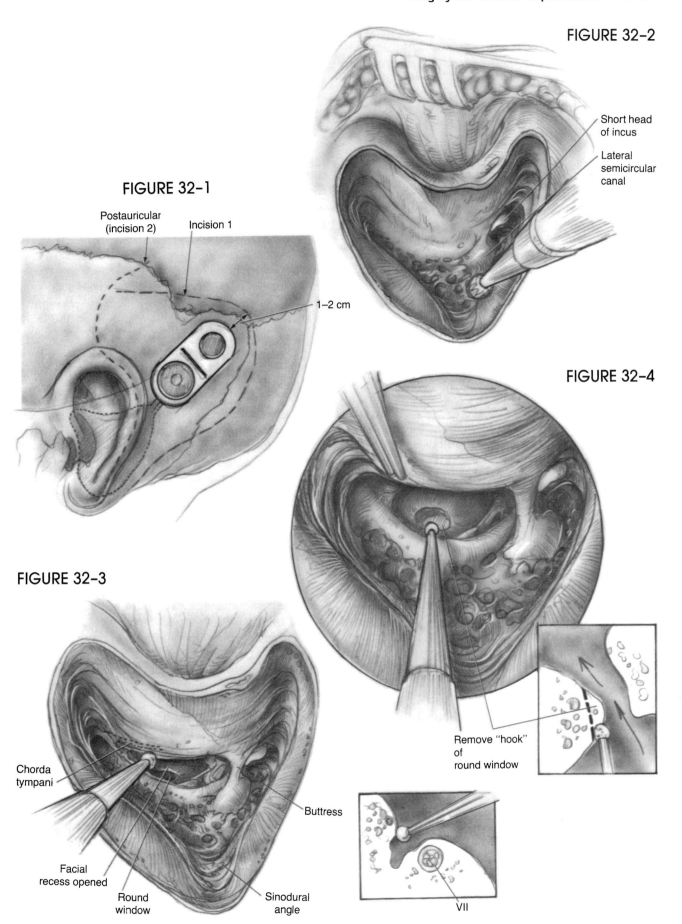

FIGURE 32-2

Short head of incus

Lateral semicircular canal

FIGURE 32-1

Postauricular (incision 2)   Incision 1

1–2 cm

FIGURE 32-4

FIGURE 32-3

Chorda tympani

Buttress

Remove "hook" of round window

Facial recess opened

Round window

Sinodural angle

VII

FIGURES 32–1 to 32–4 *See legends on opposite page*

tion of the cochlea, the surgeon may choose to perform a canal wall down mastoidectomy and close the ear canal. A trough around the modiolus is created and the electrode placed in it.[18, 19]

When drilling the round window niche or attempting to create an opening into the scala tympani through new bone growth, the surgeon must direct the burr anteriorly toward the nose (Fig. 32–4). Drilling superiorly may lead to damage to the basilar membrane and osseous spiral lamina, which may result in the loss of ganglion cells. If the surgeon directs the burr inferiorly, a hypotympanic air cell may be accidentally entered, and the active electrode will be placed improperly into this area. Postoperatively, these cases may fail to stimulate. Temporal bone imaging will show that the active electrode is extracochlear. Revision surgery with placement of the electrode array into the scala tympani will remedy this situation. If the surgeon is uncertain of the placement of the electrode, an intraoperative anteroposterior transorbital plain film can be taken to check the electrode position.

Extracochlear electrodes are usually stabilized at the round window. Short and long intracochlear electrodes are advanced carefully into the scala tympani (Fig. 32–5). Either smooth thumb forceps or small two-prong guides are used to direct the electrode tip into the scala tympani. A special electrode insertion tool has been designed to facilitate placement of the Clarion electrode. Unlike the straight electrodes of the other implant systems, the Clarion electrode is precoiled; therefore, there is a right and left cochlear implant electrode.

Most important, force must not be used when any electrode is advanced. Force may lead to insertion trauma to the inner ear structures and may distort the shape of the electrode. Both of these problems can adversely affect the outcome.

If electrocautery is used after placement of the internal receiver, bipolar electrocautery is recommended because it minimizes the possibility of current being passed through the receiver. The postauricular flap is closed in layers; a drain is rarely used. A standard mastoid dressing is placed. If a drain is used, it is usually removed the day following surgery.

Surgery routinely takes 1.5 to 2.5 hours. Patients are usually discharged by the day after surgery, returning for their first postoperative visit about 1 week later. Approximately 4 to 6 weeks after the surgery, allowing for resolution of the edema in the postauricular flap, fitting the patient with the signal processor begins.

COMPLICATIONS

The risks of the implant procedure are the same as those for chronic otitis media surgery: infection, facial paralysis, cerebrospinal fluid drainage, meningitis, and the usual risks of anesthesia. All of these risks are remote in chronic otitis media surgery and have proved to be so in implant surgery as well.[20, 21]

Failure of the incision to heal and associated minor infections are the most common problems associated with implant surgery.[22] In a few patients in whom the internal receiver has been placed too close to the wound's edge, or

in patients in whom the flap over the internal receiver is too thin, the internal receiver has extruded. As noted earlier, at least 1 to 2 cm must be maintained between the incision and the edge of the internal receiver. The ideal thickness for the flap is 6 to 7 mm. Although too thin a flap may necrose, too thick a flap may diminish device performance by decreasing the transcutaneous transmission of information.

Problems with the facial nerve can occur as the result of both surgery and stimulation.[23] Good surgical landmarks must be maintained when the facial recess is created. Although the facial nerve is identified, it usually does not have to be uncovered with the facial recess approach. Adequate irrigation at the facial recess must be maintained to help dissipate the heat generated by the turning shaft of the diamond burr used to create the exposure of the round window and entrance into the scala tympani, especially in drill-out cases. To help alleviate the problem of the drill shaft turning against the facial nerve, a drill such as the Treace Skeeter could be used. The width of the drill bit shaft is smaller, and a sleeve around most of the length of the shaft protects the surrounding tissues as well. In cases in which the heat from the rotating burr shaft has led to facial nerve problems, the paralysis has been temporary and has resolved over several weeks to several months. Facial nerve paralysis has occurred in patients with congenital malformation of the cochlea and in patients who have undergone radical mastoidectomy many years prior to their implant procedure. In these cases, the facial nerve, either because it is congenitally displaced or exposed by previous surgery, is at greater risk.[24] The use of facial nerve monitoring may decrease the chance of facial nerve trauma.

Cerebrospinal fluid drainage has occurred at both the internal receiver site and the cochlea. In some patients, the temporal squama can be quite thin. In these cases, creating an adequate seat for the internal receiver package requires bony dissection down to the dura. If small dural tears occur, they should be covered with temporalis fascia, and the fascia should be supported with the internal receiver. After insertion of the intracochlear electrode, the cochleostomy is closed with strips of temporalis fascia to prevent perilymphatic fistula development.

A gush of cerebrospinal fluid is more likely to occur in patients with congenitally malformed inner ears. In these patients, small pieces of Surgicel can be placed through the facial recess opening into the eustachian tube orifice to temporarily occlude the eustachain tube. This procedure should be done prior to opening the scala tympani. Also, closure of the wound should be done in layers, without a drain. I am unaware of any patients who have had persistent cerebrospinal fluid rhinorrhea or leakage of cerebrospinal fluid from the wound site following cochlear implantation.

In adults, the possible effects of the implant on the vestibular system and on tinnitus have been evaluated by clinical monitoring, patient questionnaires, and objective study. No evidence that the implant has significant negative impact in these areas exists.

One concern in extending the cochlear implant program to children was the risk of increased incidence or severity of otitis media, to which children are more prone than adults. Otitis media could have caused the implanted inter-

FIGURE 32–5

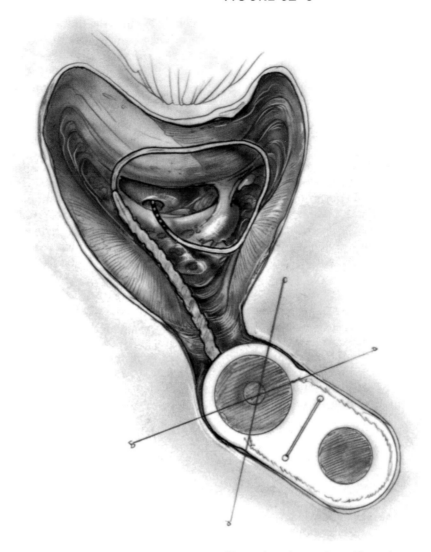

FIGURE 32–5. Electrode insertion and placement of internal receiver package. Electrodes are gently inserted into the scala tympani. After electrode placement, the internal receiver package is fixed in its seat. Soft tissue is placed around the electrode at the round window to create a seal.

nal coil and the electrode in the mastoid and middle ear to become an infected foreign body. Further, the infection might extend along the electrode into the inner ear, possibly resulting in meningitis and further degeneration of the auditory system. Information from the clinical trials with 3M/House and Nucleus 22-channel cochlear implants revealed that no increase in incidence or severity of otitis media occurred in children receiving the cochlear implant. In addition, no cases of postoperative meningitis in children have been reported. One case of meningitis in an adult patient with a cochlear implant, however, has been reported.[25]

Chronic otitis media is not a contraindication to cochlear implant surgery. In most cases, because of the prior disease and surgery, the posterior canal wall has been taken down and a radical mastoid cavity created. If no active disease exists, a one-stage surgery can be performed. The mastoid cavity is completely obliterated by everting the external auditory ear canal skin and closing the external auditory

canal meatus with a pursestring suture. Although other surgeons have performed a one-stage surgery in the presence of active disease in the middle ear and mastoid cavity, I prefer to perform a two-stage procedure in these cases. The first stage is removal of disease and obliteration of the mastoid cavity, with closure of the external ear canal meatus. Approximately 4 to 6 months later, the second stage can be performed, with placement of the cochlear implant.

REVISION SURGERY

There are two primary reasons for revision surgery: (1) to replace a failed device and (2) to upgrade a system. Revision is possible because human and animal temporal bone studies have shown the following problems either do not occur or are insignificant when the correct surgical technique for implanting electrodes of the different devices is used: degeneration of the remaining viable neural elements due to mechanical trauma to the organ of Corti during insertion or removal of the electrodes, osteogenesis, degeneration of the neural tissue by electrical stimulation, and spread of infection from the middle ear into the inner ear.

For patients undergoing revision surgery of a failed device, either a similar device or an upgrade can be reimplanted in the same ear. Most patients who have undergone revision implant surgery have had a failed device. Experience has shown that it is not difficult to remove and to reinsert a cochlear implant electrode into the scala tympani.[26] However, failure of the cochlear implant sometimes results not from a problem within the internal receiver package but from migration of the electrode out of the scala tympani and back into the mastoid cavity. In these cases, the scala tympani will fill with fibrosis, and attempting to reinsert an electrode into the tissue-filled scala is very difficult.

The facial nerve is at greater risk in revision cases than in primary cases because the tissue placed around the electrode in the facial recess in the primary case may adhere to a partially exposed facial nerve. Removal of this tissue at revision surgery to allow visualization of the middle ear and promontory must be done carefully.

In patients with functioning devices who are considering revision surgery to upgrade to a new cochlear implant, two options are available: either the ear with or the ear without an implant could be operated on. My preference in most cases with functioning devices is to place the upgrade in the ear without the implant, thus maintaining the patient's only source of hearing. Several years later, if the patient is again interested in an upgrade, I would reimplant in the worse-hearing ear, using the side that provided the lesser benefit (presumably the side with the older implant). I would reimplant an upgrade device in the ear with the currently functioning device if the ear without the implant showed changes on radiographic studies that would hinder the placement of the electrode.

Most patients who have had reimplantation for either a failed device or to upgrade are using their new devices. A few patients who were nonusers of the single-channel systems are also nonusers of the multichannel implants.

Not all of the repairs or upgrades require surgery. The external components (microphone, cables, and speech processors) are repaired or replaced as needed.

REHABILITATION

Surgical implantation of the internal receiver and electrode of the cochlear implant device is only the beginning of the treatment process:[13] Approximately 4 to 6 weeks following surgery, the patient must return to the clinic to be fitted with the external portions of the device. All of the various cochlear implant devices require adjustment of device settings to the individual patient. The more complex the device, the more complex the process for determining appropriate settings. In addition, determining the best fit for a particular patient may involve repeated changes in settings over time as the patient becomes experienced with the sound provided. In addition to setting the device, the patient must be introduced or reintroduced to sound in a manner that provides a realistic idea of the benefit and limitations of the device in relation to the patient's own personal situation. Rehabilitation must also be provided. Most cochlear implant programs include providing information on care and use of the device, simple auditory training, speech reading practice with the added sounds from the cochlear implant, and perhaps training of auditory speech reception skills. Time spent counseling the patient and family members may be considerable.

The amount of rehabilitation and training provided varies from center to center. Further, the amount of time necessary will vary depending on the particular patient and his or her needs. Each cochlear implant manufacturer recommends specific rehabilitation approaches, or provides written materials for implant training, or both. The minimum number of patient hours in the clinic following implantation is usually no less than 40. Regular follow-up visits with objective assessment of performance for the first several years are standard practice.

RESULTS

Cochlear implantation has become a standard rehabilitative approach for profoundly deaf patients who do not benefit significantly from hearing aids. Although many different cochlear implant devices are currently in use, none can provide normal hearing. Most deaf patients who receive a cochlear implant will be able to detect medium-to-loud sounds, including speech, at comfortable listening levels. Many can learn to recognize familiar sounds, such as the doorbell, car horns, telephone ringing, or even the voices of relatives or friends. For most patients, cochlear implants can aid in communication by improving speech reading ability: they are able to combine cues from the sounds and rhythms of speech with what they see. In many other patients, the implant provides some speech discrimination of words or sentences without the use of speech reading.[13, 27]

The definition of success is different from patient to patient and family to family. Several factors, including age at time of deafness, age at implant surgery, duration of deafness, status of the remaining auditory nerve fibers, training, educational setting, and type of implant, affect the benefit a patient receives from an implant. Memory of previous auditory experience appears to be one of the most important factors. Patients who have had some auditory experience and a short period of deafness may learn to use the sound information provided by the implant more quickly and effectively than those who are born with profound hearing deficit or lose their hearing very early in life.

Many professionals are concerned about whether congenitally deaf children can benefit from these devices, whether children in total communication educational programs can benefit, and whether children with cochlear implants are likely to receive the kind of training that will maximize the use of the implant. Experience indicates that, in fact, congenitally deaf children do show significant benefit from the implant, as do children in total communication programs. However, just as with hearing aids, auditory skills are not likely to be maximized without appropriate auditory training. Cost-effectiveness studies have indicated that cochlear implants are worthwhile when compared with other well-accepted medical and surgical interventions.[28]

SUMMARY

Important points about cochlear implant surgery are as follows:

- Cochlear implants are not experimental.
- Cochlear implants are not hearing aids.
- Appropriate candidates have profound bilateral sensorineural hearing loss and do not benefit from conventional amplification.
- Surgical and postoperative complications have been minimal.
- Implants increase auditory abilities and, as a result, improve speech production skills.
- Postlingually deafened adults with a short duration of deafness are excellent candidates for a cochlear implant.
- Although postlingually deafened children in aural programs demonstrate the fastest and greatest development of auditory skills as a group, congenitally and prelingually deafened children show substantial benefit from a cochlear implant.

References

1. Luxford WM, Brackmann DE: The history of cochlear implants. *In* Gray RF (ed): Cochlear Implants. London, Croom Helm, 1985, pp 1–26.
2. Clinical Bulletin: Introducing the Nucleus 24 Cochlear Implant System. Cochlear Corporation, Englewood, CO, October 1998.
3. Malton A: Recent Advances in Advanced Bionics. Presented at the Seventh Symposium on Cochlear Implants in children. Iowa City, IA, 1998.
4. Ochs DN: Current Experiences and Future Developments of the C40+ System. Presented at the 7th symposium on Cochlear Implants in Children. Iowa City, IA, 1998.
5. Luxford WM: Cochlear implant indications. Am J Otol 10: 95–98, 1989.
6. Dowell RC, Mecklenburg DC, Clark GM: Speech recognition for 40 patients receiving multi-channel cochlear implants. Arch Otolaryngol Head Neck Surg 112: 1054–1059, 1986.
7. O'Donoghue GM, Jackler RK, Jenkins WM, et al: Cochlear implantation in children: The problem of head growth. Otolaryngol Head Neck Surg 94: 78–81, 1986.
8. Marks DR, Jackler RK, Bates GJ, Greenberg S: Pediatric cochlear implantation: Strategies to accommodate for head growth. Otolaryngol Head Neck Surg 101: 38–46, 1989.
9. Gray RF, Evans RA, Freer CEL, et al: Radiology for cochlear implants. J Laryngol Otol 105: 85–88, 1991.
10. Shelton C, Luxford WM, Tonokawa LL, et al. The narrow internal auditory canal in children: A contraindication to cochlear implants. Otolaryngol Head Neck Surg 100: 227–331, 1989.
11. Slattery WH, Luxford WM: Cochlear implantation in the congenital malformed cochlea. Laryngoscope 105: 1184–1187, 1995.
12. Waltzman SB, Cohen NL, Shapiro WH, Hoffman RA: The prognostic value of round window electrical stimulation in cochlear implant patients. Otolaryngol Head Neck Surg 103: 102–106, 1990.
13. Staller SJ, Beiter AL, Brimacombe JA, et al: Pediatric performance with the Nucleus 22-channel cochlear implant system. Am J Otol 12(Suppl): 126–136, 1991.
14. Green JD Jr, Marion MS, Hinojosa R: Labyrinthitis ossificans: Histopathologic consideration for cochlear implantation. Otolaryngol Head Neck Surg 104: 320–326, 1991.
15. Novak MA, Fifer RC, Barkmeier JC, Firszt JB: Labyrinthine ossification after meningitis: Its implications for cochlear implantation. Otolaryngol Head Neck Surg 103: 351–356, 1990.
16. Balkany T, Gantz B, Nadol JB Jr: Multichannel cochlear implants in partially ossified cochleas. Ann Otol Rhinol Laryngol Suppl 135: 3–7, 1988.
17. Steenerson RL, Gary LB, Wynens MS: Scala vestibuli cochlear implantation for labyrinthine ossification. Am J Otol 11: 360–363, 1990.
18. Gantz BJ, McCabe BF, Tyler RS: Use of multichannel implants in obstructed and obliterated cochleas. Otolaryngol Head Neck Surg 98: 72–81, 1988.
19. Lambert PR, Ruth RA, Hodges AV: Multichannel cochlear implant and electrically evoked auditory brainstem responses in a child with labyrinthitis ossificans. Laryngoscope 101(1Pt1): 14–19, 1991.
20. Cohen NL, Hoffman RA: Complications of cochlear implant surgery in adults and children. Ann Otol Rhinol Laryngol 100(9Pt1): 708–711, 1991.
21. Webb RL, Lehnhardt E, Clark GM, et al: Surgical complications with the cochlear multiple-channel intracochlear implant: Experience at Hannover and Melbourne. Ann Otol Rhinol Laryngol 100: 131–136, 1991.
22. Haberkamp TJ, Schwaber MK: Management of flap necrosis in cochlear implantation. Ann Otol Rhinol Laryngol 101: 38–41, 1992.
23. Niparko JK, Oviatt DL, Coker NJ, et al: Facial nerve stimulation with cochlear implantation: VA Cooperative Study Group on Cochlear Implantation. Otolaryngol Head Neck Surg 104: 826–830, 1991.
24. House JR, Luxford WM: Facial nerve injury in cochlear implantation. Presented at the Southern Section, Triological Society, Boca Raton, FL, January 1993.
25. Daspit CP: Meningitis as a result of a cochlear implant: Case report. Otolaryngol Head Neck Surg 105: 115–116, 1991.
26. Parisier SC, Chute PM, Weiss MH, et al: Results of cochlear implant reinsertion. Laryngoscope 101: 1013–1015, 1991.
27. Parkin JL, Randolph LJ: Auditory performance with simultaneous intracochlear multichannel stimulation. Laryngoscope 101: 379–383, 1991.
28. Wyatt JR, Rothman M, Delissovoy G. Niparko J: Cost utility of the multichannel cochlear implant in 258 profoundly deaf individuals. Laryngoscope 1996; 106: 816–821.

33

Implantable Hearing Devices

William H. Slattery III, M.D. ▪ Sigfried D. Soli, Ph.D.

It is estimated that 28 million Americans have a hearing loss severe enough to cause problems with communication, and this number is expected to increase as the population ages.[1] The severity of loss ranges from mild, in which the individual may have difficulty only when significant background noise is present, to a profound loss, in which even in the quietest situation the patient is unable to understand and communicate. Most hearing loss is sensorineural in nature. Although hearing loss may affect all frequencies, it is most common for individuals to have some component of high-frequency sensorineural hearing loss. Less than 1 per cent of the hearing-impaired population have losses correctable by medical or surgical means. Patients with a mild loss may receive no treatment other than instructions on modifying their acoustic environment to diminish background noise and selecting seating arrangements for improved listening conditions. Individuals with conductive losses have the opportunity to undergo surgical therapy to have the conductive hearing loss corrected. Individuals with profound sensorineural loss may receive cochlear implants, which provide electrical stimulation directly to the cochlear nerve.

Most of the sensorineural hearing loss population must rely on amplification to provide a better means of hearing to improve communication; this is generally accomplished with conventional air-conduction hearing aids. In recent years, hearing aids have decreased in size and improved microchips have been developed, resulting in improved signal processing capabilities. Hearing aids have become easier to program with digital processors, thus providing much better individualization of amplification according to each patient's needs. Despite the improvements in conventional hearing aid technology, only 15 to 20 per cent of the hearing-impaired population who could receive benefit from amplification use these devices.[2]

There are many reasons why individuals do not wear hearing aids. One of the most prevalent reasons is that conventional air-conduction hearing aids do not provide enough amplification of sounds to which the individual wishes to listen; in addition, they produce troubling amplification of unwanted sounds, especially when background noise is present. Another major problem with conventional hearing aids is the limited high-frequency response. High-frequency output is limited by feedback of high frequencies, because the microphone and speaker of conventional air-conduction hearing aids are close together. New circuitry (feedback cancellation) has diminished some of these problems, but most conventional air-conduction hearing aid users still complain of feedback problems, especially as the ear canal changes in response to long-term use of the device. Current microchip technology has allowed these devices to become smaller, thus improving their cosmetic acceptance. The limited frequency output can cause problems with distortion, and the limitation of high-frequency amplification restricts sound localization abilities.

Patients complain about the cosmetic aspect of conventional air-conduction hearing aids because they believe that wearing such a device indicates to others a disability and carries the stigma of old age. Some patients complain of discomfort in the ear canal, especially with the smaller devices that fit more medially in the ear canal. Having a device in the ear canal may cause problems with an occlusion effect, which results in loss of low-frequency information. With the ear canal plugged, cerumen and cerumen impaction problems may increase. Wearing a device in the external ear canal increases the moisture within the ear canal; this situation requires treatment to prevent recurring external otitis. If the ear canal can be left open, a more natural sound quality may be obtained over a broad range of frequencies.

CONVENTIONAL VERSUS IMPLANTABLE HEARING AIDS

Normally, sound waves are received by the pinna, and the frequency response of this sound input is changed by the shape of the pinna. The acoustic energy is funneled toward the ear canal, stimulating vibrations of the tympanic membrane. The changes in acoustic energy that occur within the external ear and pinna provide "spectral cues" that help with sound localization. The acoustic energy is transmitted from sound wave vibrations in a gas (air) to vibrations in a solid material (tympanic membrane). This transmits vibratory information across the ossicular chain, which in turn vibrates the fluids of the cochlea. Hair cell stimulation results in response to the sound waves in liquid within the cochlea. Conventional air-conduction hearing aids amplify sound before it reaches the middle ear. A microphone converts the incoming acoustic signal into an electrical signal. The amplifier and signal processors modify the electrical signal to increase its strength. The receiver increases the amplified electrical signal into an amplified acoustic signal for presentation to the eardrum (Fig. 33–1). The amplified acoustic signal is transmitted via the middle ear to the inner ear in the normal physiologic manner.

Although conventional air-conduction hearing aids provide amplified sound to the normal auditory system, the implantable devices provide vibratory acoustic energy to the middle ear system, bypassing the external ear canal. Normal vibrations of the ossicles occur as a result of

FIGURE 33-1

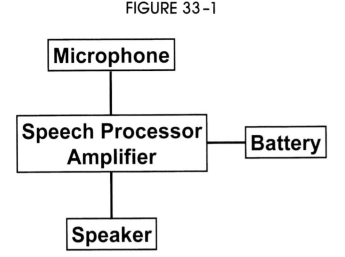

FIGURE 33–1. Conventional hearing aid components.

FIGURE 33-3

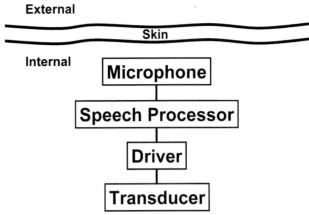

FIGURE 33–3. Fully implantable hearing aid components.

acoustical sound input. Implantable devices take advantage of the vibration of the middle ear ossicles to drive the ossicular chain. These devices may be totally implantable or partially implantable. The partially implantable device consists of a microphone speech processor connected to a transmitter with an external coil that transmits electrical energy transcutaneously to the internal device (Fig. 33–2). The internal device consists of an internal receiving coil connected to a receiver, which provides electrical energy to a mechanical driver connected to the ossicular chain. The external device also consists of a battery to power the system.

A fully implantable device contains the same elements as the partially implantable device, with the exception of the transmitter coil system and receiver (Fig. 33–3). The microphone may be placed under the skin or in the middle ear space and is connected to the internal speech processor, powered by an implantable battery. The acoustic sound wave is received by the microphone and converted into an electrical signal. This electrical signal is converted into a

mechanical vibration by the driver, which is then transmitted to the ossicular chain within the middle ear space, bypassing the external ear canal.

Current implantable devices differ primarily by the type of transducer used and the connection to the ossicular chain. These devices allow a broad frequency response with low linear and nonlinear distortion. They also have the advantage of amplifying high frequencies without the problem of acoustic feedback seen in conventional hearing aids. These devices provide the potential of better acoustic input with better hearing in background noise. A fully implantable device eliminates the perceived social stigma of conventional air-conduction hearing aids. In addition, these devices potentially could eliminate the occlusion effect and other distortions. There are, of course, disadvantages to implantable hearing aids, which include the risks of implantation surgery and general anesthesia. If the device fails, surgical intervention is required to replace the device. There is concern about the high cost of these devices and how reimbursement will occur. Battery recharging and replacement are also difficult technologic challenges to be overcome. The full benefit and limitations of these devices will not be known until further progress has been made on these issues.

REQUIREMENTS OF IMPLANTABLE DEVICES

The ideal implantable hearing aid should be easy to implant. The device should cause no trauma or damage to the normal auditory system. It is extremely important that the auditory system remain intact in case of device failure. Experience with cochlear implants has demonstrated the reliability of implantable devices in the postauricular and mastoid area.

Increased stiffness of the ossicular chain resulting from device fixation to the ossicles may impede the low-frequency response, whereas implants that increase the mass effect of the ossicular chain reduce the high-frequency responses. The ideal device is safe over a long period. Battery

FIGURE 33-2

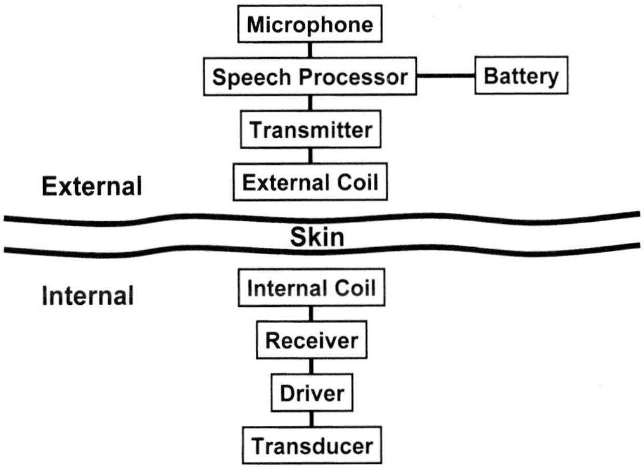

FIGURE 33–2. Partially implantable hearing aid components.

changes should be easy to perform in the office or on an outpatient basis for fully implantable devices. The device should be easy to upgrade, because it is expected that as this technology improves, better speech processing strategies will become available.

The amount of acoustic energy a device is able to deliver above the incoming signal is defined as *gain*. An implantable hearing aid must provide greater gain than conventional air-conduction devices. Amplification of high frequency is expected, and gain must be significant enough to provide adequate benefit to the patient. Most patients with sensorineural hearing loss require high gain levels in the high frequencies to receive any benefit from a device. Outputs greater than 105 dB sound pressure level (SPL) are required for patients with moderate to severe hearing loss. A flat frequency reception up through 8 kHz is desirable for maximum speech comprehension. If the device does not provide enough amplification in the high frequencies, benefit is reduced.

According to Miller and Fredrickson,[3] the maximum level of output in decibels SPL required to accommodate various levels of hearing loss is approximately the level of hearing loss in dB hearing level + 50 dB, with some adjustment in output requirements for greater degrees of hearing loss. To provide benefit to those with moderate to moderately severe hearing loss, a hearing aid needs to provide a maximum output level equivalent to 90 to 115 dB SPL (Fig. 33–4). An implanted hearing aid must provide a mechanical stimulation equivalent to this maximum output level, which we call *dBI*, for decibel implant.

TYPES OF MIDDLE EAR IMPLANTS

There are essentially two types of transducers currently used in middle ear implants: piezoelectric and electromagnetic.

Piezoelectric transducers are ceramic crystals, the shape of which is altered by the passage of electricity through the material. The change in the shape of the ceramic is not permanent, and the ceramic reverts to the original shape when the electrical current is no longer applied. There are two types of ceramic crystals: monomorph and biomorph. The monomorph crystal consists of a single layer of piezoelectric material, which expands and contracts to directly create the vibrations. The biomorph form consists of two bonded ceramic layers, the layers of which are opposing electrical polarities. When a current is passed through the bonded layers, the entire structure bends, creating the vibrations. Piezoelectric ceramic materials are limited by anatomic size restrictions (the amount of bending is proportional to the length of the crystal), reducing the amount of transductive power available.

The *electromagnetic transduction* of sound involves the creation of mechanical vibrations by passing a current through a coil proximal to a magnet. As the electricity is passed through the coil, an electromagnetic field is created, vibrating the magnet, which by direct or indirect contact will cause movement of the middle ear structures or cochlear fluids. Two methods of creating the electromagnetic field are used: attachment of a magnet directly to the middle ear (tympanic membrane, vibratory pathway, incus, or stapes) along with an induction coil or placement of the magnet and coil inside a single assembly. If the magnet and coil are housed together, a probe extending from the magnet-coil assembly is placed against the ossicular chain. As the current is passed through the assembly, the probe vibration is sent directly to the ossicular chain. This type of stimulation is also referred to as *electromechanical stimulation*.

A major limitation of the electromechanical approach is insufficient power output to derive benefit from the device. In addition, if the magnet and coil are separately placed in the middle ear space, individual anatomic differences may result in larger gaps between the magnet and coil, further reducing performance. The major limitation of a device housing both the magnet and the coil is the nature of the device-ossicle connection or coupling. If the device shifts relative to the ossicles, there may be a reduction in the optimal transduction of the auditory stimulus to the ossicular chain.

SPECIFIC DEVICES

There are a number of middle ear implantable devices currently available: Vibrant Soundbridge (manufactured by Symphonix), Totally Integrated Cochlear Amplifier (TICA, Implex American Hearing Systems), Direct Drive Hearing System (DDHS, Soundtec), Envoy (St. Croix Medical), Middle Ear Transducer (MET, Otologics), and RION (Yanagihara and Suzuki, Japan). See Table 33–1 for a summary of device characteristics.

The Vibrant Soundbridge System

The Vibrant Soundbridge, developed by Symphonix Devices, Inc., of San Jose, California, is a semi-implantable hearing aid consisting of two parts: the speech processor and the vibrating ossicular prosthesis (VORP). The VORP is surgically placed and consists of a floating mass trans-

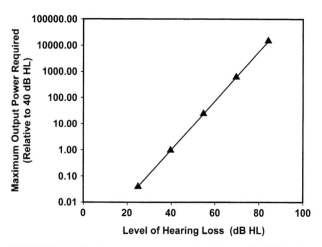

FIGURE 33–4. Maximum output power (relative to 40 dB hearing level) versus level of hearing loss (decibels of HL).

TABLE 33–1. Device Characteristics

DEVICE	TRANSDUCTION METHOD	PATIENT CHARACTERISTICS	IMPLANTABLE	SIGNAL PROCESSING
Vibrant Soundbridge	Electromechanical	No benefit from conventional hearing aids	Semi-implantable	Digital
TICA	Piezoelectric	Moderate to severe loss	Totally implantable	3-channel, digital-analog
DDHS	Electromagnetic	Moderate to severe loss	Semi-implantable	—
Envoy	Piezoelectric	Moderate to severe SNHL	Totally implantable	—
MET	Electromechanical	Bilateral moderate to severe SNHL	Semi-implantable	Digital speech processor
RION	Piezoelectric	Conductive deafness, mild to moderate loss	Semi-implantable	—

SNHL, sensorineural hearing loss.

ducer (FMT), a conductor link, and an internal receiver. The FMT is a unique electromagnetic transducer that contains a magnet of inertial mass within two electromagnetic coils. When activated, the magnet mass vibrates within the FMT, between the coils, causing the entire unit to vibrate. The unit is attached by titanium strips around the long process of the incus, and the floating mass transducer is oriented in the direction of the stapes. Vibration occurs parallel to the plane of the stapes. The external audio processor is held in place over the internal receiver by a magnet.

Placement of the internal device requires a mastoidectomy, similar to cochlear implantation. The facial recess is opened to allow visualization of the incudostapedial joint.

The facial recess must be opened widely enough to allow the FMT to pass through the facial recess easily. The FMT is crimped onto the incus after the VORP is embedded in a seat. A seat is created for the VORP to keep it in cortical bone posterior to the sigmoid sinus (Fig. 33–5).

The company began clinical trials in 1996 and approximately 70 patients have implants in the United States. This device has recently been approved by the U.S. Food and Drug Administration (FDA). The device has also been approved for implantation in the European Union. The speech processor has recently been upgraded to a digital speech processor (the Vibrant D).

A preliminary investigation of 49 patients has demonstrated that more than 94 per cent of the subjects reported

FIGURE 33-5

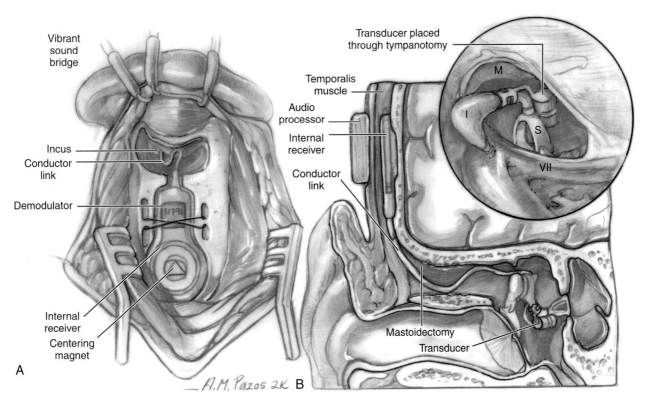

FIGURE 33–5. The Symphonix Vibrant Soundbridge system. *A,* Location of internal receiver. *B,* Position of transducer. M = Malleus; I = incus; S = stapes; VII = facial nerve.

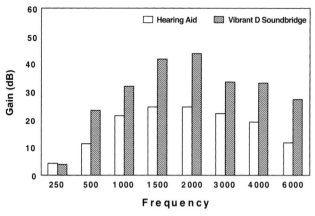

FIGURE 33–6. Gain (decibels) found in 49 patients comparing their preoperative air-conduction hearing aid with the results from the Vibrant D Soundbridge.

TABLE 33–2. Current Indications for Symphonix Vibrant Soundbridge System*

PURE-TONE AIR-CONDUCTION THRESHOLDS	FREQUENCY (kHz)					
	0.5	**1**	**1.5**	**2**	**3**	**4**
Lower limit	10	10	20	30	40	40
Upper limit	65	75	80	80	85	85

*Other indications include the following:
• Pure-tone air-conduction average thresholds for both ears within 20 dB.
• Air-bone gap at 0.5, 1, 2, and 4 kHz no greater than 10 dB at two or more of these frequencies.
• Word recognition scores of at least 50 per cent using a phonetically balanced word list (NU-6) at 40 dB sensation level or most comfortable loudness level (MCL).

improvement in their signal quality satisfaction rating with the Vibrant Soundbridge compared with their previous conventional air-conduction hearing aids. Ninety-seven per cent of the subjects who reported feedback problems with their presurgery hearing aids reported no feedback with the Vibrant Soundbridge. Eighty-eight per cent of patients improved the sound quality satisfaction rating of their own voice, and 98 per cent of the subjects reported satisfaction with the overall fit and comfort of the Vibrant Soundbridge. Figure 33–6 shows the gain in 49 patients comparing results from their preoperative air-conduction hearing aid with the results from the Vibrant D Soundbridge.

The external processor is attached approximately 6 weeks following surgery, and the device is programmed at that time. As part of the clinical trial, the patients have undergone extensive preoperative testing; postoperative testing and postprogramming testing is performed at 1 month, 3 months, 6 months, and every 6 months after activation. Current indications for use of the Soundbridge are found in Table 33–2.

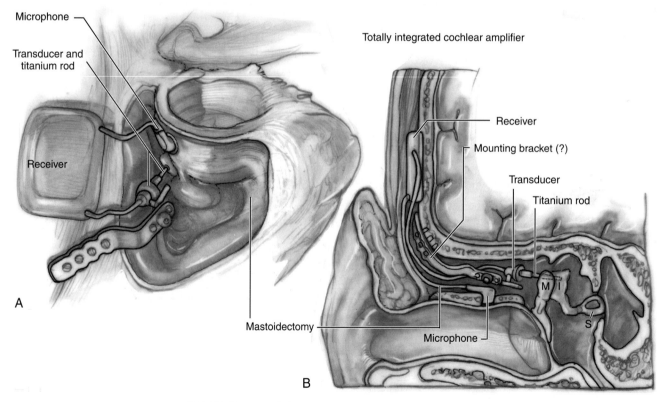

FIGURE 33–7. The TICA system. *A,* Surgical view. *B,* Coronal view showing position of transducer. M = Malleus; I = incus; S = stapes.

TICA

The TICA (total implantable cochlear amplifier) has been developed by Implex Corporation, Munich, Germany. It is a total fully implantable device, which consists of a microphone attached to an implantable speech processor, and battery. The device is placed via a postauricular incision in which a mastoidectomy is created. The ossicular chain is exposed. The microphone is placed in the ear canal. The skin of the ear canal is elevated and a hole is placed in the bony ear canal. Fascia is placed over the microphone to prevent extrusion or exposure of the microphone. The piezotransducer is fixed to the mastoid cortex and positioned to allow the stimulating rod to be in contact with the incus. A micromanipulator is used for placement of the stimulating rod on the incus body. A seat is created for the speech processing monitor and battery, which is anchored in the cortical bone, over the temporal lobe.

The TICA is controlled by a small remote control unit, which can turn the device on and off, adjust the volume, and select different programs for various listening conditions. The battery is recharged with a portable charging unit placed over the device. Transcutaneous transmission of electrical energy is delivered to the battery to allow charging at approximately 1½ hours. The battery is expected to last 3 to 5 years before requiring replacement (Fig. 33–7).

The device has been implanted in approximately 20 patients in Europe. Feedback has been a problem and has required disruption of the ossicular chain in some patients. The malleus head has been removed to prevent the feedback problem. The device has not been implanted in the United States at the time of this publication.

DDHS

The DDHS has been developed by Soundtec, Oklahoma City, Oklahoma and uses the electromagnetic approach. A tiny magnet, no bigger than a grain of rice, is attached to the incudostapedial joint. The coil, which drives the magnet, is located in the ear canal in a conventional ear mold. The signal processor and microphone are located behind the ear (BTE) and are linked to the ear mold coil.

The magnet is placed in the incudostapedial joint through a transcanal approach. This approach may be performed under local anesthesia as an outpatient. The coil and ampli-

FIGURE 33-8

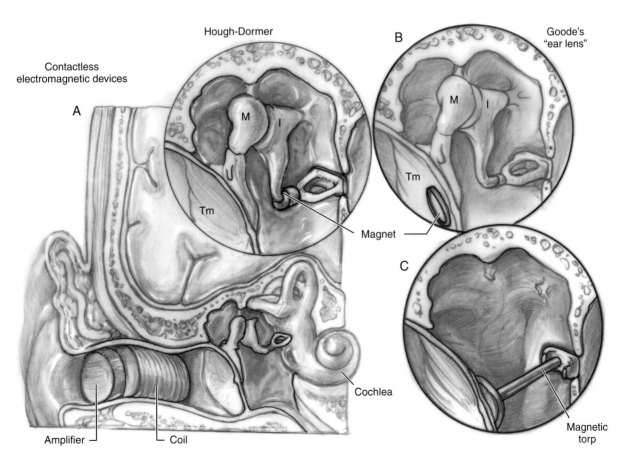

FIGURE 33–8. The Direct Drive Hearing System. A, Electromagnetic driver in ear canal. B, Magnet at incudostapedial joint or on tympanic membrane. C, Magnetic middle ear prosthesis. M = Malleus; I = incus; Tm = tympanic membrane.

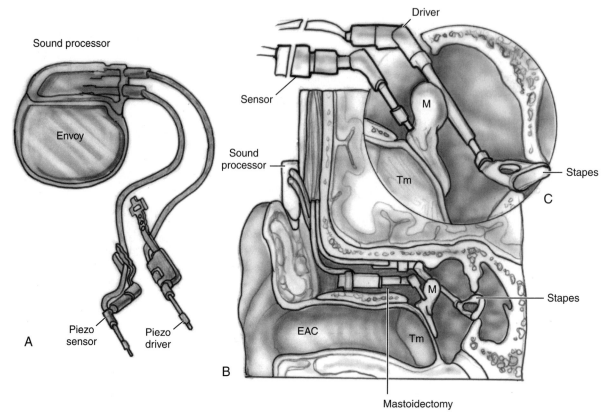

FIGURE 33–9. Envoy implant. *A,* Implant assembly. *B,* Coronal view showing position of transducer. *C,* Sensor attached to malleus, driver in contact with stapes. M = Malleus; Tm = tympanic membrane; EAC = external auditory canal.

fier are placed after complete healing has occurred. This device has been successfully tested in five patients, and the company has recently begun phase II clinical trials (Fig. 33–8).

Envoy

The Envoy has been developed by St. Croix Medical, Inc., of Minneapolis, Minnesota. It is a fully implantable system, which uses piezoelectric transducers consisting of two internal plates separated by a thin conduction material for reception and transduction. The first transducer detects movement of the malleus and responds to sound stimulation. The second piezoelectric transducer (the driver) is placed on the stapes. The piezoelectric units use the bimorph design for the sensor and the driver. One end of the sensor is fixed to the malleus to detect vibration, whereas the other is fixed to the skull cortical bone. A small amplifier in the base increases the gain. This fully implantable device contains a speech processor, powered by a lithium iodine battery (Fig. 33–9).

The device is implanted through a postauricular incision. A mastoidectomy is performed. The mastoid must be widely opened to allow adequate room in the attic area for the sensor and driver. A bed is created in the cortical bone

for the sound processor/battery module. The facial recess is opened to allow adequate visualization of the chorda tympani, facial nerve, and stapes. The bone of the posterior wall of the external auditory canal must be thinned carefully to expose the course of the chorda tympani nerve. The incudostapedial joint is severed and the long process of the incus is separated from the body. A large amount of space is created to allow the piezoelectric driver adequate space to vibrate through the facial recess area. If this is not accomplished, then full removal of the incus is necessary. The sensor may be attached to the malleus head or incus body.

The first device was implanted in March 2000 in Germany. There were no complications of the procedure. Results from this device are not yet known.

MET

The MET is a semi-implantable device produced by Otologics, LLC., of Boulder, Colorado. It consists of an external digital speech processor and an implanted unit. The external components consisting of a microphone, speech processor, battery, and transmitter are housed in a standard BTE hearing aid case. The implanted components consist of a subcutaneous electronic package with transcutaneous

TABLE 33–3. Audiometric Thresholds for the MET

THRESHOLD	FREQUENCY (kHz)					
	0.25	0.5	1	2	4	8
Lower limit	15	15	45	45	45	55
Upper limit	80	85	95	100	105	115

MET, Middle Ear Transducer system.

receiver and transducer motor in a hermetically sealed case. The electromagnetic motor drives a biocompatible probe tip, which is placed in a hole in the body of the incus. Activation of the device causes mechanical motion of the probe tip, which in turn vibrates the ossicular chain. The transducer was found to have a linear input–output curve to beyond 1000 dynes at 1 kHz. The response is linear, which is indicative of low distortion. The frequency response is relatively flat, varying only by about 10 dB and up to 10 kHz. See Table 33–3 for audiometric thresholds for the MET.

The device is placed in an outpatient procedure through a postauricular incision (Fig. 33–10). The initial procedure required an atticotomy, and that a view port be created. The attic area was opened to allow visualization of the ossicular chain. A mounting hole is then placed into the mastoid cortex, in which a mounting ring is placed. This secures the electromechanical motor. A seat is created to place the electronic housing and receiving coil. A laser-assisted fenestration is created in the incus body for the probe tip to rest. The procedure has recently been modified to allow a new mounting ring to be used, which is easier to place surgically. Six to 8 weeks after device placement, the external speech processor is attached and programmed. The patient is followed up to 3 and 6 months postimplantation.

The device has been placed in nine patients in the United States and five in Europe. There have been no complications from device placement, and all patients have received an auditory response. Results from this phase I trial are currently being compiled for FDA approval. There has been no sensorineural hearing loss or infection associated with placement of these devices. Phase II studies are expected to be started later this year.

RION

The RION was developed at Ehime University and Teikyo University in Japan, in collaboration with Rion Company. This device was developed by Dr. Yanagihara and colleagues more than 10 years ago and uses the piezoelectric transduction approach. This device is a partially implantable device, which consists of a microphone, speech

FIGURE 33-10

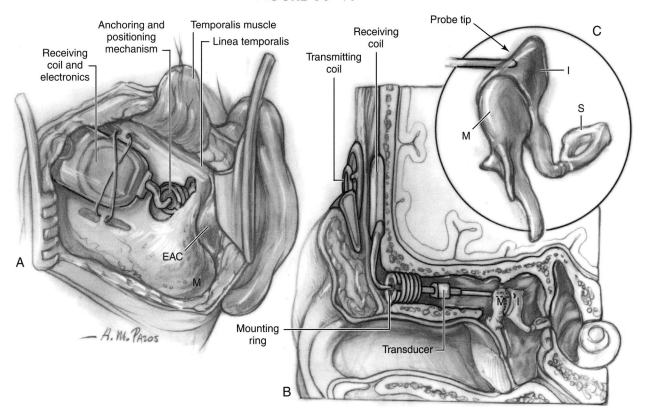

FIGURE 33–10. The Middle Ear Transducer system. A, Surgical view. B, Coronal view showing position of transducer. C, Probe tip seated in body of incus. EAC = External auditory canal; M = malleus; I = incus; S = stapes.

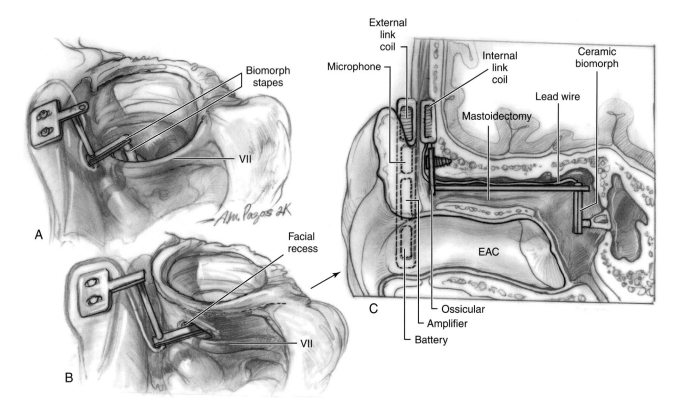

FIGURE 33–11. The RION system. *A*, Canal wall down mastoidectomy. *B*, Canal wall up mastoidectomy. *C*, Coronal cross section, canal wall up mastoidectomy. VII = Facial nerve; EAC = external auditory canal.

processor, and battery contained in an external BTE unit. The internal component consists of the ossicular vibrator and internal coil, which are coupled. The essential component is the vibrator element, consisting of a bimorph or two piezoelectric ceramic elements pasted together in opposite polarity and coated with layers of biocompatible material. The free end of the bimorph, attached to the stapes, vibrates in response to applied electrical voltage, and the ceramic bimorph is attached to a housing unit that is screwed into the mastoid cortex (Fig. 33–11).

The device is placed via postauricular incision. The device may be placed during canal wall down mastoidectomy for treatment of chronic ear disease or through a facial recess transmastoid approach. The cavity creation is the preferred method because it allows adequate exposure of the ossicles. The device is fixed to the mastoid cortex, and the bimorph container is placed over the stapes. A seat is created for the internal coil and electronic unit. With the canal wall down technique, the ear canal is closed off.

TABLE 33–4. Criteria for Selection of Candidates of the RION Device

- Average bone-conduction hearing level speech frequencies (500, 1000, 2000 Hz) do not exceed 50 dB.
- There is a moderate to severe deafness in the other ear.
- An intraoperative vibratory hearing test demonstrates the effectiveness of the unit.

The device has been primarily used for patients with conductive hearing loss from chronic otitis media. (See Table 33–4 for current criteria for selection of candidates for the RION.) Frequency responses are attenuated after approximately 5000 Hz; therefore, patients with sensorineural hearing loss may not receive as much benefit as those with conductive type of losses. The device has been implanted in Japan but is not currently available in the United States.

CONCLUSION

Multiple companies and researchers have worked diligently over the past several decades to develop the devices described within this chapter. Although there have been successes, this field must be considered in its infancy, and all of these devices should be considered investigational. Long-term results will not be known for many years. This field is developing rapidly, and further clinical trials will be conducted as the devices improve. The results from the current devices are encouraging, as patients are aware that these devices can be more beneficial than conventional air-conduction hearing aids. As signal processing improves, as battery devices become smaller, and as implantable microphones advance, so will performance of the devices.

References

1. Snik FM, Cremers WRJ: First audiometric results with the Vibrant Soundbridge, a semi-implantable hearing device for sensorineural hearing loss. Audiology 38: 335–338, 1999.

2. Fredrickson JM, Coticchia JM, Khosla S: Current status in the development of implantable middle ear hearing aids. *In* Advances in Otolaryngology, Vol 10. St. Louis, Mosby, 1996.

3. Miller DA, Fredrickson JM: Implantable hearing aids. *In* Valente M: Audiology Treatment. New York, Thieme, 2000, pp 489–510.

4. Hüttenbrink KB: Current status and critical reflections on implantable hearing aids. Am J Otol 20: 409–415, 1999.

5. Goode RL, Rosenbaum ML, Maniglia AJ: The history and development of the implantable hearing aid. Otolaryngol Clin North Am 28: 1–16, 1995.

6. Fredrickson JM, Coticchia JM, Khosla S: Ongoing investigations into an implantable electromagnetic hearing aid for moderate to severe sensorineural hearing loss. Otolaryngol Clin North Am 28: 107–120, 1995.

7. Goode RL: Current status and future of implantable electromagnetic hearing aids. Otolaryngol Clin North Am 28: 141–146, 1995.

8. Baker RS, Wood MW, Hough JVD: The implantable hearing device for sensorineural hearing impairment: The Hough Ear Institute experience. Otolaryngol Clin North Am 28: 147–153, 1995.

9. Chasin M: Current trends in implantable hearing aids. Trends Amplification 2: 84–104, 1997.

10. Update on Implant Technology, Part 2: Implantable Hearing Aids. Hearing Review, December 1999.

11. First Chronic Implant Performed. Envoy-Voices. St. Croix Medical, Minneapolis, Minnesota, March 2000.

34

The Bone-Anchored Hearing Aid

Anders Tjellström, M.D., Ph.D.

In spite of advances in middle ear reconstruction surgery, it is not possible to provide all patients with a dry ear and good hearing. Some patients need amplification. A conventional air-conduction aid is the most common choice, but some patients cannot or should not use such an aid. Bone-conduction transducers are sometimes the hearing aid of choice, but the disadvantages with the old-fashioned bone-conduction hearing aids are numerous. The sound quality is generally poor: the sound has to pass through soft tissue, and much of the sound energy is lost there. When the sound waves reach the skull bone they are transmitted with fairly low attenuation and distortion at least to the ipsilateral cochlea. The magnitude of the attenuation of the speech frequencies varies between 7 and 15 dB[1] and the greatest losses are in the important high-frequency range. The attenuation of the sound reaching the contralateral cochlea varies depending on the frequency, but there are also great interindividual differences. Due to the attenuation of the sound energy from the transducer to the inner ear, the old-fashioned bone-conduction hearing aid must be driven hard, raising the level of distortion. This problem is significant in patients with both conduction loss and cochlear dysfunction.

A direct coupling between the transducer and the skull without any soft tissue between is thus of great acoustic advantage. There are, however, other advantages with a direct coupling to the skull, namely, there is no discomfort due to the pressure of the transducer, the position of the hearing aid is stable, and no steel spring over the head, head bands, or heavy frames of glasses are needed.[2–7]

OSSEOINTEGRATION

The possibility of establishing and maintaining a direct anchorage of a hearing aid coupling to the bone of the mastoid process is based on the concept of osseointegration. The term *osseointegration* was coined by Professor Per-Ingvar Brånemark of Göteborg, Sweden in 1977 and is defined as "a direct contact between living bone and a loaded implant surface."[8, 9] Implants have been used for many years but primarily to stabilize fractures during healing. Under such circumstances, the choice of implant material is less important. For example, in orthopedic surgery, a plate and screws of different metals and alloys allow healing to take place. However, during healing, the patient is not allowed to load the fracture, which could lead to loss of implant stability and jeopardize fracture healing. When healing has been established, it is not important if the implant material is encapsulated in fibrous tissue. This does become a problem when a whole joint, for example,

a hip or a knee, has to be replaced. A zone of fibrous tissue between the implant and the bone will not stand a load in the long run. In the geriatric patient, this problem may be insignificant but in today's sport injuries in young and active patients, this is a larger problem.[10] In oral surgery, implants have been used in the treatment of patients with partial or total edentulousness for many years. The forces used during chewing could be very high (50 to 2000 N), and most implants used earlier became loose after loading.

Establishing Osseointegration

To achieve osseointegration the implant material requires careful consideration, as do several other factors, including the surgical technique, which is described in detail later. A combination of hardware and software is necessary for the operation to be successful.[11, 12]

Implant Material

The choice of implant material is important. The implant material used by the author is commercially pure titanium. This nonalloyed titanium has a purity of 99.75 per cent. The mechanical properties of this implant change even at very minor changes in its purity. One of the most common titanium implants used in surgery is an alloy called *Ti 6Al 4V*. This alloy consists of 90 per cent titanium, 6 per cent aluminum, and 4 per cent vanadium. It is possible to establish a direct contact between such an implant and living bone tissue, but the quality and the quantity of this contact are less than that of commercially pure titanium. The reason for these differences is not completely clear but probably involves aluminum ions leaking out from the implant into the tissue and competing with calcium ions at the interface. Local and general reactions of an implant material must be taken into consideration. Aluminum is known to be toxic to the central nervous system, an effect that is especially important to remember when an implant is placed in a young patient who could be expected to have his or her implant in the tissue for 60 to 80 years. Although no neoplastic changes have been reported, this possibility must be remembered when new implant materials are used in the aggressive environment of the bioliquid. The clinical follow-up with the commercially pure titanium implant material goes back to 1966.[8]

Implant Design

The implants used are screw shaped and have the same type of threads and the same diameter as the implants used by Brånemark intraorally. The implants come in two lengths, 3 and 4 mm, and have a flange that is 5.5 mm in diameter (Fig. 34–1). The rationale for having a threaded implant instead of a smooth one is to get a good initial stability. If the implant moves during healing, fibrous tissue instead of bone could result. The flange improves the initial stability but also acts as a protection against too deep penetration at the time of surgery or later if a direct trauma affects the skin-penetrating coupling.

Implant Surface

The surface of the implant has minor irregularities that improves the stability of the implant, especially against

FIGURE 34–1

FIGURE 34–2

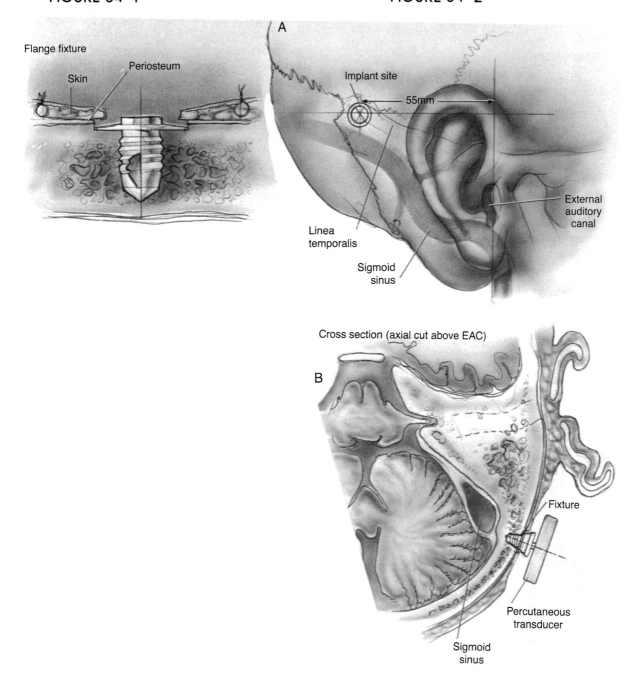

FIGURE 34–1. The flange fixture.

FIGURE 34–2. A and B, Optimal position of the implant to avoid acoustic feedback. EAC, external auditory canal.

shear forces. Perhaps an even more important point is to keep the implant surface free from foreign material. Because of the electrophysical properties of the oxide layer that covers the implant when it is machined, the surface is active and adheres to foreign material. Such foreign material could jeopardize osseointegration, even if these particles are sterile. Small metal fragments could give rise to electrical currents and induce fibrous tissue instead of bone. The surgeon and nurse must remember this during the different steps of the insertion of the implant.

Loading of the Implant

Originally, a two-stage procedure was used based on the experience from implant surgery in the oral cavity. However, the success rate with permanent implant stability in the mastoid process has been high and as the load to the implant is much less in the oral cavity, a one-stage procedure was introduced in 1989. The skin penetration was performed at the time of insertion but implants were not loaded until 2 to 3 months after surgery based on animal studies performed by Steinemann and coworkers.[13] During the last few years this time has been further reduced and the fitting of the hearing aid is today made 4 to 6 weeks after surgery. Animal studies have shown that immediately after insertion the stability is good but that it will go down during the first 3 weeks, at which time it will increase again. This is due to the fact that the inevitable tissue damage at surgery at that time has reached a maximum. The regeneration is taking over and will rapidly improve the bone quality and quantity. Our clinical experience supports these experimental data. In compromised tissue and in younger patients, 3 months between insertion and loading is still recommended.

PATIENT SELECTION

The indication for a bone-anchored hearing aid (BAHA) is the need for amplification in a patient who cannot be helped by reconstructive surgery and who cannot use an air-conduction hearing aid. There are two main groups that qualify for a BAHA: patients with chronic ear conditions and patients with bilateral external ear canal atresia. Patients with draining ears or ears that start to drain when the external ear canal is occluded with a hearing aid mold are suitable candidates. Many of these patients have a combined hearing impairment, and the better the inner ear function, the better the chances are for a good result. If the mean value for the bone conduction from 0.5 to 3 kHz is better than 45 dB and the speech discrimination score is better than 60 per cent, the chances that the patient will have satisfactory hearing are 89 per cent. As many patients have a maximum conductive loss of 60 dB, a hearing threshold of 105 dB can be helped. Patients with hearing close to the 45 dB level bone conduction are told that they probably could use the standard ear level device called the *HC 300 Classic*. However, a stronger hearing aid called *Cordelle* is available. This is a hearing aid with a strong transducer fitted with a snap coupling to a specially de-

signed body aid. Patients with a bone conduction down to 60 dB could use this aid.[14–16]

Patients with bilateral atresia often have normal or near-normal cochlear function and are the ideal patients for the BAHA. Reconstructive atresia surgery is difficult, and in patients with a Jahrsdoerfer rating of 7 or worse, we often suggest a BAHA instead of reconstructive trials.[17] One advantage with the BAHA is that it will not interfere with atresia surgery later on. The author has treated children as young as 2 years of age. When these children grow up, an evaluation of their anatomy can be made, as can the final decision about atresia surgery. The BAHA could also be used in patients with special problems, for example, patients with severe otosclerosis in the only hearing ear, patients with occlusion problems, patients with external otitis, and those who react against all different materials used for ear molds.

Patient selection is of special importance for fitting with a BAHA. The patient must have realistic expectations and be aware that the BAHA has limitations. The patient should also be able to come to regular outpatient follow-up visits and should be able to take care of the skin penetration. Because one of the main reasons for adverse skin reactions is inadequate hygiene, the need to have a high level of personal hygiene must be stressed preoperatively.

Age is not a contraindication per se. The oldest patient operated on was 82, and the youngest, 2 years of age. Psychiatric disease is considered the only contraindication, and when in doubt, a psychiatric consultation is helpful.

PREOPERATIVE EVALUATION

During the preoperative evaluation, a general ear, nose, and throat examination, audiologic testing with sound thresholds, and speech audiometry are included. In children with congenital malformations, a high-resolution computed tomographic scan is done to evaluate the level of the middle cranial fossa, the position of the sigmoid sinus, and whether the facial nerve has an abnormal route. In patients with chronic ear disease, no radiologic examination is made routinely. Even radical surgery does not interfere with the position of the implant for the hearing aid. Because the skin penetration should be in a hairless area, the skin over the mastoid process is examined. If hair follicles are present, the patient is informed that these will be removed at a radius of about 20 mm. The patient is also informed that a subcutaneous tissue reduction will be performed.

The patient must be informed about the procedure and what it means to have a skin-penetrating implant. The patient is told that he or she must come to regular follow-up visits. The importance of personal hygiene must also be stressed, especially in patients with greasy skin or seborrhea. However, these conditions and others, like psoriasis and eczema, are not considered as contraindications.[18]

A simple way to give the patient a general idea of how the BAHA will sound is to use the "test rod," a plastic rod with a hearing aid coupling glued to one end of the rod. The patient is asked to take the rod between the teeth, and the BAHA is attached to the coupling. To avoid acoustic feedback, the patient must close the lips around the rod. If the patient does not have teeth or dentures secured to osseointegrated implants, the rod can be pressed against the skin over the mastoid process. This method, however, is not as good as using the teeth. Another way to evaluate if a BAHA is a good solution for a patient is to provide him or her with an old-fashioned bone-conduction hearing aid for a couple of weeks. The patient is asked to evaluate only the sound quality and to not pay any attention to discomfort or the size of the equipment. If the patient is satisfied with the sound, the chances are good that he or she will be satisfied with the BAHA.

In patient counseling, it is also stressed that if he or she is sure of the decision and has been provided with a BAHA but for any reason does not like the arrangement, it is easy to return to the original situation before surgery. Patients may also use the BAHA in combination with other aids if they wish.

SURGICAL TREATMENT

Preoperative Preparation

The surgical procedure is simple and is generally performed under local anesthesia as an outpatient procedure.[11, 19] In children, general anesthesia is used. No antibiotics or steroids are used. The patient is placed on the operating table in the same way as for any type of ear surgery. Before the draping is made, the implant site is marked according to Figure 34–2. This marking should be made before the external ear is folded anteriorly, because the hearing aid must not touch the pinna and cause acoustic feedback. The preoperative preparation is also the same as for any other ear surgery using a postauricular approach. The patient is shaved in the posterosuperior area behind the ear a radius of 30 mm from the implant site. The field is cleaned with 70 per cent alcohol. In patients with congenital malformation, the mastoid process is outlined with surgical ink, and the expected route of the facial nerve is marked. If there is no external ear canal and the patient may be a future candidate for an auricular prosthesis retained on implants, the site for the hearing aid implant should be about 55 mm behind the anticipated external ear meatus. It is often advantageous to place the implant in the linea temporalis because the bone here is normally fairly thick. Above the linea temporalis, the bone over the middle cranial dura may be thin, especially in malformed children. Below the linea temporalis, air cells are often close to the cortical surface. In the patient with chronic otitis media, this is seldom a problem because of the reduced pneumatization of the mastoid process. In patients who have had radical surgery, the cavity is more anterior and will not interfere with the implant site. After the patient and the implant site are cleaned and draped, the area is covered with an adhesive plastic film to prevent even sterile particles from cloth from entering the implant site, which could jeopardize osseointegration. The author prefers using magnifying lenses over the otomicroscope because this method makes it easier to find the exact axis of direction for the different steps of the procedure.

Special Instruments

The instruments used consist of general surgical instruments and instruments specially designed for this implant surgery, including a drill machine with high- and low-speed functions as well as a feature to reverse the direction of rotation. The torque can also be adjusted. The instruments and the implants and the sound processors are produced by Eutipic Medical Systems AB, Göteborg, Sweden.

Standard Instruments

The standard instruments listed are placed by the scrub nurse on a sterile draped Mayo stand and consist of

5 Mosquito clamps
1 Mayo scissors
1 Curved scissors, small
1 Adson forceps
1 Needle holder
2 Bard-Parker blades
2 Skin hooks, small
2 Self-retaining retractors, small
1 Raspatory
1 Periosteal elevator

Special Instruments

The special instruments are made of either stainless steel or titanium. It is of utmost importance that these instruments are not mixed.

The stainless steel instruments are

Raspatory
Dissector
Open-ended wrench for fixture mount
Wrench for hearing aid coupling
Cylinder wrench
Screwdriver
Hexagon screwdriver
Screwdriver for hearing aid coupling
Connection to handpiece
Punch
Bowl

The titanium instruments are

Titanium organizer
Cleaning needle
Forceps
Fixture mount
Bowl

The drilling equipment consists of

Control unit with stand and foot control
Motor for high and low speeds
Shank and head

The control unit is draped with a sterile plastic bag and the motor and its cord are covered with a plastic tube.

The drills and screw taps are sterile-packed and disposable to guarantee maximum sharpness and to avoid the time-consuming cleaning procedure used earlier.

The components used are guide drills with fixed depth to 3 and 4 mm. The implants used are a flange fixture, 3 or 4 mm, and a hearing aid abutment for the sound processor. The abutment is secured to the flange fixture with an internal screw. During the healing period, a healing cap is used.

Surgical Technique

The different steps of the surgical procedure are illustrated in Figure 34–3.[11, 19] When the implant site has been marked and the surgical field draped with the plastic sheet, 10 ml of local anesthesia is injected. The author prefers 2 per cent lidocaine (Xylocaine) with adrenalin. Some of the local anesthesia should be put underneath the periosteum to get perfect anesthesia for the drilling. A U-shaped incision about 20 mm in diameter is made down to the periosteum. At the intended implant site a 6-mm-wide hole is made in the periosteum and the bone surface is exposed. The 3-mm guide drill is attached to the head of the drill, and the switch on the motor is turned to high speed, which is also indicated on the control unit. The drill speed is 1500 to 2000 rpm. During all drilling, cooling with room temperature saline is used to avoid unnecessary tissue damage. When the guide drills, which are 1.8 mm in diameter, are used, the hole is widened about 2.5 to 3.0 mm. The reasons for this step are that the surgeon gets a better view into the bottom of the hole, the irrigation will reach the site where the cutting takes place, and less bone has to be cut away when the final dimension is established with the countersink. If there is bone at the bottom of the hole when the fixed depth of the 3-mm guide drill is all the way down, the short guide drill is changed to the 4-mm guide drill. The flange of the guide drill must be down to the bony surface because the countersink is not sharp at its tip. Therefore, if there is soft tissue at the bottom, such as the wall of the sigmoid sinus or the dura of the middle cranial fossa, the hole could still be used for the implant. The next step is to change the drill countersink to the appropriate length. The drill speed is still 1500 to 2000 rpm, and generous cooling is imperative. The drill should be moved up and down, and the grooves at the side of this spiral drill should be cleaned several times during the drilling. The bone cut away will be collected in these grooves, and when they are filled with bone, the cutting will be reduced and a lot of heat produced. During this phase of the procedure, the final direction of the implant will be established. The implant should be perpendicular to the surface. If it becomes too oblique, there is a risk that the sound processor will touch the skin and cause acoustic feedback.

The hole is now ready for the tapping procedure, which is performed at low speed, 8 to 15 rpm. The low-speed mode will be available by turning the switch on the motor. When the low-speed mode is used, the torque can be adjusted on the control unit, as indicated on its window. A torque of 40 Ncm is suggested for the standard procedure. In children and in patients with soft and thin bone, 20 Ncm should be used. The exact speed is adjusted by the surgeon through the foot control. The 3- or 4-mm titanium tap is taken from its sterile glass tubing and put into the organizer without being touched with the gloved hand or with any nontitanium instruments. It could be poured into the titanium tray and transferred to its place in the organizer with the titanium forceps. The connection to the hand piece, which is made out of stainless steel and thus could be handled in the normal way, is attached to the hand piece of the motor. The tap is then picked up with the adaptor, which has a spring arrangement that will keep the tap in place. The tap is kept over the implant site, and the motor is started at a low speed. When the correct direction is established, the tap is gently pressed down into the hole. Simultaneous irrigation is essential. When the tap starts to move down, no further pressure is needed because the tap will find its own way. If the tap is stuck before coming to the bottom of the hole, the direction was not correct, and the motor is reversed by use of the knob on the control unit. When the tap is up, the direction is corrected and the tapping is made. If the tap gets stuck several times, a new implant site nearby is prepared. When the tap is removed by reversing the motor, the motor should not be lifted by its shank and head, as the tap could be dislodged.

The implant site is now ready for the implant, the flange fixture, which also comes sterilely packed in a glass cylinder. The fixture is put in the organizer without being contaminated by any nontitanium instrument. The fixture mound is lifted up with the open-ended wrench and secured to the fixture with the internal screw and screwdriver. The hexagon on the top of the fixture must be properly fitted into the hexagonal indentation of the fixture mount. If there is good cortical bone at the implant site, the screw of the fixture mount is tightened more than if the bone is thin and soft. The fixture mount, with the fixture, is picked up with the connection of the hand piece attached to the motor. The implant is kept over the implant site, and the engine is started on low speed. When the correct direction has been established, the fixture will find its way down without any pressure. The implant site should be empty when this part of the procedure is started. Irrigation should not start until the small notches at the tip of the fixture have entered the implant site so that the hole is not filled with saline. As the flange of the implant is coming close to the bone surface, the speed is reduced to get a gentle stop and to avoid damage to the threads in the bone. This step is especially important if the bone is soft. The cylinder wrench is used to manually check that the implant is securely fastened. However, this has to be done with utmost care because large forces could be produced due to the cantilever effect.

If the fixture is stable, the skin-penetrating abutment is connected directly. If it is not stable, 3 to 4 months are allowed for osseointegration to take place without any load to the implant. In most cases, the implant site is under hair-bearing skin; the coupling should penetrate skin without any hair follicles, and these should be removed from the flap. To establish a reaction-free skin penetration, the skin around the implant must not move in relation to the implant. To achieve this, a subcutaneous tissue reduction is made by use of sharp blades and skin hooks. The amount of tissue that should be removed varies among patients, but the aim is to ensure that the edges of the field around the implant site slope gently down. There should be no steps or steep slopes down to the percutaneous coupling of the sound processor. The flap is thinned as much as possible and should look almost like it had been prepared with a dermatome. The flap is folded back over the fixture and

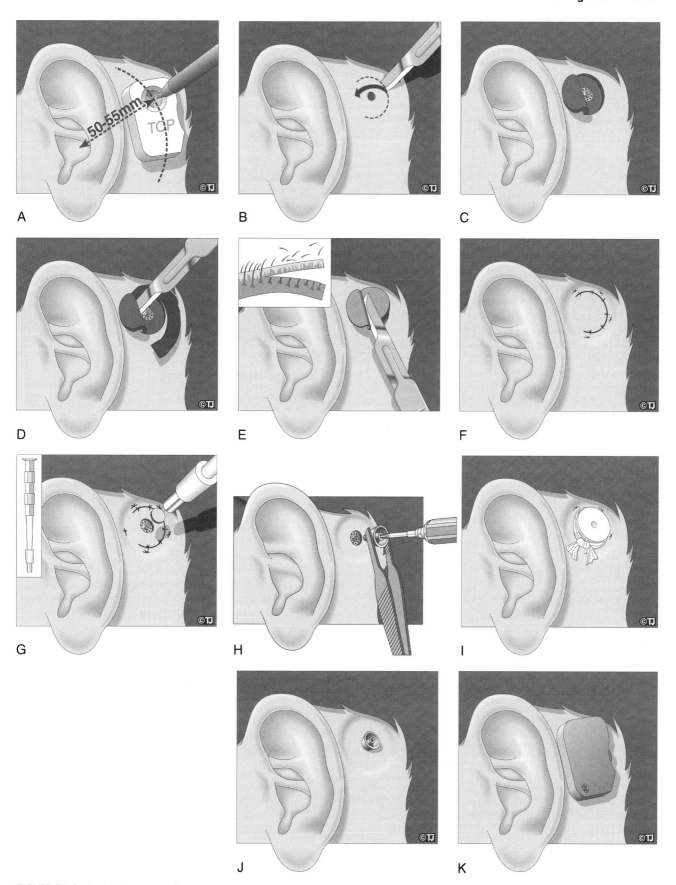

FIGURE 34–3. *A* to *K,* The steps of the surgical procedure.

kept in place with 6-0 nylon monofilament. A hole is punched in the flap for the hearing aid coupling, the abutment. The abutment with its internal screw comes sterilely packed. The abutment is picked up with a "gold" screwdriver, and is secured to the fixture. A wrench is used to reduce torque on the fixture. Finally, a healing cap is snapped onto the abutment. This cap will keep an ointment-soaked gauze down to eliminate bleeding and postoperative hematoma. An ordinary mastoid dressing with light pressure is used for 1 day. After that, only a small, light draping is necessary.

POSTOPERATIVE CARE

The day after surgery, the mastoid draping is thus removed and replaced by a light bandage, a "black patch." Five to 7 days after surgery, the patient comes back for the first dressing. The healing cap is tilted off and the gauze is removed. The area is cleaned carefully and left open for about 30 minutes. The healing cap is then put back in place, and a new ointment-soaked gauze is wound under the cap. After another 6 to 7 days, the healing cap is removed and the stitches taken out. The patient is then asked to clean the area gently with soap and water and also to use some of the same ointment once a day for a couple of weeks. When healing is completed, the patient is informed about the importance of good personal hygiene and instructed to use soap and water. If a slight irritation occurs, the patient is told to use the ointment prescribed. Having a skin-penetrating abutment will not stop the patient from taking a sauna or from dyeing or perming the hair. Of course, it is possible to go swimming and diving with the implant. The sound processor, however, must be removed! In Figure 34–4 a schematic drawing of the arrangement, including the assembly tool, is presented.

PITFALLS IN SURGERY

The surgical procedure is simple, and since its start in 1977 and after, more than 3000 implants in the mastoid process, including implants for retention of auricular prostheses, no

serious complication has been experienced by the author. In about 10 per cent of cases, the wall of the sigmoid sinus is identified at the bottom of the implant site. In a few cases, the wall has been injured, and slight bleeding has occurred. This condition, however, is easy to control. If the damage occurs within 2 mm, the site is plugged with a piece of periosteum, and another site is identified close by. If the damage occurs at the final 0.5 mm, the hole is widened and threaded, and an implant is put in place. The dura mater of the middle cranial fossa is sometimes seen but seldom damaged. Having the dura at the bottom of the implant site is not considered a contraindication for placing a fixture in that site. In the well-pneumatized mastoid process, air cells are sometimes entered. If the bone is good, contact with an air cell will not call for any special precaution, and the site can often be used. If the amount of bone is small, another implant site is looked for; good cortical bone for a 4-mm fixture may be available within a couple of millimeters. Suction in a site that is in contact with an air cell should be avoided, however, because this situation may lead to a fast retraction of the drum and could be uncomfortable.

SOUND PROCESSOR

Six to 8 weeks after surgery, the patient is fitted with the sound processor. Three sound processors are available, but their basic design is the same, and a schematic drawing is seen in Figure 34–5. The main advantage with this direct percutaneous coupling between the bone and the transducer is that the gap between the two components of the transducer can be kept short (50 μm). Because of the suspension arrangement, this distance will also be constant. Less power is needed, which means higher output and lower distortion. For a detailed description of the sound processor, a paper by Håkansson and associates[2] from 1990 is recommended. The standard sound processor is the HC 300 Classic (Fig. 34–6), which is an ear-level hearing aid that can be used by most patients with a bone conduction threshold of 45 dB pure tone average (PTA) for the speech frequencies (0.5 to 3 kHz) or better. The stronger Cordelle (Fig. 34–7)

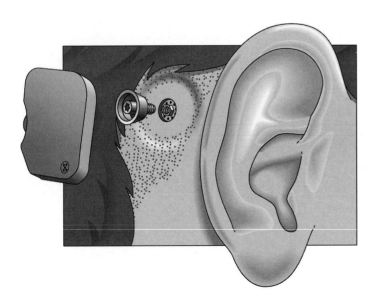

FIGURE 34–4. Schematic drawing of arrangement with fixture in the bone, skin-penetrating snap coupling and sound processor.

FIGURE 34-5

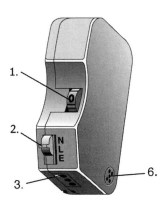

FIGURE 34–5. The principal design of the transducer. Note the small gap between the two components of the transducer and the suspension arrangement, important for the signal flux.

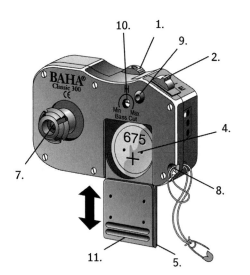

1. Volume control, on/off
2. Tone switch
3. Electrical input
4. Battery compartment
5. Battery cover
6. Microphone
7. Abutment snap
8. Attachment for safety line
9. Gain control (gain is factory preset)
10. Tone control (bass cut)
11. Serial number

FIGURE 34–6. Bone-anchored hearing aid (BAHA) Classic 300. (Courtesy of Eutipic Medical Systems AB, Göteborg, Sweden.)

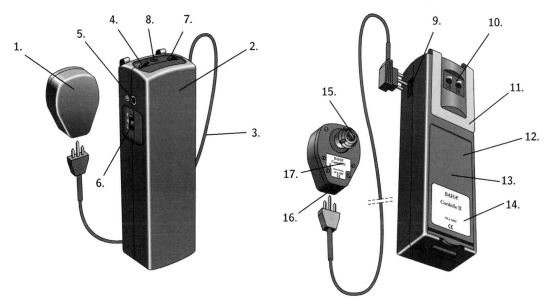

1. Transducer
2. Body worn unit
3. Cord
4. M-MT-T switch
5. Electrical input
6. Tone switch
7. Volume control
8. Microphone
9. Electrical output
10. Trim controls
11. Clip
12. Battery cover
13. Battery compartment
14. Serial number
15. Abutment snap
16. Electrical input
17. Serial number

FIGURE 34–7. Schematic drawing of the Cordelle transducer (1), sound processor (2), and rechargeable battery (3). (Courtesy of Eutipic Medical Systems AB, Göteborg, Sweden.)

is a transducer that is driven through a specially designed body aid. Patients with hearing losses as low as 60 dB for bone conduction could use this device. A BiCROS with a microphone and a telecoil function is available.

Fitting of the Soundprocessor

An improved snap coupling as illustrated in Figure 34–4 is currently used instead of the bayonet coupling. No plastic insert or O-ring is needed. This snap coupling is more stable and also gives a better transfer of the signals from the BAHA to the skull. Many patients report an improved "clarity" of the sound. No parts have to be changed with the passage of time. The audiologist can adjust the settings on the BAHA according to the patient's hearing loss and personal preferences.

RESULTS

The results in patients equipped with a BAHA were published in detail as a supplement of *Annals of Otology* by Håkansson and colleagues.[14] When direct bone conduction is compared with conventional bone conduction, the improvement for pure tones varies from 5 to 20 dB, depending on the frequency as seen in Figure 34–8. In objective testing, the speech discrimination score measured in noise improves from 50 to 71 per cent in patients who have been using a conventional bone-conduction hearing aid. In patients who had been wearing an air-conduction aid, the improvement was from 50 to 60 per cent. Many patients claimed that there was improved clarity of the sound that is hard to demonstrate in objective tests. In a questionnaire, 89 per cent of the patients with a level of bone conduction better than 45 dB and a speech discrimination score better than 60 per cent reported improved hearing.[20] Four per cent reported worse hearing, and 7 per cent,

no difference between the old aid and the BAHA. The level of comfort was also high: comfort improved in 95 per cent, was worse in 3 per cent, and was no different in 2 per cent. One of the main advantages expressed by patients with chronic ear conditions was that the drainage from the ear had diminished or disappeared. Another way to evaluate the efficacy of a hearing aid is to determine how many hours per day patients are using the aid. When a group of patients was asked this question, 94 per cent stated that they used it more than 8 hours a day. This could be compared with a study by Ovegård and Ramström who found that only 14 per cent of those patients fitted with a conventional air-conduction hearing aid used it more than 8 hours a day.[21] Another important advantage reported by patients with chronic ear conditions who had been using air-conduction aids is that the external ear meatus was no longer occluded, and the drainage from the ear canal stopped with the BAHA.

COMPLICATIONS AND MANAGEMENT

Skin

Maintaining reaction-free skin penetration over years is an important consideration with this type of hearing aid. As mentioned earlier, the reduction of subcutaneous tissue is essential and is the responsibility of the surgeon. The patient is responsible for the daily care. A high level of hygiene is important, and the patient is told to clean the implant area with soap and water regularly. In some patients, this means every day, in others, every second, third, or fourth day. The frequency depends on the general properties of the skin. A patient with greasy skin or seborrhea must be more active than an individual with dry skin free of sebaceous glands. The patient should have mild antibiotic ointment available at home in case of temporary irritation. If irritation occurs, the patient is instructed to intensify the general level of hygiene and use the ointment. If the irritation persists for a couple of days, the patient should get in touch with the treatment team. One reason for a temporary irritation is that an abutment screw that keeps the coupling secured to the flange fixture has unscrewed itself and needs tightening. These minor movements can be hard to detect without an otomicroscope. Such a loose screw can be tightened with the "gold" screwdriver and the wrench as a counterforce without any local anesthesia. If granulation tissue develops, it has to be removed and its cause investigated as described earlier. The removal is often easy with a sterile dental floss or a knife. A healing cap could be temporally placed on the coupling and a gauze with an appropriate antibiotic ointment put in place and kept for several days. In only one of more than 350 patients operated on by the author, the abutment had to be removed because of adverse soft tissue reaction.

In a study based on 1739 observations made at 6-month intervals between 1977 and 1989, no adverse skin reaction occurred in 92.5 per cent of those observations. Seventy-five per cent of the patients never had had an episode of skin reaction around the implant during the same time. A small group (4 per cent) of the patients were responsible

FIGURE 34–8

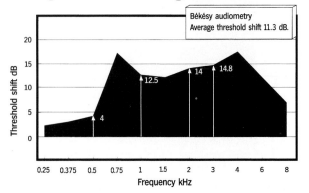

Improved hearing threshold

FIGURE 34–8. The threshold shift with and without skin penetration using Békésy audiometry. (Courtesy of Eutipic Medical Systems AB, Göteborg, Sweden.)

for more than 50 per cent of the reactions. This low frequency of adverse skin reactions has been confirmed in a recent follow-up study.[22]

A sensation of pain when the implant is touched is almost always an indication that something is loose. A loose coupling can, but will not always, cause pain. If the fixture has lost its integration, pain will almost always occur for one or more days before the implant comes out. The risk of losing an implant because of loss of integration is in the range of 2 to 4 per cent over time. Such a loss may occur before the sound processor has been fitted but may also occur as late as 10 years after insertion. Direct trauma is another cause of implant loss. In the author's series of more than 1000 patients, not a single case of osteomyelitis has been diagnosed, and there has been no other serious complication of any kind.

Hearing

A deterioration of function could result from three different causes: the patient's hearing may have diminished, the coupling arrangement between the sound processor and the bone may not function as it is supposed to, and a dysfunction of the sound processor may occur.

Patient Hearing

It is a well-known fact that as a patient gets older, the hearing gets worse, especially in the high-frequency range. A draining ear may also influence cochlear function in a negative way. Ototoxic drugs are a third hazard to inner ear function. These are some of the causes the surgeon should remember when a patient is reporting that a BAHA is not working as it used to do. Regular hearing tests are recommended for these patients.

Coupling Between Sound Processor and Bone

With the current snap coupling, one reason for suboptimal function has been eliminated because the plastic insert and O-ring are no longer needed. However, if the screw that keeps the coupling secured to the fixture has become loose, the patient may experience this as a deterioration of hearing. As mentioned earlier, a loose coupling could also result in skin irritation. If this occurs, the screws should be tightened. If the fixture has lost its osseointegration, this condition can result in decreased efficacy, but there is almost always pain associated with touching or shaking the coupling. If the flange fixture has lost its integration, the chance that it will be integrated once again is small, even if the coupling is removed and the fixture is left without any load. The insertion of a new implant is the solution to this problem.

Defect Sound Processor

The defect sound processor is a third alternative. There is a skull simulator, an artificial mastoid, available to test the sound processor, and it is a most helpful instrument in determining the reason for a deterioration of function. The

longevity for these hearing aids seems to be the same as for conventional hearing aids, ranging from 3 to 5 years.

SUMMARY

Osseointegration has been defined as a direct contact between living bone and a loaded implant surface. Establishment of a lasting anchorage of a titanium implant in the mastoid process has proved to be a safe and simple method for attaching a BAHA. It is also possible to establish and maintain a reaction-free skin penetration over many years. Of more than 1700 observations of skin reactions around the implant, less than 8 per cent had any irritation and less than 4 per cent needed active treatment. Seventy-five per cent of the patients had never had a single episode of adverse skin reaction. The cochlear function should not be worse than 45 dB for the ear-level device and not worse than 60 dB for the body aid. The degree of conductive loss added to the bone threshold is of no significance.

The BAHA is suggested as an alternative in selected hearing-impaired patients in whom reconstructive surgery has been unsuccessful or is contraindicated and in whom a conventional air-conduction hearing aid could not or should not be used.

References

1. Brandt A: On sound transmission characteristics of the human skull in vivo. Thesis, Technical report No 61L, Göteborg, Sweden: School of Electrical Engineering, Chalmers University of Technology, 1989.
2. Håkansson B, Tjellström A, Carlsson P: Percutaneous versus transcutaneous transducers for hearing by direct bone conduction. Otolaryngol Head Neck Surg 102: 339–344, 1990.
3. Håkansson B, Tjellström A, Rosenhall U: Hearing thresholds with direct bone conduction versus conventional bone conduction. Scand Audiol 13: 3–13, 1984.
4. Håkansson B, Carlsson P, Tjellström A: The mechanical point impedance of the human head, with and without skin penetration. J Acoust Soc Am 80: 1065–1075, 1986.
5. Carlsson P, Håkansson B, Rosenhall U, Tjellström A: A speech reception threshold test in noise with the bone-anchored hearing aid: A comparative study. Otolaryngol Head Neck Surg 94: 421–426, 1986.
6. Tjellström A: Percutaneous implants in clinical practice. Crit Rev Biocompatibility 1: 205–228, 1985.
7. Håkansson B, Tjellström A, Rosenhall U: Acceleration levels and threshold with direct bone conduction versus conventional bone conduction. Acta Otolaryngol (Stockh) 100: 240–252, 1985.
8. Brånemark PI, Hansson B, Adell R: Osseointegration in the treatment of the edentulous jaw: Experience from a 10-year period. Scand J Plast Reconstr Surg 16: 1–132, 1977.
9. Brånemark PI: Introduction to osseointegration. In Brånemark PI, Zarb G, Albrektsson T (eds): Tissue-integrated Prostheses. Chicago, Quintessence Publishing, 1985, pp 11–76.
10. Albrektsson T, Albrektsson B: Osseointegration of bone implants. Acta Orthop Scand 58: 567–577, 1987.
11. Tjellström A: Osseointegrated systems and their application in the head and neck. Adv Otolaryngol Head Neck Surg 3: 39–70, 1989.
12. Jacobsson M, Tjellström A: Clinical application of percutaneous implants, in high performance biomaterials. In Szycher M (ed): A Comprehensive Guide to Medical and Pharmaceutical Applications, Lancaster, Basel, Technomic, 1991, pp 207–229.
13. Steinemann SG, Eulenberger J, Maesuli PA, et al: Adhesion of bone to titanium. In Christel P, Munier A, Lee AJC (eds): Biological and Biomechanical Performance of Biomaterials. Amsterdam, Elsevier, 1986, pp 409–414.
14. Håkansson B, Lidén G, Tjellström A, et al: Ten years of experience of the Swedish bone anchored hearing system. Ann Otol Rhinol Laryngol Suppl 99: 1–16, 1990.

15. Abramson M, Fay TH, Kelly JP, et al: Clinical results with a percutaneous bone-anchored hearing aid. Laryngoscope 99: 707–710, 1989.

16. Mylanus EAM, van den Pouw CTM, Snik AFM, et al: An intraindividual comparison of the BAHA and air-conduction hearing aids. Arch Otolaryngol Head Neck Surg 124: 271–276, 1998.

17. Jahrsdoerfer RA, Yeakley JW, Aguilar EA, et al: Grading system for the selection of patients with congenital aural atresia. Am J Otol 13: 6–12, 1992.

18. Holgers K-M, Bjursten LM, Thomsen P, et al: Experience with percutaneous titanium implants in the head and neck: A clinical histological study. Invest Surg 2: 7–16, 1989.

19. Tjellström A: Surgery for the bone-anchored hearing aid. Göteborg Medical Service, Video Library, No 17/87, 1987.

20. Tjellström A, Jacobsson M, Norvell B, et al: Patient attitudes to the bone-anchored hearing aid: Results of a questionnaire study. Scand Audiol 18: 119–123, 1989.

21. Ovegård A, Ramström BB: Individual follow-up of hearing aid fitting. Scand Audiol 23: 57–63, 1994.

22. Reyes R, Tjellström A, Granström G: Evaluation of implant losses and skin reactions around extraoral bone-anchored implants: A zero- to eight-year follow-up report. Otolaryngol Head Neck Surg 122: 272–276, 2000.

35

Endolymphatic Sac Procedures

Michael M. Paparella, M.D.

Endolymphatic sac surgery for Ménière's disease has been used for more than 73 years. The objective of this operation is to preserve and, if possible, enhance labyrinthine function. Most surgical series demonstrate clinically significant control of vestibular symptoms, including vertigo. The operation has been used successfully to preserve cochlear function and to improve cochlear symptoms. The physiologic role of the endolymphatic sac in normal labyrinthine function has yet to be established, as has the physiologic basis for successful control of symptoms of intractable Ménière's disease by use of endolymphatic sac surgery, although objective and subjective evidence accumulate. Endolymphatic sac surgery offers a patient who has failed medical control of Ménière's disease a nonablative surgical procedure that in most cases results in elimination or control of vertiginous spells, preservation of hearing, and sometimes improvement of hearing along with improvement of other associated labyrinthine symptoms.

Since it was first described in 1927, endolymphatic sac surgery has stood the test of time.[1, 2] This operation, described in all textbooks of otolaryngology, is practiced widely in the United States and throughout the world by leading otologic surgeons, some of whom have very large series. It is the only conservative, nondestructive form of surgery that avoids invasion of the labyrinth. Other procedures commonly done today are destructive either to the peripheral labyrinth or to the vestibular nerve. Logically, any procedure that invades the labyrinth will cause a higher postoperative incidence of labyrinthine dysfunction and deafness. The endolymphatic sac is not part of the labyrinth and exists anterior to Trautmann's triangle within the dura, medial and inferior to the posteroinferior semicircular canal, in a remote location, with communication to the labyrinth via the vestibular aqueduct.

Controversy exists about all methods of treating Ménière's disease, both medical and surgical (including destructive and conservative methods). Indeed, on both philosophic and medical grounds, operations designed to destroy an organ or its parts (irreversible) are more controversial than conservative ones. Opinions regarding diagnosis and treatment of this disease were even stronger in 1861, the year Ménière described this syndrome, and although opinions vary to date, much understanding has developed and more agreement now exists regarding management than existed in those early years.

Endolymphatic sac surgery is now the most commonly done operation for Ménière's disease in the United States and worldwide, with large series having been established by leading otologists. Silverstein[3] sent a questionnaire regarding vestibular nerve section to members of the Otological and Neurotological Society and found that fewer than 3000 nerve sections had been done by all of the members. The majority (approximately two thirds) consider endolymphatic sac surgery a primary procedure, whereas a smaller number consider vestibular nerve section a primary procedure, even though the questionnaire was directed toward vestibular nerve section. Morrison, in England, has performed more than 2000 endolymphatic sac procedures for Ménière's disease (personal communication, 1992). Huang, a leading otologist in Asia, has performed more than 2500 sac procedures (personal communication, 1999), and Plester and Portmann also have large series (personal communications, 1992 and 1992). Many centers and individuals in the United States, including the author, have series in excess of 1000 or 2000 cases.

A study by Bretlau and associates[4] has received attention. They compared the results of sac surgery in 15 patients with the results in patients receiving a "sham" operation. In this small series, numerous questions arise, including criteria for selection of patients, techniques employed, and multiple surgeons.[5] Their findings were interpreted as being statistically flawed by Pillsbury and colleagues[6] and by four other statisticians of whom the author is aware. The author experienced more than 100 cases before considering publication, and before a sense of comfort and confidence was achieved for favorable short- and long-term results.

It is understandable that endolymphatic sac surgery is done more commonly than destructive procedures. One important reason is that Ménière's disease is bilateral in at least one in three cases, more likely closer to one of every two cases, according to Stahle and coworkers.[7] The author has encountered too many patients in whom Ménière's disease has caused deafness in one ear and then later, vertigo and deafness in the second ear. The author has also seen the tragedy of patients who have had surgical treatment resulting in deafness in one ear who would then develop Ménière's disease and deafness in the second ear at a later date.

Perhaps the ultimate trust in, and application of, this procedure is based on its ability to treat a patient who has Ménière's disease in an only-hearing ear that is in the process of developing profound hearing loss, dizziness, or both. Studies by the author on the natural history of Ménière's disease suggest that once the progressive form develops, there is an approximate 20 per cent chance that the patient will develop a profound or severe loss or even complete deafness. The author has reluctantly, but successfully, used endolymphatic sac surgery to treat the only-hearing ear in patients with Ménière's disease in 24 patients to date. It was surprising to find that many other leading otologists have a larger experience in this regard. Pulec described endolymphatic sac surgery for an only-hearing ear.[8] To date, Morrison has safely and successfully performed sac surgery in more than 100 patients with only-hearing ears.[9] Huang has performed surgery in 30 cases (personal communication, 1999), and Plester has done the same in approximately 15 cases of only-hearing ears (personal communication, 1992).

Certainly, otologists who recommend destructive surgery as a primary modality would never consider such a procedure in an only-hearing ear. An obvious question is: If endolymphatic sac surgery is useful to preserve hearing as a last-step measure, why would it not be considered earlier in the disease or preferably on the first ear involved? Because patients are seen in whom Ménière's disease and a severe hearing loss or deafness have developed in the second ear, it is conservative and prudent to do everything possible to preserve hearing in the first ear involved.

The wide application of this conservative procedure is not only for bilateral disease but also for safer treatment for the atypical forms of Ménière's disease (specified later). Endolymphatic sac surgery has had broader acceptance and appeal for otologic surgeons because it provides an opportunity to preserve and, in some instances, enhance function in the vestibular and the cochlear labyrinths. Thus, when patients have predominantly vestibular Ménière's disease with normal or relatively normal hearing, or have cochlear Ménière's disease with relatively little vestibular symptomatology, this conservative procedure can be used successfully in selected cases.

A prudent philosophy and policy for Ménière's disease are that conservative treatment should precede any consideration of surgical treatment. Medical treatment with psychologic support comes first. If cochlear or vestibular symptoms, especially vertigo, become intractable, a conservative surgical procedure, endolymphatic sac enhancement or shunt, should be considered. This procedure can be considered an "extension of conservative treatment" because it has minimal risks and appears to affect pathophysiology beneficially.[10]

The role of endolymphatic sac surgery in treatment of Ménière's disease is in treating patients who develop intractable or progressive Ménière's disease, including vestibular and/or cochlear symptoms, in spite of adequate and prolonged trials of medical, supportive, empirical management. Because the physiology of the normal labyrinth and the pathophysiology of Ménière's disease are both poorly understood, it is impossible to describe the role of endolymphatic sac surgery with any certainty. Nevertheless, objective and subjective evidence continue to suggest strongly that endolymphatic sac surgery enhances the ability of the endolymphatic sac to absorb endolymph. By focusing on what is understood, or reasonably well understood, about Ménière's disease, we are able to diagnose and treat patients conservatively.

Evidence has been reported in previous publications by the author that describes the etiology of Ménière's disease as multifactorially inherited. Occasionally, extrinsic causative factors are known, but a genetic underlying basis most likely leads to the anomalous changes, both physical and chemical, that lead to Ménière's disease. The pathogenesis of Ménière's disease is considered to be based on malabsorption of endolymph. Endolymphatic hydrops was first described by Hallpike and Cairns[11] and also by Yamakawa[12, 13] in 1938. Endolymphatic sac surgery, irrespective of the surgical technique used, likely enhances the absorption of endolymph by (1) decompression, (2) passive diffusion of nanoliters of endolymph along alloplastic material, (3) osmotic changes in pressure that result in an extracellular milieu (pump) around the sac, (4) alteration of blood supply, and (5) most likely, alteration of immune factors in the endolymphatic sac (Fig. 35–1).[10, 14]

SELECTION OF PATIENTS

Generally, indications for surgical procedures on the endolymphatic sac are the development of intractable or progressive Ménière's disease over time, and failure of medical empirical management (Fig. 35–2). Most patients with Ménière's disease have the nonprogressive form and can be managed medically indefinitely. Most patients with progressive (intractable) Ménière's disease develop progression over many years, and a few develop Ménière's disease with destruction of the labyrinth more rapidly, over a brief period—a month or a few months, for example. The latter patients therefore need more rapid consideration of intercession. Previous publications by the author indicate that the average duration of disease was approximately 6 years prior to the patient's receiving sac enhancement surgery.[15, 16]

The most common indication for sac procedures is vertigo in classic Ménière's disease, in which patients have characteristic symptoms in all three categories: vestibular symptoms, cochlear symptoms, and aural pressure. Vestibular symptoms include typical episodic attacks of vertigo occurring intermittently at variable intervals; "drop," or so-called utricular-collapse attacks; severe disequilibrium or imbalance, which also develops from Ménière's disease; frequent bouts of nausea occurring alone or sometimes with vomiting accompanying the paroxysmal attacks; visually induced vertigo, or so-called shopping center nystagmus (these patients develop dizziness when they look at a computer, read a book, or see movement in a supermarket or shopping center); and positional or motion dizziness, which invariably occurs during an attack of Ménière's but often between vertiginous episodes as well. Cochlear symptoms include hearing loss, progressive hearing loss, and fluctuating sensorineural hearing loss, which can become stable; tinnitus, which can be disabling, either constant or intermittent, and often exacerbates during attacks; intolerance of loudness (measured by recruitment studies); and diplacusis or distortion of sound, typically perceived by the patient while listening during a telephone conversation. Aural pressure, a significant component of Ménière's disease, is characteristically perceived as pressure in one (unilateral) or both ears (bilateral) but sometimes as a pressure in the head in general, or a headache or discomfort on the side of the head, or in other regions of the head and neck. In addition, pressure or a dull ache from Ménière's disease can be confused with temporomandibular joint syndrome, sinusitis, migraine headaches, or other causes of discomfort in the region.

Another indication for sac surgery is intractable vestibular Ménière's disease. Vestibular Ménière's disease does

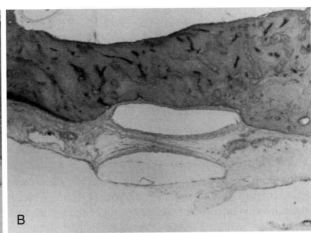

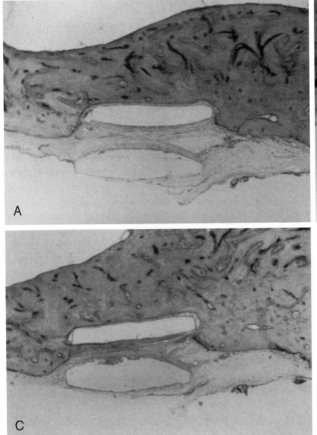

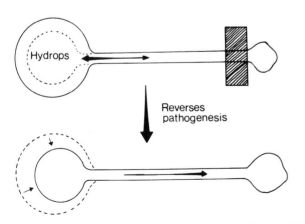

FIGURE 35–1. *A* to *C,* This patient had a sac enhancement operation and died later from unrelated causes. Please note inert silicone sheeting struts within the endolymphatic sac. There is no significant foreign body reaction.

exist, as clearly evidenced by the study of patients who have classic Ménière's disease, because 20 to 50 per cent of them (according to various studies) have vertigo and vestibular symptoms, sometimes occurring over a period of many years (as long as 45 years in one patient). Over time, many of these patients develop cochlear symptoms, allowing the diagnosis of typical Ménière's disease. The role for sac enhancement in the successful treatment of these patients has been described by Miller and Welsh,[17] Paparella and Mancini,[18] Huang,[19] and Plester (personal communication, 1992).

FIGURE 35–2. This illustration depicts progressive (intractable) Ménière's disease versus nonprogressive Ménière's disease, over time.

Cochlear Ménière's disease can occur in the absence of vestibular symptoms.[20] It can be treated successfully by sac enhancement surgery, especially when there is fluctuating hearing loss. The key is to treat the disease while there are temporary threshold shifts such as can be seen in patients who demonstrate a history of fluctuation. In those who develop a permanent threshold shift due to irrevocable damage from endolymphatic hydrops, surgery may not improve hearing. Nevertheless, many patients have preservation of hearing without progression as a result of a conservative sac procedure. Pearson and Brackmann[21] have performed sac surgery on cochlear Ménière's disease when the diagnosis has been confirmed by positive results on glycerol test and typical electrocochleography (ECoG) changes. Hearing results have been spectacular in approximately 20 such cases. Morrison has a similar experience (personal communication, 1992).

Although Ménière's disease typically strikes adults, usually occurring during the third and fourth decades, it does occur in children,[22] and the indications for treating children are identical to those for adults[23]: Conservative medical management precedes any consideration of surgery until the disease becomes intractable or progressive. Sac enhancement surgery can also be considered for elderly patients because it is a more conservative procedure, requiring typically one overnight stay in a hospital, in contrast with destructive procedures, which require longer periods of hospitalization, including care in the intensive care unit. Morrison (personal communication, 1992) and Huang (personal communication, 1992) have successfully performed this procedure for patients older than 70 years of age. The author has had a similar experience in successfully performing such a procedure in patients who are elderly, including several in their 90s who were otherwise incapacitated.

Ménière's disease can coexist with other diseases, sometimes with a causative or as a coincidental relationship. Multiple otopathologies are not rare.[24] Otosclerosis has been described in association with Ménière's disease. In selected patients, endolymphatic sac enhancement has proved to be useful.[25] Usually, a stapedectomy-sacculotomy is attempted first, particularly if there is a significant conductive component to the hearing loss. The clinical picture of syphilitically induced labyrinthine changes can be identical to Ménière's disease. After exhausting medical management, sac procedures have been used successfully in such patients by Paparella and associates[26] and by Huang and Lin.[27] Ménière's disease has also been found to develop over a period of years following chronic inactive otitis media and mastoiditis. This relationship has been clearly defined in otopathologic studies and clinically in patients.[28] Endolymphatic sac enhancement has been successful in treating a significant number of these patients, particularly those in a study by Huang and Lin.[29]

Bilateral Ménière's disease is another indication for endolymphatic sac surgery. No published author known to this author would consider destructive procedures on the second ear in patients who have bilateral Ménière's disease. The first provocative, or worst, ear is treated first, and if there is intractability in the second ear after months or a period that allows for stabilization of the first ear, sac surgery can be considered on the opposite side. Usually, bilateral surgery is unnecessary because once the offending ear with clinical presentation (hearing loss, pressure, and tinnitus) is treated successfully with endolymphatic sac surgery, the patient is comfortable, and the opposite ear often remains stable and not progressive, especially regarding sensorineural hearing loss. Bilateral sac surgery has been performed in approximately 100 patients by Morrison and colleagues,[30] in approximately 80 patients by Huang (personal communication, 1992), and in a similar number of patients by the author.

Earlier congenital anomalies of the inner ear, such as Mondini's dysplasia, were thought to be treated successfully with endolymphatic sac surgery. A more recent study, however, suggests that the results are not good; therefore, this procedure may not be indicated for patients who have congenital malformations of the inner ear, such as those resulting from Mondini's deafness.[23]

Patients can develop delayed hydrops with onset of vertigo, who have developed sudden deafness earlier in their lifetime or childhood deafness from various causes.[31] For example, in children or adults, congenital or acquired forms of deafness, such as meningogenic labyrinthitis, may develop that years later can result in severe vertigo, pressure, and tinnitus in an ear that has a profound hearing loss or that is severely deafened. The author has successfully performed sac surgery in approximately 20 patients in this group who required same-day discharge or overnight stay without severe disability resulting from destructive labyrinthectomy or nerve section, and without the difficulties in compensation that would ensue from a destructive modality.

Endolymphatic sac revision is another indication for endolymphatic sac surgery. For example, a patient may have had a successful previous endolymphatic sac procedure for a period of 3 or 4 years but subsequently may develop characteristic and disabling symptoms of Ménière's disease in the same ear. The patient is told what could be developing, and the patient is advised that often bone tissue (osteoneogenesis) or scar tissue (fibrosis) forms in the region external to the sac to cause reobstruction at that site and that aditus block can cause formation of tissue and bone in the mastoid. Frequently, scar tissue forms from the undersurface of the inferior wound (skin) contiguous with the adjacent sac.[15, 32] Of course, Ménière's disease can also exacerbate on its own accord. The patient is then advised of the condition and is provided the options of choosing between destructive procedures, such as vestibular nerve section, particularly if there is residual hearing remaining, sac revision, or both. Most patients select a sac revision procedure. Many authors have described sac revision. In the author's experience, the incidence of revision has been approximately 5 per cent, whereas many others have found the incidence of revision to be as high as 10 per cent (Huang, personal communication, 1999; Morrison, personal communication, 1992; Plester, personal communication, 1992).[32–34]

Finally, sac procedures are the only surgical procedures considered in patients who have an only-hearing ear from Ménière's disease. As mentioned, these patients have become deaf in the first ear from the disease or from a destructive procedure, such as labyrinthectomy. Once the second ear becomes intractable and develops severe, progressive, fluctuating deafness, a sac procedure can be considered. Many patients have been successfully treated, as was discussed in the previous section (Huang, personal communication, 1999; Plester, personal communication, 1992).[7, 28] The author has performed sac enhancement in 24 such patients, all of whom have preserved hearing; a few have improved hearing, whereas none, thankfully, has developed deafness over a prolonged period of time, in some instances many years.

PREOPERATIVE EVALUATION AND PATIENT COUNSELING

The method of diagnosis for Ménière's disease is documented in detail elsewhere but highlighted here.[10] The most important part of the diagnosis is the history, which perhaps contributes 90 per cent or more to the diagnosis. The history starts with the chief complaint, and specifically structured questions are asked in each of three categories (vestibular, cochlear, or aural pressure), depending on the chief complaint. The chief complaint is usually vertigo or vestibular upset; thus, the various specific questions are asked relative to vestibular symptoms of Ménière's disease. If the chief complaint originates in the cochlea, specific symptoms are reviewed regarding hearing loss, fluctuating hearing loss, tinnitus, intolerance of loudness, and diplacusis. The chief complaint may also relate to severe pressure or headache in the region of the ear or head.

Once the history is established, diagnostic studies are performed. The next most important diagnostic study is a routine audiogram consisting of air conduction, bone conduction, speech-reception thresholds, and speech discrimination. Other diagnostic tests follow, depending on indications. Routine diagnostic studies in the author's clinic include mastoid radiographs (especially lateral Law's view) to identify whether the mastoid is pneumatic, sclerotic, diploic, or otherwise pathologic. Studies indicate that hypoplasia exists in the mastoid in patients with Ménière's disease and that the sigmoid sinus occupies an anterior and deep location. Thus, inexpensive diagnostic information is quickly available in this regard. Plus, if surgery is to take place, radiographs provide a quick guide for rapid drilling in the mastoid; for example, one should be more cautious if the mastoid is sclerotic with a prominent, deep sigmoid sinus, as opposed to a pneumatic mastoid.

An audiometric study of brainstem response (ABR) is typically ordered to rule out lesions of the cerebellopontine angle, such as a vestibular schwannoma, although these two diseases result in quite different clinical presentations. ABR has been demonstrated to be 95 per cent accurate. If the possibility of a space-occupying lesion exists, magnetic resonance imaging with gadolinium or, less often, a computed tomographic study with enhancement is recommended. An electronystagmogram (ENG) is routinely ordered; ENG results can, however, be normal in up to 52 per cent of patients with Ménière's disease.[36] The patient may have incapacitating classic Ménière's disease and normal ENG (caloric) results. Posturography and sinusoidal chair testing are used in some centers and have been widely used by the author but have not proved essential or necessary in the diagnosis of Ménière's disease.

Glycerol testing was promoted earlier and continues to be practiced by some, but it is not nearly as commonly employed as it used to be because of lack of persistent relevance. This has been the experience in the author's clinic as well. ECoG can be ordered if it is available; however, it is not essential. ECoG is typically ordered in the routine battery practiced by the author. After these tests are ordered, the patient continues to be treated medically, if possible, unless the patient has been referred from a specialist, having already had prolonged medical management.

Communication, counseling, and education of the patient are the next important part of management. A patient who understands his or her problem is a far better patient to manage and will have a more positive result than a patient who is uninformed about the problem. Once a diagnosis is made, it is carefully explained to the patient. An explanation is made concerning the nature of endolymph and the fact that endolymphatic hydrops results from chemical or mechanical obstruction of the vestibular aqueduct and sac. Then, the patient is told how this procedure can reverse pathogenesis, thus allowing for an improved equilibrium of fluid, which provides an excellent opportunity to preserve and sometimes enhance function and ameliorate symptoms.

The patient is advised of the complications and risks of the disease process and benefits of the procedure. This consideration is important. The risks and complications from progressive Ménière's disease, including deafness, as well as the possibility of deafness from surgery, must be considered. Once the disease has been explained to the patient through diagrams and posters, informational reading material is provided the patient. The patient is advised that the goal of surgery is to try to preserve function and, depending on the nature of permanent damage to the labyrinth, to enhance function. The patient is advised that there is no cure for Ménière's disease but that there is always hope for improvement. Options for treatment, including continued medical conservative treatment, conservative surgical intervention, and destructive surgical intervention, are explained to the patient, reserving destructive procedures for treatment failures (which are uncommon). The patient then chooses from the conservative options.

The following statistics based on the author's published experience are then translated to the patient: the patient is advised that there is an approximate 2 per cent chance that deafness or profound hearing loss might result from the surgery. This loss is not a result of entering the labyrinth but usually relates to the healing process, which is discussed later. The patient is advised about the cause and pathogenesis of the disease process. The word "recommend" is not used; the problem or disease is described to the patient and the patient is allowed to choose freely among the various options, although destructive surgery is not considered an option at this stage. The incidence of bilaterality or the possibility that the disease may develop in the opposite ear over time is considered by the patient. Patients generally conclude that a conservative approach precedes destructive surgery. In the author's clinic, destructive surgeries, including vestibular nerve section, are not commonly done because conservative approaches have worked for most patients over a prolonged period.

The patient is advised that there is a 70 per cent chance to stop and ameliorate not only the vertigo but also the other associated vestibular symptoms that accompany Ménière's disease. An additional 20 per cent of patients continue to have vestibular symptoms, but the attacks are less severe and less intense, thus allowing continued medical management. They are advised that there is a 90 per cent or better chance that the procedure will help preserve hearing or that the hearing loss will not progress so severely over time and that there is a 30 to 40 per cent chance that the hearing might improve over preoperative threshold levels. The odds of improvement of tinnitus or pressure are slightly better than 50 per cent.[15, 16]

PREOPERATIVE PREPARATION

Antibiotics are not used preoperatively unless there is an associated condition requiring such treatment first. The patient receives general anesthesia and is encouraged to speak with the anesthesiologist ahead of time, if concerns or questions exist.

PREPARATION OF THE SURGICAL SITE, DRAPING, AND POSITIONING

The patient is positioned with the head down at a 45-degree angle on an operating table that easily moves up or down. The patient is placed in a Juers-Derlacki head holder. One inch of hair is shaved from around the ear. The site is then cleaned with alcohol to remove any oils from the skin. Next, a 2-inch Blenderm tape is used to tape the hair out of the field. A povidone-iodine (Betadine) wash is done and the area patted until dry. Then a povidone-iodine paint preparation is applied and patted until dry. The site is draped, and the complete site is washed and prepared, including the ear canal. The surgeon sits on a comfortable secretarial-type chair and has room to move to the head of the table so that he or she can visualize all aspects within the temporal bone. Sometimes, the patient requires additional Trendelenburg positioning to get the sinodural angle or posterosuperior aspect of the tympanic membrane and canal in a directly vertical position with the position of the binocular microscope.

An air drill is used. Facial nerve monitoring is not used, and in more than 1500 patients, only 2 have had a temporary nerve palsy; none has had a permanent paralysis. Monitoring by ABR is not used. Steroids and diuretics are not routinely provided.

Monitoring by ECoG is not used by the author. Some individuals have found this to be useful as a monitoring procedure during surgery. ECoG is a method of assessing cochlear function, and because the main indication for surgery in these patients is vertigo or vestibular dysfunction, this test and what it indicates over a brief period do not seem likely to provide uniformly accurate information regarding an ultimate postoperative result. Progressive Ménière's disease can be compared to a motion picture that fluctuates over a long period. Any test for function, such as ECoG, simulates a "snapshot," or an aspect of labyrinthine function at a given point and may not describe the overall course of events. Too many intangibles exist relating to healing and morphologic and physiologic considerations to provide a diagnostic test with predictive relevance. The overall clinical picture, defined primarily by the history and secondarily by audiometric information, the experience and judgment of the surgeon, and cooperation and understanding by the patient constitute the best prognosis for a favorable result.

SPECIAL INSTRUMENTS

The instruments used by the author have been developed and described elsewhere. Typical and routine instruments are used. An air drill is used and diamond burrs are available; however, the most important burrs are cutting burrs, especially those that can be reversed to provide smooth bony surfaces, stoppage of bleeding, and more cutting action than can be achieved safely with the typical diamond burr. All burrs are available and used. Special instruments are a fenestrometer to demarcate and measure the solid angle and a large Hough hoe, used first to enter the sac, followed by whirlybirds. No other special instruments are necessary to perform this operation.

SURGICAL TECHNIQUE

Historical Considerations

The first sac operation, by Portmann in 1927,[1] was an exposure of the sac, performed with mallet and gouge without benefit of modern-day magnification. The sac was simply incised with a small knife. Others tried the procedure, but relatively few publications appeared in the literature until an important publication by Yamakawa.[12] In 1954, Yamakawa and Naito published an article that dealt with an interesting modification of Portmann's operation for Ménière's disease. The method involved creating a shunt between the endolymphatic sac and cerebrospinal fluid to avoid postsurgical obliteration of the shunt due to granulation tissue, which was experienced with Portmann's method. This shunt operation also included a surgically induced permanent fistula between the endolymphatic sac and the subarachnoid space.[13, 37]

Credit for popularizing endolymphatic sac surgery deservedly goes to William House, who, because of the availability of the operating microscope and modern otologic techniques, made Portmann's operation much safer. In House's technique, the inner wall of the sac was incised, and a communication was created between the endolymphatic sac and the subarachnoid space; a polytetrafluoroethylene (Teflon) tube was placed into this aperture to ensure its patency. Because his early success with this technique showed satisfactory results, House abandoned simple drainage in favor of this shunt surgery in 1962.[38] Gardner continues to favor a modification of the endolymphatic sac to subarachnoid shunt procedure.[39]

After this development, the vast majority of published reports described sac procedures confined to the mastoid. In 1966, Shea reported on a series with promising results, in which a Teflon wick was placed from the sac to the mastoid cavity.[40] Subsequently, Shambaugh noted that even when he was unable to identify the sac, simple decompression of the dura around the sac seemed to effect satisfactory results.[41, 42] Graham and Kemink described a similar observation and experience.[43] Plester's technique included a large incision in the sac, through which a triangular piece of silicone sheeting was inserted; the sac was then covered with a free graft of muscle.[44]

The first inner ear valves were implanted in 1975 and 1976 in Sweden by Stahle and associates and in the United States by Arenberg, who developed a one-way valve placed into the endolymphatic sac with a limb of silicone sheeting extending into the mastoid.[45–47] Morrison popularized the capillary endolymphatic shunt in a large series of patients.[48] In this technique, a capillary tube is inserted into the lateral end of the endolymphatic duct, with its distal tip inserted into a silicone sheeting sponge. Paparella and Hanson described their method in 1976[16]; it included a wide exposure of the dura, avoiding the skeletonization of the posterior semicircular canal, and draining the sac via a T-strut. Spector and Smith, using a similar method, reported 122 cases over a period of 3 years.[49]

Kitahara and coworkers' method of drainage was based on an intramastoid opening of the endolymphatic sac and a folding back of the lateral wall of the sac with an insertion of absorbable gelatin sponge (Gelfoam) into its lumen.[50, 51] Futaki and Nomura used the Kitahara method, in comparison to their modified method of the vein-graft drainage procedure, which showed improved results.[52] Austin also confined his surgery to the mastoid with his method of "capillary endolymph dispersement."[53] Goldenburg and Justus,[54] Brown,[55] Chui and associates,[56] Ford,[57] Brackmann and Anderson,[58] and Maddox[59] successfully employed endolymphatic sac procedures confined to the mastoid in sizable series of cases.

In 1987, Brackmann and Nissen[60] reported their results with use of an endolymphatic subarachnoid shunt and an endolymphatic mastoid shunt, showing no statistical differences between the two procedures. Shea and colleagues,[61] through detailed examination and measurements from 40 temporal bones, established reference points by which the conservative surgeon can approach the endolymphatic sac below the level of the posterior semicircular canal. These observations make it unnecessary to risk exposure of the blue line of the posterior canal, thus minimizing risk of labyrinthine injury. Endolymphatic procedures confined to the mastoid are more common than those attempting a communication to the subarachnoid space.

Endolymphatic Sac Enhancement

The method for endolymphatic sac enhancement utilized by the author has been modified during a more than 30-year period. Current surgical principles and steps are summarized in the following paragraphs.

A curvilinear postauricular incision in the skin is placed approximately 1 inch behind the mastoid tip. This method helps avoid postoperative depression of the skin into the mastoid cavity. The posterior tip incision helps reduce scar tissue, which can grow from the subcutaneous wound into the region of the sac postoperatively, especially when accompanied by deficient aeration of the mastoid (Fig. 35–3A).

The mastoid cortex is exposed, a complete simple mastoidectomy is done, and the aditus is widened. The incus is always exposed (the only exception being when there is a lack of mastoid air cells) (Fig. 35–3B and C). The aditus ad antrum is opened widely, including a posterior atticotomy, to expose the head of the malleus. Although usually underdeveloped in patients with Ménière's disease, the facial recess (suprapyramidal recess) is enlarged (opened) contiguous with the aditus ad antrum to encourage postoperative aeration of the mastoid cavity, an important objective. The tegmen mastoideum and mastoid tip are exposed, the posterior bony wall of the external auditory canal is thinned, and the depth of drilling in the mastoid cavity is never extended below the dome of the horizontal semicircular canal or the incus, if a safer depth drilling reference is preferred. The purposes of this procedure are to gain good exposure, especially for later in the procedure; to be able to see the incus and horizontal semicircular canal for orientation; and to make possible later measurements—drilling below the dome of the horizontal canal endangers the posteroinferior semicircular canal. The enlarged aditus helps not only to promote drainage and transfer of air between middle ear and mastoid but also helps to avoid a postoperative aditus block syndrome (Fig. 35–3D) and granulation tissue, fibrosis, and osteoneogenesis in the mastoid and sac region.

By use of the fenestrometer, measurements are made from the fossa incudis 10 mm along the axis of the horizontal semicircular canal and 12 mm (approximately 45 degrees) from the linea temporalis. The zone of the solid angle (containing the canals) is demarcated so that further surgery will not enter this zone (Fig. 35–3E). These measurements, based on earlier anatomic dissections, create a demarcated zone to protect the canals and to serve as a landmark for further dissection.

The sigmoid sinus is skeletonized and decompressed throughout its length in the mastoid. Bone over Trautmann's triangle is thinned and removed with mastoid curettes or a rongeur (Fig. 35–3F and G). Because the sigmoid sinus is characteristically prominent in an anterior and medial location in Ménière's disease and is often associated with hypopneumatization of air cells and a small or nonexistent Trautmann's triangle, decompression of the sigmoid sinus enhances subsequent decompression of Trautmann's triangle and the contiguous dura below the solid angle.

Immediately below the demarcated bony zone, an infralabyrinthine cell tract is searched for. Here, a shelf of bone is preserved to contain and hold the silicone sheeting spacers to be placed later for a sustained effect of decompression. Often, infralabyrinthine cells do not exist. In restrictive mastoids (sclerotic or diploic), the anteriorly located facial nerve should be watched for and avoided. The purpose is to expose infralabyrinthine dura because the main body of the sac and its lumen often lie within this area and not posterior to the posteroinferior semicircular canal, as depicted earlier in textbooks. This step also helps dural decompression.

The dura contiguous with the decompressed sigmoid sinus is firmly decompressed (pushed down), especially below the solid angle (Fig. 35–3H). Care must be taken not to traumatize dura above the sac, which is often thin; trauma can lead to drainage of spinal fluid. Sometimes, a prominent bony shelf (operculum) exists below the dura on the side of the posterior cranial fossa and can hamper decompression of the dura. Because of anatomic factors, the dura is often tight in this region, and decompression counteracts this tightness and assists sac enhancement later.

The sac is entered beneath the solid angle. Sac epithelium is visualized by use of a sickle knife. A whirlybird or other blunt instrument helps identify the lumen, especially toward the infralabyrinthine region (Fig. 35–3H and I). The entrance to the sac should not be opened to the mastoid cavity so as to prevent fibrous or granulation tissue from invading the sac.

One or two silicone sheeting T-struts are placed within the sac. Depending on the size of the lumen, a selection is made of a preprepared small, medium, or large T-strut. The tail of the strut is placed outside the sac between dura and bone but not open to the mastoid. Small, medium, or large "spacers" or strips of silicone sheeting, as many as possible, are folded above and below the sac between the dura and the bone to decompress the dura and contiguous sigmoid sinus permanently. All silicone is placed or contained between bone and dura and not in the mastoid. Rubber strips or spacers serve as soft, springlike mechanisms for decompression of dura and sac. T-struts within the lumen enlarge the lumen and help the passive transfer of nanoliters of endolymph. It is important to open and treat the lumen of the sac as well as the surrounding region. This observation is emphasized during revisional sac surgery (Fig. 35–3J).

FIGURE 35–3

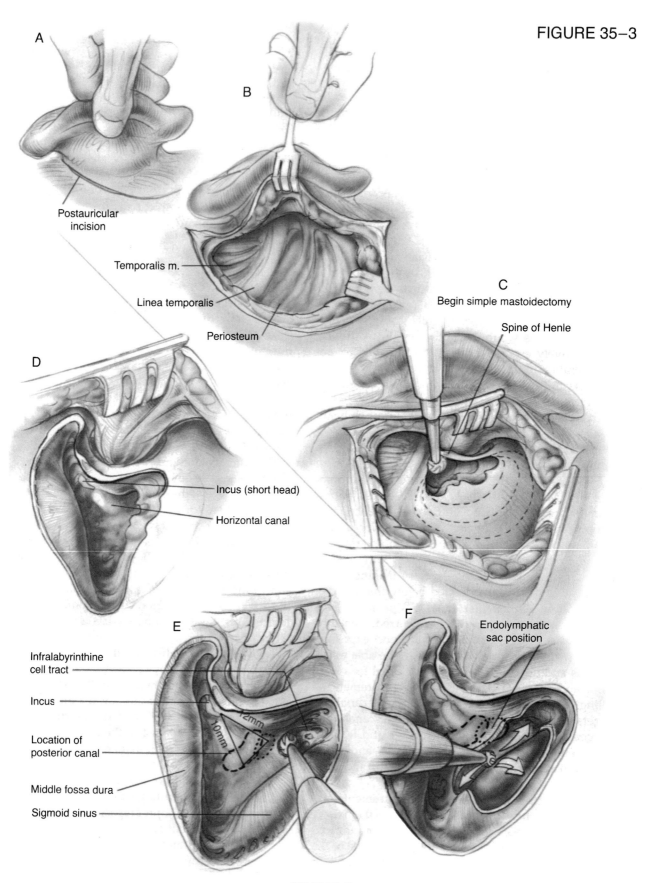

A

Postauricular
incision

B

Temporalis m.

Linea temporalis

Periosteum

C

Begin simple mastoidectomy

Spine of Henle

D

Incus (short head)

Horizontal canal

E

Infralabyrinthine
cell tract

Incus

Location of
posterior canal

Middle fossa dura

Sigmoid sinus

12mm

10mm

F

Endolymphatic
sac position

FIGURE 35–3

FIGURE 35–3 *(continued)*

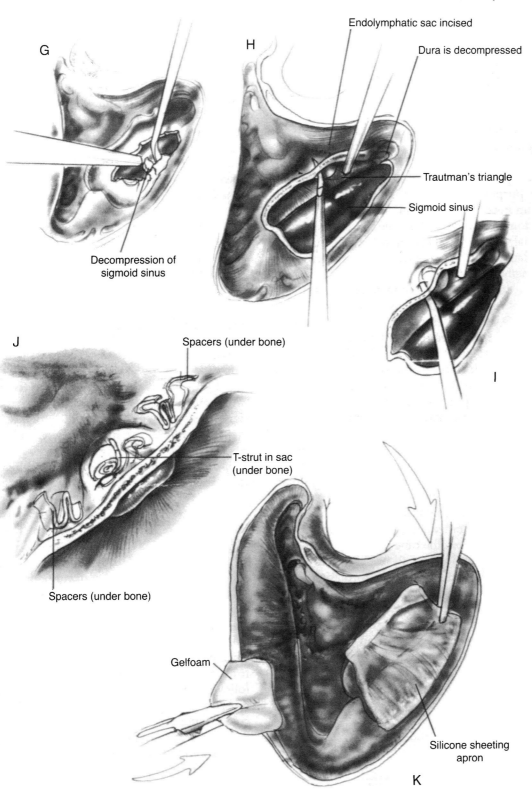

G

Decompression of
sigmoid sinus

H

Endolymphatic sac incised

Dura is decompressed

Trautman's triangle

Sigmoid sinus

I

J

Spacers (under bone)

T-strut in sac
(under bone)

Spacers (under bone)

Gelfoam

Silicone sheeting
apron

K

FIGURE 35–3 *Continued*

A silicone sheet apron is placed to cover this region, followed by a large piece or two of absorbable gelatin sponge dipped in a steroid-antibiotic solution and loosely placed to hold the apron in place (Fig. 35–3K). The purpose of this step is to help keep fibroblasts from invading the region of the endolymphatic sac. Previous techniques using pedicle grafts, temporalis fascial grafts, and protection by gold foil have been replaced by this original, more effective, and simpler method.

As was done before the lumen of the sac was opened, all bone dust and debris are removed meticulously. Bone dust routinely enters the middle ear and oval window and stapes through the aditus and should be irrigated out and removed. Failure to do so invariably leads to conductive hearing loss, osteoneogenesis, and fixation of the stapes months and years after surgery. All bleeding is stopped, and the wound is closed by use of subcutaneous absorbable sutures followed by skin sutures (vertical or horizontal mattresses) or metal staples. The purpose for this step is to ensure healthy, rapid healing and to avoid infection of the wound.

A ventilation tube is placed in the tympanic membrane, and the middle ear is suctioned through this site. The ventilation tube may not be used if drainage of cerebrospinal fluid occurs. The goal is to promote drainage of operative fluids from the middle ear and mastoid in the immediate (2 month) postoperative period. In addition, the tube promotes ventilation to the middle ear and especially the mastoid via the enlarged aditus so as to discourage formation of tissue in the mastoid, both in the short term and long term, and in particular to help avoid aditus block and long-term formation of tissue (granulations, scar, and bone) around the sac, which can lead to subsequent recurrent symptoms and signs of Ménière's disease. The tube has also been helpful in preventing otitis media and barotrauma from flying. The ventilation tube usually extrudes spontaneously in a year or so and is not replaced. The patient's symptoms are not affected when the tube extrudes.

DRESSING THE WOUND AND POSTOPERATIVE CARE

A typical mastoid dressing is applied for the first day, and if the patient has had leakage of cerebrospinal fluid (in <5 per cent), this dressing may be left on longer. Typically, the dressing is removed and the patient uses no dressing when he or she leaves the hospital the following day.

The patient is hospitalized overnight. Typically, the patient is empirically given amoxicillin or another appropriate broad-spectrum antibiotic to help avoid postoperative inflammation and infection. The patient usually does not require other medication, but if it is required, additional medication is provided. The patient is seen a week later, and the staples or sutures are removed. Although the patient is ambulatory, it takes approximately 2 months for the ear to "settle down," at which time an audiogram is usually obtained. Depending on the patient's postoperative status, more frequent visits may be needed. Even after the ear is stabilized and a good result achieved, the patient is advised to have at least an annual or, preferably, semiannual visit to monitor the status of both labyrinths.

PITFALLS OF SURGERY

In the author's experience, one pitfall of surgery is when a thorough mastoidectomy is not performed. The aditus (often narrow) should be widened to encourage aeration of the mastoid postoperatively. The sigmoid sinus is decompressed routinely; it is almost invariably found in a medial (deep) and anterior position.

Endolymphatic sac surgery can be difficult in many cases because of the pathologic and anatomic characteristics of Trautmann's triangle and surrounding structures. Trautmann's triangle may not exist or be accessible, it may exist in a vertical or horizontal orientation, and it may sometimes be located beneath the sigmoid sinus. Thus, wide decompression of the sigmoid sinus and adjacent dura of Trautmann's triangle can be difficult, depending on these variations.

One should take great care to use a blunt instrument and frequent irrigation when removing bone from the sigmoid sinus because removal of a simple spicule of bone can result in hemorrhage or bleeding from the sinus. Absorbable gelatin sponge is used, followed by adrenaline-soaked umbilical tapes and gauze packing, and pressure is applied. Then the gelatin sponge can be carefully moved aside, while pressure is still applied, to gain access to the region of the sac underneath the posteroinferior semicircular canal in Trautmann's triangle. The operation is completed.

The subarachnoid space is avoided, but sometimes simple removal of bone above the sac, and especially in elderly patients, will reveal a very thin bluish dura, and cerebrospinal fluid may drain. This is not a serious complication: reverse Trendelenburg's position takes place, pressure is applied, and the operation is completed. If cerebrospinal fluid is draining at the end of the operation, gelatin sponge is packed into this region, followed by adrenaline tapes and gauze packing. The gauze and tapes are removed, and once the ear is dry, the wound is closed and the patient is advised to keep the head in an upright position and avoid exertion postoperatively. In only one patient has it been necessary to return to the operating room for surgical closure of persistent drainage of cerebrospinal fluid. Cerebrospinal fluid can also flow from trauma to a thin medial wall of the sac. Careful blunt probing of the sac helps avoid this.

One problem can be identification of the sac. The sac is usually easily demarcated and seen, but sometimes it is diffuse without a demarcated border. The sac is typically found beneath and inferior to the posteroinferior canal and not open in the mastoid. Blunt identification of the lumen helps identify the sac beneath the solid angle. In 97 per cent of patients treated by the author, it has been possible to identify the lumen of the sac. Rarely (in approximately 3 per cent of patients), the sac is so markedly hypoplastic and small that the lumen cannot be found.

Another pitfall is injury to the posteroinferior semicircular canal. This problem has largely been resolved by the measurement, demarcation, and avoidance of the solid angle, as described herein. Key principles include thinning the posterior external auditory canal wall and depth drilling above the dome of the horizontal semicircular canal (or incus) in the solid angle. Rarely, the vertical course of the facial nerve can be injured if it is anomalous or, especially, in a tight, sclerotic mastoid. Thinning of the posterior bony canal wall and careful depth drilling, sometimes with a diamond or reverse burr, help identify the nerve and avoid injury to the nerve.

Hypoplasia of the mastoid air-cell system is commonly seen. A prominent Körner septum can reduce exposure of the antrum and aditus and must be eliminated. A small number of patients have no mastoid air cells (sclerotic), and the aditus and landmarks are not seen. The procedure can be accomplished by wide decompression and exposure of the sigmoid sinus. Then, decompression of the sinus and contiguous dura beneath the solid angle permits a narrowed, but usually adequate, exposure of the sac.

A bony shelf sometimes exists as part of the operculum beneath the sac in the posterior cranial fossa. When this happens, it is impossible to decompress the sac, and one has to accept this anatomic anomaly and somehow try to decompress widely around it. An objective is to maintain decompression. Spacers are used for this purpose, below the sac and above the sac, if the dura is not too thin.

Wound healing has been the major problem to date. This wound is treated with much greater respect than was formerly the case. Many patients have thick subcutaneous tissue, and if that tissue grows into the mastoid postoperatively, it can form a bridge of scar tissue between the postauricular wound (particularly in the region of the tip of the mastoid) and thereby cause reobstruction of the sac. Some patients have smaller mastoids and do not aerate their mastoids well postoperatively, thus encouraging subcutaneous fibrosis to grow into this region and osteoneogenesis to develop subsequently, which can lead to an inadequate result either within a short period (if this develops rapidly) or, more typically, over a prolonged period. Helpful techniques include meticulous treatment of the wound to stop all bleeding and removal of all bone dust, including bone dust that invariably enters the middle ear and oval window, where it can often result in a minor or major conductive hearing loss postoperatively.

Another problem is controlling bleeding from all bony sites. Meticulous care should be taken to stop bony bleeding before the wound is closed. Bony oozing can fill the mastoid with blood, again encouraging fibrosis, and can interfere with aeration of the mastoid, which is essential to getting a good result from this procedure. In instances of revision when the subcutaneous tissue is found to be thick, the surgeon should take time to thin it with plastic scissors to discourage fibrosis from entering the mastoid and the region of the sac from the inferior postauricular wound.

RESULTS

The sutures are removed in about a week. The ear is fairly well healed in 1 to 2 weeks, but the patient is advised that it takes about 2 months for the ear finally to settle down from the surgery. In the meantime, the patient is ambulatory and usually functions normally. Many patients are back to work only a few days after surgery. Patients' experience will be individualized because of the vagaries of the disease process and the individual psychologic characteristics, attitudes, and ability to heal postoperatively. Medication is necessary for some patients and not for others.

Patients have also been seen who have had vertigo and other symptoms during the first couple of months postoperatively who have then had a prolonged excellent result over a period of years. Thus, the fact that they have difficulty for the first month or two need not mean that they are going to have a poor result on a long-term basis. Results of this surgery are elimination of vestibular symptoms (in 70 per cent), improvement in them (in 90 per cent), preservation of hearing (in 90 per cent or better), and improvement in hearing (in approximately 30 to 40 per cent). There is a better than 50 per cent chance that the symptoms of pressure and tinnitus will be improved or eliminated as well. A smaller number of patients in the author's series had tinnitus as their chief complaint.

Some patients may require continued medical management but do not require destructive procedures. Clearly, one cannot go back and restore function after a destructive procedure, whereas the options for medical, conservative surgical (revision), or destructive procedures are still available to the patient if problems recur.

Silicone sheeting, when placed in the endolymphatic sac, does not cause severe fibrosis or a reaction. During revisional procedures, fibrosis and osteoneogenesis occurred extrinsic to the sac, as a result of wound healing and lack of mastoid aeration in Trautmann's triangle, in the region of the sac and in the mastoid, but not in the lumen of the sac. Typically, at the time of revision, the lumen is intact; there is a yellowish discoloration to the silicone sheeting, suggesting transudation of fluid relating to extracellular ions accumulating in this area, thus substantiating the concept of a change in osmotic potential concomitant with this procedure. In 1984, Belal, in a study of pathology patients who had endolymphatic sac surgery with silicone sheeting, concluded that it did not cause any difficulty.[62] Figure 35–1 shows a temporal bone from the otopathology laboratory at the University of Minnesota from a patient who received sac enhancement surgery; the silicone sheeting was inert, not causing fibrosis or difficulty in the lumen of the endolymphatic sac or around the sac.

COMPLICATIONS

The major complication of endolymphatic sac procedures in 2 per cent of patients is deafness or profound hearing loss that usually develops within the first few weeks or within a month or two after the surgery. This complication results not so much from entry into the labyrinth as from inflammation in the wound or lack of mastoid aeration postoperatively. Postoperative overt or subclinical and subcutaneous inflammation of the mastoid can invade the endolymphatic sac, causing labyrinthitis and deafness. The wound must be treated meticulously, all bony particles and dust and debris must be cleaned from the wound and its subcutaneous aspects, and all bleeding must be stopped before this wound is closed.

ALTERNATIVE TECHNIQUES

Medical management precedes consideration of conservative surgical management, namely endolymphatic sac enhancement. Vestibular nerve section is reserved for patients who fail conservative management. Destructive labyrinthectomy (rarely necessary) is a last resort. These patients represent a small minority treated in the author's clinic and hospital because the conservative methods of management suffice to control or eliminate symptoms in most patients who have Ménière's disease. Endolymphatic sac revision can be considered for those who have recurrent symptoms (5 to 10 per cent).

In recent years, in selected cases, the author has combined surgery with exposure of the open sac (7 minutes) with absorbable gelatin sponge saturated in streptomycin (or more recently, gentamicin) during endolymphatic sac revision, with successful results. Another useful adjunct to surgery is the extended approach via the facial recess, used in selected cases and in cases of revision in which the mastoid is small and there appears to be aditus block or a potential for aditus block. The facial (suprapyramidal) recess is opened contiguously with the enlarged aditus and posterior attic. This helps the flow of air into the mastoid postoperatively, which helps avoid healing problems and enhances a favorable result.

RECENT LITERATURE AND SAC SURGERY

An updated review of recent literature regarding function in the endolymphatic sac and surgery on the endolymphatic sac indicates that more basic scientific information regarding the physiology of the endolymphatic sac is developing, and surgery on the endolymphatic sac for Ménière's disease continues to be a successful treatment modality after failed medical therapy. The endolymphatic sac has several functions. In the rationale for surgery on the endolymphatic sac, its absorptive activities are probably primary. Hoshikawa and colleagues[63] studied the absorptive activity and barrier properties in the endolymphatic sac and found that both the intermediate portion and the distal portion of the sac may play a role in macromolecular absorption.

Immune reaction in the endolymphatic sac and its relationship to endolymphatic hydrops was studied by Tomiyama and coworkers.[64] Possible secretory substances were found in the endolymphatic sac by Tian and colleagues.[65] The surgical anatomy of the endolymphatic sac was studied by Bagger-Sjöbäck.[66] A large interindividual variety in the size and shape of the endolymphatic sac was found, leading the author to suggest that one possibility for surgical failure is the fact that the surgeon did not actually approach the sac. Surgical observations of the endolymphatic sac in Ménière's disease were also reported by Yazawa and coworkers.[67]

As was discussed earlier in this chapter, the etiology and pathogenesis of Ménière's disease have relevance to clinical diagnosis and treatment, including surgery on the endolymphatic sac. Ménière's disease is most commonly seen in adults, but endolymphatic hydrops has been a frequent histopathologic finding in children.[68] Traumatic endolymphatic hydrops leading to Ménière's disease was described as resulting from surgical or accidental trauma.[69] Late onset of vertigo (or a Ménière-like disease) can follow sensorineural hearing loss, sometimes many years later.[70] Progres-

sive papillary tumors can arise from the endolymphatic sac, leading to a clinical picture similar to that for Ménière's disease. Obviously, the treatment is directed to removal of the tumor.[71] Recent studies suggest that migraine headaches can be confused with Ménière's disease.[72, 73] I have treated a subset of patients with intractable Ménière's disease and severe migraine headaches for whom endolymphatic sac enhancement ameliorated the symptoms of Ménière's disease and the migraine headaches together. Using electrocochleography and history, the diagnosis of vestibular Ménière's disease, a distinct and sometimes incapacitating entity, was diagnosed in 73 to 100 per cent of patients with vestibular disease.[74]

After empirical medical management fails and patients have continued disability with intractable Ménière's disease, two categories of surgical therapy remain as options: (1) destruction and (2) conservative treatment. The definition of *destruction* refers to a purposeful attempt to destroy cellular contents of the labyrinth (surgical labyrinthectomy) or its attached vestibular nerve (intracranial vestibular neurectomy). In recent years there has been a resurgence of interest in chemical labyrinthectomy that dates back to the mid-1940s and was promoted in the 1950s. Transtympanic gentamicin is used widely for this purpose. The ototoxic drug must necessarily pass through the round window and through the cochlea to reach the vestibular labyrinth. Up to 30 per cent or more of cochlear losses have been reported, and since routine audiology does not measure at the basal turn of the cochlea (the average human cochlea is approximately 31 mm long), it is likely that damage to hair cells and high-frequency hearing losses occur in many, if not in most, of these patients. The ultimate risk-reward test for these procedures is whether they would be used for difficult, intractable unilateral or bilateral Ménière's disease, especially with reasonably good hearing. The only conservative surgical procedure that has been used for 73 years is endolymphatic sac surgery, which is directed toward the endolymphatic sac and mastoid and not to the labyrinth directly.

Recent studies confirm the efficacy of endolymphatic sac surgery for Ménière's disease. In this era of managed care, the first outcome-based assessment of endolymphatic sac surgery for Ménière's disease indicates that

Using 1995 AAO-HNS* guidelines, a 76 per cent improvement of vertigo in the most difficult population of patients with Ménière's disease was found. The SF-36 was a good measure of functional impairment and quality of life and correlated well with AAO-HNS guidelines.[75]

Pensak and Friedman also described the efficacy and the role of endolymphatic mastoid surgery in the managed care area.[76] A study and report of policy at Karolinska Hospital indicate

For patients with Ménière's disease and serviceable hearing, endolymphatic sac surgery offers good results (82 per cent total or good control of vertigo) with a low complication rate.[77]

The majority (65 per cent) of 454 endolymphatic sac procedures, including 26 patients having surgery on the

---

*AAO-HNS, American Academy of Otolaryngology—Head and Neck Surgery.

only-hearing ear, resulted in good long-term outcomes, and the authors conclude that "early endolymphatic sac surgery can substantially limit the risk of permanent hearing loss and disability in patients with Ménière's disease.[78] Gianoli and coworkers reported favorable results for sac decompression,[79] and Telischi and Luxford reported 93 per cent favorable long-term results in 234 patients following endolymphatic sac surgery for vertigo.[80]

SUMMARY

A plethora of publications regarding basic and clinical science aspects of the endolymphatic sac have appeared in the literature. Many more studies are needed and can be expected. In the future, the role of the endolymphatic sac in health and disease (e.g., Ménière's disease) will be better understood and its role in treating not only Ménière's disease but also other labyrinthine diseases will unfold.

ACKNOWLEDGMENT

This work was supported in part by NIDCD Grant No. 8P50 DC-00133 and the International Hearing Foundation.

References

1. Portmann G: The saccus endolymphaticus and an operation for draining the same for the relief of vertigo. Arch Otolaryngol 6: 309, 1927.
2. Portmann M: The Portmann procedure after sixty years. Am J Otol 8: 271–274, 1987.
3. Silverstein H: Vestibular neurectomy in the United States—1990. Trans Am Otol Soc 149–156, 1991.
4. Bretlau P, Thomsen J, Tos M, Johnsen NJ: Placebo effect in surgery for Ménière's disease: A three-year follow-up study of patients in a double-blind, placebo-controlled study on endolymphatic sac shunt surgery. Am J Otol 5: 558–561, 1984.
5. Smith WC, Pillsbury HC: Surgical treatment of Ménière's disease since Thomsen. Am J Otol 9: 39–43, 1988.
6. Pillsbury HC, Arenberg IK, Ferraro J, Ackley RS: Endolymphatic sac surgery: The Danish sham surgery study—an alternative analysis. Otolaryngol Clin North Am 92: 113–118, 1983.
7. Stahle J, Stahle C, Med B, Arenberg IK: Incidence of Ménière's disease. Arch Otolaryngol Head Neck Surg 104: 99–102, 1978.
8. Pulec JL: Endolymphatic subarachnoid shunt for Ménière's disease in the only-hearing ear. Laryngoscope 91: 772–783, 1981.
9. Morrison AW: Management of Sensorineural Deafness. London, Butterworth, 1975, pp 109–144.
10. Paparella MM, daCosta SS, Fox R, Yoon TH: Ménière's disease and other labyrinthine diseases. In Paparella MM, Shumrick DA (eds): Otolaryngology: Otology and Neurology. Philadelphia, WB Saunders, 1990.
11. Hallpike CS, Cairns H: Observations on the pathology of Ménière's syndrome. J Laryngol 53: 625–655, 1938.
12. Yamakawa K: Uber die Pathologische Varanderung bei einem Ménière-Kranken. Z Otol 44: 192–193, 1938.
13. Paparella MM, Morizono T, Matsunaga T: Kyoshiro Yamakawa and temporal bone histopathology of Ménière's patients reported in 1938. Arch Otolaryngol Head Neck Surg 118: 660–662, 1992.
14. Paparella MM: Pathogenesis of Ménière's disease and Ménière's syndrome. Acta Otolaryngol (Stockh) 406(Suppl): 10–25, 1984.
15. Liston S, Nissen RL, Paparella MM, daCosta SS: Surgical treatment of vertigo. In Paparella MM, Shumrick DA (eds): Otolaryngology, 3rd ed, Vol II, Otology. Philadelphia, WB Saunders, 1990, pp 1715–1732.
16. Paparella MM, Hanson DG: Endolymphatic sac drainage for intractable vertigo (methods and experience). Laryngoscope 86: 697–703, 1976.
17. Miller GW, Welsh RL: Surgical management of vestibular Ménière's disease with endolymphatic mastoid shunt. Laryngoscope 93: 1430–1440, 1983.
18. Paparella MM, Mancini F: Vestibular Ménière's disease. Otolaryngol Head Neck Surg 93: 148–151, 1985.
19. Huang TS, Lin CC: Endolymphatic sac surgery for Ménière's disease: A composite study of 339 cases. Laryngoscope 95: 1082–1086, 1985.
20. Williams A, Horton B, Day L: Endolymphatic hydrops without vertigo. Trans Am Otol Soc 35: 116, 1947.
21. Pearson BW, Brackmann DE: Committee on Hearing and Equilibrium: Guidelines for reporting treatment results in Ménière's disease. Otolaryngol Head Neck Surg 93: 579–581, 1985.
22. Meyerhoff WL, Paparella MM, Shea D: Ménière's disease in children. Laryngoscope 88: 1504–1511, 1978.
23. Jackler RK, Luxford WM, Brackmann DE, Monsell EM: Endolymphatic sac surgery in congenital malformations of the inner ear. Laryngoscope 98: 698–704, 1988.
24. Paparella MM, Goycoolea MV, Schachern PA: Multiple otological pathologies. Ann Otol Rhinol Laryngol 91: 14–18, 1988.
25. Paparella MM, Mancini F, Liston SL: Otosclerosis and Ménière's syndrome: Diagnosis and treatment. Laryngoscope 94: 623–629, 1984.
26. Paparella MM, Kim CS, Shea DA: Sac decompression for refractory luetic vertigo. Acta Otolaryngol (Stockh) 89: 541–546, 1980.
27. Huang TS, Lin CC: Endolymphatic sac surgery for refractory luetic vertigo. Am J Otol 12: 184–187, 1991.
28. Paparella MM, deSousa LC, Mancini F: Ménière's syndrome and otitis media. Laryngoscope 93: 1408–1415, 1983.
29. Huang TS, Lin CC: Surgical treatment of chronic otitis media and Ménière's syndrome. Laryngoscope 101: 900–904, 1991.
30. Morrison GA, O'Reilly BJ, Chevreton EB, Kenyon GS: Long-term results of revision endolymphatic sac surgery. J Laryngol Otol 104: 612–616, 1990.
31. Nadol JB Jr, Weiss AD, Parker SW: Vertigo of delayed onset after sudden deafness. Ann Otol Rhinol Laryngol 84: 841–846, 1975.
32. Paparella MM, Sajjadi H: Endolymphatic sac revision for recurrent Ménière's disease. Am J Otol 9: 441–447, 1988.
33. Gya K, Yangihara N: Endolymphatic-mastoid shunt operation: Results of the 24 cases and revision surgery with the Silastic sheet. Auris Nasus Larynx 9: 59–66, 1982.
34. House WF, Fraysee B: Revision of the endolymphatic subarachnoid shunt for Ménière's disease: Review of 59 cases. Arch Otolaryngol Head Neck Surg 105: 599–600, 1984.
35. Morrison AW: Sac surgery on the only or better hearing ear. Otolaryngol Clin North Am 16: 143–151, 1983.
36. Silverstein H: The effect of the endolymphatic subarachnoid shunt operation on vestibular function. Laryngoscope 88: 1603–1611, 1978.
37. Naito T: Notre expérience de l'opération de G. Portmann (ouverture du sac endolymphatique dans la maladie de Ménière). Rev Laryngol Otol Rhinol (Bord) 83: 643–645, 1962.
38. House WF: Subarachnoid shunt for drainage of endolymphatic hydrops. Laryngoscope 72: 713–729, 1962.
39. Gardner G: Shunt surgery in Ménière's disease: A follow-up report. South Med J 81: 193–198, 1988.
40. Shea JJ: Teflon film drainage of the endolymphatic sac. Arch Otolaryngol Head Neck Surg 83: 316–319, 1966.
41. Shambaugh GE Jr: Surgery of the endolymphatic sac. Arch Otolaryngol Head Neck Surg 83(Suppl): 305–315, 1966.
42. Shambaugh GE Jr: Effect of endolymphatic sac decompression on fluctuant hearing loss. Otolaryngol Clin North Am 8: 537–540, 1975.
43. Graham MD, Kemink JL: Surgical management of Ménière's disease with endolymphatic sac decompression by wide bony decompression of the posterior fossa dura: Technique and results. Laryngoscope 95: 680–683, 1984.
44. Plester D: Surgery of endolymphatic hydrops. J Otolaryngol Soc Aust 3: 393–395, 1972.
45. Arenberg IK, Stahle J, Wilbrand H, Newkirk JB: Unidirectional inner ear valve implant for endolymphatic sac surgery. Arch Otolaryngol Head Neck Surg 104: 694–704, 1978.
46. Arenberg IK: Results of endolymphatic sac to mastoid shunt surgery for Ménière's disease refractory to medical therapy. Am J Otol 8: 335–344, 1987.
47. Arenberg IK, Balkany TJ: Revision endolymphatic sac and duct surgery for recurrent Ménière's disease and hydrops: Failure analysis and technical aspects. Laryngoscope 92: 1279–1284, 1982.
48. Morrison AW: Cochleostomy or endolymphatic sac surgery for ad-

vanced Ménière's disease. Otolaryngol Clin North Am 16: 135–142, 1983.

49. Spector GJ, Smith PG: Endolymphatic sac surgery for Ménière's disease. Ann Otol Rhinol Laryngol 92: 113–118, 1983.

50. Kitahara M, Kitano H: Surgical treatment of Ménière's disease. Am J Otol 6: 108–109, 1985.

51. Kitahara M, Kitajima K, Yazawa Y, Uchida K: Endolymphatic sac surgery for Ménière's disease: Eighteen years' experience with the Kitahara sac operation. Am J Otol 8: 283–286, 1987.

52. Futaki T, Nomura Y: The surgical procedures and evaluation of two modifications of endolymphatic sac surgery: The epidural shunt and vein graft drainage. Acta Otolaryngol (Stockh) 468(Suppl): 117–127, 189.

53. Austin DF: Endolymphatic fistulization. Ann Otol Rhinol Laryngol 93: 534–539, 1984.

54. Goldenburg RA, Justus MA: Endolymphatic mastoid shunt for treatment of Ménière's disease: A five-year study. Laryngoscope 93: 1425–1429, 1983.

55. Brown JS: A ten-year statistical follow-up of 245 consecutive cases of endolymphatic shunt decompression with 328 consecutive cases of labyrinthectomy. Laryngoscope 93: 1419–1424, 1983.

56. Chui RT, McCabe BF, Harker LA: Ménière's disease at the University of Iowa: 1973–1980. Otolaryngol Head Neck Surg 90: 482–487, 1982.

57. Ford CN: Results of endolymphatic sac surgery in advanced Ménière's disease. Am J Otol 3: 339–342, 1982.

58. Brackmann DE, Anderson RG: Ménière's disease: Results of treatment with the endolymphatic subarachnoid shunt. ORL J Otorhinolaryngol Relat Spec 42: 101–118, 1980.

59. Maddox HE: Surgery of the endolymphatic sac. Laryngoscope 91: 1058–1062, 1981.

60. Brackmann DE, Nissen RL: Ménière's disease: Results of treatment with endolymphatic subarachnoid shunt compared with the endolymphatic mastoid shunt. Am J Otol 8: 275–282, 1987.

61. Shea DA, Chole RA, Paparella MM: The endolymphatic sac: Anatomical considerations. Laryngoscope 89: 88–94, 1979.

62. Belal A Jr: Pathology as it relates to ear surgery: IV. Surgery of Ménière's disease. J Laryngol Otol 98: 127–138, 1984.

63. Hoshikawa H, Furuta H, Mori N, Sakai SI: Absorption activity and barrier properties in the endolymphatic sac: Ultrastructural and morphometric analysis. Acta Otolaryngol (Stockh) 114: 40–47, 1994.

64. Tomiyama S, Nonaka M, Gotoh Y, et al: Immunological approach to Ménière's disease: Vestibular immune injury following immune reaction of the endolymphatic sac. ORL J Otorhinolaryngol Relat Spec 56: 11–18, 1994.

65. Tian Q, Rask-Andersen H, Linthicum FH Jr: Identification of substances in the endolymphatic sac. Acta Otolaryngol (Stockh) 114: 632–636, 1994.

66. Bagger-Sjöbäck D: Surgical anatomy of the endolymphatic sac. Am J Otol 14: 576–579, 1993.

67. Yazawa Y, Suzuki M, Tanaka H, et al: Surgical observations on the endolymphatic sac in Ménière's disease. Am J Otol 19: 71–75, 1999.

68. Bachor E, Karmody CS: Endolymphatic hydrops in children. ORL J Otorhinolaryngol Relat Spec 57: 129–134, 1995.

69. Shea JJ Jr, Ge X, Orchik DJ: Traumatic endolymphatic hydrops. Am J Otol 16: 235–240, 1995.

70. Langman AW, Lindeman RC: Sensorineural hearing loss with delayed onset of vertigo. Otolaryngol Head Neck Surg 112: 540–543, 1995.

71. Megerian CA, McKenna MJ, Nuss RC, et al: Endolymphatic sac tumors: Histopathologic confirmation, clinical characterization, and implication in von Hippel-Lindau disease. Laryngoscope 105: 801–808, 1995.

72. Savundra PA, Carroll JD, Davies RA, et al: Migraine-associated vertigo. Neurosurgery 17: 505–510, 1997.

73. Parker W: Ménière's disease: Etiologic considerations. Arch Otolaryngol Head Neck Surg 121: 377–382, 1995.

74. Dornhoffer JL, Arenberg IK: Diagnosis of vestibular Ménière's disease with electrocochleography. Am J Otol 14: 161–164, 1993.

75. Smith DR, Pyle GM: Outcome-based assessment of endolymphatic sac surgery for Ménière's disease. Laryngoscope 107: 1210–1216, 1997.

76. Pensak ML, Friedman RA: The role of endolymphatic mastoid shunt surgery in the managed care era. Am J Otol 19: 337–340, 1998.

77. Söderman A-CH, Ahlner K, Bägger-Sjöbäck D, et al: Surgical treatment of vertigo: The Karolinska Hospital policy. Am J Otol 17: 93–98, 1996.

78. Pulec JL: Permanent restoration of hearing and vestibular function by the endolymphatic subarachnoid shunt operation. Ear Nose Throat J 74: 544–559, 1995.

79. Gianoli GJ, Larouere MJ, Kartush JM, et al: Sac-vein decompression for intractable Ménière's disease: Two-year treatment results. Otolaryngol Head Neck Surg 118: 22–29, 1998.

80. Telischi FF, Luxford WM: Long-term efficacy of endolymphatic sac surgery for vertigo in Ménière's disease. Otolaryngol Head Neck Surg 109: 83–87, 1993.

36

Middle Cranial Fossa: Vestibular Neurectomy

Ugo Fisch, M.D. ▪ Joseph M. Chen, M.D.

The treatment of Ménière's disease continues to evoke controversy, as evidenced by a multitude of treatment modalities and their claims of efficacy. Medical management in an attempt to alter or stall the course of this condition has proved ineffective, with the exception of symptomatic relief of vertiginous attacks with the use of pharmacologic agents.

In light of the questionable efficacy of endolymphatic sac operation and the undesirable sequelae of a myriad of ablative procedures, vestibular neurectomy in recent years has been accepted as the most effective means to manage recalcitrant and disabling Ménière's disease.

With either the middle fossa or posterior fossa approaches, ablation of vestibular functions and vertigo is reported to be from 85 to 99 per cent,[1-4] greatly exceeding the results of other treatment protocols.

Technical difficulties have been cited by many authors as the major reason for abandoning the middle cranial fossa approach in favor of a predominantly neurosurgical approach from the posterior, especially as collaborative efforts between otoneurology and neurosurgery increase. However, many centers in Europe and South America continue to use the middle fossa approach with great success.[3-6]

The middle cranial fossa vestibular neurectomy performed at the University of Zurich is also known as the *transtemporal-supralabyrinthine approach*. In contrast to the middle fossa approach of House,[7] which involves significant elevation of the middle fossa dura and retraction of the temporal lobe, the transtemporal-supralabyrinthine access to the internal auditory canal (IAC) is gained through bony reduction, with only minimal retraction of the dura.

PATIENT SELECTION

Patients with unilateral Ménière's disease who suffer incapacitating attacks of vertigo of at least 6 months' duration despite maximal medical therapy are candidates for vestibular neurectomy. These patients usually have residual and fluctuant hearing. Patients with severe-to-profound hearing loss and extremely poor speech discrimination are better managed by a translabyrinthine cochleovestibular neurectomy. The severity of the vertiginous attacks indicative of surgical management is rather subjective and depends more on the patient's functional capacity than on the frequency of attacks.

In bilateral Ménière's disease, surgery could still be contemplated if a dominant side can be identified. Four patients at the University of Zurich underwent bilateral vestibular neurectomies in stages (separated by at least 1 year following good vestibular compensation); surprisingly, postoperative vestibular compensation was shorter and easier after the second operation. These patients have remained symptom free for 16 to 20 years since surgery. Patients with Ménière's disease suitable for a vestibular neurectomy account for approximately 10 per cent of the whole group.

Unilateral peripheral vertigo without the full spectrum of Ménière's disease may also benefit from vestibular neurectomy.[8] In these patients, it is important to confirm the side of pathology with vestibular function tests if there is no hearing loss to provide a lateralizing sign. Other indications for vestibular neurectomy are rare. Labyrinthine trauma with residual hearing and disabling vertigo after successful stapedectomy with good hearing could be considered.

Contraindications of surgery include the only-hearing ear, signs of central vestibular dysfunction, and poor medical condition. Age older than 70 years is a relative contraindication subject to individual assessment.

PREOPERATIVE EVALUATION AND COUNSELING

Prior to surgery, the patient generally undergoes a full auditory-vestibular evaluation that includes full audiometry, electronystagmography, and auditory brainstem response. Electrocochleography and dehydration tests are not part of the test battery performed at the University of Zurich. A high-resolution computed tomographic and an MRI scan are obtained to rule out a cerebellopontine angle lesion, and to determine perilabyrinthine pneumatization. A Stenvers view is routinely obtained to demonstrate the contours of the floor of the middle cranial fossa as well as the relationship of the meatal plane and superior semicircular canal with respect to the arcuate eminence.

Immunologic evaluation is obtained if autoimmune disorders or significant allergies are suspected. It is not a standard part of the test battery.

Patients are usually referred from other otologists and have been managed conservatively for a prolonged period without relief. They are made aware of the efficacy of vestibular neurectomy and its related complications, particularly those pertaining to hearing and facial nerve.

PREOPERATIVE MEDICATION

The patient is premedicated with clonidine, metoclopramide, and midazolam prior to surgery. A perioperative antibiotic, ceftriaxone (Rocephin), 2 g intravenously for 24 hours, is started at the time of surgery and continued for the duration of the intravenous infusion, usually for 5 days.

SURGICAL SITE PREPARATION, POSITIONING, AND DRAPING

The surgical site is prepared in the OR after the induction of anesthesia. Hair over the temporal region is shaved 9 cm above and 5 cm behind the pinna. The skin is then washed with Betadine.

The patient is secured on the Fisch operating table (Fig. 36–1) in supine position with the head turned to the side. Draping is standard except for a large-reservoir plastic bag, which is at the head of the table to catch excess irrigation fluid and blood.

INTRAOPERATIVE MONITORING AND ANESTHETIC CONCERNS

Intraoperative facial nerve monitoring using the Xomed nerve integrity monitor with percutaneous electromyographic needles is standard. Both unipolar and bipolar stimulating forceps are available. Intracranial pressure is controlled by deep anesthesia induced intravenously before introducing inhalation anesthetic. The P_{CO_2} is maintained between 30 and 40 mm Hg. Pharmacologic manipulation with dexamethasone (Decadron, 4 mg every 8 hours perioperatively for 4 days) and mannitol (0.5 mg/kg intravenously intraoperatively) are also standard. Furosemide is added when necessary. Lumbar cerebrospinal fluid drainage is not routinely performed. Hypotensive anesthesia with nitroglycerin and/or clonidine (Catapres) is used in most cases to maintain a systolic blood pressure between 80 and 90 mm Hg.

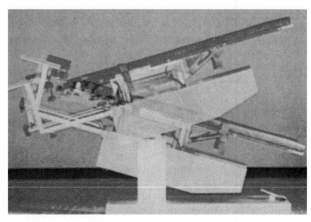

FIGURE 36–1. The Fisch table. (From Fisch U, Mattox DE: Microsurgery of the Skull Base. New York, Thieme, 1988, p 17.)

SPECIAL INSTRUMENTS

1. The Fisch operating table (Contraves/Zeiss): motorized table with the center of rotation at the temporal bone, allowing easy remote control for optimal positional changes that can be operated by the scrub nurse or the anesthetist (see Fig. 36–1)
2. Articulated middle fossa retractor (Fischer-13-18-200): a self-retaining retractor that allows adjustments in the angle of retraction, tilting, and sideways shifting of the retractor blade (Fig. 36–2)
3. Temporalis muscle retractor (Fischer-13-18-200): a strong, self-retaining retractor with a wide opening span, essential for the exposure of the zygomatic root (Fig. 36–3)
4. Angled microraspatory (Fischer-13-18-308 [left], 13-18-306 [right]): specially designed to facilitate dural elevation; its shoulder retracts the dura away, while the tip is used to separate dural attachments to bone (Fig. 36–4)

SURGICAL TECHNIQUE

The objective of the transtemporal-supralabyrinthine approach for vestibular neurectomy is to gain access to the IAC through the exenteration of the supralabyrinthine bone, while dural elevation and retraction are limited to no more than 1.5 cm. This principle is schematically illustrated in Figure 36–5.

Skin Incision

A preauricular incision is made from approximately the lower edge of the zygomatic root and extended to the temporal area at an angle for about 7 cm (Fig. 36–6). The depth of the incision is made to the temporalis fascia, and branches of the superficial temporal artery are divided and clamped. Retraction of the skin edges is provided by securing arterial clamps to the drapes.

Temporal Muscle Flap

After some undermining, the temporalis muscle is well exposed with a self-retaining retractor. Five muscle flaps designed according to Figure 36–7 are developed, elevated from the temporal squama, and retracted away with stay sutures. The temporal squama should be exposed from the root of the zygoma to the parietosquamous suture line. A temporalis muscle retractor should be used for the inferior exposure, where the identification of the zygomatic root is essential in the accurate positioning of the craniotomy.

Craniotomy

A 2 × 3 cm craniotomy (Fig. 36–8) is made perpendicular to, and at least 1 cm above, the temporal line, centered over the zygomatic root. This is performed with a 5-mm cutting burr on a straight hand piece, and when dura is blue-lined, a 4-mm diamond burr is used. Care is taken to

FIGURE 36-4

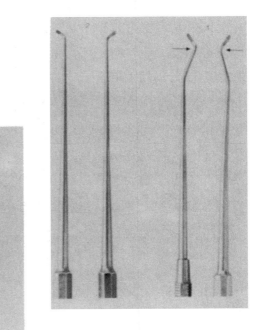

FIGURE 36-3

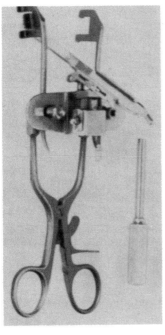

FIGURE 36-2

FIGURE 36-5

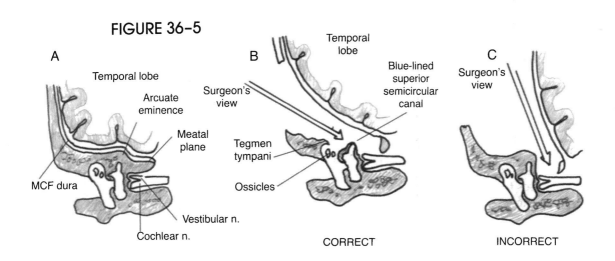

A

Temporal lobe

Arcuate eminence

Meatal plane

MCF dura

Vestibular n.

Cochlear n.

B

Temporal lobe

Surgeon's view

Blue-lined superior semicircular canal

Tegmen tympani

Ossicles

CORRECT

C

Surgeon's view

INCORRECT

FIGURE 36–2. Middle fossa retractor. (From Fisch U, Mattox DE: Microsurgery of the Skull Base. New York, Thieme, 1988, p 426.)

FIGURE 36–3. Temporal muscle retractor. (From Fisch U, Mattox DE: Microsurgery of the Skull Base. New York, Thieme, 1988, p 426.)

FIGURE 36–4. Angled raspatory. (From Fisch U, Mattox DE: Microsurgery of the Skull Base. New York, Thieme, 1988, p 427.)

FIGURE 36–5. A, Middle cranial fossa (MCF) topography. B and C, Correct and incorrect approaches, respectively. (A to C, Redrawn from Fisch U, Mattox DE: Microsurgery of the Skull Base. New York, Thieme, 1988, p 430.)

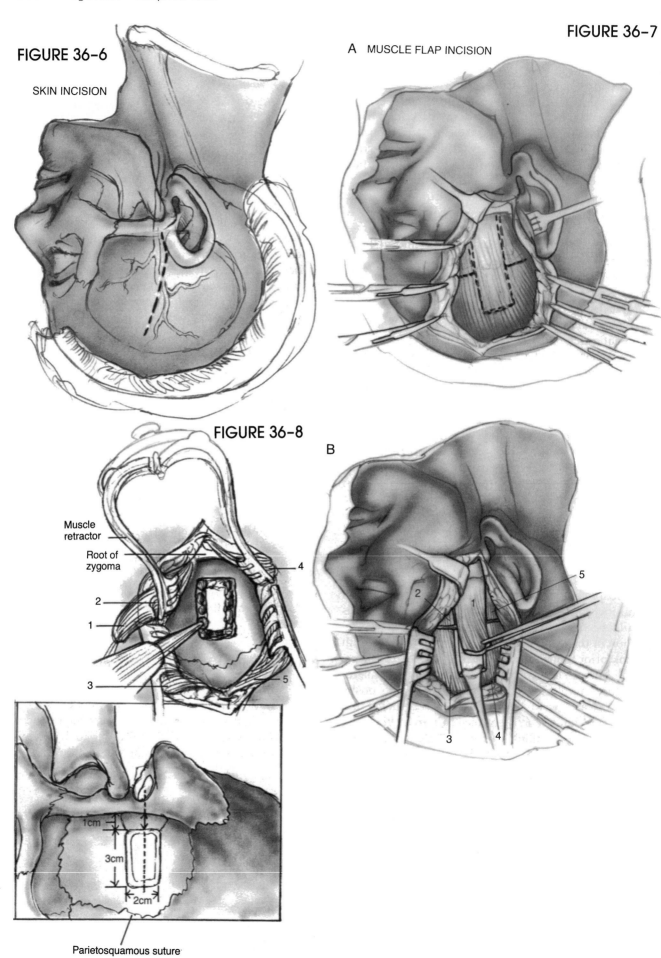

FIGURE 36–6

SKIN INCISION

FIGURE 36–7

A MUSCLE FLAP INCISION

FIGURE 36–8

B

Muscle retractor

Root of zygoma

2

1

3

4

5

1cm

3cm

2cm

Parietosquamous suture

FIGURES 36–6 to 36–8. *See legends on opposite page*

avoid injuring the dura and branches of the middle meningeal artery, which usually cross the undersurface of the bone flap in its midportion but could be variable.

The bone flap is elevated from the dura with a dura raspatory and is kept in Ringer's solution for later use. The dura is elevated from the edges of the craniotomy to facilitate the placement of the middle fossa retractor. In the region of the middle meningeal arterial branches, this step must be done with care. Sharp edges are removed with a small rongeur to prevent dural laceration.

The craniotomy is extended inferiorly toward the zygomatic arch to the floor of the middle cranial fossa. Lateral extensions of 1 cm on each side provide better visibility for the next step (Fig. 36–9).

Dural Elevation

Dural elevation is performed with the microscope. It is perhaps the most delicate part of the operation; if it is not carried out properly, troublesome hemorrhage can occur. It is important to keep the dural elevation to a minimum and to avoid the region of the middle meningeal artery anteriorly, where significant vascular channels between dura and cranium can be found around the foramen spinosum.

In addition to pharmacologic reduction of the intracranial pressure with mannitol and dexamethasone, cerebrospinal fluid decompression through a small dural incision further facilitates dural elevation. This should be done by first coagulating a small central portion of the dura and then elevating this area with a hook prior to making an incision (Fig. 36–10).

With the use of a curved suction and angled microraspatory, dural elevation is performed from posteriorly forward. Vascular channels are coagulated and cut close to bone. Persistent bleeding from bone can be controlled by drilling over it with a diamond burr. Oozing from dural vessels at the corners can be controlled with Oxycel packed beneath a cottonoid. Dural attachment to the petrosquamous suture is also coagulated and cut.

Exposure of the Meatal Plane and Arcuate Eminence

Dural elevation is extended to the superior petrosal sulcus and over the arcuate eminence. Moving anteriorly, the meatal plane is reached; this is an area bound by the arcuate eminence, superior petrosal sulcus, and facial hiatus (Fig. 36–11). When the meatal plane is not well defined because of a flat arcuate eminence, it can be identified after blue-lining the superior semicircular canal (SCC). If the attachment of the greater superficial petrosal nerve limits the exposure of the meatal plane, it can be separated from dura gently to avoid traction injury of the facial nerve.

Meticulous hemostasis in this region is important, and direct coagulation is avoided because of the proximity of the facial nerve.

Introduction of the Middle Cranial Fossa Retractor

The middle cranial fossa retractor can be introduced at this point without the use of a microscope. The self-retaining jaws are firmly attached to the edges of the craniotomy first; the multidirectional stage is slid over the self-retaining portion and loosely placed. The dura is retracted with a suction to reveal the meatal plane to allow the accurate placement of the retractor blade, which is positioned parallel to the superior petrosal sulcus, and its tip just beyond the arcuate eminence (Fig. 36–12). Once the desired position is attained, screws on the multidirectional stage are tightened. Fine adjustments thereafter are done under the microscope.

Bony Exenteration and Blue-Lining of the Superior Semicircular Canal

The operating table is now placed in Trendelenburg's position to better visualize the area over the retractor blade. Bone posterior and lateral to the arcuate eminence is removed with a cutting burr (5 mm), enabling wider access for the final exposure and the progressive identification of the superior SCC. Because of the variable relationship of the superior SCC to the arcuate eminence, its identification is best accomplished from a posterolateral approach through the pneumatic cells; the yellow compact bone of the SCC can be readily exposed. To blue-line the SCC, removal of bone should be done with small diamond burrs (2.3, 3.1, 4.0 mm) in a wide rotatory fashion (Fig. 36–13).

Exposure of the Internal Auditory Canal

Once the blue-line of the superior SCC is identified, using a 60 angle centered over the superior canal ampulla, the area of the meatal plane overlying the IAC can be defined. If the surgeon stays within this angle, there is no danger of damaging the facial nerve or the basal turn of the cochlea. The initial drilling is focused over the meatal plane, staying as close as possible to the blue-lined SCC. The axis of the drill is directed medioinferiorly, toward the superior lip of the porus and the medial roof of the IAC. These areas are progressively thinned out, until they are blue-lined (Fig. 36–14). The lateral exposure of the IAC involves the removal of bone over the meatal fundus and

---

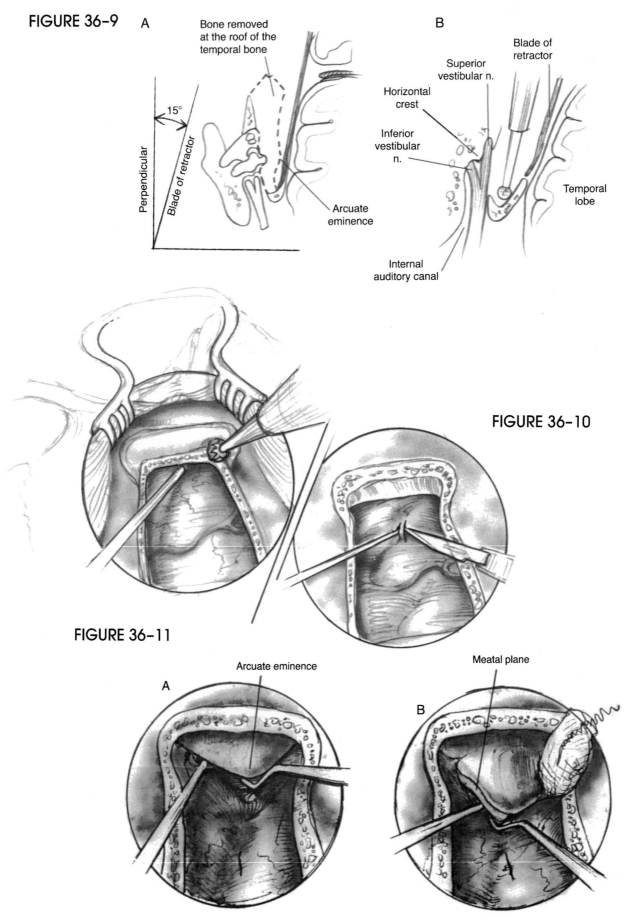

FIGURE 36-9

A

Bone removed at the roof of the temporal bone

15°

Perpendicular

Blade of retractor

Arcuate eminence

B

Blade of retractor

Superior vestibular n.

Horizontal crest

Inferior vestibular n.

Temporal lobe

Internal auditory canal

FIGURE 36-10

FIGURE 36-11

Arcuate eminence

A

Meatal plane

B

FIGURES 36–9 to 36–11. *See legends on opposite page*

tegmen tympani (Fig. 36–15). This small triangular area is bordered by the ampulla of the superior SCC, the facial nerve in its labyrinthine and tympanic portions; only 3 mm separates the superior ampulla from the genu of the facial nerve. The tegmen is opened if necessary to expose the malleus head and incus for better orientation. Bone over the meatal foramen and the distal superior vestibular nerve (SVN) is removed to clearly identify the vertical crest (Bill's bar), which gives the fundus its inverted-W shape. If this is not well defined, the SVN proximal to the ampulla should be exposed. The meatal foramen of the facial nerve should not be unroofed so as to avoid facial nerve injury.

At least one third of the upper circumference of the IAC must be exposed to properly perform a vestibular neurectomy. In particular, the posterior edge of the meatal roof deep in front of the superior SCC must be removed to adequately expose the SVN.

Vestibular Neurectomy

Once the IAC is unroofed from the fundus to the porus, dura over the SVN is opened with a 1.0-mm hook. The nerve is identified and cut sharply with a neurectomy knife distal to the vestibular crest (Fig. 36–16). Avulsion of the SVN with a hook is to be discouraged because of the high incidence of deafness associated with this maneuver as a result of either traction or vascular injury to the cochlear nerve.

The meatal dura is incised along the posterior edge toward the porus. The cut end of the SVN is retracted with a microsuction to expose the saccular and singular branches of the inferior vestibular nerve, which are then sectioned with a neurectomy knife. The entire vestibular nerve is stabilized with the suction while the vestibulofacial anastomoses are cut sharply with a neurectomy scissor. The vestibular nerve is now everted with Scarpa's ganglion in full view, which is slightly darker and has a pronounced vascular pattern over it. The vessels are coagulated, and the nerve is then resected proximal to the ganglion with neurectomy scissors (Fig. 36–17). The facial nerve should be only partially exposed, retaining most of its dural cover for protection. The cochlear nerve is hidden beneath the facial nerve and need not be exposed.

Repair of the Floor of the Middle Cranial Fossa

The IAC is covered with a free muscle plug and stabilized with fibrin glue. The tegmen defect is reconstructed with the thinner half of the craniotomy bone flap (wrapped in a gauze and fractured with a rongeur). This bony fragment usually straddles the tegmen defect perfectly and is also

fixed in position with fibrin glue (Fig. 36–18). The middle fossa retractor is now removed.

Wound Closure

The dura is elevated with a dural hook and suspended to the adjacent temporalis muscle with 4-0 Vicryl sutures (Fig. 36–19). This action obliterates the dead space between dura and bone and prevents the formation of an epidural hematoma.

The supralabyrinthine cavity is obliterated with the long, anteriorly based muscle flap (No. 1), which is then sutured to its opposing flap (No. 5). The craniotomy bone flap is then placed over the upper bony defect, and the remaining muscle flaps are sutured over it (Fig. 36–20).

A single 3.0-mm suction drain is placed over the temporalis muscle and brought out through a separate stab incision posteriorly. The skin is closed in two layers with 2-0 catgut and 3-0 nylon sutures.

DRESSING AND POSTOPERATIVE CARE

A compression dressing based over the surgical site is applied following skin closure and is left for 5 days. The patient is kept in the postanesthesia care unit for at least 24 hours following surgery, with close monitoring of routine and neurologic vital signs every 30 to 60 minutes. Adequate analgesics and antiemetics are ordered to keep the patient comfortably at bed rest. Ambulation and oral intake are started slowly in 2 or 3 days. Subcutaneous heparin is often given in the early convalescent period.

Intravenous antibiotic (ceftriaxone [Rocephin]) is discontinued when the patient no longer requires intravenous infusion. Oral sulfamethoxazole and trimethoprim (Bactrim Forte) or ciprofloxacin (Ciproxin) is prescribed for at least 5 days. The drain is removed when the daily drainage is less than 10 ml, and scalp sutures are removed after 10 days.

TIPS AND PITFALLS

- The root of the zygoma must be well identified to accurately guide the placement of the craniotomy. The craniotomy should be perpendicular to the temporal line, its width not exceeding 2 cm, because of the limited opening span of the middle fossa retractor.
- The floor of the middle fossa is usually at the level of the temporal line.
- The elevation of the dura should not exceed 1 cm. The necessary access is gained by removing bone at the floor of the middle fossa.

FIGURE 36–9. A and B, Craniotomy extension.

FIGURE 36–10. Cerebrospinal fluid decompression.

FIGURE 36–11. A and B, Dural elevation.

FIGURE 36–13

FIGURE 36–12

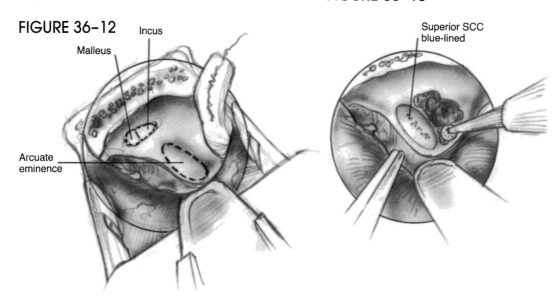

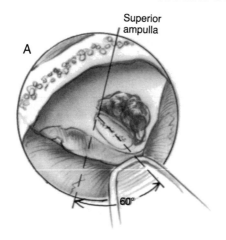

FIGURE 36–14

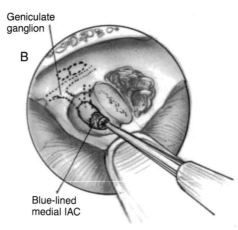

FIGURE 36–15

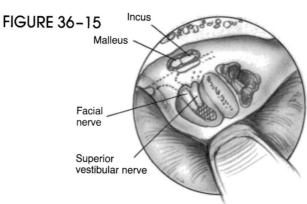

FIGURE 36–12. Retractor in position.

FIGURE 36–13. Blue lining the superior semicircular canal (SCC).

FIGURE 36–14. *A* and *B,* Medial internal auditory canal exposure.

FIGURE 36–15. Lateral internal auditory canal exposure.

FIGURE 36–16

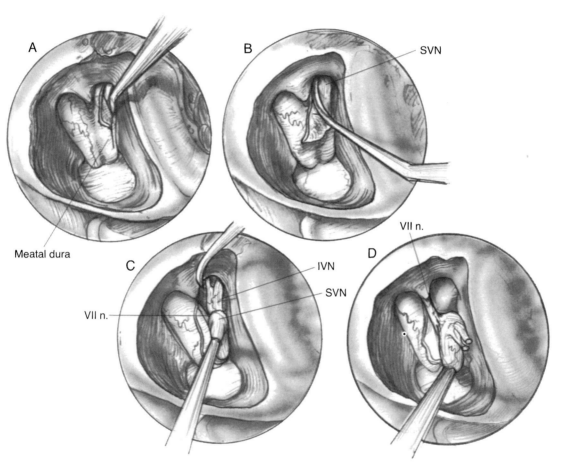

FIGURE 36–16. *A* to *D*, Superior vestibular nerve (SVN) section. IVN, inferior vestibular nerve.

FIGURE 36-17

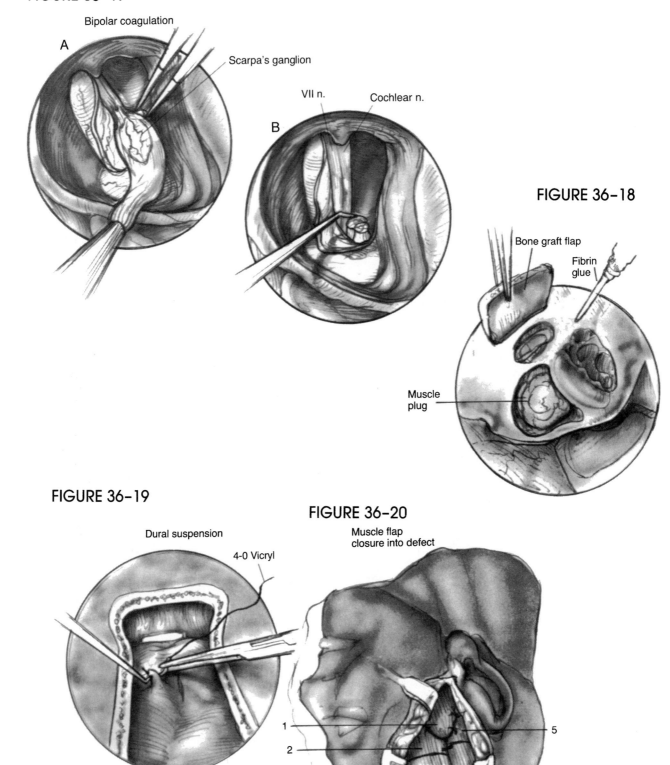

FIGURE 36-18

FIGURE 36-19

FIGURE 36-20

FIGURES 36–17 to 36–20. *See legends on opposite page*

■ If the arcuate eminence is not prominent (flattened middle fossa), the dura should be elevated in the area where it is anticipated, that is, in line with the external auditory canal. The pneumatic cells are removed posterior to this region to identify the superior SCC.

■ The meatal plane should be identified before the retractor is placed. It is often more medial than expected and may be hidden by a shelf of bone.

■ The blue-lined superior SCC is the only essential landmark for the identification of the IAC, but the surgeon should not hesitate to open the tegmen tympani to identify the malleus and incus or the tympanic portion of the facial nerve if more landmarks are needed.

■ Adequate exposure of the IAC requires lowering of bone between the superior ampulla and the geniculum of the facial nerve (genicular crest). This procedure must be performed with the utmost care.

■ When attempting to identify the blue-line of the IAC, the surgeon must work medially toward the porus rather than laterally to avoid injuring the labyrinthine segment.

■ The vertical crest (Bill's bar) should be clearly identified by thinning the bone over the meatal foramen. The meatal dura should not be opened before the completion of bone removal, because the pressure of the cerebrospinal fluid suspends the facial and vestibular nerves against the dura and thus facilitates identification.

■ The intrameatal facial nerve often appears to impinge on and partially cover the SVN. The posterior roof of the IAC close to the superior SCC must be removed to adequately expose and identify the cleavage plane between the nerves for the subsequent neurectomy.

■ The surgeon should always cut the vestibular nerve with a neurectomy knife rather than avulse the nerves with a hook. This prevents inadvertent traction on the cochlear nerve and its vascular supply, resulting in deafness.

■ One should look for a loop of the anteroinferior cerebellar artery before cutting the nerve close to the porus.

■ Lateral suspension of the dura decreases the dead space and prevents epidural hematoma formation.

■ To avoid perforation, overzealous blue-lining of the superior SCC and its ampulla is discouraged. If it does occur, however, the area of opening should be immediately covered with a piece of fascia, with bone dust pate or wax applied over it, and stabilized with fibrin glue.

■ The basal turn of the cochlea should not be encountered if the "60 rule" (see Fig. 36–14) is followed. However, one must be cautious when a change of color is observed in the bone while working anteriorly within the 60° angle. Working deep in the bone without an adequate view around the tip of the burr can be avoided by removing the lateral bone overhang between the superior ampulla, labyrinthine and tympanic segments of the facial nerve.

RESULTS

Follow-up of 3 to 15 years was available in 281 vestibular neurectomy patients operated on at the University of Zurich from 1967 to 1988.[8] Of these, 218 of the operations were for Ménière's disease, including four patients who underwent staged operations for bilateral disease, whereas 63 were for other forms of peripheral vestibular disorder. The success rate of transtemporal vestibular neurectomy to alleviate intractable vertigo was 98.2 per cent for the Ménière's group and 96.8 per cent for the peripheral vestibular disorder group.

In 61 per cent of the Ménière's group, evidence suggests a stabilizing effect of the surgery on residual hearing. An initial hearing improvement of more than 15 dB was seen in 12 per cent of patients, with some improvement lasting for as long as 7 years, but invariably hearing deterioration ensued. Although difficult to explain, this hearing improvement could be due to (1) the division of cochlear efferents traveling with the vestibular nerve, (2) the reduction in the rate of endolymph production resulting from the devascularization and destruction of the dark cell areas, or (3) a change in the parasympathetic innervation of the inner ear subsequent to the sectioning of the olivocochlear bundle in the vestibulofacial anastomosis.[9]

COMPLICATIONS

Vestibular compensation usually takes a few weeks, and most patients are back to work in a few months. Twenty per cent of the patients complain of a mild, transient dizziness after rapid head movements in the first postoperative year. Two per cent suffer from incomplete vestibular compensation and continue to experience disabling vertigo.

Complications specifically associated with this approach include a sensorineural hearing loss in 2 per cent. This complication is most likely a result of traction injury of the cochlear nerve and unrecognized perforation of the semicircular canal. Transient facial paresis is seen in 3.2 per cent of cases and occurs 5 to 7 days following surgery. Recovery is expected within 1 to 3 months.

Transient cerebrospinal fluid rhinorrhea during the first 5 to 7 days occurs in 6 per cent of patients, all successfully treated with conservative measures. One case of epidural hematoma was noted and required evacuation with no sequela. No meningitis, temporal lobe epilepsy, or atrophy was associated with this technique.

ALTERNATIVE TECHNIQUES

The indication for endolymphatic sac surgery appears to be hearing preservation only in patients with early-stage

---

FIGURE 36–17. *A* and *B,* Vestibular neurectomy.

FIGURE 36–18. Bone flap reconstruction.

FIGURE 36–19. Dural suspension.

FIGURE 36–20. Muscle closure.

disease. The long-term results at the University of Zurich have been as disappointing as those reported by others.[10–12]

Endolymph-perilymph shunting procedures and peripheral labyrinthine ablation by either medical or surgical means continue to find support in many centers.[13–17] Many are of historical interest only, whereas others, such as intratympanic injection of vestibulotoxic medications, show some promise; however, the results both in the control of vertigo and in prevention of hearing loss make them less than desirable alternatives. Vestibular neurectomy and neurotomy (nerve section) appear to offer the best control of intractable vertigo refractory to medical therapy.

Retrolabyrinthine and retrosigmoid vestibular nerve sections[1, 2, 11] have been recently proposed as alternatives to the middle fossa (transtemporal-supralabyrinthine) vestibular neurectomy. It is, however, more logical to divide the vestibular nerve fibers in the distal IAC where fibers are distinct to achieve a complete section while preserving the cochlear nerve. Also, the resection of the vestibular nerve, including Scarpa's ganglion, ensures that regeneration does not occur. Furthermore, one is less likely to encounter large vessels in the distal portion of the IAC. These three important anatomic considerations are not adequately addressed with the posterior fossa approaches and must be kept in mind when comparing long-term results of the various surgical options.

Although the surgical access to the IAC in the transtemporal-supralabyrinthine approach is narrower compared with that of the standard middle fossa approach, the dangers associated with temporal lobe retraction are practically eliminated. The posterior fossa approach entails more risks of severe cerebrospinal fluid leaks, meningitis, deafness, permanent facial paralysis, and intracranial hemorrhage, not to mention a common sequela of permanent headache[2] that is often downplayed.

We concur that the transtemporal-supralabyrinthine approach is challenging and demands a thorough knowledge of the temporal bone; however, these challenges are similar to those of other neurotologic procedures.

References

1. House JW, Hitselberger WE, Mc Elveen J, et al: Retrolabyrinthine section of the vestibular nerve. Otolaryngol Head Neck Surg 92: 212–215, 1984.
2. Silverstein H, Norrell H: Microsurgical posterior fossa vestibular neurectomy: An evolution in technique. Skull Base Surg 1: 16–25, 1991.
3. Fisch U, Mattox D: Microsurgery of the Skull Base. New York, Thieme, 1988.
4. Garcia-Ibanez E, Garcia-Ibanez JL: Middle fossa vestibular neurectomy: A report of 373 cases. Otolaryngol Head Neck Surg 88: 486–490, 1980.
5. Castro D: Transtemporal-supralabyrinthine vestibular neurectomy for Ménière's disease. *In* Fisch U, Yasargil MG (eds): Neurological Surgery of the Ear and Skull Base. Berkeley, Kugler & Ghedini Publications, 1989.
6. Portmann M, Sterkers JM, Charachon R, Chouard CH: Le Conduit Auditif Interne-Anatomie, Pathologie, Chirurgie. Paris, Librairie Arnette, 1973, pp 102–117.
7. House WF: Surgical exposure of the internal auditory canal and its contents through the middle cranial fossa. Laryngoscope 71: 1363–1365, 1961.
8. Kronenberg J, Fisch U, Dillier N: Long-term evaluation of hearing after transtemporal supralabyrinthine vestibular neurectomy. *In* Nadol JB (ed): The Second International Symposium on Ménière's Disease. Amsterdam, Kugler & Ghedini Publications, 1989, pp 481–488.
9. Chouard CH: Acousticofacial anastomosis in Ménière's disorder. Arch Otolaryngol Head Neck Surg 101: 296–300, 1975.
10. Bretlau P, Thomsen J, Tos M, Johnsen NJ: Placebo effect in surgery for Ménière's disease: Nine-year follow-up. Am J Otol 10: 259–261, 1989.
11. Glasscock ME, Jackson CG, Poe DS, Johnson GD: What I think of sac surgery. Am J Otol 10: 230–233, 1989.
12. Brown JS: A ten-year statistical follow-up of 245 consecutive cases of endolymphatic shunt and decompression with 328 consecutive cases of labyrinthectomy. Laryngoscope 93: 1419–1424, 1983.
13. Schuknecht HF: Cochleosacculotomy for Ménière's disease: Theory, technique, and results. Laryngoscope 92: 853–854, 1982.
14. Pennington CL, Stevens EL, Griffin WL: The use of ultrasound in the treatment of Ménière's disease. Laryngoscope 80: 578–581, 1980.
15. Wolfson RJ: Labyrinthine cryosurgery for Ménière's disease—present status. Otolaryngol Head Neck Surg 92: 221–227, 1984.
16. Shea J: Perfusion of the inner ear with streptomycin. Am J Otol 10: 150–155, 1989.
17. Moller C, Odkvist LM, Thell J, et al: Vestibular and audiologic functions in gentamicin-treated Ménière's disease. Am J Otol 9: 383–391, 1989.

37

Retrolabyrinthine/Retrosigmoid Vestibular Neurectomy

Herbert Silverstein, M.D., F.A.C.S. ▪ Seth I. Rosenberg, M.D., F.A.C.S.

Vestibular neurectomy (VN) is an accepted procedure to preserve hearing and relieve vertigo associated with unilateral vestibular disorders that are refractory to medical management. A survey of the American Otological Society and the American Neurotologic Society in 1990 indicated that almost 3000 VNs have been performed in the United States.[1] Ninety-five per cent of these were posterior fossa VNs, including retrolabyrinthine, retrosigmoid, or combined approaches. In this series, representing the experience of 58 surgeons, the cure rate was greater than 90 per cent, as was the reported patient satisfaction. The goals of VN are to cure vertigo by completely denervating the vestibular system while preserving the patient's hearing at the preoperative level.

Classic Ménière's disease is the most common inner ear disorder treated by VN; however, the procedure is also useful in treating selected cases of recurrent vestibular neuronitis, traumatic labyrinthitis, and vestibular Ménière's disease.

From 1978 to 1985, the retrolabyrinthine vestibular neurectomy (RVN) approach (anterior to sigmoid sinus) was used to transect the vestibular nerve in the posterior fossa. From 1985 to 1987, the retrosigmoid–internal auditory canal (RSG-IAC) approach (posterior to sigmoid sinus) was used, and from 1987 to the present, the combined retrolabyrinthine-retrosigmoid (combined RR) approach (posterior to the sigmoid sinus) has been used.[2–5] In this chapter, 218 consecutive VNs performed for the treatment of Ménière's disease using the RVN (78 cases), RSG-IAC (14 cases), and combined RR (126 cases) approaches are presented.

PATIENT SELECTION

The patient's choice is the strongest consideration in the decision of when to perform VN. Some patients may have one or two severe Ménière's attacks a month and not have their lifestyles sufficiently affected to warrant a surgical procedure to correct their problem. Other patients with only two or three attacks a year can be so severely affected that they live in constant dread of the next recurrence. In some patients the loss of a warning signal (i.e., change in hearing, tinnitus, or aural fullness) prior to their attack of vertigo is what motivates them to have surgery.

Contraindications to VN include bilateral vestibular disease, poor medical condition, ataxia or other indications of a possible significant central nervous system involvement,

and vertigo arising from an only-hearing ear. Unless a patient is experiencing an acute Ménière's attack, he or she should be able to perform a tandem gait test reasonably well. Vertigo from an ear with very poor hearing (i.e., 80-dB speech reception threshold and/or <20 per cent discrimination score) is usually more appropriately treated with a transcochlear eighth nerve section.[6, 7]

A previous endolymphatic sac operation or mastoidectomy is not a contraindication for posterior fossa VN. When the patient is healthy and has good balance function, advancing age is also not a concern. VN has been done successfully in patients older than 70 years of age with excellent results and little additional morbidity. However, elderly persons usually take longer to regain good balance function postoperatively than do younger individuals.

PREOPERATIVE EVALUATION AND PATIENT COUNSELING

Before surgery can be considered, objective evidence of unilateral inner ear disease should be provided by audiogram, electronystagmography (ENG), and/or electrocochleography. An auditory evoked brainstem response is also obtained to help rule out a central disorder and as baseline for intraoperative eighth nerve monitoring. A high-resolution computed tomographic scan is obtained before surgery primarily to identify the singular canal in the IAC and to measure the overall length of the IAC. These dimensions are significant if the posterior rim of the IAC is drilled to expose the eighth nerve within the canal. A magnetic resonance imaging study is generally not required.

Patients are told that the goals of VN are to relieve their episodic vertigo and preserve their hearing. They should expect to have vertigo that usually lasts 3 to 5 days immediately after surgery. Imbalance may last for several weeks or months, but most patients resume their normal activities within 3 weeks. All patients are encouraged to increase their activity as soon as possible after surgery.

SURGICAL ANATOMY

The surgical anatomy is described regarding the right ear as if the patient were supine and the head was turned away from the surgeon (Fig. 37–1). At the labyrinthine end of the IAC, six separate branches of the seventh and eighth

FIGURE 37-1

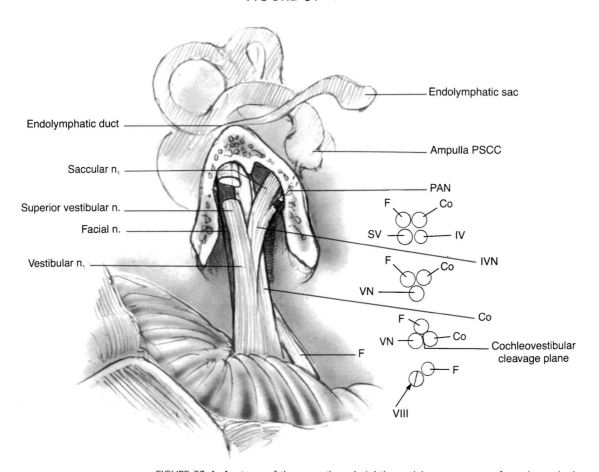

FIGURE 37-1. Anatomy of the seventh and eighth cranial nerves as seen from the otologic surgical position (right ear). Note the 90-degree rotation of cochlear and vestibular nerves. PSCC, posterior semicircular canal; PAN, posterior ampullary nerve; SV, superior vestibular nerve; IV and IVN, inferior vestibular nerve; F, facial nerve; VN, vestibular nerve; Co, cochlear nerve; VIII, eighth cranial nerve.

cranial nerves enter the temporal bone: the facial nerve (FN), nervus intermedius (NI), superior vestibular (SV), saccular, singular (posterior ampullary), and cochlear nerve (CN). The transverse (falciform) crest, which lies in a perpendicular plane, divides the lateral IAC into superior and inferior compartments. A vertical crest of bone (Bill's bar) separates the superior half of the IAC into an anterosuperior quadrant containing the FN and NI and a posterosuperior quadrant containing the SV nerve. Anterior and inferior to the transverse crest lies the CN, hidden from the surgeon by the inferior vestibular nerve. The singular nerve lies in a separate canal (singular canal) that enters the IAC in the posteroinferior quadrant, approximately 2 mm medial to the transverse crest. This reliable landmark is the point at which drilling stops when the posterior wall of the IAC is being surgically removed. The inferior vestibular nerve is formed when the saccular nerve joins the singular nerve just medial to the transverse crest.

The SV nerve innervates the superior semicircular canal, horizontal semicircular canal, utricle, and part of the saccule. The inferior vestibular nerve innervates the saccule (saccular nerve) and the posterior semicircular canal (singular nerve).

The separation between the CN and vestibular nerve, the cochleovestibular (CV) cleavage plane at the labyrinthine end of the IAC, lies in the superoinferior plane, with the vestibular nerves occupying the posterior half of the IAC. Between the transverse crest and the porus acusticus, the SV and inferior vestibular nerves fuse. Laterally, within the IAC is a constant, well-delineated cleavage between these two nerves.[8]

At the distal end of the IAC, the CN lies anterior to the inferior vestibular nerve. The CN and inferior vestibular nerve fuse within the IAC, just medial to the transverse crest. The CN and vestibular nerve then rotate 90 degrees, so that the CN, which at first lies anterior to the inferior vestibular nerve, rotates to lie caudal and inferior to the vestibular nerve as it enters the porus acusticus.[9] Most of the rotation occurs within the IAC; only slight rotation occurs in the cerebellopontine (CPA) angle (see Fig. 37-1). The CN leaves the brainstem caudal and slightly dorsal to the vestibular nerve. The flocculus of the cerebellum covers 5 mm of the eighth cranial nerve at the brainstem.

After the vestibular and CNs fuse within the IAC, the CV cleavage plane usually persists grossly and histologically.[8] The vestibular fibers remain segregated and are cephalad or superior; the cochlear fibers are caudad or inferior. Occasionally, inferior vestibular fibers run with the CN, while the efferent cochlear fibers run in the inferior vestibular nerve. Near the labyrinth, the CV cleavage plane runs in a superoinferior direction and, because of rotation, in an anteroposterior direction in the CPA. In the CPA the CV cleavage plane appears grossly as a fine septum along the eighth cranial nerve in 75 per cent of patients.[8]

In the lateral IAC, the facial nerve is positioned in the anterosuperior quadrant, anterior to the superior vestibular nerve, running proximally to a ventrocaudal position as it exits the brainstem. The FN remains ventrally positioned and hidden by the eighth cranial nerve along much of its entire course. In the IAC, the FN is connected to the SV nerve by the Rasmussen facial-vestibular anastomosing fibers, and in the CPA the FN lies adjacent to, but distinct from, the eighth nerve. Although it remains hidden from the surgeon's view by the eighth cranial nerve, the FN can easily be seen by gentle retraction of the SV nerve in the IAC or the eighth nerve in the CPA. The FN exits the brainstem 3 mm ventral and usually caudal to the eighth nerve root entry zone. In the IAC, the seventh nerve appears whiter than the eighth nerve; in the CPA it appears grayer.

The NI, which may consist of a single nerve or multiple bundles, runs between the seventh and eighth nerves through their entire course. The NI enters the brainstem closest to the eighth nerve and usually delineates the CV cleavage plane on the anterior surface of the eighth nerve.

SURGICAL TECHNIQUES

Preoperative Preparation

The shave preparation that has previously been done at the patient's bedside is examined for adequacy. Any excess hair is removed in the operating room. Perioperative intravenous antibiotics are given, usually nafcillin (2 g) in three doses: the first preoperatively, the second during surgery, and the third eight hours later. Intravenous mannitol (1.5 g/kg to a maximum of 100 g) is administered when the drilling begins, causing contraction of the cerebellum and allowing a wider exposure of the CPA.

Surgical Site Preparation and Draping and Positioning

Injections are made with 1 per cent lidocaine and epinephrine 1:100,000, into the postauricular area. A plastic Steri-Drape (No. 1010) is cut in thirds and used to border the surgical area. Benzoin is used to secure the drape. The skin prep is done using a thick gelatin-like Betadine. The area is blotted dry and a Steri-Drape II (No. 2045) is placed over the surgical site. The sterile area is covered with a split-contoured sheet. A hole is cut in the drape for placement of the Silverstein wrist rest (Diversatronics) bar; the horseshoe and bar are inserted and adjusted to the proper height, and a sterile drape tape is used to seal the opening. The wrist rest allows surgeons to comfortably support their wrists on the horseshoe during surgical manipulations.[10]

An abdominal prep is done on the left lower quadrant. Abdominal adipose tissue is obtained at the onset of the procedure; a suction drain is used to prevent hematoma formation. This tissue is used to obliterate the surgical defect in the RVN and the combined RR-VN procedures.

A magnetic mat to hold instruments is placed on the drapes across the patient's chest. A Zeiss OPMI 6 on a Neuro Contravus I base (Zeiss) microscope with a 250 lens is used for magnification. The Super Lux Light source (Dyonics) provides brilliant illumination during the surgical procedure. The 35-mm Contax camera and the Sony 3CCD camera DXC 750 MD are attached to the microscope beam splitter to document parts of the procedure. The surgeon can view one of the two television monitors in the room. The other can be seen by the scrub technician.

To reduce tangling of suction tubing and electrical cords, a polyvinylchloride (PVC) cord holster attaches by Velcro straps to the undersurface of the Mayo stand. The drill cords, the monitor cords, and the suction and irrigation tubes are placed through PVC tubes to keep them from getting tangled on the surgical field. Five-inch-long PVC tubes, glued to a flat, plastic plate and attached to the end of the Mayo stand, are used to hold drills, suction tips, and cautery tips. Two suction irrigator setups with Silastic tubing are used with Essar suction tips (Xomed-Treace). A 1000-ml saline irrigation bag is placed inside a pneumatic blood pressure cuff applying constant pressure of 150 psi to deliver a constant stream of irrigation fluid. The Essar irrigation suction tips contain a pressure-sensitive valve controlled by the thumb and forefinger. This allows the fluid to pass through the irrigation tip; the index finger applied to the regulator hole controls the suction.

The FN is monitored using a mechanical pressure sensor consisting of the WR-S8 monitor (WR Medical Electronics).[11] The hook wires and needle electrodes for the Brackmann electromyography monitors are placed in the orbicularis oris and the frontalis muscles. The strain-gauge sensor for the Silverstein WR-S8 Facial Nerve Monitor/Stimulator is placed in the patient's mouth and the set-screw is tightened. The sensor is tested by tapping on the face, which activates the alarm. The cable from the sensor is secured with a strip of Micropore tape to the patient's neck. This helps eliminate artifact created by motion of the drapes pulling the sensor wires during surgery. A molded surgical mask (3M) is placed over the sensor and taped in place to prevent the surgical drapes from putting pressure on the mouthpiece and setting off the alarm. A slit is made in the mask to allow for the endotracheal tube.

To help preserve serviceable hearing during VN, eighth nerve action potentials (8AP) in combination with brainstem auditory evoked responses and electrocochleography have been used. Electrodes are placed on the forehead (ground) and ear lobe for intraoperative monitoring of brainstem and direct 8AP using the Nicolet Pathfinder. Intraoperative eighth nerve monitoring has been found to enhance the surgeon's ability to preserve hearing and allows the surgeon to inform the family immediately after surgery whether hearing will probably be unchanged.[12, 13]

A major difficulty encountered during VN in the posterior fossa is that in approximately 25 per cent of the cases, the CV cleavage plane is not readily identifiable.[8] Recently a flush-tipped, bipolar electrode recording probe has been

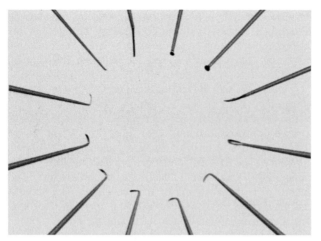

FIGURE 37–2. The series of microsurgical instruments for vestibular neurectomy in the posterior fossa.

used to directly record responses to monaural click stimuli conducted along the CN but not along surrounding tissue. This technique has been used to help identify the CV cleavage plane.[14]

Special Instruments

Several unique instruments have been developed for vestibular neurectomy (Fig. 37–2).[15] A modified Penfield elevator is used to elevate bone of the endolymphatic sac or dura, so that a small ronguer can be used to remove this bone quickly. The Silverstein lateral venous sinus retractor[16] is used to compress and retract the lateral venous sinus posteriorly to provide greater exposure of the posterior fossa during RVN. The arachnoid dissector allows the surgeon to incise arachnoid and release cerebrospinal fluid (CSF) from the CPA cistern. A long sickle knife is used to start the separation between the CN and vestibular nerve. A nerve separator is a blunt, slightly curved instrument that is used to complete the separation developed in the CV cleavage plane. A 3-mm mirror is used to view the eighth nerve complex from the anterior side. The malleable nerve hook is used when it is necessary to develop cleavage plane from the anterior aspect of the nerve. Luetje microscissors are used to transect the vestibular nerve. Round knives (1, 2, and 3 mm) are used to separate the eighth nerve from the flocculus and the FN if they are intimately related. All these instruments are manufactured by Storz Instrument Co., St. Louis, Missouri.

These instruments are also available with insulated handles, which can be attached via the SACS (Silverstein adapter for continuous stimulation) to the Silverstein WR-S8 Facial Nerve Monitor or Brackmann monitor. The instruments can then become electrical probe tips as well as dissectors.

Technique of Surgery in Detail

Middle Fossa Vestibular Neurectomy

From 1963 to 1978, the middle fossa (subtemporal) approach was exclusively used by the senior author to section the vestibular nerve. Results for vertigo relief were good, but the procedure was formidable, anatomic landmarks were difficult, and complications such as FN weakness and deafness did occur.[17, 18] Patients older than 60 years of age were generally not candidates. The procedure was technically difficult and carried a high risk of complications; thus, many patients who had significant disability were not enthusiastically offered a middle fossa VN. This procedure is discussed in greater detail in Chapter 36.

Posterior Fossa Vestibular Neurectomy

Retrolabyrinthine Approach. In 1978, the senior author developed the RVN approach to the posterior cranial fossa for vestibular neurectomy.[19, 20] Although previously used as an approach for trigeminal nerve section, its application for selective vestibular nerve section had not been described.[21]

A 4 × 5 cm anteriorly based U-shaped postauricular incision is made (Fig. 37–3). The flap is elevated with the periosteum and postauricular muscles as one layer. A simple mastoidectomy is performed, and the sigmoid sinus and posterior fossa dura just behind the sinus and in front of it are exposed. The endolymphatic sac is widely exposed, and the bone overlying the posterior semicircular canal is identified. The sigmoid sinus is collapsed with a retractor, and the dura incised in a C shape anterior to the sigmoid sinus based on the labyrinth (Fig. 37–4). A Penrose drain is placed over the cerebellum, which is gently retracted until the arachnoid is opened with a blunt instrument (arachnoid knife, Storz Instruments) to allow CSF to escape. The cerebellum will fall away from the temporal bone, allowing exposure of cranial nerves V, VII, VIII, IX, X, and XI. After the cleavage plane is visualized under high-power magnification, a longitudinal incision is made in the cleavage plane, the cochlear and vestibular fibers are separated, and the vestibular nerve is transected.

Several landmarks are helpful in finding the cleavage plane. The vestibular nerve often appears grayer and the CN is whiter; the cochlear fibers are more numerous, averaging 31,000, whereas the vestibular fibers average 18,000. A fine blood vessel frequently courses on the surface between the cochlear and vestibular fibers. A mirror can be used to view the anterior surface of the eighth nerve, because the cleavage plane is sometimes more visible from this surface. The NI, which usually lies in the cleavage plane, can also be seen anteriorly. A bipolar electrode recording probe has been developed to identify a physiologic cleavage plane while stimulating the cochlear nerve with auditory clicks.[14] The superior half of the eighth cranial nerve is transected when a cleavage plane cannot

FIGURE 37–3. The 4 × 5-cm U-shaped postauricular incision used for all approaches.

FIGURE 37–4. The posterior fossa as seen through the retrolabyrinthine approach.

FIGURE 37-4

FIGURE 37-3

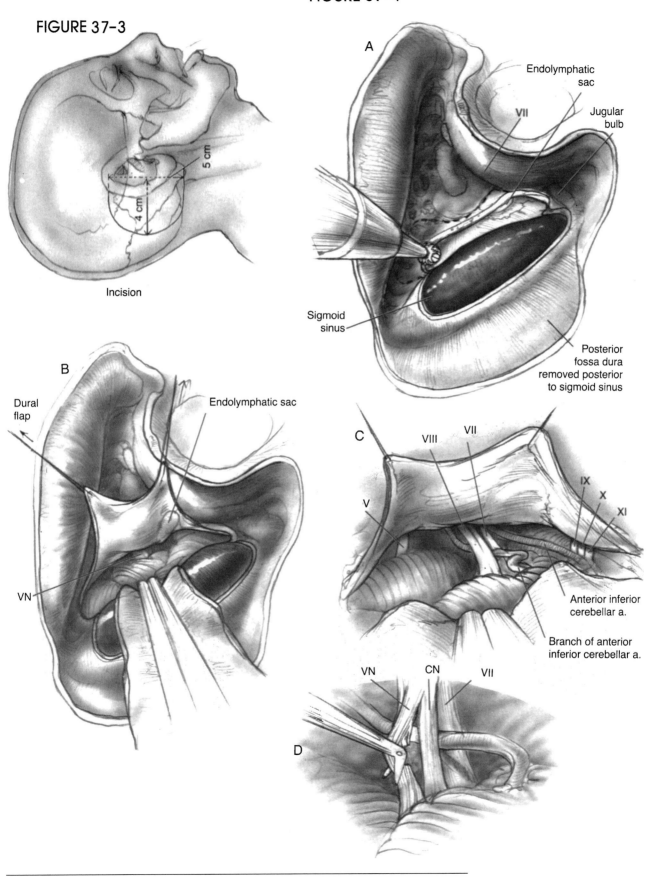

Incision

FIGURE 37–5

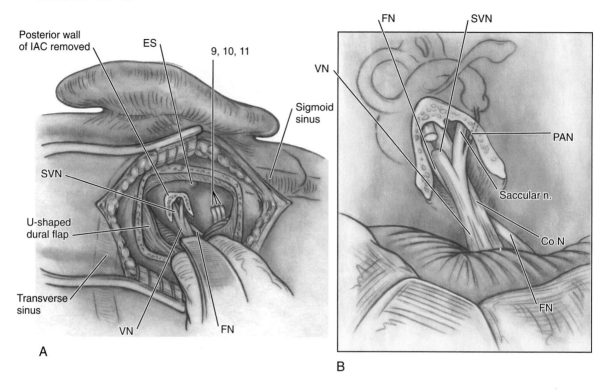

A

B

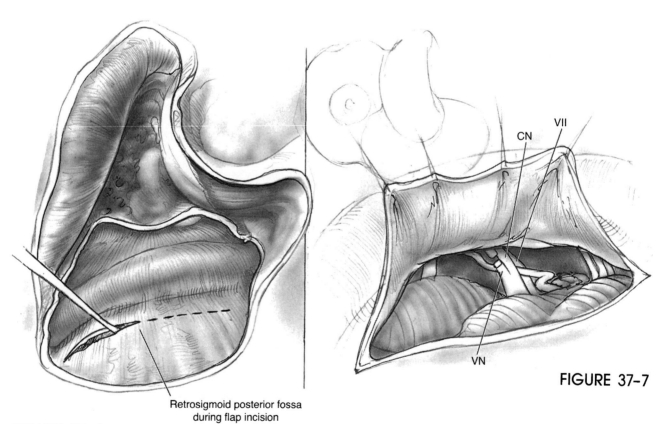

Retrosigmoid posterior fossa
during flap incision

FIGURE 37–6

FIGURE 37–7

FIGURES 37–5 to 37–7. *See legends on opposite page*

be readily identified. Most vestibular fibers will be cut, and most cochlear fibers will be spared using this technique. The dura is closed with three or four interrupted 4–0 silk sutures and the mastoid cavity is filled with abdominal adipose tissue. Unfortunately this approach resulted in a 10 per cent incidence of CSF leak.[3]

Retrosigmoid–Internal Auditory Canal Approach. In 1985, in an attempt to perform a more complete vestibular neurectomy nearer to the labyrinth, to improve vertigo relief and hearing preservation, and to decrease the incidence of CSF leak, the RSG-IAC approach was developed.[22] Because the cleavage plane between cochlear and vestibular fibers is more completely developed within the IAC, a more complete and selective VN can be performed by cutting the nerve within the IAC.

In this procedure, a posterior fossa craniotomy is performed immediately behind the lateral sinus, and the cerebellum is retracted to give exposure to the seventh and eighth cranial nerves and the IAC.

The first major landmark seen in the posterior fossa above the jugular foramen is the white linear fold of dura: the jugular dural fold (JDF, or "Herb's fold"). The JDF extends approximately 2 cm from the anterior aspect of the foramen magnum, overlying the junction of the lateral sinus and jugular bulb, and attaching to the temporal bone 7 mm medial to the endolymphatic duct. The JDF lies 7 to 9 mm lateral to the exit of the ninth nerve. The anterior aspect of the fold usually points to the eighth cranial nerve, which is 7 to 10 mm medial. Using a diamond drill bit, the posterior wall of the IAC is removed to the singular canal, thereby exposing the branches of the eighth cranial nerve (Fig. 37–5). The SV nerve and the singular nerve are sectioned. The inferior vestibular fibers that innervate the saccule are not divided because of their close association with cochlear fibers. The saccule has no known vestibular function in humans, so sparing these fibers does not result in postoperative vertigo attacks.

This procedure offers several advantages over the RVN. No abdominal fat is needed to fill the defect; thus, the procedure can be performed on thin patients. Since the exposure does not enter the mastoid, patients who have had chronic mastoiditis, a sclerotic mastoid, or an anterior-lying sigmoid sinus can be candidates for the RSG-IAC approach.

Combined Retrolabyrinthine-Retrosigmoid Approach. A further evolution of the VN procedure, the combined RR was developed in 1987.[23] The combined RR incorporates the advantages of the RVN and RSG-IAC

approaches. It also allows the surgeon to assess the CV cleavage plane in the posterior fossa and decide where the neurectomy should be performed. If a good CV cleavage plane exists, the vestibular nerve section will be done in the CPA. If not, the IAC can be opened and the SV and posterior ampullary nerves sectioned within the IAC. In this approach, a limited mastoidectomy is done. The sigmoid sinus is exposed from the transverse sinus inferiorly 3 cm, and the posterior fossa dura is exposed for 1.5 cm posterior to the sigmoid sinus. The dural incision is made 3 mm behind and parallel to the sigmoid sinus for 2.5 cm (Fig. 37–6). The sigmoid sinus is retracted anteriorly using stay sutures placed in the dural cuff. After the CPA cistern is opened, the eighth nerve is examined and, if a cleavage plane is present, the vestibular nerve section is performed in the CPA, as in the retrolabyrinthine approach (Fig. 37–7). If no cleavage plane is identified, then the dura is reflected off the temporal bone, the IAC is opened with a diamond burr, and the SV and singular nerves are divided laterally within the IAC, as in the retrosigmoid approach (see Fig. 37–5). The mastoid air cells are sealed with bone wax, the dura is closed with 4–0 braided nylon in a watertight manner, and the surgical defect is filled with abdominal adipose tissue.

Dressing

A mastoid dressing is applied in the operating room at the end of the procedure. The dressing is left in place for 48 to 72 hours unless it becomes saturated with blood or CSF.

Postoperative Care

For the first 24 hours postoperatively the patient is observed in a neurosurgical intensive care unit. On the first postoperative day the Foley catheter and arterial lines are removed. The abdominal dressing and suction drain are left in place for 24 to 48 hours. Early activity is encouraged; the patients sit up, stand, and ambulate usually on the first postoperative day and are usually discharged on the fourth to sixth postoperative day.

Patients are seen 1 week postoperatively for suture removal and audiogram. One month postoperatively a repeat audiogram and ENG with iced caloric testing are performed. The ENG is obtained to document the percentage of reduced vestibular response. All patients are encouraged

---

FIGURE 37–5. *A* and *B*, The retrosigmoid internal auditory canal (IAC) vestibular neurectomy. Note the 90-degree rotation of the eighth nerve from the ear to the brain. Most of the rotation occurs in the IAC. Note the superior vestibular nerve (SVN) and posterior ampullary nerves that are transected while the saccular nerve is spared. This allows for complete denervation of the vestibular labyrinth without damaging the cochlear nerve. FN, facial nerve; 9, 10, 11, cranial nerves IX, X, and XI; VN, vestibular nerve; ES, endolymphatic sac.

FIGURE 37–6. Combined retrolabyrinthine-retrosigmoid vestibular neurectomy. Dura is transected behind the sigmoid sinus while leaving a dura cuff for retraction purposes (right ear).

FIGURE 37–7. Combined retrolabyrinthine-retrosigmoid vestibular neurectomy in the cerebellopontine angle (CPA). There is a good cochleovestibular cleavage in the CPA and the neurectomy is done in the posterior fossa (right ear). The vestibular nerve (VN) has been transected. CN, cochlear nerve; VII, seventh cranial nerve.

to resume an active lifestyle, which we believe is the best rehabilitation program. Most patients not only maintain their preoperative lifestyle but also return to activities they had given up because of their Ménière's disease, including golf, tennis, bicycling, and running. Following recovery, more than 90 per cent of patients consider themselves to be more active than before surgery.

Pitfalls and Tips in Surgery

Bleeding from injury to the sigmoid sinus or jugular bulb is usually managed by placing an Avitene surgical pack over the bleeding site and holding it in place with a cottonoid neurosurgical sponge. Bleeding from a large mastoid emissary vein is controlled with Avitene packs; however, this can be prevented if a stump of vein, which can be cauterized, is left on the sigmoid sinus. If the emissary vein can be seen before bleeding occurs, dissection should proceed with a diamond burr. When opening the dura, small vessels can be cut inadvertently. Bleeding is controlled with microbipolar cautery set at 20. Lifting the dura and cutting with scissors helps avoid cutting these vessels.

After opening of the dura, there is a slight chance that brain swelling may occur. This is prevented by lowering the P_{CO_2} during surgery by hyperventilating the patient and by administering mannitol (1.5 g/kg to a maximum of 100 g) intravenously when bone work is begun. Damage to the cerebellum is prevented by using a Penrose drain placed against the cortex while retracting the cerebellum to gain exposure of the CPA and by releasing CSF. In younger patients, the cerebellum may be tense and protrude slightly through the dural incision. Gentle pressure against the Penrose drain lying on the cerebellum allows CSF to escape. The Penrose drain is slid along the cerebellum at the inferior margin of the wound toward the ninth cranial nerve. After CSF is released from the CPA by opening the arachnoid layer with a blunt instrument, the cerebellum will fall away from the temporal bone and allow good exposure of the CPA without cerebellar retraction. If brain swelling occurs from trauma to the cerebellum and the posterior fossa cannot be easily exposed, it is best to back out and close the wound. We have not had to do this in any case. Care must be taken not to traumatize the petrosal veins located above the fifth cranial nerve and near the tentorium. Because of the brain shrinkage from mannitol, these veins are on stretch and can easily rupture. Bleeding is controlled with Avitene or electrocautery.

When the thin arachnoid layer is dissected away from the seventh and eighth cranial nerves, bleeding from small vessels may occur. This is prevented by cauterizing the vessel with an irrigating microbipolar cautery and transecting with a microscissors. Sometimes the flocculus of the cerebellum is adherent and hides much of the eighth cranial nerve. The flocculus must be dissected away from the eighth cranial nerve using a round knife. Locating cranial nerves V, IX, and X helps orient the surgeon to the vestibular portion of the eighth cranial nerve (the superior half is closest to the fifth cranial nerve). To prevent injury to the FN, a small mirror is used to look on the anterior aspect of the eighth cranial nerve. Occasionally, the facial nerve is attached to the vestibular nerve and must also be sepa-

rated with a round knife. FN injury is avoided by seeing the nerve before the VN is performed. The cleavage between the CN and vestibular nerve is first made with a sharp sickle knife, then completed with an electrified nerve separator. This instrument, electrified at 0.05 mA with the SACS, alerts the surgeon if the FN is in proximity on the anterior side of the cleavage plane.

Unless the nerve separator can be seen emerging from the anterior aspect of the eighth cranial nerve and the FN is not near the vestibular nerve, only about 80 per cent of the vestibular nerve is transected with the Luetje microscissors. The transection is then completed with a sharp sickle knife, which is also electrified. This avoids injury to the facial nerve and the internal auditory artery. Total hearing loss can occur if the internal auditory artery is interrupted during the VN. This is more likely to occur if a 3- to 4-mm section of nerve is removed for histologic study; this is not recommended as a routine procedure. If the FN is inappropriately transected, it must be repaired at the time of surgery. Fortunately, this has not happened to any of our patients. Because this procedure is done in the posterior fossa, a neurosurgeon should be available in the event of an unusual complication with which the otologist is unfamiliar. Most intraoperative complications are prevented by using careful, gentle microsurgical techniques.

RESULTS

Retrolabyrinthine Vestibular Neurectomy

Results of the RVN procedure have been good. In reviewing 78 patients, 88 per cent were completely cured of their vertigo and 7 per cent were substantially improved; only 5 per cent noted no change postoperatively. Overall patient satisfaction with the procedure has been 93 per cent, and sensorineural hearing has been maintained to within 20 dB of the preoperative level in 70 per cent. Some patients experienced a mild conductive loss in the low frequencies probably secondary to bone dust fixing the stapes or adipose tissue impeding the ossicular chain.

Retrosigmoid–Internal Auditory Canal Vestibular Neurectomy

The RSG-IAC VN procedure produced a 90 per cent cure rate in 14 patients, and hearing results are similar to those of the RVN. This procedure was originally believed to have several advantages over the RVN. Because no abdominal fat is needed to fill the defect, the procedure can be performed on thin patients. Because the exposure does not enter the mastoid, patients who have had chronic mastoiditis or a sclerotic mastoid or those with an anterior-lying sigmoid sinus are good candidates. Complications have been infrequent, except for severe postoperative headache in 75 per cent of the patients. Fifty per cent of the patients have had significant headaches that are difficult to control with non-narcotic analgesics and last for many months. Two years after undergoing the procedure, 25 per cent still experience severe headaches requiring continuous medication. The cause for this problem is unknown. This is perplexing, particularly because this approach has been used successfully for vascular decompression or section of the fifth cranial nerve. It is speculated that drilling the bone from the IAC or bone dust may have produced arachnoiditis with resultant headache. The postoperative headaches remain a major concern and have tempered our enthusiasm for the classic RSG-IAC VN.

Combined Retrolab-Retrosigmoid Vestibular Neurectomy

The combined RR procedure is a significant improvement over the two previous procedures. Because much less bone removal is needed than in the retrolabyrinthine approach, the surgical time is shortened. In addition, the surgeon has the option of opening the IAC and cutting the vestibular nerve more laterally where the CV cleavage plane is better defined. The incidence of CSF leak (2.5 per cent) is also markedly reduced. The advantage that this procedure has over the retrosigmoid approach is that cerebellar retraction is not necessary and the bony defect is smaller. Of 126 patients, vertigo has been cured in 85 per cent, with substantial improvement in another 7 per cent. Hearing has been preserved within 20 dB of preoperative levels in 86 per cent of patients, and discrimination has been maintained to within 20 per cent of the preoperative level in 77 per cent of patients. In a 1996 study on hearing results after posterior fossa VN, 66 per cent of patients who were evaluated at 18 to 24 months after surgery had pure-tone average preserved within 20 dB of preoperative levels and discrimination maintained to within 20 per cent of the preoperative levels.[24] It appears that drilling the posterior lip of the IAC for VN results in headache complaints in 50 per cent of patients. Using the RR VN, less than 5 per cent of patients have had the IAC drilled for better exposure of the vestibular nerve. In the last 97 cases the IAC has not been drilled. The incidence of headache has been minimized.

COMPLICATIONS, INCIDENCE, AND MANAGEMENT

Postoperative Complications

Early postoperative bleeding in the posterior fossa requires assessment by a neurosurgeon. The wound may have to be opened immediately. This complication has not occurred in our series. Meningismus with mild temperature elevation occurring soon after surgery usually represents a chemical meningitis caused by small amounts of blood in the CSF. This requires no treatment.

Wound infection secondary to serum collected beneath the flap in the postauricular crease is treated by incision and drainage, culture of the pus, and appropriate antibiotic treatment. This complication is prevented by keeping the skin flap and muscle layer together when elevating the skin flap and by using perioperative antibiotics such as nafcillin. No wound infection has been seen in the last 75 cases, and, fortunately, none has ever progressed to meningitis in

our series. Several days postoperatively, if there is a spiking temperature elevation with nuchal rigidity and headache, a lumbar puncture for culture and sensitivity should be done, and the patient should be treated for meningitis. As yet we have not had to treat this complication.

Following RVN, the most common early complication is CSF leak (10 per cent) from the wound edge or through the eustachian tube. Initially, these leaks were treated by immediate re-exploration of the wound and repacking with adipose tissue. Now, a CSF leak is treated with continuous lumbar drainage for 3 or 4 days. After lumbar drainage, all acute CSF leaks have stopped without reoperation. Because the dura cannot be closed watertight using the retrolabyrinthine exposure, no method has been developed to prevent the high incidence of CSF leaks. When the dural incision can be closed watertight, as in the combined RR approach, the incidence of CSF leak is greatly reduced. In this series there have been no cases of facial paralysis or meningitis, or deaths.

Late Complications

The cause for postoperative headache (75 per cent) after RSG-IAC VN remains a mystery. Twenty-five per cent of patients continue to have headaches for years after surgery, but they eventually have improvement over several years. Using the combined RR approach and drilling the IAC only in those cases in which a cleavage plane cannot be determined helps minimize this side effect of surgery. When IAC drilling is required, the combined RR procedure, which is less extensive than the retrosigmoid approach and does not require cerebellar retraction, appears to reduce the severity of the headache.

About 5 per cent of patients continue to have some vertigo postoperatively. Usually the vertigo is mild and the patient's quality of life is greatly improved. There are several explanations for this. Some patients (1 per cent) develop bilateral Ménière's disease. These patients are offered subtotal streptomycin ablation if their symptoms warrant further treatment. Patients with vertigo secondary to some cause other than Ménière's disease have a higher failure rate than those with classic Ménière's disease. In some patients all vestibular fibers may not have been transected.[25] It is important to obtain an ENG with iced caloric testing 6 months postoperatively to document complete vestibular ablation. If some vestibular function remains and the patient continues to have severe episodic vertigo, imbalance, or tinnitus, a transcochlear eighth nerve section is recommended. This has been performed eight times (4 per cent) in our service.

References

1. Silverstein H, Wanamaker H, Flanzer J, Rosenberg S: Vestibular neurectomy in the USA, 1990. Am J Otol 13: 23–30, 1992.
2. Silverstein H, Norrell H, Rosenberg S: An evolution of approach in vestibular neurectomy. Otolaryngol Head Neck Surg 102: 374–381, 1990.
3. Silverstein H, Norrell H, Rosenberg S: The resurrection of vestibular neurectomy: A 10-year experience with 115 cases. J Neurosurg 72: 533–539, 1990.
4. Silverstein H, Norrell H, Smouha E, Jones R: Combined retrolab-

retrosigmoid vestibular neurectomy: An evolution in approach. Am J Otol 10: 166–169, 1989.

5. Silverstein H, Rosenberg S: Vestibular neurectomy via the posterior fossa. *In* Surgical Techniques of the Temporal Bone and Skull Base. Philadelphia, Lea & Febiger, 1992, pp 175–194.

6. Silverstein H: Transmeatal labyrinthectomy with and without cochleovestibular neurectomy. Laryngoscope 86: 1777–1791, 1976.

7. Jones R, Silverstein H, Smouha E: Long-term results of transmeatal cochleovestibular neurectomy: An analysis of 100 cases. Otolaryngol Head Neck Surg 100: 22–29, 1989.

8. Silverstein H: Cochlear and vestibular gross and histologic anatomy (as seen from the postauricular approach). Otolaryngol Head Neck Surg 92: 207–211, 1984.

9. Silverstein H, Norrell H, Haberkamp T, McDaniel A: The unrecognized rotation of the vestibular and cochlear nerves from the labyrinth to the brainstem: Its implications in surgery of the eighth cranial nerve. Otolaryngol Head Neck Surg 95: 543–549, 1986.

10. Silverstein H: Silverstein wrist rest. Otolaryngol Head Neck Surg 89: 305–306, 1981.

11. Silverstein H, Rosenberg S: Intraoperative facial nerve monitoring. Otolaryngol Clin North Am 24: 709–725, 1991.

12. Silverstein H, Wazen J, Norrell H, Hyman S: Retrolabyrinthine vestibular neurectomy with simultaneous monitoring of eighth nerve action potentials and electrocochleography. Am J Otol 5: 552–555, 1984.

13. McDaniel A, Silverstein H, Norrell H: Retrolabyrinthine vestibular neurectomy with and without monitoring of eighth nerve potentials. Am J Otol Nov (Suppl): 23–26, 1985.

14. Rosenberg S, Martin W, Pratt H, et al: Bipolar cochlear nerve recording technique: A preliminary report. Am J Otol 14: 369–372, 1993.

15. Silverstein H: Microsurgical instruments and nerve stimulator-monitor for retrolabyrinthine vestibular neurectomy. Otolaryngol Head Neck Surg 94: 409–411, 1986.

16. Silverstein H: Silverstein lateral venous sinus retractor. Otolaryngol Head Neck Surg 89: 303–304, 1981.

17. Glasscock M, Kveton J, Christiansen S: Middle fossa vestibular neurectomy: An update. Otolaryngol Head Neck Surg 92: 216–220, 1984.

18. Silverstein H, Norrell H, Haberkamp T: A comparison of retrosigmoid IAC, retrolabyrinthine, and middle fossa vestibular neurectomy for treatment of vertigo. Laryngoscope 97: 165–173, 1987.

19. Silverstein H, Norrell H: Retrolabyrinthine surgery: A direct approach to the cerebellopontine angle. *In* Silverstein H, Norrell H (eds): Neurological Surgery of the Ear, Vol 2. Birmingham, AL, Aesculapius, 1979, p 318.

20. Silverstein H, Norrell H: Retrolabyrinthine surgery: A direct approach to the cerebellopontine angle. Otolaryngol Head Neck Surg 88: 462–469, 1980.

21. Hitselberger WE, Pulec JL: Trigeminal nerve (posterior root) retrolabyrinthine selective section. Arch Otolaryngol 96: 412–415, 1972.

22. Silverstein H, Norrell H, Smouha E: Retrosigmoid-internal auditory canal approach versus retrolabyrinthine approach for vestibular neurectomy. Otolaryngol Head Neck Surg 97: 300–307, 1987.

23. Silverstein H, Norrell H, Smouha E, Jones R: Retrolabyrinthine or retrosigmoid vestibular neurectomy: Indications. Am J Otol 8: 414–418, 1987.

24. Rosenberg S, Silverstein H, Norrell H, et al: Hearing results after posterior fossa vestibular neurectomy. Otolaryngol Head Neck Surg 114: 32–37, 1996.

25. Rosenberg S, Silverstein H, Norrell H, White D: Audio and vestibular function after vestibular neurectomy. Otolaryngol Head Neck Surg 104: 139–140, 1991.

38

Cochleosacculotomy

Harold F. Schuknecht, M.D.† ▪ Michael J. McKenna, M.D.
K. Paul Boyev, M.D.

The surgical treatment for Ménière's disease can be classi-fied into two groups, according to mode of action: (1) procedures that have the objective of total or partial abla-tion of vestibular function and (2) procedures that are intended to enhance the drainage of endolymph by fistuli-zation of the membranous labyrinth and decompression of the endolymphatic sac. Endolymphatic drainage procedures can be further divided into (a) external shunts that attempt to drain excessive endolymph from the endolymphatic sac into the mastoid or subarachnoid space and (b) internal shunts that attempt to drain excessive endolymph into the perilymphatic space. The cochleosacculotomy operation falls into the latter group, that is, an internal shunt proce-dure.

PHYSIOLOGIC, ANATOMIC, AND PATHOLOGIC RATIONALE

Ménière's disease is characterized pathologically by pro-gressive endolymphatic hydrops that is probably related to a disturbance in endolymphatic sac function. This condition must be differentiated from nonprogressive endolymphatic hydrops in which the hydrops is the result of a single traumatic or inflammatory insult to the labyrinth, causing a permanent but not progressive endolymphatic hydrops.[1]

The symptoms of progressive endolymphatic hydrops can be correlated with two principal types of pathologic change: (1) distentions and ruptures of the endolymphatic system[2, 3] and (2) alterations in the cytoarchitecture of the auditory and vestibular sense organs, sometimes accompa-nied by atrophic changes. Coincident with rupture, there is sudden contamination of the perilymphatic fluid with neurotoxic endolymph (140 mEq/L of potassium) that causes paralysis of the sensory and neural structures and is expressed clinically as episodic vertigo, fluctuating hearing loss, or both. The American Academy of Otolaryngology—Head and Neck Surgery (AAO-HNS)[4] recommended that these episodes be designated the "definitive" symptoms of Ménière's disease. As the disease progresses, there are changes in the cytoarchitecture of the sense organs that consist of distortion and atrophy of the sensory cells and supporting cells as well as disruption and deformation of their gelatinous aprons. These alterations impair the motion mechanics of the sense organs, resulting in permanent functional deficits. The symptoms for the auditory system are hearing loss and tinnitus, and for the vestibular system

are constant or recurring sensations of unsteadiness, de-scribed as being off-balance, floating, tilting, falling, or spinning, and are often aggravated by head movement. The AAO-HNS recommended that they be known as "ad-junctive" symptoms. To be successful, surgical procedures based on facilitating drainage of endolymph should allevi-ate definitive symptoms and arrest the progression of ad-junctive symptoms.

Among the internal shunt procedures are the saccu-lotomy of Fick,[5, 6] the tack operation of Cody,[7, 8] the otic-perotic shunt of Pulec and House,[9] and the cochleosaccu-lotomy.[10] In the sacculotomy and tack procedures, picks are introduced through the footplate of the stapes to punc-ture the saccule with the hope of producing a permanent fistula in the saccular wall by which excessive endolymph can drain into the perilymphatic space. This approach, however, fails to consider the histopathologic observation that in Ménière's disease, the distended saccule often fills the vestibule; its distended wall is adherent to the footplate and could not be fistulized into the perilymphatic space by these maneuvers.[11] The otic-perotic shunt, as conceived by House and Pulec, involves the placement of a platinum tube through the basilar membrane to connect the scala media and scala tympani; however, the procedure is not surgically feasible because of the small size of the coch-lear duct.

The cochleosacculotomy operation consists of creating a fracture-disruption by impaling the osseous spiral lamina and cochlear duct with a pick introduced through the round window. The rationale is supported by two histopathologic observations and muted by a third.

1. Histologic study of the temporal bones from patients with Ménière's disease shows that the distended membra-nous labyrinth may fistulize permanently in any area. Such spontaneous fistulization may account for the long remis-sions and even permanent arrest of symptoms of episodic vertigo and fluctuating hearing loss in some patients.

2. Animal experiments have shown that surgical disrup-tion of Reissner's membrane[12] or the walls of the utricle, saccule, or semicircular canals[13] results in prompt healing of the fistulas. However, it has been shown in experimental studies on cats[14–16] and guinea pigs[17] that fracture-disruption of the osseous spiral lamina and cochlear duct can some-times result in a permanent communication between the endolymphatic and perilymphatic spaces. Furthermore, those experiments clearly demonstrate that such fistulas exist without impairing the hearing for frequencies other than those tonotopically located immediately adjacent to the fistulas.

†Deceased.

407

3. A histopathologic finding in human temporal bones of persons with Ménière's disease that militate against the success of internal shunts is that the distended membranes in some cases block the flow of endolymph toward such a fistula.[18] For this reason, a successful cochleosacculotomy fistula will not relieve symptoms in all instances.

PATIENT SELECTION

Some otolaryngologists believe that surgery is never indicated for the relief of symptoms of Ménière's disease because in the normal course of the disease, the vertigo eventually subsides. This approach has merit if the patient is not unduly handicapped. In many cases, however, the disequilibrium erodes occupational efficiency as well as recreational and family lifestyle to the extent that invasive therapy is justified. This approach applies to patients having frequent and severe vertiginous episodes unrelieved by medication and those having falling attacks (Tumarkin's otolithic catastrophe).[19]

Some general considerations need to be addressed before cochleosacculotomy is recommended. The diagnosis of Ménière's disease must be unequivocal. Other disorders that cause fluctuating hearing loss and episodic vertigo, such as otosyphilis, inner ear autoimmune disease, perilymph fistula, demyelinating diseases, and intracranial neoplasms, must be ruled out. The operation is not recommended for patients who present audiovestibular symptoms that are atypical for progressive endolymphatic hydrops. There should be no evidence of involvement of Ménière's disease or other disorders that might be progressive in the opposite ear. It is prudent to require a duration of symptoms of at least 1 year. The opposite ear becomes involved in almost 50 per cent of cases, sometimes many years after the onset of symptoms in the first ear.

Cochleosacculotomy is the procedure of choice for patients who for health reasons are at risk for the stress of postoperative vertigo and who should not have general anesthesia, as well as for elderly patients who often compensate poorly to procedures that ablate vestibular function. It has the advantage of being technically simple to perform, is almost totally free of morbidity, and carries little or no risk of mortality. Labyrinthectomy is more certain than cochleosacculotomy to relieve disabling episodic vertigo; however, it has the disadvantage of producing severe postoperative vertigo, permanent hearing loss, and in some cases, prolonged disequilibrium. For these reasons, some patients may choose to have a cochleosacculotomy as a first attempt to resolve their vertigo problem.

SURGICAL TECHNIQUE

The ear is prepared and draped similarly to any transcanal procedure. The operation is performed under local anesthesia. With the aid of a nasal speculum, the fibrocartilaginous external auditory canal is infiltrated circumferentially in four positions with 1 per cent lidocaine (Xylocaine) containing 1:100,000 epinephrine, using a 27-gauge, 1.5-inch needle. The ear canal is dilated with the nasal speculum, which also serves to diffuse the anesthetic solution uni-

formly into the tissues. An ear speculum of the surgeon's preference is introduced into the ear canal and locked in an adjustable speculum holder, thus freeing both of the surgeon's hands. The posterior aspect of the bony canal is exposed, and the skin of the bony canal is infiltrated at two sites with 1 per cent lidocaine containing 1:1000 epinephrine, using a 30-gauge, 1.5-inch needle. The beveled opening of the needle must be introduced flush against the bone at an obtuse angle, and the blanching area of infiltration should extend to the tympanic annulus from the 6 to 12 o'clock position. Adjustments of the speculum and speculum holder are made as often as necessary to achieve optimum exposure of the surgical field.

Incisions are made, and a triangular skin flap is elevated to the tympanic annulus (Fig. 38–1*A*). Bleeding must be meticulously controlled at all times. The tympanomeatal flap is elevated by lifting the tympanic annulus from its sulcus and folding the flap into the anterior tympanomeatal angle of the ear canal (Fig. 38–1*B*). The chorda tympani nerve and the ossicles are not disturbed. The ear speculum is locked into a position that exposes the round window niche and posterior aspect of the hypotympanum. In rare cases, the round window niche is partly hidden behind the posteroinferior part of the bony tympanic annulus, in which case a small burr is used to remove sufficient bony annulus to allow access to the round window niche.

Usually, the round window niche accommodates a 3-mm right-angle pick without removal of bone. The pick is advanced through the round window membrane, which may or may not be visible. The pick is guided in the direction of the oval window while hugging the lateral wall of the inner ear to ensure that the cochlear duct is traversed (Fig. 38–1*C*). When the pick has been introduced to its full 3-mm length, the end of the pick will be located beneath the footplate of the stapes. Occasionally, the subiculum, which is a ridge of bone lying in the boundary between the round window niche and sinus tympani, interferes with introduction of the pick. It can readily be shaved down with a 2-mm burr. Occasionally, the overhanging bony lip of the round window niche must be removed to accommodate the pick (Fig. 38–1*D*). In this case, a 2-mm (rather than a 3-mm) pick is used to avoid excessively deep penetration into the vestibule and possible injury to the utricular macula (Fig. 38–2). Rarely, a high jugular bulb blocks access to the round window niche, in which case it may be necessary to abort the operation (Fig. 38–3).

Occasionally, a slight loss of resistance is felt as the pick passes through the cochlear partition and causes the planned fracture-disruption of the osseous spiral lamina and cochlear duct (Fig. 38–4). Usually, the patients experience no sensation as the pick is advanced, but a few have noted momentary vertigo, and several have reported hearing a "click." The maneuver does not produce vertigo, presumably because the vestibular sense organs are not mechanically disturbed, and the endolymph from the fistulized area drains into the scala tympani rather than into the perilymphatic space of the vestibule. The pick is withdrawn, and the perforation in the round window membrane is sealed by a tissue graft of perichondrium or adipose tissue. The operation is terminated by returning the tympanomeatal flap to its original position. Strips of silk cloth are laid over the incisions, and a round synthetic rubber

FIGURE 38-1

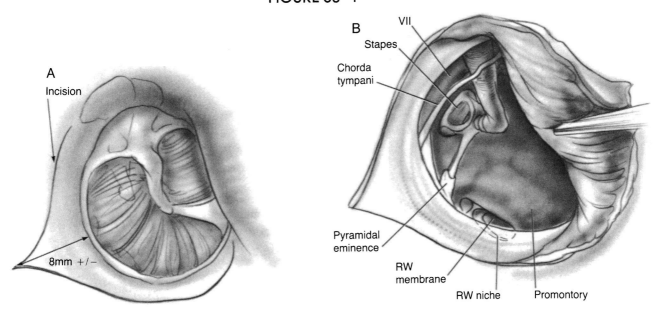

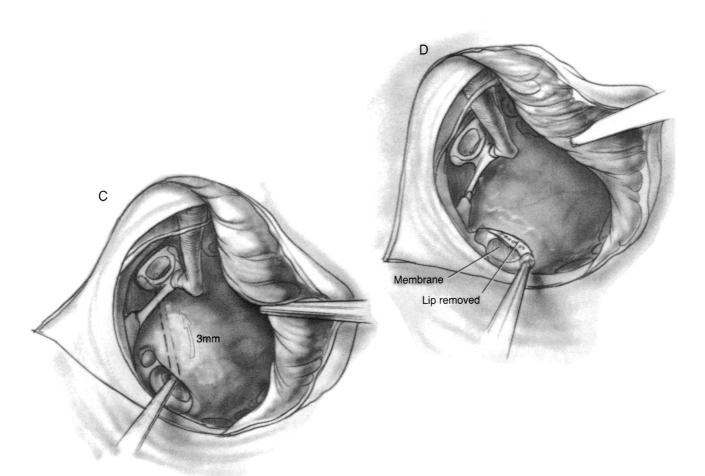

FIGURE 38-1. *A*, Skin incisions are made in the posterior wall of the bony external auditory canal. *B*, The tympanomeatal flap is elevated and reflected into the anterior tympanomeatal angle. *C*, A 3-mm right-angle pick is advanced through the round window membrane in the direction of the oval window. *D*, If the niche will not accommodate a 3-mm right-angle pick, the bony lip of the round window is removed, and a 2-mm right-angle pick is used to accomplish the cochleosacculotomy.

FIGURE 38-2

FIGURE 38-3

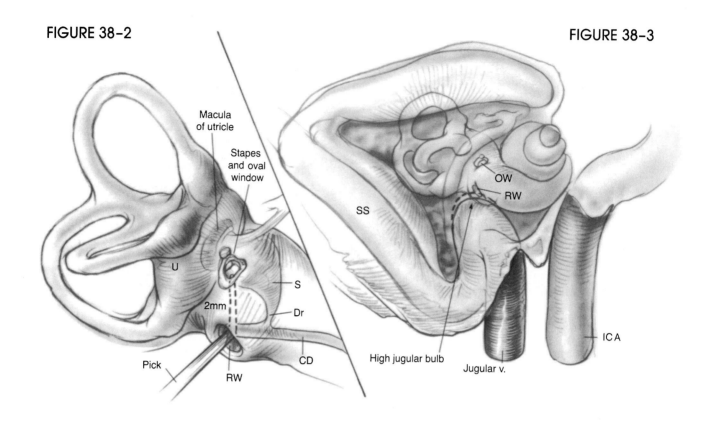

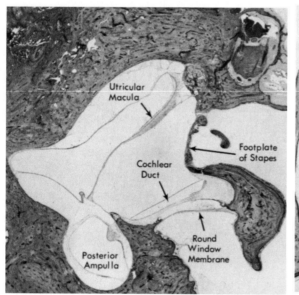

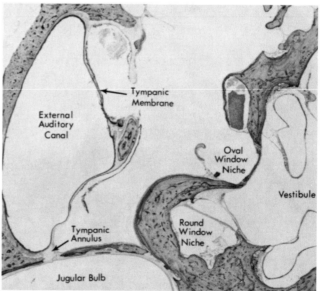

Key to abbreviations

S	Saccule	RW	Round window	OW	Oval window
Dr	Ductus reuniens	SV	Scala vestibuli	OSL	Osseous
CD	Cochlear duct	ST	Scala tympani		spiral lamina
U	Utricle	SS	Sigmoid sinus	M	Macula

FIGURES 38-2 and 38-3 *See legends on opposite page*

FIGURE 38-4

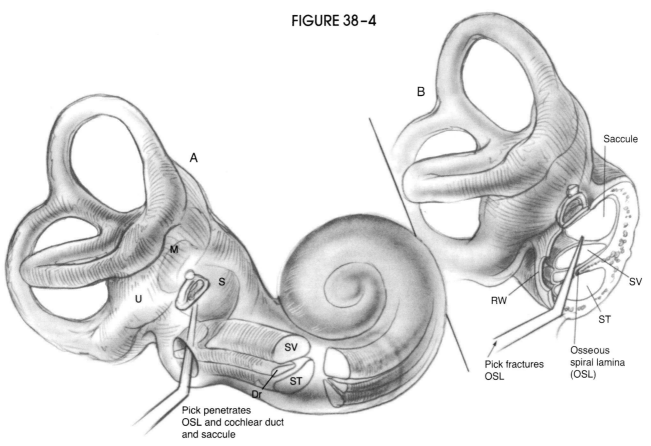

FIGURE 38–4. *A* and *B*, The 3-mm right-angle pick is shown penetrating the dilated cochlear duct and dilated saccule.

sponge of appropriate size is placed in the canal to maintain slight pressure on the skin flap. Cotton is placed in the ear canal. A few patients note slight unsteadiness for a day or two; however, all feel well enough to be discharged from the hospital on the following day. The packing is removed 1 week later, at which time the tympanic membrane and canal wall skin should be well healed.

Serial hearing tests at weekly intervals show a sensorineural hearing loss for 2 to 3 weeks, followed by recovery in most cases (Irwin Ginsberg, personal communication). The authors first test hearing 6 weeks after surgery, when the hearing has stabilized. The complications of cochleosacculotomy are about the same as those for stapedectomy and include perforation of the tympanic membrane, tears of the jugular bulb, postoperative otitis media, sensorineural hearing loss, facial nerve injury, and perilymph fistula. The only significant complication in cochleosacculotomies performed by the authors, other than sensorineural hearing loss, was one case of otitis media that resulted in profound sensorineural hearing loss in the infected ear.

RESULTS

The Massachusetts Eye and Ear Infirmary experience currently consists of 142 cochleosacculotomies performed since April 1979.[20-22] Follow-up times average 6.16 years, ranging from one month to 7.4 years. Definitive control of vertigo has been achieved in 68.3 per cent of patients. Hearing was made worse in 35.2 per cent (as defined by AAO-HNS criteria[4] of either 15-dB loss in pure tone average or 15 per cent loss in speech discrimination). Postoperative profound sensorineural hearing loss occurred in 11 per cent.

The success rates reported for either internal or external endolymphatic shunt procedures should be viewed with some caution. For example, in a review of 834 articles published on Ménière's disease between 1952 and 1975, Torok[23] found that almost without exception, advocates of either medical or surgical treatment reported success rates in the range of 60 to 80 per cent. Not only is there a strong placebo effect, but sudden prolonged remission of

FIGURE 38–2. This vertical section of a normal ear demonstrates the anatomic features of the middle and inner ears that are relevant to cochleosacculotomy. Histologic sections represent similar anatomic characteristics as drawing.

FIGURE 38–3. This vertical section of a normal ear shows a high jugular bulb abutting the tympanic annulus and encroaching on the round window niche. Other sections show a reduced orifice leading to a small niche. It is not feasible to attempt cochleosacculotomy in such cases.

symptoms are characteristic of Ménière's disease. However, some patients who had vertiginous attacks on a weekly basis (or more often) had a total cessation of attacks following cochleosacculotomy. In the management of disabling Ménière's disease, the discerning otologist will find cochleosacculotomy to be a useful alternative to vestibular nerve section and labyrinthectomy in selected cases.

References

1. Schuknecht HF, Gulya AJ: Endolymphatic hydrops: An overview and classification. Ann Otol Rhinol Laryngol 92(Suppl 106): 1–20, 1983.
2. Schuknecht HF: Ménière's disease: A correlation of symptomatology and pathology. Laryngoscope 73: 651–665, 1963.
3. Dohlman GF: On the mechanism of the Ménière attack. Arch Otorhinolaryngol 212: 301–307, 1976.
4. Committee on Hearing and Equilibrium: Report of Subcommittee on Equilibrium and its Measurement. Ménière's disease: Criteria for diagnosis and evaluation of therapy for reporting. Trans Am Acad Ophthalmol Otolaryngol 76: 1462–1464, 1972.
5. Fick IA van N: Decompression of the labyrinth: A new surgical procedure for Ménière's disease. Arch Otolaryngol 79: 447–458, 1964.
6. Fick IA van N: Ménière's disease: Aetiology and a new surgical approach—sacculotomy. J Laryngol Otol 80: 288–306, 1966.
7. Cody DTR, Simonton KM, Hallberg OE: Automatic repetitive decompression of the saccule in endolymphatic hydrops (tack operation): Preliminary report. Laryngoscope 77: 1480–1501, 1967.
8. Cody DTR: The tack operation for endolymphatic hydrops. Laryngoscope 79: 1737–1744, 1969.
9. Pulec JL: Ménière's disease: The otic-perotic shunt. Otolaryngol Clin North Am 1: 643–648, 1968.
10. Schuknecht HF: Cochleosacculotomy for Ménière's disease: Theory, technique, and results. Laryngoscope 92: 853–858, 1982.
11. Schuknecht HF: Pathology of Ménière's disease as it relates to the sac and tack procedures. Ann Otol Rhinol Laryngol 86: 677–682, 1977.
12. Duval AJ III, Rhodes VT: Ultrastructure of the organ of Corti following intermixing of cochlear fluids. Ann Otol Rhinol Laryngol 76: 688–708, 1967.
13. Kimura RS, Schuknecht HF: Effect of fistulae on endolymphatic hydrops. Ann Otol Rhinol Laryngol 84: 271–286, 1975.
14. Schuknecht HF, Neff WD: Hearing losses after apical lesions in the cochlea. Acta Otolaryngol (Stockh) 42: 263–274, 1952.
15. Schuknecht HF, Sutton S: Hearing losses after experimental lesions in basal coil of cochlea. Arch Otolaryngol 57: 129–142, 1953.
16. Schuknecht HF, Seifi A El: Experimental observations on the fluid physiology of the inner ear. Ann Otol Rhinol Laryngol 72: 687–721, 1963.
17. Kimura RS, Schuknecht HF, Ota CY, Jones DD: Experimental study of sacculotomy in endolymphatic hydrops. Arch Otorhinolaryngol 217: 123–137, 1977.
18. Schuknecht HF, Rüther A: Blockage of longitudinal flow in endolymphatic hydrops. Eur Arch Otorhinolaryngol 248: 209–217, 1991.
19. Tumarkin A: Otolithic catastrophe: A new syndrome. BMJ 2: 175–177, 1936.
20. Schuknecht HF: Cochlear endolymphatic shunt. Am J Otol 5: 546–548, 1984.
21. Schuknecht HF, Bartley M: Cochlear endolymphatic shunt for Ménière's disease. Am J Otol 6(Suppl): 20–22, 1985.
22. Schuknecht HF: Cochleosacculotomy for Ménière's disease: Internal endolymphatic shunt. Op Tech Otolaryngol Head Neck Surg 2: 35–37, 1991.
23. Torok N: Old and new in Ménière's disease. Laryngoscope 87: 1870–1877, 1977.

39

Chemical Treatment of the Labyrinth

Edwin M. Monsell, M.D., Ph.D. ▪ Stephen P. Cass, M.D.
Leonard P. Rybak, M.D., Ph.D. ▪ Julian M. Nedzelski, M.D.

Most patients with Ménière's disease can be managed satisfactorily with dietary salt restriction, diuretics, and vestibular suppressants. Only about 10 per cent of patients become disabled from work, domestic activities, travel, and the general enjoyment of life. The goals of treatment of Ménière's disease are to control the definitive spells of vertigo and to preserve hearing. Four treatments are widely used for patients who meet diagnostic criteria and who are disabled (American Academy of Otolaryngology—Head and Neck Surgery [AAO-HNS] functional levels 4 to 6).[1] In this chapter we discuss the therapeutic use of aminoglycosides and the application of corticosteroids via the middle ear.

In 1944, streptomycin was isolated from cultures of a soil organism, *Streptomyces griseolus*.[2] This drug displayed broad-spectrum antibacterial activity and was the first found to be effective against tuberculosis. Because effective treatment of tuberculosis with streptomycin required prolonged therapy, ototoxicity became evident soon after introduction of the drug. As early as 1948, streptomycin was used to treat patients with unilateral Ménière's disease specifically on the basis of its vestibulotoxic effects.[3]

Aminoglycosides exert their toxic effects on the hair cells of the inner ear by two general mechanisms. First, aminoglycosides bind to the plasma membrane and displace calcium and magnesium. This event results in acute but reversible interference with calcium-dependent mechanical-electrical transduction channels.[4] Second, aminoglycosides are transported into the cell by an energy-dependent process. Within the cell, the drug binds to phosphatidylinositol. This event is associated with progressive disruption of the plasma membrane and inhibition of the second messenger inositol triphosphate. With progressive disruption of the second messenger system and the plasma membrane, cell death occurs.[5–7]

The disruption of cell membranes and other intracellular components may be mediated by free radicals. Recent studies have shown that aminoglycosides form a complex with iron and that this complex catalyzes the production of free radicals. The combination of iron chelators and free radical scavengers in animal experiments provides complete protection from gentamicin ototoxicity.[8]

Aminoglycosides do not become concentrated in cochlear fluids, although the elimination half-life increases with chronic administration. These observations suggest that intracellular sequestration of the drug occurs.[9] Aran and associates have demonstrated that aminoglycosides undergo a rapid uptake by cochlear and vestibular hair cells and a slow clearance from these cells.[10]

Amikacin, dihydrostreptomycin, and kanamycin are primarily cochleotoxic, whereas gentamicin and streptomycin are primarily vestibulotoxic. At high doses, streptomycin is also cochleotoxic. For example, streptomycin, 25 mg/kg per day, administered systemically to cats resulted in loss of vestibular hair cells only, but at 100 mg/kg/day, both vestibular and cochlear hair cells were lost.[11]

Recent animal experiments have tried to model the pharmacokinetics of intratympanic administration of gentamicin applied in a sustained-release vehicle of liquid fibrin glue. High levels of gentamicin were measured in perilymph within 8 hours of administration. These high levels persisted for at least 24 hours, then declined rapidly by 72 hours. The elimination rate for gentamicin was 1.04 mg/ml per hour.[12]

The hair cells of the cristae, the ampullae, and the cochlea degenerate to different degrees following the administration of aminoglycosides. The primary vestibular neurons, the cochlear nuclei, and the vestibular nuclei are not directly affected, even at high doses.[11, 13] The basal turn of the cochlea is the region most susceptible to permanent loss of hair cells, resulting in an initial loss of high-frequency hearing sensitivity. Although the mechanisms of this differential toxicity are incompletely understood, several contributing factors have been identified, including the route of administration, dose variables, and the specific aminoglycoside used.

Damage to vestibular dark cells, which are thought to play a role in the production of endolymph, has been reported following administration of doses of aminoglycoside below the threshold for damage to hair cells. It is possible, but unproven, that impaired function of dark cells is beneficial in Ménière's disease.[14, 15]

INTRAMUSCULAR APPLICATION OF STREPTOMYCIN

Clinical Studies

Between 1948 and 1980, eight investigators reported a total of 49 patients treated with intramuscular streptomycin for unilateral or bilateral Ménière's disease.[16] In the first extensive studies of intramuscular streptomycin, Schuknecht administered 0.75 to 1.75 g intramuscularly (IM) every 12 hours (Table 39–1).[17, 18] Treatment continued until there were no ice water caloric responses in the diseased ear(s). The total doses ranged from 13.5 to 89 g (mean 39 g). All patients became severely ataxic and most suffered

TABLE 39–1. Review of Literature on Intratympanic Aminoglycoside Therapy

Author(s) and Reference	No. of Patients Treated	Amino-glycoside Used	Dosage	End Point	AAO-HNS Guidelines Used?	Control of Vertigo (%)	Loss of Caloric Response (%)	Hearing Preserved (%)
Schuknecht[18]	8	Streptomycin	50–300 mg/dose; 350–600 mg total dose	Vestibular ablation	No	63	63	37
Beck & Schmidt[50]	43	Gentamicin	30 mg/day	Vestibular ablation	No	91	NR	42
	40	Gentamicin	"6 doses planned"	First ototoxic reaction	No	92	NR	85
Lange[43]	92	Streptomycin Tobramycin Gentamicin	60 mg/day "typically several days"	First ototoxic reaction	No	90	NR	76
Moller et al[58]	15	Gentamicin 30 mg/ml	15–30 mg/dose	First ototoxic reaction	No	93	100	66
Sala[59]	62	Gentamicin 30 mg/ml	Up to 30 mg/day; 1–8 doses	First ototoxic reaction	No	86	51	70
Blessing & Schlenter[60]	82	Gentamicin 40 mg/ml	5–40 mg/dose 1–2 day	Ablative nystagmus or hearing loss	No	89	28	67
Laitakari[57]	20	Gentamicin 40 mg/ml	0.2 ml/day for 3 days then qod for 3–12 doses	Ablative nystagmus	Yes*	90	70	Improved 5 Unchanged 50 Worse 45 (Profound 30)
Nedzelski et al[48]	20	Gentamicin 26.7 mg/ml	3 times per day for 4 days	12 doses or first ototoxic reaction	Yes	90	85	80
Youssef & Poe[51]	37	Gentamicin 30 mg/ml	2–4 doses once/wk, then reassessment; 1–8 doses total	Loss of hearing (priority) or relief of vertigo	Yes	A 41 B 46 C D Failed 14	23 (n = 26)	Improved 14 Unchanged 23 Worse 63 (n = 35)
Minor[61]	34	Gentamicin	1–6 weekly doses	First sign of vestibular hypofunction	Yes	A 74 B 17 C 3 D 6	20	Improved 36 Unchanged 32 Worse 32 (Profound 3)
Atlas & Parnes[52]	68	Gentamicin 26 mg/ml	1–4 weekly doses	4 doses or first ototoxic reaction	Yes*	A 84 B 6 C 1 D 9	45	Improved 40 Unchanged 47 Worse 13 (Profound 0) (n = 47)
Eklund et al[62]	93	Gentamicin 30 mg/ml	1–4 daily doses	Fixed doses	Yes†	NR	NR	Improved 15 Unchanged 47 Worse 38 (Profound 11)

*Not all patients had 24-month follow-up.

†Results for vertigo control were not reported.

AAO-HNS, American Academy of Otolaryngology—Head and Neck Surgery; NR, not reported; qod, every other day.

oscillopsia early in the course of treatment, but none experienced hearing loss. Ninety-five percent of patients had no post-treatment vertigo. Thirty-five percent had persistent ataxia and 15 per cent had persistent oscillopsia. Hearing was stabilized, that is, did not change or fluctuate, in 90 per cent of patients. Thus, when a totally ablative dose of IM streptomycin was administered, vertigo was controlled and hearing was preserved.[19] Unfortunately, patients who undergo total vestibular ablation may still be disabled by chronic disequilibrium, ataxia, and oscillopsia.[20]

To attempt to limit the chronic oscillopsia and ataxia that follow total bilateral vestibular ablation, subtotal or "titration" treatment protocols with streptomycin were developed.[21, 22] Rather than giving an ablative dose, streptomycin was administered until episodic vertigo was controlled.

Treatment Method for Subtotal Vestibulectomy with Intramuscular Streptomycin

Our suggestions have been adapted from established protocols and modified by our own experience.[21, 22] *From the*

standpoint of the clinical skills required by the practitioner and the potential morbidity to patients, the administration of aminoglycosides for vertigo by any route of administration should be considered as great an undertaking as surgical treatment. Because not all the problems and pitfalls of any technique can be conveyed in a printed article, we advise that streptomycin treatment be learned under the guidance of a practitioner experienced in its use.

Indications

IM streptomycin may be considered for patients with disabling episodic vertigo caused by Ménière's disease in the following situations: (1) simultaneously active Ménière's disease in both ears, or when it is unclear from which ear the attacks of vertigo are arising, (2) Ménière's disease in an only-hearing ear, or (3) in the second ear following an ablative procedure on the opposite side, such as selective vestibular nerve section. It is essential to determine to what extent a patient may be disabled by the definitive episodic vertigo of Ménière's disease as defined by the AAO-HNS.[1] Patients disabled primarily by continuous disequilibrium, ataxia, oscillopsia, or motion intolerance are generally not good candidates for vestibular destructive procedures of any type, because their symptoms are due to a failure of central compensation, to the perception of disequilibrium in the presence of normal balance performance, or both.[23, 24]

It is important to identify patients with Cogan's syndrome, luetic hydrops, and autoimmune disease of the ear, because these patients may respond to nondestructive medical treatment, such as corticosteroids.[25] Patients with markedly reduced caloric function prior to treatment with streptomycin should be managed with additional caution, because they may develop permanent disequilibrium or oscillopsia with the loss of additional vestibular function. Consideration should be given to treating such patients with lower doses of streptomycin.

Pretreatment Evaluation and Patient Counseling

The pretreatment evaluation requires a complete history and physical examination, including a neurologic examination, observation of eye movements, and vestibulospinal examination. The vestibulospinal examination consists of observation of gait, tandem gait, Romberg, and tandem Romberg maneuvers. A simple, effective assessment of postural stability can be performed in the examination room or bedside by having a patient stand on 4 to 6 inches of dense foam with eyes closed. The foam reduces the reliability of proprioceptive input to postural control mechanisms so those subjects must depend on vestibular inputs when eyes are closed. Normal persons have no difficulty standing on the foam, but patients with bilateral loss of vestibular function or an acute vestibular loss will fall when forced to rely solely on vestibular cues to maintain posture. Baseline audiometric and laboratory vestibular function tests are performed, including electronystagmography, rotational testing, and posturography. Renal function tests are performed as indicated.

It is essential to distinguish clearly between two phenomena in patients with Ménière's disease who are undergoing IM treatment with aminoglycosides: (1) vertigo due to the disease, and (2) the syndrome of acute bilateral vestibular loss caused by vestibulotoxicity. Vertigo is the hallucination of motion, that is, the perception of motion when none is occurring. The vertigo of Ménière's disease occurs without provocation, consists of a spinning or rotating sensation always with spontaneous nystagmus, lasts 15 minutes to several hours, and is accompanied by disequilibrium and nausea that may last for hours.[1]

The syndrome of acute bilateral vestibular loss may include rotational vertigo, but the vertigo is related to treatment rather than being spontaneous. Commonly, patients experience discomfort associated with rapid head movements, a sense of disorientation in space, and ataxia. Patients may also manifest oscillopsia, a disturbing sensation of the visual field bobbling as the patient walks about or rides in car. This phenomenon is due to impairment or loss of the vestibulo-ocular reflex, which helps to maintain a stable image on the retina during head movement. Oscillopsia may be temporary or permanent following a bilateral loss of vestibular function.[19, 20, 26]

These distinctions are important because symptoms due to Ménière's disease are indications to resume treatment, whereas symptoms due to vestibulotoxicity are indications to halt treatment. Occasionally, the physician may find it difficult to make this distinction from a patient's history. In such cases, caution would dictate that treatment should be discontinued until the situation is clarified by repeated observations over time.

Patient counseling is extremely important. Patients are counseled that the purpose of the titration streptomycin is to control the recurrent episodes of vertigo typical of Ménière's disease and that disability due to disequilibrium may replace disability due to episodic vertigo. Patients need to understand that treatment may be protracted and that additional courses of streptomycin may be needed in the future. Other risks and complications include hearing loss, tenderness from the deep IM injections, nausea, perioral or peripheral numbness or tingling, rash, and fever. Renal, visual, and hematologic effects have also been reported with prolonged treatment with aminoglycosides.

Special discussion is required for patients with abnormal renal function, because renal toxicity is a potential complication of aminoglycosides. Careful monitoring of renal function and consultation with a nephrologist are recommended to ensure safe treatment of a patient with impaired renal function.

Occasionally a patient will report allergy to aminoglycosides. In this case the nature of the allergy is explored and an intradermal test dose is considered.

Treatment Technique

Therapy may start with streptomycin sulfate injected IM 1 g bid for 5 days, that is, a 10 g total cumulative dose. After this initial course, clinical reassessment is performed by interview, vestibulospinal physical examination, audiometry, and vestibular function tests. If studies remain unchanged, there is no clinical indication of decreased vestibular function, and the patient continues to suffer vertigo, then additional streptomycin may be given. For example, a second course could consist of additional streptomycin sulfate injected IM 1 g bid for 5 days, that is, 10 g in the second course and a total cumulative dose of 20 g. After administration of the first 20 g of total cumulative dose, we suggest that additional doses be smaller, such as streptomycin sulfate injected IM 1 g once per day for 5 days, that is, 5 g per increment.

Streptomycin injections should be stopped when any one of the following occurs: (1) episodic vertigo ceases or seems to abate; (2) the syndrome of acute vestibular loss appears or worsens; (3) worsening of balance performance on the vestibulospinal examination; (4) laboratory tests of vestibular function demonstrate loss of vestibular function, such as reduction of caloric responses, increase in phase or decrease in gain of the vestibulo-ocular reflex on rotational testing, and a fall on posturography when forced to rely solely on vestibular cues; or (5) decline in hearing. It is important to proceed with treatment slowly and cautiously. The effects of streptomycin can be delayed, and if the reduction of vestibular function continues to complete ablation, ataxia and oscillopsia may persist chronically. If episodic vertigo recurs, additional courses of streptomycin can be given as indicated.

Results

The long-term results of IM subtotal streptomycin therapy for bilateral Ménière's disease are known from only one report.[26] Nineteen patients were reviewed with follow-up from 2 to 9 years. Recurrent vertigo was controlled in 95 per cent of patients within the first 6 to 18 months following treatment. At last follow-up 63 per cent of patients reported having had no recurrence of vertigo. Persistent mild disequilibrium occurred in 60 per cent of patients without recurrent vertigo and oscillopsia persisted in 16 per cent of patients.[26]

APPLICATION OF STREPTOMYCIN TO THE LATERAL SEMICIRCULAR CANAL

Experimental Studies

Kimura and colleagues reported that the application of gentamicin to the lateral semicircular canal of normal guinea pigs produced a selective vestibular lesion.[27] There was sensory cell degeneration in the utricular maculae and all but one of the cristae of the superior, lateral, and posterior canals of 27 ears. The saccular maculae were less affected. All cochleas were normal except one that had a small lesion of outer hair cells at the basal turn. Fenestrated control ears were normal throughout. Kimura and coworkers repeated some of their experiments with streptomycin after producing experimental endolymphatic hydrops by occlusion of the endolymphatic duct.[28] Hydropic ears sustained substantial cochlear lesions, as well as vestibular lesions, when streptomycin was applied to the lateral semicircular canal. Fenestration of the lateral canal without drug application produced a significant cochlear lesion, but not a vestibular lesion.

Clinical Studies

The application of streptomycin to the labyrinth through the lateral semicircular canal (labyrinthotomy with streptomycin infusion [LSI]) was introduced by Shea.[29, 30] The rationale of this procedure was that application to the vestibular labyrinth might cause more drug to reach the vestibular hair cells than cochlear hair cells and produce a more selective lesion with a single treatment. Accomplishment of this route of administration requires the performance of a mastoidectomy and opening the bony otic capsule.

Surgical Method

The technique of LSI was described by Shea and Norris.[29] A simple mastoidectomy was performed and the lateral semicircular canal was identified. The bone of the dome of the semicircular canal is gradually thinned with a diamond burr. A "double blue line" technique is used to create a fenestration of the lateral semicircular canal.

A small amount of fluid containing streptomycin was slowly infused into the perilymphatic space of the lateral semicircular canal. Opening the lateral semicircular canal in Ménière's disease resulted in enhancement of the ratio of the summating potential to the action potential of the electrocochleographic recording, primarily by reduction in the amplitude of the action potential. The ratio did not change during infusion of streptomycin but sometimes declined slightly after the fenestration was closed.[31]

The volume of fluid, the composition of the diluent (lactated Ringer's solution or other physiologic solution), the amount of streptomycin in the solution delivered, the amount of time over which the fluid is introduced, and whether the streptomycin solution is followed by a "rinse" of a physiologic solution without streptomycin are important technical variables that could affect the amount of streptomycin administered and the amount of trauma to the inner ear. After the drug is infused, the fenestration is closed with a thick piece of temporalis muscle and fascia. The postauricular wound is closed in the usual manner.

On the basis of animal experiments Shea initially recommended puncturing the lateral membranous canal in hydropic ears to release endolymph, possibly decompressing endolymphatic hydrops acutely,[29, 30, 32] but has subsequently withdrawn this recommendation.

Results

In 1989 a multicenter study was initiated to produce an independent study of LSI results for hearing preservation and control of vertigo. Preliminary data from this and other studies have been reported.[31, 33]

Preoperative pure tone averages ranged from 14 to 76 dB HL with a mean of 54 dB (SD = 14). Postoperative pure tone averages ranged from 25 to 110 dB HL with a mean of 76 dB. Four patients (9 per cent) had an early postoperative hearing result that was improved over the preoperative hearing level.[34] In 11 patients (23 per cent) the hearing was unchanged, and in 32 (68 per cent) it was worse. In 27 patients (57 per cent) the postoperative pure tone level was 71 dB or worse (severe to profound hearing loss). Hearing outcome (change in pure tone average or word recognition) did not seem to be a function of patient age, sex, side of surgery, duration of hearing loss prior to surgery, or whether the patient had had a surgical procedure on the ear prior to the LSI, or which surgeon performed the procedure. A trend was identified suggesting that patients with milder preoperative losses may sustain less hearing damage from LSI. Opening the endolymphatic space of the lateral membranous canal resulted in more loss of hearing than when the membranous canal was not opened ($P = 0.05$).

The postoperative follow-up time ranged from one to 18 months, with a mean of 10 months. Eight patients (17 per cent) had secondary procedures for control of vertigo during the first few postoperative months.

Discussion

Silverstein reported that patients with good hearing seemed to be more resistant to hearing loss from streptomycin applied intratympanically.[22] There appeared to be less postoperative hearing loss from LSI when the preoperative pure tone average was 40 dB or better.

Findings in patients with vestibular disorders appear to corroborate findings in the guinea pig model; that is, the hydropic ear shows more sensitivity to aminoglycoside ototoxicity than the normal ear, and there is less selectivity of lesions between vestibular and cochlear hair cells in hydropic ears.[28]

The long-term results (≥2 years) for hearing preservation and control of vertigo by LSI have not been reported. Because of the high risk of associated hearing loss, this procedure should not be considered an established treatment.

INTRATYMPANIC GENTAMICIN THERAPY

Experimental Studies

Intratympanic injection of aminoglycosides allows treatment of unilateral Ménière's disease without producing systemic toxicity or effects on the opposite ear. Tracer studies have demonstrated that the primary route of entry into the inner ear is through the round window membrane.[35–39] A secondary route of entry into the inner ear may be through the annular ligament of the stapes.[27, 40]

Following the intratympanic application of streptomycin to guinea pigs, the cristae of the semicircular canals showed the most degeneration, followed by the utricle, then the saccule and the cochlea.[41] The selectivity of the lesion for vestibular versus cochlear hair cells after intratympanic injection was reduced at higher dosages. For example, the application of 8 mg of streptomycin to the round window membrane of the cat produced only vestibular toxicity, whereas 20 to 40 mg produced both cochlear and vestibular toxicity.[42] These experimental results emphasize the potential for cochlear toxicity when the primary route of entry into the inner ear is through the round window membrane.

Clinical Studies

The use of intratympanic aminoglycosides to induce a chemical labyrinthectomy for the treatment of unilateral Ménière's disease was introduced by Schuknecht.[17, 18] He reported the results of eight patients given large daily doses of streptomycin (150 to 600 mg/day) for 1 to 7 days. The treatment end point was the onset of signs and symptoms of vestibular ablation. The treatment was successful in controlling vertigo in five of eight patients, all of whom lost substantial hearing in the treated ear. Although hearing was preserved in the remaining three of eight patients, persistent vertigo necessitated surgical labyrinthectomy. Schuknecht found that complete control of vertigo with intratympanic streptomycin required abolition of ice water caloric responses, and that when this was accomplished, hearing was also lost.

Lange reported an extensive experience using various aminoglycosides to treat Ménière's disease.[43–45] In his group of 92 patients, Lange reported that 90 per cent had no further episodes of severe vertigo and hearing remained unchanged in 76 per cent of patients. Unfortunately, many of the studies reported from 1956 to 1990 did not use standardized reporting methods (see Table 39–1).

One of the authors (JMN) developed a fixed-dose protocol, which he applied consistently.[46–48] A catheter was attached to a tympanostomy tube, which was placed near the round window. The aminoglycoside solution used was buffered to pH 6.4 with a final concentration of 26.7 mg/ml. Three doses of 0.65 ml were instilled per day for 4 days. Bone conduction audiometry was performed daily. He studied the patients prospectively using the AAO-HNS guidelines for reporting treatment results of Ménière's disease.[1, 34] He also monitored post-treatment caloric responses as the best indicator of biologic treatment effect.

Results were reported for the first 30 patients followed for at least 2 years.[48] Complete control of vertigo was obtained in 83 per cent and substantial control (vertigo class B) in 17 per cent. Hearing was worse in 27 per cent of patients; 13 per cent sustained a profound hearing loss. Ice water caloric responses were abolished in 53 per cent of patients, all of whom had complete control of vertigo for the first 2 years at least. Complete control of vertigo was obtained in 80 per cent of patients who had persistent ice water caloric responses. Four patients required retreatment within 2 years because of persistent attacks.

In a study to characterize the delayed effects of intratympanic gentamicin, Magnusson and Padoan treated five patients with a total of two doses of gentamicin (30 mg/ml, pH 6.4), given 12 hours apart.[49] The first symptom of an ototoxic reaction noted by the patients was a sensation of unsteadiness occurring 2 to 5 days (mean 3.2 days) after the injections. Vertigo and nystagmus were noted 3 to 8 days (mean 5.1 days) after the injections. With 1 year of follow-up, vertigo was controlled (with a loss of caloric responsiveness in the treated ear) and hearing preserved in all five patients.[49]

This preliminary study raised the question of whether very low intratympanic doses of gentamicin may be effective in controlling vertigo and preserving hearing. Because this technique did not totally ablate vestibular function, vertigo may recur, but hearing was usually preserved. Additional gentamicin could be used if vertigo recurred.

Beck and Schmidt administered gentamicin 30 mg/day and stopped after 6 days or at the slightest indication of ototoxicity.[50] In 40 patients treated with their regimen, control of vertigo occurred in 92.5 per cent of patients. Eighty-five per cent of patients maintained hearing. Following the work of Beck and Schmidt, several investigators developed the hypothesis that if a "titration" dosage schedule were adopted, it might be possible to achieve satisfactory rates of control of vertigo while preserving hearing in more patients. Much of the ongoing controversy about intratympanic gentamicin treatment has been over the issue of whether such approaches achieve this goal and how various protocols compare with each other.

Studies by several authors showed remarkably similar results for control of vertigo, ranging from 86 to 93 per cent of patients treated (see Table 39–1). Some patients required additional gentamicin injections or surgery. Authors have noted an association between loss of the ice water caloric response and complete control of vertigo.[51, 52]

On the other hand, reports showed considerable variation in rates of hearing preservation, ranging from 55 to 85 per cent. The results suggest that the administration schedule and total dosage may be significant factors in hearing preservation. The variability in reports may also be due to differences in case selection, because some series have more elderly patients or patients with worse pretreatment hearing levels than other series. It is suspected, but has not been established, that there may be a trade-off between control of vertigo and preservation of hearing.

One of the authors (SPC) has developed a titration method. A full diagnostic assessment was made, including a complete history, physical examination, neurologic examination, observation of eye movements, vestibulospinal examination, vestibular function testing (electronystagmography, posturography, rotational chair testing), and audiometric evaluation.

Retrocochlear and metabolic disorders were excluded. Given the low total dose of gentamicin used, the need to withhold treatment based on abnormal renal function was rare.

Patients were counseled that the purpose of the intratympanic gentamicin injections was to control the recurrent episodes of vertigo typical of Ménière's disease. The expectation and time course of post-treatment unsteadiness or disequilibrium typical of unilateral vestibular ablation were explained. Moreover, the possibility that additional courses of gentamicin may be needed in the future or that surgical ablation may be required to control vertigo was reviewed. The possibility of increased hearing loss, including a profound loss of hearing that would be unaidable, was reviewed. Hearing preservation results from the literature and personal series were discussed. Potential positive and negative effects on aural fullness and tinnitus were explained. Intratympanic aminoglycoside therapy was considered in any patient with disabling vertigo, sensorineural hearing loss (fluctuating or fixed), tinnitus, and aural fullness consistent with unilateral Ménière's disease that was persistent and refractory to previous medical or surgical management.[1]

The gentamicin solution was buffered to a pH of 6.4 to reduce the sting associated with intratympanic injection. A buffered solution was prepared as follows: 1.5 ml of gentamicin solution (40 mg/ml) was injected into a sterile 5-ml vial. A 0.6 M sodium bicarbonate solution was prepared by combining 2 ml of 8.4 per cent sodium bicarbonate and 1.36 ml of sterile water in a 5-ml sterile vial; 0.5 ml of the 0.6 M sodium bicarbonate solution was added to the sterile vial containing 1.5 ml of gentamicin to form 2 ml of a solution of gentamicin (30 mg/ml, pH 6.4) ready for injection.

Patients were comfortably positioned supine with the head turned away from the ear to be treated (Fig. 39–1). This position was maintained for 30 minutes following the injection. Patients were instructed not to swallow or clear the middle ear during this period. A small injection site on the surface of the tympanic membrane was anesthetized with a small drop of phenol and the gentamicin was injected into the middle ear using a tuberculin syringe and a 27-gauge needle (Fig. 39–2). Typically, about 0.5 ml of solution filled the middle ear.

One intratympanic injection of approximately 0.5 ml of

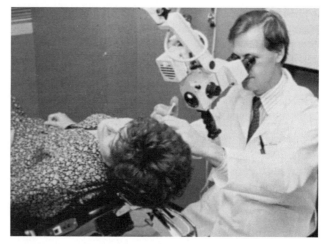

FIGURE 39–1. Patient positioning for intratympanic injection of gentamicin.

gentamicin, 30 mg/ml, pH 6.4, was given per week. If weekly audiograms were unchanged, weekly injections were continued to reach a total of four doses (40 to 60 mg total dose). Treatment was stopped early if auditory toxicity was noted. Additional doses were given if vertigo was not controlled or recurred.

Seventy-seven per cent of 48 patients followed for 2 or more years post-treatment had complete control of definitive spells of vertigo.[1] Seventeen per cent had substantial (grade B) control. Two patients (4 per cent) failed treatment and had subsequent surgical treatment. Hearing thresholds worsened by at least 10 dB in 24 per cent of patients treated; 14 per cent had nonserviceable hearing (class D).

Because intratympanic aminoglycoside therapy is a nonsurgical outpatient treatment, elderly patients and those with significant surgical or anesthetic risks may be treated safely and thus are primary candidates. Intratympanic aminoglycoside therapy can also be used to avoid additional surgery in patients with recurrent vertigo and a return of caloric function following previous ablative vestibular surgery. Patients with profound hearing loss are good candidates for intensified treatment.

The data on efficacy of intratympanic aminoglycoside therapy to control vertigo and its safety in preservation of hearing are almost exclusively from patients with Ménière's disease. Most patients with non-Ménière's vestibulopathy have normal hearing. The nonhydropic ear seems to be relatively resistant to the effects of aminoglycosides. For these reasons we do not currently recommend intratympanic aminoglycoside therapy in the primary treatment of vertigo caused by disorders other than Ménière's disease.

TREATMENT OF LABYRINTHINE DISORDERS WITH INTRATYMPANIC CORTICOSTEROIDS

Experimental Studies

Various components of the inflammatory or immune response are inhibited by glucocorticoids. Macrophages,

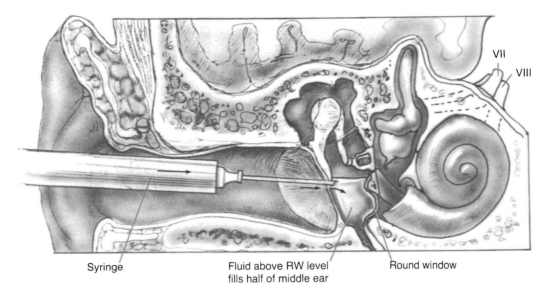

FIGURE 39–2. Intratympanic injection of gentamicin through a pinhole perforation. Gentamicin fills a middle ear space and bathes a round window (RW) membrane with antibiotic solution.

monocytes, and endothelial cells produce arachidonic acid and its metabolites, which include prostaglandins and leukotrienes. The production of these metabolites is inhibited in part by the induction of a protein, lipocortin, that is an inhibitor of phospholipase A_2, the first enzyme in the cascade of prostaglandins and leukotrienes. Macrophages and monocytes also release cytokines, including interleukins and tumor necrosis factor-α (TNF-α). These substances have multiple effects on the inflammatory response, including the activation of T cells and stimulation of the growth of fibroblasts.

The action of basophils is also affected by glucocorticoids. They inhibit the IgE-dependent release of histamine and leukotriene C4. The production of fibroblasts and the release of arachidonic acid derivatives are inhibited by glucocorticoids. Like macrophages and monocytes, lymphocytes produce cytokines and TNF-α, which are inhibited by steroids. These multiple effects all would serve to attenuate an inflammatory or autoimmune process in the middle and inner ear when glucocorticoids are administered intratympanically.

The properties of glucocorticoids vary. For example, cortisone and prednisone have an 11-keto group, which must be enzymatically reduced in the liver before they are biologically active.[53] Steroids such as prednisone and methylprednisolone have a shorter half-life than dexamethasone or betamethasone. In addition, the latter steroids are about seven times as potent as prednisone and prednisolone and about five times as potent as methylprednisolone.[53]

Clinical Studies

There is substantial clinical evidence that some otologic conditions are autoimmune in etiology and responsive to systemic immunosuppressive medications.[25] All of these have undesirable systemic side effects that limit their use. Consequently, there is considerable interest in applying immunosuppressive drugs, principally corticosteroids, intratympanically.

Much less is known about the pharmacokinetics and clinical effects of intratympanic corticosteroid administration than is known about aminoglycosides. It may be possible to achieve high concentrations in some otic tissues, but safety and efficacy in otologic disorders remain unproven. Although some benefit has been reported,[54] hearing loss attributable to treatment has also been reported.[55] One prospective, randomized, double-blind, crossover trial showed no benefit compared with placebo in Ménière's disease.[56] There are anecdotal reports of tympanic membrane perforation and even fulminant mastoiditis following instillation of corticosteroids in the middle ear. It is possible that future studies will define safe and effective protocols for intratympanic treatment with corticosteroids and perhaps other medications in certain subsets of patients.

SUMMARY

Subtotal bilateral chemical labyrinthectomy by intramuscular streptomycin administration is an accepted treatment for disabling vertigo due to bilaterally active Ménière's disease or Ménière's disease in an only-hearing ear. Long-term results show preservation of hearing and control of vertigo in most cases, although chronic disequilibrium and oscillopsia remain as problems for some patients. Consequently, this treatment should be reserved for patients who are disabled and meet criteria for treatment.

Application of streptomycin to the lateral semicircular canal appears to cause a higher rate of hearing loss than does IM intratympanic application. Long-term results for hearing preservation and efficacy of control of vertigo with standard reporting methods are not known for application to the lateral semicircular canal. Reports of early postoperative results indicate a high rate of hearing loss. Treatment by this approach is not accepted at the present time.

Intratympanic application of gentamicin frequently results in treatment-related hearing loss, although vertigo is usually well controlled. Patients with recurrent post-treatment vertigo can be treated again. A current trend in intratympanic application is to administer one or two doses rather than treating until ototoxicity is clinically evident. Just enough additional doses are applied to achieve control of attacks. The advantages of such titration protocols over fixed-dosage protocols have not been proven in long-term studies. Intratympanic gentamicin should be reserved for patients with classic Ménière's disease who meet appropriate treatment criteria. Prolonged disabling disequilibrium occurs about as frequently as following surgical labyrinthectomy or vestibular nerve section. Complete ablation and long-term control of vertigo are not achieved as reliably as with surgical labyrinthectomy or vestibular nerve section.[57]

The safety and efficacy of corticosteroid intratympanic treatment of Ménière's disease and other inner ear disorders are undefined at this time.

References

1. Committee on Hearing and Equilibrium: Committee on Hearing and Equilibrium guidelines for the diagnosis and evaluation of therapy in Ménière's disease. Otolaryngol Head Neck Surg 113: 181–185, 1995.
2. Sande M, Mandell G: Antimicrobial agents. *In* Gilman A, Rall T, Nies A, et al (eds): Goodman and Gilman's The Pharmacological Basis of Therapeutics. New York, Pergamon Press, 1999, pp 1098–1116.
3. Fowler E: Streptomycin treatment of vertigo. Trans Am Acad Ophthalmol Otolaryngol 52: 239–301, 1948.
4. Ohmori H: Mechano-electrical transduction currents in isolated vestibular hair cells of the chick. J Physiol 359: 189–217, 1985.
5. Rybak L: Ototoxic mechanisms. *In* Altschuler RA, Hoffman DW, Bobbin RP (eds): Neurobiology of Hearing. New York, Raven Press, 1986, pp 441–454.
6. Williams S, Smith D, Schacht J: Characteristics of gentamicin uptake in the isolated crista ampullaris of the inner ear of the guinea pig. Biochem Pharmacol 36: 89–95, 1987.
7. Williams S, Zenner H, Schacht J: Three molecular steps of aminoglycoside ototoxicity demonstrated in outer hair cells. Hear Res 30: 11–18, 1987.
8. Song B-B, Anderson D, Schacht J: Protection from gentamicin toxicity by iron chelators in guinea pig in vivo. J Pharmacol Exper Ther 282: 369–377, 1999.
9. Henley CI, Schacht J: Pharmacokinetics of aminoglycoside antibiotics in inner ear fluids and their relationship to ototoxicity. Audiology 27: 137–147, 1988.
10. Aran J, Chappert C, Dulon D, et al: Uptake of amikacin by hair cells of the guinea pig cochlea and vestibule and ototoxicity in comparison with gentamicin. Hear Res 82: 179–183, 1999.
11. McGee T, Olszewski J: Streptomycin sulfate and dihydrostreptomycin toxicity. Arch Otolaryngol 75: 295–311, 1962.
12. Balough A, Hoffer M, Wester D, et al: Kinetics of gentamicin uptake in the inner ear of chinchilla langier after middle-ear administration in a sustined-release vehicle. Otolaryngol Head Neck Surg 119: 427–431, 1998.
13. Berg K: The toxic effect of streptomycin on the vestibular and cochlear apparatus. Acta Otolaryngol 157: 1–77, 1951.
14. Park J, Cohen G: Vestibular ototoxicity in the chick: Effects of streptomycin on equilibrium and on ampullary dark cells. Am J Otolaryngol 6: 117–127, 1982.
15. Pender D: Gentamicin tympanoclysis: Effects on the vestibular secretory cells. Am J Otolaryngol 6: 358–367, 1985.
16. Monsell E, Cass S, Rybak L: Chemical labyrinthectomy: Methods and Results. *In* Brackmann DE, Arriaga C, Shelton C (eds): Otologic Surgery. Philadelphia, WB Saunders, 1994, pp 509–518.
17. Schuknecht H: Ablation therapy for the relief of Ménière's disease. Laryngoscope 66: 859–870, 1956.
18. Schuknecht H: Ablation therapy in the management of Ménière's disease. Acta Otolaryngol (Stockh) Suppl 132: 1–42, 1957.
19. Wilson W, Schuknecht S: Update on the use of streptomycin therapy for Ménière's disease. Am J Otolaryngol 2: 108–111, 1980.
20. "J.C.": Living without a balance mechanism. N Engl J Med 246: 458–460, 1952.
21. Graham M, Kemink J: Titration streptomycin therapy for bilateral Ménière's disease: A progress report. Otolaryngol Head Neck Surg 92: 440–447, 1984.
22. Silverstein H: Streptomycin treatment for Ménière's disease. Ann Otol Rhinol Laryngol Suppl 112: 44–88, 1984.
23. Konrad H: Intractable vertigo—when not to operate. Trans Am Acad Ophthalmol Otolaryngol 95: 482–484, 1986.
24. Monsell E, Brackmann D, Linthicum F: Why do vestibular destructive procedures sometimes fail? Otolaryngol Head Neck Surg 99: 472–479, 1988.
25. Harris J, Tomiyama S: Immunology/virology of Ménière's disease. *In* Harris J (ed): Ménière's Disease. The Hague, Kugler Publications, 1999, pp 123–138.
26. Langman A, Kemink J, Graham M: Titration therapy for bilateral Ménière's disease: Follow-up report. Ann Otol Rhinol Laryngol 99: 923–926, 1990.
27. Kimura R, Iverson N, Southard R: Selective lesions of the vestibular labyrinth. Ann Otol Rhinol Laryngol 97: 577–584, 1988.
28. Kimura R, Lee K-S, Nye C, et al: Effects of systemic and lateral semicircular canal administration of aminoglycosides on normal and hydropic inner ears. Acta Otolaryngol (Stockh) 111: 1021–1030, 1991.
29. Shea J, Norris C: Streptomycin perfusion of the labyrinth. *In* Nadol JB (ed): Second International Symposium on Ménière's Disease, Cambridge, MA, June 20–22, 1988. Amsterdam, Kugler & Ghendini Publications, 1989.
30. Shea J: Perfusion of the inner ear with streptomycin. Am J Otol 10: 150–155, 1989.
31. Monsell E: Electrocochleographic recording in patients undergoing labyrinthotomy with streptomycin infusion. *In* Arenberg IK (ed): Surgery of the Inner Ear: Proceedings of the Third International Symposium and Workshops on Surgery of the Inner Ear, Snowmass, CO, July 29–August 4, 1990. Amsterdam, Kulger & Ghedini, 1991.
32. Konishi S, Shea J: Experimental endolymphatic hydrops and its relief by interrupting the lateral semicircular duct in guinea pigs. J Laryngol Otol 89: 577–592, 1975.
33. Monsell E, Shelton C: Labyrinthotomy with streptomycin infusion: Early results of a multicenter study. Am J Otol 13: 416–422, 1992.
34. Subcommittee on Equilibrium: Ménière's disease: Criteria for diagnosis and evaluation of therapy for reporting. AAO-HNS Bulletin, 6–7. 7–1985. (Generic)
35. Smith B, Myers M: The penetration of gentamicin and neomycin into the perilymph across the round window membrane. Otolaryngol Head Neck Surg 87: 888–891, 1978.
36. Saijo S, Kimura R: Distribution of HRP in the inner ear after injection into the middle ear cavity. Acta Otolaryngol (Stockh) 97: 593–610, 1999.
37. Goycoolea M, Carpenter A, Muchow D: Ultrastructural studies of the round window membrane of the cat. Arch Otolaryngol 113: 617–624, 1987.
38. Kawauchi H, DeMaria T, Lim D: Endotoxin permeability through the round window. Acta Otolaryngol (Stockh) Suppl 457: 100–115, 1988.
39. Lundman L, Bagger-Sjöbäck D, Holmquist L, et al: Round window membrane permeability. Acta Otolaryngol (Stockh) Suppl 457: 73–77, 1988.
40. Jahnke K: Transtympanic application of gentamicin with cochlea protection, *In* Nadol JB (ed): Second International Symposium on Ménière's Disease. June 20, 1988. Cambridge, MA, Amsterdam, Kugler & Ghedini, 1988.
41. Lindeman H: Regional differences in sensitivity of the vestibular sensory epithelia to ototoxic antibiotics. Acta Otolaryngol (Stockh) 67: 177–189, 1969.
42. Cass S, Bouchard K, Graham M: Controlled application of streptomycin to the round window membrane of the cat. Otolaryngol Head Neck Surg 103: 223, 1990.
43. Lange G: Gentamicin and other ototoxic antibiotics for the transtympanic treatment of Ménière's disease. Arch Otorhinolaryngol 246: 269–270, 1989.
44. Lange G: Isolierte Medikamentose Ausschaltungeines Gleichgewichtsorganes beim Morbus Ménière mit Streptomycin-Ozothin. Arch Klin Exp Ohren-Nasen-Kehlkopfheilkd 191: 545–549, 1999.

45. Lange G: Transtympanic treatment for Ménière's disease with gentamicin sulfate. *In* Vosteen K-H, Schuknecht HF, Pfaltz CR, et al (eds): Ménière's Disease: Pathogenesis, Diagnosis, and Treatment. Stuttgart, Georg Thieme Verlag, 1981.

46. Commins D, Nedzelski J: Topical drugs in the treatment of Ménière's disease. Curr Opin Otolaryngol Head Neck Surg 4: 319–323, 1996.

47. Hone S, Nedzelski J: Selective chemical ablation as treatment for Ménière's disease. *In* Harris J (ed): Ménière's Disease. The Hague, Kugler Publications, 1999, pp 381–389.

48. Nedzelski J, Schessel D, Bryce G, et al: Chemical labyrinthectomy: Local application for the treatment of unilateral Ménière's disease. Am J Otol 13: 18–22, 1992.

49. Magnusson M, Padoan S: Delayed onset of ototoxic effects of gentamicin in treatment of Ménière's disease. Acta Otolaryngol 111: 671–676, 1991.

50. Beck C, Schmidt C: Ten years of experience with intratympanically applied streptomycin (gentamicin) in the therapy of morbus Ménière. Arch Otorhinolaryngol 221: 149–152, 1978.

51. Youssef T, Poe D: Intratympanic gentamicin injection for the treatment of Ménière's disease. Am J Otol 19: 435–442, 1998.

52. Atlas J, Parnes L: Intratympanic gentamicin titration therapy for intractable Ménière's disease. Am J Otol 20: 357–363, 1999.

53. Schimmer B, Parker K: Aminoglycoside antibiotics. *In* Harman J, Limbird L, Molinoff P, et al (eds): Goodman and Gilman's The Pharmacological Basis of Therapeutics, 9th ed. New York, McGraw-Hill, 1996, pp 1459–1488.

54. Shea J, Ge X: Dexamethasone perfusion of the labyrinth plus intravenous dexamethasone for Ménière's disease. Otolaryngol Clin North Am 29: 353–358, 1996.

55. Spandow O, Hellstrom S, Anniko M: Impaired hearing following instillation of hydrocortisone into the middle ear. Acta Otolaryngol (Stockh) Suppl 455: 90–93, 1988.

56. Silverstein H, Isaacson JE, Olds MJ, et al: Dexamethasone inner ear perfusion for the treatment of Ménière's disease: A prospective, randomized, double-blind, cross-over trial. Am J Otol 19: 196–201, 1998.

57. Laitakari K: Intratympanic gentamicin in severe Ménière's disease. Clin Otolaryngol 15: 545–548, 1990.

58. Moller C, Odkvist L, Thell J, et al: Vestibular and audiologic functions in gentamicin-treated Ménière's disease. Am J Otolaryngol 9: 383–391, 1988.

59. Sala T: Transtympanic administration of aminoglycosides in patients with Ménière's disease. Arch Otorhinolaryngol 245: 293–296, 1988.

60. Blessing R, Schlenter W: Langzeitergebnisse der Gentamicin-Therapie Des Morbus Ménière. Laryngol Rhinol Otol 68: 657–660, 1989.

61. Minor L: Intratympanic gentamicin for control of vertigo in Ménière's disease: Vestibular signs that specify completion of therapy. Am J Otol 20: 209–219, 1999.

62. Eklund S, Pyykko I, Aalto H, et al: Effect of intratympanic gentamicin on hearing and tinnitus in Ménière's disease. Am J Otol 20: 356, 1999.

40

Transcanal Labyrinthectomy

Joseph B. Nadol, Jr., M.D. ▪ Michael J. McKenna, M.D.

Labyrinthectomy is an effective surgical procedure for the management of unremitting or poorly compensated unilateral peripheral vestibular dysfunction in the presence of ipsilateral, profound, or severe sensorineural hearing loss. The physiologic rationale is that central vestibular compensation is more rapid and complete for unilateral absence of peripheral vestibular function than for unilateral abnormal function, either episodic or chronic.[1]

Unilateral vestibular ablation has been advocated for over six decades. Selective or total eighth nerve transection by the suboccipital approach was introduced by Dandy in 1928.[2] Destruction of the peripheral end organs of the vestibular labyrinth was introduced by Jansen in 1895 for complications of suppurative labyrinthitis.[3] This technique was applied to unilateral peripheral vestibular disturbance by Milligan[4] and by Lake[5] in 1904 and was reintroduced by Cawthorne[6] in 1943 as a canal wall up technique. In his original description, Cawthorne apparently ablated only the lateral semicircular canal. However, in its current form, complete vestibular ablation is accomplished by exenteration of all three of the semi-circular canals and both maculae.

The earliest report of a transcanal procedure for vertigo is credited to Crockett, who in 1903 described removal of the stapes as an effective treatment for vertigo.[7] Lempert described an endaural transmeatal approach to the oval and round windows for Ménière's disease.[8] In this procedure, the stapes was removed and the round window punctured to "decompress" the membranous labyrinth. However, there was no mention of the importance of destruction of the vestibular end organs. The modern transcanal labyrinthectomy for unilateral peripheral vestibular dysfunction was introduced by Schuknecht in 1956[9] and by Cawthorne in 1957.[10] In a series of papers, Schuknecht's technique evolved to emphasize the importance of destruction of all five vestibular end organs.[11–13] The importance of total ablation of peripheral vestibular function was also emphasized by Armstrong[14] and Ariagno.[15]

PATIENT SELECTION

The modern complete transcanal labyrinthectomy is an extremely effective treatment option for unilateral peripheral vestibular dysfunction. Rates of control of vertigo in the range of 95 to 99 per cent have been achieved by several authors. The modified Cawthorne transmastoid labyrinthectomy and the translabyrinthine vestibular or eighth nerve section are equally effective options for ablation of peripheral vestibular dysfunction. However, the transcanal labyrinthectomy has the obvious advantages of a more direct approach to the vestibular end organs, a shorter operating time, and a lower morbidity, particularly for postoperative facial nerve dysfunction and cerebrospinal fluid leak.

Medical management appropriate to the unilateral vestibular disorder, including vestibular supressants and diuretics for Ménière's disease, should be attempted prior to consideration of labyrinthectomy. These forms of medical management are less successful for poorly compensated peripheral vestibular dysfunction, such as the sequelae of vestibular neuronitis, labyrinthitis, or trauma. In these cases, rehabilitative vestibular physical therapy should be attempted prior to labyrinthectomy. Labyrinthectomy should be performed only when it has been clearly demonstrated that the vestibular dysfunction is unilateral and when the ipsilateral hearing loss is severe or profound. Although the published indications for labyrinthectomy have included hearing levels poorer than a 50 dB speech reception threshold and a 50 per cent discrimination score, in view of the incidence of bilateral Ménière's disease of 10 to 40 per cent, as reported by Greven and Oosterveld[16] and Paparella and Griebie,[17] labyrinthectomy should be reserved for cases in which the hearing loss is severe to profound, generally with a speech reception threshold of 75 dB or worse and a speech discrimination score of less than or equal to 20 per cent. This threshold for labyrinthectomy should be increased if hearing in the contralateral ear is not in the normal or near-normal range. Given the acute and often protracted vestibular disturbance following labyrinthectomy, this procedure should be done only for debilitating peripheral vestibular dysfunction. That is, the patient with only mild or infrequent attacks may be best treated nonoperatively. Obviously, the definition of handicapping vertigo also depends on many other clinical factors, such as age, intercurrent disease, and occupation of the patient.

A successful labyrinthectomy depends not only on total ablation of peripheral vestibular dysfunction but also on compensation for this unilateral vestibular loss. In general, negative indicators for successful vestibular compensation include increased age, visual disturbances, obesity, sedentary lifestyle, arthritis or other lower limb dysfunction, dependent personality, or clear indication of secondary gain.

PREOPERATIVE EVALUATION

A complete history and otolaryngologic and head and neck examination should be performed. Bilateral behavioral audiometry, including pure-tone thresholds for air and bone conduction and speech discrimination, is necessary. Vestibular testing should include at least bilateral caloric function, best done by electronystagmography. This assessment is necessary to evaluate the possibility of bilateral vestibular dysfunction and also to confirm vestibular dysfunction in the affected ear based on audiometry and history. Hallpike's positional testing and evaluation for the presence of the fistula and Hennebert's signs should be done.[18] A neurologic exam should be done to rule out concurrent cranial nerve, cerebellar, or other neurologic dysfunction that would belie the working diagnosis of a peripheral unilateral vestibular dysfunction. Radiographic assessment with computed tomography and magnetic resonance imaging (MRI) is not essential in every case. However, the symptoms and findings of longstanding unilateral Ménière's disease may be similar to those caused by lesions of the posterior fossa. In general, MRI with gadolinium enhancement is useful to rule out cerebellopontine angle or other tumors and demyelinating lesions. In summary, the ideal candidate for labyrinthectomy is an individual with unremitting or uncompensated peripheral vestibular dysfunction with severe-to-profound unilateral sensorineural hearing loss, unilateral vestibular dysfunction on electronystagmography, and lack of neurologic and radiographic evidence of central neurologic disease.

In general, the functional outcome is better in patients with unilateral Ménière's disease than in those with other peripheral vestibular dysfunction. In some patients with Ménière's disease, the electronystagmogram will be normal. In such cases, labyrinthectomy is justified if the symptoms and signs are sufficiently localizing to be convincing of unilateral peripheral dysfunction. Thus, the presence of fluctuating or severe-to-profound sensorineural loss, ipsilateral tinnitus, and aural symptoms concurrent with Ménière's attack is sufficient to warrant labyrinthectomy, even in the presence of normal caloric function if other selection criteria are met. The patient should be aware that postoperative vertigo will be more severe when preoperative function is normal or nearly so in the affected ear.

PREOPERATIVE PATIENT COUNSELING AND INFORMED CONSENT

Preoperative counseling should include a discussion of the natural history of Ménière's disease, including both the spontaneous rate of remission of approximately 70 per cent within 8 years as well as the 10 to 40 per cent incidence of involvement of the second ear.[19] In addition, the patient should be aware that all hearing will be lost in the ear receiving surgery and that the effect on tinnitus is unpredictable. The patient must be aware that immediately postoperatively there will be a period of vertigo much like a typical attack and that this episode will continue for several days. In addition, a period of protracted disequilibrium may occur, and in those with negative indicators for compensation, there may be some degree of permanent disability that requires a rehabilitative program. A discussion of alternative treatments for the vestibular symptomatology of Ménière's disease should be well understood by the patient. The discussion should include medical regimens; alterna-

tive ablative techniques, including transmastoid or translabyrinthine approaches; and selective ablative techniques through the middle or posterior fossa to save residual hearing. Particularly in the aged or in patients with other negative indicators for compensation, a round window labyrinthotomy should be considered and discussed with the patient as a possible alternative to labyrinthectomy. This procedure has the advantage of not resulting in a protracted period of disequilibrium and does not preclude a labyrinthectomy, if necessary. In addition, the usual risks of ear surgery should be discussed, including paresis or paralysis of the facial nerve, perforation of the tympanic membrane, dysgeusia, failure of the procedure to achieve the desired result, the possible need for revision or secondary procedures, spinal fluid leakage or meningitis, and the fact that harvesting of a fat graft may be necessary.

SURGICAL TECHNIQUE

General anesthesia is required because of the violent vestibular response during removal of the vestibular end organs. One exception may be in a revision labyrinthectomy in an ear with minimal residual vestibular function. In such cases, local anesthesia may allow intraoperative confirmation that the site of residual vestibular function has been located. The patient is placed in a supine position in a head holder with the head positioned similar to any transcanal procedure. Hair is shaved 0.5 inch around the auricle and prepared with an antiseptic solution. Generally, systemic antibiotics and steroids are not required.

Facial nerve monitoring is usually not done in primary labyrinthectomy but may be useful in a revision case if there is considerable scarring in the oval window area. No special instruments are necessary, but an instrument to remove the utricle from the recesses of the vestibule and a probe to mechanically destroy the cristae of the three semicircular canals should both be available. For these purposes, a 4-mm right-angle hook or a whirlybird from the Austin middle ear instrument set is useful. A microdrill is necessary to widen the oval window or to connect the oval and round windows for exposure.

Incision and Exposure

The procedure is done by the transcanal approach in most cases. Occasionally, with a very narrow meatus, an endaural incision or postauricular transcanal approach may be useful. An anteriorly based tympanomeatal flap, somewhat longer than that used for stapedectomy, is elevated to allow wide curettage in the oval and round window areas (Fig. 40–1). The horizontal segment of the facial nerve, the entire stapes footplate, and the entire round window niche should all be easily visible after elevation of the flap and curettage of the posterior aspect of the bony tympanic annulus.

Preparation for Opening the Vestibule

The incus is removed. The stapedial tendon is then sectioned and the stapes removed in a rocking motion in an

FIGURE 40-1

FIGURE 40-2

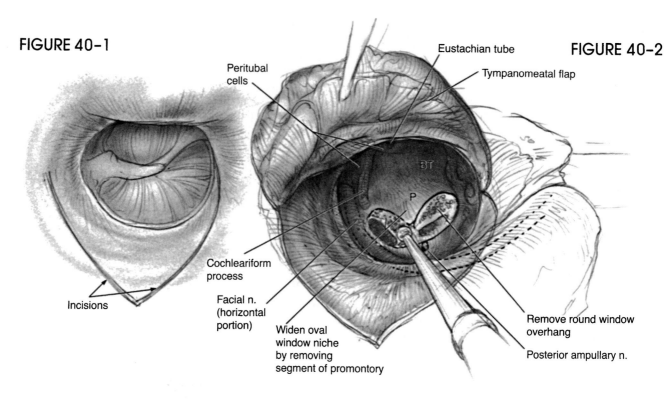

Peritubal cells

Eustachian tube

Tympanomeatal flap

Cochleariform process

Facial n. (horizontal portion)

Widen oval window niche by removing segment of promontory

Incisions

Remove round window overhang

Posterior ampullary n.

FIGURE 40-3

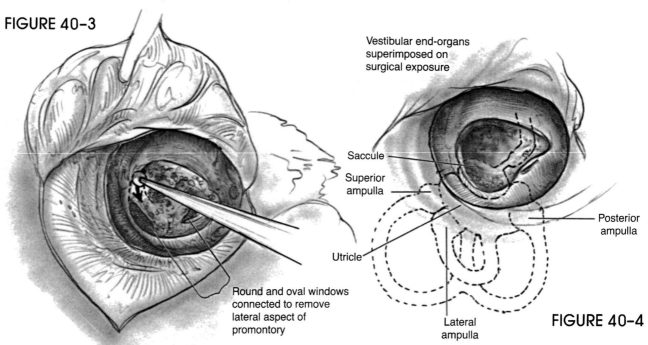

Vestibular end-organs superimposed on surgical exposure

Saccule

Superior ampulla

Utricle

Posterior ampulla

Lateral ampulla

Round and oval windows connected to remove lateral aspect of promontory

FIGURE 40-4

FIGURE 40-1. Incisions for transcanal labyrinthectomy. The anteriorly based tympanomeatal flap should be slightly wider and longer than that used for stapedectomy to allow wide curettage of the bony tympanic annulus. Curettage should allow visualization of the horizontal segment of the facial nerve and the entire oval and round window niches.

FIGURE 40-2. Access to the vestibule may be achieved by widening the oval window niche by removing a segment of promontory. At this time the posterior ampullary nerve may be located in the floor of the round window niche. This step is facilitated by removal of the round window overhang.

FIGURE 40-3. As an alternative way of exposure of the vestibule, the round and oval windows may be connected to remove the lateral aspect of the promontory.

FIGURE 40-4. The normal anatomic positions of the five vestibular end organs are superimposed on the surgical exposure.

anteroposterior direction to allow removal of the stapes without fracture. Every effort should be made to avoid aspiration of the vestibule at this time to avoid displacement of the utricle. To obtain access to the vestibular end organs, the oval window may simply be enlarged at its anterior and inferior aspects (Fig. 40–2), or the oval and round windows may be connected to remove a segment of the promontory (Fig. 40–3). At this juncture, an attempt may be made to expose the posterior ampullary nerve. It may be exposed near the posterior aspect of the round window niche (see Figs. 40–2 and 40–3), which affords the surgeon an opportunity to practice identification and section of the posterior ampullary nerve and also helps guarantee a more complete labyrinthectomy. In a study of labyrinthectomy in the cat, Schuknecht[23] reported that subtotal destruction of the vestibular end organs occurred in 10 of 24 ears and that the crista of the posterior semicircular canal was the end organ most commonly missed.

Removal of Vestibular End Organs

Total mechanical destruction of the five vestibular end organs is the goal of this surgery. The normal position of the vestibular end organs and their relationship to the oval and round windows are shown in Figure 40–4. However, endolymphatic hydrops or intraoperative loss of perilymph may cause displacement of these end organs. For example, during aspiration or loss of perilymphatic fluid, the utricle usually retracts superiorly to lie medial to the horizontal segment of the facial nerve. Before aspiration of the vestibule, the utricle should be removed with a 4-mm hook, whirlybird, or utricular hook in the superior aspect of the vestibule (Fig. 40–5). The utricle is substantial and can easily be seen under low power of the operating microscope. Avulsion of the utricle from the vestibule will usually result in avulsion of the cristae of both lateral and superior semicircular canals as well, but not that of the posterior semicircular canal. The sacule is destroyed mechanically by aspiration of the medial aspect of the vestibule in the area of the spherical recess. Manipulation of the medial aspect of the vestibule must be done with care to avoid fracture of the cribrose area, which would result in profuse leakage of cerebrospinal fluid from the internal auditory canal. Any residual neuroepithelium of the cristae of the three semicircular canals is then destroyed by mechanical probing. The surgeon can feel the 4-mm hook drop into the ampullary ends of the bony canals (Fig. 40–6). This entire technique should be practiced in the temporal bone laboratory to gain both familiarity with the anatomy and proficiency in this procedure.

After destruction of the vestibular end organs, the vestibule is usually packed with absorbable gelatin sponge (Gelfoam) or, preferably, a small fat graft from the ear lobe (Fig. 40–7). Some surgeons recommend the use of streptomycin-soaked gelatin sponge in the medial aspect of the vestibule to guarantee destruction of residual neuroepithelium. As seen in Figure 40–8, the absence of a tissue graft of the open oval window results in a pneumolabyrinth postoperatively. Generally, this result does not cause a problem, but a tissue seal with fat or fascia provides a better barrier between the middle ear and spinal fluid

spaces. Leakage of spinal fluid after aspiration of the vestibule should be repaired with a tissue seal. The tympanomeatal flap is then returned to the posterior canal wall and held in place with packing, and the procedure is terminated.

POSTOPERATIVE CARE

The degree of postoperative vestibular disturbance is positively correlated with preoperative residual vestibular function. That is, individuals with normal or near-normal caloric response preoperatively will have a more severe reaction than those with minimal or no vestibular response. Third-degree nystagmus, nausea, and vomiting can be expected. Control of the vestibular symptomatology may be achieved with promethazine or droperidol. Vestibular suppressants should be tapered as quickly as possible, given the evidence that they may impair or slow central compensation for unilateral vestibular ablation. Rapid advancement of physical activity should be encouraged, including sitting and ambulation with assistance in the first few days. The patient may be discharged when he or she is relatively self-sufficient and ambulating without assistance. This improvement may take from 3 to 7 days.

At the first postoperative visit at 1 week, the packing is removed, and progressive activity is encouraged. The patient is seen 1 month postoperatively to evaluate residual symptoms, progress, and compensation and to ascertain healing of the tympanic membrane and ear canal. At this time, there is usually no residual spontaneous nystagmus, and a caloric test of the ear that had surgery, using 20-ml of ice water and Frenzel's lenses, is used to ascertain the completeness of unilateral vestibular ablation. Further follow-up is dependent on the patient's progress.

SURGICAL COMPLICATIONS AND MANAGEMENT

Intraoperative Complications

Cerebrospinal Fluid Leakage

Fracture of the cribrose bone on the medial aspect of the vestibule results in profuse spinal fluid leakage from the internal auditory canal. The leakage can be controlled by a tissue graft using fascia, or subcutaneous fat, or both, to seal the vestibule.

Failure to Find Utricle

Identification and removal of the utricle are essential to a complete labyrinthectomy. When perilymph has been aspirated from the vestibule, the utricle may retract superiorly under the horizontal segment of the facial nerve. The use of a modified right-angled hook (utricular hook) (see Fig. 40–5) or a right-angle No. 3 Fr suction may aid in retrieval. Alternately, the utricle will remain fixed to the lateral and superior semicircular canals, which may be palpated in the depths of the vestibule. A wide exposure achieved by removing the bone from the inferior aspects

FIGURE 40–5

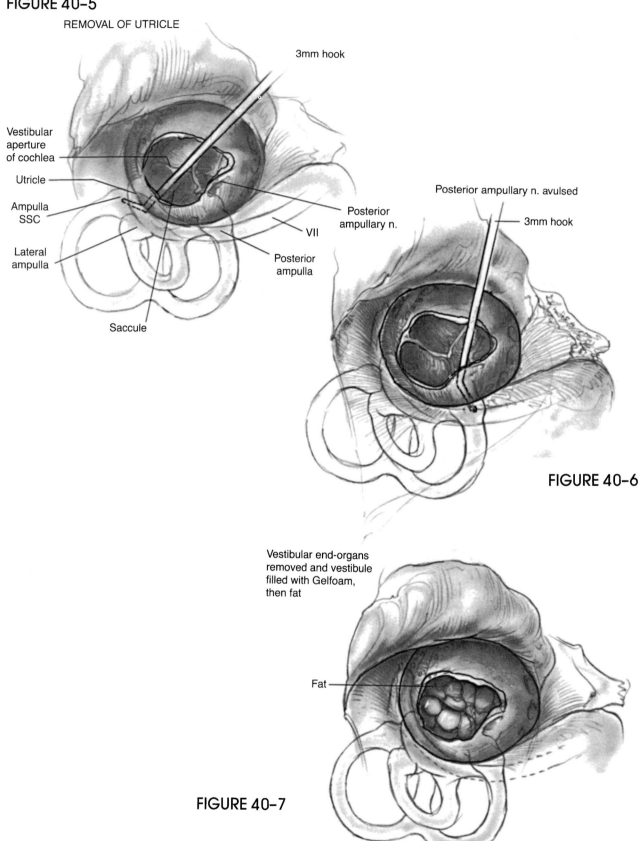

REMOVAL OF UTRICLE

3mm hook

Vestibular
aperture
of cochlea

Utricle

Ampulla
SSC

Lateral
ampulla

Saccule

Posterior
ampullary n.

VII

Posterior
ampulla

Posterior ampullary n. avulsed

3mm hook

FIGURE 40–6

Vestibular end-organs
removed and vestibule
filled with Gelfoam,
then fat

Fat

FIGURE 40–7

FIGURES 40–5 to 40–7 *See legends on opposite page*

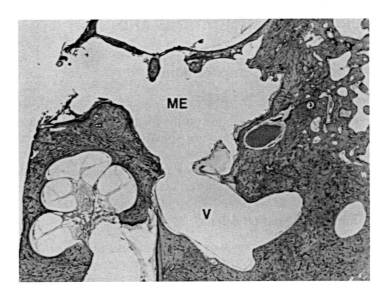

FIGURE 40–8. The vestibule (V) remains in communication with the middle ear (ME) 14 years following a transcanal labyrinthectomy.

of the oval window or by connecting the round and oval windows improves access to the vestibule and its contents.

Facial Nerve Injury

The facial nerve may be damaged in its horizontal segment. Care must be taken, particularly in retrieval of the utricle, to avoid trauma to the medial aspect of the horizontal segment of the nerve. Treatment of injury to the facial nerve should follow the usual principles of management of iatrogenic injury. A delayed facial paresis occurs infrequently and may be managed expectantly.

Postoperative Complications

Incomplete Labyrinthectomy

The incidence of incomplete labyrinthectomy in many series is less than 5 per cent. However, persistent postoperative vestibular symptoms or failure to compensate following labyrinthectomy may signal residual neuroepithelium and vestibular function in the operated ear. A postoperative ice water caloric test is valuable, if the results are positive, to confirm the presence of functional neuroepithelium. However, absence of induced symptoms or nystagmus on postoperative ice water caloric test does not necessarily indicate total destruction of the vestibular end organs. In the presence of persistent symptoms or poor compensation following surgery in the absence of contralateral disease, the possibility of an incomplete labyrinthectomy should be considered despite the absence of caloric response.

Management of suspected incomplete labyrinthectomy should include revision surgery. One option is revision transcanal labyrinthectomy with the patient under local anesthesia using the patient's response during manipulation of the vestibule as a means of localizing residual neuroepithelium. However, this is frequently a difficult procedure with fibrous tissue and, occasionally, new bone formation within the vestibule. A more certain means of ablating vestibular function in such cases is a transmastoid labyrinthectomy and translabyrinthine vestibular nerve section.

HISTOPATHOLOGY OF LABYRINTHECTOMY

Postmortem histopathology of temporal bones from patients who, in life, underwent labyrinthectomy has been reported by Belal and Ylikoski,[20] Linthicum and associates,[21] Pulec,[22] and Schuknecht,[23] and all have reported examples of incomplete mechanical disruption of the vestibular end organ after transcanal labyrinthectomy. These results underscore the importance of proper exposure, removal of the utricle, and thorough probing of the ampullae. In an animal study of labyrinthectomy, Schuknecht reported that the neuroepithelium of the posterior semicircular canal persisted in 10 of 24 ears. This fact argues for wider exposure of the vestibule by connecting the oval and round windows and for selective destruction of the posterior ampullary nerve, as recommended by Gacek, as an additional step to guarantee complete labyrinthectomy.[24] Both Linthicum and associates[21] and Belal and Ylikoski[20] reported

FIGURE 40–5. Removal of the utricle can be accomplished with a 4-mm hook (as shown), a utricular hook, or a whirlybird. Removal of the utricle often results in simultaneous avulsion of the ampullary ends of the lateral and superior canals but not of the posterior canal.

FIGURE 40–6. After removal of the utricle and aspiration of the saccule, any residual neuroepithelium of the three semicircular canals is destroyed by mechanical disruption using a 3- to 4-mm angled hook.

FIGURE 40–7. After avulsion and destruction of the vestibular end organs, the vestibule is filled with absorbable gelatin sponge soaked in gentamicin or streptomycin solution and a tissue graft, such as fat.

traumatic neuroma within the vestibule following labyrinthectomy (Fig. 40–9). Both groups interpret this finding as an indication of the superiority of the translabyrinthine vestibular neurectomy. However, in one case, a traumatic neuroma was also described after transmastoid labyrinthectomy and section of the superior vestibular nerve. In an experimental study in the cat, Schuknecht reported no evidence of regeneration of vestibular nerve fibers or formation of traumatic neuroma following labyrinthectomy.[23] In temporal bone specimens from human subjects who had undergone transcanal labyrinthectomy during life, degeneration of the vestibular nerve was seen in one, and a proliferation of nerve fibers was identified in another (Fig. 40–10). However, no evidence exists to suggest that nerve fibers, whether residual or regenerative, can contribute to afferent vestibular input if the vestibular neuroepithelium distal to it has been destroyed.

Two patients are cited by Linthicum and associates[21] as examples of failure of labyrinthectomy because of traumatic neuroma. In the first case, reported by Hilding and House,[25] the neuroma was uncovered at revision labyrinthectomy, but there was no evidence that the persistent symptoms resulted from the neuroma rather than from residual neuroepithelium.

In the second case, reported by Pulec,[22] a traumatic neuroma was identified by postmortem temporal bone histopathology in a patient with persistent vestibular symptoms for 10 years after labyrinthotomy, not labyrinthectomy. In addition, despite no response on the premortem caloric testing, the ampulla of the posterior semicircular canal was normal. In this case, the persistent vestibular symptoms probably resulted from residual vestibular neuroepithelium rather than from the traumatic neuroma.

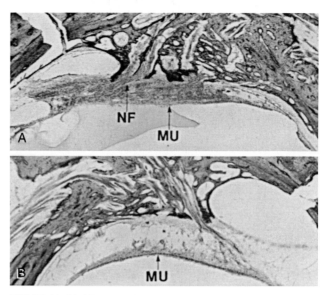

FIGURE 40–10. Histopathology 4 months after left labyrinthectomy. The macular utriculi (MU) of the ear that had surgery (A) shows atrophy. However, the stroma of the macula is intact, and there has been proliferation of nerve fibers (NF) within it. The superior vestibular nerve and macular utriculi (MU) of the unoperated side (B) appear normal.

RESULTS OF SURGERY

The reported results as measured by ablation of caloric function or cure of the patient have varied considerably. For example, Linthicum and associates[21] reported that only 17 (60 per cent) of 25 patients who underwent labyrinthectomy were cured or improved by this approach; therefore, they advocated translabyrinthine nerve section as a more reliable method of ablating vestibular function. However, Ariagno found a 98 per cent success rate in controlling peripheral vestibular disorders through transcanal labyrinthectomy, emphasizing the need for total destruction of the vestibular end organs by joining the oval and round windows.[15] Hammerschlag and Schuknecht reported a cure of episodic vertigo in 120 (96.8 per cent) of 124 patients by transcanal labyrinthectomy.[26] The remaining 4 patients had continuing disequilibrium, and 3 with persistent vestibular response by postoperative ice water caloric tests were cured by revision transcanal labyrinthectomy, resulting in an overall cure rate of 99 per cent.

SPECIAL CONSIDERATIONS

The advent of cochlear implantation as a possibility for rehabilitation of the profoundly deaf and the fact that 10 to 40 per cent of patients with Ménière's disease have bilateral involvement require consideration of the implications for eventual implantation after any surgical procedure for management of vestibular disturbance. Chen and colleagues[27] reported on three temporal bone cases from patients who in life had undergone labyrinthectomy, two by the transcanal route and one by the transmastoid approach. Based on the patency of the cochlear duct, remaining spiral ganglion, and neural elements, and maintenance of the

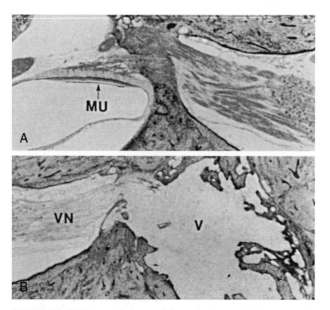

FIGURE 40–9. Histopathology of the superior vestibular nerve 36 months after transcanal labyrinthectomy in the cat. The unoperated control ear (A) at the level of the normal macular utriculi (MU). In the ear that had undergone labyrinthectomy (B) there was moderate degeneration of the vestibular nerve (VN), new bone and fibrous tissue within the vestibule (V), and no evidence of proliferation of the remaining vestibular nerves.

organ of Corti as evaluated by histopathologic study, these authors predicted that labyrinthectomy would not preclude subsequent cochlear implantation. In six patients who had undergone previous unilateral transmastoid labyrinthectomy, Lambert and coworkers[28] reported that round window electrical stimulation resulted in a psychophysical response to stimulus in all patients and electrically evoked middle latency response in five of six patients. Kveton and associates[29] reported an ear deafened by transmastoid labyrinthectomy with subsequent successful cochlear implantation resulting in speech comprehension comparable to that of patients deafened by other causes.

References

1. Stockwell CW, Graham MD: Vestibular compensation following labyrinthectomy and vestibular neurectomy. *In* Nadol JB Jr (ed): Second International Symposium for Ménière's Disease. Amsterdam, Kugler & Ghedini Publishers, 1989, pp 489–498.
2. Dandy WE: Ménière's disease: Its diagnosis and a method of treatment. Arch Surg 16: 1127–1152, 1928.
3. Jansen A.: Referat uber die operationsmethoden bei den verschiedenen otitischen gehirukoneplikationen. Verh Dtsch Otol Gesell (Jena), 1895, p 96.
4. Milligan W: Ménière's disease: A clinical and experimental inquiry. Br Med J 2: 1228, 1904.
5. Lake R: Removal of the semicircular canals in a case of unilateral aural vertigo. Lancet 1: 1567–1568, 1904.
6. Cawthorne TE: The treatment of Ménière's disease. J Laryngol Otol 58: 63–71, 1943.
7. Crockett EA: The removal of the stapes for the relief of auditory vertigo. Ann Otol Rhinol Laryngol 12: 67–72, 1903.
8. Lempert J: Lempert decompression operation for hydrops of the endolymphatic labyrinth in Ménière's disease. Arch Otolaryngol Head Neck Surg 47: 551–570, 1948.
9. Schuknecht HF: Ablation therapy for the relief of Ménière's disease. Laryngoscope 66: 859–870, 1956.
10. Cawthorne T: Membranous labyrinthectomy via the oval window for Ménière's disease. J Laryngol Otol 71: 524–527, 1957.
11. Schuknecht HF: Ablation therapy in the management of Ménière's disease. Acta Otolaryngol Suppl (Stockh) 132: 1–42, 1957.
12. Schuknecht HF: Destructive therapy for Ménière's disease. Arch Otolaryngol Head Neck Surg 71: 562–572, 1960.
13. Schuknecht HF: Destructive labyrinthine surgery. Arch Otolaryngol Head Neck Surg 97: 150–151, 1973.
14. Armstrong BW: Transtympanic vestibulotomy for Ménière's disease. Laryngoscope 69: 1071–1074, 1959.
15. Ariagno RP: Transtympanic labyrinthectomy. Arch Otolaryngol Head Neck Surg 80: 282–286, 1964.
16. Greven AJ, Oosterveld WJ: The contralateral ear in Ménière's disease. Arch Otolaryngol Head Neck Surg 101: 608–612, 1978.
17. Paparella MM, Griebie MS: Bilaterality of Ménière's disease. Acta Otolaryngol (Stockh) 97: 233–237, 1984.
18. Nadol JB Jr: Positive "fistula sign" with an intact tympanic membrane. Arch Otolaryngol Head Neck Surg 100: 273–278, 1974.
19. Silverstein H, Smouha E, Jones R: Natural history versus surgery for Ménière's disease. *In* Nadol JB Jr (ed): Second International Symposium for Ménière's Disease. Amsterdam, Kugler & Ghedini Publishers, 1989, pp 543–544.
20. Belal A, Ylikoski J: Pathology as it relates to ear surgery: II. Labyrinthectomy. J Laryngol Otol 97: 1–10, 1983.
21. Linthicum FH, Alonso A, Denia A: Traumatic neuroma. Arch Otolaryngol Head Neck Surg 105: 654–655, 1979.
22. Pulec JL: Labyrinthectomy: Indications, technique, and results. Laryngoscope 84: 1552–1573, 1974.
23. Schuknecht HF: Behavior of the vestibular nerve following labyrinthectomy. Ann Otol Rhinol Laryngol 91(5 Suppl 97): 16–32, 1982.
24. Gacek RR: Transection of the posterior ampullary nerve for the relief of benign paroxysmal positional vertigo. Ann Otol Rhinol Laryngol 83: 596–605, 1974.
25. Hilding DA, House WF: "Acoustic neuroma": Comparison of traumatic and neoplastic. J Ultrastruct Res 12: 611–623, 1965.
26. Hammerschlag PE, Schuknecht HF: Transcanal labyrinthectomy for intractable vertigo. Arch Otolaryngol Head Neck Surg 107: 152–156, 1981.
27. Chen DA, Linthicum, RH, Rizer FM: Cochlear histopathology in the labyrinthectomized ear: Implications for cochlear implantation. Laryngoscope 98: 1170–1172, 1988.
28. Lambert PR, Ruth RA, Halpin CF: Promontory electrical stimulation in labyrinthectomized ears. Arch Otolaryngol Head Neck Surg 116: 197–201, 1990.
29. Kveton JF, Abbott C, April M, et al: Cochlear implantation after transmastoid labyrinthectomy. Laryngoscope 99: 610–613, 1989.

41

Overview of Transtemporal Skull Base Surgery

Moisés A. Arriaga, M.D.

OBJECTIVE

The objective of neurotologic skull base surgery is exposure of the skull base through precise management of the temporal bone. In the following chapters, a series of procedures are presented that accomplish ample surgical exposure and minimize brain retraction in posterior, medial, and lateral skull base lesions.

The modern era of neurotologic transtemporal skull base surgery began in 1961 when William House introduced the operating microscope and multidisciplinary surgery for removal of acoustic neuromas. The conceptual advantage of this transtemporal technique was a wide exposure of the lesion with substantially less cerebellar retraction than the techniques available at that time in addition to direct facial nerve preservation. With its low mortality and enhanced facial nerve preservation rates, House established the translabyrinthine (TL) procedure as a technique to which all other microsurgical approaches to the cerebellopontine angle (CPA) are compared.

Neurotologic skull base surgery includes a variety of techniques that permit the surgeon to tailor the procedure to a particular patient's pathology and physiologic status. An array of neurotologic procedures provides safe exposure of the mid brain, clivus, CPA, vertebrobasilar junction, petrous apex, and infratemporal fossa. This chapter presents an anatomic framework for organizing and planning transtemporal neurotologic skull base approaches. In addition, the difficulties of terminology and classification of approaches are discussed. The emphasis is on anatomic descriptions rather than eponyms.

Figure 41–1 presents an organizational framework for transtemporal surgery based on management of the otic capsule. The otic capsule is selected as the organizational center both on a functional and a locational basis. Functionally, anatomic preservation of the otic capsule is the requirement for preservation of audiovestibular function (although exceptions to this principle are developing). Anatomically, the paired petrous pyramids encompass the center of lateral skull base exposure. The approaches listed in Figure 41–1 can be used individually; however, in certain cases combinations of these approaches offer the ideal exposure.

Approaches that traverse the otic capsule (transcapsular) permit wide exposure by sacrificing hearing: translabyrinthine (Chapter 50), transcochlear (Chapter 53), and transotic (Chapter 52). The posterior approaches that spare the otic capsule (retrocapsular) provide varying degrees of CPA exposure with an opportunity for hearing preservation: retrolabyrinthine (Chapter 37) and retrosigmoid (Chapter 51). Superior approaches (supracapsular) permit unroofing the internal auditory canal with varying degrees of petrous apex exposure and an opportunity for hearing preservation: middle fossa (Chapter 49) and middle fossa transpetrous (Chapter 54).

Combined approaches permit the widest transtemporal exposure with varying opportunities for preservation of neurologic function: retrolabyrinthine petrosal (Chapter 56), and translabyrinthine petrosal (Chapter 56), and transcochlear petrosal (Chapter 56). The inferior approaches (infracapsular) permit minimally invasive access for drainage of cystic lesions of the petrous apex: infracochlear and infralabyrinthine (Chapter 46). The anterior approaches (precapsular) such as the infratemporal fossa (Chapter 55) techniques permit exposure to the middle skull base, including the region of the foramen ovale, foramen spinosum, foramen lacerum, pterygoid space, and avenues to the nasopharynx and paranasal sinuses. These lateral approaches can even be combined with facial disassembly and endoscopic sinus approaches in selected cases.

Neurotologic skull base surgery is not a hodgepodge of unrelated techniques. Instead, when considered in the context of the management of the otic capsule, these approaches are a spectrum of techniques for three-dimensional surgical exposure of the cranial base.

NOMENCLATURE

There has been a rapid expansion of terminology describing skull base surgical approaches. The techniques and their applications have evolved extensively. There have been many variations, some minor and some major. Unfortunately, in the context of this rapid expansion of application and techniques, there has been a conflicting development of terminology for these approaches. Not only are various eponyms attached to the approaches, but the same terms are used for different surgical techniques. Because of the potential conflict and debate over attribution, in general, eponyms for the description of surgical approaches should be avoided. Instead, anatomic terminology should be selected. Considering transtemporal surgical approaches to the skull base, even this concept becomes confusing. Conceptually most of these transtemporal approaches involve management of the petrous bone. Accordingly, these approaches all have rightfully been described as petrosal

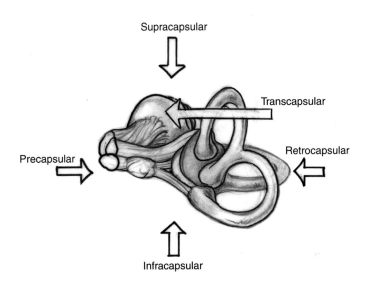

Supracapsular

Transcapsular

Retrocapsular

Precapsular

Infracapsular

Transcapsular: TL, TO, TC, TP
Retrocapsular: RL, RS, ERS
Supracapsular: MF, MFT
Infracapsular: IL, IC
Precapsular: ITF

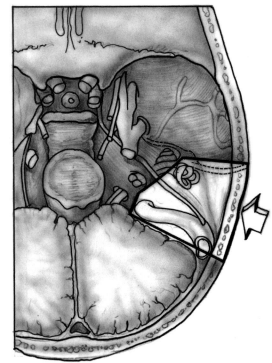

FIGURE 41-1. Transtemporal neurologic skull base approaches, based on management of the otic capsule. TL, translabyrinthine; TO, transotic; TC, transcochlear; TP, transpetrous; RL, retrolabyrinthine; RS, retrosigmoid; ERS, extended retrosigmoid; MF, middle fossa; MFT, middle fossa transpetrous; IL, infralabyrinthine; IC, infracochlear; ITF, infratemporal fossa.

approaches in various modifications at different times. The terminology in Figure 41-1 is anatomically descriptive based on the structures of the otic capsule itself. In general, we use the term *petrosal approaches* for combined posterior fossa and subtemporal surgical techniques that include division of the superior petrosal sinus (Chapter 56).

The following chapters summarize the current state of the art in neurotologic skull base surgery. Although the terminology is the same, a number of these approaches have been modified from their original description. For example, the standard translabyrinthine approach includes removal of bone posterior to the sigmoid sinus and along the tegmen mastoideum. As these techniques have evolved, it is not necessary to refer to this as an extended translabyrinthine technique. Similarly, with the transcochlear approach, the original description by William House described an anterior extension of the translabyrinthine approach without transection of the ear canal and removal of the middle ear contents. In the current context, the transcochlear approach usually includes transection of the ear canal, removal of the skin of the ear canal, and removal of the tympanic membrane and ossicular chain as well as cochlear removal.

COLLABORATION IN TRANSTEMPORAL SURGERY

Multidisciplinary transtemporal approaches for posterior fossa skull base neoplasms are an adjunct and not a substi-

tute for standard neurosurgical techniques in managing these lesions. The neurotologist and neurosurgeon are truly cosurgeons in the management of these lesions, each having intimate familiarity with the other's role. The reader will notice that many chapters are coauthored by otolaryngologists and neurosurgeons, reflecting the true collaborative nature of modern skull base surgery. Precise temporal bone management offers the operative team flexibility to tailor the management to a patient's specific anatomic and functional needs.

As a team considers an individual patient's management, it is useful to systematically consider each of the basic categories of surgical approaches in terms of otic capsule management. A lesion can be managed in many different ways; however, systematic consideration of these approaches and their respective merits ensures that all surgical options are being considered.

OVERVIEW

The fundamental prerequisite for success in transtemporal skull base surgery is complete, three-dimensional understanding of temporal bone anatomy and its surgical and functional applications. The chapters that follow demonstrate the indications, contraindications, and technical details of neurotologic skull base surgery.

42

Translabyrinthine Vestibular Neurectomy

Ralph A. Nelson, M.D., M.S.

Successful surgery for vertigo is predicated on three conditions, the first of which is altering or denervating the peripheral end organ. If the symptoms do not originate in the end organ, surgery is unlikely to be of value. Second, surgery is warranted only when dysequilibrium is significantly disabling. Because major surgery for vertigo often produces minor but noticeable sequelae, such as poor post-denervation central compensation, we must ensure that the cure is not worse than the disease. Third, medicinal or noninvasive measures must have failed to produce a response in the patient. If all these criteria are met, surgery may be considered.

The type of surgical intervention considered depends on several criteria, including surgical expertise and experience, residual hearing in the ear to be operated on, condition of the opposite ear, auditory needs of the patient, and site of lesion. If the surgeon does not have the knowledge, training, and facilities to perform certain procedures, choices become limited. The levels of residual hearing also dictate which procedures are best suited because a destructive labyrinthectomy may be quite appropriate when no residual hearing exists, but a hearing conservation procedure will be used in most other circumstances. Last, the specific site of a peripheral lesion may have some influence on the procedure selected. As an example, a labyrinthectomy may not help patients with dizziness originating from a vestibular nerve tumor located medial to the end organ.

The translabyrinthine vestibular nerve section is the gold standard for denervation procedures. It is both a postganglionic nerve section, because of the labyrinthectomy used to access the internal auditory canal (IAC), and a preganglionic procedure, because of the vestibular nerve section. Some controversy surrounds the significance or even existence of traumatic neuromas in postganglionic procedures. Numerous traumatic neuromas have been documented in the House Ear Institute temporal bone collection,[1] and persisting balance problems in some patients have been attributed to these neuromas. Because of these histologic findings and the symptoms accompanying them, we prefer preganglionic surgical procedures whenever feasible.

The single largest drawback to the translabyrinthine vestibular nerve section is the sacrifice of residual hearing. In the past, a hearing level of 50 per cent speech discrimination and 50 dB loss was thought to be the dividing line between serviceable and nonserviceable hearing; however, with the advent of better hearing aids and greater understanding of the role of binaural hearing in central processing, the parameters of serviceability have been expanded. This is especially true in situations in which the remaining ear is marginal or could become diseased, such as in Ménière's syndrome.[2]

Preoperative radiologic, auditory, vestibular, and metabolic testing is not specific for translabyrinthine vestibular nerve section. Such testing is performed as a part of the dizziness evaluation done to determine the origin of symptoms. Surgery is not scheduled until these problems have been addressed.[3] These studies ensure that unrecognized pathology has not been missed, and in the case of vestibular function tests, that the proper end organ is operated on. It is necessary to point out, however, that in a large series of translabyrinthine eighth nerve sections, there was no direct correlation between success or failure of surgery and the degree of reduced vestibular response, as seen on electronystagmography.[4] This finding undoubtedly results from the inability of standard electronystagmography to test the function of the inferior vestibular nerve.

SURGICAL TECHNIQUE

Surgery is performed with the patient under general anesthesia and placed on the table in reverse to allow for table manipulations and to permit the surgeon to sit comfortably with knees under the table. The patient is supine, and the head is turned to the side facing away from the surgeon. The anesthesia machine is at the foot of the table and is connected to the endotracheal tube by extended tubing (Fig. 42–1). A sterile, hairless area is prepared 2 cm above and 5 cm behind the ear, and the field is draped off. The high-speed drill with various cutting burrs and suction-irrigation with sterile saline are on the field. Monopolar and bipolar electrocautery are available. If it is to be used, seventh cranial nerve monitoring equipment is set up and the electrodes are inserted.

An incision is made approximately 1 cm above and behind the postauricular crease and follows the contour of the auricle (Fig. 42–2). A plane is established in the galea-aponeurotic layer lateral to the temporalis muscle, and the auricle is turned forward. A thick periosteal flap is created by incising this tissue along the linear temporalis just anterior to the incision line and then inferior to the mastoid tip. This flap is elevated off the mastoid cortex and retracted forward with a large self-retaining retractor. The staggered two-layer incision provides better closure to prevent cerebrospinal fluid leaks.

The high-speed drill with a large cutting burr and constant suction-irrigation is used to perform a cortical mastoidectomy. The posterior external bony canal wall is thinned, the bone over the tegmen is thinned, and the sigmoid sinus is skeletonized (Fig. 42–3). We frequently "eggshell" the bone over the sinus and decompress it by collapsing it with thumb pressure, leaving tiny, fragmented

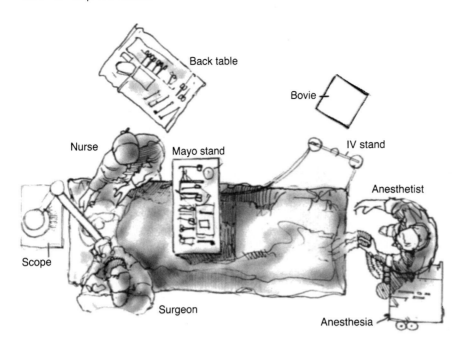

FIGURE 42–1. Room setup.

pieces of bone, similar to the armor of medieval chain mail, over the highly vulnerable sigmoid sinus to protect it from damage from instruments entering and exiting the wound (Fig. 42–4). The sinus is easily collapsed and gives needed exposure medially. The sinodural angle is opened as far back on the cortex as possible. Because the vestibule lies under the facial nerve anteriorly, an angulated view via the sinodural angle is necessary to visualize the contents of the vestibule and eventually identify landmarks used to excise the superior vestibular nerve.

Bone over the posterior fossa dura is thinned out but not removed. The labyrinth is skeletonized and the cells of the mastoid tip are opened. The labyrinthectomy is performed by opening the crown of the lateral (horizontal) semicircu-

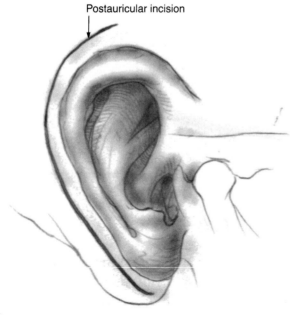

FIGURE 42–2. Postauricular incision.

lar canal on its posterior border and following the half-opened canal posteriorly to the posterior canal. The lateral canal is only half opened to protect the external genu of the facial nerve until careful trimming can be done. The posterior canal, having been opened, can be traced to its confluence with the superior semicircular canal, where the two canals combine to become the common crus (Fig. 42–5). The common crus may then be followed directly forward to the vestibule (Fig. 42–6).

The posterior surface of the facial nerve over the external genu is now thinned carefully, and the anterior limb of the posterior canal is followed to its ampulla at the inferior pole of the elliptical recess. The lateral canal is opened anteriorly and medially to its ampullated end, and the ampulla of the superior canal identified next to that of the lateral is opened. The superior canal is opened along the tegmen throughout its course, which curves back to the common crus.

With all the canals and the vestibule opened, all soft tissue elements of the membranous labyrinth should be removed. This step would be the normal end point of the postauricular, postganglionic labyrinthectomy but only sets the stage to skeletonize the IAC in a translabyrinthine vestibular nerve section and preganglionic denervation (Fig. 42–7).

A key factor in successful exploration of the IAC is clear identification of the IAC contents. Identification is possible only if the soft tissue contents are not violated in the removal of bone during IAC skeletonization. Loss of part or all of any of the soft tissue landmarks places all of the other contents at great risk because of the difficulty in differentiating the nerves from one another. The purpose in using the facial nerve–vestibular nerve tissue plane when dissecting the IAC is to enable identification of the facial nerve in its normal position and extend the dissection into the diseased area, where those relationships are sometimes more difficult to ascertain.

A useful technique for IAC skeletonization is blue-lining

FIGURE 42-3

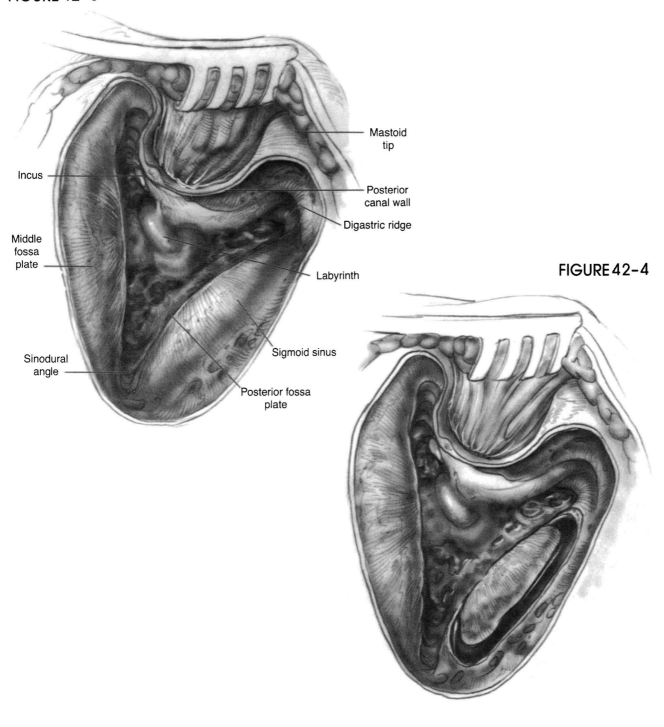

FIGURE 42-4

FIGURE 42-3. Cortical mastoidectomy.

FIGURE 42-4. Sigmoid sinus decompression—"Bill's island."

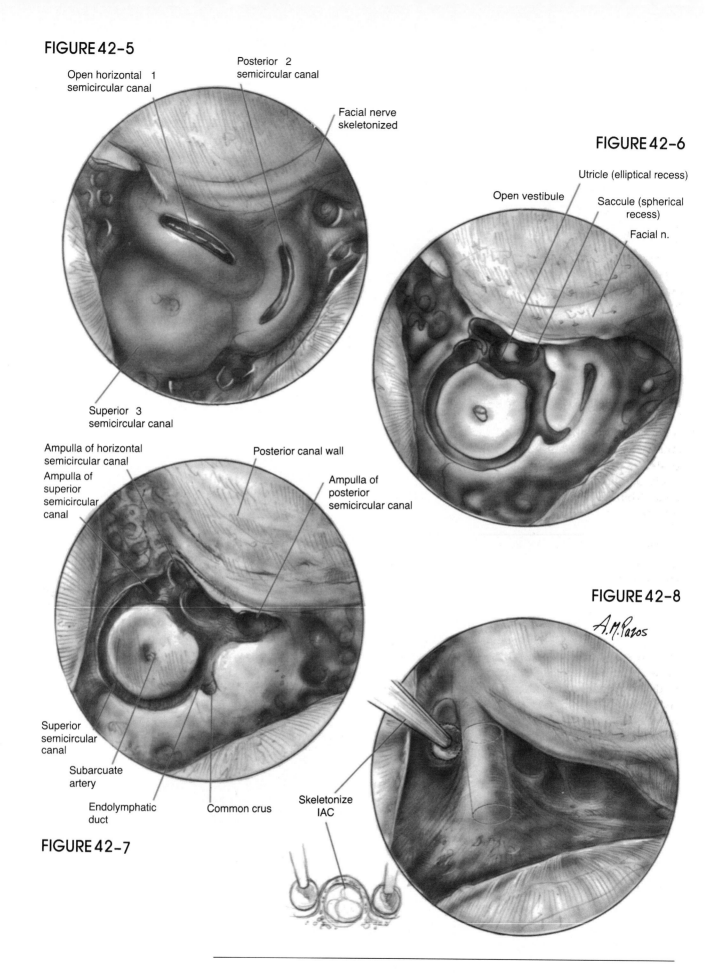

FIGURE 42-5

Open horizontal 1
semicircular canal

Posterior 2
semicircular canal

Facial nerve
skeletonized

FIGURE 42-6

Open vestibule

Utricle (elliptical recess)

Saccule (spherical
recess)

Facial n.

Superior 3
semicircular canal

Ampulla of horizontal
semicircular canal

Ampulla of
superior
semicircular
canal

Posterior canal wall

Ampulla of
posterior
semicircular canal

FIGURE 42-8

A.M.Pazos

Superior
semicircular
canal

Subarcuate
artery

Endolymphatic
duct

Common crus

Skeletonize
IAC

FIGURE 42-7

FIGURES 42–5 to 42–8. *See legends on opposite page*

436

the IAC throughout the area to be opened. The thin bony cover protects the soft tissue structures within the IAC. Blue-lining actually starts at the vestibule because this is where the bone is thinnest. The nerves of the IAC exit into the bony labyrinth through perforations in the thin bone separating the fundus of the IAC from the vestibule. This naturally blue-lined area can be used as a starting point for skeletonization of the remainder of the canal. Removal of bone should extend to the porus acusticus and should cover 180 degrees of the lateral side of the canal. The general orientation of the IAC is that the fundus is lateral just medial to the vestibule. The superior border is along a line drawn between the superior semicircular canal ampulla and the sinodural angle, and the inferior border is along the line starting at the posterior semicircular canal ampulla drawn posteriorly parallel to the superior border. The IAC angles away from the surgeon in an anterolateral to a posteromedial direction very deep to the sigmoid sinus (Fig. 42–8).

Once the IAC is adequately skeletonized, the irrigation fluid is changed to a solution of 0.25 per cent bacitracin in saline, and the wound is thoroughly rinsed. The thin bone over the canal is lifted away with a small right-angle pick. The perforated area where the superior vestibular nerve enters both the lateral and the superior ampullae is thinned carefully, and a 1-mm hook is used to avulse the superior vestibular nerve from the vestibular nerve recess that it makes in the labyrinthine bone lateral to the fallopian canal. As the superior vestibular nerve is reflected, the facial nerve comes into view deep to the plane of dissection (Fig. 42–9). If the facial nerve is not immediately visible, the hook can be used to palpate the bone of the vestibular nerve recess ("Bill's bar," or the lateral wall of the fallopian canal) until the edge of the fallopian canal is found and the hook is easily (and gently!) inserted into this labyrinthine segment of the canal.

With the superior vestibular nerve separated from the facial nerve (vestibulofacial fibers have to be lysed), the inferior vestibular nerve is also avulsed with the singular nerve to the posterior semicircular canal. Because the singular nerve frequently leaves the inferior nerve midway out of the IAC, the surgeon must be careful to check for it. Failure to include the singular nerve may spell failure for the entire operation.

Scarpa's ganglion lies midway out of the IAC. The avulsed ends of the two vestibular nerves are reflected and the fused nerves sectioned medial to the ganglion. The specimen is sent to a pathologist for examination (Fig. 42–10).

Although the cochlear nerve may also be sectioned, this action would preclude its use in a cochlear implant if that opportunity arises. Generally, implantation is not a strong consideration, but sometimes a cochlear nerve section may be entertained as a possible solution to overwhelming tinnitus symptoms. Because elimination of tinnitus is not guaranteed, this approach is rarely encouraged.

Hemostasis is achieved through bipolar cautery and the application of bovine collagen (Avitene). Control of cerebrospinal fluid leak is achieved through dural closure with 4-0 silk sutures when possible, but primarily through packing. The IAC and labyrinthine defects are sealed with strips of adipose tissue obtained from the abdominal wall, and the mastoid incision is closed with interrupted, slow-absorbing sutures in a two-layer fashion: first, the thick periosteal flap, and then a subcuticular closure of the skin. Steri-Strips are placed over the incision, and a bulky mastoid dressing is applied. The abdominal wall incision is usually drained. The patient is watched in intensive care for a day with hourly neurologic checks and then is moved to a step-down room when neurologic stability is assured. The abdominal drain is removed in 1 day and the Steri-Strips in 1 week.

Complications seen with translabyrinthine neurectomy in order of frequency include cerebrospinal fluid leak, meningitis, and facial nerve paralysis. Facial paralysis can be considered the consequence of working in an area in which the nerve is anatomically at risk. Avoidance is the best solution to this problem: the surgeon should be certain of the nerve's location and treat it with respect. Postoperative steroids or limited decompression of the nerve, particularly in the labyrinthine segment, may be useful in preventing sequelae when the nerve is known to have been abused. We do not routinely employ perioperative antibiotics other than the bacitracin irrigation because of the fear of encouraging subclinical infections, which might become apparent only after release from the hospital. When fever and meningismus occur, a spinal tap is performed and appropriate antibiotic coverage is instituted.

Cerebrospinal fluid leaks are aggressively pursued within 2 to 3 days to prevent retrograde contamination and meningitis. Initially, a tight head dressing is applied, and the patient is placed on carbonic anhydrase inhibitors, such as acetazolamide (Diamox). The patient is placed at bed rest in a semi-Fowler position. If resolution of the leak is not seen within 2 days, the wound is explored, usually with the patient under local anesthesia, and the adipose plug readjusted.

Patients are encouraged to sit up and dangle their legs on the first or second postoperative day and to begin ambulation with help as soon as possible thereafter. Discharge from hospitalization occurs between the fifth and eighth days. Patients are checked in the office within the

---

FIGURE 42–5. Opening the semicircular canals.

FIGURE 42–6. Opening the vestibule.

FIGURE 42–7. Cleaning the vestibule.

FIGURE 42–8. Skeletonizing the internal auditory canal (IAC).

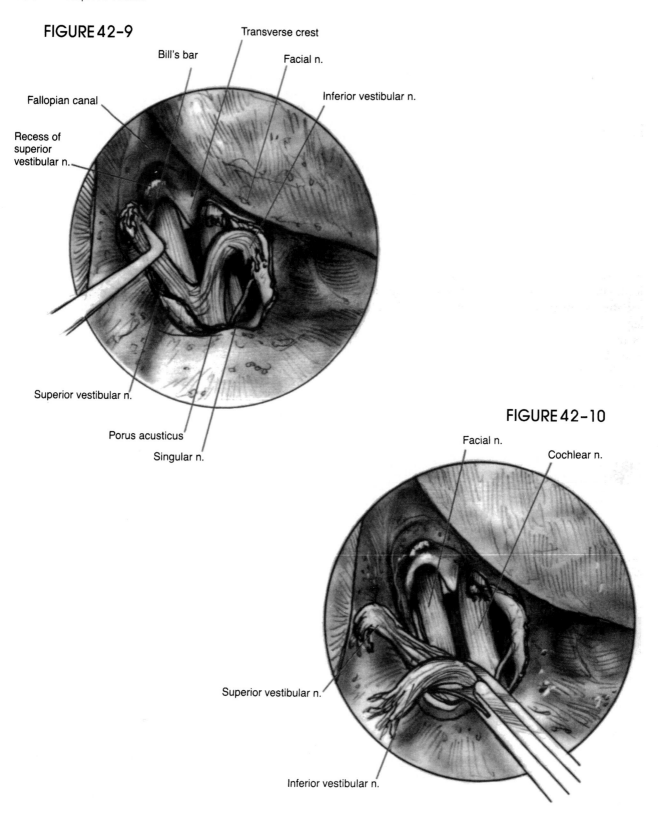

FIGURE 42-9

Fallopian canal

Recess of
superior
vestibular n.

Bill's bar

Transverse crest

Facial n.

Inferior vestibular n.

Superior vestibular n.

Porus acusticus

Singular n.

FIGURE 42-10

Facial n.

Cochlear n.

Superior vestibular n.

Inferior vestibular n.

FIGURE 42–9. Establishing the plane between the seventh and eighth nerves.

FIGURE 42–10. Section of the vestibular nerves medial to
Scarpa's ganglion.

next 7 days to be certain that the postoperative progress is satisfactory.

Results of translabyrinthine vestibular nerve section indicate that our ability to properly diagnose the etiology of vertigo is imperfect. If complete denervation of the end organ is accomplished (and translabyrinthine neurectomy is the most complete denervation theoretically possible), vertigo should be absent postoperatively. However, we find that with the exception of Ménière's syndrome, which has a 93 per cent cure, our ability to control vertigo is 80 per cent or higher. Inability to properly diagnose the origin of the vertigo or inability of the central nervous system to compensate for the denervation is a logical explanation for these statistics.[4]

References

1. Linthicum FH, Alongso A, Denia A: Traumatic neuroma: A complication of transcanal labyrinthectomy. Arch Otolaryngol Head Neck Surg 105: 654–655, 1979.
2. Shelton C, Hitselberger WE, House WF, Brackmann DE: Hearing preservation after acoustic tumor removal: Long-term results. Laryngoscope 100: 115–119, 1990.
3. Nelson RA, Brackmann DE: Clinical Problems in Diagnosis and Documentation of Ménière's Disease. Immunobiology, Histophysiology, and Tumor Immunology in Otolaryngology. Proceedings of 2nd International Academic Conference, Utrecht, The Netherlands. Berkeley, CA, Kugler, 1987, pp 3–8.
4. Nelson RA: Labyrinthectomy and translabyrinthine nerve section. *In* Brackmann DE (ed): Neurological Surgery of the Ear and Skull Base. New York, Raven Press, 1982.

43

Posterior Ampullary Nerve Section for Benign Paroxysmal Positional Vertigo

Richard R. Gacek, M.D. ▪ Mark R. Gacek, M.D.

Benign paroxysmal positional vertigo (BPPV), or cupulolithiasis, is a disorder of the semicircular canal system, usually the posterior semicircular canal.[1] Transformation of the cupula into a gravity-sensitive receptor that initiates the brief but severe vestibulo-ocular response has been generally accepted as the responsible pathophysiology for BPPV. High specific gravity deposits, fixed to the cupula or free floating in the endolymph, are probably derived from the otoconial blanket in the utricular macula.[2] These deposits presumably are dislodged by trauma, viral labyrinthitis, aging, or ear surgery.

However, there are features of BPPV that are not explained on a purely mechanical basis. These are the limited (15- to 25-second) duration of the response provoked by the Hallpike position and its fatigability on repeat provocation. Recent observations in temporal bone specimens from three patients who exhibited the typical signs and symptoms of BPPV before death revealed focal degeneration of primary afferent neurons in the inferior vestibular division, particularly the posterior ampullary nerve.[3] This indicates a neural component to the pathophysiology in BPPV, which may shed light on the features of the provoked vestibuloocular response.

Based on vestibular anatomy and physiology, the following explanation may explain the vigorous, short-lasting burst of nystagmus that fatigues on repeated provocation. The partial loss of afferent neurons to the posterior canal crista removes their contact with vestibular efferent neurons in the brainstem, thus depleting efferent inhibitory control of neural transmission in the neuroepithelium of the posterior canal crista. When the gravity-sensitive cupula is displaced in the Hallpike position, the intact afferent neurons to the sense organ receive a burst of excitatory neurotransmitter (probably glutamate) and produce a nystagmus that is brisk and short because the neurotransmitter substance is depleted at the hair cell–afferent terminal interface. A limited response is observed even though the cupula remains deflected. Repeat provocation after return to the sitting position produces a weak or absent response because the neurotransmitter has been insufficiently replenished to excite afferent neurons.

The focal axonal degeneration of vestibular afferents to the posterior canal crista suggests a loss of clusters of vestibular ganglion cells. Several morphologic and clinical factors suggest that these ganglion cell lesions are induced by a neurotropic virus acquired early in life and reactivated from a latent state by a stressful event such as trauma, upper respiratory infection, emotional stress, surgical insult to the body, and pregnancy. A likely viral agent is the herpes simplex I or varicella zoster virus.

Patients with this disorder complain of a rotatory experience when the head is placed in either the head-back or the to-the-side positions.[4] The vertiginous experience typically has a duration of less than 1 minute and reappears briefly when the original position is resumed. In severe cases, nausea and vomiting may accompany the vertiginous experience. Repeat positioning results in decreased signs and symptoms.

The Hallpike maneuver[5] is used diagnostically to reproduce the patient's symptoms and nystagmus (Fig. 43–1). The direction of nystagmus is typically a rotatory one that occurs in a counterclockwise direction when the right ear is nearest the floor and clockwise when the left ear is downmost. The type and direction of nystagmus are determined by the anatomic projections of the posterior canal sense organ.[1] These projections are diagrammed in Figure 43–2 and summarize the input of the posterior semicircular canal to the inferior rectus and the superior oblique muscles, which on excitation produce the rotatory type of nystagmus described with Hallpike's positioning maneuver. Because many patients with this disorder have normal hearing, a selective denervation of the posterior canal sense organ without invading the labyrinthine capsule is desirable to preserve hearing. The nerve to the ampullary posterior canal crista travels in a separate canal (singular canal) and can be approached from a middle ear direction.

There is another group of patients with balance symptoms, not typically paroxysmal positional vertigo, resulting from incomplete ablation of labyrinthine function, which had been attempted either by labyrinthectomy or vestibular nerve transection. Because the posterior canal sense organ and its nerve supply are anatomically inaccessible in these procedures, they may escape ablation. This residual function of the posterior canal sense organ may be responsible for persistent symptoms following vestibular ablation procedures. In these patients, transection of the singular nerve can be performed to provide relief of their symptoms.

PATIENT SELECTION

Because the vast majority of patients with BPPV undergo spontaneous resolution within a 6- to 12-month period or may be only mildly disabled by their symptoms, surgical treatment is not frequently employed.[6] Exercise programs that use the head and neck and upper trunk muscles may

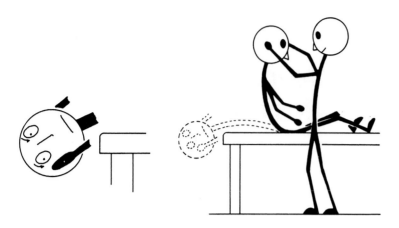

FIGURE 43–1. Diagram of the maneuver used to demonstrate nystagmus in positional vertigo. (From Carmichael EA, Dix MR, Hallpike CS: Pathology, symptomatology, and diagnosis of the organic affections of the eighth nerve system. Br Med Bull 12: 146–152, 1956.)

be helpful in reducing the severity of symptomatology and promoting spontaneous resolution.[7] However, for a small group of patients who demonstrate chronic positional vertigo for more than 1 year and are sufficiently disabled from their normal activities, singular neurectomy (SN) has provided an effective means of relief from the disabling symptoms.[1, 8] Some patients with chronic BPPV continue to live with their symptoms by avoiding the provocative position and changing their lifestyle. Surgical relief is offered only to those who request it and are willing to accept a less than 3 per cent risk of hearing loss.

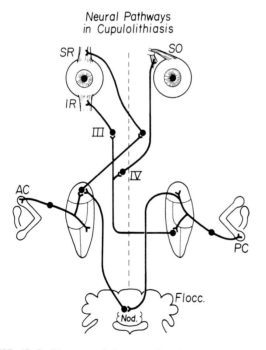

FIGURE 43–2. Diagram of the neural pathways responsible for nystagmus during provocative test and following singular neurectomy. AC, anterior canal; PC, posterior canal; SR, superior rectus; IR, inferior rectus; SO, superior oblique; III, oculomotor nucleus; IV, trochlear nucleus; Nod., nodulus; Flocc., flocculus. (Modified from Baloh RW, Spooner JW: Downbeat nystagmus: A type of central vestibular nystagmus. Neurology 31: 304–310, 1981, as in Gacek RR: Pathophysiology and management of cupulolithiasis. Am J Otolaryngol 6: 66–74, 1985.)

PREOPERATIVE EXAMINATION

The evaluation and diagnosis of BPPV consists of an accurately obtained history documenting labyrinthine trauma, such as head injury, viral labyrinthitis, inner ear or general surgery, or aging. All of these may be considered stressors capable of reactivating a latent virus (i.e., herpes simplex) located in vestibular ganglion cells. Tests of auditory and vestibular function are essential. Most patients with this syndrome are middle aged (mean age is in the sixth decade). There is a 2:1 female predominance. The vast majority of patients have a normal ear examination, although an occasional patient with chronic middle ear inflammatory disease experiences BPPV. The patients with chronic inflammatory disease should undergo surgical eradication of the inflammatory disease to control vestibular symptoms. The functional evaluation consists of pure tone and speech audiometry as well as electronystagmographic assessment of the vestibular sensitivity by the caloric method. Auditory brainstem response and electrocochleographic examinations are not necessary in the evaluation of a patient with this disorder.

The most important diagnostic test is the Hallpike maneuver properly performed with or without Frenzel's glasses with the patient on an examining room table (see Fig. 43–1). The test has been well described in the literature[5] and consists of the examiner taking the patient to a head-hanging position, first right and then left, from the sitting position and observing the patient's ocular response along with his or her subjective vestibular experience. Posterior canal BPPV typically produces a rotatory nystagmus either clockwise or counterclockwise after a latency of a few seconds. The nystagmus builds to a crescendo and then disappears over a period of 25 to 30 seconds but reappears when the sitting position is again assumed. Repeat testing produces less nystagmus and subjective symptoms, supporting the peripheral location of the pathology (fatigability). It is important to test both right and left head-down positions because approximately 15 to 18 per cent of patients with BPPV have bilateral disease[9] that is usually worse in one ear than the other. In patients with cupulolithiasis, a nystagmus response is not seen when the contralateral (noninvolved) ear is placed geotropically because the gravity-sensitive cupula is deflected utriculopetally (opposite to hair cell polarization). When the involved ear is geotropic, cupular deflection is utriculofugal and in the direction of hair cell polarization, thereby causing depolarization (Fig. 43–3). Occasionally, the Hallpike test may reveal a horizontal nystagmus with the same time characteristics and fatigability observed with the rotatory nystagmus.[10] These patients are not candidates for singular neurectomy, because their symptoms may be caused by pathology in other labyrinthine sense organs, such as the lateral canal crista.

Because a central nervous system lesion has been identified rarely in patients with similar findings, an imaging study, such as enhanced magnetic resonance imaging or computed tomographic scan, of the posterior fossa is recommended to rule out the slim chance of a central lesion being responsible for the positional vertigo.

Once a patient has been identified as having BPPV of the peripheral type, the degree of disability from the positional vertigo must be determined from an evaluation of the patient's work and lifestyle. If the patient is willing to risk a sensorineural hearing loss for relief of the positional vertigo, it is considered sufficiently disabling to warrant surgical intervention. The goal of SN is to eliminate the BPPV and to preserve hearing.

SURGICAL TECHNIQUE

The preoperative preparation is similar to that for any transcanal middle ear surgery: Preoperative or intraoperative antibiotics are not used. Postoperative antibiotics are routinely used to prevent ascending infection through the singular canal. However, such infection has not occurred in our series of more than 187 patients. The surgical site is prepared with a sterilized solution, such as providone-iodine (Betadine) and draped for transcanal surgery. A bifenestrated drape with an opening for the patient's face and one that fits around the auricle is available commercially. The patient is in a prone position with the head turned so that the operated ear is facing up toward the surgeon and the head is in a somewhat dependent position; the ear canal is then on a straight line with the surgeon's view. A small amount of hair is shaved around the post-auricular area so that the drape can adhere to the skin surface. The surgical procedure is carried out with the patient under local anesthesia with 1 per cent lidocaine (Xylocaine) with 1:100,000 dilution of adrenaline injected into the external auditory meatus and the posterior and inferior canal wall skin. A 27-gauge needle is helpful to successfully place the local anesthetic in the subperiosteal layer of the ear canal and dissect down to the level of the tympanic annulus. Medically assisted anesthesia with intravenous medication from an anesthesiologist helps allow local anesthesia to be effective.

Instruments

The instruments for this procedure are the same as those used for routine middle ear surgery, including various-sized speculae, speculum holder, angled canal wall elevators, and hooks and picks used in oval window surgery. The most essential instrument for this procedure is an electric-powered microdrill for use through an ear speculum with diamond burrs of 1- and 0.5-mm diameters. The drill is preferably angled so that the visualization around the drill in the transcanal speculum approach is permitted to remove the round window niche overhang and to approach the singular canal in the floor of the round window niche. Monitoring of hearing or facial nerve is not included in our experience, although monitoring of auditory function may be useful in determining any untoward event in auditory function from the surgical procedure. With the patient under local anesthesia, the surgeon can monitor the patient's subjective symptoms of vertigo and pain when the singular nerve is transected and can observe a vertical or rotatory nystagmus at this transection.

SURGERY

After elevation of the tympanomeatal flap, the drill is used to remove the overhang of the round window niche so that the entire round window membrane can be visualized from anteriorly to posteriorly (Fig. 43–4). Often, a mucous membrane fold will cover the aperture of the round window niche and should not be confused with the round window membrane (Fig. 43–5). This membrane fold is dissected free with small hooks and picks so that the round window membrane can be clearly identified by its dark gray appearance and by its displacement when the ossicular chain is depressed. After the round window membrane has been satisfactorily exposed, the drill is used to create a depression in the floor of the round window niche just inferior to the bony attachment of the posterior segment of the round window membrane. This bony depression is deepened to a level of 2 mm, at which point the singular canal is usually encountered and is recognized by the white myelinated nerve bundle that runs slightly at an angle to the alignment of the round window membrane (Fig. 43–6). If the singular

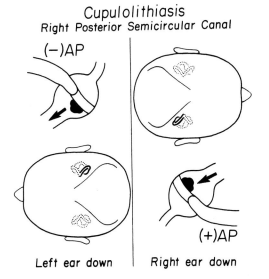

Cupulolithiasis
Right Posterior Semicircular Canal

(−)AP

(+)AP

Left ear down | Right ear down

FIGURE 43–3. Explanation for different responses of right posterior semicircular canal in right ear down and left ear down position tests. AP, action potentials. (From Gacek RR: Pathophysiology and management of cupulolithiasis. Am J Otolaryngol 6: 66–74, 1985.)

FIGURE 43-4

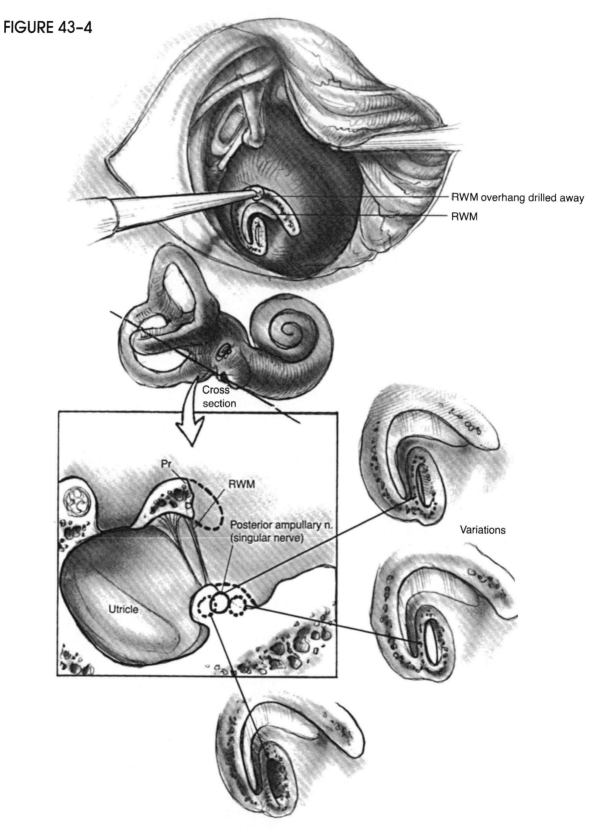

FIGURE 43-4. Surgical view of the right middle ear with a corresponding vertical section taken through the round window niche. The three most common variations in the anatomy of the singular canal are shown. RWM, round window membrane; Pr, promontory. (Redrawn from Gacek RR: Pathophysiology and management of cupulolithiasis. Am J Otolaryngol 6: 66–74, 1985.)

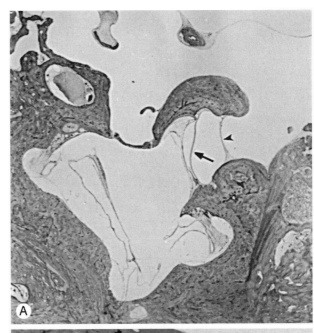

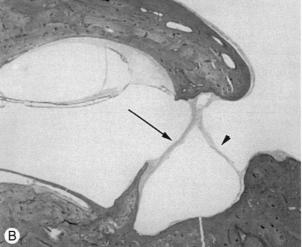

FIGURE 43–5. *A* to *C*, Variations in anatomy of the round window niche. A mucous membrane curtain *(arrowheads)* may shield the round window membrane *(arrows)* at various positions.

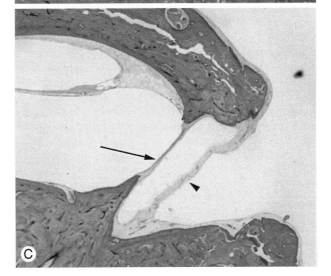

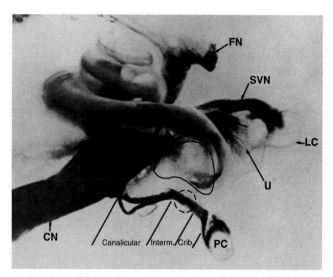

FIGURE 43–6. Dissection of human labyrinth and its nerve supply shows the relationship of the singular nerve to the round window membrane *(solid line)*. *Dashed circular line* indicates the point for transection of the nerve. The three divisions of the singular canal are explained in the text. (From Gacek RR: Transection of the posterior ampullary nerve for the relief of benign paroxysmal positional vertigo. Am Otol Rhinol Laryngol 83: 596–605, 1974.)

canal is not identified at the level of 2 mm or more, the singular canal may be superiorly located under the attachment of the round window membrane. The drill can then be used to enlarge the base of the bony depression in the floor of the niche to reach the singular canal from the inferior direction by undercutting the attachment of the round window membrane. In these cases, identification of the nerve in the singular canal is highlighted by the patient's abrupt response of vertigo or pain.

The canal is then probed with a small, right-angle hook, probing only the proximal end of the singular canal. Probing the distal end of the canal is not advised because of the proximity to the posterior canal ampulla. After repeated probing of the canal with destruction of the nerve tissue, the bony defect is drilled lightly to place bone dust into the canal lumen. This dust should form a bony barrier to regeneration of nerve fibers. Absorbable gelatin sponge (Gelfoam) may then be used to fill the bony defect. Because the segment of singular canal exposed is either the intermediate or cribrose segment, cerebrospinal leak is not usually encountered. The nerve is surrounded by cerebrospinal fluid in the proximal canalicular segment, which lies inferior to the floor of the vestibule. Rarely, a leak of spinal fluid may be seen if the singular canal is probed too far proximally. In these cases, a small piece of adipose tissue will satisfactorily control the leak. On a few occasions, the SN was exposed at its entrance into the recess for the posterior canal ampulla (Fig. 43–7). After the tympanic membrane and flap are returned to their original position, a small pack is used to hold them into position for approximately 1 week while healing occurs. A small cotton ball in the external auditory meatus and a small outer ear dressing is applied for the first 24 hours. Beyond that, a sterile cotton ball is placed in the external auditory meatus and the pack is removed in 1 week's time at an outpatient visit.

POSTOPERATIVE CARE

Oral antibiotics are used routinely for 1 week. Postoperatively, patients have varying degrees of ataxia and dizziness; some patients are able to leave the hospital 1 day after surgery; others require from 2 to 4 days. The Hallpike maneuver, when carried out on the first postoperative day, does not demonstrate a rotatory nystagmus as in the preoperative positional test but instead will demonstrate a downbeat vertical nystagmus reflecting the imbalance between eye muscles supplied by the complimentary vertical canals. There is an unopposed pull of the superior rectus from the contralateral anterior canal following denervation of its coplaner posterior canal. This nonfatiguing positional downbeat nystagmus will be observed for 1 to 3 days and usually parallels the patient's ability to leave the hospital. Vestibular exercises are not necessary but may help to allow some patients to complete the compensatory process necessary to overcome the vestibular deficit created by singular neurectomy.

PITFALLS OF SURGERY

The primary risk of this surgery is injury to the cochlea through the round window membrane. This injury can be prevented by carefully identifying the round window membrane and avoiding injury to it with instrumentation, particularly the drill. Maintaining a ridge of bone between the attachment of the round window membrane and the site created for exposing the singular canal is helpful in avoiding this undesirable result. Another significant complication of the procedure is not finding the singular canal and the nerve. Because of variability in the anatomic position of the canal, this may occur when the singular canal is located superiorly under the round window membrane attachment. The use of local anesthesia to permit the pa-

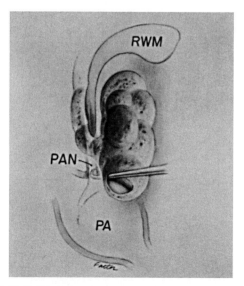

FIGURE 43–7. Diagram of the surgical exposure and probing of singular canal aperture into the recess for posterior canal ampulla. RWM, round window membrane; PAN, posterior ampullary nerve; PA, posterior canal ampulla. (From Gacek RR: Pathophysiology and management of cupulolithiasis. Am J Otolaryngol 6: 66–74, 1985.)

tient's response when the canal is exposed and probed is crucial in avoiding this pitfall of surgery.

RESULTS

From 1972 through 1998, 187 patients have undergone SN for disabling, chronic (>1 year) positional vertigo. One hundred seventy-seven patients had a unilateral singular neurectomy and 10 patients underwent sequential SNs at intervals of 6 months to 1 year for bilateral paroxysmal positional vertigo. The incidence of BPPV in this group of patients was 18 per cent.

There were 131 women and 56 men with an age range from 21 years to 86 years. The peak incidence was in the sixth decade. The etiology for the BPPV was idiopathic in 131, head trauma in 38, surgery (other than otologic) under general anesthesia 17, and cerebrovascular accident 1.

Complete relief from positional vertigo was obtained following 189 (96 per cent) singular neurectomies and partial relief from vertigo after 3 (1.5 per cent) SNs. No relief was experienced in 5 patients (2.5 per cent). In this group of failures, clear exposure of the singular canal was lacking. Sensorineural hearing loss of various levels in severity was encountered in 5 patients (2.5 per cent).

COMPLICATIONS

Infection and delayed healing of the tympanic membrane should not occur in the hands of a trained otologic surgeon. The primary problem following this surgery is a recurrence of symptoms.

Recurrence of vertigo following singular neurectomy may be caused by incomplete transection of the singular nerve in the operated ear or by BPPV involving the contralateral ear. Carefully performed Hallpike's maneuvers with documentation of the nystagmus response are necessary to determine the presence of positional vertigo in either ear. Approximately 15 to 18 per cent of patients may exhibit bilateral cupulolithiasis. Other forms of disequilibrium may be experienced by patients following singular neurectomy and are related to inadequate vestibular compensation to the ablation procedure.

ALTERNATIVE TECHNIQUES

Patients with chronic, disabling BPPV that is not responsive to conservative methods of management may be considered for other methods of surgical ablation. The procedure of posterior canal occlusion through a mastoidectomy approach has been recently described by Parnes and McClure,[11] who cited a high percentage of effective relief from positional vertigo and no apparent significant incidence of sensorineural hearing loss. Although the proce-

dure is based on the theory that compression of the membranous canal will immobilize the endolymph fluid compartment, preventing the cupular displacement, a more plausible explanation for the relief of positional symptoms by the surgical procedure is degenerative effect on the posterior canal sense organ sensitivity as a result of surgical labyrinthitis. The delay (up to 8 weeks) in the disappearance of the positive Hallpike response following surgery as well as the reversible sensorineural hearing loss that usually occurs following the procedure are clinical signs that suggest labyrinthitis. Careful observation over time and reporting of results will be necessary to decide on the efficacy of this procedure. Furthermore, this procedure requires a mastoidectomy performed under general anesthesia and poses some risk of injury to the facial nerve.

Total ablation of the vestibular input from the labyrinth by selective vestibular nerve section is another approach to ablating the posterior canal activity. Unfortunately, this procedure also ablates remaining vestibular labyrinth function, thus unnecessarily denervating the input from important sense organs, such as the utricular macula, the saccule, and the two cristae supplied by the superior vestibular division. In addition, the morbidity associated with vestibular nerve section is significantly higher than with singular neurectomy.

In the rare patient who may have cupulolithiasis involving the posterior canal in an only-hearing ear, a SN by an experienced otologic surgeon is the preferred management since the remaining four sense organs remain functional. A less favored approach is to ablate vestibular function with titrated parenterally administrated streptomycin sulfate. We have successfully managed BPPV in an only-hearing ear by performing SN.

References

1. Gacek RR: Pathophysiology and management of cupulolithiasis. Am J Otolaryngol 6: 66–74, 1985.
2. Schuknecht HF: Cupulolithiasis. Arch Otolaryngol Head Neck Surg 90: 113–126, 1969.
3. Gacek RR: The pathology of facial and vestibular neuronitis. Am J Otolaryngol 20: 202–210, 1999.
4. Barany R: Diagnose von Krankheitserscheinungen im Bereiche des Otolithenapparates. Acta Otolaryngol (Stockh) 2: 434–437, 1921.
5. Carmichael EA, Dix MR, Hallpike CS: Pathology, symptomatology, and diagnosis of the organic affections of the eighth nerve system. Br Med Bull 12: 146–152, 1956.
6. Barber HO: Positional nystagmus, especially after head injury. Laryngoscope 74: 891–944, 1964.
7. Brandt T, Daroff RB: Physical therapy for benign paroxysmal positional vertigo. Arch Otolaryngol Head Neck Surg 106: 484–485, 1980.
8. Gacek RR: Singular neurectomy update: II. Review of 102 cases. Laryngoscope 101: 855–862, 1991.
9. Longridge NS, Barber HO: Bilateral paroxysmal positioning nystagmus. J Otolaryngol 7: 395–400, 1978.
10. McClure JA: Horizontal canal BPV. J Otolaryngol 14: 30–35, 1985.
11. Parnes LS, McClure JA: Posterior semicircular canal occlusion for intractable benign paroxysmal positional vertigo. Ann Otol Rhinol Laryngol 99: 330–334, 1990.

44

Posterior Semicircular Canal Occlusion for Benign Paroxysmal Positional Vertigo

Lorne S. Parnes, M.D.

Benign paroxysmal positional vertigo (BPPV) is the most common vestibular end-organ disorder: in one busy vestibular clinic, BPPV accounted for 17 per cent of diagnoses.[1] Patients complain of brief vertigo spells, often accompanied by nausea but rarely vomiting. The actual duration of the spells (5 to 15 seconds) is usually much shorter than what the patient describes (10 seconds to 5 minutes). Spells are induced by characteristic head movements, such as rolling to the affected side while supine or extending the neck while upright. Less common precipitating movements include bending forward, arising from a supine position, and rotating the head. When the disease is very active, in addition to the brief positional vertigo episodes, patients may complain of protracted, nonspecific imbalance and dizziness accompanied by mild lassitude.

BPPV is most often an idiopathic disorder. The most common identifiable cause is head or temporal bone trauma.[2] Other less common causes include viral labyrinthitis, vestibular neuronitis, stapedectomy, perilymph fistula, Ménière's disease, and chronic otitis media.[3–8]

Three factors provide conclusive evidence that BPPV is a disorder of the posterior semicircular canal of the undermost ear during the provocative Hallpike maneuver, the diagnostic test for BPPV. First, various combinations of rotatory, vertical, and oblique nystagmus may be seen in response to the Hallpike maneuver, depending on the position of the globe within the orbit during the nystagmus. However, the nystagmus profile correlates with the known neuromuscular pathways arising from the crista of the undermost posterior canal.[9–12] Second, in a postmortem temporal bone study, Schuknecht and Ruby[13] identified large basophilic deposits attached to the posterior canal cupula in three specimens. These three patients had premortem documentation of BPPV affecting the same ear. They coined the term *cupulolithiasis* to describe this finding. Third, when successful, selective denervation of the undermost posterior canal (singular neurectomy) cures this condition.[14]

The Hallpike maneuver begins by quickly rotating the patient back from a sitting to a head-hanging position with the head turned 45 degrees and the affected ear facing down toward the floor. This maneuver serves to rotate the undermost posterior semicircular canal in the earth's vertical plane, thereby inducing a characteristic oculomotor response of rotatory nystagmus, which from the examiner's viewpoint has its fast phase beating clockwise with the left ear down and counterclockwise with the right ear down. There is a brief latent period (usually 2 to 5 seconds but as long as 10 to 20 seconds) between the patient's assuming the head-hanging position and the onset of the nystagmus. The patient complains of accompanying vertigo and often nausea. The vertigo and nystagmus briefly crescendo, plateau, and then gradually decrescendo with a typical limited total duration of 10 to 30 seconds. Once the nystagmus stops, the patient is returned to the sitting position, where after a short latent period, a milder reverse-direction nystagmus occurs with a less intense sensation of vertigo. Fatigability occurs whereby the nystagmus and vertigo responses decrease in intensity and duration with each repeated maneuver at the same sitting. Because standard electronystagmography does not record rotational eye movements, normal electronystagmographic positional testing should not preclude the diagnosis of BPPV. The necessity for direct visualization of the eyes during the Hallpike maneuver cannot be overstated.

BPPV must be differentiated from other causes of vertigo and nystagmus. The history is usually quite typical, and a positive response to the Hallpike maneuver is virtually diagnostic, assuming that all features are present. Typical posterior canal BPPV, which produces a positive response to the Hallpike maneuver, must be differentiated from the much less common lateral canal BPPV.[15] This latter disorder gives rise to more severe and prolonged vertigo spells. It is brought on by head movements that produce gravitational forces on the affected lateral canal and is therefore diagnosed by rolling the patient from one lateral supine position to the other and observing the eyes for horizontal nystagmus. Fortunately this variant usually resolves within days to weeks of onset. The remainder of this chapter deals solely with the management of typical posterior canal BPPV.

BPPV has three types of clinical courses. Most common is the self-limited variety that subsides spontaneously over weeks to months. A second group of patients experience remissions and recurrences ranging from weeks to years. A still smaller group seem to have the more permanent form of this disorder. In one busy vestibular clinic, about 30 per cent of untreated patients had symptoms lasting longer than 1 year.[8]

PATHOPHYSIOLOGY

Under normal physiologic conditions, the cupula has the same density as the surrounding endolymph. Therefore, the semicircular canals are normally not sensitive to gravity (linear acceleration). However, a fixed cupular deposit would render the posterior canal crista gravity sensitive.[16] Rotation of the canal in the earth's vertical plane during the Hallpike maneuver produces cupular displacement through the gravitation pull on the deposit, resulting in nystagmus and vertigo. This condition, so-called cupulolithiasis, may represent the extremely rare, more permanent form of this disorder.

The more common self-limited form and the form with remissions and recurrences likely has a different pathophysiologic mechanism. Free-floating endolymph particles within the posterior canal produce a Hallpike response identical to that of a fixed cupular deposit.[17] Because the posterior canal is the most dependent part of the vestibular labyrinth, free-floating endolymph particles have a predilection for settling in the posterior canal endolymph. With the head upright, the most dependent part of the canal is the area just posterior and inferior to the ampulla on the side of the cupula opposite the utricle. As the posterior canal rotates during the Hallpike maneuver, the particles initially rotate upward because of their inertia. After a short latent period, gravity pulls them down and away from the cupula (utriculofugal) to a more dependent position. Their hydrodynamic drag creates an endolymph current in the same direction, thereby displacing the cupula away from the utricle. Utriculofugal displacement of the posterior canal cupula increases the resting discharge rate of the first-order neurons. As known from previous animal studies, this action produces excitation of the ipsilateral superior oblique and contralateral inferior rectus muscles,[9] which causes counterclockwise eye rotation with stimulation of the left posterior crista and clockwise rotation with right-sided stimulation. However, the fast component of the induced nystagmus is in the opposite direction, corresponding with the clinical features of typical BPPV. These free-floating posterior canal particles have in fact been identified in vivo in patients undergoing surgery for BPPV.[18, 19] This theory of free-floating particles is an important concept as it relates to the treatment of this condition.

PREOPERATIVE PATIENT COUNSELING AND CONSERVATIVE MANAGEMENT

First and foremost, the patient must be reassured that BPPV is an inner ear disorder that is relatively benign and most often self-limited. To date, effective medical management for BPPV remains unproven experimentally.[20] The most efficacious means of vertigo control is avoidance of the specific provocative head movements that induce the attacks. Most patients already use this approach by not lying on the affected side and by not extending the neck to look upward. Patients who stringently avoid these movements may have more prolonged courses because the absence of provocative movements prevents dispersement of the particles from the canal.

Most cases of BPPV resolve spontaneously over weeks to months without any treatment. Brandt and Daroff[21] recommended a rigorous course of physiotherapy under heavy sedation during several days of hospitalization. They felt that the exercises shook free the otolithic debris from the cupula. Unfortunately, other clinicians could not reproduce

their excellent results (personal communication). Semont and associates[22] reported excellent results using a technique called the *liberatory maneuver*. They theorized that this technique liberated deposits from the cupula and reported a 92 per cent success rate following two maneuvers.

The liberatory maneuver is difficult to perform in elderly, frail patients. The particle-repositioning maneuver[23–25] provides the same benefits as the liberatory maneuver but is simpler to accomplish. It is based on the free-floating particle pathophysiologic theory of BPPV and is adapted from Dr. John Epley's canalith repositioning procedure.[26] For the purpose of this discussion, it is important to remember that the cupula forms a complete barrier across the ampullated end of the canal that is impermeable to endolymph and free-floating particles. Therefore, free-floating posterior canal endolymph particles can enter and exit the canal only through the common crus.

The current particle-repositioning technique (Fig. 44–1) begins with the patient seated lengthwise on the examining table. The Hallpike maneuver is then performed by rotation of the posterior semicircular canal of the undermost (affected) ear in the earth vertical axis (Fig. 44–1B). The examiner should observe the classic nystagmus response, which confirms the diagnosis, and then reassure the patient as the vertigo subsides. The patient maintains this position for 2 to 3 minutes after resolution of the nystagmus, thereby allowing the particles to settle in their new dependent position closer to the common crus. In the second stage, the patient rolls laterally through position C into position D onto the opposite side with the head turned 45 degrees downward. This stage is performed in a smooth, continuous motion, and the neck is kept extended throughout. This method serves to rotate the posterior canal 180 degrees in the plane of gravity, allowing the free-floating particles to follow the natural curve of the canal and continue their relative course through the common crus into the utricle.

While the examiner supports the patient's head in position D, a secondary nystagmus response is usually noted, once again following a short latent period. A nystagmus response that replicates the initial nystagmus (positive response) during the Hallpike maneuver can result only from further passage of the particles in the same ampullofugal direction. Such passage would lead them through the common crus into the utricle, where they would no longer induce a pathologic response. Conversely, a secondary nystagmus that reverses direction from that of the Hallpike maneuver may occur through two possible mechanisms. In one, the particles reverse their direction of movement because of an improperly performed maneuver, resulting in a utriculopetal endolymph current. This usually happens when the neck is not hyperextended enough during the roll. Cupulolithiasis is the other possible mechanism underlying reversal nystagmus. The gravitational effect on a fixed cupular deposit results in utriculofugal cupular deflection during the Hallpike maneuver (Fig. 44–1B), as would be seen with free-floating particles. The position assumed during the second stage of the particle-repositioning maneuver effectively rotates the posterior canal 180 degrees in the earth's vertical plane (Fig. 44–1D). This action reverses the gravitational pull on the cupula, resulting in utriculopetal cupular displacement and a reversal of the nystagmus response.

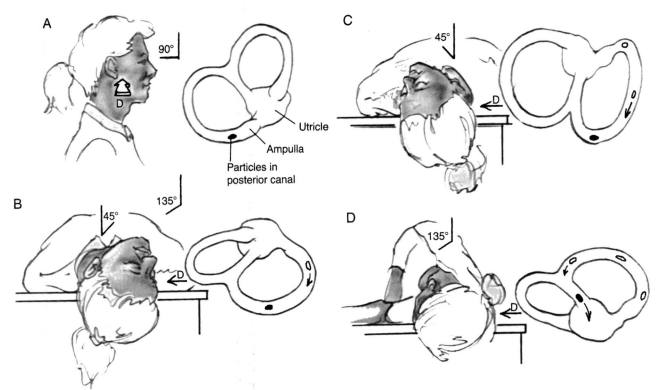

FIGURE 44–1. Particle-repositioning maneuver, four positions, right ear. Schematic representation of patient and concurrent movement of labyrinth, specifically the posterior and superior semicircular canals. In each position, the dark oval represents the new position of the particle conglomerate in the most dependent part of posterior canal, and the open oval represents the previous position. *A,* Patient seated. *B,* Patient in Hallpike head position. Particles gravitate in ampullofugal direction, causing counterclockwise rotatory nystagmus (right ear). Position is maintained for 2 to 3 minutes. *C,* Mid position. *D,* Final position of second stage of maneuver performed in one steady continuous motion. Particles continue gravitating in ampullofugal direction through common crus into utricle. Eyes are observed for nystagmus response. Position is maintained for 1 to 2 minutes; then patient sits up. D, Direction of view of labyrinth.

After another 1 to 2 minutes, the patient sits back up and is observed for nystagmus. With a successful maneuver, no nystagmus occurs when the patient returns to the upright position because the particles have been removed from the canal. This result is in contrast with that of the conventional Hallpike maneuver, in which one notes a reversal nystagmus. Patients are then instructed to maintain an upright position for 48 hours, theoretically to prevent particle re-entry into the posterior canal. Patients are then reassessed 1 month later, and if necessary, the maneuver is repeated. When appropriately administered, repositioning maneuvers should alleviate BPPV in the vast majority of cases (>95%).[27]

Several other clinical findings help support the free-floating particle theory as the mechanism underlying most cases of BPPV. In some patients with classic histories of BPPV, an initial Hallpike maneuver often fails to induce a positive response. I have noted that in many of these patients, a vigorous headshake or application of a skull oscillator may often elicit a latent response. In these cases, the vibration may overcome the particle conglomerate's inertia or its minor adherence to the membranous canal wall, allowing for its mobilization.

Free-floating particles may also explain the fatigability of a conventional Hallpike maneuver. Each maneuver likely causes increased endolymph dispersion of the particle con-glomerate, resulting in a smaller mass effect with each subsequent maneuver and reducing the degree of hydrodynamic drag and endolymph current. In several patients, a repeat Hallpike maneuver 30 to 60 minutes after a fatigued response often elicits the same maximal response seen during the initial Hallpike maneuver. Theoretically, the particles have had time to reassemble into the large conglomerate mass within the endolymph of the posterior canal.

PATIENT SELECTION

Operative intervention is offered for intractable cases in which symptoms are severe enough to significantly affect the patient's occupation or lifestyle and failure to respond to the particle-repositioning maneuver. Since I started using the particle-repositioning maneuver, the number of surgical cases has decreased dramatically. Until the advent of posterior canal occlusion, singular neurectomy was the gold standard of operative treatment.[14, 28–30] However, the procedure is technically difficult, is performed by very few surgeons, and yields variable rates of failure and sensorineural hearing loss.[31, 32] Furthermore, Ohmichi and colleagues[33] showed that the singular nerve is inaccessible through a tympanotomy approach in 14 per cent of human temporal bones.

The newer procedure of posterior semicircular canal occlusion evolved to circumvent the shortcomings of singular neurectomy. Money and Scott[34] initially used this technique in feline vestibular physiology experiments. Plugging individual semicircular canals blocked their receptivity to angular acceleration without influencing the responses of the other ipsilateral vestibular receptors. Although posterior canal occlusion was at first a theoretical remedy for BPPV, the main concern in applying this technique to humans was its possible detrimental effect on hearing. This problem was not addressed in the original cat studies. Therefore, Parnes and McClure[35] carried out a study in guinea pigs to measure the effect of canal occlusion on hearing using brainstem auditory evoked responses. The hearing responses remained relatively unchanged during follow-up times as long as 6 months.

To test the hypothesis that canal occlusion would indeed abolish BPPV, two patients fortuitously presented with intractable BPPV in ears with coexisting profound sensorineural hearing losses. With no hearing to lose, both agreed to undergo what at that time was an experimental procedure. Both patients were relieved of their BPPV and have remained symptom-free for at least 4 years, when they were lost to follow-up.[36, 37] In addition, both maintained postoperative lateral semicircular canal function as measured by caloric responses. This important finding supports the postulate that the procedure's success results from its isolated direct effect on the posterior canal and not from a generalized destructive process of the vestibular labyrinth.

The theoretical intent of the procedure is to compress the membranous labyrinth closed against the opposite bony wall, thereby creating a closed, fluid-filled (endolymph) space between the plug and cupula, both of which are impermeable to endolymph. Because fluid cannot expand or compress without a change in temperature, this action eliminates all endolymph movement within the posterior canal, effectively fixing the cupula. The canal no longer responds to the gravitational effect on a fixed cupular deposit, eliminating the BPPV. In addition, the canal no longer responds to physiologic angular acceleration. However, because the deficit is constant and permanent, gradual compensation occurs through central adaptation.

Singular neurectomy eliminates the resting discharge from the posterior semicircular canal crista, creating a static vestibular asymmetry[38] between the two posterior canals. This effect results in immediate postoperative vertigo at rest and spontaneous rotatory nystagmus. However, posterior canal occlusion does not disturb the resting neuronal discharge from the occluded canal; therefore, most patients do not have spontaneous postoperative vertigo or nystagmus at rest unless their conditions are complicated by other factors. Both singular neurectomy and posterior canal occlusion result in a dynamic vestibular asymmetry,[38] itself resulting in motion sensitivity. The dynamic asymmetry gradually resolves because of central adaptation, as does the static vestibular asymmetry.

PREOPERATIVE EVALUATION

Preoperative evaluation includes a routine audiogram. The procedure is not recommended in an only- or significantly better–hearing ear. Preoperative electronystagmography and evoked response audiometry are not necessary. A high-resolution computed tomographic scan of the temporal bone defines the anatomy and ensures that the posterior canal is indeed accessible through a transmastoid approach. To date, all posterior canals have proven to be accessible.

SURGICAL TECHNIQUE

Perioperative broad-spectrum antibiotic coverage is necessary only for ears with a past history of otitis media. Obviously, the procedure is contraindicated during acute or subacute episodes of otitis media. The patient is placed in the supine position with the head turned 45 degrees toward the opposite side. The surgical site, preparation, and draping are performed in a routine fashion. Intraoperative auditory and facial nerve monitoring are not necessary.

With the patient under general anesthesia, a limited mastoidectomy is performed through a postauricular incision (Fig. 44–2A). The antrum is opened, providing exposure of the lateral canal. Identification of the tegmen and digastric ridge is not necessary. The sigmoid sinus is identified, from which bone removal proceeds anteriorly along the cerebellar plate toward the posterior canal. Once the posterior canal otic capsule is identified, the bone is blue lined with progressively smaller diamond burrs and copious suction irrigation. The target zone for the occlusion is the area at, or just inferior to, a line extending posteriorly from the lateral semicircular canal. Because this part of the posterior semicircular canal is furthest from the ampulla and vestibule, manipulation in this region is theoretically least likely to induce other vestibular or cochlear damage.

Using an 0.8-mm diamond burr, a 3-mm segment of canal is skeletonized 180 degrees around the outer circumference down to endosteum, creating a 1×3-mm endosteal island (Fig. 44–2B). Bone removal should proceed evenly along the circumference so that once the endosteum is violated and perilymph is exposed, all drilling can cease. The endosteal island is removed with a fine 90-degree pick to expose the perilymph (Fig. 44–3). Great care must be taken not to suction directly on the perilymph and especially the membranous labyrinth. At this stage, the exact outline and limits of the membranous labyrinth are usually not clearly discernible. Although not essential, perilymph may be gently "wicked" away with a cottonoid to expose the membranous labyrinth, at which time the membranous duct collapses. In canals with particles, perilymph removal allows for confirmation that these are indeed free-floating particles within the endolymph. Particles have been identified in 10 canals to date, eight of which were previously reported.[19] In three of these more recent cases, the exposed membranous labyrinths with particles were isolated and resected. Although two of these specimens are awaiting analysis, one underwent scanning electromicroscopy, which demonstrated that the particles were degenerating otoconia.[19]

Dry bone chips previously gathered from the mastoidectomy are mixed with one drop of a two-component fast-acting human fibrinogen glue (Tisseel, Immuno, Vienna, Austria). Once set (about 30 seconds), it forms an easily workable but malleable plug with a firm consistency (Fig. 44–4). The plug is gently and firmly inserted through the fenestra with the intention of completely filling the canal lumen and thereby compressing the membranous labyrinth closed (Fig. 44–5). The membranous labyrinth is surpris-

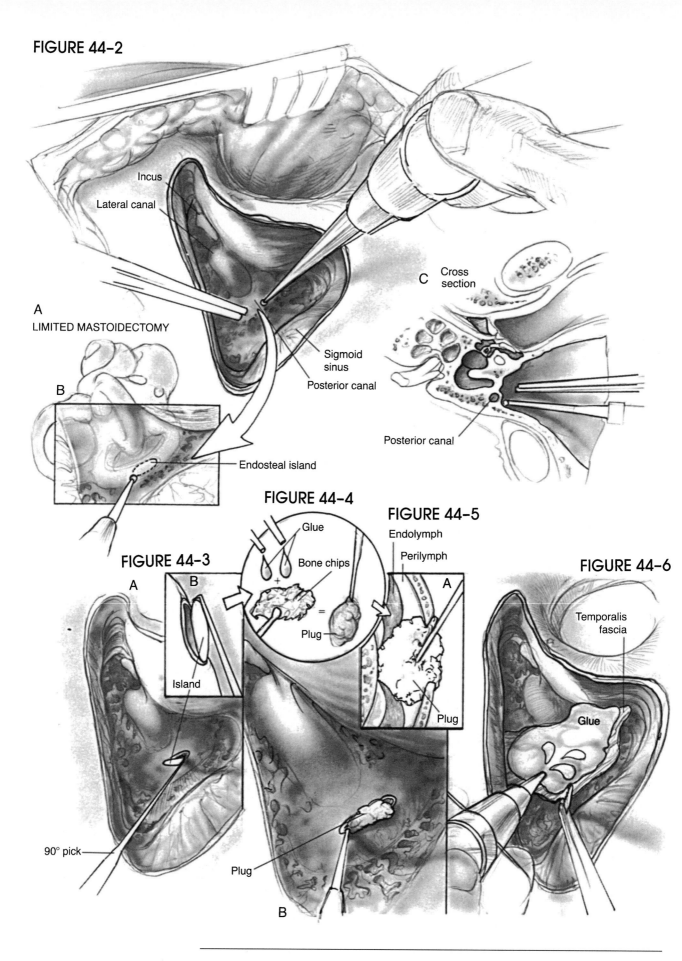

FIGURE 44-2

Incus

Lateral canal

A

LIMITED MASTOIDECTOMY

B

Endosteal island

Sigmoid sinus

Posterior canal

C   Cross section

Posterior canal

FIGURE 44-4

Glue

Bone chips

+

=

Plug

FIGURE 44-5

Endolymph

Perilymph

A

Plug

FIGURE 44-3

A

B

Island

90° pick

Plug

B

FIGURE 44-6

Temporalis fascia

Glue

FIGURES 44–2 to 44–6. *See legends on opposite page*

ingly resistant to tearing, providing that no shearing forces are applied. The bone chips within the plug cause intracanal ossification that leads to complete permanent occlusion of the canal.

If commercially prepared fibrinogen glue is not available, autologous glue may be fashioned from the patient's own serum. Alternatively, some surgeons have successfully used plugs made from periosteum or fascia.

After completing the plug insertion, the fenestra and surrounding bone are covered with a piece of temporalis fascia, which is maintained in place by several more drops of fibrinogen glue (Fig. 44–6). A good tissue seal is necessary to prevent a postoperative perilymph fistula.

The incision is closed in two layers, and a standard mastoid dressing is applied. A drain is not necessary. The dressing is maintained for 1 or 2 days.

In a variation of this technique, Anthony[39] successfully treated BPPV by applying an HGM argon laser to the blue-lined posterior canal. The laser burns are purported to create fibrous bands within the canal, leading to obstruction of the membranous duct. Alternatively, Kartush and Sargent used a CO_2 laser–assisted occlusion technique.[40]

RESULTS

To date, 44 posterior canals in 42 patients have been occluded, 2 patients having successive bilateral occlusions. The average age at surgery was 59 years, with a range of 28 to 83 years. Surprisingly, there were 33 females and 11 males, and 28 left ears and 16 right ears. The average duration of symptoms was 6.3 years, ranging from 1 to 35 years. The follow-up times ranged from 1 to 12 years.

All 44 ears remain completely free of BPPV. Four ears had profound preoperative deafness. Of the 40 ears with normal preoperative hearing, most demonstrated an initial postoperative mixed hearing loss that in all cases recovered to the preoperative level. One patient had a delayed sudden hearing loss accompanied by a 7-day vertigo spell during the fourth postoperative month. The symptoms were preceded by an intense 2-day headache. Unfortunately, she did not return for follow-up until 1 month later, at which time her audiogram showed a 70-dB sensorineural hearing loss with only 32 per cent discrimination. This hearing loss persisted on subsequent audiograms. The working diagnosis was labyrinthitis, but the exact causal relationship to the canal occlusion was unknown. Interestingly, she had undergone two previous unsuccessful attempts at singular neurectomy in the same ear. One other patient had a 20-dB drop in bone conduction levels at 1-year follow-up audiogram and no change in speech discrimination score.

All 44 cases were followed by an initial 1- to 4-week period of imbalance, giddiness, and motion sensitivity. Six cases had more protracted courses, and five were thought to have had labyrinthitis. Four of these were thought to have aseptic labyrinthitis, the other, postoperative otitis media–mastoiditis. This patient had a history of chronic otitis media and had undergone a prior cortical mastoidectomy. Fortunately, her sensorineural hearing loss recovered following antibiotic therapy. The sixth developed BPPV in the contralateral ear, but there also appeared to be some functional overlay.

Three other cases deserve brief but special mention. As noted previously, two patients underwent successive bilateral posterior canal occlusions. Both remain symptom-free with no other adverse effects from the surgery. As expected, the intact superior semicircular canals provide the complementary vestibular input of their contralateral posterior canal counterparts, which were rendered nonfunctional by surgical occlusion. The other notable patient had her canal occluded under local anesthesia due to multiple other medical problems. Surprisingly, she had no intraoperative complaints of vertigo or dizziness.

The average duration of postoperative hospitalization is 2 to 5 days in an uncomplicated case. As expected, the older patients have longer recovery periods and tend to require longer hospital stays. The degree of postoperative motion sensitivity determines the length of stay. Although postoperative vestibular suppressants may provide early short-term relief, their use is discouraged because they tend to prolong the overall recovery. All patients are now provided with early postoperative vestibular physiotherapy.

SUMMARY

Most typical BPPV cases appear to result from free-floating posterior semicircular canal endolymph particles. Most of these patients may be cured with the particle-repositioning maneuver. Fortunately, intractable cases are rare. For this small subset of patients, posterior semicircular canal occlusion is a safe, curative procedure.

References

1. Nedzelski JM, Barber HO, McIlmoyl L: Diagnoses in a dizziness unit. J Otolaryngol 15:101–104, 1986.
2. Barber HO, Leigh RJ: Benign (and not so benign) postural vertigo: Diagnosis and treatment. In Barber HO, Sharpe A (eds): Vestibular Disorders. Boca Raton, FL, CRC Press, 1988, pp 215–232.
3. Lindsay JR, Hemenway WG: Postural vertigo due to unilateral sudden partial loss of vestibular function. Ann Otol Rhinol Laryngol 65:692–706, 1956.

FIGURE 44–2. *A,* Exposing the right posterior semicircular canal otic capsule. *B,* Creating the 1 × 3-mm endosteal island with a small diamond burr. *C,* Cross-sectional view.

FIGURE 44–3. *A,* Lifting out the endosteal island with a fine 90-degree pick. *B,* Magnified lateral view.

FIGURE 44–4. Creating the plug with two-component fibrinogen glue and mastoid cortex bone chips.

FIGURE 44–5. *A,* Tamping plug through fenestra into the canal. *B,* Cross-section schematic of canal shows intact but occluded membranous canal.

FIGURE 44–6. Covering fenestra and surrounding bone with fascia and glue.

4. Spector M: Positional vertigo after stapedectomy. Ann Otol Rhinol Laryngol 70:251–254, 1961.
5. Stahle J, Terins J: Paroxysmal positional nystagmus. Ann Otol Rhinol Laryngol 74:69–83, 1965.
6. Barber HO: Positional vertigo and nystagmus. Otolaryngol Clin North Am 6:169–187, 1973.
7. McClure JA, Rounthwaite J: Vestibular dysfunction associated with benign paroxysmal vertigo. Laryngoscope 87:1434–1442, 1977.
8. Baloh RW, Honrubia V, Jacobson K: Benign positional vertigo: Clinical and oculographic features in 240 cases. Neurology 37:371–378, 1987.
9. Cohen B, Suzuki J, Bender MB: Nystagmus induced by electrical stimulation of ampullary nerves. Acta Otolaryngol (Stockh) 60:422–436, 1965.
10. Harbert F: Benign paroxysmal positional vertigo. Arch Ophthalmol Head Neck Surg 84:298–302, 1970.
11. Baloh RW, Sakala S, Honrubia V: The mechanism of benign paroxysmal positional nystagmus. Adv Otorhinolaryngol 25:161–166, 1979.
12. Katsarkas A, Outerbridge JS: Nystagmus of paroxysmal positional vertigo. Ann Otol Rhinol Laryngol 92:146–150, 1983.
13. Schuknecht HF, Ruby RRF: Cupulolithiasis. Adv Otorhinolaryngol 20:434–443, 1973.
14. Gacek R: Transection of the posterior ampullary nerve for the relief of benign paroxysmal positional nystagmus. Ann Otol Rhinol Laryngol 83:596–605, 1974.
15. Fife TD: Recognition and management of horizontal canal benign positional vertigo. Am J Otol 19:345–351, 1998.
16. Schuknecht HF: Pathology of the Ear. Cambridge, MA, Harvard University Press, 1974.
17. Hall SF, Ruby RRF, McClure JA: The mechanics of benign paroxysmal vertigo. J Otolaryngol 8:151–158, 1979.
18. Parnes LS, McClure JA: Free-floating endolymph particles: A new operative finding during posterior semicircular canal occlusion. Laryngoscope 12:988–992, 1992.
19. Welling DP, Parnes LS, O'Brien B, et al: Particulate matter in the posterior semicircular canal. Laryngoscope 107:90–94, 1997.
20. McClure JA, Willett JM: Lorazepam and diazepam in the treatment of benign paroxysmal vertigo. J Otolaryngol 9:472–477, 1980.
21. Brandt T, Daroff RB: Physical therapy for benign paroxysmal positional vertigo. Arch Otolaryngol Head Neck Surg 106:484–485, 1980.
22. Semont A, Freyss G, Vitte E: Curing the BPPV with a liberatory maneuver. Adv Otorhinolaryngol 42:290–293, 1988.
23. Parnes LS, Price-Jones G: Particle-repositioning maneuver for benign paroxysmal positional vertigo. Ann Otol Rhinol Laryngol 102:325–331, 1993.
24. Parnes LS, Robichaud J: Further observations during the particle-repositioning maneuver for benign paroxysmal positional vertigo. Otolaryngol Head Neck Surg 116:238–243, 1997.
25. Fung K, Hall SF: Particle-repositioning maneuver: Effective treatment for benign paroxysmal positional vertigo. J Otolaryngol 25:243–248, 1996.
26. Epley JM: The canalith-repositioning procedure: For treatment of benign paroxysmal positional vertigo. Otolaryngol Head Neck Surg 107:399–404, 1992.
27. Epley JM: Positional vertigo related to semicircular canalithiasis. Otolaryngol Head Neck Surg 112:154–161, 1995.
28. Gacek R: Further observations on posterior ampullary nerve transection for positional vertigo. Ann Otol Rhinol Laryngol 87:300–305, 1978.
29. Epley JM: Singular neurectomy: Hypotympanotomy approach. Otolaryngol Head Neck Surg 88:304–309, 1980.
30. Gacek R: Singular neurectomy update. Ann Otol Rhinol Laryngol 91:469–473, 1982.
31. Silverstein H: Singular neurectomy: A treatment for benign positional vertigo. In Brackmann DE (ed): Neurological Surgery of the Ear and Skull Base. New York, Raven Press, 1982, pp 331–335.
32. Meyerhoff WL: Surgical section of the posterior ampullary nerve. Laryngoscope 95:933–935, 1985.
33. Ohmichi T, Rutka J, Hawke M: Histopathologic consequences of surgical approaches to the singular nerve. Laryngoscope 99:963–970, 1989.
34. Money KE, Scott JW: Functions of separate sensory receptors of nonauditory labyrinth of the cat. Am J Physiol 202:1211–1220, 1962.
35. Parnes LS, McClure JA: Effect on brainstem auditory evoked responses of posterior semicircular canal occlusion in guinea pigs. J Otolaryngol 14:145–150, 1985.
36. Parnes LS, McClure JA: Posterior semicircular canal occlusion for intractable benign paroxysmal positional vertigo. Ann Otol Rhinol Laryngol 99:330–334, 1990.
37. Parnes LS, McClure JA: Posterior semicircular canal occlusion in the normal hearing ear. Otolaryngol Head Neck Surg 104:52–57, 1991.
38. McClure JA, Lycett P: Vestibular asymmetry. Arch Otolaryngol Head Neck Surg 109:682–687, 1983.
39. Anthony P: Partitioning the labyrinth: Application in benign paroxysmal positional vertigo. Am J Otol 12:388–393, 1991.
40. Kartush JM, Sargent EW: Posterior semicircular canal occlusion for benign paroxysmal positional vertigo—CO_2 laser–assisted technique: Preliminary results. Laryngoscope 105:268–274, 1995.

45

Operations for Vascular Compressive Syndromes

Peter J. Jannetta, M.D. ▪ Elad I. Levy, M.D.

Only in recent years has microvascular decompression become a recognized treatment for a number of idiopathic disorders of the cranial nerves. These cranial rhizopathies have long defied categorization, clarification of pathophysiology, and effective treatment despite efforts by clinicians in several disciplines. Though the clinical presentation of disorders such as trigeminal neuralgia, hemifacial spasm, glossopharyngeal neuralgia, tinnitus, spasmodic torticollis, disabling positional vertigo, and Ménière's disease are quite different, these problems all share a common underlying pathology: vascular compression of the respective cranial nerve exit zone near the brainstem. Most recently, several studies have demonstrated improved systolic blood pressure control in severe, medically refractory hypertensive patients following microvascular decompression of the left lateral medulla oblongata.[1, 2]

Beginning in 1966, a patient with known trigeminal neuralgia was noted to have compression of the trigeminal nerve by a small artery near the brainstem.[3] That same year, a patient with hemifacial spasm was cured following coagulation of a small vein that was distorting the facial nerve exit zone. Following several more operations to relieve vascular compression of the trigeminal and facial nerves, it became apparent that pulsatile, mechanical forces from a blood vessel were the pathophysiologic mechanism responsible for these cranial hyperactive syndromes. These later included glossopharyngeal neuralgia, tinnitus, and vertigo. In fact, all the cranial nerves are subject to the forces of vascular compression, such as arteriosclerosis, dolichoectasia, and parenchymal atrophy.

In this chapter, we describe the patient selection criteria, operative technique, perioperative management, results, and complications following more than 4500 microvascular decompressions for the aforementioned cranial rhizopathies.

PREOPERATIVE EVALUATION

Prior to microvascular decompression for any cranial rhizopathy, all patients at our institution are required to give a detailed history followed by a physical examination. Preoperative testing for every patient involves otologic examination, audiometry (pure tone and speech), acoustic middle ear reflexes, and brainstem auditory evoked potentials (BAEPs). All patients have preoperative magnetic resonance imaging (MRI) and computed tomographic scans to rule out tumors, cysts, vascular, and/or bony anomalies.

The audiometric tests are performed preoperatively to obtain a baseline for quantitatively determining deteriorations or improvement in hearing function. The pure tone audiogram often shows anomalies represented by small dips in the frequency range of 1500 to 2000 Hz.[4] Additionally, preoperative BAEPs provide baseline information for the neurophysiology team so that they may warn the surgeon of any deviations that are observed during monitoring of the intraoperative auditory evoked potentials. Typical changes observed in the BAEP are an increased interpeak latency between peaks I and III ipsilaterally or prolongation of interpeak latency between III and V contralaterally (Figs. 45–1 to 45–4). These findings are based on our knowledge of neural generators of BAEPs.[5–8]

Audiometric tests are typically repeated on postoperative day 6 to detect any hearing changes due to surgery. Some patients may experience transient conductive hearing loss due to effusions in the mastoid air cells. Nearly all spontaneously resolve within 2 to 5 weeks. Audiometry may be repeated 3 months postoperatively in such cases.

TRIGEMINAL NEURALGIA

Patient Selection

Patients with trigeminal neuralgia are selected for microvascular decompression on the basis of their symptoms, history, ability to undergo a general anesthetic, and refractoriness to medical management. Patients with contraindications to general anesthetics or intracranial procedures are often treated with percutaneous glycerol rhizotomies, percutaneous radiofrequency rhizotomies, trigeminal balloon microcompression, stereotactic radiosurgery, and peripheral neurectomy.[9, 10] A brief discussion of these other surgical techniques is imperative for understanding why microvascular decompression is the surgical procedure of choice for most patients.

Peripheral neuroectomies, though less invasive, typically have a short duration of tic relief and thus may be indicated for those with a shortened life expectancy.[11] Radiofrequency gasserian lesions, created by percutaneous passage of a needle into the gasserian ganglion, have an initial success rate of 90 per cent or greater, with long-term results ranging from 20 to 78 per cent of patients who are pain free.[12–15] Approximately 10 per cent of patients suffer from facial dysesthesias following radiofrequency rhizotomies. Glycerol rhizotomies cause facial dysesthesias less fre-

455

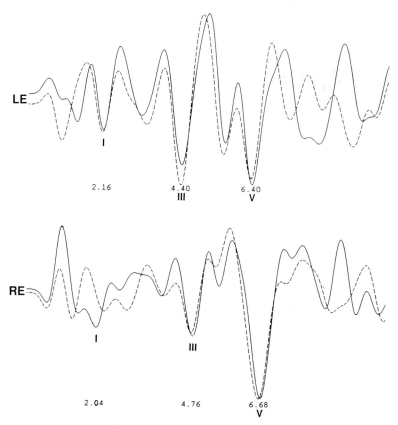

FIGURE 45–1. Brainstem auditory evoked potentials recordings from a patient with normal hearing and with hemifacial spasm of 8 years' duration on the right side. The recordings from the left ear (LE) show a normal response, whereas those from the right ear (RE) show an increased interpeak latency I–III and a double-peak II.

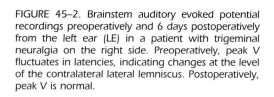

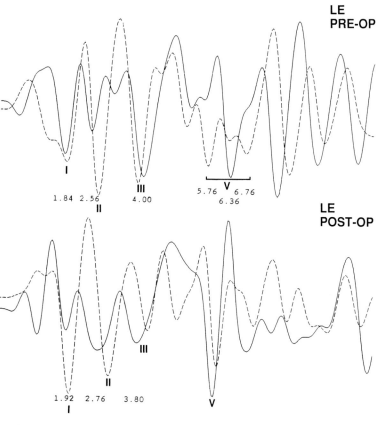

FIGURE 45–2. Brainstem auditory evoked potential recordings preoperatively and 6 days postoperatively from the left ear (LE) in a patient with trigeminal neuralgia on the right side. Preoperatively, peak V fluctuates in latencies, indicating changes at the level of the contralateral lateral lemniscus. Postoperatively, peak V is normal.

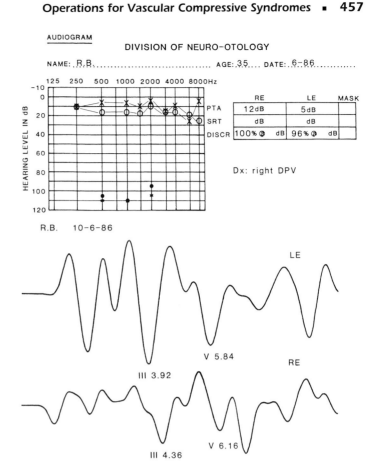

FIGURE 45–3. Results of audiometry and recordings of brainstem auditory evoked potentials (BAEPs) in a patient with a 10-year history of disabling positional vertigo (DPV) on the right side. There is a slight decrease in pure-tone threshold in the right ear (RE) and bilateral increased thresholds of the acoustic middle ear reflex responses. BAEPs show low amplitude and increased interpeak latency I–III for the right ear. Initial vestibular tests showed canal paresis on the right side, and 4 years later directional preponderance to the right; tests prior to operation show a normal electronystagmographic result. LE, left ear. (From Møller MB: Results of microvascular decompression of the eighth nerve as treatment for disabling positional vertigo. Ann Otol Rhinol Laryngol 99: 724–729, 1990.)

quently than do radiofrequency rhizotomies. Though glycerol rhizotomies have initial success rates reported between 80 and 90 per cent,[16] reported median time to recurrence varies from 16 to 36 months.[17–20] Balloon microcompression of the trigeminal ganglion has initial success rates ranging from 78 to 100 per cent,[16, 21] with mean time to recurrence of 3.5 years.[22] Minor dysesthesias occur in approximately 20 per cent of patients,[22] and mild temporary masseter weakness is seen in the majority of those treated with balloon microcompression.[21] Stereotactic radiosurgery for trigeminal neuralgia, the least invasive of the aforementioned procedures, targets the nerve root entry zone with 60 to 90 Gy of single-dose radiation.[23–25] Benefits are seen within 1 to 8 weeks of initial treatment, and approximately 60 per cent of patients are pain free. The choice between microvascular decompression and other procedures should be governed by the patient preference and ability to tolerate a craniotomy under general anesthesia. Advantages of microvascular decompression include consistently higher long-term success rates with a substantially lower incidence of facial dysesthesias. These advantages are quite substantial in that the average life expectancy of the patients treated by the authors was 32 years from the initial onset of symptoms.[26]

The classic symptom of typical trigeminal neuralgia is lancinating pain in one or more distributions of the trigeminal nerve. Talking, eating, shaving, and feeling the wind blowing often precipitate symptoms. Patients typically have an abrupt and memorable onset of symptoms, with a variable duration of remission. A burning, aching pain without specific trigger points characterizes atypical trigeminal neuralgia, unlike typical trigeminal neuralgia. Though surgical success with these patients is less than that with typical symptoms, no other reasonable alternative treatments currently exist. Many patients have initial success with medical management using agents such carbamazepine, phenytoin, baclofen, valproic acid, clonazepam, and gabapentin (Neurontin). Carbamazepine historically has been most effective, yet only 56 per cent of patients maintain satisfactory pain relief after 10 years.[27] Often, side effects, allergies, and the development of refractory symptoms to medications necessitate the need for early surgical intervention.

Operative Technique

As in any operation, patient positioning is crucial for surgical success. The patient is placed on the operating table such that the head is at the foot of the bed, thus providing maximal room for the surgeon during the microscopic portion of the case. A three-point head fixation device is then applied and the patient is placed in the lateral decubitus position. An axillary roll and padding to other pressure points is then placed. The head is then flexed, always maintaining two fingerbreadths between the patient's chin

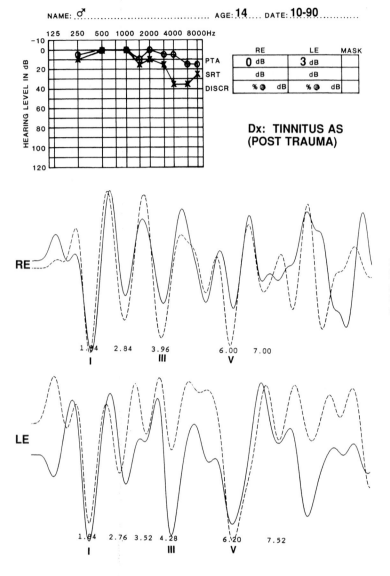

NAME: ♂ .... AGE: **14** .... DATE: **10-90** ....

Dx: **TINNITUS AS (POST TRAUMA)**

	RE	LE	MASK
PTA	**0** dB	**3** dB	
SRT	dB	dB	
DISCR	% @ dB	% @ dB	

RE — I 1.94 · 2.84 · III 3.96 · V 6.00 · 7.00

LE — I 1.94 · 2.76 · 3.52 · III 4.28 · V 6.20 · 7.52

FIGURE 45–4. Results of audiometry and recordings of brainstem auditory evoked potentials in a patient with severe tinnitus, such as that occurring after trauma. An increased interpeak latency I–III occurs on the left side and there is a double-peak II. LE, left ear; RE, right ear.

and sternum. The patient is then secured to the bed appropriately and the head fixation device is fastened into position. The patient's shoulder is taped caudally for maximal working room[28] (Fig. 45–5).

Following satisfactory positioning, a 3 × 3-cm area behind the ear is shaved and prepped in usual sterile fashion. The incision, approximately 3 to 5 cm long, is placed 0.5 cm posterior to the hairline, extending one fourth above the iniomeatal line and three fourths below.[28] Electrocautery is used to dissect and clear soft tissue until the mastoid eminence is adequately visualized. Often the occipital artery and mastoid emissary vein are encountered, and they may be used as landmarks. The artery is typically sacrificed.

Before beginning the craniectomy, the digastric groove should be visualized. The burr hole is placed over the mastoid emissary vein, which is a good landmark for the junction between the sigmoid and transverse sinuses. The craniectomy is expanded until the junction of the transverse and sigmoid sinuses is definitively appreciated, with the apex of the triangular craniectomy pointed at this junction (variations are discussed with other cranial nerve syn-

dromes) (Fig. 45–6). All air cells are then waxed diligently, after which a curvilinear or T-shaped durotomy is performed, exposing a direct corridor along the petrotentorial bone down to the brainstem.[28]

Once the dura is sutured back, the operating microscope is used to "turn the corner," or expose the cerebellopontine angle. While gently retracting on the cerebellum with a cottonoid on a sterile piece of latex (rubber dam), the surgeon must allow adequate cerebrospinal fluid to drain so that the cerebellum falls away, minimizing the need for much cerebellar retraction. Penetration of the trigeminal cistern and sharp dissection of arachnoid adhesions greatly reduce the need for significant cerebellar retraction medially. The cottonoid and a precisely flexible, curved self-retaining brain retractor are placed on the supralateral portion of the cerebellum for trigeminal exposures. The cerebellum is then retracted up and medially. Often, the first vessels encountered are the petrosal vein complex, which are coagulated and cut.[28]

Prior to performing microvascular decompression of the trigeminal nerve, the surgeon must be cognizant of the fact that the dorsal root exit zone of the trigeminal nerve extends to a more distal portion of the nerve. Therefore, the nerve must be meticulously inspected from the brainstem to Meckel's cave, and all offending vessels must be decompressed. When performing the actual decompression, all arachnoid over the nerve must be dissected away. Shredded Teflon felt is placed between the vessel and the nerve. The most frequent vessel found is the superior cerebellar artery. Often multiple pieces of shredded Teflon felt are used to decompress looping arteries affecting more than one side of the trigeminal nerve.[28]

Before closing, a Valsalva maneuver is performed to ensure hemostasis. The durotomy is closed carefully with a watertight closure to prevent cerebrospinal fluid leakage. If a watertight closure cannot be obtained, cadaveric, synthetic, or muscle (if the leak is small) is used to patch the leak. The bone edges are waxed for a second time and a cranioplasty is performed using wire mesh or methylmethacrylate placed over a piece of Gelfoam. Fascia, subcutaneous tissue, and skin are closed in standard manner.

Results

The most frequent operative finding was trigeminal compression by the superior cerebellar artery in 76 per cent of the patients (Fig. 45–7). Veins were involved in 68 per cent of patients but were the sole offending vessel in only 13 per cent.[29, 30] In a report by Barker and associates,[29] of 1204 patients who underwent initial microvascular decompression at the University of Pittsburgh, 80 per cent were pain free at 1 year, and an additional 8 per cent had greater than 75 per cent relief, for a total success rate of 88 per cent. At 10 years, 70 per cent remained pain free and 4 per cent had greater than 75 per cent relief. Persistent postoperative facial numbness was noted in only 17 per cent, of which only 1 per cent was severe. Postoperative facial dysesthesias were reported in less than 5 per cent of the patients after single microvascular decompression in the absence of ablative procedures.[29] Repeat microvascular decompression was performed in 11 per cent of the patients for persistent or recurrent pain.[29] Of these, 96 per cent were either pain free or had greater than 75 per cent pain relief a year after surgery (89 per cent at 10 years).

Microvascular decompression for pediatric-onset trigeminal neuralgia has a lower success rate than that for adults. At time of discharge 73 per cent of patients had complete pain relief, with an additional 18 per cent having greater than 75 per cent diminution of pain.[31] At last follow-up (mean of 105 months), 57 per cent of patients had either complete relief or greater than 75 per cent relief of pain. The lower therapeutic response is likely due to the fact that the pathophysiology of the disease is different in this population. Venous compression was noted in 86 per cent of the cases and was the sole offending vessel in 18 per cent. This is markedly greater than for the adult population. Additionally, venous compression often results in recurrence of pain due to venous revascularization. In 393 cases of trigeminal neuralgia due to veins, 31 per cent developed recurrence (most within 1 year of initial operation) after initial improvement of pain.

Complications

In a recent review by McLaughlin and colleagues, hearing loss was noted in 31 of 3196 patients following microvascular decompression for trigeminal neuralgia (0.97 per cent).[28] Prior to 1990, the incidence of hearing loss was 1.33 per cent. Since 1990, that number has decreased to 0.59 per cent.[28] This decline in hearing loss is greatly attributed to the use of brainstem auditory evoked response monitoring by our neurophysiologists. The incidence of other complications is quite rare, with death occurring in 0.14 per cent of cases.[30]

HEMIFACIAL SPASM

Patient Selection

Hemifacial spasm is more than simply a cosmetic problem. Although relatively uncommon (prevalence of 7/100,000),[32] it has significant psychosocial consequences and may interfere with the patient's ability to read, drive, or work. In the pediatric population, hemifacial spasm may retard reading ability, causing significant and profound educational difficulties.[33] Unlike some disorders that may mimic hemifacial spasm, this disorder is characterized by paroxysmal contractions of the facial muscles on one side. The contraction typically begins around the orbicularis oculi muscles and progresses inferiorly to involve the lower portion of the face and even the platysma. Approximately 15 per cent of the patients have frontalis involvement. Atypical hemifacial spasm differs from the more common form in that contractions start in the buccal muscles and progress rostrally. The tonus phenomenon, or sustained contracture, is common in both atypical and typical hemifacial spasm resulting in eye closure and ipsilateral abduction of the corner of the mouth. Response to microvascular decompression is similar between these two groups.

In contrast with patients with trigeminal neuralgia, those with hemifacial spasm rarely receive temporary benefit from medications such as baclofen, carbamazepine, phenytoin, clonazepam, and other antianxiety medications.[34, 35] Botulinum toxin has been reported to be successful in 80 to 100 per cent of treated patients.[36–38] These benefits are transitory, with recurrence following in 12 to 16 weeks.[36, 37] Obvious facial weakness occurs in nearly 75 per cent of patients treated with repeated injections for at least 3 years.[39] A previous analysis showed that the mean life expectancy for patients with hemifacial spasm is 35 years from symptom onset.[26] In such patients, botulinum toxin may be less cost effective and potentially debilitating if given over such a protracted period.

Operative Technique

Microvascular decompression for hemifacial spasm is quite similar in several respects to that of trigeminal neuralgia (described earlier). However, there are several important differences. As previously mentioned, the patient's position is crucial for maximizing surgical success. For hemifacial spasm, the patient's head is rotated away 10 degrees (as in

FIGURE 45-5

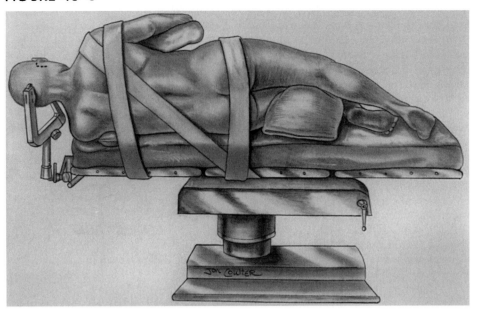

FIGURE 45-6

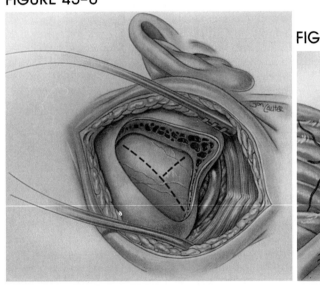

FIGURE 45-7

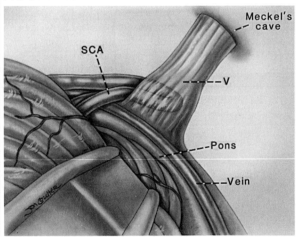

FIGURE 45-8

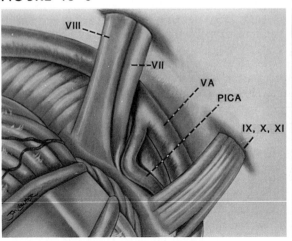

FIGURE 45-9

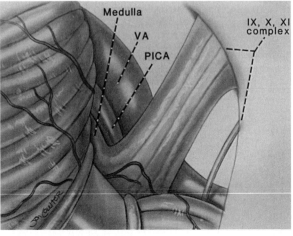

FIGURES 45–5 to 45–9. *See legends on opposite page*

trigeminal neuralgia), and then the vertex is lowered 15 degrees toward the floor.[28] This important maneuver rotates the vestibulocochlear complex cephalad while exposing the proximal portion of cranial nerve VII. Failure to tilt the vertex down results in poor visualization of the facial nerve and failure to achieve adequate decompression. The patient is then positioned and fixed in the standard lateral position (as previously described).

A second important difference is that the patient must not be given muscle relaxants or paralytics because these interfere with intraoperative monitoring of electromyographic potentials recorded from muscles innervated by cranial nerve VII. In patients with hemifacial spasm, stimulation of the temporal or zygomatic branch of the facial nerve electrically produces electromyographic potentials in the mentalis muscle. This muscle response, specific for hemifacial spasm, has a latency of 10 milliseconds.[40] These abnormal electromyographic recordings, known as *lateral spread*, disappear following decompression of the offending vessel. Failure to see disappearance of the lateral spread necessitates further inspection of the nerve by the surgical team.

The skin incision and soft tissue dissection are the same for hemifacial spasm and trigeminal neuralgia. The bone work differs slightly in that more of the craniectomy extends inferiorly and laterally. The dura is opened in a curvilinear or T-shaped fashion and affixed with sutures. As cerebrospinal fluid drains, the operating microscope is employed, and the brain retractor is placed on the inferolateral portion of the cerebellum, elevating both the cerebellum and the tonsils. Next, the cisterna magna is opened, sharply exposing cranial nerves IX, X, XI, and, more superiorly, VII and VIII.[28]

Most commonly, a loop of the posterior inferior cerebellar artery is the offending vessel in typical hemifacial spasm (Fig. 45–8). The surgeon typically finds this loop anterior and caudal to the root entry zone. The posterior inferior cerebellar artery is found in 68 per cent of patients, the anterior inferior cerebellar artery in 35 per cent, and the vertebral artery in 24 per cent (in some cases multiple offending vessels were found).[41] In atypical hemifacial spasm, the surgeon should first look for the offending vessel rostrally, lying between cranial nerves VII and VIII.

Failure to recognize one or all offending vessels is most common when attempting microvascular decompression of cranial nerve VII.

Results

Many clinicians report high success rates with microvascular decompression for hemifacial spasm. Iwakuma and co-workers reported a 97 per cent success rate after treating 74 patients.[42] Auger and associates reported complete relief of spasm in 81 per cent of their patients after nearly 4 years.[43] In an analysis of 16 series, Loeser and Chen reported an 84 per cent rate of complete spasm relief and an additional 4 per cent relief after a second operation.[44] In a review of the author's series, 86 per cent had excellent relief of spasm, with an additional 5 per cent claiming greater than 75 per cent improvement in spasms.[41] These results remained stable at 10-year follow-up. Of 12 patients without any improvement, 11 underwent repeat microvascular decompression and 10 achieved excellent long-term results.[41] We recommend that patients without any symptomatic improvement in the initial postoperative period undergo repeat exploration. For patients with even slight improvement in spasm, however, close follow-up is recommended because these patients tend to experience continued improvement.

The most common offending vessel following the author's series of 648 consecutive microvascular decompressions was the posterior inferior cerebellar artery, found in 68 per cent of the cases. The anterior inferior cerebellar artery was compressing cranial nerve VII in only 25 per cent of the cases.[41] The pathology for pediatric hemifacial spasm is quite different in that venous compression (alone or with another artery) was noted in 75 per cent of the pediatric cases.[33] As venous compression is known to recur following microvascular decompression, the rate of excellent outcomes is 67 per cent (mean follow-up 125 months) in the pediatric population.[33]

Complications

In the author's series of 782 operations for hemifacial spasm, only 3.2 per cent of patients experienced transient

---

FIGURE 45–5. A three-point head fixation device is applied to the patient's head, and the patient is placed in a lateral park bench position with the affected side up. An axillary roll is placed to prevent brachial plexus injury, and all other pressure points are padded appropriately. The head is then elevated and distracted, then rotated 10 degrees away from the surgeon. The head is then locked into place, and the ipsilateral shoulder is distracted caudally and rotated medially, giving the surgeon maximal working area. The patient is taped securely at the hips and chest to allow rotation of the table during surgery.

FIGURE 45–6. The junction of the transverse and sigmoid sinuses must be exposed at the superior margin of the craniectomy. The edge of the sigmoid sinus must be identified along the lateral margin of the craniectomy. To minimize cerebellar retraction, the craniectomy is extended caudally and laterally for procedures involving the lower cranial nerves.

FIGURE 45–7. Intraoperative view of the superior cerebellar artery (SCA) and a vein causing compression of the trigeminal nerve in a patient with trigeminal neuralgia.

FIGURE 45–8. Intraoperative view of cranial nerve VII compressed by the posterior inferior cerebellar artery (PICA) in a patient with hemifacial spasm. VA, vertebral artery.

FIGURE 45–9. Intraoperative view of the left lateral medulla and fascicles of cranial nerves IX and X compressed by the left posterior inferior cerebellar artery (PICA) and left vertebral artery (VA).

TABLE 45–1. Complications Following 782 Consecutive Microvascular Decompressions for Hemifacial Spasm[41]

COMPLICATION	PERCENTAGE
Permanent facial weakness	3.3
Transient facial weakness	3.2
Complete ipsilateral hearing loss	2.7
CSF leak	2.4
Wound infection	1.2
Pseudomeningocele	0.5
Bacterial meningitis	0.5
Cerebellar hematoma	0.5
Infarct	0.3
Operative death	0.1
Other	<1.0

CSF, cerebrospinal fluid.

facial weakness.[41] In McLaughlin and colleagues' report of 1069 operations, the incidence of hearing loss was 2.99 per cent.[28] Following 1990, when the use of intraoperative brainstem evoked potentials was routine, the incidence of hearing loss was 1.59 per cent.[28] Cerebrospinal fluid leaks were noted in 2.4 per cent of patients, and 1.2 per cent had wound infections. Other complications were extremely rare (Table 45–1).

DISABLING POSITIONAL VERTIGO AND TINNITUS

Patient Selection

Patients with compression of cranial nerve VIII may present with a myriad of symptoms, which include tinnitus, hearing loss, Ménière's disease, paroxysmal vertigo, and persistent dysequilibrium. Patients with compression of only the cochlear portion or the vestibular portion of the eighth cranial nerve present with isolated auditory or vestibular dysfunction, respectively.

Patients with disabling positional vertigo have a characteristic pattern of symptoms, the most common of which is persistent vertigo augmented with activity but mitigated with bed rest. This is distinct from patients with Ménière's disease characterized by aural fullness, violent attacks of vertigo, tinnitus, and hearing loss lasting for several hours with the patients asymptomatic between attacks.[45] In contrast with patients with benign paroxysmal positional vertigo, patients with disabling positional vertigo often complain of associated nausea and occasional vomiting, or they may say that they walk as if they "had a few drinks too many." Patients often stagger, are unable to make quick turns, and tend to fall to the affected side. Over time, 20 per cent of afflicted patients develop associated cochlear compression resulting in a slowly progressive loss of hearing in the mid- to high-frequency range. Occasionally, patients may develop symptoms from adjacent cranial nerves such as hemifacial spasm, ear pain (geniculate neuralgia), or trigeminal neuralgia (V2 distribution).

As previously mentioned, patients with eighth nerve compression may present with isolated auditory symptoms. Typically, these patients have hearing loss in the high-frequency range that does not fluctuate.[45] Differences in pure tone hearing threshold and tinnitus are also common signs of cochlear nerve compression (see Fig. 45–4).

Patients with eighth nerve compression differ from patients with other vestibular syndromes in that their symptoms are often unresponsive to common vestibular suppressants such as meclizine (Antivert) or dimenhydrate (Dramamine). Some patients report intermittent success with medical therapy involving benzodiazepines such as diazepam and clonazepam.

Operative Technique

The position of the patient is similar to that of hemifacial spasm, with the head rotated away 10 degrees and the vertex lowered 15 degrees towards the floor.[28] The bony opening is shaped like an isosceles triangle, with the apex pointed at the junction of the sigmoid and transverse sinuses.[28] The durotomy is similar to that of a hemifacial spasm approach. The intradural approach, however, is different in that the retractor blade and cottonoid are placed supralaterally over the cerebellum, elevating it off the eighth nerve. The root entry zone must be dissected free from the flocculus of the cerebellum more medially than in hemifacial spasm. This allows for greater exposure of the veins along the brainstem, which may be the offending vessels.[46–48]

Patients with vertigo and/or dysequilibrium are likely to have compression of the superior vestibular nerve at or just distal to the root entry zone. Recalcitrant nausea, however, is typically associated with compression of the inferior vestibular nerve. In patients with tinnitus, the surgeon must inspect the cochlear nerve from the root entry zone to the internal auditory meatus. Patients with tinnitus and associated deep ear pain with or without vertigo often have compression of the intermediate nerve and the cochlear nerve. Typically, the offending vessel is running between cranial nerves VII and VIII. Intrafascicular compression by arteries is often a difficult problem to treat and may require division of the intermediate nerve.[48]

Results

The group with cranial nerve VIII dysfunction was composed of 281 patients with disabling positional vertigo, tinnitus, hearing loss, and/or dysequilibrium. Patients with predominantly vestibular symptoms were noted to have proximal compression at the root entry zone. Cochlear dysfunction was associated with more peripheral compression. Of the patients with vestibular pathology, 79 per cent were markedly improved or symptom free following surgery, whereas only 40 per cent of the patients with pure cochlear disturbance were significantly better.[45] Improvement in tinnitus is delayed and may take up to 2 years.

Complications

Hearing was damaged in 11 (4.7 per cent) of 235 patients operated on for disabling positional vertigo and/or tinnitus. Two patients developed worsened tinnitus. Additionally, there was 1 patient with transient vocal cord weakness, 1 with trochlear nerve palsy, and 2 with transient facial weakness.[45]

GLOSSOPHARYNGEAL NEURALGIA

Patient Selection

Glossopharyngeal neuralgia is characterized by sharp, lancinating, intermittent pain involving the posterior tongue, pharynx, and deep ear structures. Once other etiologies are eliminated, these patients are excellent candidates for microvascular decompression.[49] Glossopharyngeal neuralgia is due to vascular compression of cranial nerves IX and X. In patients with associated brainstem compression, associated symptoms may include sleep apnea, syncope, ataxia, autonomic dysreflexia, and hypertension (discussed separately).

Some patients find relief with carbamazepine, phenytoin, or baclofen. The efficacy of pharmacotherapy has not been well defined. Attempted medical management, however, may be indicated for some patients given the higher operative morbidity for glossopharyngeal neuralgia than for trigeminal neuralgia.

Operative Technique

Microvascular decompression of cranial nerves IX and X requires a more extensive craniotomy. Once the patient is positioned, prepped, and draped as is usual, the skin incision is made from the level of the iniomeatal line to the level of the inferior portion of the mastoid tip 0.5 cm behind the hairline. This provides an area large enough to extend the craniectomy inferiorly to the floor of the posterior fossa, and laterally exposing the sigmoid sinus as it approaches the jugular bulb. The durotomy is opened with a curvilinear or T-shaped incision and is more extensive than for the approaches previously described.

The surgeon places the retractor and rubber dam over the inferolateral portion of the cerebellum, thus elevating the flocculus off cranial nerves IX and X. If bridging veins are encountered, they may be coagulated and cut. The cisterna magna is then sharply opened, allowing cerebrospinal fluid to drain and the cerebellum to relax, minimizing the need for extensive retraction.

Prior to the microvascular decompression, arachnoid trabeculae must be meticulously dissected off the cranial nerves and cerebellum, allowing for maximal exposure. If the offending vessel is venous, it may be moved off the nerve and coagulated. If arterial compression is identified, it must be moved away from the nerves and held in place with shredded Teflon felt. Although the craniectomy for glossopharyngeal neuralgia is more extensive than for the aforementioned cranial nerves, closure of the surgical site is identical.

Results

The prognosis for patients with glossopharyngeal neuralgia is quite good following microvascular decompression. Of the patients operated on by the senior author (PJJ), 79 per cent had at least 95 per cent relief and another 10 per cent had at least 50 per cent relief, with the remaining 10 per cent considered failures.[49] Based on intraoperative observations, the posterior inferior cerebellar artery was the most common cause of neural compression (39 per cent).[49]

Complications

There were two postoperative deaths (5 per cent), both from sequelae of iatrogenic intraoperative hypertension. Three patients had permanent cranial nerve IX and X palsies (8 per cent), and four others had transient palsies (10 per cent).[49]

NEUROGENIC HYPERTENSION

Patient Selection

Elevated arterial pressure not caused by well-described pathologic findings such as renal artery stenosis, pheochromocytoma, or renal disease has been termed *essential hypertension.*[1] In 1979, Jannetta and Gendell first introduced the concept of neurogenic hypertension.[50] They reported on 16 consecutive hypertensive patients with vascular compression of the left rostral ventrolateral medulla (RVLM). During the past three decades, there has been an abundance of scientific evidence in the forms of animal experimentation,[51–54] postmortem anatomic dissection,[55, 56] operative observations,[1, 2, 50] and radiographic findings[57–59] demonstrating that pulsatile compression of the left RVLM elicits sympathetically mediated hypertension.

Hypertensive candidates for microvascular decompression are refractory to oral antihypertensive medication, have pressure lability interfering with activities of daily living, have associated autonomic dysreflexia, or have intractable side effects from the medication. All patients must be screened for carcinoid, renal artery stenosis, pheochromocytoma, and renal diseases. Additionally, a minimum of three blood pressure measurements confirming hypertension must be documented while adhering to pharmacologic management. Though many patients had demonstration of brainstem compression by ectatic vessels on preoperative MRI, current MRI techniques have been shown to be insufficiently sensitive as a screening tool for neurogenic hypertension.[60] Postoperatively, continuous blood pressure measurements are obtained for 24 hours, followed by blood pressure recordings every 6 to 8 hours for 48 hours. Daily measurements are then required for 2 weeks.

Operative Technique

The operation for neurogenic hypertension is similar to that of glossopharyngeal neuralgia with respect to positioning, craniectomy, durotomy, and approach. The surgeon should expect to find the vertebral artery, the posterior inferior cerebellar artery, or the basilar artery causing RVLM compression.[1, 51, 58] Mobilization of the larger vessels, especially if dolichoectactic or calcified, may be quite difficult. Multiple pieces of shredded Teflon felt are usually required to mobilize the vessel away from the point of maximal compression. Great care must be taken to avoid injury to all perforators in this region, because inadvertent tearing of small arteries may cause irreversible neurologic deficits.

Results

After observing an association between hypertension and left RVLM compression, Jannetta and coworkers reported such compression in 51 of 53 hypertensive patients undergoing microvascular decompression for either trigeminal neuralgia or hemifacial spasm.[61] Several years later, two papers were published within a few months of each other from different groups describing outcomes of patients with medically intractable hypertension treated with microvascular decompression of the RVLM.[1, 2] Not surprisingly, the results were similar. Levy and associates[1] showed improvement in 72 per cent of the patients treated, with 54 per cent achieving normotensive pressures. Additionally, 54 per cent of the patients with severe medically intractable hypertension were regulating their pressure with fewer medications. Similarly, Geiger and colleagues showed that 50 per cent of the patients in their study were normotensive after a 1-year follow-up.[2] The posterior inferior cerebellar artery was compressing the brainstem in 92 per cent of the patients[1] (Fig. 45–9). These studies by Geiger and Levy and their colleagues demonstrate the potential for operative intervention prior to irreversible end-organ damage typical of poorly controlled hypertensive patients. Current randomized, multicenter, prospective trials are investigating the efficacy of microvascular decompression for neurogenic hypertension.

Complications

In our recent study, complications were noted in two patients (17 per cent). These included ipsilateral deafness in one patient after re-exploration for intractable autonomic dysreflexia. A second patient had transient congestive heart failure and paraparesis (of unknown etiology).

SUMMARY

The cranial nerves all are susceptible to the forces that cause cranial rhizopathies. These forces, such as atherosclerosis, elongation of vessels, and cerebellar atrophy, place an aging population at significant risk for developing any one of the syndromes discussed in this chapter. An understanding of the cerebellopontine angle anatomy with respect to the cranial nerves enables trained microsurgeons the opportunity to offer patients a nondestructive cure for their disease with long-term success. Favorable outcomes are primarily dependent on patient selection, preoperative and intraoperative monitoring, and surgical experience. In experienced hands, the morbidity of microvascular decompression is quite low and the cure rate ranges from 70 to 90 per cent for most cranial rhizopathies.

References

1. Levy EI, Clyde B, McLaughlin MR, Jannetta PJ: Microvascular decompression of the left lateral medulla oblongata for severe refractory neurogenic hypertension. Neurosurgery 43: 1–6, 1998.
2. Geiger H, Naraghi R, Schobel HP, et al: Decrease of blood pressure by ventrolateral medullary decompression in essential hypertension [see comments]. Lancet 352: 446–449, 1998.
3. Jannetta PJ, Rand RW: Transtentorial retrogasserian rhizotomy in trigeminal neuralgia by microneurosurgical technique. Bull Los Angeles Neurol Soc 31: 93–99, 1966.
4. Møller MB, Møller AR: Audiometric abnormalities in hemifacial spasm. Audiology 24: 396–405, 1985.
5. Møller AR, Jannetta PJ: Comparison between intracranially recorded potentials from the human auditory nerve and scalp recorded auditory brainstem responses (ABR). Scand Audiol 11: 33–40, 1982.
6. Møller AR, Jannetta PJ: Compound action potentials recorded intracranially from the auditory nerve in man. Exp Neurol 74: 862–874, 1981.
7. Møller AR, Jannetta PJ, Sekhar LN: Contributions from the auditory nerve to the brainstem auditory evoked potentials (BAEPs): Results of intracranial recording in man. Electroencephalogr Clin Neurophysiol 71: 198–211, 1988.
8. Møller AR, Jannetta PJ: Auditory evoked potentials recorded from the cochlear nucleus and its vicinity in man. J Neurosurg 59: 1013–1018, 1983.
9. Sweet WH, Poletti CE: Problems with retrogasserian glycerol in the treatment of trigeminal neuralgia. Appl Neurophysiol 48: 252–257, 1985.
10. Mullan S, Lichtor T: Percutaneous microcompression of the trigeminal ganglion for trigeminal neuralgia. J Neurosurg 59: 1007–1012, 1983.
11. Møller MB, Møller AR: Brainstem auditory evoked potentials in patients with cerebellopontine angle tumors. Ann Otol Rhinol Laryngol 92: 645–650, 1983.
12. Laha RK, Jannetta PJ: Glossopharyngeal neuralgia. J Neurosurg 47: 316–320, 1977.
13. Broggi G, Franzini A, Lasio G, et al: Long-term results of percutaneous retrogasserian thermorhizotomy for "essential" trigeminal neuralgia: Considerations in 1000 consecutive patients. Neurosurgery 26: 783–786, 1990.
14. Taha JM, Tew JMJ, Buncher CR: A prospective 15-year follow-up of 154 consecutive patients with trigeminal neuralgia treated by percutaneous stereotactic radiofrequency thermal rhizotomy. J Neurosurg 83: 989–993, 1995.
15. Taha JM, Tew JMJ: Treatment of trigeminal neuralgia by percutaneous radiofrequency rhizotomy. Neurosurg Clin North Am 8: 31–39, 1997.
16. Zakrzewska JM: Surgery at the level of the gasserian ganglion. In Zakrzewska JM: Trigeminal Neuralgia. London, WB Saunders, 1995, pp 125–156.
17. Lunsford LD, Bennett MH: Percutaneous retrogasserian glycerol rhizotomy for tic douloureux: I. Technique and results in 112 patients. Neurosurgery 14: 424–430, 1984.
18. Lunsford LD, Apfelbaum RI: Choice of surgical therapeutic modalities for treatment of trigeminal neuralgia: Microvascular decompression, percutaneous retrogasserian thermal, or glycerol rhizotomy. Clin Neurosurg 32: 319–333, 1985.
19. Burchiel KJ: Percutaneous retrogasserian glycerol rhizolysis in the management of trigeminal neuralgia. J Neurosurg 69: 361–366, 1988.
20. Slettebo H, Hirschberg H, Lindegaard KF: Long-term results after percutaneous retrogasserian glycerol rhizotomy in patients with trigeminal neuralgia. Acta Neurochir (Wien) 122: 231–235, 1993.
21. Lichtor T, Mullan JF: A 10-year follow-up review of percutaneous microcompression of the trigeminal ganglion. J Neurosurg 72: 49–54, 1990.
22. Brown JA, Gouda JJ: Percutaneous balloon compression of the trigeminal nerve. Neurosurg Clin North Am 8: 53–62, 1997.
23. Kondziolka D, Lunsford LD, Flickinger JC, et al: Stereotactic radiosurgery for trigeminal neuralgia: A multi-institutional study using the gamma unit. J Neurosurg 84: 940–945, 1996.
24. Kondziolka D, Flickinger JC, Lunsford LD, Habeck M: Trigeminal neuralgia radiosurgery: The University of Pittsburgh experience. Stereotact Funct Neurosurg 66(Suppl 1): 343–348, 1996.
25. Kondziolka D, Lunsford LD, Flickinger JC: Gamma knife radiosur-

gery as the first surgery for trigeminal neuralgia. Stereotact Funct Neurosurg 70(Suppl 1): 187–191, 1998.

26. Vital statistics of the United States, 1987, Vol II, part A—mortality. Hyattsville, MD, U.S. Department of Health and Human Services, 1990.

27. Taylor JC, Brauer S, Espir ML: Long-term treatment of trigeminal neuralgia with carbamazepine. Postgrad Med J 28: 16–18, 1981.

28. McLaughlin MR, Jannetta PJ, Clyde BL, et al: Microvascular decompression of cranial nerves. J Neurosurg 90: 1–8, 1999.

29. Barker FG, Jannetta PJ, Babu RP, et al: Long-term outcome after operation for trigeminal neuralgia in patients with posterior fossa tumors. J Neurosurg 84: 818–825, 1996.

30. Barker FG, Jannetta PJ, Bissonette DJ, et al: The long-term outcome of microvascular decompression for trigeminal neuralgia [see comments]. N Engl J Med 334: 1077–1083, 1996.

31. Resnick DK, Levy EI, Jannetta PJ: Microvascular decompression for pediatric onset trigeminal neuralgia. Neurosurgery 43: 804–807, 1998.

32. Auger RG, Whisnant JP: Hemifacial spasm in Rochester and Olmstead County, Minnesota, 1960 to 1984. Arch Neurol 47: 1233–1234, 1990.

33. Levy EI, Resnick DK, Jannetta PJ, et al: Pediatric hemifacial spasm: The efficacy of microvascular decompression. Pediatr Neurosurg 27: 238–241, 1997.

34. Alexander GE, Moses H III: Carbamazepine for hemifacial spasm. Neurology 32: 286–287, 1982.

35. Sandyk R, Gillman MA: Clonazepine in hemifacial spasm. Int J Neurosci 33: 261–264, 1987.

36. Dutton JJ, Buckley EG: Long-term results and complications of botulinum A toxin in the treatment of blepharospasm. Ophthalmology 95: 1529–1534, 1988.

37. Taylor JDN, Kraft SP, Kazdan MS, et al: Treatment of blepharospasm and hemifacial spasm with botulinum A toxin: A Canadian multicentre study. Can J Ophthalmol 26: 133–138, 1991.

38. Yoshimura DM, Aminoff MJ, Tami TA, et al: Treatment of hemifacial spasm with botulinum toxin. Muscle Nerve 15: 1045–1049, 1992.

39. Park YC, Lim JK, Lee DK, et al: Botulinum A toxin treatment of hemifacial spasm and blepharospasm. J Korean Med Sci 8: 334–340, 1993.

40. Møller AR, Jannetta PJ: Microvascular decompression in hemifacial spasm: Intraoperative electrophysiological observations. Neurosurgery 16: 612–618, 1985.

41. Barker FG, Jannetta PJ, Bissonette DJ, et al: Microvascular decompression for hemifacial spasm. J Neurosurg 82: 201–210, 1995.

42. Iwakuma T, Matsumoto A, Nakamura N: Hemifacial spasm: Comparison of three different operative procedures in 110 patients. J Neurosurg 57: 753–756, 1982.

43. Auger RG, Piepgras DG, Laws ER Jr: Hemifacial spasm: Results of microvascular decompression of the facial nerve in 54 patients. Mayo Clin Proc 61: 640–644, 1986.

44. Loeser JD, Chen J: Hemifacial spasm: Treatment by microsurgical facial nerve decompression. Neurosurgery 13: 141–146, 1983.

45. Møller MB, Møller AR, Jannetta PJ, et al: Microvascular decompression of the eighth nerve in patients with disabling positional vertigo: Selection criteria and operative results in 207 patients. Acta Neurochir (Wien) 125: 75–82, 1993.

46. Jannetta PJ: Trigeminal neuralgia [letter]. Neurosurgery 18: 677, 1986.

47. Jannetta PJ: Neurovascular cross-compression in patients with hyperactive dysfunction symptoms of the eighth cranial nerve. Surg Forum 26: 467–469, 1975.

48. Jannetta PJ: Neurovascular cross compression of the eighth nerve in patients with vertigo and tinnitus. In Samii M, Jannetta PJ (eds): The Cranial Nerves. Heidelberg, Germany, Springer-Verlag, 1981.

49. Resnick DK, Jannetta PJ, Bissonnette D, et al: Microvascular decompression for glossopharyngeal neuralgia. Neurosurgery 36: 64–68, 1995.

50. Jannetta PJ, Gendell HM: Clinical observations on etiology of essential hypertension. Surg Forum 30: 431–432, 1979.

51. Granata AR, Ernsberger P, Reis DJ: Hypotension and bradycardia elicited by histamine into the C1 area of the rostral ventrolateral medulla. Eur J Pharmacol 136: 157–162, 1987.

52. Morrison SH, Milner TA, Reis DJ: Reticulospinal vasomotor neurons of the rat rostral ventrolateral medulla: Relationship of sympathetic nerve activity and the C1 adrenergic cell group. J Neurosci 8: 1286–1301, 1988.

53. Segal R, Gendell HM, Canfield D, et al: Cardiovascular response to pulsatile pressure applied to ventrolateral medulla. Surg Forum 30: 433–435, 1979.

54. Segal R, Jannetta PJ, Wolfson SKJ, et al: Implanted pulsatile balloon device for simulation of neurovascular compression syndromes in animals. J Neurosurg 57: 646–650, 1982.

55. Naraghi R, Gaab MR, Walter GF: Neurovascular compression as a cause of essential hypertension: A microanatomical study. Adv Neurosurg 17: 182–186, 1989.

56. Naraghi R, Gaab MR, Walter GF, Kleineberg B: Arterial hypertension and neurovascular compression at the ventrolateral medulla: A comparative microanatomical and pathological study. J Neurosurg 77: 103–112, 1992.

57. Kleineberg B, Becker H, Gaab MR: Neurovascular compression and essential hypertension: An angiographic study. Neuroradiology 33: 2–8, 1991.

58. Kleineberg B, Becker H, Gaab MR, Naraghi R: Essential hypertension associated with neurovascular compression. Neurosurgery 30: 834–841, 1992.

59. Naraghi R, Geiger H, Crnac J, et al: Posterior fossa neurovascular anomalies in essential hypertension. Lancet 344: 1466–1470, 1994.

60. Colon GP, Quint DJ, Dickenson LD, et al: Magnetic resonance imaging of ventrolateral medullary compression in essential hypertension. J Neurosurg 88: 226–231, 1998.

61. Jannetta PJ, Segal R, Wolfson SKJ: Neurogenic hypertension: Etiology and surgical treatment: I. Observations in 53 patients. Ann Surg 201: 391–398, 1985.

46

Drainage Procedures for Petrous Apex Lesions

Derald E. Brackmann, M.D. ▪ Neil A. Giddings, M.D.

With the help of cranial computed tomography (CT) and magnetic resonance imaging (MRI), petrous apex lesions can be correctly diagnosed preoperatively. Consequently, cystic lesions requiring drainage should be approached with procedures designed for drainage, not total en bloc removal. Although the transmastoid infralabyrinthine procedure has been the usual approach for these lesions, transcanal infracochlear drainage offers a more dependent drainage site. The eventual role of the various approaches for petrous apex drainage will depend on the long-term follow-up of these patients.

Advances in radiologic imaging during the past decade have made it possible to reliably differentiate lesions of the petrous apex preoperatively. The development of CT scanning was the first major step in imaging the temporal bone since the development of polytomography. CT scanning gives the surgeon the ability to visualize the size of the lesion and its relationship to vital structures, including the internal auditory canal, cochlea, vestibular labyrinth, carotid artery, and jugular bulb. It also helps characterize the border of the lesion as expansile or invasive, which may differentiate between benign lesions and malignant neoplasms. MRI of the temporal bone added the capability of characterizing the substance of the lesion rather than its effect on bony interfaces, allowing the surgeon to distinguish between mucus, fat, cholesterol granuloma, cholesteatoma, and neoplasm. The combination of CT, with its superior bone imaging algorithms, and MRI, with its enhanced tissue-imaging capabilities, allows the surgeon to differentiate accurately and reliably among benign cystic lesions, normal anatomic variants, and neoplastic lesions of the petrous apex.

Patients with petrous apex lesions present with various symptoms and physical findings. The most widely recognized finding is Gradenigo's syndrome, consisting of retro-orbital pain, otorrhea, and ipsilateral sixth cranial nerve paresis. The signs and symptoms of noninflammatory or neoplastic lesions may be more subtle. Hearing loss and vestibular abnormalities are frequently associated with lesions of the petrous apex as they enlarge and compress the internal auditory canal. The facial nerve is relatively resistant to paresis from slowly expansile lesions but may be involved early with neoplastic lesions of the petrous apex or non-neoplastic lesions compressing the internal auditory canal.

Pain may be present with benign or cystic lesions but is more common in neoplastic lesions. Its distribution is dependent on the region involved. The mastoid cavity is innervated by cranial nerve IX and may radiate pain into the neck. Middle fossa and superior petrosal regions are innervated by cranial nerve V and may be perceived as retro-orbital or facial pain. Lesions extending into the posterior fossa may cause pain along the routes of distribution of cranial nerves IX and X and the first three cervical nerves.[1] Although 80 per cent of adult mastoid bones are aerated, only 30 per cent of petrous bones have air cells extending to the apex, and up to 7 per cent may have asymmetric pneumatization of the petrous apex.[2, 3] The increasing use of MRI of the head and neck makes it imperative that the clinician can differentiate pathology from normal variant in the temporal bone. Common lesions of the petrous apex and their associated radiologic findings are summarized in Table 46–1.

Asymmetric pneumatization is clearly seen on CT scanning, but supplementary MRI may be needed to rule out pathologic lesions in a symptomatic ear. Normal bony architecture can be seen on CT scanning, with hyperintensity on MRI T1W scans and hypointensity on T2W because of the large fat content in marrow. Retained mucus in the air cells also presents with normal bony architecture on CT scan but is hypointense on T1W and hyperintense on T2W MRI scans. Cholesteatoma is usually associated with chronic otitis media but may arise from congenital rest cells in the petrous apex. Because of its high water content, cholesteatoma is isointense with cerebrospinal fluid on CT and displays a hypointense T1W and hyperintense T2W image on MRI. Cholesterol granuloma is isointense with brain on CT scanning and presents a classic image on MRI with hyperintensity on T1W and T2W. Radiologic descriptions of other, less common lesions are also summarized in Table 46–1. Differentiating between chordoma, chondroma, and chondrosarcoma of the temporal bone remains difficult, even with the scanning techniques currently available. The area of origin and the age of the patient must be considered when the pathology of destructive lesions of the petrous apex is determined.[4–6]

PATIENT SELECTION

Most surgical approaches to the petrous apex were developed in the preantibiotic era for drainage of petrous apex abscesses and cure of Gradenigo's syndrome. With the arrival of modern antibiotics, infectious processes of the petrous apex have severely declined in frequency, but these same approaches may be equally effective in draining cystic lesions of the petrous apex.

TABLE 46–1. Radiologic Appearance of Common Petrous Apex Lesions

| LESION | COMPUTED TOMOGRAPHY | MAGNETIC RESONANCE IMAGING | | |
		T1W	T2W	Enhancement
Retained mucus	Normal bony architecture, nonenhancing	Hypointense	Hyperintense	No
Mucocele	Hypodense, expansile smooth border, nonenhancing Normal bony architecture,	Hypointense	Hyperintense	No
Asymmetric pneumatization	Normal bony architecture, nonenhancing	Hyperintense	Hypointense	No
Cholesteatoma	Loss of normal air cells, nonenhancing, isointense with CSF	Hypointense	Hyperintense	No
Cholesterol granuloma	Expansile smooth border, occasional rim enhancement, isointense with brain	Hypointense	Hyperintense	No
Metastatic lesion	Destructive, indistinct border	Isotense	Hyperintense	Yes
	Aggressive bone destruction, calcification	Isointense: 75% Hypointense: 25%		
Chondroma	Aggressive bone destruction, calcification	Hypointense to isointense	Hyperintense	Yes

CSF, cerebrospinal fluid.

Air cell tracts extend above, below, and anterior to the otic capsule, allowing the potential of safe passage to the petrous apex. Approaches that follow superior air cell tracts include middle fossa,[7] through the superior semicircular canal,[8] the attic, and the root of the zygomatic arch.[9] Approaches below the inner ear include the infralabyrinthine and the infracochlear.[10–13] Anterior approaches have been described by Ramadier,[14] Eagleton,[15] and Lempert,[16] who used the triangle between the anterior border of the cochlea, the carotid artery, and the middle fossa dura. All these approaches are used for drainage of inflammatory disease processes that are not responsive to antibiotic therapy or simpler operations for chronic ear disease (Fig. 46–1).

Infralabyrinthine, infracochlear, and trans-sphenoidal approaches are most commonly chosen for drainage of cystic lesions of the petrous apex in an ear with serviceable hearing. These lesions are frequently detected at an asymptomatic stage with today's imaging techniques. Because the natural history of small benign cystic lesions is not well documented, surgical drainage should be reserved for patients with larger lesions or with symptoms, including pain, visual changes, diplopia, hearing loss, vertigo, or facial nerve weakness. For patients without serviceable hearing, these lesions should be drained through a translabyrinthine approach. Because other vital structures may be affected by enlargement of the cyst, delaying surgery in symptomatic patients provides no advantage.

Cholesterol granuloma is the most common cystic lesion of the petrous apex, occurring 30 times less frequently than acoustic neuroma.[17] It may develop in any aerated portion of the temporal bone but most commonly occurs in the mastoid air cells distant to a lesion that prevents normal aeration. Cholesterol granuloma of the petrous apex probably develops when a pathologic process or trauma obstructs the air-cell tracts to a well-pneumatized petrous apex.

The treatment for cholesterol granuloma of the temporal bone is drainage and re-establishment of adequate aeration to the involved area. The cyst wall is composed of a fibrous connective tissue. It is free of keratinizing squamous epithelium that characterizes cholesteatoma, and complete removal of the cyst is not necessary.

Solid tumors of the temporal bone and cholesteatoma are removed when first identified rather than after further symptoms develop because these symptoms frequently reveal further involvement of other vital structures. Drainage procedures are obviously inadequate treatment for these lesions, and all reasonable efforts should be made to remove them entirely. Total removal may require the sacrifice of cranial nerves and major vascular structures.

PREOPERATIVE EVALUATION AND PATIENT COUNSELING

Preoperative evaluation of these patients is based on their symptoms. Patients presenting with hearing loss are evaluated initially with audiometric testing, including air, bone, and speech reception thresholds and speech discrimination scores. Electronystagmography is performed in patients who complain of imbalance or vertigo. In patients with otherwise normal results on physical examination, asymmetric hearing is next evaluated with auditory brainstem response testing. If these results are abnormal, an MRI scan is indicated. In patients with cranial nerve involvement other than the eighth nerve, with asymmetric hearing, auditory brainstem response testing is not performed, and the physician proceeds directly to an MRI scan.

Patients who have normal hearing but have other cranial nerve deficits that may be referable to the petrous apex may be screened with either a high-resolution, thin-section CT of the temporal bone or an MRI with gadolinium. If an abnormality is found, all patients undergo air, bone, and speech reception thresholds and speech discrimination audiometric testing before surgery to document hearing levels before a procedure that jeopardizes hearing.

Preoperatively, patients are counseled to expect resolution of pain, if present, and the possibility of improvement in cranial nerve function if it is decreased preoperatively. Cranial nerves that have been affected for shorter periods seem to have a better prognosis and fewer long-standing deficits than those affected longer. Patients are reminded that this is a drainage procedure with the goal of decompressing the lesion and providing an aerated cavity, if

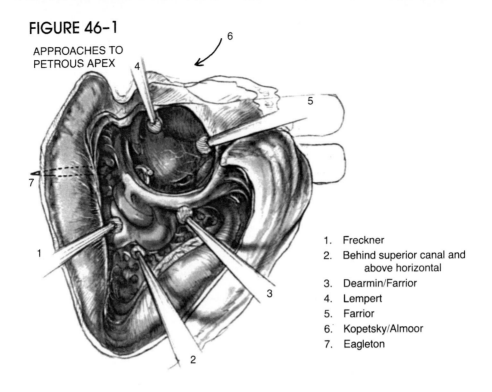

FIGURE 46-1

APPROACHES TO
PETROUS APEX

1. Freckner
2. Behind superior canal and
   above horizontal
3. Dearmin/Farrior
4. Lempert
5. Farrior
6. Kopetsky/Almoor
7. Eagleton

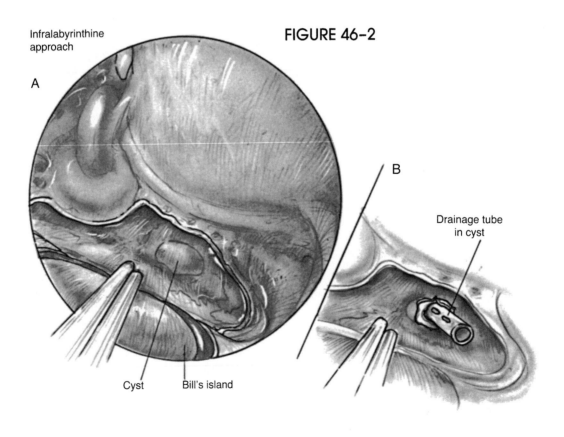

Infralabyrinthine
approach

FIGURE 46-2

A

B

Drainage tube
in cyst

Cyst   Bill's island

FIGURE 46–1. Surgical approaches for drainage of the petrous apex.

FIGURE 46–2. A, Exposure of the cyst in the infralabyrinthine cell tract. An island of bone protects the retracted sigmoid sinus (Bill's island). B, A silicone tube placed into the interior of the cavity drains into the inferior mastoid cavity.

possible. The goal is not the removal of the lesion, and close follow-up may be necessary. Recurrence of the lesion secondary to inadequate drainage is usually heralded by the return of preoperative symptoms. Follow-up MRI frequently reveals a cholesterol granuloma cyst that remains full of fluid, but the T1W image is hypointense, compared with the preoperative hyperintense image on T1W views. A return of hyperintensity on the T1W image suggests inadequate drainage in a symptomatic lesion.[18]

SURGICAL TECHNIQUES

Infralabyrinthine Drainage of the Petrous Apex

In preparation for infralabyrinthine drainage of the petrous apex, the patient is prohibited from eating and drinking for at least 8 hours preoperatively. Unless an infectious process is suspected, no preoperative antibiotics are used.

The surgical ear is prepared similarly to any other chronic otitis media case operated on through a postauricular approach. Hair is shaved to one fingerbreadth above the auricle and two fingerbreadths behind the postauricular crease. Surgical preparation is an antibacterial scrub followed by painting with antibacterial solution. Sterile Mastisol is applied around the auricle and allowed to dry. An adhesive aperture drape is placed over the ear, and sterile sheets cover the patient. Routine chronic otitis media instruments and drill are the only equipment required.

1. The patient is placed in a supine position with the involved ear facing up. The surgeon sits at the side of the patient with the patient's head turned away.

2. A postauricular incision is made 1 cm behind the postauricular crease down to the temporalis fascia superiorly, and through the periosteum below the temporal line. A second incision is made through the temporalis muscle and fascia at the temporal line, beginning above the external auditory canal and ending posteriorly at the postauricular incision, allowing the periosteum to be raised and the ear reflected anteriorly. Temporalis muscle is reflected superiorly.

3. A simple mastoidectomy is performed, removing all air cells from Trautmann's triangle (bordered by the middle fossa dural plate superiorly, the semicircular canals anteriorly, and the sigmoid sinus posteriorly) (Fig. 46–2A).

4. The facial nerve should be identified in its vertical portion but need not be exposed.

5. Mastoid air cells are removed from the mastoid tip, and the sigmoid sinus is followed until the jugular bulb is identified. The superior aspect of the jugular bulb forms the most inferior portion of the opening into the petrous apex.

6. The posterior half of the horizontal and the inferior portion of the posterior bony semicircular canal are skeletonized, and care is taken not to expose the membranous portions of the canals.

7. Once the semicircular canals and the jugular bulb are clearly defined, the infralabyrinthine air-cell tract is followed toward the petrous apex with a diamond burr or curette until the cystic lesion is encountered and opened.

8. Once the lesion is entered, it is evacuated with suction and copious irrigation. All fluid and loose debris are removed. Removal of tissue lining the cavity is neither necessary nor possible with this approach.

9. The largest silicone sheeting catheter that fits into the newly created opening is placed and retained by friction to prevent stenosis of the drainage site (Fig. 46–2B).

10. The periosteum is reapproximated with absorbable suture, and the subcutaneous tissue and skin are closed in layers, followed by the placement of a mastoid pressure dressing.

The mastoid pressure dressing is formed by placing Telfa over the postauricular incision. One half a cotton ball is placed in the concha and two 4 × 4 gauze pads are folded in half and placed in the postauricular crease. A soft, absorbent bolster is then placed over the auricle and the mastoid region. A 4-inch Kling bandage is then wrapped anteriorly to posteriorly and secured by cinching down with a tracheotomy tie 1 inch posterior to the lateral orbital rim.

Most patients are admitted to the hospital for 1 night after this surgery. The dressing is removed the following day, and the incision is cleaned, if necessary. If skin sutures were used, they are removed 1 week later. The patient is allowed to get the postauricular incision wet at this time and should be instructed to clean the incision once per day for the next 2 weeks with hydrogen peroxide to reduce crusting on the incision.

Pitfalls

Infralabyrinthine drainage has been the most commonly employed procedure in the United States for drainage of these cystic lesions. However, it is not without risk to the facial nerve, jugular bulb, and otic capsule. Surgeons attempting this procedure should be intimately familiar with the neural and major vascular anatomy of the petrous bone. When a large cystic lesion expands along the infralabyrinthine cell tracts, this approach may be the simplest. With a small lesion, following this cell tract to the area of pathology may be difficult. Probably the greatest limitation to this approach is its extreme difficulty when used in patients with a high jugular bulb. The drainage opening may be narrowed significantly, even if it is possible to decompress the jugular bulb and retract it inferiorly during the surgical procedure. Consequently, this approach should not be chosen when the jugular bulb is high or narrows the surgical approach to the apex. Injury to the jugular bulb can be temporarily controlled with external packing and light pressure. At this time, the surgeon should arm himself or herself with adequate suction and large sheets of Surgicel. The Surgicel is removed, and the damaged jugular bulb inspected as well as possible. For small lacerations, a small sheet of Surgicel is placed over the bulb and packed in place with absorbable gelatin sponge (Gelfoam). A large defect in the jugular bulb requires that a large piece of Surgicel be placed through the defect into the lumen of the vein. Small pieces should not be placed near the defect or into the lumen because of the possibility of embolization to the lung. Absorbable gelatin sponge is packed over the Surgicel, usually controlling the bleeding with light pressure.

Injury to the posterior or horizontal semicircular canal

requires early recognition of the surgical misadventure. Little or no suction should be used to inspect the fenestration. A small piece of temporalis fascia is placed over the defect, and bone wax is used to secure the fascia and provide a watertight seal. If recognized early, hearing may be preserved, although vertigo will be present for several weeks in the postoperative period.

Transcanal Infracochlear Approach to the Petrous Apex[12]

In 1984, Farrior described a transcanal approach to small glomus jugulare tumors of the hypotympanum.[11] The infracochlear approach to the petrous apex is a combination of this technique and the subcochlear approach described by Ghorayeb and Jahrsdoerfer.[13]

1. A postauricular incision is made, and the auricle is reflected anteriorly.

2. The membranous external auditory canal is completely transected laterally (Fig. 46–3A).

3. A tympanomeatal flap is elevated from 2 to 10 o'clock, leaving the tympanic membrane attached at the umbo and the superior canal wall.

4. The external auditory canal is enlarged anteriorly and inferiorly to expose the hypotympanum. The chorda tympani is followed inferoposteriorly to laterally to define the extent of posterior dissection possible without injury to the facial nerve (Fig. 46–3B).

5. Air cells are removed below the cochlea in the hypotympanum to expose the course of the carotid artery and the jugular bulb. The round window provides the superior line of dissection, and Jacobson's nerve leads to the "crutch" of the carotid and jugular bulb (Fig. 46–3C).

6. Removal of air cells continues medially. If the plane of dissection remains below the round window, the internal auditory canal structures will not be at risk (Fig. 46–3D).

7. The cholesterol granuloma cyst is entered and drained. The newly created "window" is enlarged as far anteriorly as possible to the carotid artery, as far inferiorly as the jugular bulb, and superiorly to the inferior aspect of the basal turn of the cochlea (Fig. 46–3E).

8. A silicone catheter of appropriate size is introduced, if necessary, to stent the opening (Fig. 46–3F).

9. The soft tissue of the external auditory canal is returned to its normal position, gelatin sponge is packed within the membranous external auditory canal, and bone pate (previously obtained during initial drilling) is placed between the canal wall and the newly enlarged bony canal (Fig. 46–3G).

10. The postauricular incision is closed, and a mastoid dressing is applied (Fig. 46–3H).

Postoperative dressings, care, and length of hospitalization are similar to those used for the infralabyrinthine approach, except in the care of the external auditory canal. The patient is seen 1 week postoperatively to check the postauricular incision and to ensure that excessive drainage is not occurring from the external auditory canal. The packing should be moist without evidence of active drainage. If excessive drainage or evidence of infection is present, the patient is prescribed antibiotic ear drops (Cor-

tisporin otic suspension) three times a day. If the packing is dry, the patient begins using the ear drops 2 weeks after surgery, 2 drops three times a day, until the packing is removed 1 month postoperatively. At this point, the tympanic membrane should be intact and the canal skin healing well. Small areas of exposed bony external auditory canal will epithelialize within 1 to 2 months.

This procedure is similar to the infralabyrinthine approach, in that both involve an area of the temporal bone to which most otolaryngologists have little exposure. The surgery need not be difficult, but surgeons must spend time in the temporal bone laboratory familiarizing themselves with the relative positions of the basal turn of the cochlea, the jugular bulb, and the carotid artery. After the soft tissue of the canal is reflected superiorly, a large amount of the bone lateral to the annulus can be removed with a cutting burr. Once the hypotympanum is entered, the surgeon should switch to successively smaller diamond burrs until the cyst is entered.

Injury to the jugular bulb is treated as was described for the infralabyrinthine approach. Injury to the basal turn of the cochlea is more serious than opening into a semicircular canal. It should be approached with minimal suction, and the placement of temporalis fascia should be secured by bone wax. Despite early recognition, the prognosis for hearing is much poorer when the cochlea is violated than when the semicircular canals are violated.

This approach may cause injury to the infratemporal portion of the carotid artery. The carotid arterial wall may be thinner in the temporal bone than in the neck. Every effort should be made to leave a thin wall of bone over the carotid artery. If the artery is violated, immediate control can usually be achieved with packing and pressure to the middle ear and external auditory canal. This injury is potentially life-threatening and requires the expertise of a vascular surgeon. Distal control may be achieved with an intra-arterial catheter threaded past the point of injury, and proximal control is achieved in the neck. Once proximal and distal control are achieved, the injury can be directly repaired. Obviously, occlusion of the carotid artery runs the risk of cerebral infarct.

RESULTS

No large series documenting the superior effectiveness of any one procedure exists. All procedures would be expected to relieve pain, if it was present preoperatively, and may allow the recovery of some cranial nerve dysfunction. Gherini and associates[17] reported that hearing was preserved in 83 per cent of patients who had useful preoperative hearing, but no improvement occurred in those with preoperative hearing impairment. Vertigo, if present preoperatively, usually resolves with adequate decompression.[19] Several patients displayed recovery of cranial nerve function other than the cochlear nerve, but this return of function is not universal, even after adequate decompression.[17, 19, 20]

COMPLICATIONS AND MANAGEMENT

All procedures that approach the petrous apex may cause injury to major vessels and cranial nerves. Each approach has its own set of risks. Table 46–2 compares the common procedures used for drainage of petrous apex lesions. The experience of the surgeon, the position of the lesion, and the needs of the patient all need to be addressed.

The infralabyrinthine approach is the most familiar to otolaryngologists and head and neck surgeons. It is a direct extension of the simple mastoidectomy that may be accomplished with minimal morbidity in patients with a large cyst that has expanded between the labyrinth and the jugular bulb. Smaller cysts that are more medially based become more challenging, and a high jugular bulb may preclude this approach entirely. Care must be taken not to disturb the endolymphatic sac or damage the endolymphatic duct during this dissection. Damage to these areas may lead to endolymphatic hydrops. This technique drains the cyst farther from the eustachian tube than any other otologic technique and, consequently, may be more prone to failure. Because of the debris that is never completely removed from these cysts, the mastoid itself may become poorly aerated, leading to the potential for long-term failure.

The transcanal infracochlear approach has the advantage of a direct approach to the petrous apex and the maintenance of normal ear anatomy. It requires familiarity with the surgical anatomy of the hypotympanum, but the surgical landmarks are easily identified. The round window is easily seen, and careful removal of bone with a diamond burr reveals the location of the jugular bulb and carotid artery. If major vessel damage occurs, it is easily temporized with direct pressure until the situation can be controlled with direct vessel repair or permanent packing. It also drains the cyst close to the opening of the eustachian tube into the middle ear space, which makes obstruction less likely. Complete transection of the soft tissue external auditory canal may lead to mild stenosis in the postoperative period. If this occurs, it is easily managed and corrected with the placement of a foam ear insert used by audiologists for routine audiometric testing. The insert maintains gentle pressure on the area of stenosis while allowing passage of sound down the central lumen.

ALTERNATIVE TECHNIQUES

Several other techniques are available for exposure of the petrous apex.

Trans-Sphenoidal Approach to Petrous Apex Lesions

Trans-sphenoidal drainage of petrous apex cysts may be the most simple and straightforward approach to large cysts that have a large surface area against the posterior wall of the sphenoid sinus. This technique is obviously not useful when the cyst does not impinge on the sphenoid sinus. The risk of damage to the cochlea and labyrinth is decreased with this technique, but the risk to the carotid artery increases, and an added risk of damage to the optic nerve exists (a frequently reported complication of endoscopic sinus surgery). This technique also has a high failure rate when compared with otologic drainage procedures for cholesterol granuloma of the petrous apex. Thedinger and colleagues[19] reported that 80 per cent of patients who had a trans-sphenoidal initial approach for drainage eventually required one or more procedures to effectively drain the lesion. In their series, the only patient who required revision surgery after an otologic procedure had had a middle fossa attempt that did not provide dependent drainage.

1. An external ethmoidectomy, sphenoidotomy, intranasal sphenoethmoidectomy, intranasal sphenoidotomy, transseptal sphenoidotomy, or transpalatal approach may be used to expose the posterior and lateral walls of the sphenoid sinus.[19–22]

2. Indentations in the lateral and superior walls may reveal the location of vital nervous and vascular structures, including the pituitary gland, optic nerve, maxillary nerve, carotid artery, and cavernous sinus.

3. A cruciate incision is made in the posterior sphenoid sinus mucosa, and flaps are elevated from the bony posterior wall.

TABLE 46–2. Common Drainage Approaches to the Petrous Apex

PROCEDURE	STRUCTURES AT RISK	ADVANTAGES	DISADVANTAGES
Infralabyrinthine	Jugular bulb, bony labyrinth, facial nerve	Direct approach that is more familiar to most otolaryngologists	Difficult with high jugular bulb Drainage into mastoid cavity far from eustachian tube
Transcanal infracochlear	Jugular bulb, carotid artery, cochlea	Direct drainage near the mouth of the eustachian tube Can be revised with transtympanic procedure	Anatomy may be challenging to those not familiar with hypotympanum and major vessels of temporal bone
Trans-sphenoidal	Carotid artery, optic nerve, cavernous sinus, maxillary nerve, pituitary gland	Direct approach to large cysts that are in contact with posterior wall of sphenoid sinus Opening into cyst may be directly observed in clinic with endoscope	Sphenoid anatomy is highly variable Can only be used for "giant" cysts in contact with sphenoid High rate of failure
Translabyrinthine or subtotal petrosectomy	Labyrinth, jugular bulb, internal auditory canal	Cyst and wall can be removed if desired	Profound postoperative sensorineural hearing loss
Middle fossa	Temporal lobe, cochlea, labyrinth, internal auditory canal, greater superficial petrosal nerve	Drains cyst directly into bony eustachian tube	Middle fossa craniotomy poorly tolerated in elderly Drainage is not dependent Temporal lobe may obstruct drainage path

FIGURE 46-3

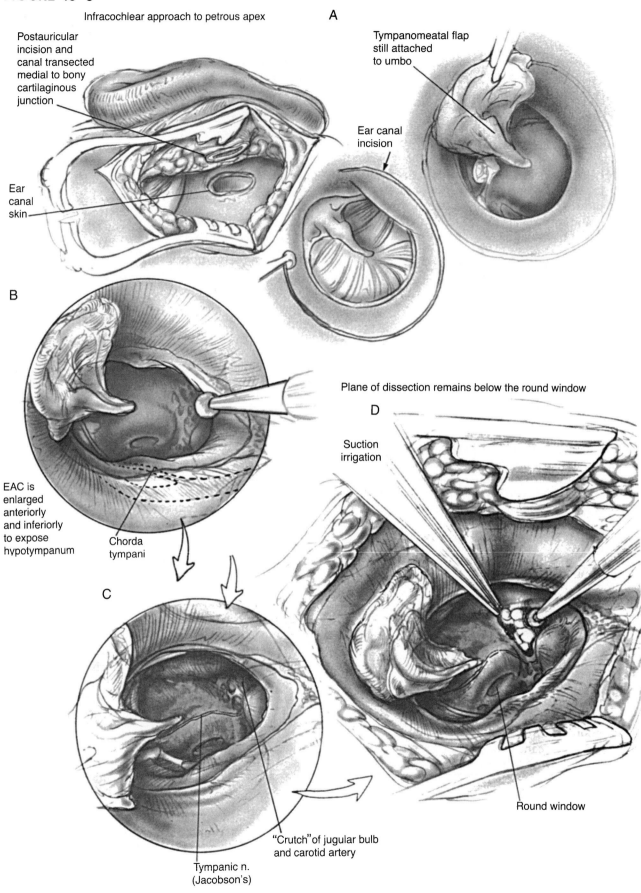

Infracochlear approach to petrous apex

A

Postauricular incision and canal transected medial to bony cartilaginous junction

Tympanomeatal flap still attached to umbo

Ear canal incision

Ear canal skin

B

EAC is enlarged anteriorly and inferiorly to expose hypotympanum

Chorda tympani

Plane of dissection remains below the round window

D

Suction irrigation

Round window

C

"Crutch" of jugular bulb and carotid artery

Tympanic n. (Jacobson's)

FIGURE 46-3. *Illustration continued on opposite page*

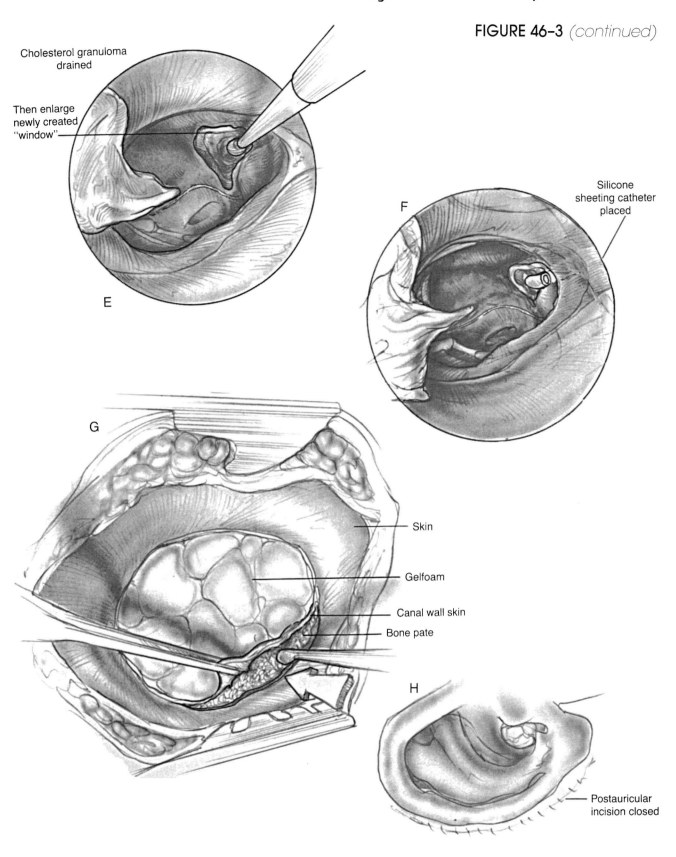

Cholesterol granuloma drained

Then enlarge newly created "window"

E

Silicone sheeting catheter placed

F

G

Skin

Gelfoam

Canal wall skin

Bone pate

H

Postauricular incision closed

FIGURE 46-3. *A* to *H,* Transcanal infracochlear approach to the petrous apex. EAC, external auditory canal.

4. Based on preoperative CT scanning, a diamond burr or sharp chisel is used to remove a small portion of the posterior bony wall of the sphenoid sinus. Pituitary rongeurs are used to enlarge the bony orifice as much as possible without violating vital structures, exposing the cystic lesion.

5. The cyst wall is opened, and the contents are drained. The cyst is irrigated, and all debris is removed. The mucosal flaps previously raised are laid into the cavity, and no synthetic drain is used.

6. A large sphenoidotomy is performed for postoperative inspection and cleaning.

7. If an intranasal approach was used, the sphenoid sinus should remain unpacked, but the nasal cavity may be lightly packed. If an external approach was chosen, the wound is closed in layers.

With the increased interest in endoscopic sinus surgery, the trans-sphenoidal approach to the petrous apex is gaining in popularity. Unfortunately, this approach does not work in smaller lesions that do not directly abut the posterior wall of the sphenoid sinus. Many endoscopists have gained a great deal of expertise with the surface anatomy of the sphenoid and other paranasal sinuses. This procedure should not be confused with routine sinusotomy or removal of infected mucosa from the sinus walls. This approach to draining the petrous apex requires bone removal from the posterior wall of the sphenoid sinus, placing the carotid artery and optic nerve at risk. Skilled endoscopists perform this procedure with a low complication rate, but those with less experience would do well to note that the sphenoid sinus is the most variable in form of any bilateral cavity or organ in the human body. The sphenoid sinus may vary in length from 4 to 44 mm, in width from 2.5 to 34 mm, and in height from 5 to 33 mm.[23]

Subtotal Petrosectomy

Fisch and Mattox[24] describe a subtotal petrosectomy in combination with removal of the otic capsule to gain full exposure of the petrous apex. This technique offers the advantage of direct exposure from the carotid artery to the sigmoid sinus in an anteroposterior direction and exposure from the hypotympanum to the middle fossa dura in an inferosuperior direction. The contents of the internal auditory canal are left undisturbed, and the facial nerve does not require transposition, making possible complete removal of benign lesions of the petrous apex, including cystic structures with their lining matrix. Unfortunately, this increased exposure results in total sensorineural hearing loss with the removal of the otic capsule.

1. A postauricular incision is made down to the temporalis fascia superiorly and through the periosteum posteriorly and inferiorly. A second incision is made along the temporal line through the temporalis muscle, the auricle is reflected anteriorly, and the cartilaginous canal is tran-

Subtotal petrosectomy

A

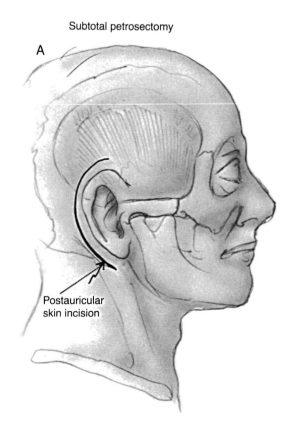

Postauricular
skin incision

FIGURE 46–4. *Illustration continued on opposite page*

FIGURE 46-4 (continued)

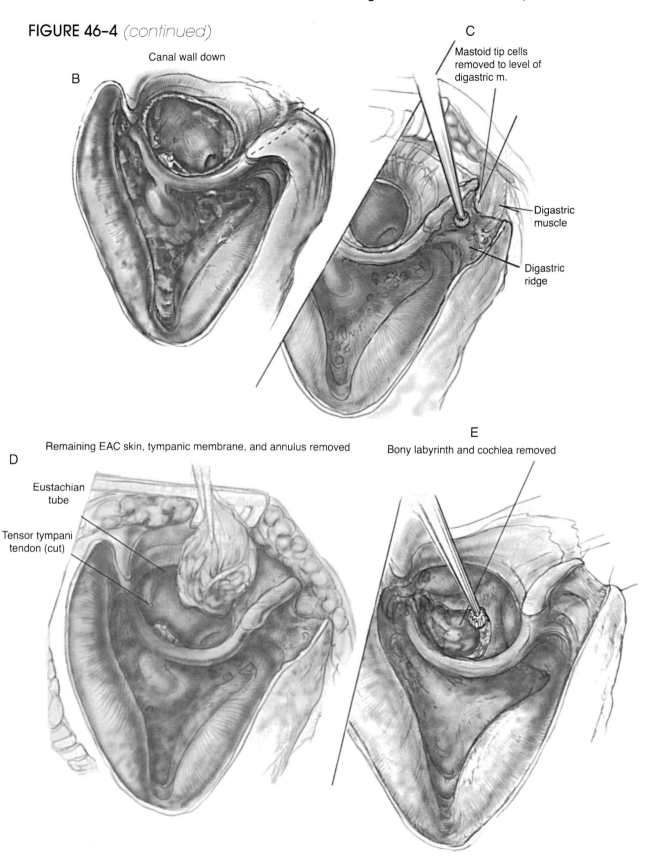

B

Canal wall down

C

Mastoid tip cells removed to level of digastric m.

Digastric muscle

Digastric ridge

D

Remaining EAC skin, tympanic membrane, and annulus removed

Eustachian tube

Tensor tympani tendon (cut)

E

Bony labyrinth and cochlea removed

FIGURE 46-4. *Illustration continued on following page*

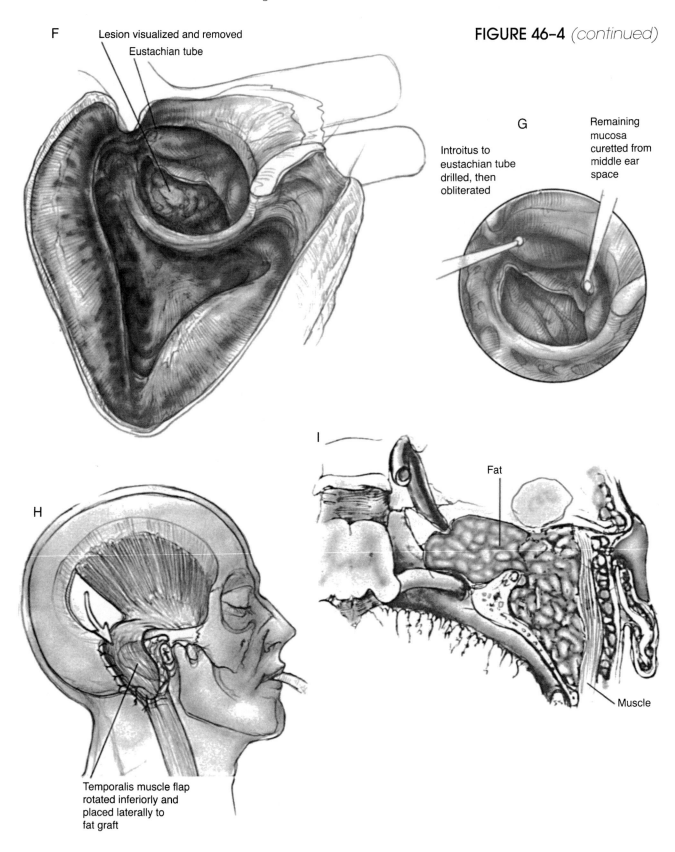

FIGURE 46–4 *(continued)*

F — Lesion visualized and removed
Eustachian tube

G — Introitus to eustachian tube drilled, then obliterated

Remaining mucosa curetted from middle ear space

I — Fat

Muscle

H — Temporalis muscle flap rotated inferiorly and placed laterally to fat graft

FIGURE 46–4. *A* to *I,* Subtotal petrosectomy approach to the petrous apex. EAC, external auditory canal.

sected. External auditory canal epithelium is everted, and the canal is sutured closed with a layer of periosteum sutured medially to form a two-layer closure (Fig. 46–4*A*).

2. A canal wall down tympanomastoidectomy is performed, and the posterior canal wall is lowered to the level of the facial nerve (Fig. 46–4*B*).

3. The mastoid tip cells are removed to the level of the digastric muscle (Fig. 46–4*C*).

4. The remaining external auditory canal skin, tympanic membrane, and annulus are removed after section of the incudostapedial joint and tensor tympani muscle (Fig. 46–4*D*).

5. Retrolabyrinthine, supralabyrinthine, supratubal, infralabyrinthine, and retrofacial air cells are then removed under direct vision. The bony labyrinth and cochlea are also removed without transposition of the facial nerve (Fig. 46–4*E*).

6. The lesion and its matrix or capsule are then removed under direct vision (Fig. 46–4*F*).

7. The remaining mucosa is gently curetted from the middle ear space. The introitus from the middle ear to the eustachian tube is drilled with a diamond burr, and the remaining mucosa is cauterized. The tube is obliterated with bone wax, muscle, and then fibrin glue (Fig. 46–4*G*).

8. The cavity is obliterated with abdominal fat, and a temporalis muscle flap is rotated inferiorly, then sutured lateral to the fat graft (Fig. 46–4*H* and *I*).

9. The incision is closed in layers, and a mastoid dressing is applied.

CONCLUSIONS

The combination of high-resolution CT and MRI makes it possible to reliably predict the character of petrous apex lesions preoperatively. Solid tumors and cholesteatoma may require destructive procedures, with cranial nerve and major vessel sacrifice for complete removal. Cystic lesions may be approached conservatively. Providing long-term adequate drainage frequently relieves all symptoms and provides long-term control. We prefer the transcanal infracochlear approach to the petrous apex for cystic lesions because of its direct approach, dependent drainage, universal applicability, and simplified revision, if necessary.

References

1. Hollinshead WH: The ear. *In* Anatomy for Surgeons, Vol 1. Philadelphia, Harper & Row, 1982, pp 159–221.

2. Myerson MC, Rubin J, Gilbert JG: Anatomic studies of the petrous portion of the temporal bone. Arch Otolaryngol Head Neck Surg 20: 195–210, 1934.

3. Roland PS, Meyerhoff WL, Judge LO, Mickey BE: Asymmetric pneumatization of the petrous apex. Otolaryngol Head Neck Surg 103: 80–88, 1990.

4. Lipper MH, Cail WS: Chordoma of the petrous bone. South Med J 84: 629–631, 1991.

5. Sekhar LN, Pomeranz S, Janecka IP, et al: Temporal bone neoplasms: A report on 20 surgically treated cases. J Neurosurg 76: 578–587, 1992.

6. Bourgouin PM, Tampieri D, Robitaille Y, et al: Low-grade myxoid chondrosarcoma of the base of the skull: CT, MR, and histopathology. J Comput Assist Tomogr 16: 268–273, 1992.

7. Hendershot EL, Wood JW: The middle fossa approach in the treatment of petrositis. Arch Otolaryngol Head Neck Surg 98: 426–427, 1973.

8. Frenckner P: Some remarks on the treatment of apicitis (petrositis) with or without Gradenigo's syndrome. Acta Otolaryngol (Stockh) 17: 97–120, 1932.

9. Mawson SR: Complications of otitis media. *In* Ludman H (ed): Mawson's Diseases of the Ear. Baltimore, William & Wilkins, 1963, pp 347–352.

10. Dearmin RM: A logical approach to the tip cells of the petrous pyramid. Arch Otolaryngol Head Neck Surg 26: 314–320, 1937.

11. Farrior JB: Anterior hypotympanic approach for glomus tumor of the infratemporal fossa. Laryngoscope 94: 1016–1020, 1984.

12. Giddings NA, Brackmann DE, Kwartler JA: Transcanal infracochlear approach to the petrous apex. Otolaryngol Head Neck Surg 104: 29–36, 1991.

13. Ghorayeb BY, Jahrsdoerfer RA: Subcochlear approach for cholesterol granulomas of the inferior petrous apex. Otolaryngol Head Neck Surg 103: 60–65, 1990.

14. Ramadier J: Exploration de la pointe du rocher par la voie du canal carotidien. Ann Otolaryngol 4: 422–444, 1933.

15. Eagleton WP: Unlocking the petrous apex for localized bulbar (pontile) meningitis secondary to suppuration of the petrous apex. Arch Otolaryngol Head Neck Surg 13: 386–422, 1931.

16. Lempert J: Complete apicectomy (mastoidotympanoapicectomy). Arch Otolaryngol Head Neck Surg 25: 144–177, 1937.

17. Gherini SG, Brackmann DE, Low WW, Solti-Bohman LG: Cholesterol granuloma of the petrous apex. Laryngoscope 95: 659–664, 1985.

18. Jackler RK, Parker DA: Radiographic differential diagnosis of petrous apex lesions. Am J Otol 13: 561–574, 1992.

19. Thedinger BA, Nadol JB, Montgomery WW, et al: Radiographic diagnosis, surgical treatment, and long-term follow-up of cholesterol granulomas of the petrous apex. Laryngoscope 99: 896–907, 1989.

20. Graham MD, Kemink JL, Latack JT, Kartush JM: The giant cholesterol cyst of the petrous apex: A distinct clinical entity. Laryngoscope 95: 1401–1406, 1985.

21. Davis AE, Robin PE: Transpalatal approach to the petrous apex. J Laryngol Otol 103: 94–96, 1989.

22. Congdon E: The distribution and mode of origin of septa and walls of the sphenoid sinus. Anat Rec 18: 97, 1920.

23. Van Alyea OE: Sphenoid sinus: Anatomic study, with consideration of the clinical significance of the structural characteristics of the sphenoid sinus. Arch Otolaryngol Head Neck Surg 34: 225, 1941.

24. Fisch U, Mattox D: Microsurgery of the Skull Base. New York, Thieme, 1988.

47

Surgery for Glomus and Jugular Foramen Tumors

Derald E. Brackmann ▪ Moisés A. Arriaga

SURGERY FOR GLOMUS TUMORS
(and Other Lesions of the Jugular Foramen)

The therapy for glomus tumors of the temporal bone continues to be controversial. Because the clinical characteristics and growth rates of these tumors are variable, the full gamut of management has been recommended from observation alone through radiation therapy and surgical management. Although there are isolated case reports of prolonged survival without treatment, these lesions can be quite deadly. The studies of Rosenwasser, Brown, Spector and associates, and others have documented mortality rates from 5 to 13 per cent for glomus jugulare tumors.[1-5] This chapter outlines the diagnostic and preoperative evaluation, surgical techniques, and results and complications in the management of glomus tumors of the temporal bone. In addition, the application of these surgical techniques for other lesions of the jugular foramen is reviewed.

PATIENT SELECTION

Temporal bone glomus tumors are neoplasms of the normal paraganglioma in the temporal bone that principally occur in the adventitia of the dome of the jugular bulb but are also found in the submucosa of the cochlear promontory within the tympanic plexus. Numerous classification schemes have been proposed for these lesions, primarily by their origin (tympanic plexus versus jugular bulb) and the anatomic extent of lesion. The clinical surgical classification proposed by Antonio De La Cruz is particularly useful in planning the clinical management of patients with glomus tumors. The extent of the tumor is described by the involvement of structures of the temporal bone and skull base. A series of operations that correspond to the extent of the tumor is used (Table 47–1). Other schemes include the Fisch (Table 47–2) and the Glasscock-Jackson classifications (Table 47–3).

Tympanic Tumor. This lesion arises from the glomus body of the promontory along Jacobson's nerve. The tumor is confined entirely to the mesotympanum, and all of its borders can be seen with routine otoscopy. This small tumor could not arise from the jugular bulb or it would extend beyond the inferior margins of the tympanic annulus. Although no additional studies are necessary to define the extent of the tumor, any vascular tumor of the middle ear must be differentiated from an aberrant carotid artery or a dehiscent jugular bulb. The aberrant carotid artery lies more anteriorly and is paler than the glomus tumor. The jugular bulb lies more posteriorly and is darker blue. If there is any question about the existence of either of these lesions, cranial computed tomography (CT) must be done to exclude them.

Tympanomastoid Tumor. Like the tympanic tumor, this lesion arises from the glomus body on the promontory. However, it extends beyond the tympanic annulus inferiorly or posteriorly. Because there is no way clinically to delineate the tumor's extent, any patient with a tumor that extends beyond the tympanic annulus must have a thorough radiographic evaluation. The key feature of this tumor category is that studies will show that the lesion does not involve the jugular bulb itself. However, tympanomastoid tumors may extend into the mastoid and into the retrofacial air cells.

Jugular Bulb Tumor. This lesion arises from the glomus body of the dome of the jugular bulb. It may extend into the middle ear and also into the bulb itself. This lesion is limited to involvement of the middle ear, the mastoid, and the jugular bulb. By definition, it does not extend onto the carotid artery or medially into the skull base or intracranially.

Carotid Artery Glomus Tumor. This lesion arises from the jugular bulb but extends beyond the confines of the jugular bulb and vein and contacts the carotid artery. Small tumors of this category may involve only the carotid artery at the skull base, whereas larger tumors may extend far medially and may also involve the horizontal portions of the internal carotid artery and the petrous apex.

Transdural Tumor. These lesions arise from the jugular bulb and extend not only to the internal carotid artery but also through the jugular foramen intracranially.

Glomus Vagale Tumor. These lesions arise from the glomus body along the vagus nerve at the base of the skull.

TABLE 47–1. De La Cruz Glomus Tumor Classification with Associated Surgical Approach

CLASSIFICATION	SURGICAL APPROACH
1. Tympanic	Transcanal
2. Tympanomastoid	Mastoid–extended facial recess
3. Jugular bulb	Mastoid-neck (possible limited facial nerve rerouting)
4. Carotid artery	Infratemporal fossa ± subtemporal
5. Transdural	Infratemporal fossa/intracranial
6. Craniocervical	Transcondylar
7. Vagale	Cervical

478

TABLE 47–2. Fisch Glomus Tumor Classification

TYPE	CRITERIA
A	Tumors limited to the middle ear cleft
B	Tumors limited to the tympanomastoid area with no infralabyrinthine compartment involvement
C1, 2, 3	Tumors involving the infralabyrinthine compartment of the temporal bone and extending into the petrous apex
D1	Tumors with an intracranial extension < 2 cm in diameter
D2, 3	Tumors with an intracranial extension > 2 cm in diameter

Because glomus vagale tumors do not begin within the temporal bone, they are often larger than glomus tumors of the temporal bone itself because they later produce symptoms of pulsatile tinnitus and hearing loss. Clinically, these lesions produce vocal cord paralysis prior to the onset of hearing loss or tinnitus or the appearance of a vascular middle ear mass. In contrast, glomus tumors of the temporal bone produce otologic symptoms prior to the onset of vocal cord paralysis.[6]

Jugular Foramen Schwannoma. Schwannomas of the jugular foramen are extremely rare even though they are the second most frequently occurring tumor of the jugular foramen. They arise from the Schwann cells of the cranial nerves IX, X, and XI. The most common cranial nerve to be affected is the vagus nerve.[7, 8] The clinical distinction between glomus vagale tumors and vagale schwannomas is that glomus vagale tumors develop vocal cord paralysis early in their course.[9]

Presentation of the jugular foramen schwannoma depends on the growth pattern. Kaye categorized three different patterns: A, B, and C. The type A tumors present primarily in the posterior fossa. Type A tumors with intracranial extension may present with ninth, tenth, or eleventh cranial nerve palsies. However, like most cerebellopontine angle tumors, hearing loss and/or imbalance may be the only significant presenting symptoms. Type B tumors remain confined to the skull base with extension often into the clivus. Type C tumors begin in the jugular foramen and extend inferiorly into the neck. Type B and C tumors

TABLE 47–3. Glassock-Jackson Glomus Tumor Classification

TYPE	PHYSICAL FINDINGS
Glomus Tympanicum	
I	Small mass limited to the promontory
II	Tumor completely filling middle ear space
III	Tumor filling middle ear and extending into mastoid
IV	Tumor filling middle ear, extending into mastoid or through tympanic membrane to fill external auditory canal; may also extend anterior to internal carotid artery
Glomus Jugulare	
I	Small tumor involving jugulare bulb, middle ear, and mastoid
II	Tumor extending under the internal auditory canal; may have intracranial extension
III	Tumor extending into petrous apex; may have intracranial extension
IV	Tumor extending beyond petrous apex into clivus or infratemporal foss; may have intracranial extension

present more frequently with lower cranial neuropathies than type A tumors.[10]

Radiologic assessment is performed with magnetic resonance imaging (MRI) and computed tomographic (CT) scanning. MRI of the jugular foramen schwannoma demonstrates a smooth, contoured mass isodense on T1W, high signal intensity is usually noted on T2W, and significant enhancement occurs on T1W gadolinium scans. CT is helpful in differentiating schwannoma from glomus jugulare tumors. Schwannomas tend to produce smooth erosion of the jugular foramen. Glomus tumors tend to show an irregular bone margin at the jugulare foramen. The third most common lesions in this area are meningiomas of the jugulare foramen. These lesions may be difficult to distinguish from schwannomas preoperatively. An enhancing "dural tail" on MRI is helpful. They also tend to infiltrate the bone around the jugular foramen rather than smoothly enlarge it.

PREOPERATIVE EVALUATION

Thorough preoperative evaluation permits surgical planning for complete and safe tumor removal. Advances in imaging technology now permit accurate preoperative assessment of tumor involvement within the temporal bone. The following tests are routinely used in the evaluation of patients with glomus tumors of the temporal bone.

Routine Hearing Tests

Air, bone, and speech audiometry are performed to assess the degree of conductive and sensorineural hearing impairments.

Cranial Computed Tomography

The mainstay of assessment of glomus tumors of the temporal bone is thin-section (1.5-mm-thick) cranial CT using the bone algorithm. Tumors confined to the middle ear and mastoid are distinguished from tumors that involve the jugular bulb. Extensive lesions that extend onto or medial to the internal carotid artery and those that extend transdurally are also defined by this technique. In many cases, cranial CT is the only examination necessary for planning treatment. Because the jugular bulb is the major consideration in preoperative planning, cranial CT has supplanted retrograde jugular venography in assessing involvement of the jugular bulb.

Magnetic Resonance Imaging

Because bone involvement by tumor is not clearly demonstrated on MRI, this technique provides only adjunctive information regarding the extent of tumor involvement. If the diagnosis is at all in question, MRI combined with CT provides exquisite preoperative guidance in the differential diagnosis of petrous apex lesions.[11] MRI can indicate occlusion of the jugular bulb and vein because the normal flow signals are altered. In intradural tumors, MRI can more clearly delineate the tumor-brain interface and the relationship of the lesion to the intradural structures. MRI must be interpreted cautiously because T1W images of glomus tumors may overestimate the degree of tumor involvement. Marrow-containing bone of the petrous apex is hyperintense and indistinguishable from enhancing tumor in the petrous apex. MR angiography and MR venography offer another diagnostic tool in evaluating glomus tumors. In their present form, however, MR angiographic techniques cannot provide adequate imaging resolution to define feeding vessels to the tumor. The role of these techniques in the preoperative assessment of glomus tumors has not been fully clarified.[12, 13]

Arteriography

Four-vessel angiography is necessary when cranial CT demonstrates a glomus tumor involving the jugular bulb, carotid artery, or intradural structures. The principal indication for angiography is assessment of the involvement of the internal carotid artery by tumor. Additionally, this technique ensures preoperative identification of additional glomus lesions, if present. Although estimates vary, paragangliomas are multicentric in approximately 10 per cent of nonfamilial cases and 33 per cent in familial cases.

Brain Perfusion and Flow Studies

For tumors that abut the internal carotid artery, it is necessary to assess the adequacy of the cerebral cross-perfusion from the contralateral internal carotid artery. Cross-compression angiography, stump-pressure measurements, and clinical evaluation during test occlusion of the involved carotid are basic guides to the risk of stroke in the event that the affected carotid artery must be sacrificed. Xenon blood flow and radioisotope studies offer much more precise quantification of the risk of stroke and the possible need for surgical replacement of the internal carotid artery.[14] In certain cases with extensive invasion of the carotid artery and acceptable results on the perfusion studies of the contralateral artery, the involved carotid artery may be permanently occluded with a detachable balloon. We generally do not recommend carotid sacrifice. Despite excellent advances in diagnostic flow studies, an appreciable risk (about 5 per cent) of stroke exists with carotid artery sacrifice even in cases with favorable functional and perfusion characteristics or test occlusion studies. If possible, repair or graft replacement of the carotid is recommended if the carotid is injured during tumor removal.

Embolization

Large glomus tumors may result in significant intraoperative blood loss. We have found that preoperative embolization of feeding vessels can significantly reduce such loss.[15] The embolization is usually performed with Ivalon and is done at the time of angiography, 1 or 2 days before surgery. A longer interval between embolization and surgery may result in collateral blood flow to the tumor that may paradoxically increase tumor perfusion and intraoperative blood loss.

Biopsy

Biopsy of vascular middle ear masses is not recommended. The clinical and radiographic appearance of glomus tumors is characteristic enough to permit definitive management without a tissue diagnosis. Efforts at obtaining a tissue diagnosis prior to completion of the radiologic evaluation can result in injury to an aberrant carotid artery or a high jugular bulb as well as significant bleeding from the tumor itself.

PATIENT COUNSELING

Patients with tympanic and tympanomastoid glomus tumors are advised of the routine risks of exploratory tympanotomy and tympanomastoidectomy surgery. However, as discussed later in this chapter, the prognosis for these patients is excellent if total tumor removal is accomplished.

Patients with jugular bulb, carotid artery, or transdural tumors should be aware of the additional risk inherent in complete removal of their tumors. Specifically, facial nerve transposition is generally necessary and carries the attendant risk of facial paresis. Furthermore, these patients should be aware of the risk of lower cranial nerve injury and possible vascular complications as well. Any patient with intradural tumor extension must be aware of the risks of craniotomy, including postoperative hemorrhage, cerebrospinal fluid leakage, meningitis, and stroke.

SURGICAL APPROACHES

The following surgical techniques are used for removal of glomus tumors of the temporal bone. Notice that the specific approaches described correspond to the tumor classification system described earlier.

Transcanal Approach

The transcanal approach is used for small glomus tympanicum tumors that are limited to the mesotympanum. Because the entire circumference of the tumor is visible within the middle ear, preoperative imaging studies are not necessary. However, if there is any doubt of the possibility of an aberrant internal carotid artery, preoperative CT scanning should be obtained to exclude this possibility. The tympanomeatal flap is modified with the inferior incision extending more anteriorly so that the inferior aspect of the tympanic membrane can be elevated. The tumor is identified on the promontory (Fig. 47–1).

The inferior tympanic branch of the ascending pharyngeal artery supplies the glomus tympanicum tumor. The vessel may be controlled with bipolar cautery or a small piece of oxidized cellulose (Surgicel) to occlude the bony canaliculus from which the vessel arises. It is critical to

FIGURE 47-1

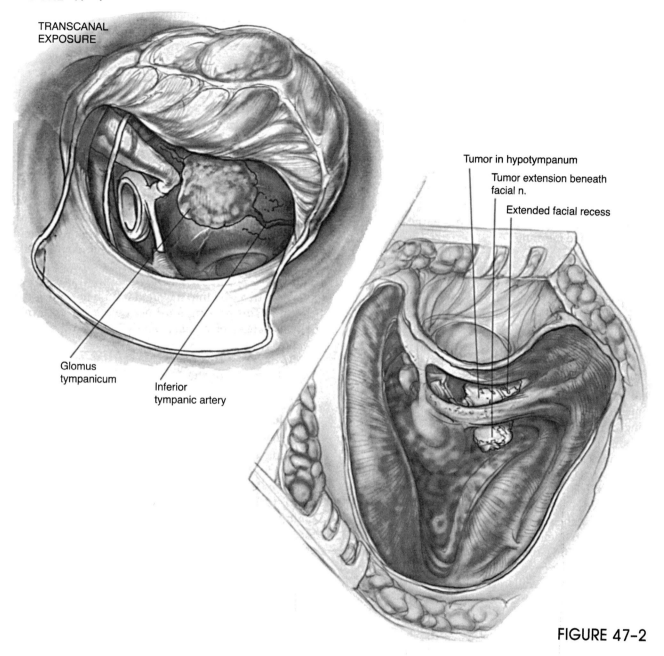

TRANSCANAL
EXPOSURE

Glomus
tympanicum

Inferior
tympanic artery

Tumor in hypotympanum

Tumor extension beneath
facial n.

Extended facial recess

FIGURE 47-2

FIGURE 47–1. Transcanal exposure of glomus tympanicum tumor limited to the promontory.

FIGURE 47–2. The facial recess has been opened widely and extended inferiorly to expose tumor in the hypotympanum. Tumor extension beneath the facial nerve is exposed by removing the retrofacial air cells and skeletonizing the facial nerve.

avoid unipolar cautery on the tympanic promontory, because this may severely injure the cochlea.

The tumor is then removed with cup forceps. The brisk bleeding from the distal end of the artery anterior to the stapes (near the cochleariform process) is difficult to control directly; however, it usually clots readily. Small pledgets of oxidized cellulose assist in hemostasis, and the tympanomeatal flap is replaced and the ear canal packed. No specific dressing is necessary, and the patient is ready for hospital discharge the following day. Accurate preoperative assessment is crucial for success with the transcanal approach for glomus tympanicum tumors. If the entire circumference of the lesion is not visible through the meatus, the hypotympanotomy or mastoid-extended facial recess approach should be considered.

Tumors with limited hypotympanic extension without posterior involvement on CT scan may be removed by a modified transcanal (hypotympanic) approach.[16] After a postauricular incision is performed with transection of the ear canal, a superiorly based tympanomeatal flap is elevated to permit access to the inferior aspect of the tympanic ring. This bone is progressively drilled until the inferior limit of the tumor is identified. The drilling involved with this exposure is usually much less than the drilling required for the transcanal infracochlear drainage procedures for the petrous apex described in Chapter 46.

Mastoid–Extended Facial Recess Approach

The mastoid–extended facial recess approach is used for tympanomastoid glomus tumors. The tumor may extensively involve the middle ear and mastoid but has arisen from the glomus tympanicum body and does not involve the jugular bulb. Preoperative CT evaluation is critical before this approach is undertaken. Because the limits of the tumor are not visible through the tympanic membrane, CT provides an assessment of the extent of tumor involvement. Patient preparation and draping are performed as for a routine tympanomastoidectomy. A wide shave is performed, and the incision is made 1.5 cm posterior to the postauricular sulcus. After a complete mastoidectomy, the facial recess is opened. The extended facial recess exposure is performed by further bone removal inferiorly accomplished by severing the chorda tympani nerve and following the fibrous annulus of the tympanic membrane as a landmark. Such an approach allows complete exposure of the middle ear and the hypotympanum. After the tumor is exposed, bipolar cautery is helpful in shrinking the tumor and in controlling the blood supply. Oxidized cellulose packs are used to further tamponade the main arterial supply in the hypotympanum, and the tumor is removed with cup forceps. The tumor can be stripped from the ossicles if necessary.

Extension of glomus tympanicum tumors into the retrofacial air cells is managed by direct exposure. A cutting burr is used to remove the air cells inferior to the labyrinth and beneath the facial nerve, thereby leaving the facial nerve suspended with a thin layer of bone to allow the surgeon access to the entire hypotympanum (Fig. 47–2). A small curette is used to remove bits of the tumor from crevices in the hypotympanum. The dome of the jugular bulb can be inspected to be certain that it is free of the tumor.

Extensive tumor involvement may necessitate removal of the ossicles and tympanic membrane. In such circumstances, a tympanoplasty and ossicular reconstruction may be accomplished in the routine manner. Similarly, if the tumor has produced extensive destruction of the posterior canal wall, such cases may be managed with a canal wall down technique combined with tympanoplasty and mastoid obliteration after complete tumor removal. At the conclusion of the procedure, a mastoid dressing is applied, and the patient is usually ready for discharge by the first postoperative morning.

Mastoid and Neck Approach

The mastoid and neck approach is used for small glomus jugulare tumors. These tumors involve the jugular bulb but do not extend onto the internal carotid artery or into the neck or posterior fossa. The preoperative evaluation of these patients may include angiography because involvement of the jugular bulb raises the question of possible carotid artery involvement. Continuous intraoperative facial nerve monitoring is used. Additionally, electromyographic electrodes in the sternocleidomastoid muscle are useful for monitoring cranial nerve XI, electrodes in the lateral pharyngeal wall can monitor cranial nerve IX, and electrodes in the vocalis muscle can monitor cranial nerve X. Specially designed endotracheal tubes with attached electromyographic electrodes are particularly useful for monitoring lower cranial nerve function. The procedure is performed by initially completing the same exposure as that described in the mastoid–extended facial recess approach (see Fig. 47–2), then amputating the mastoid tip. The periosteum of the digastric groove is followed anteriorly until it turns abruptly laterally at the stylomastoid foramen. Drilling laterally along the digastric ridge both anteriorly and posteriorly frees the entire mastoid tip. The incision is then carried into the neck along the anterior border of the sternocleidomastoid muscle. This muscle is freed from the mastoid tip and retracted posteriorly. The mastoid tip can then be removed by grabbing it with a Kocher clamp and cutting with a curved Mayo scissors along the bone. The posterior belly of the digastric muscle is identified and freed from the digastric groove and retracted anteriorly to allow exposure of the major neurovascular structures of the neck. Once the internal jugular vein is identified and dissected free from surrounding tissues, it is occluded with multiple 2-0 silk sutures. The jugular vein is followed over the transverse process of the first cervical vertebra into the base of the skull. In this fashion, the eleventh cranial nerve is identified (usually lateral to the vein) and preserved.

In limited tumors that do not extend into the neck or skull base, it is usually possible to preserve the ninth, tenth, and eleventh cranial nerves. The neck exposure is necessary to permit ligation of the jugular vein.

Exposure of the sigmoid sinus and jugular bulb is then completed with diamond burrs. Although limited tumors do not involve the medial wall of the jugular foramen, the tumor arises from the dome of the jugular bulb, and the bulb must be resected in continuity with the tumor. The proximal sigmoid sinus is controlled with extraluminal packing of oxidized cellulose. Preservation of the bone over the midportion of the sigmoid sinus permits extraluminal packing of this portion of the sigmoid sinus. Because the jugular vein has been tied in the neck, the sigmoid sinus may be opened just distal to the proximal packing. Bleeding occurs at this point from the patent inferior petrosal sinus and condylar vein. Oxidized cellulose is advanced into the jugular bulb to control this bleeding. This packing must not be placed too firmly, because a weakness of cranial nerves IX, X, and XI may result.

The tumor is now ready for resection in continuity with the dome of the jugular bulb. Bipolar cautery helps in hemostasis and shrinkage of the tumor bulk. Once the tumor and dome of the jugular bulb are excised, hemostasis is completed with oxidized cellulose packing (Fig. 47–3). Complete tumor resection is accomplished, and if the tympanic membrane or ossicles are involved, reconstruction may be performed as described earlier. It is usually possible to preserve the ninth, tenth, and eleventh cranial nerves with these limited tumors unless there is preoperative involvement of these structures. Postoperatively, these patients are cared for in the intensive care unit because the possibility of an acute lower cranial neuropathy or major postoperative hemorrhage exists. Usually, minimal morbidity is associated with this approach, and patients are stable and may be discharged from the hospital within a few days. The major pitfall associated with this approach is related to inaccurate preoperative assessment of tumor extent. The mastoid-neck approach is too limited if the tumor extensively involves the carotid artery.

Mastoid and Neck with Limited Facial Nerve Rerouting

A useful modification of the mastoid-neck approach adds a limited facial nerve rerouting to the procedure. Additional exposure in the mastoid-neck approach may be achieved by totally decompressing the facial nerve from the second genu throughout the entire vertical segment. The periosteum of the facial nerve at the stylomastoid foramen is preserved, but the fibrous attachments to the nerve in its vertical portion are sharply transected. The mobilized nerve can be transposed laterally along with the periosteum at the stylomastoid foramen and the attached posterior belly of the digastric muscle. A suture through the stylomastoid periosteum can be used to hold the nerve laterally and prevent traction on this structure. Such transposition of the facial nerve will permit further bone removal in the area of the vertical facial canal and retrofacial air cells along the infralabyrinthine air-cell tract (Fig. 47–4). This modification of the mastoid and neck approach with limited facial nerve rerouting is ideal for neuromas of the jugular foramen because they are not as intimately involved with the carotid artery as are glomus tumors. The surgeon should be cautious about applying this approach for glomus tumors that involve the carotid artery. The annulus and posterior canal wall still limit the surgeon's view of the vertical

portion of the carotid artery if extensive manipulation is necessary in this area.

Infratemporal Fossa Approach

The development of the infratemporal fossa approach by Fisch has been a significant advance in our ability to totally remove large glomus jugulare tumors.[17] Previous approaches that did not remove the external auditory canal or reroute the facial nerve did not allow adequate exposure of the tumor or internal carotid artery (Fig. 47–5). There are eight distinct steps in the infratemporal fossa exposure: (1) patient preparation; (2) management of the ear canal and tympanic ring; (3) mastoidectomy; (4) initial preparation of the jugular vein and neck exposure; (5) transposition of the facial nerve; (6) completion of the neck exposure and identification of the lower cranial nerves and skull base carotid artery; (7) tumor removal including intracranial extension; and (8) wound closure. Continuous facial nerve monitoring and electromyographic monitoring of the lower cranial nerves are employed as previously described.

A wide shave is performed, and a large postauricular incision is made in a C-shaped fashion. The incision is carried anteriorly, and the ear canal is transected slightly medially to the bone-cartilage junction of the ear canal. Cartilage is removed from the ear canal to permit fashioning of the ear canal skin as a cuff that can be everted. The skin of the meatus is closed with 4-0 nylon sutures. The periosteum of the postauricular area is elevated as a flap and sutured behind the opening in the meatus to further reinforce the closure (see Chapter 59, Figs. 59–4 and 59–5). Next, a mastoidectomy is completed, and the facial recess is opened to allow separation of the incudostapedial joint. The posterior wall of the ear canal can then be removed with rongeurs and cutting burrs. The remaining skin of the ear canal as well as the tympanic membrane, malleus, and incus are removed. Next, the facial nerve is decompressed from the geniculate to the stylomastoid foramen. An eggshell-thin layer of bone is left over the nerve itself. By use of cutting and diamond burrs, the bone of the tympanic ring is progressively removed, the level of the jugular bulb is identified, and the bone over the temporomandibular joint and vertical segment of the petrous carotid artery is removed anteriorly (Fig. 47–6).

Attention is then focused on the neck. The incision is continued vertically along the anterior border of the sternocleidomastoid muscle, the mastoid tip is removed as previously described, the jugular vein is identified, and ligatures are placed around the vein but are not yet tied at this point. The carotid artery is identified and marked with a ligature. The posterior belly of the digastric muscle is transected.

Next, the facial nerve is transposed. The transposition technique originally described by Fisch has been modified because of temporary and sometimes permanent residual facial weakness.[18] Rather than exposing the facial nerve in the parotid, the surgeon transposes the nerve with periosteum of the stylomastoid foramen and elevates the entire tail of the parotid.[19] After the nerve is decompressed, the remaining eggshell-thin bone over the facial nerve is removed with a blunt instrument. The multiple fibrous con-

FIGURE 47–3

Facial nerve in
fallopian canal

Digastric muscle and parotid
gland retracted

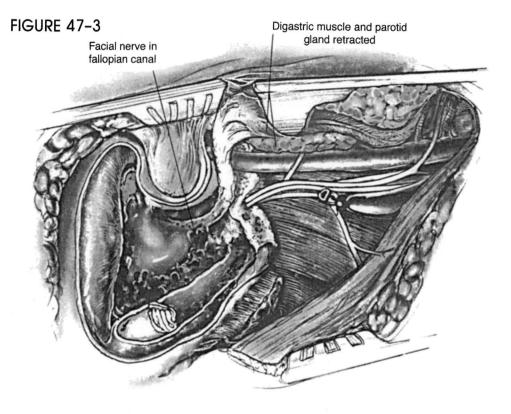

FIGURE 47–4

Tumor

Facial nerve
transposed from
bony canal and
elevated against
external auditory canal

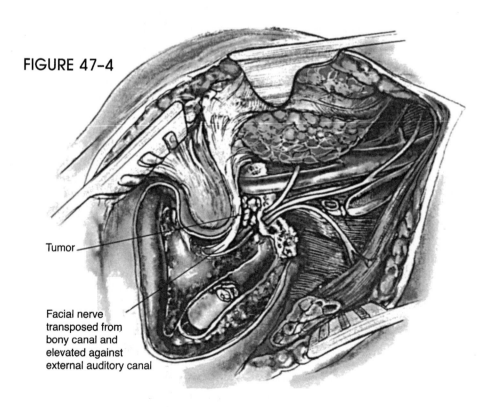

FIGURE 47–3. Completed procedure using mastoid-neck approach. The jugular bulb is resected along with the tumor after proximal and distal vessels are controlled.

FIGURE 47–4. Mastoid-neck approach with limited facial nerve rerouting. Displacement of the facial nerve exposes larger tumors of the jugular bulb.

nections along the descending portion of the nerve are sharply transected. The tympanic portion of the nerve does not have such adhesions, and this section elevates readily. The posterior belly of the digastric muscle is moved anteriorly because the fascia of this muscle contributes to the stylomastoid foramen periosteum. The nerve can then be transposed anteriorly along with the tail of the parotid. A large suture is placed through the periosteum of the stylomastoid foramen and attached to the soft tissues in the area of the root of the zygoma (Fig. 47–7), thereby elevating the facial nerve and preventing it from being stretched when retractors are placed. The use of continuous facial nerve monitoring during this maneuver has significantly improved postoperative facial nerve function.[20]

After the facial nerve is decompressed and elevated, a large Perkins retractor is placed beneath the angle of the mandible, and the entire mandible is retracted forward. This exposure avoids the need to resect the mandibular condyle, even in large tumors that extend into the infratemporal fossa extensively. The remaining bone over the distal sigmoid sinus, jugular bulb, and vertical portion of the petrous carotid artery can be removed with diamond burrs. Attention is once again focused in the neck, where the internal carotid artery is followed through the skull base into its intratemporal course. The lower cranial nerves (IX to XI) are followed into the jugular foramen as well. The twelfth cranial nerve is also identified and followed to its foramen.

The jugular vein is doubly ligated and transected between ligatures, and the external carotid artery is ligated. If the tumor extends intradurally, the proximal sigmoid sinus is double-ligated with silk sutures passed through openings in the dura with an aneurysm suture passer (Fig. 47–8). If the tumor is not intradural, then the sigmoid can be packed with Surgicel without violating the dura. The jugular vein is then elevated, and the tumor in the area of the jugular bulb is freed inferiorly to superiorly following the jugular vein into the jugular bulb. The tumor is freed from the carotid artery anteriorly, and bleeding from the caroticotympanic vessels is controlled with bipolar cautery. If the tumor is adherent to the internal carotid artery, it is best to leave a portion of it on the artery and remove the bulk of the tumor. Lower cranial nerve preservation is enhanced if the medial wall of the jugular bulb is left in situ protecting the pathway of the lower cranial nerves through the pars nervosa in the anteromedial portion of the jugular bulb. Tumor hemostasis is continued with bipolar cautery and oxidized cellulose packing of the inferior petrosal sinus; the tumor can be removed in continuity with the dome of the jugular bulb. If the last bit of the tumor from the carotid artery is not removed until the conclusion of the procedure, a small entry into the carotid artery that may occur at the location of the caroticotympanic artery can be repaired directly (Fig. 47–9).

Small intracranial tumor extensions are usually removed at the time of removal of the jugular bulb because this is the usual location of dural penetration. If there is extensive intracranial extension, however, a decision must be made about whether to attempt total removal of the tumor. The decision is largely based on the amount of blood lost to this point. If blood loss has been limited to less than 2000 ml, as is almost always the case, removal of the intracranial

extension of the tumor may proceed. However, if the amount of blood loss has been greater, problems with bleeding may occur despite the replenishment of the known clotting factors with fresh frozen plasma and platelet packs. In such cases, a two-stage procedure with removal of the intracranial portion of the tumor at a later date is planned.

The removal of the intracranial portion of the tumor is often easier than the removal of tumor within the temporal bone. By the time one is ready for the removal of the intracranial extension, the blood supply has often been controlled. The blood supply to the intracranial portion of the tumor is often discrete and can be controlled with bipolar cautery as with other cerebellopontine angle tumors (Fig. 47–10). If tumor has been left along the internal carotid artery, it is now removed. Closure is accomplished by closing the eustachian tube with oxidized cellulose, muscle, and strips of abdominal fat (Fig. 47–11). If cerebrospinal fluid has been encountered, continuous lumbar drainage is used for approximately 5 days until the wound is sealed (see Chapter 59). A drain is left in the neck wound and removed on the first postoperative morning. A pressure dressing is placed for 4 postoperative days.

One technique with encouraging results in cases with large blood loss has been the use of a Cell Saver (which is commonly used in cardiovascular surgery). By use of a special irrigating suction device with a heparinized reservoir, intraoperative blood loss can be salvaged and prepared for replacement to the patient during the same procedure. Additionally, we routinely counsel patients on preoperative autologous donation of blood to minimize the need for banked blood replacement. With these techniques, it is unusual to require banked blood transfusion even in large tumors.

Fallopian Bridge Technique

A new strategy for minimizing postoperative facial nerve dysfunction as well as enhancing preservation of the middle ear in jugular foramen surgery is the fallopian bridge technique (Fig. 47–12). In this technique, the facial nerve is left in situ but the bone surrounding the nerve is almost completely removed.[21] This technique can be utilized with the mastoid neck approach as an alternative to partial mobilization. It is even applicable with the full infratemporal fossa technique. Although the technique is relatively new, it promises to decrease the number of cases requiring facial nerve translocation with beneficial outcomes for postoperative facial nerve function and preservation of the conductive hearing mechanism.

Transcondylar Approach

In certain recurrent glomus jugulare tumors, the intracranial tumor may extend significantly toward the foramen magnum. In those situations, a wider exposure of the cranial cervical junction is necessary. Although the transigmoid translabyrinthine exposure combined with the intratemporal fossa approach offers a wide view, the cranial cervical junction itself is not fully exposed with this procedure. In this case, the transcondylar exposure is helpful with the

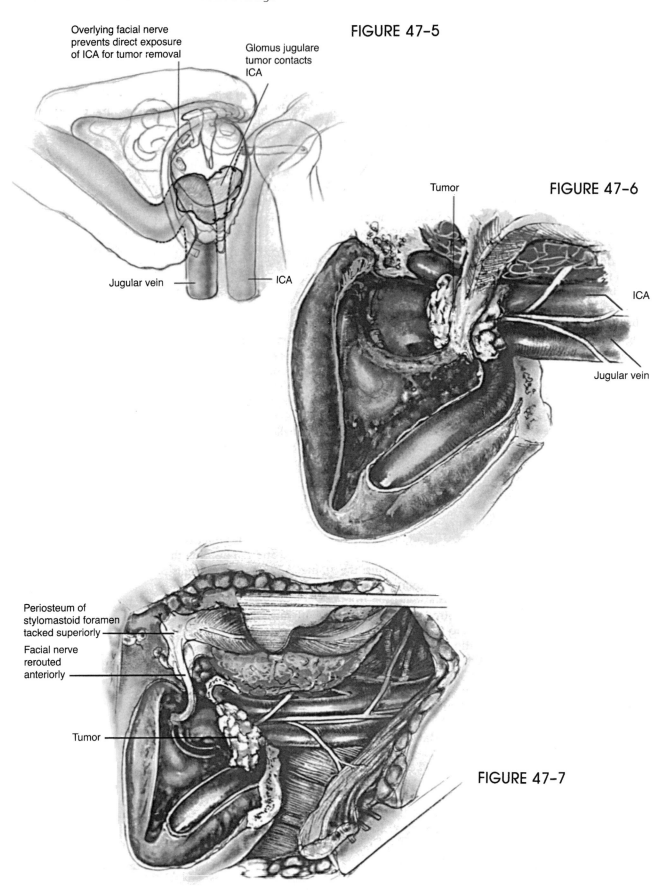

FIGURE 47-5

Overlying facial nerve
prevents direct exposure
of ICA for tumor removal

Glomus jugulare
tumor contacts
ICA

Jugular vein

ICA

FIGURE 47-6

Tumor

ICA

Jugular vein

Periosteum of
stylomastoid foramen
tacked superiorly

Facial nerve
rerouted
anteriorly

Tumor

FIGURE 47-7

FIGURES 47–5 to 47–7. *See legends on opposite page*

infratemporal fossa approach. The steps involved in the transcondylar approach[22] are initially extension of the muscular incisions of the posterior superior aspect of the neck to identify the vertebral artery posterior and inferior to the mastoid tip on the transverse process of C1. Once this landmark is clearly identified, wide exposure of the occipital condyle and jugular tubercle permits full exposure of the hypoglossal nerve and an unlimited view of the cranial cervical junction (Fig. 47–13). If more than one half of the occipital condyle is resected, careful consideration should be given to a simultaneous cervical stabilization procedure. When transcondylar exposure is needed in addition to standard otologic exposure, we find the use of head-holding pins in the lateral position helpful for access to the posterosuperior skull base.

Complete Carotid Mobilization

In rare cases of recurring glomus jugulare tumors following previous surgery and radiation, the tumor may actually completely encase the petrous carotid artery with significant extension into the far anterior infratemporal fossa. In these cases, we have found the combination of the standard otologic (posterior) infratemporal fossa approach with the preauricular infratemporal fossa approach quite useful. Specifically, an orbital zygotomy in continuity with the glenoid fossa is performed following a temporal craniotomy. In this fashion, the glenoid can be reconstructed at the conclusion of the procedure. The carotid canal can then be followed directly and fully from the base of the skull all the way to the cavernous sinus. In this way the carotid artery can be mobilized anteriorly and inferiorly if necessary for complete tumor resection. Furthermore, this approach facilitates any carotid reconstruction if necessary.

RESULTS

Glomus Tympanicum Tumors. O'Leary and associates reviewed the results of glomus tympanicum surgery at the House Ear Clinic.[23] Seventy-three glomus tympanicum tumors (tympanic tumor or tympanomastoid tumor) were managed at the Clinic between 1957 and 1990. Eighty per cent of these required a mastoid–facial recess approach, and in 20 per cent, a transcanal removal was possible. Although significant intraoperative blood loss occurred (average, > 500 ml), the morbidity was minimal. Hearing levels remained stable: the mean speech reception threshold increased 1 dB postoperatively. Of the five complications, three were residual tympanic membrane perforations requiring a secondary tympanoplasty. One patient developed

a cholesteatoma postoperatively. Another patient developed a facial nerve weakness requiring re-exploration and facial nerve decompression with an ultimately good outcome (II/VI on the House-Brackmann scale). This series demonstrated that the crucial feature of glomus tympanicum management is total tumor resection. The three cases in which an incomplete resection was performed resulted in tumor recurrence. Overall, the recurrence rate in this series was less than 5 per cent.

Glomus Jugulare Tumors. Green and colleagues reviewed the House Ear Clinic experience with glomus jugulare tumors (jugular bulb, carotid artery involvement tumors, and intradural tumors) between 1980 and 1991.[24] During this interval, 52 patients were surgically treated for glomus jugulare tumors who had undergone no prior radiotherapy or surgery. The techniques involved were the infratemporal fossa approach in 83 per cent, the mastoid-neck approach in 7 per cent, and the mastoid-neck with limited facial nerve mobilization in 10 per cent. Complete surgical removal was possible in 85 per cent of the patients. Eight patents required transection of the facial nerve for complete tumor removal. These patients underwent segmental grafting or greater auricular nerve reconstruction and achieved a grade III/VI facial nerve recovery. The mean intraoperative blood loss was 1500 ml. Long-term facial function was good: 95 per cent of patients who had facial nerve rerouting had grade I/VI or II/VI facial function at 1-year follow-up or later. Nearly 20 per cent of patients required a vocal cord augmentation procedure. However, no patient required a tracheotomy in the immediate postoperative period. Four patients required prolonged nasogastric tube feeding, and two ultimately required gastrostomy temporarily. None required long-term gastrostomy. Eighty-five per cent of the patients were able to resume the same activity level as before surgery.

COMPLICATIONS

Glomus Tympanicum Tumors. Glomus tympanicum surgery risks the same morbidity as that involved in tympanomastoid surgery. The management of associated facial nerve, tympanic membrane, sigmoid sinus, and healing complications is identical to that in tympanomastoid surgery for chronic otitis media.

Glomus Jugulare Tumors. As illustrated earlier (Results), the categories of morbidity in glomus jugulare surgery include facial nerve injury, lower cranial nerve dysfunction, carotid artery injury, bleeding problems, and intracranial complications. Direct tumor infiltration of the facial nerve necessitates transection of the involved segment and replacement of that segment with a nerve graft

Text continued on page 492

FIGURE 47–5. The overlying facial nerve prevents exposure of the internal carotid artery for tumor removal.

FIGURE 47–6. Temporal bone dissection completed. The facial nerve is skeletonized and the tympanic ring removed. The carotid artery and jugular bulb with tumor are exposed.

FIGURE 47–7. Facial nerve transposed anteriorly. A large suture tacks the periosteum of the stylomastoid foramen and facial nerve superiorly to avoid tension on the transposed nerve.

FIGURE 47-8

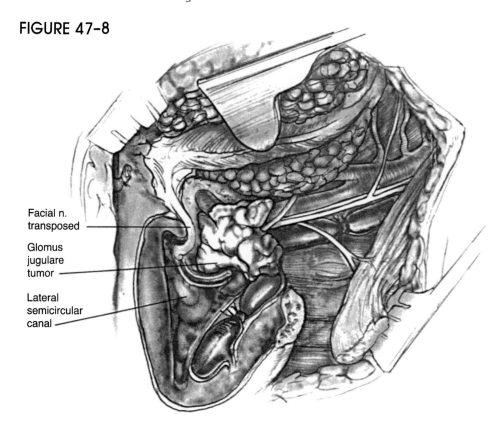

Facial n. transposed

Glomus jugulare tumor

Lateral semicircular canal

FIGURE 47-9

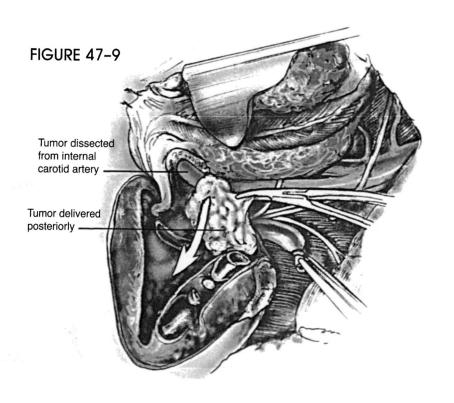

Tumor dissected from internal carotid artery

Tumor delivered posteriorly

FIGURE 47–8. The jugular vein and sigmoid sinus are doubly ligated. If the tumor does not extend intradurally, the sigmoid is occluded with extraluminal packing.

FIGURE 47–9. Final piece of tumor removed from carotid artery. The artery may be repaired with vascular suture if injury occurs with total tumor removal.

FIGURE 47-10

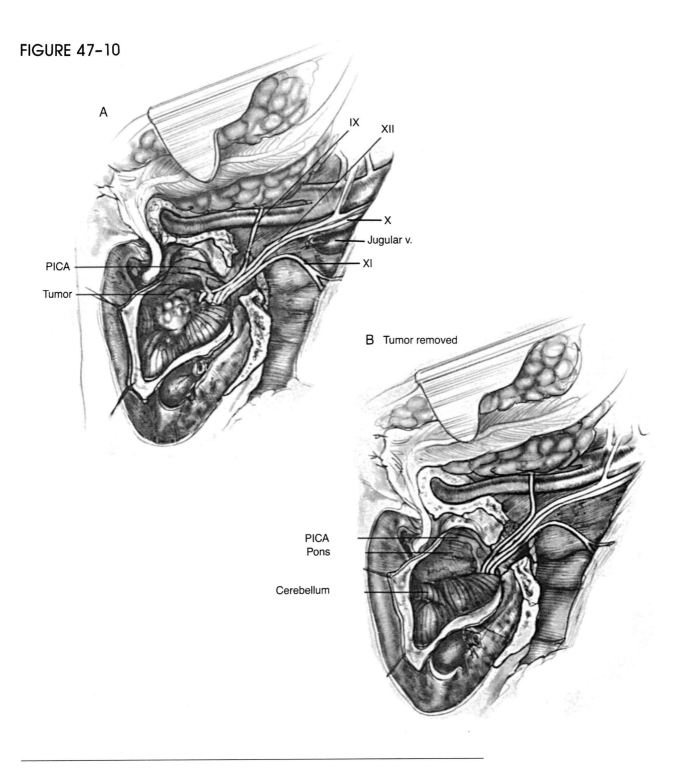

FIGURE 47–10. Removal of the intracranial extension of tumor. Intracranial feeding vessels are controlled by bipolar cautery.

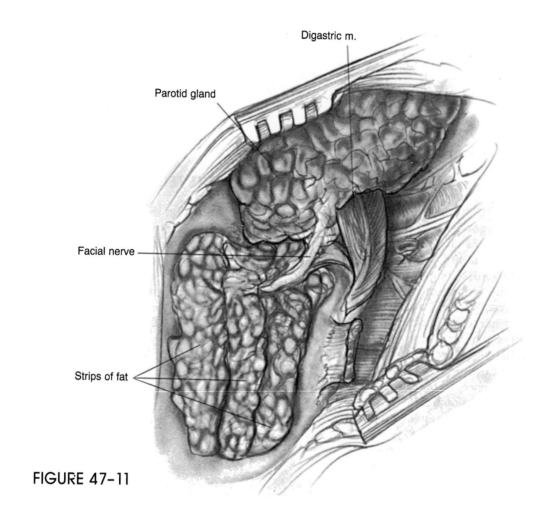

Digastric m.

Parotid gland

Facial nerve

Strips of fat

FIGURE 47-11

FIGURE 47–11. The eustachian tube is closed with oxidized cellulose and muscle. For intracranial tumors, the dura is sutured to the extent possible. Strips of abdominal fat obliterate the middle ear and mastoid.

FIGURE 47-12

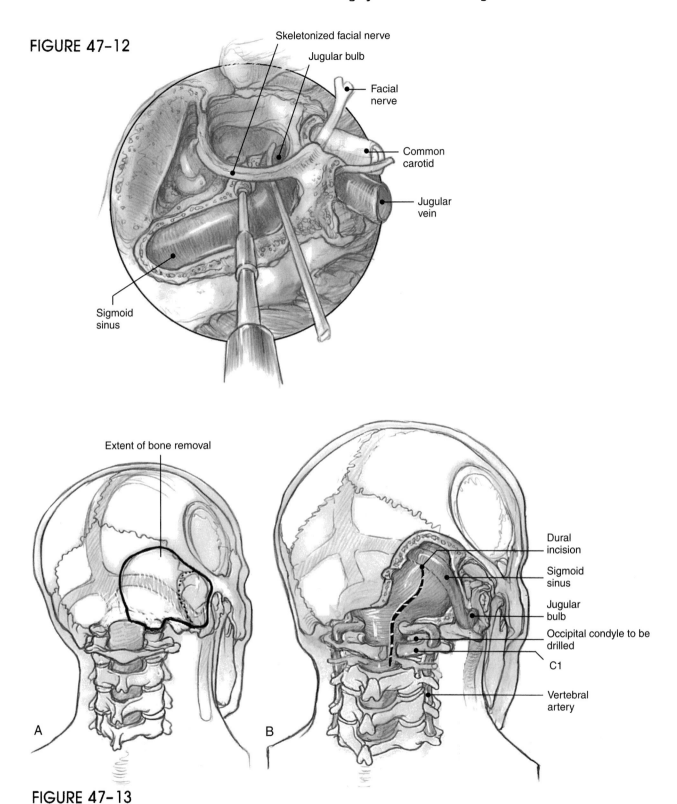

FIGURE 47-13

FIGURE 47-12. Fallopian bridge technique. In this modification the facial nerve is left in situ with only an island of bone to permit tumor dissection both lateral and medial to the facial nerve.

FIGURE 47-13. Transcondylar exposure. Once the vertebral artery is identified, the occipital condyle can be progressively removed to provide wide exposure of the craniocervical junction. A, Schematic of transcondylar approach. B, Dural incision and details of the transcondylar exposure.

using standard techniques. The advent of continuous intra-operative facial nerve monitoring has significantly improved postoperative facial nerve function in infratemporal fossa surgery.[20] In our experience, the need for tracheotomy or gastrostomy has been infrequent (<4 per cent). We recommend early vocal cord augmentation for vagal paralysis.[25]

The possibility of carotid artery injury must be anticipated. Careful preoperative imaging, including CT scans and angiography, are helpful in defining the anatomic relationships of the tumor to the internal carotid artery. Preoperative flow studies (i.e., balloon occlusion or xenon or technetium blood flow studies) are helpful in predicting how well a patient will tolerate total occlusion of the internal carotid artery. The indications for replacement versus permanent occlusion have been summarized elsewhere.[26] The possibility of significant intraoperative blood loss must be anticipated. Autologous blood donation has been helpful in avoiding transfusions of banked blood. In the weeks preceding surgery, the patient donates his or her own blood for possible autologous transfusion intraoperatively. Similarly, the Cell Saver, which recycles the patient's intraoperative blood loss, may reduce the requirement for banked blood transfusions. Finally, the surgeon must be cognizant of the extent of blood replacement and be certain that the appropriate ratio of platelets and fresh frozen plasma is replaced in addition to the red blood cell products themselves.

Intracranial glomus tumor extension should be managed cooperatively with a neurosurgeon. The techniques for tumor removal are similar to those employed for other posterior fossa neoplasms. Specifically, the possibility of intracranial hemorrhage, wound infection, and cerebrospinal fluid leakage may require neurosurgical expertise. In our experience, patients with cerebrospinal fluid fistulas respond to conservative management with pressure dressing and lumbar drainage.

ALTERNATIVE TECHNIQUES

The role of radiation therapy in the management of glomus jugulare tumors is still controversial. Histologic studies have proved that the effects of irradiation appear to be on the blood vessels and fibrous elements of the tumor rather than on the tumor cells themselves.[27] These tumors often begin growing after 10 to 15 years of control. In addition, the malignant-transformation potential of radiating benign tumors must not be underestimated. Fatal malignant transformations of benign jugular foramen tumors following radiation therapy have been reported. Accordingly, we favor radiation therapy in elderly patients with symptomatic glomus tumors or in patients who otherwise could not withstand a surgical removal. We recommend surgery as definitive therapy for patients who are medically stable enough to undergo an operative procedure.

SUMMARY

Modern imaging studies accurately delineate the extent of glomus tumors of the temporal bone. Microsurgical techniques allow total removal of even the largest tumors with acceptable morbidity and virtually no mortality. We favor surgical management of glomus tumors except in the elderly or infirm, in whom radiation therapy is a reasonable alternative.

References

1. Rosenwasser H: Carotid body–like tumor of the middle ear and mastoid bone. Arch Otolaryngol 41: 64–67, 1945.
2. Bickerstaff ER, Howell JS: The neurological importance of tumors of the glomus jugulare. Brain 76: 576–693, 1953.
3. Steinberg N, Holz WG: Glomus jugulare tumors. Arch Otolaryngol Head Neck Surg 82: 387–394, 1965.
4. Brown JS: Glomus jugulare tumors revisited: A ten-year statistical follow-up of 231 cases. Laryngoscope 95: 284–285, 1985.
5. Spector GJ, Fierstein J, Ogura JH: A comparison of therapeutic modalities of glomus tumors in the temporal bone. Laryngoscope 86: 690–969, 1976.
6. Leonetti JP, Brackmann DE: Glomus vagale tumors: The significance of early vocal cord paralysis. Otolaryngol Head Neck Surg 100: 533–537, 1989.
7. Horn KL, Hankinson H: Tumors of the jugular foramen. *In* Brackmann DE, Jackler RK (eds): Neurotology. Philadelphia, Mosby, 1994, pp 1059–1068.
8. Horn KL, House WF, Hitselberger WE: Schwannomas of the jugular foramen. Laryngoscope 95: 761–765, 1985.
9. Leonetti JP, Brackmann DE: Glomus vagale tumors: The significance of early vocal cord paralysis. Otolaryngol Head Neck Surg 100: 533–537, 1989.
10. Kaye AH, Hahn JF, Kinney JE: Jugular foramen schwannomas. J Neurosurg 60: 1045–1053, 1984.
11. Arriaga MA, Brackmann DE: Differential diagnosis of primary petrous apex lesions. Am J Otol 12: 470–474, 1991.
12. Arriaga MA, Lo WWM, Brackmann DE: Imaging case study of the month: Magnetic resonance angiography of synchronized bilateral carotid body paragangliomas and bilateral vagal paragangliomas. Ann Otol Rhinol Laryngol 101: 955–957, 1992.
13. Rogers GP, Brackmann DE, Lo WWM: Magnetic resonance angiography—a technique for evaluation of skull base lesions. J Otol 14: 56–62, 1993.
14. Janecka IP, Sekhar LN, Horton JA: General blood flow evaluation. *In* Cummings CW, Frederickson JM, Harker LA (eds): Otolaryngology Head and Neck Surgery Update II. St. Louis, Mosby–Year Book, 1990, pp 54–63.
15. Murphy TP, Brackmann DE: Effects of preoperative embolization on glomus jugulare tumors. Laryngoscope 99: 1244–1247, 1989.
16. Farrior JB: Glomus tumors—postauricular hypotympanotomy. Arch Otolaryngol Head Neck Surg 86: 367–373, 1967.
17. Fisch U: Infratemporal fossa approach for glomus tumors of the temporal bone. Ann Otol Rhinol Laryngol 91: 474–479, 1982.
18. Fisch U, Faga P, Valvanis A: The infratemporal fossa approach for the lateral skull base. Otolaryngol Clin North Am 17: 513–552, 1984.
19. Brackmann DE: The facial nerve in the infratemporal approach. Otolaryngol Head Neck Surg 97: 15–17, 1987.
20. Leonetti JP, Brackmann DE, Prass RC: Improved preservation of facial function in the infratemporal fossa approach to the skull base. Otolaryngol Head Neck Surg 101: 74–78, 1989.
21. Pensak ML, Jackler RK: Removal of jugular foramen tumors. Otolaryngol Head Neck Surg 117: 586–591, 1997.
22. Fukushima T: Manual of Skull Base Dissection. Pittsburgh, AF Neurovideo, 1996.
23. O'Leary MJ, Shelton C, Giddings N, et al: Glomus tympanicum tumors: A clinical perspective. Laryngoscope 101: 74–78, 1989.
24. Green JD, Brackman DE, Nguyen CD, et al: Surgical management of previously untreated glomus jugulare tumors. Laryngoscope 104: 917–921, 1994.
25. Netterville JD: Primary Thyroplasty in Glomus Jugulare Surgery. Oral presentation, American Neurotology Society Fall Meeting, Washington DC, September 13, 1992.
26. deVries EJ: A new method to predict safe resection of the internal carotid artery. Laryngoscope 100: 85–89, 1990.
27. Brackmann DE, House WF, Terry R, et al: Glomus jugulare tumors: Effects of irradiation. Trans Am Acad Ophthalmol Otolaryngol 76: 1423–1431, 1972.

48

Rehabilitation of Lower Cranial Nerve Deficits After Neurotologic Skull Base Surgery

James L. Netterville, M.D. ▪ Christopher A. Sullivan, M.D.

Before the advent of modern skull base surgery, the treatment of cranial base lesions was associated with significant perioperative complications and long-term morbidity. Rapid advances in medical imaging have made possible early detection of lesions and thus preservation of vital structures at the time of surgery. The development of advanced microsurgical techniques has made the removal of most skull base tumors not only possible but also feasible. Today, the major source of short- and long-term morbidity results from the loss of cranial nerves at the time of resection. Innovative approaches to cranial nerve rehabilitation have allowed many of these patients productive and enjoyable lives after cranial base surgery.

The lower cranial nerves function in concert to facilitate speech, swallowing, and airway protection (Fig. 48–1). Interruption of the complex interactions of these nerves results in articulation deficits, inanition, and aspiration. With speech and swallowing therapy, most patients are able to compensate for the loss of a single lower cranial nerve. The loss of multiple nerves, particularly in an elderly patient, may result in permanent inability to swallow despite intensive therapy. Paradoxically, preoperative loss of cranial nerve function from tumor compression will allow most patients to compensate slowly over time and may predict better postoperative speech and swallowing rehabilitation. Patient age and preoperative cranial nerve function are important factors in the decision to proceed with complete surgical resection, partial resection, or radiation therapy.

PATIENT EVALUATION

When lateral skull base surgery is elected, cranial nerves V3 to XII as well as the sympathetic trunk are at risk. A careful head and neck examination including cranial nerve evaluation and flexible fiber optic examination of the hypopharynx and larynx should be performed at the bedside on the first postoperative day to confirm known deficits and to determine the extent of any additional cranial nerve deficits. The state of the airway, vocal fold function and cord position, pooling of secretions, and the ability to clear secretions by coughing should be noted. A modified barium swallow is the gold standard for evaluating aspiration and should be performed as soon as the patient is awake and alert enough to cooperate with the study. Identification of

the level of oropharyngeal dysphagia may be identified and addressed by the speech and language pathologist at the time of this study. Flexible videoendoscopic evaluation has been described to evaluate swallowing at the bedside but is not the study of choice because it cannot identify aspiration during the pharyngeal phase of swallowing, which is the most significant component of swallowing dysfunction in lateral skull base surgery.[1] After thorough evaluation has been completed, efforts are directed at rehabilitation. The remainder of this chapter describes the pertinent regional cranial nerve anatomy and function,[2, 3] associated postoperative deficits, and methods for rehabilitation.

LOWER CRANIAL NERVE DEFICITS AND REHABILITATION

Trigeminal Nerve: Mandibular Division (Cranial Nerve V3)

The mandibular division of the trigeminal nerve (V3) carries both a branchial motor and a general sensory component. The sensory pathway travels by way of five orocutaneous nerves: auriculotemporal, meningeal, buccal, lingual, and inferior alveolar. Loss of the first two nerves leaves little functional deficit and compensation readily occurs; however, severe burns to the cutaneous distribution of these nerves may occur with the use of curling irons and other heated hair grooming devices. Therefore, patients are instructed to take care in daily hairdressing.

Loss of the buccal, lingual, and inferior alveolar nerves affects the sensory feedback loop of the initial aspects of swallowing. The food bolus is not detected in the nonsensate area, thus affecting the preparatory phase of oral swallowing. Grafting of these nerves is recommended when possible; however, because these nerves are usually resected intracranially as the nerve exits the dura, it is impossible to identify the appropriate proximal fibers for nerve grafting. Swallowing therapy is the mainstay of rehabilitation and will allow compensation in most patients.

The motor division of V3 provides function to six muscles: tensor veli palatini, tensor tympani, medial pterygoid, lateral pterygoid, masseter, and temporalis. The medial pterygoid nerve is the first branch off V3 after it exits the foramen ovale. Before it reaches the medial pterygoid muscle, it gives a branch to the tensor veli palatini and to

FIGURE 48-1

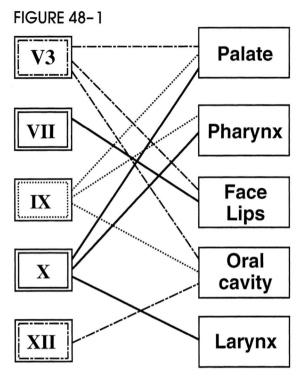

FIGURE 48–1. The function of the upper aerodigestive tract is coordinated by the complex interaction of the lower cranial nerves in speech and swallowing.

the tensor tympani, both of which pass through the otic ganglion without synapsing. Isolated tensor veli palatini paralysis is compensated for by the action of the levator palatini muscle with minimal palatal dysfunction. Aural attenuation is decreased with loss of tensor tympani function but is adequately compensated for by the action of the stapedius muscle as long as cranial nerve VII has been preserved. Therapy for loss of tensor tympani or stapedius function is usually not necessary.

Just past the otic ganglion, V3 gives off branches to the lateral pterygoid and the masseter muscle. Two or three deep temporal nerve branches arise in the same region and pass up into the temporalis muscle. As the inferior alveolar nerve enters its canal in the mandible, the final motor branches of V3 depart from it and go to the mylohyoid muscle and anterior belly of the digastric. If the contralateral muscles of mastication are intact, patients usually compensate with little trismus or chewing dysfunction. Often, early trismus associated with exposure of the temporomandibular joint during surgery in this region may be overcome by propping the mouth open with a stack of tongue depressors for several minutes two or three times daily. The number of tongue depressors is gradually increased until adequate opening is achieved. Shifting of the mandibular arch is usually corrected over time with this therapy and increasing use of the mandible.

Atrophy of the temporalis muscle is an inevitable sequela of V3 sacrifice. For this reason, attempts at masseter or temporalis transfer for facial nerve rehabilitation are doomed to failure and should not be attempted. By 1 year, noticeable temporalis wasting occurs and results in a significant cosmetic defect. Most patients will desire

placement of a silicone or methyl methacrylate implant beneath the residual temporalis muscle (Fig. 48–2). Care must be taken to contour the implant where it abuts the lateral orbital rim or else a residual crease will result in this region.

Abducens Nerve (Cranial Nerve VI)

During lateral transtemporal approaches to the cranial base, the abducens nerve is often encountered in its course along the clivus and medial aspect of the petrous apex. Its sole function is to supply somatic motor innervation to the lateral rectus muscle. After exiting the brainstem, the abducens nerve lies along the clivus and enters Dorello's canal inferomedial to the root of the trigeminal nerve. It then passes beneath (rarely above) the superior sphenopetrous ligament in a sulcus on the petrous apex. It courses through the cavernous sinus lateral to the carotid into the superior orbital fissure. Injury may occur anywhere along this course and result in lateral rectus muscle dysfunction with limitation of lateral gaze with associated diplopia. Cranial nerve VI is exquisitely sensitive to pressure injury in the cavernous sinus, and great care must be taken not to vigorously pack the cavernous sinus to control bleeding because this may result in permanent lateral rectus palsy despite anatomic integrity of the nerve. If the nerve is known to be intact, treatment is conservative; prism glasses will allow compensation until function returns, usually within 3 to 4 months. Botulinum toxin injection into the ipsilateral medial rectus has been used successfully to relieve diplopia by weakening the antagonist action of the medial rectus muscle.[4] When it appears that permanent palsy has oc-

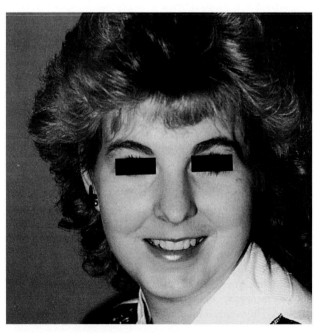

FIGURE 48–2. Significant atrophy of the temporalis has occurred 1 year after infratemporal fossa dissection with sacrifice of V3 and mobilization of the temporalis muscle. (From Netterville JL, Civantos FJ: Rehabilitation of cranial nerve deficits after neurotologic skull base surgery. Laryngoscope 103(Suppl 60):45–54, 1993.)

curred, superior and inferior rectus muscle transposition may be performed to improve lateral gaze function.[4]

Glossopharyngeal Nerve (Cranial Nerve IX)

The glossopharyngeal nerve has branchial motor, visceral motor, visceral sensory, general sensory, and special sensory components. Its branchial motor component is limited to the stylopharyngeus muscle, which elevates the pharynx during swallowing and speech. Isolated loss of motor fibers to this muscle results in little swallowing dysfunction; however, when combined with the loss of general sensory fibers of the glossopharyngeal plexus as well as vagal motor fibers, severe swallowing deficits result.

The visceral motor component of the glossopharyngeal nerve exerts parasympathetic control over parotid salivary secretion. As the ninth cranial nerve exits the skull base through the pars nervosa of the jugular foramen, it forms superior and inferior ganglia that contain nerve cell bodies that mediate general, visceral, and special sensory function. Parasympathetic fibers leave the inferior ganglion and pass into the middle ear as the tympanic nerve. In the middle ear these fibers form the tympanic plexus; branches from the tympanic plexus form the lesser petrosal nerve, which passes back up through the floor of the middle cranial fossa, travels intracranially, and then descends through the foramen ovale in the greater wing of the sphenoid bone where it synapses at the otic ganglion. Postganglionic fibers travel with the auriculotemporal nerve to reach the parotid gland. Injury to these fibers may occur at many levels and lead to decreased parotid salivary flow; rarely, this leads to chronic parotitis.

The general sensory component provides afferent feedback from the base of tongue and lateral pharyngeal wall as well as the external ear and inner aspect of the tympanic membrane. The sensory fibers to the base of tongue and pharynx run in a plexus on the undersurface of the stylopharyngeus muscle and pierce the middle constrictor to reach the mucosa of the base of tongue. Disruption of this glossopharyngeal plexus causes significant delay in the oropharyngeal phase of swallowing on the ipsilateral side. In glomus tumor surgery, the glossopharyngeal nerve is taken at the pars nervosa in the jugular foramen precluding nerve grafting. Isolated, unilateral ninth cranial nerve deficits are well compensated for with swallowing therapy that focuses on maintaining passage of the food bolus adjacent to the contralateral sensate side of the pharynx using a chin-tuck and head-turn maneuver toward the side of the deficit. When this deficit is combined with the loss of cranial nerves X and XII at the skull base, dysfunction becomes severe. Rehabilitation of this combined loss involves correction of glottal incompetence with thyroplasty and intensive swallowing therapy.

The final function of the ninth cranial nerve is visceral sensory from the carotid body and carotid sinus by way of the nerve of Hering. Disruption of the ninth cranial nerve at the skull base causes loss of the carotid sinus reflex on the ipsilateral side and was originally described for the treatment of carotid sinus syndrome.[5] Unilateral loss does not interfere with the control of blood pressure and pulse,

presumably due to the presence of an intact reflex on the contralateral side. When there is bilateral alteration of this system, acute elevation of blood pressure to greater than 220 mm Hg may be seen within a 60-second period. Preoperatively, one should consider the potential for a bilateral deficit in any patient who has had surgery on the contralateral neck where ninth cranial nerve fibers may have been disrupted, such as in carotid endarterectomy. Appropriate intraoperative management of this scenario includes administration of a pure alpha blocker such as phenoxybenzamine hydrochloride. Sodium nitroprusside may be added for further control. The patient is weaned to clonidine hydrochloride in the postoperative period. Permanent maintenance of blood pressure may be required. Consultation with an intensivist in the preoperative period is strongly recommended if a bilateral loss is anticipated.

Vagus Nerve (Cranial Nerve X)

Of the lower cranial nerves, the vagus is most intimately involved in control of the airway and swallowing function. Isolated loss of vagal function will yield a far greater deficit than the loss of any other single lower cranial nerve. The vagus nerve carries general sensory, visceral sensory, visceral motor, and branchial motor fibers. The general sensory component provides afferent signals from the external auditory canal, tympanic membrane, supraglottic larynx, and lateral pharyngeal wall. Two ganglia are formed as it exits the skull base through the pars nervosa of the jugular foramen: the superior (jugular) ganglion lies in the jugular foramen and the inferior (nodose) ganglion is located 1 to 2 cm outside the foramen. The sensory fibers from the supraglottic larynx form the superior laryngeal nerve, which passes deep to the external and internal carotid arteries to join the vagus at the level of the inferior ganglion. Isolated loss of this nerve can result in swallowing difficulties; therefore, it is grafted on rare occasions in selected patients. Most often, the vagus is resected so proximally at the skull base that grafting is technically impossible. With time and swallowing therapy, compensation for the sensory loss will occur.

The visceral sensory and branchial motor components of cranial nerve X provide afferent sensory and parasympathetic function, respectively, to the pharynx, larynx, trachea, esophagus, thoracic viscera, and abdominal viscera distally to the level of the splenic flexure of the colon. Unilateral loss of vagal function may cause decreased gastroesophageal motility, loss of lower esophageal sphincter tone, and delayed gastric emptying due to inadequate pyloric sphincter function. Subsequent regurgitation during the early postoperative period is not uncommon and may limit adequate nutrition, cause transient increases in intracranial pressure and potential for cerebrospinal fluid leak, and lead to life-threatening aspiration pneumonia. Pain medication and anticholinergic drying agents add further to gastric stasis. Treatment consist of administration of a motility agent such as metoclopramide hydrochloride and a temporary decrease in feeding rate. Over time, these symptoms will gradually improve. If feeding intolerance continues, a jejunal feeding tube may be necessary. On rare occasions, usually in cases of bilateral vagal injury, total loss of lower esophageal sphincter tone can occur and may require Nissen fundoplication.

The branchial motor component of cranial nerve X provides motor function to the palate, pharynx, and larynx, with the exception of the stylopharyngeus muscle (IX) and the tensor veli palatini muscle (V3). These fibers depart the vagus in three distinct bundles: the pharyngeal branch, the external branch of the superior laryngeal nerve, and the recurrent laryngeal nerve. The pharyngeal branch departs the vagus as the inferior (nodose) ganglion passes over the internal carotid, deep to the external carotid artery, and enters the pharynx at the upper border of the middle constrictor. Damage to this branch results in unilateral palatal and pharyngeal paralysis, which causes a loss of lateral wall motion on the affected side and an ineffective sphincter for closing the nasopharyngeal port. This leads to nasal regurgitation and hypernasal speech. In the early postoperative period, unilateral palatal paralysis causes no significant morbidity relative to more immediate concerns regarding airway and swallowing function. The pharyngeal dysfunction responds well to swallowing therapy. Subsequent velopharyngeal insufficiency (VPI) resulting in nasal regurgitation and hypernasal speech is embarrassing and quite bothersome to most patients.

Nonsurgical approaches to VPI have included speech and swallowing therapy, palatal lift prostheses, and palatal obturators. A variety of surgical procedures have been described for the treatment of VPI secondary to cleft palate, including pharyngeal augmentation and pharyngoplasty. The most popular of the pharyngoplasty techniques is the superiorly based pharyngeal flap as described by Jackson.[6] Vagal injury at or above the jugular foramen causes paralysis of not only the palate but also the pharyngeal constrictors, resulting in loss of lateral wall motion on the affected side. Superiorly based flaps and pharyngeal augmentation are used to address VPI in cleft palate patients and are designed to leave an open lateral port. Lateral pharyngoplasty techniques[7] are adynamic and do not recreate lateral pharyngeal wall movement. A simple alternative technique that addresses the palatal and pharyngeal component of VPI in skull base patients is to close the lateral port by adhering the palate on the affected side to the posterior pharyngeal wall. The chief advantage of this procedure in patients who may already have multiple cranial nerve deficits and abnormal swallowing is that it does not alter pharyngeal anatomy with long mucosal flaps and does not carry the risk of pharyngeal stenosis. Unilateral palatal adhesion successfully eliminates hypernasality and nasal regurgitation and has become the procedure of choice for the correction of velopharyngeal incompetence in neurotologic skull base patients.[8, 9]

Palatal adhesion is usually performed several months after resection when swallowing function has stabilized and when it is certain that an injured but intact vagus nerve has not recovered. Preoperative assessment by nasopharyngoscopy with either a rigid or flexible scope demonstrates unilateral closure of the nasopharynx. Under general anesthesia, the palate is exposed with a Dingman mouth gag. The paralyzed hemipalate and posterior pharyngeal wall are injected with epinephrine. Care is taken to inject just below any residual adenoid tissue. A transpalatal incision is performed in the area of the palatal crease that forms

with normal palatal elevation, and the posterior pharyngeal wall is viewed through this incision (Fig. 48–3). A similar incision is created into the posterior pharyngeal wall down to the prevertebral fascia. The pharyngeal mucosa is elevated for just a few millimeters all around to create an edge to which the nasopharyngeal mucosa of the palate is sewn. Multiple deep mattress sutures are used to suture the nasopharyngeal surface of the palate to the posterior pharyngeal wall (Fig. 48–4). The oral surface of the palate is closed on itself, creating a unilateral palatal adhesion (Figs. 48–5 to 48–7).

Postoperatively, the patient is immediately allowed to take a liquid diet and discharged from the hospital as soon as pain control is adequate. The only complication that has occurred from this procedure is a wound dehiscence that granulates in over several months, producing a secondary adhesion with minimal VPI. Sleep apnea has not been seen as a complication of this procedure. Improvement of nasal regurgitation and reduction in hypernasal speech occur in all patients.[8, 9]

The effect of paralysis of the superior, middle, and inferior constrictor muscles causes more morbidity than the palatal dysfunction. As the food bolus passes into the oropharynx, the paralyzed side dilates laterally and forms a pseudopocket that collects the bolus. The normal contraction on the contralateral side pushes the bolus into this region rather than down into the hypopharynx. This delay interrupts the normal timing of the swallowing event so that when the larynx reopens, the food bolus, which should have been in the esophagus, is still partially in the hypopharynx, where it is then aspirated. Treatment is centered around an intensive swallowing therapy program in which a head positioning technique is used to physically obliterate the paralyzed side and force the food bolus onto the normal side. Avoidance of a tracheotomy, if possible, further hastens recovery of swallowing function because the tracheotomy would interfere with laryngeal elevation. Loss of cricopharyngeal relaxation combined with an indwelling tracheotomy tube (particularly a cuffed tube) further hinders the passage of the food bolus through the esophageal inlet and encourages aspiration.

The second motor branch of cranial nerve X is the superior laryngeal nerve. It provides motor control to the ipsilateral cricothyroid muscle. Loss of this nerve results in decreased vocal range, which is usually a problem only for professional voice patients. Because the vagus is usually resected or injured at the skull base, patients will have both superior and recurrent laryngeal nerve paralyses which are rehabilitated at the same time with Silastic medialization thyroplasty and arytenoid adduction.

The third motor branch of the vagus is the recurrent laryngeal nerve, which provides innervation to the intrinsic laryngeal musculature and the cricopharyngeus muscle. True vocal fold paralysis and lack of cricopharyngeal relaxation result from resection or neural injury at the time of surgery. The resultant glottal incompetence results in a weak, breathy voice and an inefficient cough. This deficit combined with lack of cricopharyngeal relaxation results in aspiration and poor pulmonary hygiene. Tracheotomy has been universally performed to protect the airway until early swallowing rehabilitation can be accomplished. From an airway perspective, most patients with high vagal injury

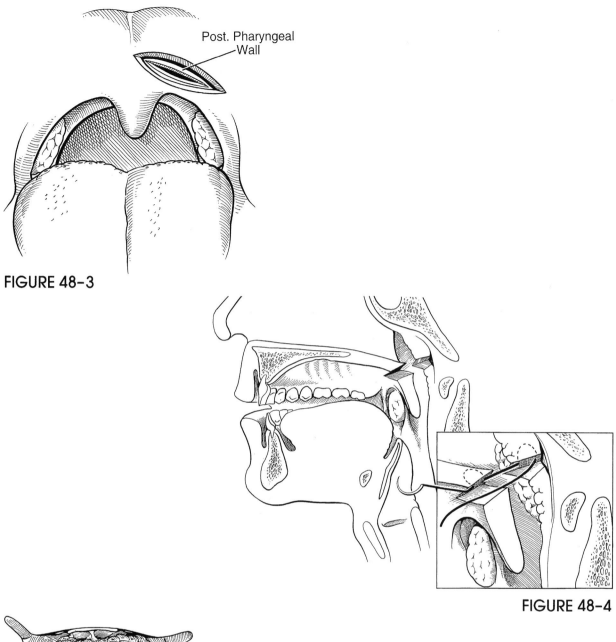

Post. Pharyngeal Wall

FIGURE 48–3

FIGURE 48–4

FIGURE 48–5

FIGURE 48–3. A transpalatal incision is made in the area of the palatal crease that forms with normal palatal elevation and the posterior pharyngeal wall is viewed.

FIGURE 48–4. Incisions are made in the palate Land the posterior pharyngeal wall. Multiple mattress stitches are placed to complete the adhesion.

FIGURE 48–5. Superior endoscopic view of left-sided palatal adhesion.

will tolerate a unilateral vocal fold paralysis, making tracheotomy generally unnecessary; for the reasons discussed earlier, tracheotomy prolongs swallowing rehabilitation and adds morbidity to the postoperative course. Silastic medialization with arytenoid adduction has been the procedure of choice for addressing vocal fold paralysis in this population.[10] Although cricopharyngeal myotomy is not routinely necessary in these patients, it has been shown to decrease aspiration and promote early swallowing.[11]

The primary goal for vocal fold medialization in skull base patients is (1) to provide glottal competence, (2) to provide an efficient mechanism for coughing, and (3) to give support and volume to the voice. Generally, most patients with a unilateral vocal fold paralysis undergo a Gelfoam injection postoperatively regardless of whether the nerve was taken. This injection lasts approximately 6 to 8 weeks and greatly facilitates speech and swallowing rehabilitation while the nerve regains function or until Silastic medialization and arytenoid adduction may be performed. It is prudent to wait 2 to 3 months before proceeding with thyroplasty because denervation vocal fold atrophy will occur over several weeks, which will alter both the size of the Silastic implant and the degree of arytenoid adduction necessary to achieve good voice and airway results. Several weeks postoperatively, the patient should return for airway evaluation, videostroboscopy, and airflow measurements. A Silastic medialization under local anesthesia is then performed. The technique is outlined in the following paragraphs and has been described elsewhere.[10, 12–14]

Under local anesthesia, a midline horizontal incision or an extension of the cervical portion of the skull base incision is made overlying the midpoint of the thyroid cartilage. The sternohyoid muscle is divided at its medial attachments to the hyoid bone superiorly. A perichondrial flap is created from the midline back to the posterior edge of the thyroid cartilage, elevating the remaining attachments of the sternohyoid muscle and the thyrohyoid muscle with the flap and exposing the inferior edge of the thyroid ala. A rectangular window is outlined so that the anterior extent lies 5 mm back from the anterior commissure in women and 7 mm back in men. The window is placed as low as possible, leaving an inferior 3-mm thyroid cartilage strut that is wide enough not to fracture when the implant is placed (Fig. 48–8). The final outline of the window is usually 6 mm in height by 13 mm in length. The location of the implant relative to the anterior commissure is based on the angle of the thyroid alae. With an increased thyroid cartilage angle as seen in women, the implant must be brought closer to the anterior commissure and must have an increased slope to compensate for the wider angle. If the implant is placed too far anteriorly, overmedialization of the anterior commissure will occur, producing a strained

quality to the voice. Using 4× loupes, a high-speed drill with a 2-mm cutting burr is used to drill away the outline of the window. The cartilage may be partially ossified, particularly inferiorly and posteriorly. The window is usually 3 to 4 mm thick anteriorly and 5 to 7 mm thick posteriorly.

Next, the long and short phonosurgery intralaryngeal elevators (Xomed, Jacksonville, MS) are used to elevate the inner perichondrium in all directions except anteriorly. Medialization is attempted, but rarely is it possible to achieve the required medialization with the inner perichondrium intact. The superior, posterior, and inferior margins of the perichondrium are incised discretely without injuring the lateral fascia of the thyroarytenoid muscle just deep to this. Branches of the superior laryngeal artery and vein can usually be seen lying just under this fascia. Although some fear that dividing the perichondrium leads to implant extrusion, this has not occurred in several hundred medialization procedures using this technique.[13] The depth gauge (Xomed, Jacksonville, MS) is used to medialize the cord, and voice quality and cord position are assessed (Fig. 48–9). Based on this visual and auditory data, an implant is carved to appropriate dimensions from a preformed Silastic block (Xomed, Jacksonville, MS) (Fig. 48–10). Its inferior border is thicker than the superior border, and the posterior border is thicker than the anterior border. This creates an even medialization of the vocal fold with the point of maximum medialization at the lower edge of the window. Good alignment of the true vocal cord in the midline is usually obtained with little medialization of the false cord. All edges of the Silastic block are beveled to allow ease of insertion through the window. The average size of the block that is used when performing this under general anesthesia is 2 to 3 mm thick anteriorly and 5 to 7 mm at the point of maximal medialization, with an overall length of 13 to 18 mm. The block is inserted in the window by placing the lower flange behind the lower window strut while compressing the upper flange until it expands under the cartilage. Some 4-0 Prolene sutures are used to stabilize the implant to the inferior strut of thyroid cartilage (Fig. 48–11). All patients are given 10 mg of dexamethasone at the time of the procedure and at least three doses every 6 hours postoperatively. Patients are treated with glycopyrolate 0.2 mg every 6 hours for 3 days postoperatively to decrease salivary secretions.

High vagal injury with loss of the superior laryngeal nerve is usually best addressed with both medialization and arytenoid adduction. Arytenoid adduction has been described elsewhere[15, 16] and is performed at the time of Silastic medialization. Once the cartilage window has been created, the voice is assessed using the depth gauge as described earlier, and the decision to proceed with arytenoid adduction is made. Exposure of the arytenoid cartilage

---

FIGURE 48–6. Sagittal view of completed palatal adhesion.

FIGURE 48–7. Endoscopic view from above of right-sided palatal adhesion during quiet respiration *(A)* and showing complete closure during production of pressureconsonant *(B)*.

FIGURE 48–8. The alar window is positioned as shown, taking care to preserve an inferior alar strut.

FIGURE 48–9. The depth gauge is used to medialize the true vocal fold based on auditory and visual feedback.

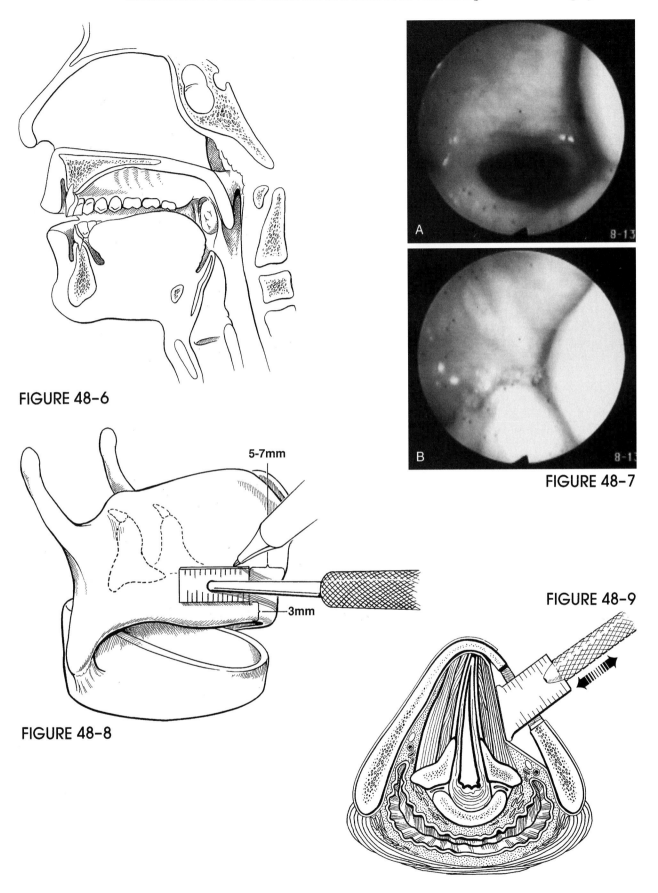

FIGURE 48-6

FIGURE 48-7

FIGURE 48-8

FIGURE 48-9

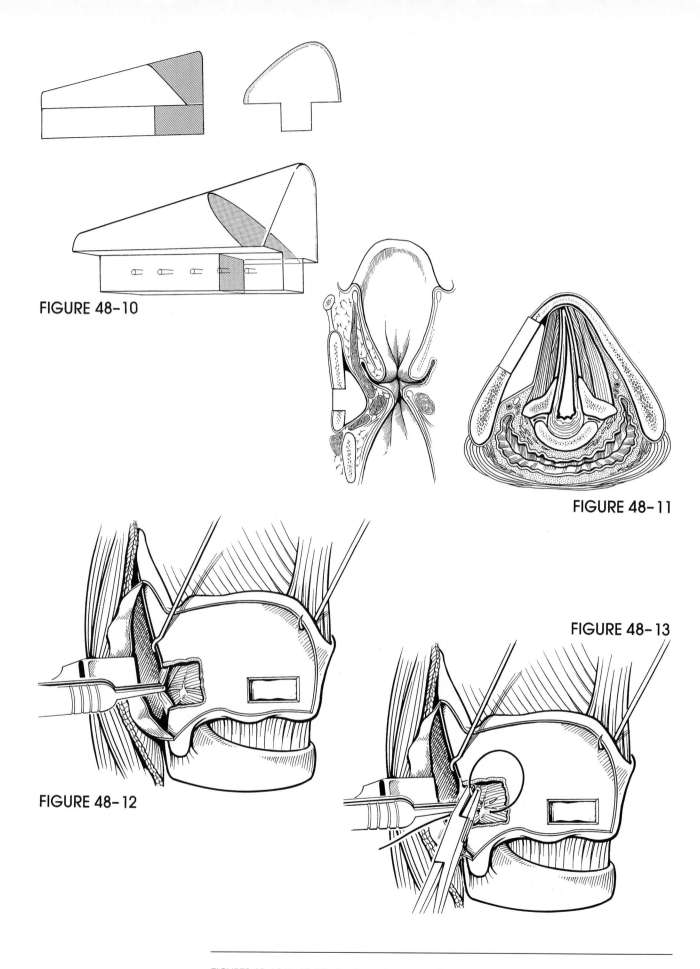

FIGURE 48-10

FIGURE 48-11

FIGURE 48-13

FIGURE 48-12

FIGURES 48–10 to 48–13. *See legends on opposite page*

is achieved by first placing a hook beneath the posterior border of the thyroid cartilage and rotating the larynx forward. The perichondrium at the posterior border is divided and the pyriform sinus mucosa is elevated away from the inner surface of the thyroid cartilage. A 5-mm Kerrison rongeur is used to remove the posterior border of the thyroid cartilage, exposing the paraglottic space lateral to the muscular process of the arytenoid. The patients are then asked to purse their lips and blow out to confirm the location of the pyriform mucosa so that dissection may be carried out anteriorly to expose the posterior cricoarytenoid muscle. The muscular process is then palpated and moved in its plane of abduction and adduction while observing the monitor (Fig. 48–12). A double-armed 4-0 Prolene suture is then passed through the lateral edge of the muscular process in a figure-eight fashion to secure the arytenoid (Fig. 48–13). The goal of this stitch is to mimic the vector of force that rotates the vocal process of the arytenoid down (inferior) and in (medial) during phonation. To accomplish this, one end of the suture is brought through the paraglottic space and out through the cartilage just anterior to the window. The other end of the suture is passed from the window below the lower cartilage strut and then through the cricothyroid membrane soft tissue in the midline. Gentle traction is applied to the arytenoid and its motion observed on the monitor. The implant is then carved and placed. Both arytenoid sutures pass deep to the implant. Final adjustments are made to the arytenoid stitch and it is tied down. The perichondrium and strap muscles are laid back into position and the wound is closed with absorbable suture.

Spinal Accessory Nerve (Cranial Nerve XI)

The spinal accessory nerve has only a branchial motor component. Its lower motor neuron cell bodies arise in the spinal cord, and its motor fibers ascend into the cranium and then descend through the pars nervosa of the jugular foramen, passing superficial to (70 per cent), posterior to (27 per cent), or through (3 per cent) the jugular vein to innervate the sternocleidomastoid and trapezius muscles.[17] Loss of sternocleidomastoid function results in weakness when turning the head away from the operated side, although this is rarely noticed by most patients. Loss of trapezius function results in downward and lateral rotation of the scapula with a shoulder droop. This causes severe shoulder disability secondary to weakness and pain. Whether the nerve may be grafted successfully or not, a shoulder exercise program that emphasizes strengthening of the levator, scalene, and rhomboid muscles should be administered by a qualified physical therapist. This program should continue indefinitely to maintain the strength and support of the shoulder girdle.

Hypoglossal Nerve (Cranial Nerve XII)

The hypoglossal nerve provides somatic motor control to all the intrinsic and extrinsic muscles of the tongue except the palatoglossus. The nerve exits the skull base through the hypoglossal canal medial to the jugular foramen. As it passes laterally, it shares fibers with the vagus nerve near the inferior (nodose) ganglion. Separation of these fibers leads to vocal fold paresis or paralysis and should be avoided.[18] In time, most patients can compensate for unilateral tongue paralysis. The deficit is characterized by difficulty in positioning the bolus during the oral phase of swallowing. Often the bolus becomes lodged beneath the tongue on the paralyzed side. With swallowing therapy and lingual exercise, patients learn to position the bolus on the nonparalyzed side.

Cervical Sympathetic Chain

The sympathetic innervation to the head and neck structures originates in the upper thoracic segment of the spinal column. The preganglionic fibers ascend in the sympathetic chain to exit through one of its four ganglia (superior, middle, vertebral, and stellate). The superior cervical ganglion lies on the surface of the longus capitus muscle at the level of the second or third cervical vertebra, deep to the internal carotid artery at the most distal or superior point of the cervical sympathetic chain. From this ganglion, postganglionic fibers typically reach the first three or four cervical rootlets. They also communicate with cranial nerves IX, X, XI, and XII as part of the pharyngeal plexus. Finally, they form the sympathetic plexus that ascends along the internal carotid artery.[2, 19] Damage to the superior cervical ganglion or the internal carotid plexus results in Horner's syndrome, consisting of ptosis, miosis, and anhidrosis. For most patients, there is little functional deficit. Rarely, visual fields may be partially obstructed due to the ptosis. More commonly it is a cosmetic nuisance. Elevation of the eyelid to its normal open position can be accomplished by either levator shortening or resection of Müller's muscle.[20]

The other significant sequela from injury to the cervical sympathetics at the skull base is loss of sympathetic innervation to the parotid gland. This is frequently seen with resection of high vagal paragangliomas where the sympathetic chain is either resected or damaged. In this

---

FIGURE 48–10. The preformed Silastic block is trimmed to fit the auditory and visual feedback.

FIGURE 48–11. The final position of the vocal cord after placement of the Silastic implant.

FIGURE 48–12. Exposure is achieved by rotating the thyroid cartilage upward with a hook. A Kerrison rongeur is used to remove the posterior thyroid ala. The muscular process is palpated and moved on its plane of abduction and adduction.

FIGURE 48–13. The arytenoid stitch is placed to mimic the vector of force that will rotate the vocal process downward and inward.

setting, a prolonged course of cramping pain is associated with the first bite of each meal and has been named "first-bite syndrome."[18] Patients usually describe this pain as a spasm over the parotid region that begins with the first bite and subsides within the next several bites. The intensity of the pain is increased with strong sialogogues such as vinegar or lemon. In the early postoperative period, the pain can be so severe as to limit oral intake. Early management consists of dietary modification with bland foods and oral carbamazepine (100 to 200 mg twice daily). Slowly, over time, the symptoms improve.

SUMMARY

Damage to any single lower cranial nerve results in sufficient morbidity to warrant therapy; however, most patients compensate for isolated loss of function. Multiple cranial nerve deficits (IX, IX, XII) as seen in glomus tumor surgery utilize the full efforts of the rehabilitative team. After vocal cord medialization, arytenoid adduction, palatal adhesion, and speech and swallowing therapy, most younger (<55-year-old) patients will resume adequate oral intake; however, the time it takes to return to a reasonable, enjoyable diet often extends up to 1 year postoperatively. Some never attain the goal of enjoyable intake and continue to struggle to maintain adequate nutrition. This is generally the rule in elderly patients, and careful consideration should be given to the slow growth potential of certain tumors, the resulting postoperative cranial nerve deficits, and the patient's age before proceeding with aggressive surgical management of lateral skull base tumors.

References

1. Bastian RW: Videoendoscopic evaluation of patients with dysphagia: An adjunct to the modified barium swallow. Otolaryngol Head Neck Surg 104: 339, 1991.
2. Hollinshead WH: Anatomy for Surgeons: The Head and Neck, 3rd ed. Philadelphia, JB Lippincott, 1982.
3. Wilson-Pouwels L, Akesson EJ, Stewart PA: Cranial Nerves: Anatomy and Clinical Comments. Philadelphia, BC Decker, 1988.
4. Rosenbaum AL, Kushyner B: Vertical rectus muscle transposition and botulinum toxin after abducens nerve palsy. Arch Ophthalmol 107: 820, 1989.
5. Ray BS, Stewart HJ: Role of the glossopharyngeal nerve in the carotid sinus reflex in man: Relief of carotid sinus syndrome by intracranial section of the glossopharyngeal nerve. Surgery 23: 411, 1948.
6. Jackson I: Discussion: A review of 236 cleft palate patients treated with dynamic muscle sphincter. Plast Reconstr Surg 71: 187, 1983.
7. Orticochea M: A review of 236 cleft palate patients treated with dynamic muscle sphincter. Plast Reconstr Surg 71: 180, 1983.
8. Netterville JL, Vrabec JT: Unilateral palatal adhesion for paralysis after high vagal injury. Arch Otolaryngol Head Neck Surg 120: 218, 1994.
9. Netterville JL, Civantos FJ: Rehabilitation of cranial nerve deficits after neurotologic skull base surgery. Laryngoscope 103: 45, 1993.
10. Netterville JL, Jackson CG, Civantos FJ: Thyroplasty in the functional rehabilitation of neurotologic skull base surgery patients. Am J Otol 14: 460, 1993.
11. Montgomery WW, Hillman RE, Varvares MA: Combined thyroplasty type I and inferior constrictor myotomy. Ann Otol Rhinol Laryngol 103: 858, 1994.
12. Isshiki N: Recent advances in phonosurgery. Folia Phoniatr Logop 32: 119, 1984.
13. Netterville JL, Stone RE, Lukens LS, et al: Silastic medialization and arytenoid adduction: The Vanderbilt experience—a review of 116 phonosurgical procedures. Ann Otol Rhinol Laryngol 102: 413, 1993.
14. Wanamaker JR, Netterville JL, Ossoff RH: Phonosurgery: Silastic medialization for unilateral vocal fold paralysis. Operative Tech Otolaryngol Head Neck Surg 4: 207, 1993.
15. Isshiki N, Tanabe M, Sawada M: Arytenoid adduction for unilateral vocal fold paralysis. Arch Otolaryngol 104: 555, 1978.
16. Miller FR, Bryant GL, Netterville JL: Arytenoid adduction in vocal fold paralysis. Operative Tech Otolaryngol Head Neck Surg 10: 36, 1999.
17. Parsons FG, Keith A: Seventh report of the Committee of Collective Investigation of the Anatomical Society of Great Britain and Ireland, for the year 1896–97: Question III. The position of the spinal accessory nerve. Whether it passes outward between the jugular vein and internal carotid artery, or between the jugular vein and the atlas? Whether it perforates the sterno-mastoid or not: If so does the whole nerve perforate or only part? Which division of the sterno-mastoid does it perforate? J Anat Physiol 32: 177, 1897.
18. Netterville JL, Reilly KM, Robertson D, et al: Carotid body tumors: A review of 30 patients with 46 tumors. Laryngoscope 105: 115, 1995.
19. Collins SL: Cervical sympathetic nerves in the surgery of the neck. Otolaryngol Head Neck Surg 105: 544, 1992.
20. Dortzbach RK: Superior tarsal muscle resection to correct blepharoptosis. Ophthalmology 86: 1883, 1979.

49

Middle Fossa Approach

Clough Shelton, M.D. • Derald E. Brackmann, M.D.
William F. House, M.D.

The middle fossa approach for vestibular nerve section was reported as early as 1904; however, hammer and chisel were used at that time, which put the facial nerve at risk.[1] The middle fossa approach did not have widespread application until refined by the senior author (WFH) in 1961.[2] The approach was used initially for decompression of the internal auditory canal in cases of extensive otosclerosis. That therapy was later abandoned, but it became evident that this approach was suitable for removal of acoustic tumors. Initially, the middle fossa approach was used for tumors of all sizes. However, further experience demonstrated that it was most suitable for small tumors[3–5] and that preservation of hearing and facial nerve function was possible in a significant proportion of operated patients.[6] The middle fossa approach was used infrequently until the development of gadolinium-enhanced magnetic resonance imaging (MRI). With this development, a larger number of acoustic tumors are diagnosed when they are small and before hearing has been significantly affected, making an attempt at hearing preservation desirable.

The middle fossa approach provides complete exposure of the contents of the internal auditory canal, allowing removal of laterally placed tumors without the need for blind dissection.[7] This exposure ensures total removal and is well suited for the removal of very small acoustic tumors.[8] The facial nerve can be located in its bony canal, allowing positive identification in a location not involved by tumor.

The middle fossa approach is technically difficult because of the lack of robust landmarks and the limited exposure. Bleeding in the posterior fossa can be difficult to control because of the limited access. Because of its location in the superior aspect of the internal auditory canal, the facial nerve is subjected to more manipulation in this approach than in other approaches.[9, 10] In the past, facial nerve results in middle fossa cases have not been as good as those from the translabyrinthine approach for similar-sized tumors.[11] However, the routine use of the facial nerve monitor has helped improve these results.

Several authors use an extended middle fossa approach for large tumors.[12–14] The tentorium is divided to give wider access to the posterior fossa. Some also perform a labyrinthectomy to enlarge the exposure when hearing preservation is not attempted.[15–17]

INDICATIONS

The primary indications for the middle fossa approach are a small acoustic tumor, with moderate extension into the cerebellopontine angle, and good preoperative hearing. For hearing conservation surgery, we use the arbitrary audiometric criteria of speech reception threshold of better than 50 dB and speech discrimination score of better than 50 per cent, although these indications must be individualized to the needs of the patient.[18] Some advocate attempting hearing preservation in the removal of small acoustic tumors if any measurable preoperative hearing exists.[19] Patients older than 65 years of age do not tolerate the middle fossa approach as well as younger patients because of the fragility of the dura and retraction of the temporal lobe.

PREOPERATIVE EVALUATION

Several preoperative factors may predict postoperative hearing preservation. The most obvious is tumor size. Intuitively, the smaller the tumor, the easier it is to remove and the more likely that hearing will be saved. This trend has been substantiated by several authors.[11, 20, 21] Some have also found that the better the preoperative hearing, the more likely it will be preserved,[22, 23] whereas others have failed to identify such a relationship.[11, 21, 24] Also, an intact preoperative stapedial reflex has been associated with successful postoperative hearing preservation.[22]

Several authors have reported a relationship between preoperative auditory brainstem response (ABR), and audiometry and hearing preservation.[16, 21] In one report, hearing was preserved in 78 per cent of patients with an intra-aural wave V latency difference of 0.4 msec or less.[11] For latency differences of 0.5 to 2.0 msec, the hearing preservation rate dropped to 58 per cent. In patients with no response on the ABR, postoperative measurable hearing remained in only 50 per cent. Thus, patients with a more normal preoperative ABR result apparently have a greater success rate for postoperative hearing preservation. This result may reflect less tumor involvement of the cochlear nerve. However, others do not find preoperative ABR to be predictive of hearing outcome.[25, 26]

Tumors arising from the superior vestibular nerve have a higher rate of hearing preservation than those arising from the inferior vestibular nerve. Acoustic tumors developing in the inferior portion of the internal auditory canal may involve the cochlear nerve earlier and more severely.[26, 27] In a series of middle fossa acoustic tumor removals, 68 per cent of patients whose tumors were found intraoperatively to arise from the superior vestibular nerve had measurable hearing preservation, whereas only 43 per cent of patients whose tumors originated from the inferior

503

vestibular nerve had measurable postoperative hearing.[11] This difference was statistically significant. Preoperative electronystagmography (ENG) may predict tumor origin and, thus, hearing preservation. The caloric response reflects superior vestibular nerve function. In the presence of a small acoustic neuroma, a normal caloric response indicates an inferior vestibular nerve tumor, whereas a decreased response suggests a tumor arising from the superior vestibular nerve. Of a group of 54 patients who had preoperative ENG, hearing was preserved in 64 per cent with hypoactive caloric responses, whereas postoperative hearing remained in only 45 per cent of those with normal caloric responses.[11] The association of normal caloric tests with nonpreservation of hearing has also been reported by others,[10, 16] although some series have not found this correlation.[28]

For intracanalicular tumors, the radiographic appearance may predict success at hearing preservation. Small tumors that enlarge the internal auditory canal have a poorer prognosis for hearing preservation (Jackler, personal communication, 1990). In our experience, these small tumors that expand the canal are very adherent to the cochlear nerve, which adversely affects the hearing outcome. Fast spin echo MRI provides ultra-high-resolution images of internal auditory canal anatomy.[29] With this imaging technique, it is possible to determine the nerve of origin for small tumors.

PATIENT COUNSELING

After a thorough discussion of the relevant anatomy and the necessity to treat acoustic tumors, the options regarding surgical approaches to remove acoustic tumors are described to the patient. For those with small tumors and relatively good preoperative hearing, the issues of hearing preservation are discussed. We tell such patients that there is an approximate 70 per cent chance of saving some measurable hearing and a 50 to 60 per cent chance of saving the hearing to near the preoperative level. If the preoperative ENG and ABR data are available and are favorable (see earlier), they are informed that the prognosis for hearing preservation is above average.

The patient is told that there is an approximate 90 per cent chance that normal or nearly normal facial nerve function will be obtained in the long term but that there is a 20 to 30 per cent chance of having temporary facial paralysis in the early postoperative period. Although the facial nerve results for either the middle fossa or retrosigmoid approach are excellent, our best and most consistent facial nerve results occur with the translabyrinthine approach.

Patients with preoperative tinnitus are counseled that the problem will likely get better but probably will not disappear. Patients with no preoperative tinnitus have an approx-

imate 25 per cent chance of developing it postoperatively.[30] Other important possible but rare complications are discussed, including cerebrospinal fluid leak, meningitis, serious brain complications, death, and blood transfusion options. The patient can donate 1 unit of autologous blood prior to surgery, although transfusion is rarely needed.

Recuperation can take weeks to months, and most patients are back at work within 6 weeks. The patient should expect to be dizzy postoperatively, and the rapidity of the central compensation greatly influences the time course of the recuperation.

SURGERY

Preoperative Preparation

Intraoperative furosemide and mannitol are given to allow easier temporal lobe retraction. A single dose of corticosteroid such as dexamethasone (Decadron) is routinely used intravenously at the beginning of surgery. This single dose of steroid does not seem to adversely affect wound healing. Long-acting muscle relaxants are avoided during surgery so as not to interfere with facial nerve monitoring. Preoperative antibiotics are administered. (Chapter 1 of this text details surgical site preparation and draping, along with the instruments used, including the House-Urban middle fossa retractor.)

Intraoperative ABR is routinely used, and one of us (DEB) also uses direct eighth nerve recordings.[31]

Surgical Anatomy

The surgical anatomy of the temporal bone from the middle fossa approach is compact but complex (Fig. 49–1). Landmarks are not as apparent as with other approaches through the temporal bone, so laboratory dissection is useful for the surgeon to become familiar with the anatomy from above.

Anteriorly, the limit of the dissection is the middle meningeal artery, which is lateral to the greater superficial petrosal nerve. The arcuate eminence marks the position of the superior semicircular canal and may be readily apparent in some patients but obscure in others. Kartush and coworkers cautioned that the relationship between the arcuate eminence and the superior semicircular canal may be variable in some patients, but the superior canal tends to be perpendicular to the petrous ridge.[32] Medially, the superior petrosal sinus runs along the petrous ridge.

Surgical tolerances are very tight in the area of the lateral internal auditory canal. The labyrinthine portion of the facial nerve lies immediately posterior to the basal turn of the cochlea. Bill's bar separates the facial and superior vestibular nerves. Slightly posterior and lateral to this area

---

FIGURE 49–1. Surgical anatomy of the temporal bone as viewed from the middle fossa approach.

FIGURE 49–2. Incision begins in the pretragal area and extends 7 to 8 cm superiorly in a gently curving fashion.

FIGURE 49–3. Two thirds of the craniotomy window is located anterior to the external auditory canal (EAC).

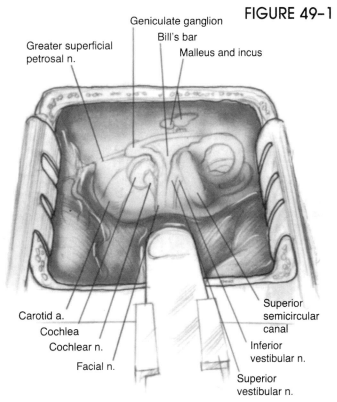

FIGURE 49-1

Greater superficial petrosal n.

Geniculate ganglion

Bill's bar

Malleus and incus

Carotid a.
Cochlea
Cochlear n.
Facial n.

Superior semicircular canal

Inferior vestibular n.

Superior vestibular n.

FIGURE 49-2

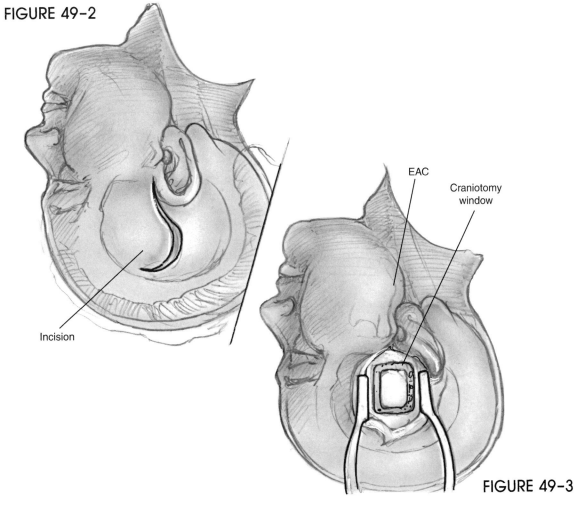

Incision

EAC

Craniotomy window

FIGURE 49-3

FIGURES 49–1 to 49–3. *See legends on opposite page*

is the vestibule and ampullated end of the superior semicircular canal.

Identification of the geniculate ganglion can be accomplished by tracing the greater superficial petrosal nerve posteriorly to it. If the tegmen is unroofed, the geniculate is found to be slightly anterior to the head of the malleus.

The internal auditory canal lies approximately on the same axis as the external auditory canal; this relationship is useful in orienting the surgical field.[12] The more medial one progresses along the internal auditory canal, the more space exists around it,[33] allowing for safe dissection in this area.

Several methods can be used to locate the internal auditory canal and are reviewed in detail elsewhere.[12, 32] The technique of Garcia-Ibañez and Garcia-Ibañez[34] provides a reliable and safe method to locate the internal auditory canal. It involves drilling on the bisection of the angle formed by the superior semicircular canal and greater superficial petrosal nerve. The internal auditory canal can be initially located in the "safe" medial area of the temporal bone and followed laterally.

Surgical Technique

The patient is placed in the supine position with the head turned to the side. The surgeon is seated at the head of the table and the anesthesiologist is at the foot. An incision is made in the pretragal area and extended superiorly in a gently curving fashion (Fig. 49–2). The midportion of the incision curves posteriorly, which keeps it in the hair of most patients with male pattern baldness. An inferiorly based U-shaped flap is fashioned of the temporalis muscle and fascia and is reflected inferiorly.

By use of a cutting burr, a craniotomy opening is made in the squamous portion of the temporal bone (Fig. 49–3). It is located approximately two thirds anterior and one third posterior to the external auditory canal and is approximately 5×5 cm². Anterior placement of the craniotomy is important for adequate exposure, especially for a left ear. This bone flap is based on the root of the zygoma as close to the floor of the middle fossa as possible. During creation of this flap, care is taken to avoid laceration of the underlying dura. The bone flap is set aside for later replacement.

The dura is elevated from the floor of the middle fossa. The initial landmark is the middle meningeal artery, which marks the anterior extent of the dissection. Frequently, venous bleeding will be encountered from this area and can be controlled with oxidized cellulose (Surgicel). Dissection of the dura proceeds in a posterior-to-anterior manner. In approximately 5 per cent of cases, the geniculate ganglion of the facial nerve will be dehiscent, but injury can be avoided with dural elevation. The petrous ridge is identified, and care is taken not to injure the superior petrosal sinus. The arcuate eminence and greater superficial petrosal nerve are identified. These are the major landmarks to the subsequent intratemporal dissection. Once the dura has been elevated, typically with a suction-irrigator and a blunt dural elevator, the House-Urban retractor is placed to support the temporal lobe. To maintain a secure position, the teeth of the retaining retractor should be locked against the bony margins of the craniotomy window and the tip of the retractor placed beneath the petrous ridge (Fig. 49–4).

The greater superficial petrosal nerve is located medial to the middle meningeal artery (Fig. 49–5). Using a large diamond drill and continuous suction-irrigation, the superior semicircular canal is identified. Bone is removed at the medial aspect of the petrous ridge at the bisection of the angle formed by the greater superficial petrosal nerve and the superior semicircular canal. The internal auditory canal is identified in this medial location and traced laterally. The dura of the posterior fossa is widely exposed (2 cm) and the circumference of the porus acusticus is exposed for approximately 270 degrees (Fig. 49–6). As the dissection proceeds laterally, it must narrow to about 90 degrees due to the encroachment of the cochlea and superior semicircular canal. At the lateral end of the internal auditory canal, Bill's bar and the labyrinthine facial nerve are exposed.

The dura of the internal auditory canal is divided along the posterior aspect (Fig. 49–7). The facial nerve is clearly identified in the anterior portion of the internal auditory canal.

The superior vestibular nerve is divided at its lateral end and the tumor is separated from the facial nerve using high magnification (Figs. 49–8). The tumor is separated initially at Bill's bar, but all dissection along the facial nerve is from medial to lateral. Intracapsular debulking is performed, if needed, using microscissors and cup forceps. Tumor removal is accomplished from a medial to lateral direction to prevent traction on the cochlear nerve and blood supply as it enters the modiolus. If uninvolved, the inferior vestibular nerve is left in an effort to preserve the labyrinthine artery. Persistent unsteadiness from a partial vestibulopathy can occur in patients with a retained inferior vestibular nerve.

After irrigation of the tumor bed (Fig. 49–9) and establishment of hemostasis, papaverine-soaked Gelfoam is placed on the cochlear nerve to prevent vasospasm. The first author (CS) also places steroid (Solu-Medrol)-soaked Gelfoam on the facial nerve to decrease postoperative edema. Abdominal fat is used to close the defect in the internal auditory canal. The House-Urban retractor is removed, and the temporal lobe is allowed to re-expand. The craniotomy flap is replaced.

The wound is closed with absorbable subcutaneous sutures over a Penrose drain, if indicated. This drain is typically removed on the first postoperative day. A mastoid-type pressure dressing is maintained for 4 days postoperatively.

The patient is observed in the intensive care unit overnight and typically is hospitalized for 5 days. Once the patient leaves the intensive care unit, ambulation is encouraged. We believe that early ambulation is important for rapid vestibular compensation.

Although not severe, postoperative pain after the middle fossa approach is more intense than that from the other approaches. This pain results from muscle spasm from division of the temporalis muscle. Some degree of temporary trismus may also result. Routine postoperative analgesics are usually sufficient to control this pain.

FIGURE 49-4

FIGURE 49-5

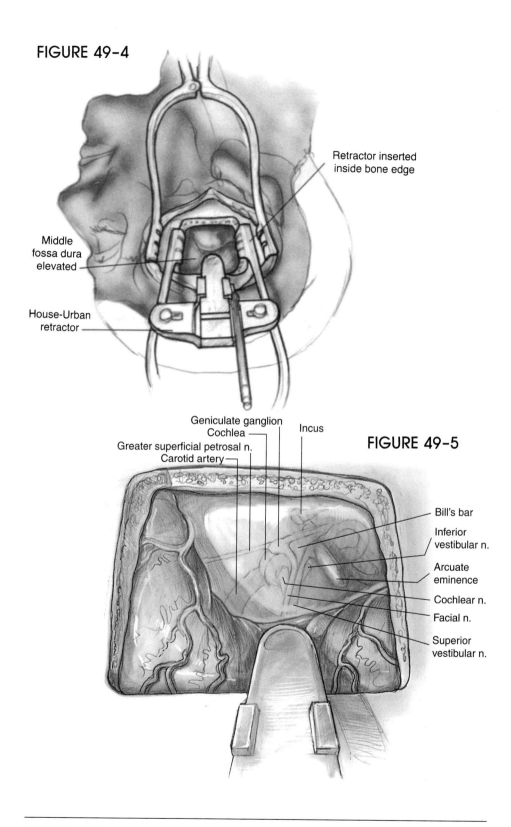

Retractor inserted inside bone edge

Middle fossa dura elevated

House-Urban retractor

Geniculate ganglion
Cochlea
Greater superficial petrosal n.
Carotid artery

Incus

Bill's bar

Inferior vestibular n.

Arcuate eminence

Cochlear n.

Facial n.

Superior vestibular n.

FIGURE 49–4. Temporal lobe is supported by House-Urban retractor.

FIGURE 49–5. The greater superficial petrosal nerve is identified medial to the middle meningeal artery.

FIGURE 49-6

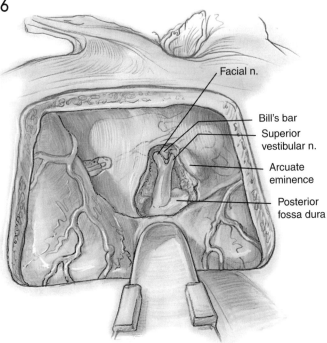

Facial n.

Bill's bar
Superior
vestibular n.

Arcuate
eminence

Posterior
fossa dura

FIGURE 49-7

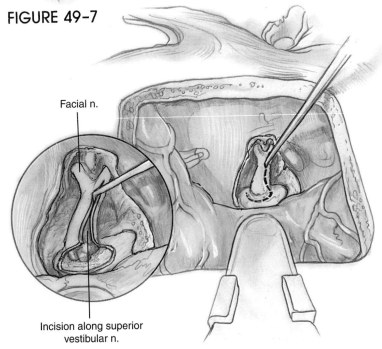

Facial n.

Incision along superior
vestibular n.

FIGURE 49–6. The geniculate ganglion is found by following the superficial petrosal nerve posteriorly. Bill's bar separates the facial from the superior vestibular nerve at the lateral end of the internal auditory canal. The internal auditory canal is skeletonized through the entire length. Bone is removed around the porus acusticus, uncovering dura of the posterior fossa.

FIGURE 49–7. The dura of the internal auditory canal is incised along the posterior aspect.

FIGURE 49-8

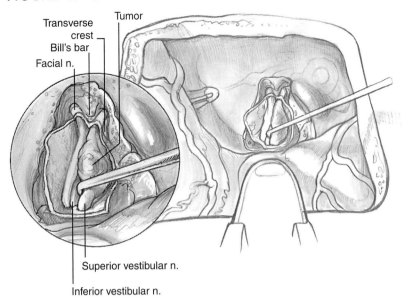

Transverse crest
Bill's bar
Facial n.
Tumor

Superior vestibular n.

Inferior vestibular n.

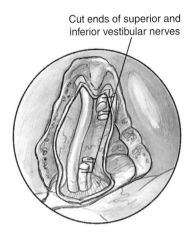

Cut ends of superior and inferior vestibular nerves

FIGURE 49-9

FIGURE 49–8. The intracanalicular acoustic tumor is dissected from the facial and cochlear nerves.

FIGURE 49–9. Divided vestibular nerves are visible after tumor removal.

RESULTS

Course of Healing

Postoperative dizziness varies with the amount of remaining vestibular function in the ear preoperatively. The more function remaining, the greater the postoperative dizziness and the longer the time for central compensation to occur. Patients tend to have the most severe dizziness the first day or two postoperatively, and by the end of the first week they are left with unsteadiness. By this time, they generally can ambulate without assistance.

The middle fossa and abdominal incisions are usually well healed, and patients are able to get them wet 1 week after surgery. Other postoperative instructions include avoidance of vigorous activity and heavy lifting for 6 weeks after surgery. When the patients no longer feel dizzy, they may begin driving.

Success Rate

In a series of 106 patients over a 25-year span with tumors removed through the middle fossa approach, hearing was preserved in 59 per cent and preserved near the preoperative level in 35 per cent of cases.[11] Hearing preservation rates have improved as a result of technical improvements (wider bony exposure of medial internal auditory canal, medial to lateral tumor dissection, use of high magnification, and use of topical papaverine)[35] and increased experience due to more frequent diagnosis of smaller tumors because of improved imaging. A recent series of 333 middle fossa acoustic tumor removals performed over a 7-year period yielded a hearing preservation rate of 80 per cent with hearing preserved near the preoperative level (within 15 dB pure tone average and 15 per cent speech discrimination score [SDS]) in 50 per cent.[28] At 1 year, 95 per cent of patients had normal or near-normal facial results (House-Brackmann I or II).[26]

Complications

Complications occurred in 18 per cent of patients.[11] Two patients had cerebrospinal fluid leaks that required surgical closure. No patient had postoperative seizures or hydrocephalus. Six patients had meningitis that responded to antibiotic therapy.

Serious complications were rare. There were two postoperative deaths, both in the 1960s, early in our experience. The middle fossa approach was used then for tumors that were larger than we would now consider appropriate. One patient died after a posterior fossa hemorrhage; the other patient died from anteroinferior cerebellar artery thrombosis.

Postoperative seizures have been reported in only two patients from one series.[21] Electroencephalographic studies in both of these patients were consistent with an ipsilateral temporal lobe source for the epileptic activity, which was felt to result from temporal lobe retraction. These complications are best avoided by limited temporal lobe retraction of short duration (1 to 1.5 hours).

Patient Selection Pitfalls

For the middle fossa approach, the most important limitation in patient selection is tumor size. Because of the limited access to the posterior fossa, this approach is best suited for intracanalicular tumors and tumors with moderate cerebellopontine angle extension. With larger tumors, difficulty in controlling bleeding in the posterior fossa may be encountered.

SUMMARY

The middle fossa approach is well suited for the removal of small acoustic tumors and may preserve hearing. The most appropriate candidates have tumors with moderate extension into the cerebellopontine angle and good preoperative hearing. Measurable postoperative hearing can be preserved in 80 per cent of patients, and normal or near-normal facial function occurs in 95 per cent. Serious postoperative complications are rare with this approach.

With the advent of gadolinium-enhanced MRI, it is now possible to reliably diagnose acoustic tumors when they are small and before hearing has been significantly affected. The middle fossa approach provides excellent access for the removal of these small tumors.

References

1. Parry RH: A case of tinnitus and vertigo treated by division of the auditory nerve. J Laryngol Otol 19: 402, 1991.
2. House WF: Surgical exposure of the internal auditory canal and its contents through the middle cranial fossa. Laryngoscope 71: 1363, 1961.
3. House WF: Middle cranial fossa approach to the petrous pyramid: Report of 50 cases. Arch Otolaryngol Head Neck Surg 78: 460, 1963.
4. House WF, Gardner G, Hughes RL: Middle cranial fossa approach to acoustic tumor surgery. Arch Otolaryngol Head Neck Surg 88: 631, 1968.
5. Kurze T, Doyle JB Jr: Extradural intracranial (middle fossa) approach to the internal auditory canal. J Neurosurg 19: 1033, 1962.
6. House F, Hitselberger WE: The middle fossa approach for removal of small acoustic tumors. Acta Otolaryngol (Stockh) 67: 413, 1969.
7. Wade PJ, House WF: Hearing preservation in patients with acoustic neuromas via the middle fossa approach. Otolaryngol Head Neck Surg 92: 184, 1984.
8. Shelton C, Hitselberger WE: The treatment of small acoustic tumors: Now or later? Laryngoscope 101: 925, 1991.
9. Brackmann DE: Middle cranial fossa approach. *In* House WF, Luetje CM (eds): Acoustic Tumors, Vol 2: Management. Baltimore, University Park Press, 1979, p 15.
10. Glasscock ME, Poe DS, Johnson GD: Hearing preservation in surgery of cerebellopontine angle tumors. *In* Fisch U, Valavanis A, Yasargil MG (eds): Neurological Surgery of the Ear and Skullbase. Amsterdam, Kugler & Ghedini, 1989, p 207.
11. Shelton C, Brackmann DE, House WF, et al: Middle fossa acoustic tumor surgery: Results in 106 cases. Laryngoscope 99: 405, 1989.
12. Dautheribes M, Migueis A, Vital JM, et al: Anatomical basis of the extended subtemporal approach to the cerebellopontine angle: Its value and limitations. Surg Radiol Anat 11: 187, 1989.
13. Rosomoff HL: The subtemporal transtentorial approach to the cerebellopontine angle. Laryngoscope 81:1448, 1971.

14. Wigand ME, Haid T, Berg M: The enlarged middle cranial fossa approach for surgery of the temporal bone and of the cerebellopontine angle. Arch Otorhinolaryngol 246: 299, 1989.
15. Bochenek Z, Kukwa A: An extended approach through the middle cranial fossa to the internal auditory meatus and the cerebellopontine angle. Acta Otolaryngol (Stockh) 80: 410, 1975.
16. Kanzaki J, Ogawa K, Shiobara R, et al: Hearing preservation in acoustic neuroma surgery and postoperative findings. Acta Otolaryngol (Stockh) 107: 474, 1989.
17. Shiobara R, Ohira T, Kanzaki J, et al: A modified extended middle cranial fossa approach for acoustic nerve tumors: Results of 125 operations. J Neurosurg 68: 358, 1988.
18. Shelton C, Brackmann DE, House WF, et al: Acoustic tumor surgery: Prognostic factors in hearing conservation. Arch Otolaryngol Head Neck Surg 115: 1213, 1989.
19. Gantz BJ, Parnes LS, Harker LA, et al: Middle cranial fossa acoustic neuroma excision: Results and complications. Ann Otol Rhinol Laryngol 95: 454, 1986.
20. Frerebeau PH, Benezech J, Uziel A, et al: Hearing preservation after acoustic neurinoma operation. Neurosurgery 21:197, 1987.
21. Glasscock M III, McKennan KX, Levine SC: Acoustic neuroma surgery: The results of hearing conservation surgery. Laryngoscope 97: 785, 1987.
22. Josey AF, Glasscock ME, Jackson CG: Preservation of hearing in acoustic tumor surgery: Audiologic indicators. Ann Otol Rhinol Laryngol 97: 626, 1988.
23. Nadol JB Jr, Levine R, Ojemann RG, et al: Preservation of hearing in surgical removal of acoustic neuromas of the internal auditory canal and cerebellar pontine angle. Laryngoscope 97: 1287, 1987.
24. Mangham CA, Skalabrin TA: Indications for hearing preservation in acoustic tumor surgery. Presented at the Annual Meeting of the American Neurotology Society, Kona, Hawaii, May 4, 1991.
25. Kemink JL, LaRouere MJ, Kileny RP, et al: Hearing preservation following suboccipital removal of acoustic neuromas. Laryngoscope 100: 597, 1990.
26. Slattery WH, Brackmann DE, Hitselberger WE: Middle fossa approach for hearing preservation with acoustic neuromas. Am J Otol 18: 596–601, 1997.
27. Glasscock ME, Woods CI, Jackson CG, et al: Management of bilateral acoustic tumors. Laryngoscope 99: 475, 1989.
28. Brackmann DE, Owens RM, Friedman RA, et al: Prognostic factors for hearing preservation in vestibular schwannoma surgery. Am J Otol 21: 417–424, 2000.
29. Shelton C, Harnsberger HR, Allen R, King B: Fast spin echo magnetic resonance imaging: Clinical application in screening for acoustic neuroma. Otolaryngol Head Neck Surg 114: 71–76, 1996.
30. Berliner KI, Shelton C, Hitselberger WE, Luxford WM: Acoustic tumors: Effect of surgical removal on tinnitus. Am J Otol 13: 13, 1992.
31. Roberson J, Senne A, Brackmann D, et al: Direct cochlear nerve action potentials as an aid to hearing preservation in middle fossa acoustic neuroma resection. Am J Otol 17: 653–657, 1996.
32. Kartush JM, Kemink JL, Graham MD: The arcuate eminence: Topographic orientation in middle cranial fossa surgery. Ann Otol Rhinol Laryngol 94: 25, 1985.
33. Parisier SC: The middle cranial fossa approach to the internal auditory canal: An anatomical study stressing critical distances between surgical landmarks. Laryngoscope 87(Suppl 4): 1, 1977.
34. Garcia-Ibanez E, Garcia-Ibanez JL: Middle fossa vestibular neurectomy: A report of 373 cases. Otolaryngol Head Neck Surg 88: 486, 1980.
35. Brackmann DE, House JR, Hitselberger WE: Technical modifications to the middle fossa craniotomy approach in removal of acoustic neuromas. Am J Otol 15: 614–619, 1994.

50

Translabyrinthine Approach

John W. House, M.D. ▪ Rick A. Friedman, M.D., Ph.D.

Since William F. House first began removing acoustic tumors through the translabyrinthine approach in 1960,[1, 2] we at the House Ear Clinic have been using this approach for most of our acoustic tumor removals. To date, we have removed about 2750 acoustic neuromas with this approach. The translabyrinthine procedure allows excellent access to the cerebellopontine angle (CPA) and exposure of the entire facial nerve from the brainstem to the stylomastoid foramen. The approach is extradural through most of the surgery. The primary disadvantage is sacrifice of hearing.

In patients with poor or no hearing, the translabyrinthine approach is ideal for acoustic neuromas; facial nerve lesions, such as neuromas; trauma due to operative injury; or head trauma. The approach has many advantages: It is the most direct route to the structures of the CPA (Figs. 50–1 and 50–2).[3] The lateral end of the internal auditory canal (IAC) can be dissected to ensure complete tumor removal from this area and allow consistent anatomic identification of the facial nerve.[4] The approach also offers exposure of the mastoid, tympanic, and labyrinthine portions of the facial nerve. Identification of the facial nerve in the mastoid is possible after removal of the semicircular canals (Fig. 50–3). Because the labyrinth has been removed, the labyrinthine segment of the nerve is readily followed into the IAC. The IAC and CPA can be exposed widely if the lesion involves the facial nerve in the posterior fossa. The facial nerve is readily accessible from the brainstem to the stylomastoid foramen and beyond into the parotid gland. Many procedures other than acoustic tumor removal can be performed through this approach, including excision of other tumors (e.g., meningiomas, cholesteatomas involving the petrous bone and posterior fossa, cholesterol granulomas, glomus tumors, and adenomas), decompression of the facial nerve, and repair of the nerve by either direct end-to-end anastomoses or nerve grafting (Fig. 50–4).

For tumors involving the area anterior to the internal auditory nerve at the clivus, the standard translabyrinthine approach is modified to allow anterior exposure (Fig. 50–5). The facial nerve is removed from the fallopian canal in the tympanic and mastoid segments and is reflected anteriorly. The cochlea is then removed to provide excellent exposure anterior to the IAC (see Chapter 53 on the transcochlear approach).

A major advantage of the translabyrinthine approach is that the patient is in the supine position with the head turned away from the surgeon (Figs. 50–6 and 50–7). This position eliminates some of the possible complications of the classic suboccipital approach to the CPA in which the sitting position is used, including risks of air embolism and injury to the cerebellum from retraction. In addition,

quadriplegia has been reported in association with the sitting position.[5] The translabyrinthine approach poses no danger of air embolism and does not require retraction of the cerebellum. The brain and surrounding structures are less likely to be injured because much of the surgery is extradural.

PATIENT SELECTION

Tumor size and residual hearing are the principal factors influencing the choice of the translabyrinthine approach. We use the translabyrinthine approach in most cases if the tumor extends into the CPA more than 1 cm and in all cases of nonserviceable hearing in the tumor ear. When tumors are confined to the IAC in an ear with serviceable hearing, we use the middle cranial fossa approach in an attempt to save hearing. In some patients with good hearing, the retrosigmoid approach is chosen, primarily for tumors in the CPA with minimal extension into the IAC.

Our definition of serviceable hearing is a pure tone average threshold better than 50 dB, a speech discrimination score of greater than 50 per cent, or both. This definition is referred to as the *50/50 rule*. Of course, exceptions exist if the hearing in the contralateral ear is poor or if bilateral tumors are present. In such cases, we may attempt tumor removal through the middle fossa approach, even if the tumor extends up to 1 cm into the CPA. We may use the retrosigmoid approach in an attempt to save hearing if the tumor is smaller than 1.5 or 2 cm and does not extend into the lateral half of the IAC.

SURGICAL PROCEDURE

The procedure is performed with general endotracheal anesthesia with inhalation agents. Muscle relaxants are used only for the induction because they may interfere with facial nerve monitoring, which is used in all cases. A nasogastric tube and Foley catheter are placed. A generous amount of hair is shaved from the postauricular and temporal areas. The skin is cleaned with povidone-iodine (Betadine) and a plastic Vi-Drape placed to cover the entire area. Because facial nerve monitoring is routine during all of our translabyrinthine procedures, needle electrodes are inserted into the orbicularis oris muscles before the drape is applied. The lower abdomen is also prepared and draped to allow for the harvesting of fat.

Lidocaine (Xylocaine) 1 per cent with epinephrine 1:100,000 is injected into the postauricular region. The

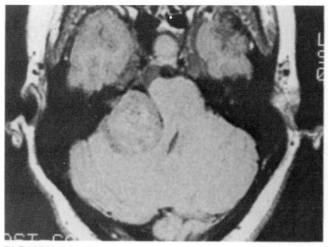

FIGURE 50-1

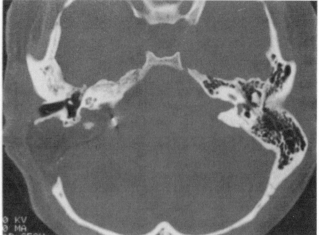

FIGURE 50-2

FIGURE 50-3

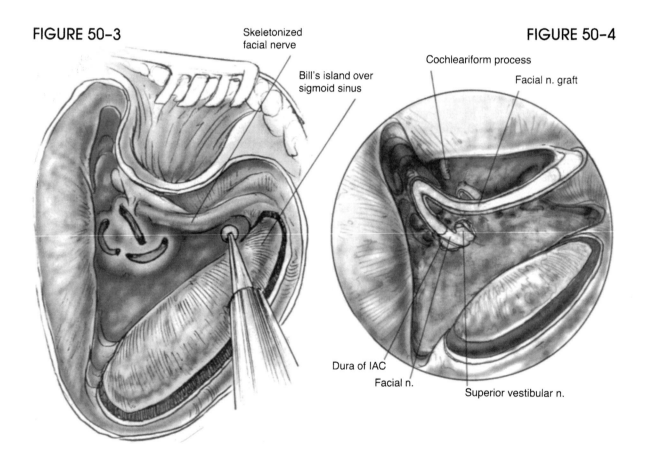

FIGURE 50-4

Skeletonized facial nerve

Bill's island over sigmoid sinus

Cochleariform process

Facial n. graft

Dura of IAC

Facial n.

Superior vestibular n.

FIGURE 50–1. Magnetic resonance image of large acoustic neuroma, illustrating the direct route to the cerebellopontine angle through the mastoid and labyrinth.

FIGURE 50–2. Postoperative computed tomographic scan of patient shown in Figure 50–1. Note the extent of removal of bone from the mastoid and labyrinth.

FIGURE 50–3. Facial nerve identified in mastoid portion after removal of semicircular canals. Note the island of bone over the sigmoid sinus.

FIGURE 50–4. Facial nerve graft through the translabyrinthine approach. A greater auricular nerve graft has been placed from the internal auditory canal to the proximal mastoid facial nerve.

FIGURE 50-5

Meningioma

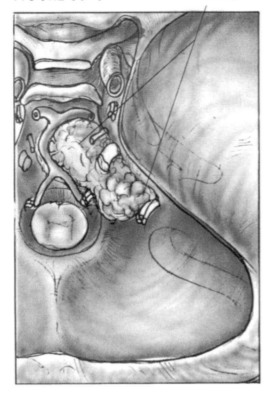

FIGURE 50–5. Meningioma involving the internal auditory canal and extending anterior to the clivus can be removed through the translabyrinthine-transcochlear approach.

FIGURE 50–6. Patient placed in the supine position with head turned away from surgeon. Anesthesiologist is at foot of table.

FIGURE 50–7. The surgeon is seated with the operating microscope. The nurse is across the table. Note the facial nerve monitor at lower left.

FIGURE 50-6

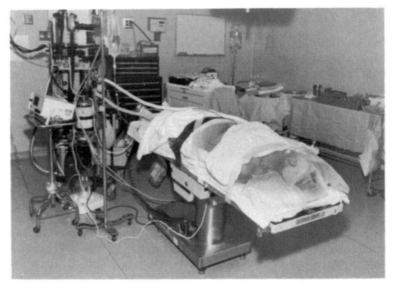

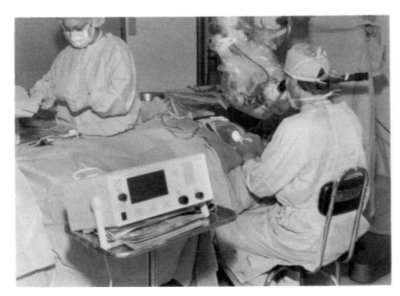

FIGURE 50-7

epinephrine assists with homeostasis. The incision is performed about 2 to 4 cm posterior to the postauricular sulcus. The incision is curved anteriorly to allow anterior retraction of the pinna. The posterior curve of the incision allows exposure of the area posterior to the sigmoid sinus. This exposure is important to allow access to the CPA. The Lempert elevator is used to elevate the periosteum off the bone of the mastoid. Soft tissue must be removed from the posterior edge of the external auditory canal to an area far posterior to the sigmoid sinus. Care must be taken not to tear the skin of the external auditory canal. We use a self-retaining retractor with rings to hold a small suction catheter that helps remove blood and irrigation fluid from the wound.

A complete mastoidectomy is performed with a high-speed drill with various sizes of cutting and diamond burrs. Removing bone 2 cm posterior to the sigmoid sinus is crucial for adequate exposure of the dura of the posterior cranial fossa. A small bony island of bone ("Bill's island" named for William F. House, who first suggested it) is left over the otherwise exposed sigmoid sinus (Fig. 50–8). This bony cover protects the sigmoid sinus from the shaft of the burr as the drilling proceeds medially to remove the labyrinth. The dissection continues with the removal of all bone covering the posterior fossa dura medial to the sigmoid sinus and down to the labyrinth. It is important to remove all bone over the sinal dural angle and a small amount of bone over the middle fossa dura adjacent to the angle. In larger tumors or contracted mastoids, we recommend removal of 2 to 3 cm of bone from temporal squama. We prefer to perform all of the lateral bone work before beginning the labyrinthectomy to obtain better exposure of the deep structures.

After the complete mastoidectomy is performed and the bone is removed from posterior fossa dura, sigmoid sinus, and some of the middle fossa dura, the deepest point of dissection shifts to the sinal-dural angle. The labyrinthectomy begins with the removal of the lateral semicircular canal and extends posterior to the posterior canal. The bone removal is continued inferior and anterior toward the ampullated end of this canal (Fig. 50–9). The ampulla of the posterior canal is the landmark for the inferior border of the internal auditory canal. The inferior extent of bony removal is the jugular bulb. The posterior semicircular canal is opened inferiorly to the vestibule and superiorly to the common crus. The facial nerve is identified in its descending portion in the mastoid and skeletonized to just proximal to the stylomastoid foramen. We prefer to identify the facial nerve after the posterior semicircular canal has been removed to use the side of the diamond burr rather than the end of it. This helps reduce the possibility of injury to the nerve. The mastoid segment of the facial nerve serves as the anterior limit of dissection. With this portion of the facial nerve identified, the remainder of the bone of the inferior IAC is removed to the vestibule. After opening the vestibule widely, the removal of the superior portion (nonampullated end) of the posterior canal is carried to the common crus, which is composed of the nonampullated ends of the posterior and superior semicircular canal.

The common crus is opened to the vestibule. The superior canal is now opened and removed to its ampullated end in the vestibule. This portion of the superior canal identifies the area where the superior vestibular nerve exits the lateral end of the IAC and is in close proximity to the labyrinthine segment of the facial nerve. Similarly, the singular nerve exits the IAC at the posterior semicircular canal ampulla and the inferior vestibular nerve exits the canal at the saccule and the spherical recess. Identification of these structures delineates the superior and inferior extent of the IAC. As the bone posterior to the IAC is removed, the vestibular aqueduct and the beginning of the endolymphatic sac are removed. An eggshell thickness of bone is left over the dura of the IAC to avoid injury to the underlying structures until all of the bony dissection is completed (Fig. 50–10).

The IAC is not entered at this time because bone must be removed medially to the porus acusticus. It is important to keep in mind that the IAC runs deep from the vestibule and away from the surgeon. A great deal of bone must be removed to properly expose the contents of the IAC and the CPA. Bone is removed around the canal superiorly and inferiorly to expose at least 270 degrees in circumference. The inferior limit of bone removal is the cochlear aqueduct and the jugular bulb. The cochlear aqueduct enters the posterior fossa directly inferior to the midportion of the IAC, superior to the jugular bulb (Fig. 50–11).[6] It identifies the location of the neural compartment of the jugular foramen anterior to the jugular bulb. By not removing bone from anterior and deep to the cochlear aqueduct, injury to cranial nerves IX, X, and XI is avoided. Bone is removed from the inferior portion of the IAC and particularly the inferior lip, thereby affording access to the inferior poll of the tumor in the CPA.

The bone is removed from the superlateral IAC last because of its close proximity to the facial nerve. Bone should be removed from the superior lip of the IAC. This dissection is tedious because the facial nerve often underlies the dura along the anterosuperior aspect of the IAC. The surgeon must be careful not to allow the burr to drop into the canal and possibly injure the nerve. As with the inferior lip, all of the bone must be removed from the

---

FIGURE 50–8. Mastoidectomy with exposure of the sigmoid sinus. Note that a small bony island is left over the sinus to protect it from the shaft of the burr.

FIGURE 50–9. Completed labyrinthectomy with ampullated ends of posterior and superior semicircular canals.

FIGURE 50–10. All bone has been removed, exposing the dura of the posterior fossa and the internal auditory canal.

FIGURE 50–11. Bone has been removed from the internal auditory canal (IAC) and the posterior fossa. The cochlear aqueduct can be seen inferior to the IAC and superior to the jugular bulb.

FIGURE 50-8

MASTOIDECTOMY

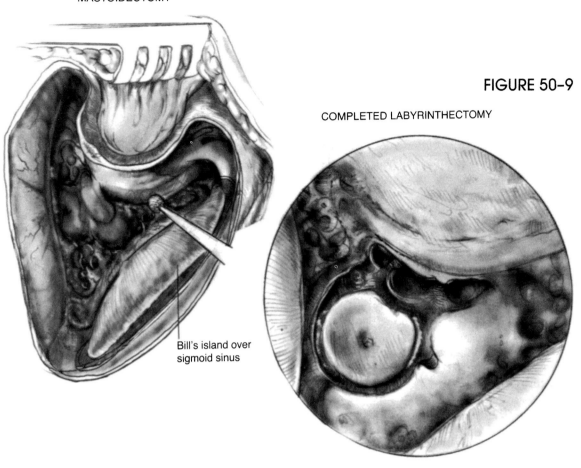

Bill's island over
sigmoid sinus

FIGURE 50-9

COMPLETED LABYRINTHECTOMY

FIGURE 50-10

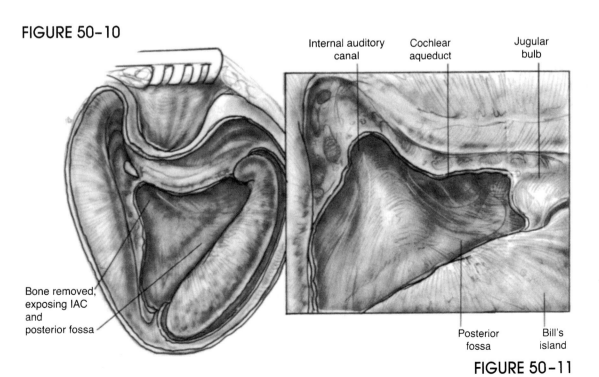

Bone removed,
exposing IAC
and
posterior fossa

Internal auditory
canal

Cochlear
aqueduct

Jugular
bulb

Posterior
fossa

Bill's
island

FIGURE 50-11

superior lip to allow access to the superior pole of the tumor. With the superior lip, the facial nerve may be close to the surface, making this part of the removal laborious.

The facial nerve is identified as it exits the lateral end of the IAC at the vertical crest of bone ("Bill's bar") with a sharp 3-mm hook. The facial nerve may be further identified in its proximal labyrinthine segment by additional bone removal. The hook is passed carefully along the inside of the superior distal IAC until Bill's bar is palpated (Fig. 50–12). It is not unusual for the facial nerve monitor to sound a warning as the hook passes along the nerve at the proximal portion of the fallopian canal.

All of the dissection thus far has been extradural, and morbidity should be minimal. Once the facial nerve has been positively identified, the dura of the posterior fossa over the midportion of the IAC is opened with sharp scissors. The length of the incision depends on the size of the tumor. For smaller tumors and nerve sections, the incision is made close to the IAC. For larger tumors it is started closer to the sigmoid sinus. The incision extends to the IAC, and then curves superiorly and inferiorly around the porus acusticus. The surgeon must take care to avoid blood vessels on the surface of the tumor and adjacent to the dura. Posteriorly the petrosal vein lies close to the dura. The IAC is opened over the inferior vestibular nerve and reflected superiorly to avoid injury to the facial nerve. Cottonoids are placed posteriorly between the tumor and the cerebellum. It is important to develop this plane accurately because doing so separates the major vessels of the CPA from the tumor.

With larger tumors the size of the tumor is reduced by the use of the House-Urban dissector (Fig. 50–13). The surface of the tumor is carefully inspected first to identify nerves. Occasionally the facial nerve is deflected posterior. The tumor capsule is incised, then the dissector is inserted to begin the intracapsular removal of the bulk of the tumor. Excessive manipulation of the tumor must be avoided because it can cause traction of the facial nerve. The capsule of the tumor is then collapsed toward its center, greatly facilitating its dissection from the CPA. The tumor is then followed medially to the brainstem. The plane between the tumor and the brainstem is developed with sharp and blunt dissection. Cottonoids are placed between the brainstem and the tumor. At this point, attempts are made to identify the facial nerve superiorly. It is usually anterior to the tumor but may be draped over the top of it. The ninth cranial nerve is identified inferiorly. In large tumors the ninth cranial nerve may be stretched over the surface of the tumor. Manipulation of the tumor may cause a change in the pulse rate or blood pressure. During this phase of the tumor removal avoidance of injury to surrounding structures is greatly facilitated by the use of the fenestrated neurotologic suction tip.[7]

The vestibular nerve and tumor are separated from the facial nerve in the IAC and carefully dissected medially to the porus acusticus and into the CPA (Fig. 50–14). Some tumors involve the lateral end of the IAC, complicating identification of the facial nerve in the canal. In these cases, bone is removed from the proximal fallopian canal to allow positive identification of the facial nerve where it is not involved with tumor. This maneuver greatly reduces injury to the facial nerve.

It may be necessary to identify the facial nerve at the brainstem and to begin to separate the tumor from the facial nerve medially to laterally. Careful, patient dissection results in complete separation of the facial nerve from the tumor as the tumor is dissected out of the posterior fossa. Continuous intraoperative facial nerve monitoring has greatly facilitated this process. It has demonstrated that use of scissors to carefully free the nerve from the tumor causes less trauma than the use of blunt dissection to establish this plane.

As the tumor is dissected free, bleeding is controlled with bipolar cautery and, in rare instances, clips. Only the vessels that enter the tumor capsule are coagulated. The other vessels are freed from the tumor capsule. A small blood vessel may accompany the eighth cranial nerve. As the nerve is cut, control of bleeding with bipolar cautery or a clip may be necessary. Careful control of bleeding produces minimal blood loss. With an average blood loss of about 250 ml our patients rarely need transfusions. As a precaution, we offer patients the opportunity to withdraw 1 or 2 units of their own blood up to 1 month prior to the scheduled surgery.

During the drilling, the wound is periodically irrigated with a solution containing bacitracin to reduce the chance of infection. After the drilling has been completed, the bacitracin irrigant is attached to the suction-irrigator used during the dissection of the tumor. This solution cannot be used during drilling because it tends to produce foam. Using this technique, we have reduced the rate of meningitis in our patients.

Closure involves the use of abdominal fat, and if the opening is large, a partial closure of the dura. Fat is obtained from the lower abdomen through a small transverse incision. The wound is closed with subcuticular sutures and a Penrose drain inserted. The fat is cut into strips and soaked in the bacitracin irrigant. The dura is closed with 4-0 silk along the posterior fossa incision. The strips of fat are inserted through the dural opening and the IAC, extending about 2 cm into the angle. These strips are tightly packed into the defect, and they expand on both sides of the dura to prevent leakage. Additional fat is packed into the attic. The incus may be removed to pack the eustachian tube and the middle ear with muscle. The mastoid is also filled with fat. The wound is closed in layers with 0 chromic and 3-0 Vicryl. Steri-Strips are applied to both wounds. A head dressing and abdominal pressure dressings are applied.

Management of the Contracted Mastoid

There are few absolute contraindications to the use of translabyrinthine approach in acoustic tumor removal. One absolute contraindication is active infection in the affected ear. In addition, there has been controversy regarding the use of this approach in anatomically constricted mastoids: A low-lying tegmen, an anterior sigmoid sinus, or a high jugular bulb are individually and/or collectively considered contraindications to this approach.

Utilizing several critical manuevers, we have never altered our approach to the CPA based on anatomic varia-

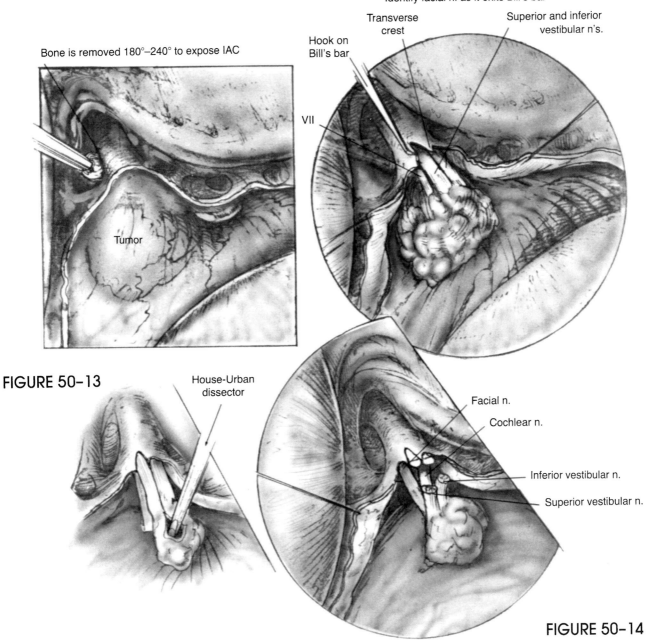

FIGURE 50-12

Bone is removed 180°–240° to expose IAC

Identify facial n. as it exits Bill's bar

Transverse
crest

Superior and inferior
vestibular n's.

Hook on
Bill's bar

VII

Tumor

FIGURE 50-13

House-Urban
dissector

Facial n.

Cochlear n.

Inferior vestibular n.

Superior vestibular n.

FIGURE 50-14

Figure 50-12. The internal auditory canal (IAC) is skeletonized, and bone is removed to expose 180 to 240 degrees of the canal. The facial nerve is identified as it exits the IAC at Bill's bar.

FIGURE 50-13. The House-Urban dissector is used for intracapsular removal of tumor bulk.

FIGURE 50-14. The vestibular nerve and tumor are separated from the facial nerve in the internal auditory canal and dissected to the porus acusticus and the cerebellopontine angle.

tions.[8] Wide removal of the bone of the temporal squama and presigmoid and postsigmoid posterior fossa dura overcomes the limitations imposed by a low-lying tegmen and anterior-placed sigmoid sinus, respectively. For a high jugular bulb, we recommend skeletonization along its anteromedial, medial, and posterior surfaces without compression. This, combined with the ability to retract the widely exposed temporal lobe dura superiorly, provides improved line of sight in the deep field of the CPA.

POSTOPERATIVE CARE

The abdominal drain is removed the following day. To prevent vomiting and aspiration, a nasogastric tube is inserted at anesthesia induction in the operating room and is attached to suction. This tube is also removed the following day. In addition, the urinary catheter inserted at the beginning of the procedure is removed on postoperative day 1 or 2. The head dressing remains for 3 days, and the Steri-Strips remain for 1 week.

The patient stays in the intensive care unit for 1 or 2 days after surgery and then is transferred to a standard room. Progressive ambulation starts the day after surgery. The patient sits on the side of the bed, stands by the bed, and is encouraged to sit in a chair. We believe that early ambulation helps reduce complications and speeds recovery.

Vital signs and temperature are monitored frequently during the first 2 or 3 days after surgery. In addition, the nurses are instructed to observe the patient for possible cerebrospinal fluid leak and neurologic changes. If the patient has drainage from the nose, the nurses test it for glucose and alert the physician.

COMPLICATIONS

Facial Nerve

Facial nerve weakness or paralysis is not a complication but a risk that cannot be entirely eliminated. The primary concern of most patients undergoing tumor removal is the ultimate facial nerve result. Continuous intraoperative facial nerve monitoring and meticulous dissection of the tumor from the facial nerve usually yield good facial nerve results. Eighty per cent of the results of surgery on all tumor patients are House-Brackmann grade I or II. Only about 5 per cent of patients have a grade VI outcome. If the facial nerve is intimately involved with the tumor or if the tumor is a facial neuroma, preservation of the anatomic continuity of the facial nerve may not be possible. We believe that repairing the nerve during the initial surgery is important. With the translabyrinthine approach, the nerve can be identified in the labyrinthine segment, exposed in the tympanic and mastoid portions, and either rerouted or an interposed graft sutured to the proximal and distal portions of the nerve. Suturing the nerve in the CPA is difficult; if this is possible, usually only one suture can be placed. The result allows for normal facial tone and good emotional and voluntary motion. Mass action or synkinesis

is always present. Grade III is the best result that can be expected.

When a primary anastomosis or nerve graft is not possible, or if facial nerve function does not return after 1 year, we perform a facial-hypoglossal (VII-XII) anastomosis. It gives good resting tone, fair voluntary motion with synkinesis, and usually a grade IV recovery. If the nerve has been paralyzed for several years and the patient has poor tone, we combine the VII-XII anastomosis with a temporalis muscle transposition to the orbicularis oris. This procedure gives an immediate cosmetic improvement to the face at rest and gradual return of voluntary motion over 6 to 12 months.

Bleeding

The most dramatic and potentially fatal complication is an early postoperative hematoma in the CPA. This complication is manifested by signs of increased central nervous system pressure, such as loss of consciousness and nonreactive pupils. It is managed by immediate opening of the wound and removal of the fat while the patient is in the intensive care unit. This is an advantage of the translabyrinthine approach, in that the angle may be rapidly decompressed for this uncommon complication. The patient is taken back to surgery, and the bleeder is identified and controlled.

Bleeding is part of the procedure. The most dramatic bleeding occurs if the sigmoid sinus is entered. Opening of the sinus produces profuse bleeding, and because the bleeding is venous, it is easy to stop with light pressure over the sinus. Bleeding is controlled with extraluminal packing with Surgicel, and great care is taken to prevent the packing from entering the lumen of the sinus. If this occurs, the packing will enter the pulmonary circulation, resulting in a pulmonary embolism.

If the lumen of the jugular bulb is opened, the jugular vein is ligated in the neck, and the bulb is packed to control bleeding. This complication is rare.

Arterial bleeding is seldom a problem. Great care is taken to identify and avoid the anterior cerebellar artery because thrombosis or injury to this artery can be fatal. Fortunately, this is extremely rare with modern microsurgical techniques.

Cerebrospinal Fluid Leak

Before 1974, we used temporalis muscle to close the dura, and our incidence of cerebrospinal fluid leak was as high as 20 per cent.[2] Since we began using abdominal fat instead, this incidence has been reduced to less than 7 per cent in translabyrinthine acoustic tumor removals.[9]

Most leaks can be stopped with a pressure head dressing and bed rest with the patient's head elevated. Typically, we leave the dressing in place for 3 or 4 days. If the leak continues with the dressing in place, or if it recurs when the dressing is removed, a lumbar spinal drain is inserted, and the patient is placed at bed rest for 3 to 4 days. If the leak still persists, the patient is taken back to surgery, the wound is reopened, the leak is located, and additional fat is placed. Usually, we harvest additional fat. If excess fat is harvested at the original surgery, it can be frozen and used in case of a later leak. Spinal fluid leaks usually occur in the first 5 days, if at all.

Meningitis

The incidence of meningitis has been falling with the use of bacitracin irrigation and reduced surgical time. In the past few years, only about 3 per cent of postoperative patients have had meningitis,[9] for which a causative agent is rarely identified. A spinal tap is performed when the patient has a fever, elevated white blood cell count, and a stiff neck. If the cerebrospinal fluid white blood cell count is greater than 100, we use high doses of intravenous antibiotics. In addition to the cell count, the spinal fluid is cultured for both anaerobic and aerobic bacteria, and total protein and glucose levels are measured. In typical meningitis patients, the cerebrospinal fluid protein level is elevated, and the glucose level is reduced. Antibiotics are altered if the cultures so indicate. The usual response to treatment is reduction in fever, drop in white blood cell count, and reduction in headache. The spinal tap is repeated on the fourth or fifth treatment day. Treatment is continued until the cerebrospinal fluid cell count is below 100 and the cerebrospinal fluid is composed mostly of monocytes.

RESULTS

The total number of acoustic neuromas removed at the House Ear Clinic now approaches 3000. With experience and refinements of technique, the results have progressively improved. A recent review from our database of acoustic tumor cases provides data from 1302 patients who underwent a translabyrinthine acoustic tumor removal between 1982 and 1993. Their mean age was 50.0 years, and 46 per cent were male and 54 per cent were female. Tumor size varied from 0.5 to 6.5 cm, with a mean size of 2.4 cm. Operating time averaged 3.3 hours. Three (0.2 per cent) deaths occurred in this series.

Data on long-term (6-month) facial nerve function as determined by the House-Brackmann scale were available on 889 cases, with a mean follow-up time of 2.1 years. Of these, 58.2 per cent had a grade I function; 12.6 per cent, grade II; 13.2 per cent, grade III; 7.8 per cent, grade IV; 3.3 per cent, grade V; and 5.1 per cent, grade VI. For cases undergoing surgery since the advent of facial nerve monitoring in 1988 and with at least 1 year follow-up, 59 per cent of the 312 patients had grade I facial nerve function; 15.4 per cent had grade II; 9.3 per cent, grade III; 7.7 per cent, grade IV; 4.2 per cent, grade V; and 4.5 per cent, grade VI.

Postoperative Follow-Up

In our experience, vestibular schwannomas rarely recur after translabyrinthine removal. Our recurrence rate for unilateral tumors removed through the translabyrinthine approach treated between 1961 and 1995 was 0.3 per cent.[10] The average interval to recurrence was 10 years. Based on these findings we have recommended a single gadolinium-enhanced magnetic resonance imaging 5 years postoperatively.

SUMMARY

The translabyrinthine approach to tumors involving the temporal bone and CPA offers excellent and safe exposure. We have used this approach for more than 30 years to remove over 2700 tumors. Our experience has yielded many refinements of the original procedure, and we continue to seek improvements to lower the morbidity. Mortality now approaches zero. We continue to believe that the translabyrinthine approach is the approach of choice for most acoustic neuromas.

References

1. House WF: Acoustic neuroma (Monograph). Arch Otolaryngol Head Neck Surg 80:598–757, 1964.
2. House WF: Translabyrinthine approach. *In* House WF, Luetje CM (eds): Acoustic Tumors, Vol 2: Management. Baltimore, University Park Press, 1979, pp 43–87.
3. Brackmann DE: Translabyrinthine removal of acoustic neurinomas. *In* Brackmann DE (ed): Neurological Surgery of the Ear and Skull Base. New York, Raven Press, 1982, pp 235–241.
4. House WF, Leutje CM (eds): Acoustic Tumors, Vol 1. Baltimore, University Park Press, 1979.
5. Hitselberger WE, House WF: A warning regarding the sitting position for acoustic tumor surgery (Editorial). Arch Otolaryngol Head Neck Surg 106: 69, 1980.
6. Brackmann DE, Green D: Translabyrinthine approach for acoustic tumor removal. Otolaryngol Clin North Am 25:311–329, 1992.
7. Brackmann DE: Fenestrated suction for neuro-otologic surgery. Trans Am Acad Ophthalmol Otolaryngol 84: 975, 1977.
8. Friedman RA, Brackmann DE, van Loveren HR, Hitselberger WE: Management of the contracted mastoid in the translabyrinthine removal of acoustic neuroma. Arch Otolaryngol Head Neck Surg 123: 342–344, 1997.
9. Rodgers GK, Luxford WM: Factors affecting the development of cerebrospinal fluid leak and meningitis after translabyrinthine acoustic tumor surgery. Laryngoscope 103: 959–962, 1993.
10. Shelton C: Unilateral acoustic tumors: How often do they recur after translabyrinthine removal? Laryngoscope 105: 958–966, 1995.

Editorial Comment

Neurotologic approaches to cranial base tumors are a team endeavor in which the neurotologist and the neurosurgeon must be fully familiar with the other members' techniques. A frequent comment by former clinical fellows after completing training at the House Ear Clinic is that differences exist in the removal of acoustic tumors, especially larger tumors, between neurosurgeons familiar with the translabyrinthine approach and those who are adjusting to this anterior exposure.

The editors have invited William E. Hitselberger, M.D. to provide the neurosurgical perspective on tumor removal through the translabyrinthine approach. With a personal experience of more than 3000 acoustic tumors removed with this technique, Dr. Hitselberger has insights that are particularly relevant for neurotologic teams in the early phases of collaboration.

Neurosurgical Techniques in Acoustic Tumor Surgery

William E. Hitselberger, M.D.

The strategy for the removal of an acoustic neuroma depends on whether the tumor is large or small. The techniques used in each of these situations, although similar, vary enough in important details that differences are described and emphasized here. The slight variation in technique is necessary because of the variation in the difficulty in preserving neurologic structures in each of these situations. Although variations exist in the technique used, the size of an acoustic neuroma is not a limiting factor in the choice of the translabyrinthine approach. In 30 years and more than 3000 acoustic neuromas, I have never found a tumor that was too large to take out through this approach.

REMOVAL OF THE SMALL ACOUSTIC TUMOR

In the removal of both the small and the large acoustic neuroma through the translabyrinthine approach, the importance of exposure cannot be overemphasized. Adequate exposure of the tumor is the sine qua non of the procedure. Bone removal should include the bone over the middle fossa dura, the sigmoid sinus should be skeletonized so that it can be easily compressed, and bone removal should extend down to the jugular bulb. The posterior fossa dura should be cleared and easily retractable. The internal auditory canal should be skeletonized for at least 180 degrees from the posterior presentation. The labyrinthine portion of the facial nerve should be identified and uncovered.

During the drill-out of the internal auditory canal, the rotation of the drill is important because the facial nerve is near the surface of the canal and exposed to a greater degree when the tumor is small than when it is larger. In a larger tumor, the tumor usually acts as a buffer between the facial nerve and the drill. If the drill is rotating into the internal auditory canal, the bit can catch on the bony edge, and the fast-moving burr may injure the nerve.

The dura should be opened over the end of the internal auditory canal, and the facial nerve should be positively identified both visually and with the facial nerve stimulator. The nerve at the end of the canal is anterior and superior to the superior vestibular nerve. The plane between these nerves can be readily developed if the bony dissection of the internal auditory canal has been completed at its lateral extent. After division of the facial-vestibular anastomosis, the plane between the superior vestibular nerve and the facial nerve leads the surgeon into the plane between the facial nerve and the tumor. This latter plane is then carried medially down to the porus acusticus.

At this point, the nerve may be bound down in adhesions and tumor. High magnification ($\times 40$) may be necessary to keep the facial nerve plane delineated from the adhesions and tumor. Facial nerve dissection may be facilitated if the nerve is identified at the brainstem. The facial nerve arises anterior and medial to the cochleovestibular nerve. The anteroinferior cerebellar artery usually crosses between the seventh and eighth nerves near the brainstem. The facial nerve is generally quite distinct and has a whiter color than the eighth nerve because of a heavier concentration of myelin.

Developing the facial nerve plane from medial to lateral leads to the medial extent of the tumor. Sometimes, the tumor will then "shell out" from the bed of the eighth nerve. More important, the continuing plane of the facial nerve can be developed back to the porus. Thus, the facial nerve plane is developed from both the medial brainstem side and the lateral internal auditory canal side. Usually, once the facial nerve has been cleared from the surface, the tumor can be easily delivered. Thus, the importance of facial nerve dissection lies both in the preservation of the facial nerve and in the delineation and ultimate removal of the tumor.

Blood vessels lying on the surface of the tumor should be dissected free without coagulation, if possible. This method preserves the blood supply to the adjacent brainstem as well as the facial nerve. A very fine bayonet forceps and scissors can be used to free the vessels from the surface of the tumor without coagulation.

After the tumor has been removed, the tumor bed is carefully evaluated for any small bleeders. Bipolar coagulation set at a low level and oxidized cellulose are generally sufficient to treat such bleeding.

REMOVAL OF THE LARGE ACOUSTIC NEUROMA

The bony removal for a large acoustic neuroma, although similar to that for a small neuroma, varies enough that important variations should be mentioned. Wide, adequate exposure is the key and is accomplished by thorough removal of bone over the middle fossa, posterior fossa, and internal auditory canal. Additionally, bone should be removed for at least 1 cm posterior to the sigmoid sinus over the subocciput. Even with a contracted mastoid, adequate exposure can be obtained for removal of any-sized neuroma if the bone removal has been exploited to the maximum. Another key for removal of a large acoustic neuroma from the cerebellopontine angle is extradural retraction. If the bone removal is inadequate, this retraction against the residual bone is impossible. Bony overhangs at the external genu of the facial nerve and the overhang of the posterior external auditory canal should also be removed.

The facial nerve is identified at the end of the internal auditory canal, as in a smaller tumor. This dissection can be more difficult if the end of the canal is distorted by an impacted tumor, which is occasionally invasive into the otic capsule. After identification of the facial nerve at the end of the internal auditory canal, the dura is opened over the posterior fossa anterior to the sigmoid sinus. The tumor may bulge into the dural opening. A rapid decompression of the interior of the tumor can be carried out with the House-Urban rotary dissector, starting from the posterosuperior compartment of the tumor adjacent to the tentorium. At this point, I am not concerned with moderate venous bleeding; rather, the goal is rapid debulking of the tumor. Coagulating small bleeding vessels is unnecessary; these stop bleeding when the tumor is removed.

Once the tumor has been decompressed, the cisterna lateralis is emptied of spinal fluid. This step further adds to the available space and allows even greater room for retraction. The position of the facial nerve should be ascertained with the facial nerve monitor before radical resection of the tumor is undertaken. Usually, the facial nerve is anterior to the tumor, but it may be superiorly placed. Rarely, it can even be in a posterior position, which is an especially dangerous position for the facial nerve because the surgeon must operate past the facial nerve to remove the tumor, subjecting it to increased risk.

After decompression of the tumor, the facial nerve dissection can be started. High magnification ($\times 40$) and sharp dissection are best suited for this process. The nerve is usually stretched and attenuated by the tumor. The facial nerve monitor is invaluable in delineating the nerve when it has been thinned out over the surface of the tumor. The facial nerve dissection proceeds from both the medial and lateral ends of the tumor.

Vascular radicles are removed from the surface of the tumor, avoiding coagulation whenever possible. A large branch of the petrosal vein is usually positioned on the posterior medial surface of the tumor and should be sought after, identified, and dealt with, either with preservation, if easily accomplished, or with bipolar coagulation.

After tumor removal, all bleeding points in the tumor bed should be controlled with bipolar coagulation. The smallest bipolar coagulating tips possible should be used to avoid excessive heat and facial nerve injury.

51

Retrosigmoid Approach to Tumors of the Cerebellopontine Angle

Robert K. Jackler, M.D. ▪ David W. Sim, F.R.C.S.Ed. (URL)

The retrosigmoid approach is a versatile type of craniotomy that creates a panoramic view of the posterior fossa from the tentorium cerebelli to the foramen magnum. Indications for the retrosigmoid approach include (1) resection of extra-axial lesions, such as schwannoma, meningioma, and epidermoid; (2) cranial nerve neurectomy (e.g., cranial nerves V, VIII, and IX); (3) vascular decompression of cranial nerves (e.g., cranial nerves V, VII, and IX); (4) vascular disorders of the vertebrobasilar system; and (5) parenchymal lesions of the brainstem and cerebellum.

The primary advantages of the retrosigmoid approach are the potential for hearing preservation and an unhindered exposure of the inferior portion of the cerebellopontine angle (CPA). Its principal disadvantages are a substantially higher incidence of persistent postoperative headache and a somewhat higher incidence of cerebrospinal fluid (CSF) leakage than those resulting from transtemporal approaches. Although the retrosigmoid approach is technically capable of addressing most lesions involving the CPA, it is best used selectively to gain optimal benefit from its advantages while avoiding its occasional disadvantages.

This chapter concentrates on the use of the retrosigmoid approach for tumors of the CPA, with an emphasis on acoustic neuroma resection.

SURGICAL ANATOMY

Historically, the earliest approach to the posterior fossa was undertaken through the suboccipital convexity. Krause and others first employed this technique during the latter portion of the nineteenth century.[1] Until the 1970s, the technique in widespread use was the so-called suboccipital approach. In this procedure, a large bone window is removed, and the anterior limit of the craniectomy is the first mastoid air cell encountered. Curtailment of the anterior opening at the first contact with pneumatization was predicated on the assumption that the mastoid was bacterially contaminated and that opening its air cell tracts created an increased risk of meningitis. Because of its more posterior angle of view, the suboccipital approach required a greater degree of cerebellar retraction and, at times, even necessitated a partial cerebellar resection. In recent years, as a result of increased experience with CPA surgery, the classic suboccipital approach has been modified to become the retrosigmoid approach, which is now the preferred method for exposing the CPA behind the sigmoid sinus. In this technique, bone is removed anteriorly up to the level of

the posterior border of the sigmoid sinus and superiorly to the inferior margin of the transverse sinus (Fig. 51–1). Although mastoid air cells are frequently transected during this maneuver, experience has not demonstrated an increased incidence of postoperative infection. The slightly higher risk of CSF leak associated with this more anterior exposure is more than offset by its more favorable angle of view into the CPA and the markedly reduced need for cerebellar retraction with this approach.

The anatomic exposure of the posterior fossa provided by the retrosigmoid approach is bounded superiorly by the tentorium cerebelli and inferiorly by the jugular foramen and foramen magnum (Fig. 51–2).[2–5] Access to the central nervous system includes the lateral cerebellar hemisphere and the lateral surface of the pons and upper medulla. Cranial nerves V through XI are visible both at their root entry zones and over their cisternal courses. Although the theoretical anterior limit of exposure is the clivus and the apical portion of the petrous pyramid, in practice, access to these ventral structures is usually limited by cranial nerves VII and VIII superiorly and IX through XI inferiorly, which bridge across the CPA, restricting ventral access to relatively narrow intervals. Exposure of the prepontine cistern is largely obstructed by the lateral aspect of the pons, which does not tolerate medial retraction well.

Anatomic variations may affect the CPA exposure provided by the retrosigmoid approach. A posteriorly placed sigmoid sinus course results in the anterior edge of the craniectomy being placed relatively more posteriorly. This creates a deeper field of action and a less favorable angle of view with the consequent need for more cerebellar retraction. This disadvantageous exposure may be further compromised by a low transverse sinus course, particularly if the patient also has a short neck and a prominent shoulder. This problem of restricted exposure may be overcome by combining the retrosigmoid approach with an anterosigmoid, retrolabyrinthine decompression to allow anterior retraction of the sigmoid sinus.[6] A highly placed jugular bulb restricts access to the internal auditory canal (IAC) and can make the dissection of the inferior bony trough between the canal and the bulb difficult. Occasionally, the bulb may even extend superiorly to overlap the IAC, partially obscuring access to the medial aspect of the canal.[7]

PREOPERATIVE EVALUATION AND PATIENT COUNSELING

Clinical history, physical examination, pure tone and speech audiometry, and an imaging study (preferably, gadolinium-enhanced magnetic resonance imaging [MRI]) constitute the minimal preoperative evaluation for a patient with a CPA tumor. In nonacoustic tumors, computed tomographic (CT) scanning for evaluation of the osseous characteristics of the cranial base and angiography to address vascular anatomy and possibly to perform embolization are occasionally indicated. Neither vestibular diagnostic testing nor auditory evoked responses are routinely obtained in patients already diagnosed with an acoustic neuroma.[8]

Numerous factors affect the selection of posterior fossa craniotomy for tumors of the CPA.[7, 9, 10] As advocates of selective management of these lesions according to the unique attributes of each tumor and the potential surgical options, we involve the patient in the discussion of the relative advantages and disadvantages of each technique. In most cases, an obvious choice can be made, whereas in others, patient preference is important. Our customary preoperative counseling includes the anticipated and potential risks to hearing, balance, and facial motor function. Less common complications discussed include CSF leak, meningitis, cerebrovascular accident, and death.[11] Although blood transfusion is seldom required, we encourage the patient to donate a unit of autologous blood.

PATIENT SELECTION

Common Indications in Neurotology

Hearing Preservation

The primary aim of acoustic neuroma management is removing the threat of progressive tumor growth while avoiding injury to the central nervous system. Preservation of cranial nerve function (facial movement, facial sensation, and hearing), which has become the primary focus of acoustic neuroma surgery in recent years, is a secondary goal. Acoustic tumors lie in three groups in terms of potential for hearing preservation. Those for whom hearing preservation is highly improbable generally undergo translabyrinthine removal. Criteria that place an individual into this group include poor hearing (< 30 per cent speech discrimination, > 70 dB speech reception threshold); large CPA component (> 3 cm), and deep penetration of the IAC. Conversely, individuals with good hearing (> 70 per cent speech discrimination, < 30 dB speech reception threshold), small CPA component (< 1 cm), and shallow IAC involvement are considered excellent candidates for a hearing conservation approach.[7] It is difficult to codify a set of rules concerning selection of a hearing conservation approach for the substantial group of patients who lie between these parameters. Each surgical team must rely on its own criteria, based on experience, together with the patient's wishes in coming to a selection of surgical approach. Undoubtedly, neurotologists would always favor undertaking a hearing conservation approach, even when the chances of success were remote, were there not potential adverse consequences from the endeavor. The lower morbidity of the translabyrinthine approach, especially in terms of persistent headache and CSF leak, leads the clinician away from the retrosigmoid hearing conservation approach when the chances of success are limited.

The concept of useful hearing is context dependent. In a patient with a normal contralateral ear, imperfect residual hearing in the tumor ear is often of little practical benefit. When hearing in the contralateral ear is impaired or threatened, such as in cases of bilateral acoustic neuromas associated with neurofibromatosis type 2, a conservative approach to hearing conservation is prudent, occasionally even at the expense of complete tumor excision.[12]

Hearing preservation is seldom achieved when tumors with a CPA component exceeding 2 cm in diameter are removed.[13] However, this rule should not be applied in nonacoustic CPA tumors (e.g., meningiomas), because hearing preservation is frequently achieved even with large tumors.[14]

The retrosigmoid approach is able to expose a variable amount of the IAC without violating the inner ear while the canal is being drilled open. Two factors should be considered in the decision of whether hearing conservation via the retrosigmoid approach is feasible: the depth to which the tumor penetrates the IAC and the degree of IAC exposable in that patient. The relationship between the inner ear and the lateral-most extension of the tumor into the IAC may be predicated by preoperative gadolinium-enhanced MRI.[15]

Acoustic Neuroma in a Patient with Chronic Otitis Media

Although patients with acoustic neuromas rarely have concomitant chronic middle ear infection, in those who do the translabyrinthine approach for acoustic neuroma resection is contraindicated. However, the retrosigmoid approach may also open into potentially contaminated mastoid air cells lying behind the sigmoid sinus as well as into air cells that may surround the IAC. To avoid potential intracranial infection, chronic middle ear infection should be controlled with tympanoplasty, antibiotics, or both, before tumor surgery whenever possible.[7]

Tumors Extending into Inferior Portion of the Cerebellopontine Angle

The retrosigmoid approach provides the best access to the lower portion of the CPA and is readily extendible to expose the foramen magnum when required. Transtemporal approaches to the CPA are limited in their inferior exposure by the sigmoid sinus and the jugular bulb. Acoustic neuromas seldom extend into the inferior reaches of the CPA. Even when they do, the capsular peel is readily mobilized superiorly after tumor debulking. However, meningiomas and other extra-axial tumors usually do not mobilize easily and are often entwined with the lower cranial nerves (IX through XII) and vital vascular structures (e.g., posteroinferior cerebellar and vertebral arteries). In such cases, the retrosigmoid approach is chosen for its superior ability to expose this region. In neurofibromatosis type 2 patients, concurrent schwannomas on the lower cranial nerves are a common finding at the time of acoustic neuroma surgery. The retrosigmoid approach permits a thorough inspection of the jugular foramen contents as well as the dural lining of the posterior cranial base for possible early meningioma formation. Small, asymptomatic schwannomas on the lower cranial nerves are typically left alone, whereas early meningiomas are excised.

Tumors with Limited Extension into Meckel's Cave

The retrosigmoid approach is also useful in approaching extra-axial posterior fossa tumors that possess minor extensions into Meckel's cave (cavum trigeminale). The majority of such tumors are trigeminal schwannomas and petroclival meningiomas. Added exposure is obtained by removing the apical petrous bone between the internal auditory canal and the tentorium. This maneuver provides access to approximately 1 to 2 cm of the posterior aspect of Meckel's cave for tumor removal.[16–18]

Revision Surgery

The retrosigmoid approach is favored in cases of recurrence following a previous translabyrinthine removal of an acoustic neuroma to avoid the dural scar from the prior procedure and to allow identification of the facial nerve as it emerges from the fat graft located in the surgical defect.

Relative Contraindications

Deep Extension into the Internal Auditory Canal

Generally, tumors extending into the lateral one third of the IAC are not resectable by the retrosigmoid approach without destroying hearing. In such cases, the translabyrinthine approach ensures complete resection and reduces operative morbidity.[7]

Extension into the Cranial Base

Tumor penetration into the posterolateral cranial base is a relative contraindication to the retrosigmoid approach. CPA tumors that invade the temporal bone (other than the medial two thirds of the IAC), the jugular foramen, or the hypoglossal canal are generally best addressed via a lateral, transbasal craniotomy.

Large Tumors

Although large CPA tumors (> 3 cm) may be approached through either the retrosigmoid or translabyrinthine technique, we prefer to use the latter because it provides ample exposure and minimizes the need for cerebellar retraction. In addition, when the pons and the cerebellar peduncle are substantially displaced medially and posteriorly, the translabyrinthine approach, by virtue of its more anterior placement, provides a more favorable angle of view posteriorly toward the brainstem interface. In cases of facial nerve disruption, which is more common in large tumors, the translabyrinthine approach affords more reconstructive options through mastoid meatal rerouting.[7]

PATIENT PREPARATION AND POSITIONING

At the University of California, San Francisco (UCSF), the operation is carried out by a multidisciplinary team consisting of a neurotologist, neurosurgeon, neuroanesthesiologist, neurophysiologist, and specialized operating room nurses. The operation is carried out with the patient under general anesthesia. A short-duration muscle relaxant is used to facilitate endotracheal intubation. Thereafter, anesthesia is maintained with inhalational agents alone, avoiding the use of muscle relaxants, which would prevent effective intraoperative cranial nerve electrophysiologic monitoring. In addition to the routine neuroanesthesia monitoring equipment, antithrombotic stockings and a urinary catheter are used. The retrosigmoid approach may be carried out in one of three surgical positions: supine, lateral supine ("park bench position"), and sitting.[10] Supine is the favored position because it affords excellent exposure and carries the lowest risk of complication, as is discussed later.

The patient is secured in the optimal operating position by means of a headholder attached to the bed frame (e.g., Mayfield). This apparatus facilitates exposure of the suboccipital region while the patient is in the supine position. Optimal surgical field exposure is obtained by a combination of head rotation, neck flexion, and ipsilateral shoulder elevation. Excessive neck torsion should be avoided to prevent cervical injury as well as to reduce the risk of cerebellar swelling secondary to compromised flow through the vertebral venous system. The cranial nerve–monitoring electromyographic electrodes are placed into the muscles supplied by cranial nerves V, VII, and XI. When intraoperative auditory brainstem monitoring is indicated, scalp electrodes are placed, and an earphone is inserted into the ipsilateral external auditory canal.[19]

We favor using an operating room table with enhanced lateral rotation capability (up to 30 degrees), which permits optimal visualization of the lateral end of the IAC at a comfortable working angle. When the surgeon works at relatively extreme rotations, the patient must be securely supported on the operating table by a lumbar support and placed on the contralateral side to the operative exposure, with both chest and thigh safety straps. The bed is reversed,

FIGURE 51–1. The incision used in the retrosigmoid approach is located approximately 6 cm behind the postauricular sulcus. Following craniectomy and retraction of the cerebellum, the tumor becomes visible within the cerebellopontine angle. Note that the anterior edge of the craniotomy is placed immediately behind the sigmoid sinus and just inferior to the lower margin of the transverse sinus.

FIGURE 51–2. Operative view of the cerebellopontine angle as seen through the retrosigmoid approach. Superiorly is the trigeminal nerve (V) and the petrosal vein. Inferiorly are the lower cranial nerves (IX, X, and XI). In the midsection of the exposure, a medium-sized acoustic neuroma is seen in relation to the facial and audiovestibular nerves.

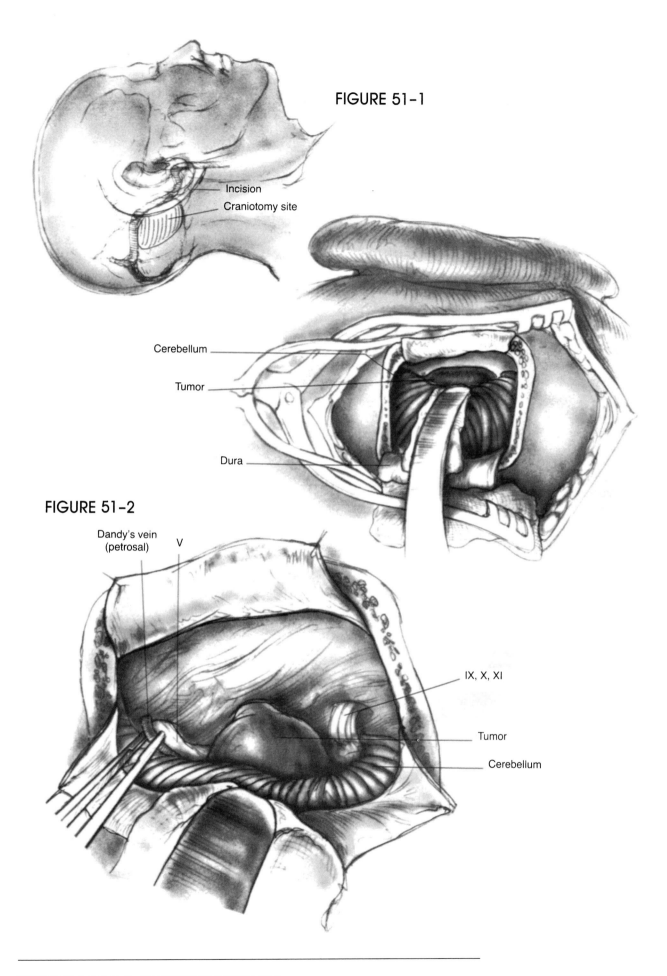

FIGURE 51-1

Incision
Craniotomy site

Cerebellum

Tumor

Dura

FIGURE 51-2

Dandy's vein
(petrosal)   V

IX, X, XI

Tumor

Cerebellum

FIGURES 51–1 and 51–2. *See legends on opposite page*

525

with the patient's head on the foot section to allow the surgeon to sit during the microsurgical portion of the procedure.

A perioperative prophylactic antibiotic with good CSF penetration (e.g., ceftizoxime, 2 g administered intravenously) is administered. Mannitol (1 gm/kg) is administered intravenously when the scalp incision is made so that its effectiveness in reducing brain swelling coincides with dural entry. We do not routinely give corticosteroids, except in patients with larger tumors (> 3 cm) or in those with peritumoral brain edema, when dexamethasone (10 mg) is administered intravenously. To reduce the risk of CSF fistulization, an indwelling lumbar CSF drain is used when extensive peri-IAC pneumatization is encountered.

SURGICAL SITE PREPARATION

We ask the patient to wash his or her hair thoroughly either the morning of surgery or on the evening before with an antiseptic shampoo. In the operating room, after induction of anesthesia, the hair over the suboccipital area is removed with electric clippers. The upper neck is included in the operative site, thereby allowing potential access to the great auricular nerve in case a graft is required for facial nerve reconstruction. The scalp is washed with providone-iodine soap, and the clipped area is shaved. To improve attachment of adhesive drapes, the surgical site is defatted with alcohol and dried. Sterile drapes are placed 1 cm from the hair edge around the prepared scalp and held in place with surgical adhesive (e.g., Mastisol). The field is then prepared with providone-iodine solution and dried. Sterile towels are placed around the operative field and held into position by an adhesive plastic sheet.

SPECIAL INSTRUMENTS

Various instruments are used for the retrosigmoid approach to the CPA, including craniectomy instruments, retractors, a high-speed surgical drill with a selection of cutting and diamond burrs, suction and suction-irrigation tips of both the fenestrated and nonfenestrated types, bipolar cautery, microdissection instruments, and a binocular operating microscope.

We perform the craniectomy with an Acra-Cut disposable cranial perforator burr-hole maker in a Hudson brace, a system that allows rapid bone removal while minimizing the chance of dural or venous sinus injury. The craniectomy is completed with rongeurs. To retract the thick suboccipital musculature, a deep-bladed Weitlaner-type retractor is used. For brain retraction, several sizes of malleable blades are used that may be held in position in several ways. We prefer to use the Apfelbaum base, which combines a Weitlaner-type retractor with a moveable arm to affix the retractor. Other options for basing the brain retractors during retrosigmoid craniotomy include a C-clamp placed on the headholder frame or a table-based system (e.g., Greenberg).

Either an electric or air-powered drill is suitable to use for this approach. When the exposure is narrow, an angled handpiece is advantageous because it is less obstructing to

the surgeon's point of view. An operating microscope with an inclinable optical pathway is desirable to accomodate the variety of exposure angles required during the procedure while maintaining a comfortable operating position. Insulated bipolar cautery forceps are essential for obtaining hemostasis during CPA tumor surgery. Both large tips for handling substantial vessels and slender, fine tips for use when the coagulation must be confined to a narrow region are needed. We have found that a self-irrigating system (e.g., Malis bipolar irrigating system) is valuable because it discourages tissue adhesion to the forcep tips.

We use a microsurgical instrument set that includes sharp and blunt dissectors in various shapes and sizes, needles, and small bone curettes (e.g., Rhoton microneurosurgical instruments). A set of sharp scissors of different sizes and angles is also important. Many special tools are available to facilitate rapid intracapsular debulking of the tumor. We prefer to use a Cavitron ultrasonic surgical aspirator (CUSA), which allows debulking without traction or torsion, minimizes hemorrhage, and respects tumor capsular planes, thereby avoiding inadvertent neural or vascular injury. Other options include the surgical laser and a rotatory surgical aspirator (House-Urban).

Operating room electrical circuitry and neuroanesthesia electrical monitoring equipment should be grounded and electronically quiet to minimize 60 Hz noise production, which interferes with the cranial nerve electrophysiologic monitoring setup. The specialized equipment for intraoperative cranial nerve monitoring used in our institution has been described elsewhere in detail.[19]

SURGICAL TECHNIQUE

Acoustic neuroma excision by the retrosigmoid approach to the CPA can be subdivided into seven stages: (1) craniectomy, (2) exposure of the CPA, (3) exposure of the IAC, (4) tumor resection, (5) hemostasis, (6) IAC closure, and (7) craniotomy closure.

Craniectomy

A curvilinear paramedian incision 3 cm behind the postauricular sulcus is made down to bone. The cervical muscles are detached anteriorly and posteriorly, exposing the mastoid and suboccipital areas. Emissary venous bleeding is controlled with bone wax. The mastoid tip is exposed, and the posterior belly of digastric muscle is elevated from its groove. Dissection directly on the bone preserves the occipital nerves and vessels. A posterior fossa craniotomy window of approximately 3 × 3 cm is made in the retrosigmoid approach. Anteriorly it is bounded by the sigmoid sinus and superiorly it is bounded by the transverse sinus. The craniectomy begins with two or three closely approximated burr holes. The burr holes are joined up with ronguers, thus creating a craniotomy window. The bone fragments are collected and stored in sterile antibiotic-saline solution for replacement in the cranial defect at the end of the procedure. Development of the craniectomy anteriorly usually opens the mastoid air cell system to a variable degree. Once the bony craniectomy is complete, the opened mastoid air cells are sealed with bone wax. Wax is also used to control bleeding from diploic bone at the craniotomy margins. Many styles of dural opening are described in the literature. We use a posteriorly based dural flap to enter the posterior fossa. The posterior fossa dura is opened 2 to 3 mm from its junction with the sigmoid and transverse sinus dura and at a similar distance from the inferior bony margin. The dural flap is then reflected posteriorly. Small, relaxing incisions are made superiorly and inferiorly in the marginal dura to create small anterior and superior dural flaps, which are then retracted with stay sutures, thereby completing the dural opening.

Exposure of the Cerebellopontine Angle

Once the dural flap has been reflected posteriorly, it and the craniotomy margins are covered with moist Telfa strips. To drain CSF from the cisterna magna, the cerebellum is gently retracted superiorly with a polytetrafluoroethylene (Teflon)-coated malleable retractor. The arachnoid of the cistern is then lanced with a bayoneted suction tip, which decompresses the posterior fossa, relaxes the cerebellum, and allows it to fall away medially. Premature medially directed cerebellar retraction, before draining the cisterna magna, risks inducing massive cerebellar swelling. After this maneuver, the retractor is withdrawn and repositioned anteriorly to develop posteromedial cerebellar retraction. Retraction in this manner, accompanied by division of arachnoid bands and bridging veins, opens the CPA. The degree of CPA exposure required varies with the size and location of the tumor being addressed. Superiorly, the petrosal veins (or Dandy's veins), which lie just below the tentorium cerebelli and run parallel to the course of the trigeminal nerve, may hinder exposure or appear to be in jeopardy of tearing with retraction. When necessary, these may be coagulated and divided. After their division, the superior pole of the cerebellar hemisphere falls posteromedially away from the tentorium, thereby providing access to the superior aspect of the CPA.

The cerebellar flocculus often overlies the brainstem root entry zones of cranial nerves VII and VIII and must be gently mobilized from the cerebellar peduncle and lateral pontine surfaces. A tuft of choroid plexus, emanating from the lateral recess of the fourth ventricle, is also frequently encountered in this area. Mobilizing these structures from the root entry zone need not necessarily be performed during hearing conservation procedures when the proximal portion of the nerves are not involved with tumor, because this maneuver places the internal auditory artery at risk. The cranial nerve electrophysiologic monitoring circuitry is then tested by stimulating cranial nerve XI, which is usually readily accessible at the inferior pole of the exposure. Particular attention is paid to the location of the anteroinferior cerebellar artery (AICA) and its branches. Inferiorly, the posteroinferior cerebellar artery may be seen in relation to the lower cranial nerves, and superiorly the superior cerebellar artery may be identified coursing through the region of the tentorial notch. In acoustic neuroma surgery, we prefer to begin the drill excavation of the IAC at a relatively early stage, before extensive opening

of the arachnoid planes above and below the CPA component. This method helps reduce bone debris contamination of the subarachnoid space.

Exposure of the Internal Auditory Canal

Exposure of the IAC and its contents involves removal of the bone surrounding the posterior, superior, and inferior aspects (Figs. 51–3 to 51–6). Optimal canal visualization may be obtained through a combination of rotation of the operating table away from the side of the surgeon and microscope positioning. These maneuvers bring the posterior petrous face into view centered over the region of the IAC. To locate the canal, the opening of the meatus is gently probed with a blunt, right-angle hook. Before IAC opening begins, the operative field is set up to contain as much bone debris as possible and to prevent its dissemination into the subarachnoid space. Absorbable gelatin sponge (Gelfoam) pledgets are placed into the superior and inferior portions of the CPA. A rectangular-shaped rubber dam is fashioned from a surgical glove, placed over the occluding pledgets, and held in place with the cerebellar retractor. An H-shaped dural incision, centered on the long axis of the IAC, is outlined on the posterior petrous face by use of a bipolar cautery. Once the dura has been incised with the tip of a No. 11 blade, superior and inferior dural flaps are elevated with a small Lempert mastoid elevator. The surgeon should exercise caution when incising inferiorly because the jugular bulb is occasionally dehiscent on the posterior petrous face. Similarly, the incision should not be carried too far laterally because laceration of the sigmoid sinus can occur. Care is taken to identify and preserve the endolymphatic sac and duct, which are located posterolaterally. The dura can usually be elevated off the endolymphatic sac. The entry point of the vestibular aqueduct into bone is a useful anatomic landmark. When the bony dissection of the IAC does not extend lateral to the operculum of the aqueduct, the labyrinth is unlikely to be breached.

The posterior IAC wall is then rapidly removed by the drilling of a trough over the posterior petrous face. Drilling from medial to lateral in the line of the IAC reduces the risk of the burr slipping into the CPA. The canal should be opened only as much as required to expose the lateral-most aspect of the tumor. Excessive bony opening does not further enhance exposure but may increase the risk of CSF leak through the opening of additional petrous air cells. Initially, the bone is removed with a cutting burr until the IAC dura is identified through a thin bony plate. To expose the dura of the posterior aspect of the IAC, the dural cuff of the meatus is first elevated from the thin residual plate. Then, the remaining bony shell over the posterior aspect of the IAC is drilled away. To reduce the risk of traumatizing the IAC dural lining or its neural structures, removal of the last eggshell of bone is accomplished with diamond burrs. Diamond burrs are more controllable by virtue of their reduced tendency to run and are less likely to cause injury if they come into contact with soft tissue structures.

Bony troughs, 3 to 4 mm in diameter, are then developed above and below the canal. These troughs are important

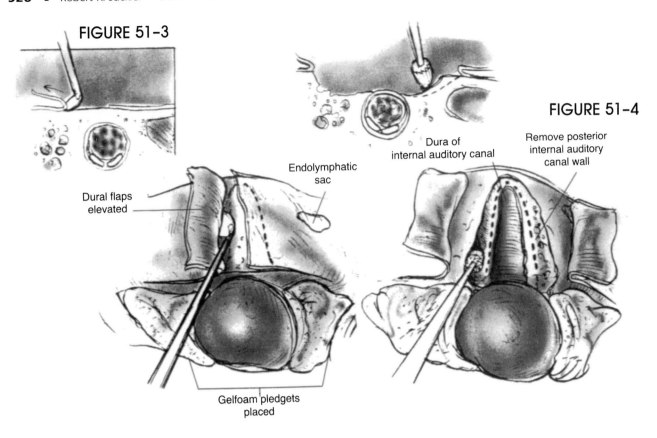

FIGURE 51-3

FIGURE 51-4

Dural flaps elevated

Endolymphatic sac

Dura of internal auditory canal

Remove posterior internal auditory canal wall

Gelfoam pledgets placed

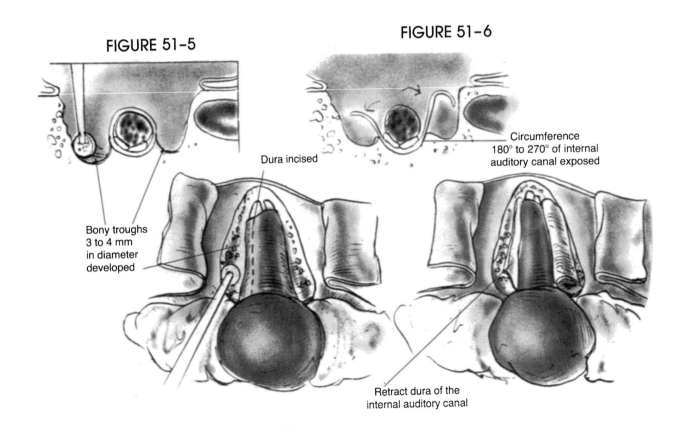

FIGURE 51-5

FIGURE 51-6

Bony troughs 3 to 4 mm in diameter developed

Dura incised

Circumference 180° to 270° of internal auditory canal exposed

Retract dura of the internal auditory canal

FIGURES 51-3 to 51-6. *See legends on opposite page*

for three reasons: (1) to provide working space for the insertion of angled instruments needed to establish a plane of dissection between the tumor and the facial and cochlear nerves, (2) to permit visualization of the facial nerve when it is acutely angled superiorly or inferiorly as a result of tumor displacement, and (3) to enhance exposure of the anterior aspect of the CPA. In preparation for the drilling of bony troughs around the canal, the IAC dura is elevated from the upper and lower canal walls with a blunt dissector. The troughs, which should be widest at the level of the porus, are then excavated with a cutting burr. As the troughs are developed, a thin shell of bone is left over the dura of the superior and inferior walls of the IAC. Once the troughs are fully developed, the remaining bony shells are progressively thinned with the side of the diamond burr until the dura is exposed. Copious irrigation is used to prevent thermal injury to neural structures. Often, the IAC dura can be gently retracted with a fenestrated suction, permitting completely atraumatic removal of the remaining bony eggshell fragments, which can then be elevated from the exposed IAC dura. This technique exposes between 180 and 270 degrees of the IAC circumference. Caution must be exercised in development of the superior and inferior troughs because of the proximity of the facial nerve and the jugular bulb, respectively. The width of the inferior trough varies with the location of the jugular bulb. When the jugular bulb is unusually high, creating an inferior bony trough at the level of the meatus may be impossible, although exposure of the fundus is typically unhindered. Compensating for the limited inferior access associated with a high jugular bulb is usually possible through creation of an unusually wide and deep superior trough. Additional exposure of the IAC from above may also be gained through retraction of the tentorium.

In hearing conservation attempts, the lateral extent of the IAC opening should be restricted to approximately the medial two thirds of the IAC because opening of the lateral one third to expose the fundus may result in a breach of the vestibule or crus commune, militating against hearing conservation. The decision as to how far laterally the IAC is opened depends on the lateral intracanalicular extent of the tumor, which may be predicted with considerable accuracy from the preoperative gadolinium-enhanced MRI.[15, 20] Alternatively, the lateral opening can be limited on the premise that an indirect inspection and clearance of the tumor from the lateral IAC can be satisfactorily achieved. However, this method has the attendant risk of leaving residual tumor in the lateral IAC. To avoid this problem, some have advocated blind curettage using special right-angle curettes followed by inspection of the fundus with a small mirror or endoscope to validate the extent of tumor resection.[21, 22] We have found that with these methods, distinguishing residual tumor from the transected vestibular nerves and traumatized dura is sometimes difficult. Dissection of tumor from the fundus without direct visualization risks leaving well-vascularized residual tumor with the potential for clinically significant recurrence.[23, 24] We advocate exposure of the IAC laterally to a point beyond the tumor interface, where the naked seventh and residual eighth cranial nerves may be visualized. At times, this process may require opening the canal to the fundus, with resultant entry into labyrinthine structures and sacrifice of residual hearing. It has been proposed that enhanced visualization of the fundus can be achieved by skeletonization of the posterior and superior semicircular canals.[25] Similarly, it has been shown that partial resection of the posterior semicircular canal may be helpful in augmental fundal exposure.[26]

After completion of the IAC exposure, the rubber dam and gelatin sponge pledgets are removed. The dura of the IAC is opened along the long axis of the canal with sharp, upturned, right-angle microscissors working from a medial to lateral direction. This incision is placed slightly eccentrically and is biased to the superior side to avoid the creation

---

FIGURE 51–3. Step 1 of exposure of the internal auditory canal during the retrosigmoid approach. After localization of the porus acusticus through palpation with a ball hook, an H-shaped dural incision is created over the long axis of the internal auditory canal. Dural flaps are then reflected anteriorly and posteriorly to expose the posterior aspect of the petrous pyramid. The dura can usually be dissected from the posterior surface of the endolymphatic sac. To maximize the possibility of hearing preservation, care must be exercised to avoid avulsion of the sac from its aqueduct. Prior to the commencement of drilling, Gelfoam pledgets are positioned above and below the 7 to 8 neurovascular bundle in the posterior fossa in an effort to minimize the spread of bone dust onto arachnoidal surfaces.

FIGURE 51–4. Step 2 of exposure of the internal auditory canal during the retrosigmoid approach. A cutting burr is used to rapidly excavate the bone overlying the internal auditory canal. Once the canal dura is encountered, a diamond burr is used. Drilling is carried out from medial to lateral (from porus to fundus), in part to minimize the possibility that the drill could accidentally run into the posterior fossa.

FIGURE 51–5. Step 3 of exposure of the internal auditory canal during the retrosigmoid approach. A diamond burr is used to create deep troughs around the internal auditory canal that should extend well deep to the canal plane to provide adequate room for microdissection with the angled instruments needed to safely remove the facial nerve from the tumor. Particular care should be exercised while the superior trough is developed because the facial nerve may lie immediately beneath the dura in this location.

FIGURE 51–6. Step 4 of exposure of the internal auditory canal during the retrosigmoid approach. In preparation for tumor removal, the dura of the internal auditory canal is incised. After an incision along the length of the canal is created with upbiting scissors, two small relaxing incisions are created at both the porus and the fundus to develop dural flaps. These are then reflected anteriorly and posteriorly to expose the canal contents.

of a long flap over the facial nerve course. The dural flaps are then reflected superiorly and inferiorly, exposing the IAC contents.

Acoustic Neuroma Resection
(Figs. 51–7 to 51–9)

Attention is now turned to planning the actual resection of the tumor, the size of the tumor largely dictating the actual sequence and pattern of removal. We prefer to initially dissect the IAC because this step helps ascertain the probable course of the facial nerve outside of the porus into the CPA and allows early identification of the facial nerve. Then, a test run of the neural monitoring system can be performed in which positive identification of the nerve by its anatomic relationships is possible. In many cases, ascertaining whether the tumor has arisen from the superior or inferior vestibular nerve is possible. When only one of these nerves is visible on the posterior surface of the tumor, it may be assumed that the other was the nerve of origin. Dissection is commenced laterally by identification of the plane between the facial nerve and the tumor. A fine-tipped dissector is insinuated between the superior dural leaf of the canal and the tumor while gentle downward pressure and a rotating motion are applied. Gradually, this process brings into view the interface between the facial nerve and the lateral end of the tumor. Once this plane has become established, a sharp, right-angle instrument is used to dissect the tumor from the posterior surface of the facial and cochlear nerves. All tissue superficial to this plane, including the tumor and both vestibular nerves, is then transected either with curved microscissors or through an upward motion with the sharp edge of the dissector. When the intracanalicular tumor component is bulky, it may require debulking to a variable degree to permit microdissection of the capsular peel from the facial and cochlear nerves. This initial dissection of the intracanalicular portion should proceed only to the lip of the porus acusticus or just beyond it, to avoid dissection of the typically most adherent section at this stage. It is important to avoid inducing neuropraxic injury, which might impair later electrical identification of the facial nerve medially at its brainstem exit.

After removal of the intracanalicular portion of the tumor, the CPA component is addressed. The posterior capsule is swept with the neural monitoring probe to ensure that the facial nerve is not on this surface (a rarity in acoustic neuroma). A rectangular incision is made in the posterior capsule with the point of a No. 11 blade, and the peel is then resected with scissors. Intracapsular debulking may be carried out with cupped forceps, sharp dissection with scissors, an ultrasonic aspirator (e.g., Cavitron), a rotatory aspiration device (e.g., House-Urban), or the surgical laser. We favor using the CUSA because it efficiently removes the tumor core while respecting its capsule, thus avoiding potential injury of adherent nerves and vessels. Tumor resection then proceeds with alternate intracapsular debulking, followed by microdissection of the thin capsule from the brain surface and cranial nerves, and, ultimately, resection of the liberated capsular segment.

The most crucial aspect of CPA tumor removal is identification and preservation of the cranial nerves and blood vessels that lie draped on the capsular surface. In larger tumors, the medial tumor brain dissection plane commences posteriorly along the middle cerebellar peduncle. Once this arachnoid plane has become established, it is gradually developed onto the lateral surface of the pons. Attention is turned inferiorly to the probable root entry zone of the seventh and eighth nerve complexes. As an aid to facial nerve identification, electrical stimulation is periodically performed along the meniscus of dissection. The course and appearance of the nerve vary depending on its displacement by the tumor. It may be thinned and fanned to a variable degree, making it difficult to delineate from surrounding thickened arachnoid tissue without the use of the microneural stimulator.

The brainstem entry of the eighth nerve is usually encountered lateral to and immediately above the seventh nerve entry zone. A small branch of AICA typically passes between the two nerves and may be a useful guide in orienting the surgeon. In hearing conservation approaches, the vestibular fibers must be separated from the cochlear fibers and divided proximally to establish a tumor dissection plane. When no effort is being made at hearing preservation, the eighth nerve may simply be transected, a maneuver that simplifies identification of the proximal seventh nerve. Once the proximal plane over these two nerves is established, an arachnoid plane can be developed between them and the tumor capsule. While the tumor capsule is dissected, both large and small arteries, potential AICA branches, are meticulously preserved. Vessels directly entering the tumor capsule can generally be safely coagulated and divided at the capsular surface without adverse consequences.

While the tumor neural plane is dissected, use of the microneural stimulator (e.g., Xomed Treace-Yingling) with a curved, pliable wire allows blind stimulation of the yet undissected anterior capsule. By localizing the facial nerve course before dissecting the tumor nerve interface, the surgeon may rapidly resect uninvolved capsule and direct meticulous efforts along the actual course of the nerve. Although the course of the facial nerve varies, it characteristically lies anterior to the tumor, occasionally with a somewhat anterosuperior or anteroinferior bias. In small tumors, the entire dissection may be accomplished from a medial to lateral direction. In larger tumors, however, medial-to-lateral dissection becomes difficult when the nerve is anteriorly angulated toward the porus acusticus. When this occurs, we return to the lateral tumor nerve interface at the end of the IAC and work medially. Alternatively, the anterior tumor capsule with attached nerve may be lifted and rotated to bring the facial nerve course into the surgeon's view. However, this action is quite traumatic to the facial nerve and risks disruption of its attenuated fibers. We prefer to dissect the tumor from the facial nerve in situ without mobilizing it from its bed, where it lies supported by an arachnoidal mesh. When the facial nerve is both splayed and tightly adherent to the tumor capsule, removing the last remnant of capsule may not be possible without disruption of the nerve.[27] In such cases, we prefer to perform a near-total removal, leaving a thin velum of capsule, only 1 to 2 mm thick, attached to the nerve. We believe that this minuscule residual capsule, hanging free in the CPA, is unlikely to generate a recurrent tumor.[23] By contrast, tumor left in the distal IAC or in contact with brainstem possesses a vascular supply and the possibility of regrowth is greater.

Several modifications in the strategy of tumor removal are used during hearing conservation approaches. The direction of dissection should be from medial to lateral, whenever possible, to reduce the risk of traumatic avulsion of the delicate cochlear nerve fibers from their entry into modiolus. Throughout the cochlear nerve dissection, changes in auditory brainstem responses relative to the previously recorded baseline waveforms obtained at the start of the procedure are reported. Continuity of the cochlear nerve is maintained if possible; however, tumor adherence to it may necessitate its resection. Even when the cochlear nerve is well preserved during dissection, hearing is often lost because of interruption of the cochlear blood supply. This may occur either in the CPA, where the labyrinthine artery branches from a loop of AICA, or in the IAC, where it courses between the inferior vestibular and cochlear nerves.

After tumor resection, anatomic and electrical continuity of the cochlear and facial nerves are checked. The facial nerve stimulation threshold voltage at the root entry zone and the intraoperative auditory brainstem response waveform pattern and latencies are recorded. We believe that electrophysiologic monitoring of the auditory nerve is not clearly beneficial, other than in the prognostic sense, in the maintenance of hearing. However, monitoring of the facial nerve is indispensable if an optimal outcome is to be obtained.

Hemostasis

After the tumor resection is completed, the wound is irrigated with bacitracin-saline solution, the blood clot is removed, and all bleeding points are identified and controlled with bipolar cautery or by application of thrombin-soaked gelatin sponge. As a means of detecting subtle or intermittent bleeding, the anesthesiologist gives the patient a Valsalva maneuver for 20 seconds. Because postoperative hemorrhage into the CPA is a potentially devastating complication, hemostatic efforts should be diligent.

Internal Auditory Canal Closure
(Fig. 51–10)

The bony troughs developed for the IAC exposure are inspected for opened air cells by palpation with a ball hook. Inspection of the cut bony edge may also be carried out through use of a 90-degree–angled rigid endoscope. Bone wax is applied to a small cottonoid and smeared over the exposed bony trough surfaces to seal overtly and covertly opened air cells to prevent CSF leakage. A small muscle graft is harvested from the exposed cervical muscles and is used to seal the IAC. A 7-0 monofilament nylon suture is placed through the dural flaps of the posterior petrous face. The muscle plug is then positioned in the IAC and the suture tied. Auditory and facial nerve monitoring are maintained until the muscle plug is secured in

place so that any possible neural irritation induced by its placement can be identified.

Craniotomy Closure

After removal of all the cottonoids and Telfa strips, the dural flap is sutured back into place with multiple, closely positioned, interrupted 4-0 braided nylon (Surgilon) sutures. At closure of the dura, bacitracin-saline solution is instilled into the subarachnoid space. The margins of the craniectomy are then reinspected for opened air cells and smeared with bone wax as indicated. When the transected air cells are large, rather than merely impacting the wax into the exposed cavities, a thin sheet of wax is applied. A gelatin sponge pad cut in the shape of the craniectomy defect is placed over the dura, and the previously preserved bone chips are replaced. In our experience, the bone regenerates over several months into a strong, bony plate that restores the cranial contour. After removal of the remaining retractors, the soft tissues of the neck are closed in a series of layers with interrupted 2-0 braided nylon (Surgilon) sutures, closing any potential dead space, after the wound is irrigated with antibiotic solution. The skin is sutured with interrupted 4-0 nylon sutures. Electromyographic electrodes, ground pads, and the external auditory canal earphone are removed after completion of wound closure and dressing.

DRESSING

After closure of the wound, it is cleaned, dried, and covered with a Telfa strip, to which a sterile adhesive, Op-Site, or similar dressing is applied. To discourage subcutaneous accumulation of CSF, a mastoid-type padded pressure bandage is applied. The dressing is removed 48 hours after surgery, and the wound is inspected and left open to the air. The skin sutures are removed 7 to 10 days after surgery.

POSTOPERATIVE CARE

The anesthesiologist awakens the patient, ideally with a smooth extubation that avoids straining and coughing. Antiemetics are given prophylactically to prevent vomiting, which could cause aspiration and associated pneumonitis during recovery from anesthesia. Postoperative monitoring is carried out initially in the postanesthesia care unit and then in the neurosurgical intensive care unit for 24 hours after surgery. After the initial 24-hour period, patients spend an average of 5 to 6 days on a hospital unit staffed by nurses experienced in postcraniotomy care. In addition to the monitoring of temperature, cardiorespiratory status, consciousness level, and fluid balance, both the nursing staff and patients are instructed to identify and report any CSF wound leakage or rhinorrhea.

Should a postoperative facial palsy be present, its grade is recorded according to the House-Brackmann scale, and preventive eye care is instituted. When eye closure is incomplete, artificial tears are applied hourly, or more often as needed, while the patient is awake. During sleep, a

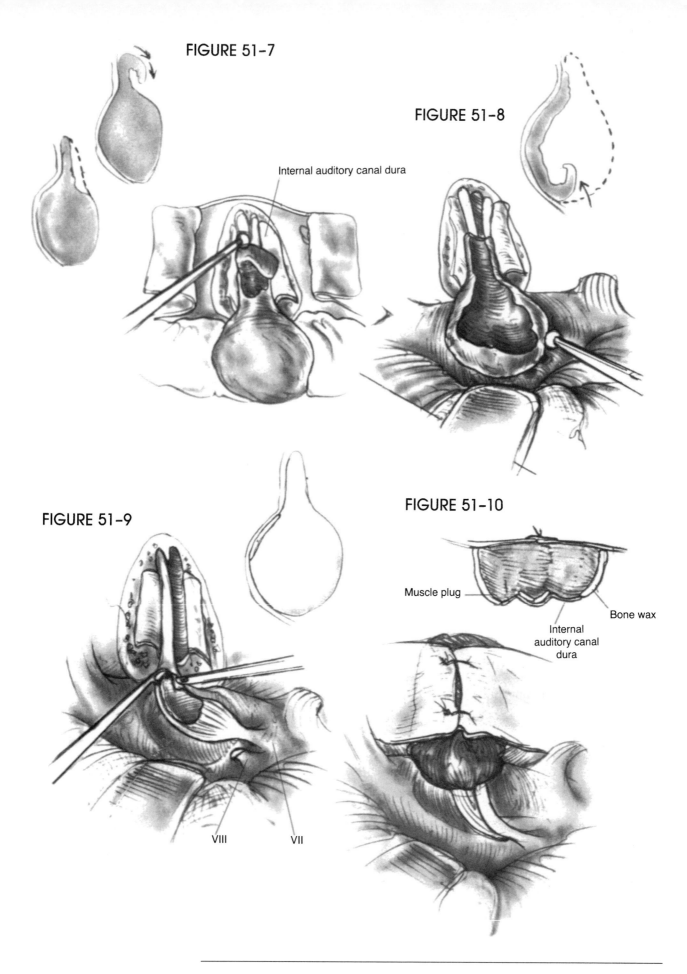

FIGURE 51-7

FIGURE 51-8

Internal auditory canal dura

FIGURE 51-9

FIGURE 51-10

Muscle plug

Bone wax

Internal
auditory canal
dura

VIII   VII

FIGURES 51-7 to 51-10. *See legends on opposite page*

plastic eye shield is placed to prevent drying and development of corneal abrasion. Special attention needs to be directed toward patients with dysfunction of both the facial and trigeminal nerves. When the cornea is dry, exposed, and insensitive, early gold weight placement is performed even when facial nerve recovery is expected.

Moderate-to-severe headache for several days is typical and may require narcotic analgesia for a variable period. Global headache that is delayed in onset by several days may signify the evolution of meningitis, either aseptic or bacterial, and is discussed later. We try to wean the patients from narcotics quickly and try to get their headaches under control with simple nonsteroidal anti-inflammatory preparations. In those relatively few cases in which corticosteroids have been used, they are tapered over a 7- to 10-day period. Vertigo can be controlled with parenterally administered antivertiginous agents, if the condition is severe, and with oral agents, if it is mild. In general, we prefer avoiding vestibular suppressants in the postoperative period because they may retard vestibular compensation.

Both diet and increasingly independent mobilization are encouraged under the guidance of a dietitian and physical therapist. We usually restrict the fluid intake for 3 days to a total of 1.5 L/24-hour period. Most patients are able to start a light diet 24 to 48 hours after surgery. Constipation and straining are avoided by the administration of stool softeners to prevent aggravation of headache and possible development of CSF leakage. Most patients begin mobility around 48 hours after surgery, although they have been encouraged to actively exercise their legs while they are recumbent in bed to reduce the risk of deep venous thrombosis. Antiembolism stockings are used until the patient is mobile. Mobilization usually takes the form of initially sitting at the bedside chair, followed by accompanied walks to the bathroom and then farther afield to the hospital corridors, and then onto a trial of practice on the stairs. Walking aids are provided by the physical therapist as required by the patient, depending on his or her progress. We usually discourage hair washing until 1 week after surgery to prevent the wound from getting wet and macerated. Patients may use a dry shampoo if desired.

Most patients are usually ready for discharge 5 to 7 days after surgery. Even when all other functions have recovered fully, easy fatigability often persists for 1 to 3 months postoperatively. The convalescent period required before returning to full-time employment and all the previous activities of daily living varies but is usually 2 to 3 months.

RESULTS

Historically, the primary issue in acoustic neuroma surgery was the survival of the patient. Fortunately, with the evolution of microsurgical techniques, mortality from acoustic neuroma surgery has become very low: less than 2 per cent in most recent series. Contemporary emphasis includes tumor control and, particularly, functional preservation. However, before the data from our own experience and the data published in the literature are addressed, it is important to appreciate that limited international standardization exists in the criteria used for reporting results on degree of resection,[28] facial nerve function,[29] and hearing preservation.[30]

In our opinion, the goal of acoustic neuroma resection should be tumor control and not necessarily complete resection in every case. Nevertheless, we perform a complete removal in most cases. Incomplete removal can be considered in two categories: subtotal and near-total excision. Subtotal removal, in which a substantial bulk of tumor remains, is seldom performed except in elderly or infirm individuals of short anticipated lifespan in whom shortening of the operative procedure is thought to be in the patient's interest. We have encountered several symptomatic recurrences in this group of patients, especially in individuals with cystic tumors. As previously discussed, near-total excision, in which a thin peel of capsule is left on the most adherent portion of the facial nerve, is occasionally used. Although few data are published on the

FIGURE 51–7. Step 1 of removal of an acoustic neuroma via the retrosigmoid approach. After the intracanalicular portion of the tumor is debulked, the lateral-most extension of the tumor is reflected medially, and a plane between the tumor capsule and the facial nerve is developed. This maneuver ensures complete removal of the tumor from the fundus. It also affords an early opportunity to confirm the function of the cranial nerve monitoring system by stimulation of the distal facial nerve under direct vision in a region where it is characteristically not especially adherent to the tumor surface.

FIGURE 51–8. Step 2 of removal of an acoustic neuroma via the retrosigmoid approach. The main portion of the tumor in the cerebellopontine angle is rapidly debulked. To facilitate rapid and safe tumor removal, we use a Cavitron ultrasonic aspirator. The tumor capsule is first liberated from the cerebellum and middle cerebellar peduncle. The pontine surface, including the root entry zones of cranial nerve VII and VIII, can then be exposed. In larger tumors, the lesion must also be microdissected from the trigeminal and lower cranial nerves (IX and X) as well.

FIGURE 51–9. Step 3 of removal of an acoustic neuroma via the retrosigmoid approach. Characteristically, the facial nerve is most adherent to the tumor capsule between the brainstem surface and the anterior lip of the porus acusticus. Liberation of the nerve from the tumor surface in this location often requires particularly delicate microdissection techniques.

FIGURE 51–10. Closure of the internal auditory canal defect at the completion of a retrosigmoid craniotomy. After waxing of the cut bony walls to seal any transected air cells, a muscle graft harvested from the nuchal area is mortised into the bony defect. The graft is retained in position by sutures, which are anchored in the dural flaps previously developed from the posterior petrous surface.

recurrence risk for this group of patients, we have observed many individuals with serial gadolinium-enhanced MRI and have yet to encounter a recurrence. The decision to undertake a near-total resection depends on the patient's age (i.e., less desirable in a younger individual) and preference as to whether the slightly higher risk of recurrence is justified by the improved facial nerve outcome.

Numerous papers appear in the literature on the subject of facial nerve preservation in acoustic neuroma surgery citing varying degrees of success. Because these are difficult to compare and draw conclusions from, we confine our commentary to our own series at UCSF. In our experience, facial nerve outcome from the retrosigmoid approach is similar to that from the other methods of removing acoustic neuromas for tumors of similar size.[31] In UCSF acoustic neuroma patients, anatomic continuity of the facial nerve was maintained in 99.2 per cent of cases. Of course, anatomic continuity does not necessarily imply functional integrity. The probability of a grade 1 or 2 facial function at 1 year after surgery in the context of tumor size was 100 per cent for tumors less than 1 cm; 90 per cent for those 1 to 3 cm; and 82 per cent for those greater than 3 cm.

With regard to hearing preservation, most published series address residual "measurable" hearing in contrast with the much more relevant concept of "useful" hearing.[32] For a patient with a unilateral acoustic neuroma, it could be argued that unless the conserved hearing maintains an interaural difference of less than 30 dB hearing loss with good speech discrimination (> 50 per cent), then it would be likely to be benefit. Preservation of useful hearing has been reported to be achieved in 25 to 58 per cent of hearing conservation candidates.[13] Very little information is available on the long-term follow-up of patients with preserved hearing. In two published series, significant late decline occured in 22 to 56 per cent of ears with successful hearing conservation.[33, 34] Factors relevant to success in hearing conservation approaches to acoustic neuroma include tumor size in the CPA, the depth to which the tumor penetrates the IAC, pure tone hearing level, and auditory brainstem response results. A full discussion of these criteria is beyond the scope of this chapter. It is not yet well established whether intraoperative auditory monitoring materially improves hearing conversation results. In one study using auditory brainstem response monitoring, it was found to be of marginal benefit overall, with the possible exception of tumors less than 1 cm in diameter.[35]

Several restrospective studies have compared hearing preservation rates following the retrosigmoid and middle fossa approaches.[36–38] In each study, the middle fossa approach yielded significantly better hearing results. Although that choice has not yet been universally accepted, the trend among centers undertaking a large volume of acoustic neuroma surgical procedures is to use the middle fossa approach as the preferred means of attempting bearing conservation. In our institution, the upper limit on the use of the extended middle fossa approach is a tumor in the 15- to 18-mm range of extracurricular diameter. The retrosigmoid approach is reserved for acoustic neuromas when three conditions are met: (1) excellent hearing, (2) a cisternal component between 15 and 20 mm, and (3) no tumor involvement of the distal one third of the IAC. The

retrosigmoid approach is still used for selected non–acoustic tumors of the CPA (such as meningiomas and epidermoids). Incomplete resection also has a potential role in hearing preservation, particularly in patients with neurofibromatosis type 2 or in those with a tumor in an only-hearing ear.[12, 39]

COMPLICATIONS

The common complications of the retrosigmoid approach to the CPA are persistent headache and CSF leakage.[11, 40, 41] Less common complications include (aseptic or bacterial) meningitis, hydrocephalus, cerebellar dysfuntion, vascular compromise (thrombosis and hemorhage), and problems associated with patient malpositioning during surgery. Of course, medical complications, such as pulmonary thromboembolism and pneumonia, may also occur but are not specific to surgery of this region. Although the potential complications of acoustic neuroma surgery are similar among the various operative approaches, their relative incidence varies considerably. In the retrosigmoid approach, both persistent headache and CSF leakage occur more frequently than with the other technique used in approaching CPA tumors.

Vascular Complications

Hemorrhage

Vascular complications may be extra-axial or intra-axial. The main extra-axial problem is bleeding into the CPA. CPA hematomas may cause brainstem compression and acute obstructive hydrocephalus. The incidence of acute CPA hematomas has been reported as varying from 0.5 to 2 per cent; however, with modern hemostatic techniques, the incidence is probably considerably less frequent.[11] This diagnosis should be suspected when a patient does not promptly awake after surgery or has a delayed deterioration in the level of consciousness. The diagnosis may be made by noncontrast CT scan in which fresh blood appears as a hyperdense mass in the CPA and extrinsic pontine compression is noted. If serious neurologic sequelae or even death are to be avoided, prompt surgical evacuation of the hemorrhage is essential. Intra-axial pontine hemorrhage may occur, particularly after removal of very large tumors that have greatly deflected the brainstem. Although major parenchymal hemorrhage is rare, minor amounts of intrinsic pontine bleeding are quite often evident radiographically after extirpation of giant tumors. Presumably, these result form the sudden re-expansion of the deeply compressed parenchyma. Supratentorial intra-axial hemorrhages have been reported after retrosigmoid approaches performed with the patient in the sitting position. These hemorrhages were associated with hypertension and may have resulted from subcortical venous tearing resulting from mechanical stress induced by the sitting position.[42–44] Extradural hematoma formation, a concern in the middle fossa approach, is uncommon after the retrosigmoid approach.

Anteroinferior Cerebellar Artery Syndrome

Brainstem infarction may occur after damage to the AICA, the vascular supply to the pons and cerebellar peduncle. Mechanisms of injury include disruption, cauterization, and arteriospasm with thrombosis. A full-fledged AICA syndrome is extremely serious and is often fatal because it results in the loss of respiratory center control.[45] Partial interruption of flow in the AICA system, avulsion of one or more of its branches, or obstruction of a nondominant AICA may result in an incomplete AICA syndrome. We have recently recognized several patients operated on for acoustic neuromas greater than 3 cm in diameter in whom gadolinium-enhanced MRI detected an infarction in the region of the middle cerebellar peduncle. These patients had unilaterally impaired cerebellar function and required prolonged physical therapy rehabilitation.[46]

Nonvascular Complications

Complications from Patient Positioning

As with any craniotomy, air embolism through breach of the major venous sinuses is a potential hazard. However, this risk is minimal when a supine or lateral patient position is used.[47] Air embolism is the main complication of the sitting position and has been reported in up to 30 per cent of cases.[48] When the sitting position is used, intraoperative monitoring with precordial Doppler ultrasonography alerts the anesthesiologist to venous air entry. The initial maneuvers to perform when air embolism has been detected are to flood the field with fluid and lower the head of the bed.

Quadriplegia (in four cases) and paraplegia have also been reported after acoustic neuroma resection in the sitting position. The degree of cervical flexion in the absence of protective spinal reflexes during anesthesia was thought to have caused spinal cord compression and infarction.[49, 50] In both the supine and lateral supine positions, the unconscious patient must be handled carefully, especially when the headholder is positioned. Excessive head rotation risks cervical injury and may obstruct vertebral venous drainage and contribute to cerebellar swelling. Excessive downward displacement of the shoulder risks traction injury on the brachial plexus.

As with any prolonged surgical procedure, adequate padding under pressure points is important to avoid pressure ulceration. Despite the best of precautions, patients frequently complain of discomfort over the ischium or other bony prominences for a few weeks postoperatively.

Cerebrospinal Fluid Leakage

CSF leakage is the most common postoperative complication, occurring in approximately 15 per cent of patients who undergo retrosigmoid approaches for acoustic neuroma. The patient must be counseled to recognize and report CSF leakage so that steps can be taken to rapidly control it to prevent infectious meningitis. CSF leak occurs either directly through the wound or indirectly through the ear and auditory tube to the nasopharynx, where it presents as a watery rhinorrhea or salty postnasal discharge. CSF escape into the ear may occur through opened and unsealed mastoid air cells in the region of the craniectomy or through air cells opened and unsealed in the bony IAC dissection.[51] CSF drainage often stops spontaneously with simple fluid restriction and avoidance of straining. The use of acetazolamide, a carbonic anhydrase–inhibiting diuretic, may also be of benefit. Alternatively, the early use of a lumbar CSF drain for 48 to 72 hours may halt the drainage. Some have advocated (1) wound re-exploration with re-waxing of the bone to close covert open air cells, (2) replacement of the muscle graft plug to close CSF leakage, and (3) continued lumbar drainage.[47] We prefer to address persistent, intractable CSF otorhinorrhea transtemporally. When useful residual hearing is present, a canal wall up mastoidectomy is performed, perilabyrinthine cells are copiously waxed, the fossa incudis is occluded with a fascia graft, and fat is used to obliterate the cavity. When the operated ear is deaf, a canal wall down mastoidectomy is performed. The external auditory canal is sutured closed, and the auditory tube is sealed under direct vision with bone wax and muscle. The mastoid air cells are also waxed, and the cavity is obliterated with fat. Lumbar CSF drainage is maintained for approximately 72 hours after surgery.

Aseptic and Bacterial Meningitis

Entry of blood and bone dust into the subarachnoid space can result in aseptic meningitis. Care is taken during the drilling of the posterior petrous face during the IAC exposure to prevent contamination of the subarachnoid space with bone dust. Gelatin sponge is placed in the CPA superior and inferior to the tumor and seventh-eighth nerve complex, and a rubber dam is placed over the cerebellum. After completion of the bone work, the wound is thoroughly irrigated and the bone debris is removed. Similarly, throughout the tumor dissection and at its completion, a combination of suction and irrigation is used to prevent the build-up of blood and clots because both blood and bone debris produce an irritative or chemical aseptic meningitis.[11]

To reduce the risk of bacterial meningitis, intravenous prophylactic antibiotics are administered at the start of surgery and bacitracin is added to the irrigant solution used to flush the CPA at the end of the procedure. This complication should be suspected if the patient develops headache, fever, and malaise in the first postoperative week. Nuchal rigidity, usually considered a sign of meningeal irritation, is of limited information following retrosigmoid craniotomy, because the neck muscles may be in spasm owing to direct surgical trauma. Bacterial meningitis may also occur in the late postoperative period, particularly when a CSF leak is present. The clinician is wise to maintain a high degree of suspicion about bacterial meningitis and, when in doubt, obtain a sample of CSF via lumbar puncture for analysis. In patients in whom the clinical picture is suggestive, intravenous antibiotics should be instituted pending results of culture and sensitivity testing.

Hydrocephalus

Hydrocephalus can occur as a result of blood and bone debris contamination of the posterior fossa subarachnoid space. Particulate and proteinaceous debris becomes ingested by arachnoid granulations, impairing their absorptive capabilities, which results in raised intracranial pressure. Cerebellar retraction with subsequent swelling at release may also result in the development of hydrocephalus.[11]

Cerebellar Dysfunction

Prolonged cerebellar retraction may result in edema and swelling and possibly contusion, with resultant dysmetria and impaired balance in the postoperative period.

Persistent Headache

Headache is encountered more frequently after the retrosigmoid approach than after other types of posterior fossa craniotomy.[52] In our experience, nearly all retrosigmoid patients have substantial headache during the first postoperative month. By 3 months after surgery, approximately one third continue to complain of this symptom. By 1 year, around 15 per cent of patients continue to have chronic moderate-to-severe headaches, compared with very few headaches for those who underwent the translabyrinthine procedure. Some individuals are unable to return to work or resume other life activities because of this symptom. Of interest, the highest incidence of persistent headache in our series has been in patients with small tumors who underwent the retrosigmoid approach in an effort to preserve hearing. Although the headache may have myriad presentations, it is most commonly either frontal or referred to the area of surgery and is often triggered by cough. Numerous potential underlying causes exist for chronic headache after retrosigmoid craniotomy, including aseptic meningitis, coupling of the suboccipital dura to the nuchal musculature, occipital neuralgia, and even exacerbation of an underlying headache tendency, such as migraine. Although numerous mechanisms are possible, we believe that most are a result of chronic arachnoiditis incited by contamination with bone dust and blood at the time of surgery. One apparent risk factor for the development of chronic headaches is retrosigmoid craniectomy in which the calvarial bony defect is left unreconstructed.[53, 54] Replacement of the retrosigmoidal bone either as a flap, bone chips, or even with alloplastic material somewhat diminishes the incidence of persistent headache.

Residual or Recurrent Tumor

We prefer to revise recurrent tumors after retrosigmoid craniotomy using a translabyrinthine approach. This method avoids the previously scarred dural areas and tends to present more favorable arachnoid dissection planes during the early portion of the procedure.[55]

ACKNOWLEDGMENT

Figures 51–1 to 51–10 were adapted from artwork produced by the authors for Jackler RK: Atlas of Neurotology and Skull Base Surgery. St. Louis, Mosby–Year Book, 1995. The original drawings in this chapter were produced by Christine Gralapp, MA.

References

1. Krause F: Zur Freilegung der hinteren Felsenbeinfläche und des Kleinhirns. Beitr Klin Chir 37: 728–764, 1903.
2. Rhoton AL Jr, Tedeschi H: Microsurgical anatomy of acoustic neuroma. Otolaryngol Clin North Am 25: 257–294, 1992.
3. Lang J: Clinical Anatomy of the Posterior Cranial Fossa and its Foramina. New York, Thieme, 1991.
4. Lang J Jr, Samii A: Retrosigmoidal approach to the posterior cranial fossa: An anatomical study. Acta Neurochir (Wien) 111: 147–153, 1991.
5. Camins MB, Oppenheim JS: Anatomy and surgical techniques in the suboccipital transmeatal approach to acoustic neuromas. Clin Neurosurg 38: 567–588, 1992.
6. Silverstein H, Morrell H, Smouha E, Jones R: Combined retrolab-retrosigmoid vestibular neurectomy: An evolution in approach. Am J Otol 10: 166–169, 1989.
7. Jackler RK, Pitts LH: Selection of surgical approach to acoustic neuroma. Otolaryngol Clin North Am 25: 361–387, 1992.
8. Selesnick SH, Jackler RK: Clinical manifestations and audiologic diagnosis of acoustic neuromas. Otolaryngol Clin North Am 25: 521–551, 1992.
9. Cohen NL, Hammerschlag P, Berg H, Ransohoff J: Acoustic neuroma surgery: An eclectic approach with an emphasis on hearing preservation. Ann Otol Rhinol Laryngol 95: 21–27, 1986.
10. Cohen NL: Retrosigmoid approach for acoustic tumor removal. Otolaryngol Clin North Am 25: 295–310, 1992.
11. Wiet RJ, Teixido M, Liang JG: Complications in acoustic neuroma surgery. Otolaryngol Clin North Am 25: 389–412, 1992.
12. Glasscock ME III, Hart MJ, Vrabec JT: Management of bilateral acoustic neuroma. Otolaryngol Clin North Am 5: 449–469, 1992.
13. Shelton C: Hearing preservation in acoustic tumor surgery. Otolaryngol Clin North Am 25: 609–621, 1992.
14. Nassif PS, Shelton C, Arriaga MM: Hearing preservation following surgical removal of meningiomas affecting the temporal bone. Laryngoscope 102: 1357–1362, 1992.
15. Blevins N, Jackler RK: Exposure of the lateral extremity of the internal auditory canal via the retrosigmoid approach: A radioanatomic study. Otolaryngol Head Neck Surg 11: 81–90, 1994.
16. Cheung SW, Jackler RK, Pitts LP, Gutin PH: Interconnecting the posterior and middle fossa for tumors which traverse Meckel's cave. Am J Otol 16: 200–208, 1995.
17. Seoane E, Rhoton AL Jr: Suprameatal extension of the retrosigmoid approach: Microsurgical anatomy. Neurosurgery 44: 553–560, 1999.
18. Samii M, Tatagiba M, Carvalho GA: Retrosigmoid intradural suprameatal approach to Meckel's cave and the middle fossa: Surgical technique and outcome. J Neurosurg 92: 235–241, 2000.
19. Yingling CD, Gardi JN: Intraoperative monitoring of facial and cochlear nerves during acoustic neuroma surgery. Otolaryngol Clin North Am 25: 413–448, 1992.
20. MacDonald CB, Hirsch BE, Kamerer DB, Sekhar L: Acoustic neuroma surgery: Predictive criteria for hearing preservation. Otolaryngol Head Neck Surg 104: 128, 1991.
21. Goksu N, Bayazit Y, Kemaloglu Y: Endoscopy of the posterior fossa and dissection of acoustic neuroma. J Neurosurg 91: 776–780, 1999.
22. Wackym PA, King WA, Poe DS, et al: Adjunctive use of endoscopy during acoustic neuroma surgery. Laryngoscope 109: 1193–1201, 1999.
23. Lye RH, Pace-Balzan A, Ramsden RT, et al: The fate of tumour rests following removal of acoustic neuromas: An MRI Gd-DTPA study. Br J Neurosurg 6: 195–201, 1992.
24. Thedinger BS, Whittaker CK, Luetje CM: Recurrent acoustic tumor after a suboccipital removal. Neurosurgery 29: 681–687, 1991.
25. Mazzoni A, Calabrese V, Danesi G: A modified retrosigmoid approach for direct exposure of the fundus of the internal auditory canal for hearing preservation in acoustic neuroma surgery. Am J Otol 21: 98–109, 2000.
26. Arriaga M, Gorum M: Enhanced retrosigmoid exposure with posterior semicircular canal resection. Otolaryngol Head Neck Surg 115: 46–48, 1996.
27. Kemink JL, Langman AW, Niparko JK, Graham MD: Operative management of acoustic neuromas: The priority of neurologic function over complete resection. Otolaryngol Head Neck Surg 104: 96–99, 1991.
28. Moffat DA: Synopsis on near-total, subtotal, or partial removal:

Acoustic neuroma. *In* Tos M, Thomsen J (eds): Proceedings of the First International Conference on Acoustic Neuroma, Copenhagen, August 25–29, 1991. New York, Kugler Publications, 1992, pp 983–984.

29. Baer S, Tos M, Thomsen J, Hughes G: Synopsis on grading of facial nerve function after acoustic neuroma treatment: Acoustic neuroma. *In* Tos M, Thomsen J (eds): Proceedings of the First International Conference on Acoustic Neuroma, Copenhagen, August 25–29, 1991. New York, Kugler Publications, 1992, pp 993–995.

30. Sanna M, Gamoletti J, Tos M, Thomsen J: Synopsis on hearing preservation following acoustic neuroma surgery: Acoustic neuroma. *In* Tos M, Thomsen J (eds): Proceedings of the First International Conference on Acoustic Neuroma, Copenhagen, August 25–29, 1991. New York, Kugler Publications, 1992, pp 985–987.

31. Lalwani A, Butt FY, Jackler RK, et al: Facial nerve outcome after acoustic neuroma surgery: A study from the era of cranial nerve monitoring Otolaryngol Head Neck Surg 111: 561–570, 1994.

32. Hinton AE, Ramsden RT, Lye RH, Dutton JE: Criteria for hearing preservation in acoustic schwannoma surgery: The concept of useful hearing. J Laryngol Otol 106: 500–503, 1992.

33. Shelton C, Hitselberger WE, House WF, Brackmann DE: Long-term results of hearing after acoustic tumor removal: Acoustic neuroma. *In* Tos M, Thomsen J (eds): Proceedings of the First International Conference on Acoustic Neuroma, Copenhagen, August 25–29, 1991. New York, Kugler Publications, 1992, pp 661–664.

34. McKenna MJ, Halpin C, Ojemann RG, et al: Long-term hearing results in patients after surgical removal of acoustic tumors with hearing preservation. Am J Otol 13: 134–136, 1992.

35. Slavit DH, Harner SG, Harper CM Jr, Beatty CW: Auditory monitoring during acoustic neuroma removal. Arch Otolaryngol Head Neck Surg 17: 1153–1157, 1991.

36. Staecker H, Nadol JB, Ojeman R, et al: Hearing preservation in acoustic neuroma surgery: Middle fossa versus retrosigmoid approach. Am J Otol 21: 399–404, 2000.

37. Irving RM, Jackler RK, Pitts LH: Hearing preservation in patients undergoing vestibular schwannoma surgery: Comparison of middle fossa and retrosigmoid approaches. J Neurosurg 88: 840–845, 1998.

38. Arriaga MA, Chen DA, Fukushima T: Individualizing hearing preservation in acoustic neuroma surgery. Laryngoscope 107: 1043–1047, 1997.

39. Wigand ME, Haid T, Goertzen W, Wolf S: Preservation of hearing in bilateral acoustic neurinomas by deliberate partial resection. Acta Otolaryngol (Stockh) 112: 237–241, 1992.

40. Mangham CA: Complications of translabyrinthine versus suboccipital approach for acoustic tumor surgery. Otolaryngol Head Neck Surg 99: 396–400, 1988.

41. Ebersold MJ, Harner SG, Beatty CW, et al: Current results of the retrosigmoid approach to acoustic neurinoma. J Neurosurg 76: 901–909, 1991.

42. Haines JH, Maroon JC, Janetta PJ: Supratentorial intracerebral hemorrhage following posterior fossa surgery. J Neurosurg 49: 881, 1978.

43. Harders A, Gilbach J, Weigel K: Supratentorial space-occupying lesions following infratentorial surgery: Early diagnosis and treatment. Acta Neurochir (Wien) 74: 57, 1985.

44. Seiler RW, Zurbrugg HR: Supratentorial intracerebral hemorrhage after posterior fossa operation. Neurosurgery 18: 472, 1986.

45. Atkinson J: The anterior cerebellar artery: Its variations, pontine distribution, and significance in the surgery of cerebellopontine angle tumours. J Neurol Neurosurg Psychiatry 12: 137–151, 1949.

46. Sim DW, Jackler RK, Pitts LH: Cerebellar peduncle infarction after acoustic neuroma surgery. 1994.

47. Harner SG, Beatty CW, Ebersold MJ: Retrosigmoid removal of acoustic neuroma: Experience 1978–1988. Otolaryngol Head Neck Surg 103: 40–45, 1990.

48. Duke DA, Lynch JJ, Harner SG, et al: Venous air embolism in sitting and supine patients undergoing vestibular schwannoma resection. Neurosurgery 42: 1282–1286, 1998.

49. Hitselberger WE, House WF: A warning regarding the sitting position for acoustic tumor surgery. Arch Otolaryngol Head Neck Surg 106: 69, 1980.

50. Samii M, Turel KE, Penker G: Management of seventh and eighth nerve involvement by cerebellopontine angle tumors. Clin Neurosurg 32: 242, 1985.

51. Smith PG, Leonetti JP, Grubb RL: Management of cerebrospinal fluid otorhinorrhea complicating the retrosigmoid approach to the cerebellopontine angle. Am J Otol 11: 178–180, 1990.

52. Schessel DA, Nedzelski JM, Rowed Feghali JG: Headache and local discomfort following surgery of the cerebellopontine angle: Acoustic neuroma. *In* Tos M, Thomsen J (eds): Proceedings of the First International Conference on Acoustic Neuroma, Copenhagen, August 25–29, 1991. New York, Kugler Publications, 1992, pp 899–904.

53. Koperer H, Deinsberger W, Jodicke A, Boker DK: Postoperative headache after the lateral suboccipital approach: Craniotomy versus craniectomy. Minim Invasive Neurosurg 42: 175–178, 1999.

54. Feghali JG, Elowitz EH: Split calvarial graft cranioplasty for the prevention of headache after retrosigmoid resection of acoustic neuromas. Laryngoscope 108: 1450–1452, 1998.

55. Beatty CW, Ebersold MJ, Harner SG: Residual and recurrent acoustic neuromas. Laryngoscope 97: 1168–1171, 1987.

52

Transotic Approach

Ugo Fisch, M.D. ▪ Joseph M. Chen, M.D.

The transotic approach to the cerebellopontine angle (CPA) was first introduced in 1979 by one of us (U.F.) in response to the limitations of the translabyrinthine technique. The objective of this approach is to obtain a direct lateral exposure and the widest possible access to the CPA through the medial wall of the temporal bone, from the superior petrosal sinus to the jugular bulb, and from the internal carotid artery to the sigmoid sinus. The tympanic and mastoid portions of the fallopian canal are left in situ. This transtemporal access is achieved at the expense of bony exenteration rather than cerebellar retraction.

In spite of well-documented technical details,[1] there is a general misconception equating the transotic approach with the transcochlear approach[2] of House and Hitzelberger. Significant differences exist between the two approaches in the extent of exposure, the management of the facial nerve, and the obliteration of the surgical cavity.

As a natural extension of subtotal petrosectomy, which forms the basis of lateral and posterior skull base surgery at the University of Zurich,[1] the transotic approach was initially designed for acoustic neuromas and has since expanded to include other pathology. Several modifications were also made over the years to optimize its use.[3–5]

INDICATIONS

Acoustic Neuroma

Although the transotic approach, like the translabyrinthine approach, can be used for tumors of all sizes, it is ideal for tumors of 2.5 cm or less in their medial-lateral extent, in patients with *no* serviceable hearing. In this clinical setting, the transotic approach offers the best possible exposure for tumor extirpation and the preservation of facial nerve and with minimal morbidity.

Tumors larger than 2.5 cm that cause significant brainstem compression are managed by the neurosurgery department as a matter of departmental policy at the University of Zurich. Small intracanalicular tumors in patients with good hearing (using the 50/50 rule of at least 50 dB hearing loss and 50 per cent discrimination score) are managed through a middle cranial fossa (transtemporal-supralabyrinthine) approach (see Chapter 36).

Other Lesions

Other lesions involving the CPA or the temporal bone with invasion of the internal auditory canal (IAC) or the otic capsule could also be approached via the transotic technique. They include the following:

- Epithelial cysts (congenital cholesteatoma)
- Arachnoid cysts
- Hemangiomas
- Giant cholesterol and mucosal cysts
- Jugular foramen schwannomas
- Temporal paragangliomas (glomus tumors)

These lesions can be quite extensive and may require a combined infratemporal fossa type A or B approach for added exposure.

PREOPERATIVE EVALUATION

The evaluation for retrocochlear lesions, such as acoustic neuromas, is fairly standard at the University of Zurich and includes routine audiometry, auditory brainstem response, electronystagmography, and magnetic resonance imaging (MRI) with gadolinium enhancement. High-resolution computed tomography is still performed for bony assessment of lesions within or invading the temporal bone. Facial nerve status is recorded clinically using the Fisch grading system[6] and quantified by electroneuronography prior to surgery.

In addition to a candid discussion of surgical and postoperative complications, patients are made aware of the advantages of the transotic approach specifically with regard to the preservation of the facial nerve and the complete obliteration of the surgical cavity, with blind sac closure of the external auditory canal to minimize cerebrospinal fluid leak. The option of conservative management by close monitoring with serial MRI to follow tumor growth is presented to all patients and is recommended for patients with nonprogressive long-standing symptoms (especially the elderly), patients with small tumors and normal hearing, patients with significant medical illnesses, or those who refuse to undergo surgery. These patients are made aware that rapid tumor growth will ultimately require surgical attention and that facial nerve function and hearing preservation may be compromised as a result of the delay in surgery.

SURGICAL TECHNIQUES

Preoperative Preparation

The patient is premedicated with clonidine, metoclopramide, and midazolam before surgery. Perioperative antibiotic, ceftriaxone (Rocephin), 2 q intravenously for 24 hours is given at the time of surgery until the removal of intravenous infusion, usually by the third day after surgery.

Surgical Site Preparation, Positioning, and Draping

The surgical site is prepared in the OR after induction of anesthesia. Hair over the temporal area is shaved 9 cm above and 5 cm behind the pinna. The skin is then washed with povidone-iodine. The abdomen and the contralateral leg are also shaved and prepared for fat harvesting and the possible need of a sural nerve graft.

The positioning and draping for this procedure are similar to those described in Chapter 1, with some minor differences. The patient is secured in supine position on the Fisch operating table (see Chapter 36), with the head turned away from the surgeon. A large plastic bag is incorporated into the draping to catch excess irrigation and blood.

Intraoperative Monitoring and Concerns

Intraoperative facial nerve monitoring using the Xomed nerve integrity monitor (NIM-II) and percutaneous electromyographic needles is standard with this approach. Intracranial pressure is controlled by deep anesthesia induced intravenously before introduction of inhalation anesthetics. The P_{CO_2} is maintained between 30 and 40 mm Hg. Pharmacologic manipulation with dexamethasone (Decadron, 4 mg every 8 hours perioperatively and 4 days postoperatively) and mannitol (0.5 mg per kg intravenously intraoperatively) are also standard. Furosemide is added when necessary. Lumbar cerebrospinal fluid drainage is not routinely performed. Hypotensive anesthesia with nitroglycerin and/or clonidine (Catapres) is used in most cases to maintain a systolic blood pressure between 80 and 100 mm Hg.

Techniques of Surgery

Skin Incision

A postauricular incision is placed along the hairline to keep it behind the operative cavity (Fig. 52–1). The incision is made from the mastoid tip to the temporal region for the surgical approach; its superior extension (dotted lines) is made at the time of wound closure for the exposure of the temporalis muscle flap.

Blind Sac Closure of the External Auditory Canal

A mastoid periosteal flap is developed while the postauricular skin flap is elevated. The external auditory canal is transected and its skin elevated, everted externally, and closed as a blind sac. A second layer of closure using the mastoid periosteal flap ensures a complete seal (Fig. 52–2).

Subtotal Petrosectomy: Exposure of Jugular Bulb and Petrous Carotid

A complete mastoidectomy is performed, and the remaining external auditory canal skin, tympanic membrane, and ossicles are removed in a stepwise fashion. The tympanic bone is progressively thinned out, and a complete exenteration of the pneumatic spaces (retrofacial, retrolabyrinthine, supralabyrinthine, hypotympanic, infralabyrinthine, and pericarotid) is carried out. Figure 52–3 shows the surgical cavity at the completion of this step. The middle fossa dura, sigmoid sinus, and jugular bulb are blue-lined; the fallopian canal and the vertical portion of the petrous carotid artery are skeletonized. The mastoid tip is removed to reduce the depth of the surgical cavity.

Obliteration of the Eustachian Tube

The mucosa of the membranous eustachian tube orifice is coagulated and the bony canal obliterated with bone wax at the isthmus. An additional muscle plug is used prior to closure.

Exenteration of the Otic Capsule

With the completion of subtotal petrosectomy, the surgical cavity is divided into two compartments by the fallopian canal (Fig. 52–4). Because the enlarged IAC lies mostly deep within the anterior compartment, the advantage of the transotic approach to fully access this region is clear.

To begin this step, the semicircular canals are removed and the vestibule is opened as in the translabyrinthine approach. The posterior aspect of the IAC is exposed from the fundus to the porus, leaving a thin layer of bone over the meatal dura. The posterior fossa dura of the posterior compartment is exposed caudal to the superior petrosal sinus and anterior to the sigmoid sinus. Retrofacial cells are subsequently removed to gain access over the inferior aspect of the IAC.

Attention is now focused on the anterior compartment. The cochlea is drilled away to expose the enlarged IAC, which lies predominantly within this compartment, and as the dissection is carried forward, the dura anterior to the porus is also exposed to the level of the vertical segment of the ICA. Bony reduction between the jugular bulb and the inferior aspect of the IAC requires working beneath and over the fallopian canal, which is left in its anatomic position across the surgical field. Sufficient bone is left surrounding the canal to prevent accidental fracture. The cochlear aqueduct is identified between the jugular bulb and the IAC. The arachnoid of the aqueduct is opened to allow the outflow of cerebrospinal fluid, thereby decompressing the lateral cistern before the posterior fossa dura is opened.

The tensor tympani muscle and bone medial to it are removed to gain more anterior access; likewise, bone medial to the vertical carotid artery is removed as much as possible.

Unroofing of the Labyrinthine Portion of the Facial Nerve

Since 1988, the unroofing of the labyrinthine segment of the facial nerve from the meatal foramen to the geniculate

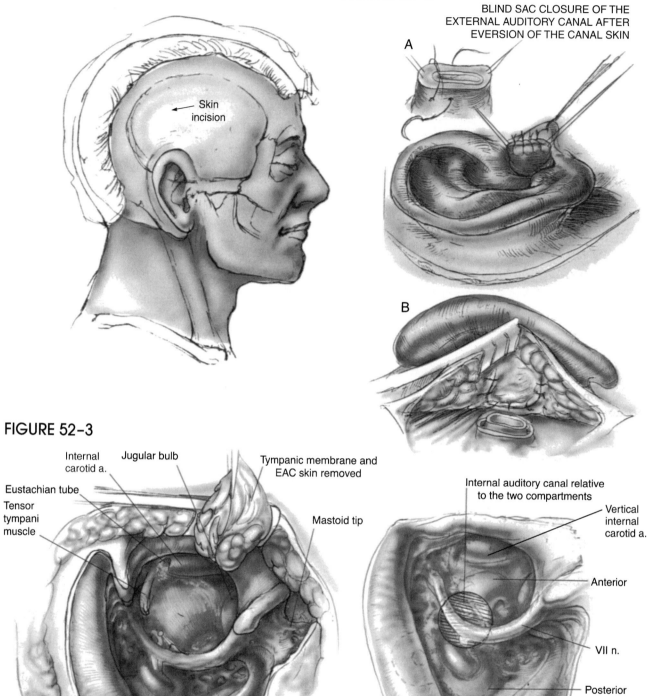

FIGURE 52-1

Skin incision

FIGURE 52-2

BLIND SAC CLOSURE OF THE
EXTERNAL AUDITORY CANAL AFTER
EVERSION OF THE CANAL SKIN

A

B

FIGURE 52-3

Internal carotid a.

Jugular bulb

Tympanic membrane and
EAC skin removed

Eustachian tube

Tensor
tympani
muscle

Mastoid tip

Sigmoid sinus

Emissary v.

Internal auditory canal relative
to the two compartments

Vertical
internal
carotid a.

Anterior

VII n.

Posterior

FIGURE 52-4

FIGURES 52-1 to 52-4. *See legends on opposite page*

ganglion has been incorporated as a standard step in the transotic approach. The meatal foramen can be found approximately 2 mm anterior and superior to the meatal fundus. This exposure will provide additional room for that portion of the facial nerve most likely to suffer traction injury and edema subsequent to tumor manipulation. Also, the labyrinthine portion of the facial nerve serves as an important landmark while further access over the porus is gained along the superior petrosal sinus.

The completed exposure is shown in Figure 52–5. The posterior fossa dura surrounding the porus is circumferentially exposed from the carotid artery to the sigmoid sinus, and from the jugular bulb to the level of the superior petrosal sinus.

Tumor Removal

A few instruments are required for tumor removal. Bayonet and angled bipolar forceps, cup forceps, microraspatories, and a long suction with finger control are the most essential.

The intrameatal portion of the tumor is approached first and is separated from the facial nerve until the level of the porus. Figure 52–6 illustrates the advantage of the additional space obtained with the transotic exenteration, whereby the intrameatal portion of the tumor can be easily displaced and mobilized during its removal.

The posterior fossa dura is incised between the sinodural angle and the posterior edge of the porus. The incision is extended superiorly and inferiorly along the porus (Fig. 52–7). It is important to elevate the dura with a hook prior to making an incision to prevent the inadvertent injury of vessels over the cerebellum. The dural edges must be cauterized before extending the incision to facilitate hemostasis. One must also be acutely aware of the variations of the course of the anteroinferior cerebellar artery (AICA) and its branches.

The superior and inferior dural flaps are retracted with 4-0 Vicryl sutures, which are clipped to the wound edges (Fig. 52–8). The full extent of the tumor can usually be demonstrated: the posterior pole of the tumor abuts against the cerebellum, the petrosal vein, and the AICA courses anteroinferior to the tumor.

Intracapsular reduction of the tumor can now commence and is continued until tumor margins can be seen without tension being placed on the facial nerve. During this step, the meatal dura at the superior pole of the porus is not detached, so as to render some stability to the tumor. It is of utmost importance to handle the tumor meticulously; manipulations should be carried out with suction over a cottonoid, and the displaced facial nerve should always be in view to avoid undue traction (Fig. 52–9).

Bleeding is diminished by coagulation of all visible vessels over the tumor capsule. The main blood supply to the tumor generally runs along the eighth nerve, and some may come from branches of the AICA: they should be coagulated, cut on the tumor, and gently pulled away.

With sufficient reduction, separation of the facial nerve can now be attempted. The advantage of the transotic approach is now easily appreciated because the displaced facial nerve can be followed in its entirety. The dural attachments of the tumor at the porus are cut, and the nerve can be gently grasped with bipolar forceps and teased away from the tumor (Fig. 52–10). Likewise, the AICA can be separated from the nerve by using the tips of the forceps or by pulling on the coagulated branches.

At the inferior pole of the tumor, the origin of the eighth nerve and the course of the AICA looping around it are identified. In many instances, the root exit zone of the facial nerve, always anterior to the eighth nerve, is identified only after the eighth nerve is cut.

The anterior access of the transotic approach offers an unparalleled view to an area that is usually partially hidden from the surgeon during suboccipital or translabyrinthine surgery.[7, 8] In this exact region, the facial nerve is most tenuous and frequently appears as a thin, transparent band. Any manipulation not under direct vision can easily rupture the nerve. Once it is completely detached from all vital structures, the tumor can now be removed. The CPA and all its structures are exposed in Figure 52–11.

The facial nerve is stimulated electrically to obtain a threshold response. Despite a normal response intraoperatively, the patient may still demonstrate an immediate or delayed facial paralysis due to impaired vascular supply and the inevitable trauma to the nerve during dissection. If stimulation fails to produce a response or facial contraction, and if the anatomic integrity of the nerve is precarious, it is best to proceed with nerve grafting immediately. Failure to do so while waiting for the improbable return of facial function may delay reinnervation for up to 2 years. The details of intracranial-intratemporal and hypoglossal-facial crossover grafting techniques are beyond the scope of this chapter and are documented elsewhere.[1, 9]

Wound Closure

A musculofascial graft that is slightly larger than the dural defect is taken from the temporalis muscle. It is placed under the dura and fixed in place with the two 4-0 Vicryl sutures used previously as stay sutures (Fig. 52–12). These sutures are passed through the edges of the graft and secured to the dura. A second temporalis fascial graft is used to cover the opened internal auditory canal. A small muscle graft is also used as a plug to supplement the prior wax obliteration of the eustachian tube. Both grafts are stabilized with fibrin glue.

A second layer of closure with abdominal fat grafts is to follow. A large piece of fat is first passed under the fallopian canal and firmly anchored (Fig. 52–13). Several

---

FIGURE 52–1. Skin incision.

FIGURE 52–2. A and B, Blind sac closure of the external auditory canal.

FIGURE 52–3. Subtotal petrosectomy. EAC, external auditory canal.

FIGURE 52–4. Position of the internal auditory canal in relation to the anterior and posterior compartments of the operative cavity.

FIGURE 52–5

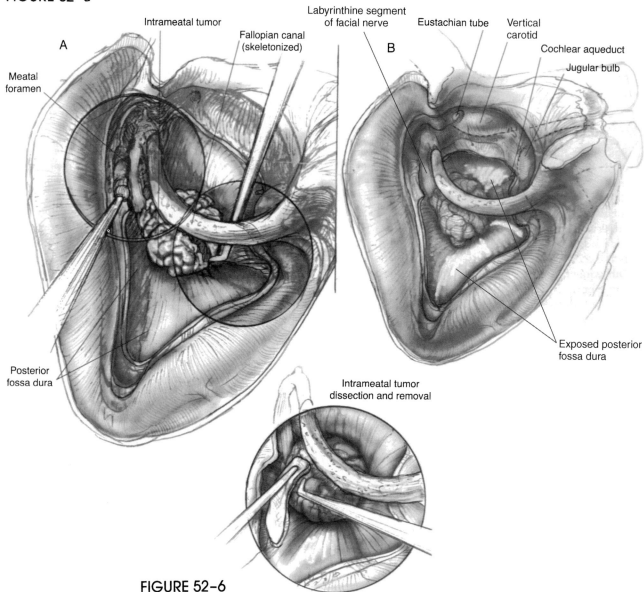

Meatal foramen

Intrameatal tumor

Fallopian canal (skeletonized)

Labyrinthine segment of facial nerve

Eustachian tube

Vertical carotid

Cochlear aqueduct

Jugular bulb

A

B

Posterior fossa dura

Exposed posterior fossa dura

Intrameatal tumor dissection and removal

FIGURE 52–6

FIGURE 52–5. *A* and *B*, Exposure of the internal auditory canal and posterior fossa dura.

FIGURE 52–6. Intrameatal tumor dissection.

FIGURE 52–7. Dural incisions. CSF, Cerebrospinal fluid; PFD, posterior fossa dura.

FIGURE 52–8. Initial cerebellopontine angle (CPA) exposure. AICA, anteroinferior cerebellar artery.

FIGURE 52–9. Intracapsular tumor reduction.

FIGURE 52–10. Intracranial facial nerve dissection. AICA, anteroinferior cerebellar artery.

FIGURE 52–11. View of cerebellopontine angle (CPA) after tumor removal. AICA, anteroinferior cerebellar artery.

FIGURE 52-7

DURAL INCISIONS

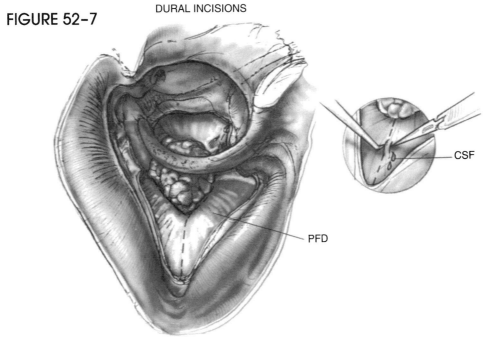

CSF

PFD

FIGURE 52-8

INITIAL CPA EXPOSURE

AICA

Petrosal v.

Facial nerve

FIGURE 52-9

Intracapsular
tumor reduction

IC VII
Anterosuperiorly
displaced

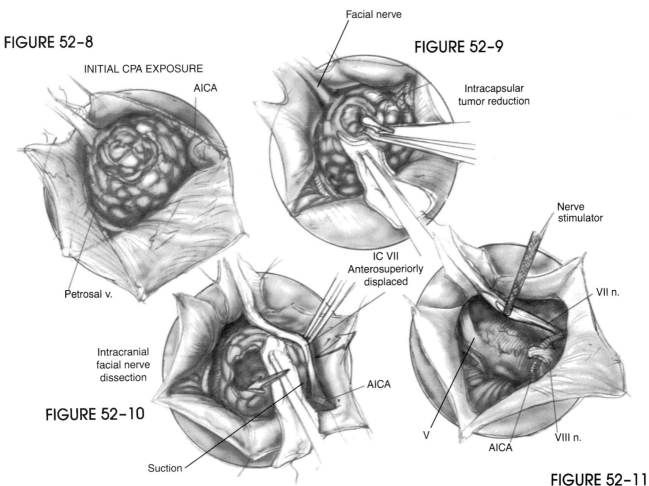

Intracranial
facial nerve
dissection

FIGURE 52-10

Suction

AICA

Nerve
stimulator

VII n.

V

AICA

VIII n.

FIGURE 52-11

FIGURES 52–7 to 52–11. *See legends on opposite page*

FIGURE 52-12

DURAL CLOSURE FASCIA

Fascia over IAM

Dura

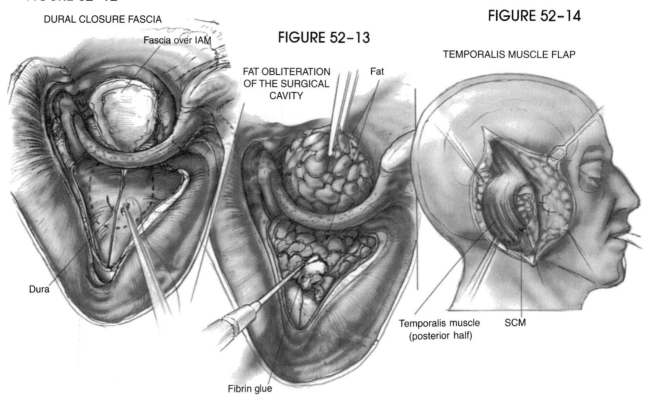

FIGURE 52-13

FAT OBLITERATION
OF THE SURGICAL
CAVITY

Fat

Fibrin glue

FIGURE 52-14

TEMPORALIS MUSCLE FLAP

Temporalis muscle
(posterior half)

SCM

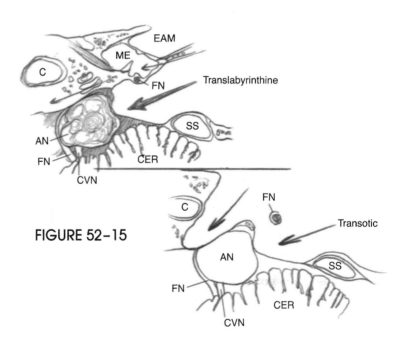

FIGURE 52-15

EAM

ME

C

FN

Translabyrinthine

SS

AN

FN

CER

CVN

C

FN

Transotic

AN

FN

SS

CER

CVN

FIGURE 52–12. Dural closure.

FIGURE 52–13. Fat obliteration of the surgical cavity.

FIGURE 52–14. Temporalis muscle flap. SCM, Sternocleidomastoid.

FIGURE 52–15. Cross-sectional views of the transotic approach versus the translabyrinthine approach. C, carotid; EAM, external auditory meatus; FN, facial nerve; SS, sigmoid sinus; ME, middle ear; AN, acoustic neuroma; CER, cerebellum; CVN, cochleovestibular nerve.

small pieces of fat are used to fill out the surgical cavity and are also stabilized with fibrin glue.

The posterior half of the temporalis muscle is now transposed and sutured in place with 2-0 Vicryl sutures. Additional fat is placed under the muscle flap to create a slight compressive tension (Fig. 52–14). This type of closure has consistently minimized the incidence of postoperative cerebrospinal fluid leaks and demonstrates another advantage of the transotic approach. A small plastic suction drain is inserted over the muscle flap while the skin incision is closed in two layers with 2-0 Dexon and 3-0 nylon sutures.

DRESSING AND POSTOPERATIVE CARE

The suction drain is removed as soon as a compression dressing is applied. Dressing is left in place for 5 days, and if there is any evidence of cerebrospinal fluid leak or subcutaneous cerebrospinal fluid accumulation, the compression dressing is reapplied.

The patient is transferred to the postanesthesia care unit extubated and fully awake. Routine and neurologic vital signs are closely monitored every 30 to 60 minutes. Adequate analgesics and antiemetics are ordered to keep the patient comfortably at bed rest, usually for 72 hours after surgery. Ambulation and oral intake are started slowly thereafter. Subcutaneous heparin is often given during the early convalescent period. An oral antibiotic, trimethoprim and sulfamethoxazole (Bactrim Forte) or ciprofloxacin (Ciproxin), is prescribed for at least 5 days after intravenous fluid and ceftriaxone therapy are discontinued.

Head and abdominal wound sutures are removed on day 12 and leg sutures after 2 weeks. The patient is discharged from hospital at this time, barring any complication.

TIPS AND PITFALLS

The transotic approach is more than a combination of the translabyrinthine and transcochlear approaches. It uses the complete infralabyrinthine compartment of the temporal bone, from the carotid artery to the sigmoid sinus, and from the jugular bulb to the superior petrosal sinus. It provides the largest possible transtemporal access to the CPA, which can be best appreciated by comparing the cross-sectional surgical exposure of the transotic approach with the translabyrinthine approach shown in Figure 52–15.

The preservation of the facial nerve in its anatomic position within the fallopian canal does not limit the visibility or illumination. Enough bone must be kept surrounding the canal initially during subtotal petrosectomy and subsequently while the otic capsule is exenterated. Skeletonization of the fallopian canal must be done progressively as the surgical cavity enlarges, and with only diamond burrs. Bone surrounding the proximal tympanic segment of the facial nerve and of the superior aspect of the IAC should be left intact to support the facial nerve.

If the fallopian canal is inadvertently fractured during dissection, it will most likely remain undisplaced and will not impede surgery. If no significant torsion or traction has occurred, no major adverse effects should result, provided that no further manipulation occurs. The fractured edges can be supported with fibrin glue, and at the time of closure, abdominal fat will adequately render support from beneath. If the fracture is displaced and unstable, a small, malleable aluminum strip can be used as a retractor and can maintain the fallopian canal in position. If this is not possible, the nerve may have to be fully unroofed and transposed anteriorly as in infratemporal fossa type A approach. This situation, however, has not occurred in our hands. The three fundamental principles for the removal of acoustic neuromas are as follows:

1. Perform intracapsular reduction of the tumor to progressively gain better visibility around the circumference of the tumor

2. Expose tumor from lateral to medial; coagulate all visible vessels over the tumor capsule and remove the devascularized portion in a piecemeal fashion

3. Separate the facial nerve from the tumor and not vice versa

Cerebrospinal fluid outflow following the opening of the cochlear aqueduct decompresses the lateral cistern before the dural incision is made. It also indicates that the pars nervosa of the jugular foramen and the lower cranial nerves have not yet been reached by the tumor.

Even in the presence of a high jugular bulb, a few millimeters of exposure can be obtained between it and the IAC to allow adequate access to the inferior pole of the tumor. Unroofing and compressing the jugular bulb to gain more exposure are unnecessary and dangerous. If access to the CPA is severely limited by the jugular bulb, the facial nerve can be unroofed and transposed anteriorly, as in the infratemporal fossa type A approach.

Bony exenteration to expose the posterior fossa dura should be done in a stepwise manner, gaining as much exposure of the posterior fossa dura around the porus as possible. The time spent in the initial bony exenteration may be tedious at first, but it is well rewarded by muchexpanded access and improved illumination, which facilitate tumor removal dramatically.

The dura should not be opened until all bony work has been completed and hemostasis perfectly controlled. While incising the dura, the surgeons should beware of the AICA, which may loop underneath, and make the initial cut in the center of the exposure to avoid this artery, which usually lies in the inferior half of the CPA. Intracapsular reduction of the tumor is performed while it is still attached to the meatal dura at the superior pole of the porus to prevent excessive traction on the facial nerve. It also stabilizes the tumor during reduction. The major blood supply of acoustic tumors runs along the eighth nerve; one should always check for vessels on the undersurface of the tumor prior to removal. The most delicate portion of the facial nerve is just proximal to the acoustic porus, where the nerve can be flattened to a thin transparent band. It is most frequently pushed anteriorly and superiorly. Keep an eye on this area while working deeper in the CPA.

If the facial nerve appears to be significantly traumatized and cannot be stimulated at the end of surgery, one must proceed directly to an intracranial-intratemporal grafting or XII-VII cross-innervation procedure, depending on the clinical setting. Spontaneous return of function with conser-

TABLE 52–1. Two-Year Postoperative Facial Function

TUMOR SIZE (cm)	N	\multicolumn{5}{c}{PER CENT RECOVERY}				
		100	80–99	60–79	40–59	0–39
1.0–1.4	14	100	—	—	—	—
1.5–2.5*	52	61	19	12	4	4
Total	66	70	15	9	3	3

*No difference in facial function following removal of tumors of 1.5–1.9 cm vs. 2.0–2.5 cm.

vative treatment is not likely to occur. Posterior fossa dura should not be resected to gain exposure; the dural edges are retracted with stay sutures. One should not forget to obliterate the eustachian tube with both bone wax and a muscle plug to prevent cerebrospinal fluid rhinorrhea. Fat graft anchored under the fallopian canal will support the musculofascial repair and prevent lateralization of these autogenous tissues.

RESULTS

Between 1979 and 1990, 147 consecutive transotic approaches were performed for the removal of unilateral acoustic neuromas by the senior author (UF). Tumors in this series were limited in size from 1.0 to 2.5 cm in their medial-lateral extension. Tumors may fill the lateral cistern, abutting but without significantly compressing the brainstem.

Complete tumor removal was achieved in all cases. Optimal visualization of the facial nerve was obtained, and the anatomic preservation of the nerve was possible in 139 cases (94.6 per cent). In eight cases in which facial nerve integrity could not be preserved, intracranial-intratemporal nerve grafting resulted in an average of 66 per cent return of facial function by the Fisch facial nerve grading system (or House-Brackmann grade III+), during a mean follow-up of 4 years.

Sixty-six patients in this series were available for follow-up of at least 2 years. Tumors of 1.0 to 1.4 cm were removed with no incidence of permanent facial injury, and 80 per cent of patients with tumors of 1.5 to 2.5 cm had normal or near-normal facial function (Table 52–1). Since 1988, the unroofing of the labyrinthine portion of the facial nerve has been a standard step in the transotic approach, which is believed to be a major contributing factor in the diminished incidence of delayed facial palsy in acoustic neuroma surgery.

COMPLICATIONS AND MANAGEMENT

The obliteration of the surgical cavity and eustachian tube, along with the blind sac closure of the external auditory canal, has significantly lowered the incidence of cerebrospinal fluid leak. In the series mentioned earlier, 4 per cent of patients developed a subcutaneous cerebrospinal fluid collection without leakage, and the collections usually resolved within 3 to 4 weeks with conservative management, including bed rest and prolonged compressive dressing over the surgical site.

Three patients (4 per cent) developed either immediate or delayed cerebrospinal fluid leaks and were treated with lumbar drainage and bed rest; only one required surgical revision. One patient had meningitis and responded to antibiotic treatment without sequelae. Most notably is the lack of any other central nervous system complication in this series. One unfortunate death occurred as a result of postoperative pulmonary embolism and cardiorespiratory failure. Wound infection with necrosis of the abdominal fat graft or temporalis muscle flap was a rare complication and was thought to be the inciting cause in the case of meningitis.

ALTERNATIVE TECHNIQUES

When and how acoustic neuromas should be operated on are issues of ongoing and often emotional debates. If surgery is contemplated, the aim is obviously to try to obtain the safest and best possible exposure that will allow complete tumor extirpation and the preservation of facial nerve. Hearing preservation is of secondary concern if the opposite ear is functional.

Translabyrinthine and suboccipital approaches are perhaps the most established and popular techniques, whereas the middle fossa approach has traditionally been reserved for small tumors in patients with serviceable hearing; an extended version of the middle fossa approach has gained popularity in some centers to remove tumors up to 4.5 cm,[10, 11] despite a seemingly high morbidity.[12] The relative efficacy of each of these approaches is difficult to quantify without a randomized multi-institutional study.

Our own experience with the translabyrinthine removal of acoustic neuromas prior to 1979 was unsatisfactory in many respects, and those problems were subsequently rectified with the transotic approach.[1] There are three advantages of the transotic approach over the translabyrinthine approach

1. A wider surgical access with a near circumferential exposure of the IAC and the porus acusticus; this added exposure is particularly important in the presence of a high-riding jugular bulb and an anteriorly positioned sigmoid sinus
2. The direct visualization and access to the anterior CPA where the facial nerve is most tenuous and vulnerable
3. A much reduced rate of cerebrospinal fluid leakage as a result of permanent closure of the ear canal and eustachian tube and complete obliteration of the surgical cavity

References

1. Fisch U, Mattox D: Microsurgery of the Skull Base. New York, Thieme, Publishers, 1988.
2. House WF, Hitzelberger WE: The transcochlear approach to the skull base. Arch Otolaryngol Head Neck Surg 102: 334–342, 1976.
3. Jenkins HA, Fisch U: The transotic approach to resection of difficult acoustic tumors of the cerebellopontine angle. Am J Otol 2: 70–76, 1980.
4. Gantz BJ, Fisch U: Modified transotic approach to the cerebellopon-

tine angle. Arch Otolaryngol Head Neck Surg 109: 252–256, 1983.

5. Chen JM, Fisch U: The transotic approach in acoustic neuroma surgery. J Otolaryngol 22:331–336, 1993.

6. Burres S, Fisch U: The comparison of facial grading systems. Arch Otolaryngol Head Neck Surg 112: 755–758, 1986.

7. Whittaker CK, Leutje CM: Translabyrinthine removal of large acoustic neuromas. Am J Otol 7(Suppl): 155–160, 1985.

8. Gardner G, Robertson JH: Transtemporal approaches to the cranial cavity. Am J Otol 7(Suppl): 114–120, 1985.

9. Fisch U, Lanser MJ: Facial nerve grafting. Otolaryngol Clin North Am 24: 691–708, 1991.

10. Wigand ME, Haid T: Extended middle cranial fossa approach for acoustic neuroma surgery. Skull Base Surg 1: 183–187, 1991.

11. Kanzaki J, Ogawa K, Yamamoto M, et al: Results of acoustic neuroma surgery by the extended middle cranial fossa approach. Acta Otolaryngol Suppl (Stockh) 487: 17–21, 1991.

12. Kanzaki J, Ogawa K, Tsuchihashi N, et al: Postoperative complications in acoustic neuroma surgery by the extended middle cranial fossa approach. Acta Otolaryngol Suppl (Stockh) 487: 75–79, 1991.

53

Transcochlear Approach to Cerebellopontine Angle Lesions

Antonio De la Cruz, M.D. ▪ Jose N. Fayad, M.D.
Sujana S. Chandrasekhar, M.D.

The transcochlear approach is the most direct surgical route to excise midline intradural lesions arising from the clivus and cerebellopontine angle masses anterior to the internal auditory canal. These lesions often extend around the verte-brobasilar arteries and, because traditional surgical approaches were limited by the cerebellum and the brainstem, they used to be considered inoperable by many surgeons. The transcochlear approach was designed primarily for meningiomas arising from the petroclinoid ridge, intradural clivus lesions, chordomas, congenital petrous apex cholesteatomas, and primary intradural epidermoids anterior to the internal auditory canal.

Evolution of the transcochlear approach resulted from an inability to excise the base of implantation and control the blood supply of these near-midline and midline tumors. A wide mastoidectomy and labyrinthectomy are performed, exposing the internal auditory canal. The external auditory canal may be removed, and the meatus may be closed. The facial nerve is completely skeletonized, with transection of the greater superficial petrosal and chorda tympani nerves, and is rerouted posteriorly out of the fallopian canal. The cochlea and the fallopian canal are completely drilled out, and the internal carotid artery is identified and dissected. A large triangular window is created into the skull base. Its superior boundary is the superior petrosal sinus; inferiorly, it extends below and medial to the inferior petrosal sinus into the clivus. Anteriorly is the region of the intrapetrous internal carotid artery, and the apex of the triangle is just beneath Meckel's cave. When the dura is opened, this window gives excellent access to the midline without need of any retraction. After tumor removal, the dura is reapproximated, and abdominal fat is used to fill the dura and mastoidectomy defects and to cushion the facial nerve.

Total removal of these lesions through a suboccipital approach is often not possible because of the interposition of the cerebellum and the brainstem.[1, 2] The transpalatal-transclival approach was tried for these intradural midline lesions, with little success.[3] The exposure is inadequate, the field is at quite a distance from the surgeon, the blood supply is lateral, away from the surgeon's view, and intracranial problems with oral contamination can occur. The retrolabyrinthine approach is limited in its forward extension by the posterior semicircular canal. Tumor access with the translabyrinthine approach is limited anteriorly by the facial nerve, which impedes removal of the tumor's base of implantation, which is anterior to the internal auditory canal, around the intrapetrous carotid artery, or anterior to

the brainstem. The more recent development of the extended middle fossa approach and combined transpetrous approaches enables complete removal of petroclinoid meningiomas, and we used it in patients with useful hearing.[4–6] The primary limitation with this approach is poor access to tumors with inferior or midline extensions.[7, 8]

The transcochlear approach was developed by William House and Hitselberger in the early 1970s as an anterior extension of the translabyrinthine approach.[2, 3] It involves complete rerouting of the facial nerve posteriorly and the removal of the cochlea and petrous bone, which exposes the intrapetrous internal carotid artery. This approach affords wide intradural exposure of the anterior cerebellopontine angle, cranial nerves V, VII, VIII, IX, X, and XI, both sixth cranial nerves, the clivus, and the basilar and vertebral arteries, without any retraction. The contralateral cranial nerves and the opposite cerebellopontine angle are also visible.[9] It used to be the only approach during which the tumor base and its arterial blood supply from the internal carotid artery are removed.[2] The addition of excision and closure of the external auditory canal, as advocated by Brackmann (Personal communication, 1987), further increases the anterior exposure for lesions of the petroclival regions and prepontine cistern. Pellet and associates described the widened transcochlear approach for large tumors of the jugular foramen with intrapetrous, intracranial, and infratemporal extensions.[10]

Advantages of the Transcochlear Approach. This approach requires no cerebellar or temporal lobe retraction. Exposure and dissection of the petrous apex and clivus facilitate complete removal of the tumor, its base of implantation, and its blood supply. This is of particular importance in meningiomas.[11, 12]

Careful handling and constant monitoring of the facial nerve during rerouting prevent injury to the intratemporal portion of the nerve. However, meningiomas often invade the nerve, and cholesteatomas tend to wrap themselves around it. If the facial nerve is lost during tumor removal, we recommend immediate repair by end-to-end anastomosis with Avitene or one 8-0 suture or nerve graft interposition.

Disadvantages of the Transcochlear Approach. The main disadvantages of this approach are sacrifice of residual hearing in the operated ear and risk of temporary facial palsy. This technique is used when no serviceable hearing exists in the involved ear or when the tumor is too far anterior for the extended middle fossa craniotomy approach. With the use of continuous facial nerve monitoring, the incidence of permanent facial nerve paralysis is low.

PATIENT EVALUATION AND PREOPERATIVE COUNSELING

Individuals with tumors that require transcochlear surgery may have minimal symptomatology, with tumors that are quite large at the time of diagnosis.[1, 13] Petrous apex cholesteatomas usually present with unilateral hearing loss and tinnitus in 80 per cent of the cases. Facial twitch is also common. Imbalance, ataxia, and parietal or vertex headaches may be the only complaints in 20 per cent.[14] Seizures, dysarthria, and late signs of dementia from hydrocephalus were common presenting symptoms in the past.[14] Patients with meningiomas and intradural epidermoids may be nearly symptom free until they present with fifth cranial nerve findings and signs of increased intracranial pressure.[15, 16] There is a relatively high rate of jugular foramen syndrome in patients with meningiomas.[1]

Hearing and vestibular functions are frequently normal, and acoustic reflex decay or abnormal auditory brainstem response audiometric results may be the only anomalies.[2]

Radiographic evaluation using high-resolution computed tomography (CT) with contrast enhancement, magnetic resonance imaging (MRI), or both, is essential for diagnosis and surgical planning.[17] Petrous apex and intradural epidermoids are expansile, spherical, or oval lesions, with scalloping of a bony edge on CT. They are isodense to cerebrospinal fluid on CT, with capsular enhancement. On MRI, they are hypointense on T1W and hyperintense on T2W images. Meningiomas enhance on MRI, and present with a "dural tail." Some tumors may also require MRI angiography. In tumors surrounding or invading the intrapetrous carotid artery, preoperative balloon occlusion of the carotid artery and selective embolization are performed 1 day before surgery. Radioisotope, xenon, or positron emission tomography studies are used to assess cerebral perfusion during occlusion studies.

The natural history of petrous apex epidermoids is that they grow and may become infected. Treatment is difficult when such infection occurs, and meningitis, sepsis, and death may result. Intracranial epidermoid tumors spread through the cisterns and subarachnoid planes to neighboring regions; petrous ridge meningiomas grow and are space-occupying lesions that increase intracranial pressure. After surgery, intracranial pressure is reduced, and cranial nerve symptoms improve. Risks and complications in the immediate postoperative period include transient vertigo, complete hearing loss, and temporary facial nerve paresis, as well as infection, bleeding, swallowing difficulties, aspiration pneumonia, cerebrovascular accidents, and death.

SURGICAL TECHNIQUE

Setup

General endotracheal anesthesia with arterial blood pressure monitoring is used, and a urinary catheter and a nasogastric tube are inserted. Long-acting muscle relaxants

are avoided. Intraoperative facial nerve monitoring is used in all cases. Prophylactic third-generation cephalosporin antibiotics and steroids are used routinely before the skin incision is made. Venous antiembolism compression boots are placed on the patient's legs before the procedure begins.

The patient is placed supine on the operating room table, with the head turned to the opposite side, and is maintained in a natural position without fixation. This position avoids air embolization, minimizes surgeon fatigue, and allows stabilization of the surgeon's hands during the microsurgical procedure.

Incision

A retroauricular incision is made 3 cm behind the postauricular fold, starting 1 cm above the ear and ending at the level of the mastoid tip. This incision can easily be extended inferiorly into the neck to provide control of the great vessels and of the lower cranial nerves, if necessary. The scalp flap is lifted anteriorly uncovering the temporalis fascia. The periosteum is incised just above the linea temporalis from the zygomatic root anteriorly to a level posterior to the sigmoid sinus. Another periosteal incision perpendicular to the previous one is carried inferiorly in the direction of the mastoid tip. The periosteal flap is elevated forward to the spine of Henle and to the level of the external auditory canal. The skin of the external auditory canal is usually left in place. In some cases of far anterior–placed lesions, a blind closure of the external auditory canal is necessary. In this case the skin, tympanic membrane, and malleus are removed, and the meatus is closed in three layers.

Mastoidectomy

An extended mastoidectomy (Fig. 53–1) is carried out with microsurgical cutting and diamond burrs and continuous suction-irrigation. Bone removal is started along two lines: one along the linea temporalis and another tangential to the external canal. The mastoid antrum is opened, and the lateral semicircular canal is identified. The lateral semicircular canal is the most reliable landmark in the temporal bone and allows the dissection to proceed toward delineating the fallopian canal and the osseous labyrinth.

The external opening of the mastoid cavity must be as large as possible and is extended posterior to the sigmoid sinus, exposing 1 to 2 cm of suboccipital dura. Mastoid emissary veins are dissected and bleeding is controlled using bipolar cautery and Surgicel packing. Removal of bone over the sigmoid sinus is performed with diamond burrs, leaving an island of bone (Bill's island) over the dome of the sinus. This eggshell of bone protects the sinus from being injured by the shaft of the burr. Bone is removed from the sinodural angle along the superior petrosal sinus. The mastoid air cells are exenterated from the sinodural angle, thereby skeletonizing the dura of the posterior and the middle fossae.

Labyrinthectomy and Exposure of the Internal Auditory Canal

Dissection of the perilabyrinthine cells down to the lateral semicircular canal is completed (Fig. 53–2). The facial nerve is identified in its vertical portion between the non-ampullated end of the lateral semicircular canal and the stylomastoid foramen.

The lateral semicircular canal is fenestrated superiorly, and the membranous portion is identified and followed anteriorly to its ampullated end and posteriorly to the posterior semicircular canal. All three membranous and bony semicircular canals are removed, and the saccule and utricule in the vestibule are identified and removed.

The dissection proceeds along the sinodural angle and the superior petrosal sinus. The dura of the posterior fossa is exposed anteriorly. The cells over the jugular bulb are removed, skeletonizing it, and the cochlear aqueduct is also removed. The internal auditory canal is identified, beginning inferiorly and then around the porus acusticus. The falciform crest (transverse) and vertical crest (Bill's bar) are used as identifying landmarks for the superior and inferior vestibular nerves as well as the facial nerve. The roof of the internal auditory canal is skeletonized.

Facial Nerve Dissection
(Figs. 53–3 and 53–4)

After removal of the incus, an extended facial recess opening is created. The facial nerve is completely skeletonized from the internal auditory canal to the stylomastoid foramen, including the geniculate ganglion, with diamond burrs. An area comprising 180 degrees of the bony fallopian canal is uncovered. The greater superficial petrosal nerve is cut at its origin from the geniculate ganglion. The nerve is then reflected posteriorly out of the fallopian canal, and care is taken to avoid traction on the nerve, especially near the mastoid genu, which is the site of several branches to the stapedius muscle. Care is also taken to avoid kinking of the nerve at the stylomastoid foramen when reflecting it posteriorly. The facial nerve is protected at all times and kept wet.

Closure of the External Auditory Canal

When further anterior exposure is required, removal and closure of the external auditory canal are included. The canal skin is transected at the bony-cartilaginous junction and is undermined laterally. Extra cartilage is removed, and the skin is closed with interrupted nylon sutures in a dimple-like fashion at the external auditory meatus. A periosteal flap is used to oversew the undersurface of the canal skin. After removal of all the canal skin, the tympanic membrane, and the malleus, the bony external auditory canal is drilled out and excised circumferentially. Care is taken to avoid entering the glenoid fossa.

Transcochlear Drill-Out (Fig. 53–5)

The fallopian canal is then removed, the promontory is now exposed, and the ossicles have been removed. Starting with the basal coil, the cochlea is completely drilled out. Bone removal is carried forward around the internal carotid artery, and the inferior extent of bone removal extends to the inferior petrosal sinus and jugular bulb. Superiorly, the superior petrosal sinus is followed to Meckel's cave. Medially, bone removal extends to the clivus. At this stage, a large triangular window, covered by dura, has been created into midline of the skull base. Its boundaries are superiorly, the superior petrosal sinus; inferiorly, below and medial to the inferior petrosal sinus into the clivus; anteriorly, the region of the internal carotid artery; and medially, the lateral clivus. The apex of the triangle is just beneath Meckel's cave.

Tumor Removal (Fig. 53–6)

With meningiomas, arterial feeder vessels from the internal carotid artery were encountered and eliminated during the approach. The diamond burr is used to excise these vessels and the base of implantation at the petroclival area. The dura is opened anterior to the internal auditory canal, and the opening is extended as far forward as is necessary for complete tumor exposure. The dural opening extends from the superior petrosal sinus superiorly to the inferior petrosal sinus inferiorly.

The facial nerve is kept on the posterior surface of the tumor. The junction of the intracranial portion of the facial nerve and the skeletonized intratemporal portion is now identified. The nerve is protected and kept moist.

The tumor pseudocapsule is opened, and the center of the main mass of the tumor is removed with the House-Urban rotatory dissector. As the dissection proceeds forward and medially, the basilar artery and sixth cranial nerves are identified anterosuperiorly. The vertebral arteries appear posteroinferiorly. The tumor is removed from these vessels and their major tributaries under direct vision. In tumors extending across the midline, the basilar artery and its major branches can be dissected posteriorly off the tumor capsule. When the lesion is removed in this fashion, the cranial nerves and the internal auditory canal in the opposite cerebellopontine angle come into view. No brain retractors are needed to allow for this exposure.

For dumbbell-shaped tumors, the tentorium can be opened to excise the part of the tumor that is lying in the middle fossa. Care is taken not to injure the vein of Labbé or the fourth cranial nerve at the edge of the tentorium.

Closure

After the tumor has been removed, hemostasis is secured. The dura is reapproximated, and the facial nerve is reflected forward. The eustachian tube orifice is plugged with Surgicel, bone wax, and bone paté. Abdominal fat strips are used to fill the dural defect, the mastoid and skull base defect, as well as to form a bed for the facial nerve. The postauricular incision is closed in three layers, and a

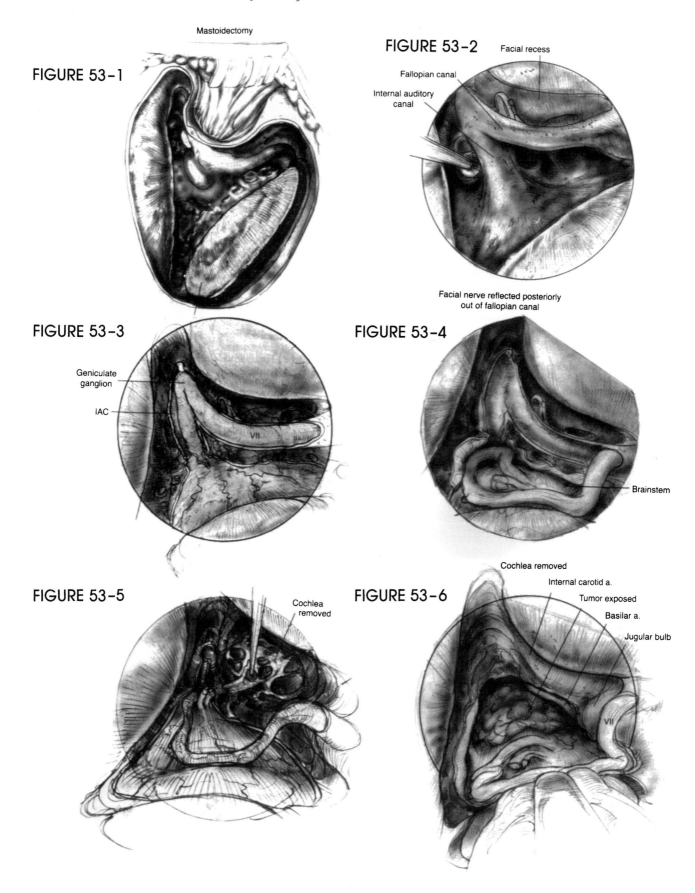

FIGURE 53-1

Mastoidectomy

FIGURE 53-2

Facial recess

Fallopian canal

Internal auditory canal

Facial nerve reflected posteriorly out of fallopian canal

FIGURE 53-3

Geniculate ganglion

IAC

VII

FIGURE 53-4

Brainstem

FIGURE 53-5

Cochlea removed

FIGURE 53-6

Cochlea removed

Internal carotid a.

Tumor exposed

Basilar a.

Jugular bulb

VII

FIGURES 53–1 to 53–6. *See legends on opposite page*

compressive dressing is placed securely about the head. Lumbar drainage is used for 5 days.

POSTOPERATIVE CARE

The patient is observed in the intensive care unit for 48 hours after surgery and remains in the hospital for 5 days. Steroids are continued for 48 hours. Antibiotics are not routinely used after the perioperative period. Early mobilization and ambulation allow for avoidance of thromboembolism and speedy return of balance.

RESULTS

In 1982, De la Cruz reviewed the results of 16 patients in whom the transcochlear approach was used.[1] A combination transcochlear–middle fossa approach was used in the three cases involving dumbbell-shaped tumors in both the posterior and middle cranial fossae. Total tumor removal was possible in 13 of the 16 patients. Each of the other 3 patients has had surgery elsewhere and presented with large recurrent meningiomas and extensive neurologic deficits preoperatively. During the transcochlear approach, scraps of tumor were left behind on the vertebral artery in 2 of these cases. None of these patients has tumor recurrence.

Four patients had facial paresis or twitch preoperatively; of the other 12, 4 had permanent facial paralysis due to tumor involvement of the nerve, and 7 had temporary paresis with good-to-excellent recovery of facial function. This paresis was attributed primarily to the excessive manipulation necessary for total tumor removal, and these patients were operated on before facial nerve monitoring was available.

Two deaths occurred in this series. One individual had bleeding from the vertebral artery 1 week postoperatively, requiring clipping of the vessel, with subsequent infarction of the brainstem; the other was diabetic and succumbed 1 month postoperatively to gram-negative shock from pyelonephritis. He was one of the patients reported as having a "permanent" facial paralysis. Autopsy revealed no evidence of residual tumor on the facial nerve or elsewhere.

Yamakawa and colleagues[16] reported results with the suboccipital approach revealing subtotal tumor removal in 17 of 29 patients with intracranial epidermoids and tumor recurrence in 7 patients. One of 14 patients with cerebello-pontine angle tumors had postoperative seventh nerve paralysis, 6 had abducens palsy, 4 had dysphagia, and 2 had deafness.

The report by Yasargil and coworkers[18] published in the same year analyzed results in 43 patients, 35 with epidermoid tumors and the rest with intracranial dermoid tumors. No recurrences were seen. Aseptic meningitis and transient cranial nerve palsies were the most common complications. Two deaths were reported.

Angeli and associates in 1995 reviewed a second series of 24 patients operated on at the House Ear Clinic using the transcochlear approach or one of its modifications.[19] In one case a modified transotic approach was used (small melanoma); in two other cases the transcochlear approach was extended inferiorly with an infratemporal and upper neck dissection (one glomus and one meningioma). The majority of the tumors (16 of 24) were meningiomas. The other tumors included four cholesteatomas, two melanomas, one glomus, and one ependymoma. The external auditory canal was closed in 12 patients. A total tumor removal was achieved in 19 (80 per cent) of 24 patients. In 2 cases (8 per cent), it was elected intraoperatively to do a subtotal tumor resection either due to excessive blood loss (intracranial glomus jugulare tumor) or unresectability (melanoma invading the brainstem).

Ninety-five per cent of the patients had some degree of facial dysfunction following surgery. About one half of the patients had total facial paralysis during their hospital course. This paralysis subsequently improved and 60 per cent had obtained a grade III or better by the last follow-up visit.

Early postoperative complications included brain edema, hydrocephalus, meningitis, sigmoid sinus thrombosis, pneumonia, and brainstem infarct in one patient. Fifty-nine per cent of the patients had neurologic sequelae as a result of their disease or the surgical procedure. The most common neurologic deficit was diplopia (27 per cent). Cranial nerves IV and VI are at risk when retracting or cutting the tentorium at the incisura. Other complications included dysphagia, facial numbness, unsteadiness, hoarseness, hemiparesis, and dysarthria.

COMPLICATIONS AND THEIR MANAGEMENT

Temporary facial nerve paresis is the most common complication. If facial paresis occurs, prompt eye care is essen-

---

FIGURE 53–1. Transcochlear approach: mastoidectomy. There is wide exposure of the posterior and middle fossa dura, with identification of the bony labyrinth and skeletonization of the sigmoid sinus, preserving Bill's island over the dome.

FIGURE 53–2. Transcochlear approach: exposure of the internal auditory canal (IAC), skeletonization of the facial nerve from the IAC to the stylomastoid foramen, and extended facial recess. The labyrinthectomy has been completed.

FIGURE 53–3. Transcochlear approach: bone over the facial nerve is removed. At this point, the greater superficial petrosal nerve is sectioned. IAC, internal auditory canal.

FIGURE 53–4. Transcochlear approach: location of the facial nerve after it is completely reflected posteriorly out of the bony fallopian canal.

FIGURE 53–5. Transcochlear approach: cochlear drill-out.

FIGURE 53–6. Transcochlear approach: tumor removal.

tial: adequate lubrication with drops, night-time ointments, and a moisture shield prevent corneal complications. Unless the facial nerve has been severed, surgical intervention for facial reanimation is not indicated. The best approach in individuals with even complete paralysis after transcochlear surgery, if the facial nerve is anatomically intact, is eye care that includes soft lenses, spring and gold weights, sometimes canthoplasty, and "watchful waiting" because the great majority of these patients recover to an acceptable grade of facial function within the first year after surgery.

Other cranial nerve palsies may occur and should be addressed individually. The neurotologist must attain a good working relationship not only with a neurosurgeon but also with an ophthalmologist and a laryngologist to help in the management of these cranial nerve deficits.

Intracranial bleeding is controlled at the time of surgery. Close observation of the patient in the intensive care unit for the initial 48 hours postoperatively allows early recognition of delayed postoperative intracranial hemorrhage. In these cases, treatment consists of immediate reopening of the surgical wound and removal of the fat in the intensive care unit while the operating room is being prepared, and then operative evacuation of the hematoma and control of the bleeding site or sites.

Meningitis may occur after complete excision of intracranial epidermoids, and the incidence increases when the tumor capsule is left in place.[18, 20, 21] Meningitis may be fatal if it is infectious and requires early, aggressive antibiotic therapy. More commonly, however, it is a chemical aseptic meningitis, and the patient is treated with dexamethasone. Postoperative pain is not as severe as that seen with the suboccipital approach and is managed adequately with oral analgesics.

With this approach, tumor recurrence is rare when all visible tumor has been removed. Patients with recurrences do not present typically and may have vague complaints of unsteadiness or trigeminal neuropathy several years after the initial resection.[1] Biannual follow-up with gadolinium-enhanced MRI is necessary. In cases of suspected tumor regrowth or recurrence, complete re-evaluation is performed, and removal of the recurrent tumor is advised.

SUMMARY

Access to midline intradural lesions, intradural clival tumors, and cerebellopontine angle tumors arising anterior to the internal auditory canal has been dissected. With the transcochlear approach the facial nerve is mobilized, the cochlea removed, and the petrous apex dissected around the internal auditory artery, allowing direct exposure of these lesions and of midline and contralateral structures, without using retraction. Total removal of the tumor and its base and blood supply is accomplished with this approach.[22] The transcochlear approach is recommended for these lesions in patients with poor hearing. Its safety and efficacy encourage its use.

References

1. De la Cruz A: The transcochlear approach to meningiomas and cholesteatomas of the cerebellopontine angle. *In* Brackmann DE (ed): Neurological Surgery of the Ear and Skull Base. New York, Raven Press, 1982, pp 353–360.
2. House WF, De la Cruz A: Transcochlear approach to the petrous apex and clivus. Trans Am Acad Ophthalmol Otolaryngol 84: 927–931, 1977.
3. House WF, Hitselberger WE: The transcochlear approach to the skull base. Arch Otolaryngol Head Neck Surg 102: 334–342, 1976.
4. Hitselberger WE, Horn KL, Hankinson H, et al: The middle fossa transpetrous approach for petroclival meningiomas. Skull Base Surg 3: 130–135, 1993.
5. Spetzler RF, Daspit CP, Pappas CT: The combined supratentorial and infratentorial approach for lesions of the petrous and clival regions: Experience with 46 cases. J Neurosurg 76: 588–599, 1992.
6. Daspit CP, Spetzler RF, Pappas CT: Combined approach for lesions involving the cerebellopontine angle and skull base: Experience with 20 cases—preliminary report. Otolaryngol Head Neck Surg 105: 788–796, 1991.
7. Shiobara R, Ohira T, Kanzaki J, Toya S: A modified extended middle cranial fossa approach for acoustic nerve tumors: Results of 125 operations. J Neurosurg 68: 358–365, 1988.
8. Wigand ME, Haid T, Berg M: The enlarged middle cranial fossa approach for surgery of the temporal bone and the cerebellopontine angle. Arch Otol Rhinol Otolaryngol 246: 299, 1989.
9. Jackler RK, Sim DW, Gutin PH, Pitts LH: Systematic approach to intradural tumors ventral to the brain stem. Am J Otol 16: 39–51, 1995.
10. Pellet W, Cannoni M, Pech A: The widened transcochlear approach to jugular foramen tumors. J Neurosurg 69: 887–894, 1988.
11. Arriaga M, Shelton C, Nassif P, Brackmann DE: Selection of surgical approaches for meningiomas affecting the temporal bone. Otolaryngol Head Neck Surg 107: 738–744, 1992.
12. Thedinger BA, Glasscock ME III, Cueva RA: Transcochlear transtentorial approach for removal of large cerebellopontine angle meningiomas. Am J Otol 13: 408–415, 1992.
13. Brackmann DE, Anderson RG: Cholesteatomas of the cerebellopontine angle. *In* Silverstein H, Norrell H (eds): Neurological Surgery of the Ear. Birmingham, Aesculapius Publishing Company, 1979, pp 340–344.
14. De la Cruz A, Doyle KJ: Epidermoids of the cerebellopontine angle. *In* Jackler RA, Brackmann DE (eds): Neurotology. York, PA, Spectrum, 1994, pp 823–834.
15. Nager GT: Epidermoids involving the temporal bone: Clinical, radiological, and pathological aspects. Laryngoscope 2(Suppl): 1–22, 1975.
16. Yamakawa K, Shitara N, Genka S, et al: Clinical course and surgical prognosis of 33 cases of intracranial epidermoid tumors. Neurosurgery 24: 568–573, 1989.
17. Mafee MF: MRI and CT in the evaluation of acquired and congenital cholesteatomas of the temporal bone. J Otolaryngol 22: 239–248, 1993.
18. Yasargil MG, Abernathy CD, Sarioglu AC: Microneurosurgical treatment of intracranial dermoid and epidermoid tumors. Neurosurgery 24: 561–567, 1989.
19. Angeli SI, De la Cruz A, Hitselberger WE: The transcochlear approach revisited. Submitted for publication.
20. Cantu RC, Ojemann RG: Lucosteroid treatment of keratin meningitis following removal of a fourth ventricle epidermoid tumor. J Neurol Neurosurg Psychiatry 31: 75, 1968.
21. Guidetti B, Gagliardi FM: Epidermoid and dermoid cysts. J Neurosurg 47: 12–18, 1977.
22. De la Cruz A: Transcochlear approach to lesions of the cerebellopontine angle and clivus. Rev Laryngol Otol Rhinol (Bord) 102: 33–36, 1981.

54

Middle Fossa Transpetrous Approach for Access to the Petroclival Region (Extended Middle Fossa Approach)

Karl L. Horn, M.D. ▪ Hal L. Hankinson, M.D.
William E. Hitselberger, M.D.

Removal of petroclival neoplasms remains one of the most formidable challenges to skull base surgeons for numerous reasons. Lesions of the petrous apex and clivus are uncommon, and this region is not commonly frequented by either neurotologists or neurosurgeons. The nuances of surgical anatomy of this area are therefore less familiar to most surgeons than are other regions of the skull base that are more commonly involved with pathologic processes. Access to lesions of the petroclival region through any surgical approach is difficult because of interposed vital structures, including the cerebellum, brainstem, cranial nerves, vascular structures, and temporal bone. Surgical approaches to this area require the surgeon to make difficult decisions about working around these structures or removing vital structures to improve exposure. These problems have led to the use of numerous surgical approaches to the petroclival region.

SURGICAL APPROACHES TO THE REGION

For many years, the petroclival area has been approached through the conventional suboccipital craniotomy. In this procedure, the surgeon's view of the petrous tip and clivus is obscured by the brainstem, branches of the anteroinferior cerebellar artery, and cranial nerves V through IX. Overhanging cerebellum requires at least minimal retraction, and the surgeon must work at an uncomfortable distance from the lesion.

Although midline transclival approaches have proved helpful for extradural tumors, these procedures have limitations for intradural lesions.[1] The surgeon must work at a considerable distance from the operative field once the tumor is exposed. Tumor manipulation is difficult because of the restricted surgical field. Hemostasis and cerebrospinal fluid leakage are difficult to manage, and the potential for postoperative meningitis is significant.

The infratemporal approach offers excellent exposure of structures inferior to the otic capsule, but exposure of the clivus requires removal of the otic capsule, displacement of the internal carotid artery, or both. This procedure always requires rerouting of the facial nerve and obliteration of the middle ear.[2]

The widest exposure of the petroclival area is provided by the transcochlear approach, which is an anterior extension of the translabyrinthine approach. In this exposure, bone removal is carried anterior to the internal auditory canal after rerouting of the facial nerve posteriorly and removal of the cochlea. In its modified form, the complete petrous apex is removed, and dissection may be continued into the clivus.[3] The major advantage of this approach is wide exposure of the cerebellopontine angle and the petroclival area. The major disadvantages to this technique are unilateral deafness and transient facial weakness and synkinesis.

The disadvantages of hearing loss and transient facial weakness have led several authors to avoid removal of the otic capsule. The petrosal approach extends the retrolabyrinthine or presigmoid approach by transection of the superior petrosal sinus and the tentorium.[4] This approach provides wide exposure of the petroclival region but often obviates removal of bone that may be involved with tumor. The subtemporal-preauricular infratemporal approach provides removal of bone of the petrous apex and clivus; however, it entails removal of the carotid artery from its bony canal, transection of the eustachian tube, and, often, removal of the mandibular condyle.[5] Spetzler and associates have organized many of these concepts into three supratentorial and infratentorial approaches in which the superior petrosal sinus and tentorium are always cut.[6] The amount of bone removed varies and may include retrolabyrinthine, translabyrinthine, or transcochlear techniques. Ligation and section of the sigmoid sinus may be done when deemed necessary and safe.

Although all of these techniques may be used to approach petroclival lesions, they are formidable procedures that may not be required for many lesions anterior to the internal auditory canal. The middle fossa transpetrous approach, which is more anteriorly centered than most other techniques, provides access to the petroclival region anterior to the internal auditory canal and requires removal of few if any vital structures. This technique is a modification of the middle fossa approach that has been used for many years in acoustic tumor surgery. Most of the anatomy and technique are therefore familiar to skull base surgeons.

In 1931, Eagleton was the first to approach the petroclival region through a middle fossa transpetrous approach.[7] However, interest in this approach has been renewed only recently by Kawase[8] and House[9] and their colleagues. In the middle fossa transpetrous approach, the anterior cerebellopontine angle is entered through a middle fossa or subtemporal craniotomy by removal of bone medial to the petrous carotid artery and cochlea. Kawase and colleagues used this approach for access to lower basilar aneurysms in two patients, whereas House and coworkers used the approach for removal of a fifth cranial nerve schwannoma in one patient and petroclival meningioma in a second patient. The roughly triangular area of bone removed medial to the carotid artery has become known as Kawase's triangle.

Pensak and associates presented a combined retrolabyrinthine and middle fossa transpetrous approach for petroclival meningioma removal.[10] In this approach, all of the petrous bone except the otic capsule is removed, thus avoiding removal of the cochlea and rerouting of the facial nerve. Of course, the great advantage to this approach is preservation of hearing and facial nerve function.

SURGICAL ANATOMY

The underlying principle of the operation described in this chapter is to provide access to the posterior fossa through a middle fossa approach. This concept is not new and has been used in acoustic tumor surgery for many years. This technique differs from the traditional and more recently discussed widened middle fossa techniques for acoustic tumor surgery by virtue of its anterior dissection.[11-13] In the middle fossa transpetrous technique, the petrous apex anterior to the internal auditory canal and medial to the carotid artery is removed (Fig. 54–1). The opening into the anterior portion of the posterior fossa may be significantly enlarged by transection of the tentorium over the area of petrous bone removal. A sound understanding of the anatomy of the petrous apex and the tentorium attached to the petrous apex is necessary to safely perform this procedure.

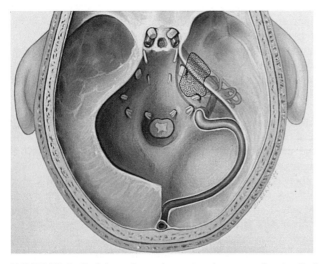

FIGURE 54–1. Skull base from above showing area of petroclival bone removal.

PETROUS APEX

As noted by Paullus and others, the petrous apex has both superior (middle fossa) and posterior (posterior fossa) surfaces.[14-16] The tentorium is attached to the temporal bone at the angle of intersection of these two surfaces. The superior petrosal sinus runs in a sulcus along the edge of the petrous bone roughly at the angle of intersection of the superior and posterior surfaces in the area of dural attachment.

The superior surface of the petrous apex forms the posterior medial floor of the middle fossa. The petrosquamous suture separates the petrous and squamous portions of the temporal bone and is often a site of dural attachment to the middle fossa floor. The most important clinical significance of the petrosquamous suture line is its relationship to the greater superficial petrosal nerve. The greater superficial petrosal nerve is always medial to the petrosquamosal suture and runs in a groove on the superior surface of the petrous apex from the facial hiatus toward the foramen lacerum.

The arcuate eminence lies posterior to the facial hiatus, and the bone between these two structures overlies the internal auditory canal. Fisch and Mattox have termed this surface of bone the *meatal plane*.[17] Anterior and lateral to the greater superficial petrosal nerve is the foramen spinosum and the middle meningeal artery. Anterior and medial to the foramen spinosum is the foramen ovale for the third division of the trigeminal nerve. The foramen ovale represents the most anterior portion of surgical dissection for the middle fossa transpetrous approach. A line connecting the foramen spinosum and the foramen ovale is parallel to the horizontal petrous carotid artery.

The posterior surface of the petrous bone is roughly triangular in shape. Anterior to the internal auditory canal, this surface is bounded above by the superior petrosal sinus and the tentorium. Inferiorly, this triangle is bounded by the inferior petrosal sinus and the petro-occipital synchondrosis. Anterior to the internal auditory canal, no structures pass through the dura on the posterior surface of the petrous apex.

Within the petrous apex anterior to the internal auditory canal are two important structures: the cochlea and the internal carotid artery. The basal turn of the cochlea lies beneath the geniculate ganglion and the labyrinthine segment of the facial nerve. The posterior loop of the petrous carotid artery is anterior to the cochlea, and the basal turn is usually separated from the artery by 1 to 2 mm of bone. The course of the greater superficial petrosal nerve on the floor of the middle cranial fossa is roughly parallel to the course of the horizontal petrous carotid artery within the petrous apex.

TENTORIUM

The tentorium is attached to the petrous ridge, posterior clinoid process, and anterior clinoid process. Transection and retraction of the tentorium above the area of petrous bone removal greatly improve the exposure of the middle fossa transpetrous approach. Several structures are in close relationship to the tentorium in this area. The most significant structure is the petrosal vein (Dandy's vein), which usually enters the superior petrosal sinus just posterior to Meckel's cave. However, the site of entry of the petrosal vein into the superior petrosal sinus is variable, and it may be inadvertently injured as the tentorium and superior petrosal sinus are sectioned.[16] In addition, the tentorium may be laced with a plexus of otherwise un-named veins that may complicate section of the structure.

The tentorium receives arterial supply from several sources. In approximately one fourth of cases, the superior cerebellar artery sends a branch to the undersurface of the free edge of the tentorium.[19] Such a vessel may be encountered as the tentorium is divided above the anterior petrous ridge.

The trochlear nerve enters the free edge of the tentorium in the posterior portion of the oculomotor trigone. Although the nerve is not in the tentorium that is sectioned above the petrous apex, this nerve may be injured as the anterior dural leaf is retracted for exposure. The extended course and delicate nature of the trochlear nerve make it particularly susceptible to injury. The trigeminal nerve is less vulnerable but may be injured by injudicious trauma caused by procedures such as cautery.

SURGICAL TECHNIQUE

The patient is placed in the supine position and given general anesthesia. Electrodes for monitoring the sixth and seventh cranial nerves are inserted. The hemicranium is shaved, the skin is cleaned with povidone-iodine (Betadine), and self-adhering plastic drapes are applied. The incision begins at the tragal notch and extends 7 to 8 cm anterosuperiorly (Fig. 54–2). The plane between the skin and temporalis fascia is developed with blunt dissection. The temporalis fascia is opened, and the exposed temporalis muscle is reflected inferiorly over the zygomatic arch. We have not found it necessary to transect the zygomatic arch to improve exposure or to displace the temporalis muscle out of the field. A self-retaining retractor is placed beneath the remaining temporalis muscle, exposing the squamous temporal bone. A 3 × 5 cm bone flap is removed, thereby exposing the temporal dura (Fig. 54–3). The craniotomy is located two thirds anterior and one third posterior to the external auditory canal. Bone is removed to the floor of the middle cranial fossa with rongeurs and drill. Hyperventilation, osmotics, and spinal drainage are used when appropriate.

The dura is elevated from the floor of the middle cranial fossa by posterior-to-anterior dissection. This direction of dissection is used to avoid injury to an exposed geniculate ganglion or inadvertent elevation of the greater superficial petrosal nerve with resultant traction of the facial nerve. The dura is firmly adherent to the petrosquamosal suture and may require cauterization and sharp dissection. The greater petrosal nerve is medial to this structure. The temporal lobe is elevated with a self-retaining retractor.

The middle meningeal artery, the greater superficial nerve, and the arcuate eminence are identified (Fig. 54–4). A diamond burr is used to expose the geniculate ganglion and to blue line the superior semicircular canal. The labyrinthine segment of the facial nerve is followed into the

fundus of the internal auditory canal (Fig. 54–5). The internal auditory canal is skeletonized but not opened. The middle meningeal artery is clipped or cauterized at the foramen spinosum and transected. The third division of the trigeminal nerve (V3) is identified at the foramen ovale, which lies anteromedial to the foramen spinosum.

Bone within Glasscock's triangle is removed (Fig. 54–6). This triangle is bordered laterally by a line from the arcuate eminence to the foramen spinosum, anteriorly by the third division of the fifth nerve, and medially by the groove for the greater superficial petrosal nerve. The greater superficial petrosal nerve lies over the horizontal petrous carotid artery. The nerve may be sacrificed to prevent traction of the geniculate ganglion and to allow wide exposure of the carotid artery. The horizontal petrous carotid artery is skeletonized from the posterior loop to V3. Dissection should not be extended behind the posterior loop of the internal carotid artery because of close proximity of the cochlea. Dissection may be extended medial to V3 by transection of the nerve or by bone removal from the anterolateral foramen ovale and mobilization of V3 anterolaterally.

Removal of bone medial to the horizontal carotid canal and cochlea is continued inferiorly to the level of the inferior petrosal sinus (Kawase's triangle). The posterior fossa dura has thus been exposed from the internal auditory canal to Meckel's cave and from the superior petrosal sinus above to the inferior petrosal sinus below. The dura is opened through an inferiorly based flap.

The dissection may be extended medially into the clivus by transection of the inferior petrosal sinus in the petro-occipital synchondrosis. Dissection above the level of the tentorium may be accomplished by transection of the superior petrosal sinus and tentorium. This is performed by an incision in the middle fossa dura just lateral to the superior petrosal sinus from the internal auditory canal to the third root of the trigeminal nerve. The superior petrosal sinus is clipped or coagulated, and the tentorium is transected in the midportion of this incision (Fig. 54–7). Special care is taken to avoid injury to the petrosal vein or trochlear nerve. The tumor is debulked with mechanical techniques or the fiber optic argon laser. After tumor removal, the defect is obliterated with abdominal adipose tissue, and the bone flap is wired in place. The wound is closed in layers.

For selected lesions that extend posterior to the internal auditory canal, the middle fossa transpetrous approach may be combined with a retrolabyrinthine or presigmoid approach. Several modifications are necessary to combine these approaches. An S-shaped incision is used that incorporates the supra-auricular portion of the middle fossa incision with a lower postauricular retrolabyrinthine incision. The lower component of the incision is made 2 cm behind the postauricular sulcus and passes 1 cm above the pinna to join the upper component. The middle fossa craniotomy is enlarged posteriorly to include the squamous temporal bone above the retrolabyrinthine craniectomy. The increased subtemporal exposure may require a double-armed system, such as the Greenberg, to adequately elevate the temporal lobe. The posterior fossa dura may be opened along the superior petrosal sinus from V3 to the sigmoid sinus. Increased exposure may also be accomplished by continuing the dural incision inferiorly into the presigmoid

FIGURE 54-2

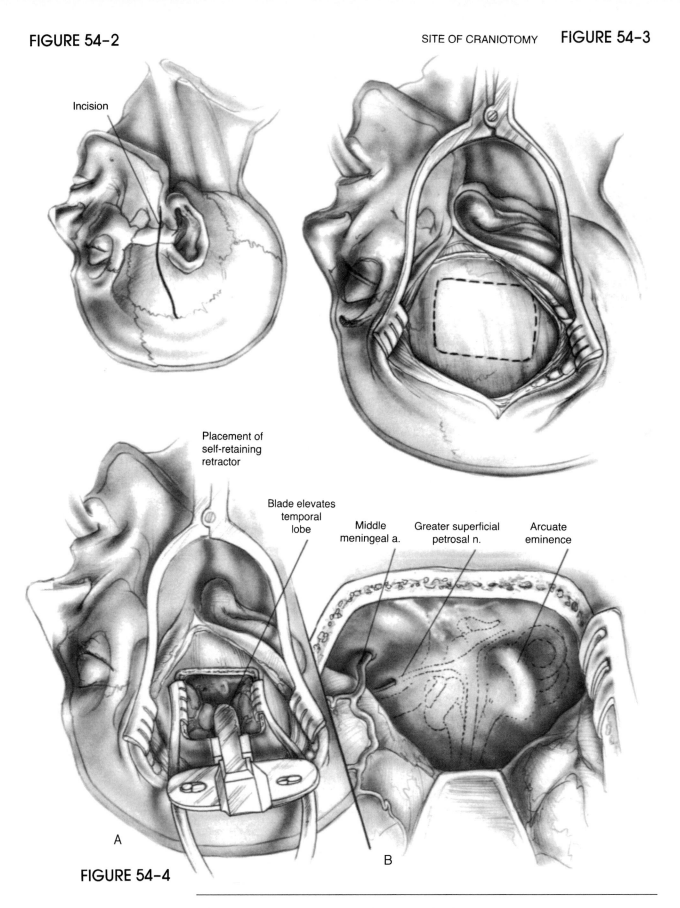

Incision

Placement of
self-retaining
retractor

Blade elevates
temporal
lobe

Middle
meningeal a.

Greater superficial
petrosal n.

Arcuate
eminence

A

B

FIGURE 54-4

FIGURE 54–2. Skin incision extending from tragus 7 to 8 cm superiorly.

FIGURE 54–3. Reflection of temporalis muscle flap and 3 × 5 cm craniotomy.

FIGURE 54–4. A and B, Elevation of dura from middle fossa floor with identification of the middle meningeal artery, greater petrosal nerve, and arcuate eminence.

FIGURE 54-5

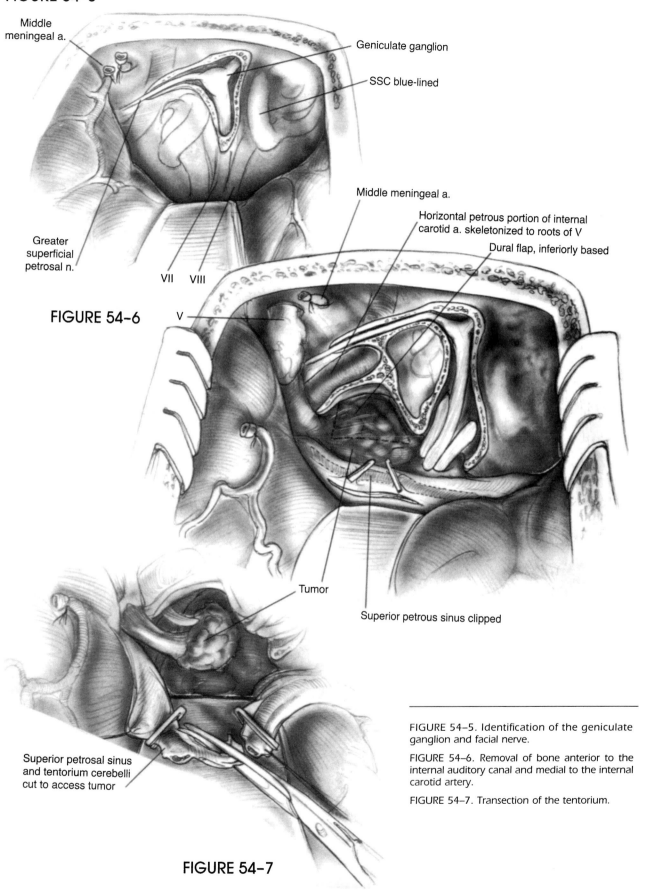

Middle meningeal a.

Geniculate ganglion

SSC blue-lined

Greater superficial petrosal n.

VII   VIII

FIGURE 54-6

V

Middle meningeal a.

Horizontal petrous portion of internal carotid a. skeletonized to roots of V

Dural flap, inferiorly based

Tumor

Superior petrous sinus clipped

Superior petrosal sinus and tentorium cerebelli cut to access tumor

FIGURE 54-5. Identification of the geniculate ganglion and facial nerve.

FIGURE 54-6. Removal of bone anterior to the internal auditory canal and medial to the internal carotid artery.

FIGURE 54-7. Transection of the tentorium.

FIGURE 54-7

region. This enlarged exposure allows the surgeon to work either anterior or posterior to the otic capsule. Although one might anticipate easier retraction of the tentorium with this combined approach, the tentorium is unyielding to superior retraction without transection of the superior petrosal sinus and the lateral two thirds of the tentorium. However, complete tentorial transection is necessary only to remove lesions extending above the incisura. Double tentorial incisions permit broad-based tentorial retraction.

MIDDLE FOSSA TRANSPETROUS APPROACH

The middle fossa transpetrous approach provides exposure to petroclival lesions anterior to the internal auditory canal. This approach, through Kawase's triangle, accesses the posterior fossa anterior to the internal auditory canal, posterior to Meckel's cave, inferior to the superior petrosal sinus, and superior to the inferior petrosal sinus (Fig. 54–8). It has been used for removal of petroclival neoplasms and for access to basilar artery aneurysms.[8–10] Large meningiomas have been removed through this approach by us and others.[20, 21] The technically limiting factor of this procedure is not tumor size alone. Indeed, tumors extending well across the midline and above the anterior tentorial incisura have been removed through this approach. However, because hearing preservation is a primary objective of the procedure, dissection is limited anatomically by the internal auditory canal and the contents of the otic capsule. Lesions that extend posterior to the internal auditory canal require use of different technique, such as the transcochlear approach, or the addition of second technique, such as the suboccipital and extended retrolabyrinthine approaches. The addition of the retrolabyrinthine approach to the mid-

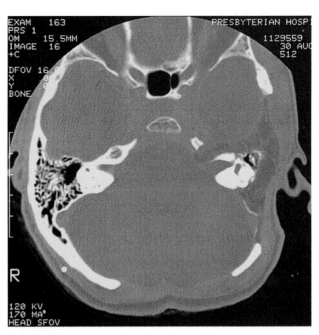

FIGURE 54–9. Axial CT scan demonstrating bone removal with combined transpetrous middle fossa and retrolabyrinthine approaches.

dle fossa transpetrous approach results in removal of considerable bone anterior, inferior, and posterior to the otic capsule and middle ear without loss of hearing or facial nerve function (Fig. 54–9).

The most significant disadvantage of the middle fossa transpetrous approach is the occasional necessity of transecting the third division of the fifth nerve for bone removal at the petrous tip. Except for numbness of the chin, transection of this nerve has caused little functional disability. Another disadvantage to this technique is temporal bone retraction. Although not reported by other authors, we have one patient with temporary expressive aphasia that was attributed to temporal lobe retraction.

References

1. Miller E, Crockard HA: Transoral transclival removal of anteriorly placed meningiomas at the foramen magnum. Neurosurgery 20: 966–968, 1987.
2. Fisch U, Pillsbury HC: Infratemporal fossa approach to lesions in the temporal bone and base of the skull. Arch Otolaryngol Head Neck Surg 105: 99–107, 1979.
3. Horn KL, Hankinson HL, Erasmus MD, et al: The modified transcochlear approach to the cerebellopontine angle. Otolaryngol Head Neck Surg 104: 37–41, 1991.
4. Al-Mefty O, Fox JL, Smith RR: Petrosal approach for petroclival meningiomas. Neurosurgery 22: 510–517, 1988.
5. Sekhar LN, Schramm VL, Jones NF: Subtemporal-preauricular infratemporal fossa approach to large lateral and posterior cranial base neoplasms. J Neurosurg 67: 488–499, 1987.
6. Spetzler RF, Daspit CP, Pappas CTE: Combined approach for lesions involving the cerebellopontine angle and skull base: Experience with 30 cases. Skull Base Surg 1: 226–234, 1991.
7. Eagleton WP: Unlocking the petrous pyramid for localized bulbar (pontile) meningitis secondary to suppuration of the petrous apex. Arch Otolaryngol Head Neck Surg 13: 386–422, 1931.
8. Kawase T, Toya S, Shiobara R, et al: Transpetrosal approach for aneurysms of the lower basilar artery. J Neurosurg 63: 857–861, 1985.
9. House WF, Hitselberger WE, Horn KL: The middle fossa transpetrous

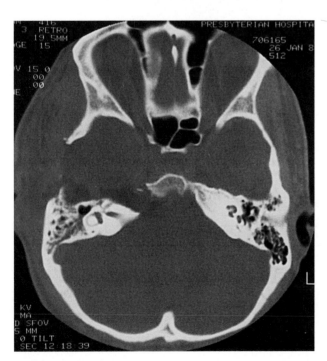

FIGURE 54–8. Axial CT scan demonstrating bone removal in the middle fossa transpetrous approach.

approach to the anterior-superior cerebellopontine angle. Am J Otol 7: 1–4, 1986.

10. Pensak ML, Loveren HV, Tew JM, et al: Transpetrosal access to meningiomas juxtaposing the temporal bone. Laryngoscope 104:814–820, 1994.
11. House WF: Surgical exposure of the internal auditory canal and its contents through the middle cranial fossa. Laryngoscope 71: 1363–1385, 1961.
12. House WF: Middle cranial fossa approach to the petrous pyramid: A report of 50 cases. Arch Otolaryngol Head Neck Surg 78: 406–469, 1963.
13. Wigand ME, Haid T, Berg M, et al: Extended middle cranial fossa approach for acoustic neuroma surgery. Skull Base Surg 1: 183–187, 1991.
14. Paullus WS, Pait TG, Rhoton AL: Microsurgical exposure of the petrous portion of the carotid artery. J Neurosurg 47: 713–726, 1977.
15. Leonitti JP, Smith PG, Linthicum FH: The petrous carotid artery:

16. Andrews JC, Martin NA, Black K, et al: Middle cranial fossa trans-temporal approach to the intrapetrous internal carotid artery. Skull Base Surg 1: 142–146, 1991.
17. Fisch U, Mattox D: Microsurgery of the Skull Base. New York, Thieme, 1988.
18. Lang J: Clinical Anatomy of the Posterior Cranial Fossa and Its Foramina. New York, Thieme, 1988.
19. Ono M, Ono M, Rhoton AL, et al: Microsurgical anatomy of the region of the tentorial incisura. J Neurosurg 60: 365–399, 1984.
20. Velut S, Jan M: Anterior petrosectomy during approach to the pe-troclival area. *In* Schmidek HH (ed): Meningiomas and Their Surgical Management. Philadelphia, WB Saunders, 1991, pp 435–450.
21. Hitselberger WE, Horn KL, Hankinson HL, et al: The middle fossa transpetrous approach for petroclival meningiomas. Skull Base Surg 3: 130–135, 1993.

Anatomic relationships in skull base surgery. Otolaryngol Head Neck Surg 102: 3–12, 1990.

55

Anterior and Subtemporal Approaches to the Infratemporal Fossa

Ricardo L. Carrau, M.D. ▪ Amin Kassam, M.D. ▪ Moisés Arriaga, M.D.

The infratemporal fossa (ITF) is a potential space bounded superiorly by the greater wing of the sphenoid and the temporal bone. Neurovascular foramina, including the carotid canal, jugular foramen, foramen spinosum, foramen ovale, and foramen lacerum, communicate the ITF with the middle cranial fossa. Medially, the ITF is contained by the superior constrictor muscle, the pharyngobasilar fascia, and the pterygoid plates. Medially, the ITF communicates with the pterygopalatine fossa via the pterygomaxillary fissure, which is continuous with the inferior orbital fissure, and thus the orbit. Laterally, the ITF is bounded by the zygoma, mandible, parotid gland, and masseter muscle. The pterygoid muscles comprise the anterior boundary, whereas posteriorly the ITF is confined by the articular tubercle of the temporal bone, glenoid fossa and styloid process. Therefore, using this definition, the ITF contains the parapharyngeal space (i.e., internal carotid artery [ICA], internal jugular vein [IJV], cranial nerves IV to XI), and the masticator space (i.e., internal maxillary artery, pterygoid venous plexus, and pterygoid muscles).

The presence of neurovascular structures within the ITF (e.g., ICA) or adjacent to it (e.g., cranial nerve VII) is the limiting step for designing a surgical approach to the ITF. Therefore, surgical approaches often center on the preservation and identification of these neurovascular entities.

The first report in the English literature of a surgical approach to the ITF is attributed to Fairbanks-Barbosa, who in 1961 described his approach for advanced tumors of the maxillary sinus.[1] Transtemporal approaches described by Fisch and preauricular approaches by Schramm and Sekhar are the basis for other modifications.[2–9] Other subsequent approaches follow the surgical and anatomic principles demonstrated by these authors.

PATIENT SELECTION

Tumors may originate within the confines of the ITF or may invade this area by direct extension from any of its boundaries—namely, the upper aerodigestive tract, the parotid gland, the temporal bone, the greater wing of the sphenoid, and structures within the cranial cavity. Accurate assessment of the nature, origin, and extension of the tumor is crucial for the therapeutic-surgical plan. Other factors affecting the selection of the surgical approach include patient needs and demands, the biologic behavior of the tumor or other coexistent diseases, and the training and experience of the surgeon. Furthermore, most pathologies affecting the ITF require a multidisciplinary approach to stage, diagnose, and extirpate the tumor, and at the same time to provide an acceptable cosmetic and functional reconstruction.

PREOPERATIVE EVALUATION

Diagnostic and Staging Work-up

Owing to the inaccessibility of the ITF to physical examination, radiographic imaging is a vital component of the evaluation. Computed tomography (CT) and magnetic resonance imaging (MRI) scan provide valuable information and are obtained using standard skull base protocols. CT is superior to MRI, demonstrating the remodeling or erosion of neurovascular foramina or other bones of the skull base. MRI better delineates the soft tissue planes, the tumor–soft tissue interface, and the presence of tumor along neural and vascular structures (Fig. 55–1). Therefore, CT and MRI are often complementary.

Another critical question is the relationship of the tumor to the ICA. MR angiography (MRA) provides a noninvasive assessment of the vasculature of the ITF and brain. If preoperative embolization of the tumor is indicated (e.g., juvenile nasopharyngeal angiofibromas, paragangliomas), angiography is preferred over MRA. Angiography provides important information regarding the vascularity of the tumor, its relationship to the ICA, and the cerebral circulation and its collateral blood supply. Neither study, however, is adequate to reliably predict the adequacy of the collateral intracranial circulation if sacrifice of the ICA is necessary.

If the risk for injury or sacrifice of the ICA is high, the collateral cerebral blood flow may be evaluated using angiography-balloon occlusion with xenon CT (ABOX-CT). A nondetachable balloon is inserted in the ICA via the femoral artery. The balloon is inflated for 15 minutes while the awake patient is monitored for any neurologic deficit. If the patient does not develop any deficit, the balloon is deflated and the patient is transferred to a CT suite. A mixture of 32 per cent xenon/68 per cent O_2 is administered via facial mask for 4 minutes. CT demonstrates the distribution of xenon, which reflects the blood flow within the cerebral tissue, providing a quantitative assessment of milliliters of blood flow per minute, per 100 gm of brain tissue. Then the process is repeated after reinflation of the arterial balloon. A computer calculates the differential of the xenon diffusion in the brain before

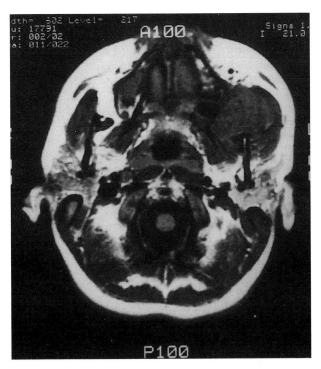

FIGURE 55-1. MRI demonstrates a soft tissue tumor involving the left infratemporal fossa (ITF). Even malignant tumors of the ITF may reach a large size before they are visible or palpable on physical examination. Such tumors may present with facial numbness, pain, or difficulty with mastication.

and after the balloon inflation, identifying those patients at risk for an ischemic stroke secondary to reduced blood flow after occlusion of the ipsilateral ICA (Table 55-1).[9]

Despite a negative finding from the ABOX-CT testing, patients can suffer ischemic brain injury due to the loss of collateral vessels that are not assessed by balloon occlusion testing ("watershed area"), or due to embolic phenomena. In addition, this test is performed under ideal and controlled circumstances and does not account for the possibility of episodes of hypoxia, hypotension, or electrolyte and acid-base disturbances that may alter the brain's hemodynamics. Thus, every effort should be made to preserve or reconstruct the ICA and to diminish the possibility of embolus formation during the surgery. Other techniques that provide information regarding collateral cerebral blood flow include single-photon emission CT (SPECT) with balloon occlusion and transcranial Doppler.

TABLE 55-1. Xenon Computed Tomography

CEREBRAL BLOOD FLOW (ml/min/100 gm of tissue)	RISK	IMPLICATION
>35	Low	Carotid may be sacrificed
21–35	Moderate	Patient will tolerate occlusion under controlled circumstances; reconstruction is recommended
≤20	High	Patient will not tolerate occlusion of the internal carotid artery

Histologic diagnosis should be obtained before the extirpative surgery whenever possible. Tumors amenable to a punch or open biopsy are approached in this manner. Those tumors that are in deeper planes may be sampled by fine-needle aspiration biopsy (FNAB). Rarely, a histologic diagnosis cannot be obtained prior to the approach due to the intrinsic limitations of FNAB. Under these circumstances, a frozen section analysis, obtained via a skull base approach, may be sufficient to justify the resection of the tumor. Vital neurovascular structures such as the ICA, the eye, and cranial nerves, however, should not be sacrificed based on a frozen section analysis.

The extent of the evaluation to rule out regional or distant metastasis or to determine that the ITF tumor is a metastasis is dictated by the histologic type and stage of the tumor. CT of the neck is more sensitive than physical examination for the detection of regional lymphadenopathy. Patients presenting with tumors that metastasize hematogenously (sarcoma, melanoma) should undergo a CT scan of the chest and abdomen and a bone scan. Cerebrospinal fluid (CSF) cytology is advised for patients with tumors that have invaded the dura. These patients are also at risk for "drop metastasis," which should be ruled out by a spinal MRI.

Rehabilitation Considerations

Functional and/or neurologic deficits that are identified preoperatively should be taken into consideration during the surgical planning, as well as during postoperative care. These deficits often have a significant impact on the recovery and functional rehabilitation of the patient.

Dysfunction of the trigeminal nerve and/or the masticator muscles is commonly underdiagnosed. Cutaneous and corneal sensation should be assessed preoperatively. Corneal anesthesia associated with concomitant facial nerve palsy requires aggressive measures to prevent corneal injury.

Lateral deviation of the jaw on opening may reflect weakness or paralysis of the ipsilateral pterygoid muscles, invasion of the muscles, or dysfunction of the temporomandibular joint (TMJ). Likewise, trismus may be due to mechanical restriction caused by the bulk of the tumor, ankylosis of the TMJ, scarring, tumor tethering, or pain. The nature of the trismus is an important consideration in the perioperative management of the airway. Trismus due to pain resolves with the induction of general anesthesia, allowing safe oral endotracheal intubation. In patients with mechanical trismus, an awake nasotracheal intubation may be performed if it is anticipated that surgery will correct the trismus. Otherwise, a tracheostomy, performed under local anesthesia, is the safest perioperative airway.

Neoplastic invasion of the facial nerve may present with facial weakness or paralysis, facial spasms, epiphora, facial spasms, and dysgeusia. Significant destruction of the facial nerve by tumor may occur before the patient develops these clinical signs. A gold weight, implanted in the upper eyelid, or surgical tightening of the lower lid may be necessary to protect the cornea.

Hearing loss caused by a tumor of the ITF may be either *conductive,* resulting from eustachian tube dysfunction, or *sensorineural,* resulting from tumor involvement of the temporal bone or posterior cranial fossa. A myringotomy or amplification or both facilitate communication with the patient.

Deficits of the lower cranial nerves (IX, X, XI, XII) are associated with tumors that originate in the parapharyngeal space and/or those that extend to the jugular foramen. Patients with deficits of cranial nerves IX, X, and XII present varying degrees of swallowing or speech problems, such as hypernasal or slurred speech, nasal regurgitation, dysphagia, aspiration, and dysphonia. Findings on physical examination reflect the involvement of specific cranial nerves and include decreased elevation of the palate, decreased mobility and strength of the tongue with deviation to the involved side on protrusion, decreased supraglottic sensation, pooling of secretions in the hypopharynx, ipsilateral vocal cord paralysis, and decreased bulk and strength of the sternocleidomastoid and trapezius muscles. Patients with partial deficits of the lower cranial nerves (paresis) often suffer a complete deficit (paralysis) after surgery, resulting in increased dysphagia and aspiration. Consequently, a tracheostomy for tracheal toilet and a gastrostomy tube for nutrition and hydration are often necessary during the perioperative period.

Laryngeal framework surgery (thyroplasty) performed during the extirpative surgery or the early postoperative period improves the glottic closure and decreases the risk for aspiration, often obviating the need for a tracheotomy for the sole purpose of tracheopulmonary toilet.[10–12] It should be remembered, however, that laryngeal framework surgery allows the patient to compensate for the deficits using the remaining function (contralateral side) more effectively. Laryngeal framework surgery does not restore the motor or the sensory function. Thus, these patients remain at a higher risk for aspiration and nutritional deficiencies. Collaboration with an experienced speech and language pathologist, who can assist with the monitoring of the patient and the diet modifications and provide intensive swallowing therapy, is crucial to prevent the pulmonary and nutritional complications of aspiration. In patients with severe deficits or in those with cognitive problems, strong consideration should also be given to placement of a gastrostomy tube to facilitate postoperative feeding and decrease the risk of prandial aspiration.

Velopharyngeal insufficiency may be ameliorated by a palatal lift prosthesis that pushes the soft palate against the posterior pharyngeal wall. Alternatively, a pharyngeal flap or a palatopexy may be performed in those patients who do not tolerate the prosthesis.

Reconstructive Considerations

Most commonly, a temporalis muscle transposition flap is adequate to separate the cranial cavity from the upper aerodigestive tract and obliterate the dead space. Microvascular free flaps such as the rectus abdominis flap (for soft tissue defects), latissimus dorsi flap (for myocutaneous or massive defects), or iliac composite flaps (for defects requiring bone reconstruction) are indicated when the temporalis muscle or its blood supply will be sacrificed as part of the oncologic resection, when the patient requires a complex resection involving composite tissue flaps with skin and/or bone, or when the extirpative surgery leads to a massive soft tissue defect and dead space. These needs are usually anticipated during the surgical planning, and the patient and consultants (e.g., the microvascular surgeon) are informed accordingly.

Ideally, functional and cosmetic deficits created by the tumor or the surgery should be addressed in a single stage, concomitant with the oncologic resection. When a temporary facial palsy is anticipated, corneal protection using lubricants and/or a temporary lateral tarsorrhaphy are usually adequate. Grafting of the facial nerve, however, involves a longer recovery period. Thus, insertion of a gold weight implant into the upper eyelid is advisable. When an immediate reconstruction of the facial nerve is not possible, static fascial slings or muscle transpositions are indicated. Lower cranial nerve deficits may be ameliorated by laryngeal framework surgery, tracheotomy, or laryngotracheal separation, as previously discussed.

Other Perioperative Considerations

Preoperatively, the patient's blood is typed and cross-matched for 2 to 6 units of packed red blood cells (PRBCs), according to the extent and nature of the tumor and surgery. Autologous blood banking is used when feasible, although it is frequently impractical. A Cell Saver autologous device may be used during the resection of benign vascular tumors.

Perioperative antibiotic prophylaxis with a wide spectrum against the flora of the skin and upper aerodigestive tract and that exhibits good penetration of the blood-brain barrier is administered before the surgery and is continued for 48 hours after the surgery. The use of a broad-spectrum cephalosporin with good CSF penetration (e.g., ceftriaxone) appears to be as effective as multiple antibiotic regimens.

Somatosensory evoked potential (SSEP) monitoring using the median nerve is indicated whenever surgical manipulation of the ICA is anticipated. Lower cranial nerve monitoring is not routinely employed. It may be useful for the identification and preservation of nerve function when the tumor is in close proximity to these nerves. Conversely, facial nerve monitoring is routinely used for transparotid or transtemporal approaches. Monitoring electrodes and lines for vascular access should be secured with sutures, staples, or adhesive dressings.

The choice of anesthetic agent is influenced by the extent of intracranial dissection, potential for brain injury, systemic hemodynamics, the need for monitoring of cortical and brainstem functions (e.g., brainstem-evoked response, SSEPs, electroencephalography), and the need for cranial nerve monitoring (VII, X to XII). Henceforth, all these factors should be thoroughly discussed with the anesthesiologist.

When changes of the head position during surgery are anticipated, the endotracheal tube should be secured with a circumdental or circum-mandibular wire ligature (No. 26 stainless-steel wire). The operating table is positioned perpendicular to the anesthesia staff, and, if intradural dissection is anticipated, a spinal drain is inserted and secured with sutures and adhesive dressing (e.g., Tegaderm, Op-Site). Other measures to diminish the intracranial pressure, such as hyperventilation, osmotic diuresis, and corticosteroids, are used as needed throughout the surgery.

A nasogastric tube and Foley catheter are passed and secured after adequate placement is corroborated. Antiembolic sequential compression stockings are recommended to prevent deep venous thrombosis.

SURGICAL APPROACHES

The head of the patient is positioned on a horseshoe headrest or, if necessary for intracranial neurovascular or neurosurgical work, on a three-pin head fixation system. When the horseshoe headrest is used, it is important to use additional "egg-crate" foam padding since the scalp may develop a pressure ulcer during prolonged surgery. If the ICA is at risk, the head should be positioned in slight extension to provide access to the neck for proximal control of the ICA. Tarsorrhaphy sutures are placed for protection of the eyes. The scalp is shaved following the planned incision line (e.g., bicoronal), and the incision line is infiltrated with a solution of lidocaine and epinephrine (1:100,000 to 1:400,000).

Preauricular (Subtemporal) Approach[10, 11]

The preauricular approach is suited for tumors that originate in the ITF and intracranial tumors that originate at the anterior aspect of the temporal bone, or greater wing of the sphenoid bone, and that extend into the ITF. It may also be combined with other approaches such as a subfrontal approach to expose massive tumors that extend to both the anterior and middle skull base. The preauricular approach, however, does not provide an adequate exposure for the resection of tumors that invade the tympanic bone and does not provide control of the intratemporal facial nerve or jugular bulb.

An incision, following a hemicoronal or bicoronal line, is carried through the subcutaneous tissue, galea, and pericranium (Fig. 55–2). Over the temporal area, the incision extends down to the deep layer of the temporal fascia. The anterior branches of the superficial temporal artery are preserved, ensuring adequate blood supply to the scalp flap. Ipsilateral to the tumor, the incision is extended following into the preauricular crease down to the level of the tragus. When proximal control of the ICA is warranted, the incision is extended into the neck using a "lazy S" pattern or, alternatively, a separate cervical incision is performed. The scalp is dissected following a subpericranial plane, separating the attachments of the pericranium to the deep layer of the temporal fascia. The scalp flap is elevated from the deep temporal fascia using a broad periosteal elevator.

Above the zygoma, the deep temporal fascia splits into superficial and deep layers, which attach to the lateral and medial surfaces of the zygomatic arch, respectively. To continue the surgical exposure, the superficial layer of the deep temporal fascia is incised following an imaginary line that joins the superior orbital rim to the zygomatic root. The dissection continues deep to this plane, elevating the

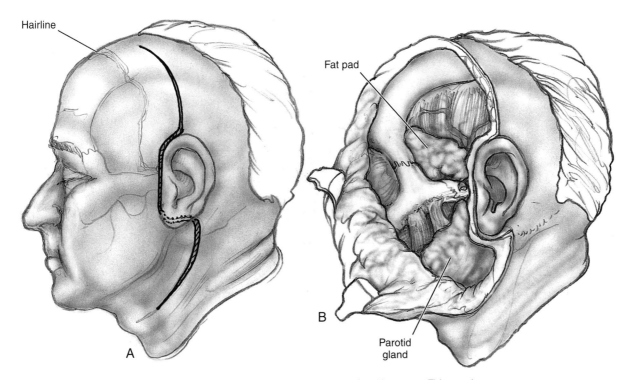

FIGURE 55–2. *A,* A bicoronal scalp incision is extended along a preauricular skin crease. This may be continued into the upper cervical region as a lazy S incision or a separate cervical incision may be made for exposure of the vessels and nerves. *B,* The scalp flap is elevated from the underlying cranium, fascia, lateral orbital rim, zygomatic arch, and masseteric fascia. The plane of dissection is deep to the superficial layer of the deep temporal fascia (incised) and deep to the parotid masseteric fascia.

superficial layer of the deep temporal fascia off the zygomatic arch (see Fig. 55–2). Fascia and periosteum are reflected anteriorly with the scalp flap. This maneuver protects the frontal branches of the facial nerve that are just lateral to the superficial layer of the deep temporal fascia. Elevation of the periosteum from the lateral surface of the zygomatic arch and malar eminence complete exposure of the orbitozygomatic complex. The periorbita is elevated from the lateral orbit using a Penfield No. 1 dissector, exposing the roof and lateral wall of the orbit down to the inferior orbital fissure.

The fascial attachments of the temporalis and masseter muscles to the zygomatic arch are transected using electrocautery. The attachments of the temporalis muscle to the cranium are transected with the electrocautery, and the muscle is elevated off the temporal fossa. If the temporalis muscle will be returned to its original position at the completion of the surgery, a curved titanium plate (1.5 to 1.7 mm) is screwed at the temporal line, leaving some screw holes empty to facilitate suturing from the plate to the muscle (Fig. 55–3). Then, the masseteric fascia is dissected from the masseter muscle, thus elevating the overlying parotid gland with a broad periosteal elevator (see Fig. 55–2). To increase the arc of rotation of the scalp flap, any soft tissue anterior to the tympanic bone can be transected from superior to inferior, down to the level of the facial nerve. The facial nerve is identified and preserved using a standard technique. It is helpful to preserve a cuff of soft tissue around the main trunk of the facial nerve to prevent a traction injury to the main trunk of the facial nerve.

Using the caudal limb of the incision, the sternocleidomastoid muscle is dissected laterally and the carotid sheath is exposed. When necessary, the contents of the carotid sheath, including the ICA and common and external carotid arteries, as well as the IJV, are exposed, dissected, and controlled. Cranial nerves X to XII are also identified and preserved. Vessel loops are placed around these structures and secured with hemoclips rather than hemostats to avoid inadvertent traction.

Orbitozygomatic osteotomies are performed at the zygomatic root posteriorly, the zygomaticofrontal suture superiorly, and the zygomaticomaxillary buttress at the level of the zygomaticofacial nerve, medially (see Fig. 55–3). Prior periorbital elevation off the lateral and inferior walls is necessary to identify the inferior orbital fissure and to complete the osteotomies of the orbitozygomatic complex. The tip of the reciprocating saw is then placed in the most lateral aspect of the inferior orbital fissure; an osteotomy is performed through the malar eminence following a vertical imaginary line medial to the zygomaticofacial foramen. This osteotomy separates the zygoma from the maxilla. Accidental entry into the maxillary sinus may occur, requiring closure of the defect using fascia and/or pericranium free grafting. These free tissue grafts are held in place by compression against the opening when orbitozygomatic bone graft is replaced and plated at the completion of the surgery. All osteotomies are completed with a reciprocating saw transecting the bone in beveled and/or V-shaped manner in such a way that maximizes the exposure and facilitates replacement of the bone graft at the completion of the surgery. If tumor involvement of the orbit is present, the osteotomies are modified to secure a complete resection.

In cases requiring both intracranial and extracranial exposure, the superior and lateral osteotomies are made through the superior and lateral orbital walls after the craniotomy is completed and the brain is separated from the skull base. This way, the orbital walls can be incorpo-

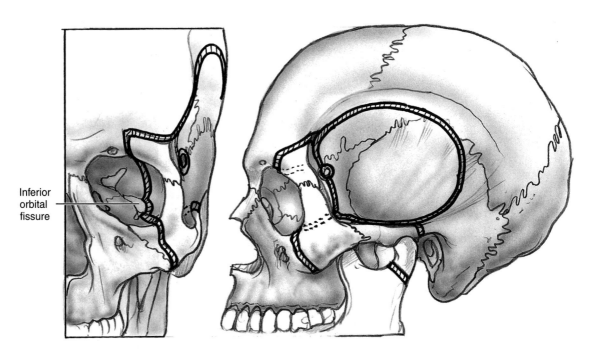

Inferior orbital fissure

FIGURE 55–3. The areas of bone removal are noted with dark stippling. A temporal craniotomy is performed in conjunction with an orbitozygomatic osteotomy. Additional exposure of the infratemporal skull base may be achieved by removal of subtemporal cranium *(striped area)* and resection of the mandibular condyle *(lightly stippled area)*.

rated in the orbitozygomatic graft. Using both intracranial and extracranial exposures, osteotomies are made through the superior and lateral orbital walls to remove the orbitozygomatic bone segment. This approach provides excellent access to the infratemporal skull base, orbital apex, and lateral maxilla.

The temporalis muscle is then reflected inferiorly until the infratemporal crest is fully visualized. A subperiosteal plane is then followed to dissect the soft tissues from the infratemporal cranium. Bleeding from the underlying bone is controlled by the application of bone wax.

Fracturing or removal of the coronoid process increases the arc of rotation of the temporalis muscle. Care should be exercised when dissecting the medial aspect of the temporalis muscle, especially near its insertion (coronoid process) because the blood supply to the muscle (deep temporal artery from the internal maxillary artery) penetrates the muscle at this area. Likewise, the soft tissue at the sigmoid notch should be dissected carefully to prevent accidental injury to the internal maxillary artery that travels adjacent to the medial surface of the mandibular ramus.

Dissection of the soft tissues from the infratemporal skull base is usually associated with troublesome bleeding arising from the pterygoid plexus. Bleeding is controlled with the use of bipolar cautery and/or cottonoids moistened in oxymetazoline 0.05 per cent. Unipolar cautery is seldom used because it stimulates V3, causing contraction of the mastication muscles and occasional cardiac arrhythmias.

A subtemporal craniectomy may aid in the identification of neurovascular structures piercing the infratemporal skull base and to augment the exposure. The most lateral bone is removed using rongeurs. The origin of the lateral pterygoid plate at the skull base is identified anteriorly. Ana-

tomic relationships that are useful for the identification of infratemporal skull base structures are seen in Figure 55–4, including the posterior curve of the attachment of the lateral pterygoid plate that is in alignment with the foramen ovale, foramen spinosum, and the spine of the sphenoid bone. These structures lie in a straight "line of sight" that is lateral to the canal of the ICA. The inferolateral aspect of the sphenoid sinus may be accessed removing the bone (i.e., pterygoid plates) between the second and third divisions of the trigeminal nerve. The extirpation of the tumor can now proceed, including the involved soft tissue and bone.

To continue the subtemporal exposure, the middle meningeal artery is clipped or cauterized using bipolar electrocautery and transected. Bleeding from the venous plexus that accompanies V3 through the foramen ovale may be controlled with Surgicel packing.

Lesions that do not involve the temporal bone or petrous portion of the ICA are adequately exposed with this stepwise approach. However, dissection of the petrous ICA is necessary; the glenoid fossa is removed as part of the orbitozygomatic bone graft. It is first necessary to perform a temporal craniotomy for exposure of the superior aspect of the glenoid fossa (Fig. 55–5). The capsule of the TMJ is dissected free from the fossa and displaced inferiorly. If possible, the capsule and meniscus are preserved. With use of a reciprocating saw, osteotomies are then made through the glenoid fossa, incorporating the lateral two thirds of the fossa (see Fig. 55–5). This maneuver avoids potential injury to the ICA that is located medial to the fossa. In addition, this modification provides stability for the mandibular condyle following reconstruction, although it can be prone to anterior dislocation. Injury to the cochlea

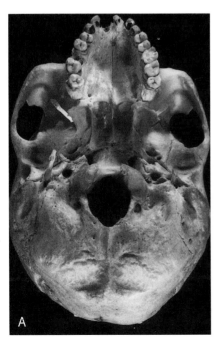
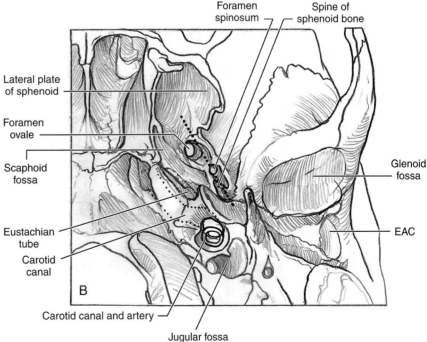

FIGURE 55–4A and B. Base of the skull demonstrating the anatomic relationships of the carotid canal. The foramen ovale and the foramen spinosum are in a direct line from the lateral pterygoid plate to the spine of the sphenoid.

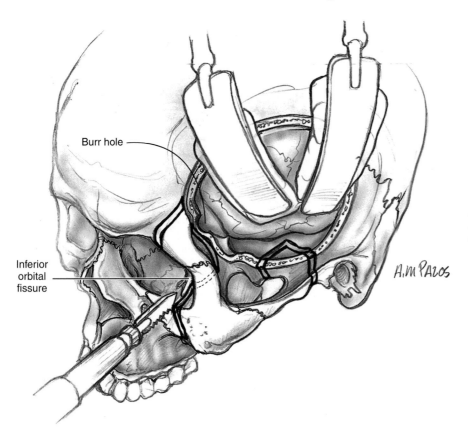

Burr hole

Inferior orbital fissure

A.M PAZOS

FIGURE 55–5. Using intracranial and extracranial approaches, osteotomies of the superior orbital roof, lateral orbital wall, and glenoid fossa are performed.

is possible if the osteotomies are made too posteriorly. If additional exposure is necessary (i.e., carotid canal and extratemporal ICA), the condylar neck and contents of the condylar fossa can be transected at the level of the sigmoid notch and removed (Fig. 55–6).

To dissect the petrous segment of the ICA, it is necessary to transect the mandibular division of the trigeminal nerve at the foramen ovale (see Fig. 55–6). Once the ICA is mobilized from its horizontal canal, it can be transposed and/or retracted to facilitate the resection of tumor or to gain access to the petrous apex.

Approaches to the ITF are modified according to the extent of the tumor and other clinical circumstances. Tumors that invade the mandible mandate a partial mandibulectomy to obtain negative margins. In the pediatric age group patient, the distance from the body of the mandible to the infratemporal skull base is greatly foreshortened. Adequate exposure of the infratemporal skull base can often be achieved using a transcervical approach with superior transposition of the facial nerve.

Following extirpation of the tumor, it is necessary to close any communication with the upper aerodigestive tract. If viable, a temporalis muscle flap is used to obliterate the dead space and protect the ICA (Fig. 55–7). Because of the branching pattern of the blood supply to the temporalis muscle, the muscle can be divided vertically and the anterior half of the muscle may be transposed with an intact blood supply. The remaining posterior half of the muscle is transposed anteriorly to fill the temporal fossa defect.

Defects of the orbital floor may be reconstructed with titanium mesh, which is then covered with a temporalis muscle transposition flap or temporoparietal fascia flap.

Likewise, defects of the lateral orbital wall can be reconstructed with titanium mesh. In selected patients, anteriorly or posteriorly based pericranial scalp flaps may be elevated to provide protection of the infratemporal skull base. When the temporalis muscle is not available, massive soft tissue defects are best reconstructed with microvascular free tissue flaps.

The orbitozygomatic bone graft is then replaced and fixated in its original position with titanium alloy adaptation plates, wire, or braided nylon sutures. Plating of the bone grafts is preferred because it provides greater stability. To avoid compression of reconstructive flaps, it is sometimes necessary to remove a portion of the zygomatic arch.

If resection of the mandibular condyle was necessary to expose the petrous ICA, reconstruction of the TMJ is not attempted. Reconstruction of the TMJ after oncologic exenteration of the ITF does not improve the postoperative function significantly and may actually lead to scarring, ankylosis, and trismus.

Periosteal and muscular attachments to the craniofacial skeleton must be repaired to prevent retraction and/or sagging of the muscles and other soft tissues. The skin and mucosal incisions are closed using a multilayered technique

Postauricular (Transtemporal) Approach[10, 11]

The postauricular approach is designed to expose and resect lesions involving the temporal bone and extending into the ITF. A "question mark" or C-shaped incision is started in the temporal area and extended, postauricularly, into the

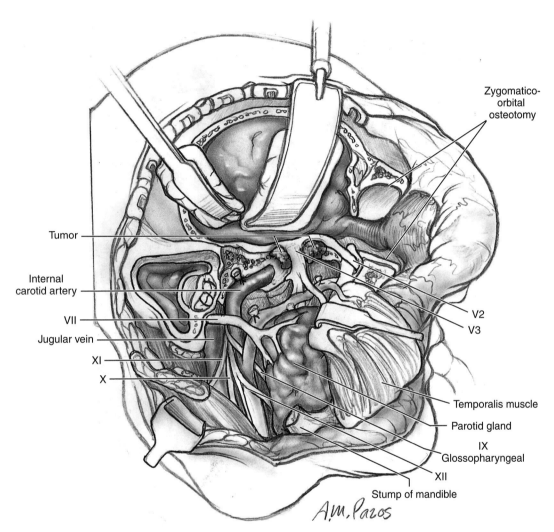

FIGURE 55–6. This illustration demonstrates a tumor medial to the mandibular division of the trigeminal nerve and in close proximity to the petrous portion of the internal carotid artery (ICA). Additional exposure of the ICA and removal of the tumor often necessitate transection of the mandibular division of the trigeminal nerve. This illustration demonstrates a postauricular approach.

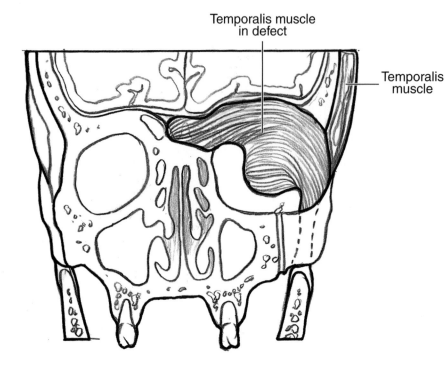

Temporalis muscle
in defect

Temporalis
muscle

FIGURE 55–7. The anterior portion of the muscle may be transposed to fill an infratemporal skull base defect as illustrated with this left temporalis muscle.

mastoid region, curving down to follow one of the midneck horizontal skin creases (Fig. 55–8A).

If the middle ear will be sacrificed as part of the approach or the tumor resection and there is a risk of a postoperative CSF leak (intradural work), the external auditory canal is closed permanently to prevent CSF otorrhea. The external auditory canal is divided at the bony-cartilaginous junction and then closed using everting stitches. This closure is reinforced with a myoperiosteal U-shaped flap based on the posterior margin of the external auditory canal. Alternatively, if the middle ear will be spared, the canal may be preserved by placing the incisions in the conchal area (Fig. 55–8B). The incision follows the margin of the conchal bowl and tragus so that the scar will be hidden. In the conchal area, the skin, cartilage, and perichondrium are incised to communicate with the retroauricular plane of dissection. These incisions, placed laterally, facilitate the anastomosis of the external auditory canal to the pinna at the end of the extirpative procedure. An incision inside the external auditory canal is not recommended because it is difficult to suture in a watertight manner and tends to stenose. A Penrose drain can be inserted through the conchal defect in the skin-auricle flap to facilitate its retraction.

Elevation of the cervicofacial flap is carried in a subplatysmal plane in the cervical area, suprasuperficial musculoaponeurotic system plane over the parotid area, and following the deep layer of the deep temporal fascia over the cranium.

The main trunk of the facial nerve is identified anterior to the external auditory canal just distal to the stylomastoid foramen, as is described for a parotidectomy. If circumferential mobilization of the main trunk is not necessary, a cuff of soft tissue is preserved around its main trunk to minimize the possibility of a traction injury when the facial flap is retracted anteriorly. In selected cases, a "tail"

parotidectomy may enhance the access to the retromandibular area. A total parotidectomy is indicated when facing a epithelial malignancy of the parotid gland. Skeletonization of the main trunk of the facial nerve and its branches facilitates their retraction and thus the access to the ITF (Fig. 55–6). Resection of the main trunk of the facial nerve and its branches (radical parotidectomy) is indicated when the nerve is invaded by the tumor.

Attention is then directed to the cervical exposure to obtain proximal control of the common, internal, and external carotid arteries, as well as the IJV. Cranial nerves X to XII are identified and preserved. The sternocleidomastoid and digastric muscles are transected at their insertion to the mastoid bone. The stylohyoid and stylopharyngeus muscles are transected and the styloid process is removed. Cranial nerve IX can usually be identified at this time, as it crosses lateral to the ICA.

A mastoidectomy and dissection of the vertical portion of the facial nerve allows the transposition of the facial nerve, thus providing a wider access to the infratemporal fossa (see Figs. 55–6 and 55–9). In patients who require a radical parotidectomy, a mastoidectomy provides the means to obtain proximal control of the neural margins and to graft the nerve. It also provides access to the jugular bulb and adjacent lower cranial nerves.

Orbitozygomatic osteotomies may be performed as previously described (preauricular approach). After the orbitozygomatic complex is removed, the anterior, superior, medial, and posterior boundaries of the infratemporal fossa are well exposed, and all major vessels are "controlled." Completion of the infratemporal skull base approach, including a temporal craniotomy, is performed as described in the previous section. The extirpation of the tumor can now proceed, including the involved soft tissue and bone. Reconstruction of the defect follows the principles outlined in previous sections.

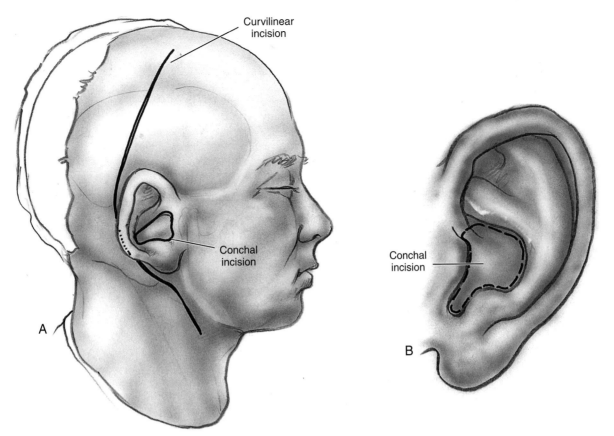

FIGURE 55–8. *A*, A curvilinear incision is made from the temporal area to the mastoid bone and upper cervical region. The flap is elevated superficial to the deep temporal fascia, deep to the mastoid periosteum, and deep to the platysma muscle. *B*, A conchal incision is preferable to an incision of the external auditory canal when permanent obliteration of the ear is not indicated.

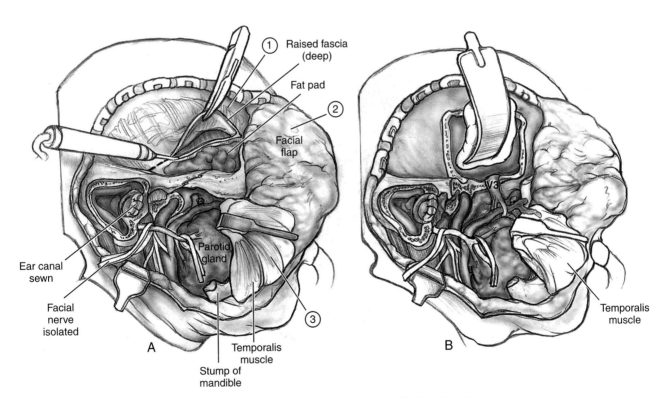

FIGURE 55–9. *A*, The deep temporal fascia is split to expose the temporal fat pad (1). The fascia is then elevated with the facial flap, thus protecting the frontal branches of the facial nerve (2). The temporalis muscle can then be retracted inferiorly allowing the exposure and resection (B) of the subtemporal skull base. The drawing demonstrates a postauricular approach after a temporal craniotomy.

Lateral Fisch Infratemporal Fossa Approaches

Ugo Fisch has described an array of lateral infratemporal fossa approaches that are the prototypic otologic approaches to the ITF (Fig. 55–10). The hallmark of these approaches is temporal bone management emphasizing facial nerve rerouting and subtemporal dural exposure for wide access to the lateral skull base. Figure 55–10 illustrates the anatomic regions appropriate for the Fisch A, B, and C approaches. The Fisch A approach has been described in detail in Chapter 47 regarding its application in glomus jugulare surgery. The Fisch B and C approaches are designed to approach more anterior pathology involving the petrous apex and clivus. The type C approach is an extension of the type B approach and used for lesions of the anterior ITF, sella, and nasopharynx. The type D is a preauricular ITF approach using an orbitozygotomy and resection of the floor of the middle fossa for medial dural exposure without a lateral temporal craniotomy.

Type B

The principal exposure maneuver in the type B ITF approach is reflection of the zygomatic arch and temporalis muscle inferiorly and removal of the bone of the skull base floor to provide access to the ITF.

The incision is wide and C-shaped beginning at the angle of the mandible and extending retroauricularly and anterior laterally to the eyebrow. The ear canal is transected and closed in the same manner as described in Chapter 47 in a two-layer technique.

The main trunk of the facial nerve is identified using standard landmarks at the stylomastoid foramen. The superior division is followed to the level of the frontalis branch. With this direct visualization, the periosteum attached to the zygomatic arch is reflected down to protect the frontalis branch of the facial nerve. At this point, the osteotomies of the zygomatic arch can be completed anteriorly as close as possible to the orbital rim and posteriorly at the root of the zygoma. The masseter muscle is left attached at the zygomatic arch to be reflected inferiorly. The temporalis muscle is then completely reflected inferiorly, carefully protecting its blood supply.

A key to this extradural exposure is the subtotal "petrosectomy." This step includes a canal wall down mastoidectomy including complete skeletonization of the labyrinth, facial nerve, sigmoid sinus, middle fossa, and posterior fossa dura and the jugular bulb as well as exenteration of all hypotympanic air cells and skeletonization of the ICA. The unique aspect is that by removing the ossicular chain and middle ear structures, the carotid artery can be skeletonized completely beyond the genu to the foramen lacerum.

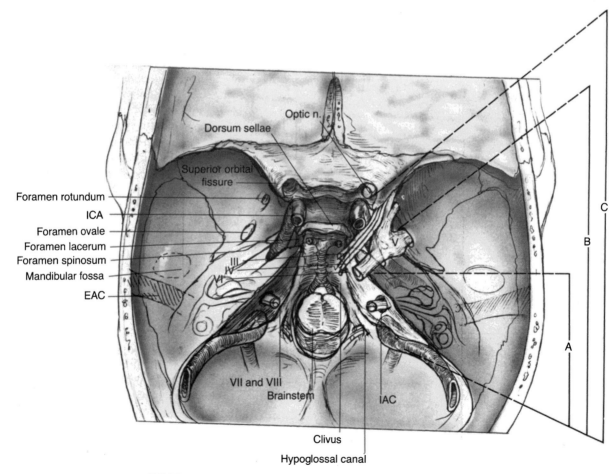

FIGURE 55–10. The different exposures obtained with the Fisch types A, B, and C approaches to the infratemporal fossa.

The TMJ is disarticulated by incising the capsule and removing the articular disc. At this point, the bone of the glenoid fossa and the root of the zygoma are completely removed with cutting and diamond burrs. Middle fossa dura in the subtemporal region is completely skeletonized. By placing the infratemporal fossa retractor over the mandibular condyle, additional skeletonization of the middle fossa dura can be accomplished medially until reaching the middle meningeal artery and V3 at the foramen ovale. Cauterization of the middle meningeal artery and transection of the mandibular nerve permit greater exposure. At this point, further skeletonization of the carotid artery is possible along the lateral and anterior wall of the ICA. Complete exposure of the carotid artery permits its mobilization out of the carotid canal, providing free access to the petrous apex and clivus. The eustachian tube must be sutured closed to prevent infection of the nasal cavity. While the bone defect is filled with abdominal fat, temporalis muscle is used to cover the fat and is placed inferior to the skeletonized middle fossa dura and mandibular condyle. The zygomatic arch can be secured with microplates, and the skin can be closed in a standard fashion.

Fisch C

The principal distinguishing feature of the type C in comparison to the type B approach is resection of the pterygoid plates. This permits exposure of the lateral wall of the nasopharynx, eustachian tube orifice, posterior maxillary sinus, and posterior nasopharyngeal wall past the midline.

Following completion of the type B approach, the lateral surface of the pterygoid process is identified and soft tissues are elevated. In this manner, the base of both medial and lateral plates of the pterygoid processes can be drilled away, exposing the lateral wall of the nasopharynx. Thus, the nasal cavity can be entered. The exposure permits full visualization of the peritubal area, which can be resected

en bloc. Inferiorly, the excision can extend to the upper surface of the palate. Superiorly, the dissection can extend to the carotid artery and the cavernous sinus.

The wide communication between the nasopharynx and the operative field makes closure in type C ITF surgery more difficult than in type B. Although mobilization of the entire temporalis muscle into the wound is one technique, vascularized free flaps are often necessary to provide adequate closure. Abdominal fat should be avoided because of the possibility of contamination.

Type D

The Fisch D ITF exposure is a new preauricular modification of the Fisch infratemporal approach. D1 addresses tumors of the anterior infratemporal fossa, whereas the D2 is designed for lateral orbital wall lesions and high pterygopalatine fossa tumors. The distinguishing feature of the D approach from the B and C approach is that the middle ear and eustachian tube area is not obliterated and conductive hearing is not sacrificed. In addition, the intratemporal facial nerve is not rerouted and the petrous ICA is not fully exposed. Although these preauricular approaches do not include a temporal craniotomy, the floor of the skull base can be drilled away to allow full access to the ITF.

Anterior Transfacial Approach (Facial Translocation)[10, 11]

The anterior transfacial technique is best used to approach sinonasal tumors invading the ITF, the masticator space, or the pterygomaxillary fossa and for tumors of the nasopharynx extending into the ITF (Fig. 55–11). A bicoronal incision with an ipsilateral preauricular extension is performed and extended through the subcutaneous tissue (see the

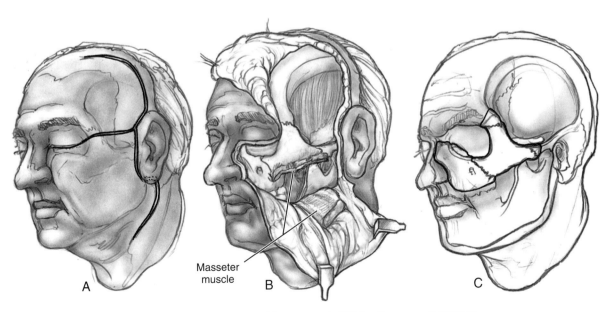

Masseter muscle

A   B   C

FIGURE 55–11. A hemicoronal incision is combined with an extended Weber-Fergusson incision in the anterior transfacial approach. The incision may be made through the conjunctiva or through the skin several millimeters inferior to the ciliary line. The orbitozygomatic complex is then exposed and osteotomies are performed to expose the infratemporal fossa.

section on preauricular approach). A Weber-Fergusson incision is completed and extended down to the periosteum of the maxilla, nasal bones, and orbital rim. During a "traditional" translocation approach, a horizontal incision is carried over the superior edge of the zygomatic bone, extending into the lateral canthus, to meet the Weber-Fergusson incision (see Fig. 55–11). The frontal branches of the facial nerve are identified and dissected as they cross over the zygomatic arch. They are then entubulated with silicone tubing and transected. These nerve branches will be reanastomosed at the end of the case, using an entubulation technique. Subperiosteal dissection of the anterior maxilla exposes the infraorbital nerve that is then transected and tagged to facilitate its identification and reanastomosis at the end of the case. Then, an inferiorly based flap including the upper third of the upper lip, entire cheek, lower eyelid, parotid gland, and the facial nerve is reflected inferiorly. The frontotemporal scalp flap is elevated in a subpericranial plane. This flap is reflected anteriorly, exposing the superior orbital rims (see Figure 55–11). Alternatively, the exposure can be achieved without the temporal incision by combining the preauricular approach with the anterior exposure provided by the Weber-Fergusson incision.

Orbitozygomatic osteotomies are performed and joined with the maxillary osteotomies to free the anterior face of the ipsilateral maxilla en bloc with the orbitozygomatic complex. Alternatively, the maxillary bone graft can be elevated as a vascularized graft attached to the cheek flap, as described by Catalano and Biller.[8] The temporalis and masseter muscles are dissected from the zygomatic bone with electrocautery. Osteotomies are completed and the bone graft is removed. The temporalis muscle is reflected inferiorly. Removal of the coronoid process increases the caudal arc of rotation of the temporalis muscle. After completion of these steps, the anterior, medial, and lateral boundaries of the ITF are well exposed.

In selected cases, the pterygoid plates can be excised to provide further access to the medial ITF or nasopharynx. A temporosubtemporal craniotomy provides additional exposure superiorly and allows dissection of intracranial structures (Fig. 55–12). Following the tumor resection, the temporalis muscle may be used to obliterate the surgical defect and provide separation of the cranial cavity from the upper aerodigestive tract, as previously described.

Periosteal and muscular attachments are repaired and the incisions are closed using a multilayer technique. The conjunctiva is repaired with running 6-0 fast-absorbing suture. The lacrimal canaliculi are stented with Crawford silicone tubing that is tied to itself in the nasal cavity. The eye is closed with a temporary tarsorrhaphy for 10 to 14 days to prevent a lower lid ectropion.

Transorbital Approach

In selected cases, a transorbital approach may be used to complement the exposures obtained with one of the previous approaches enhancing the exposure of the orbital apex and cavernous sinus. This approach consists of transection

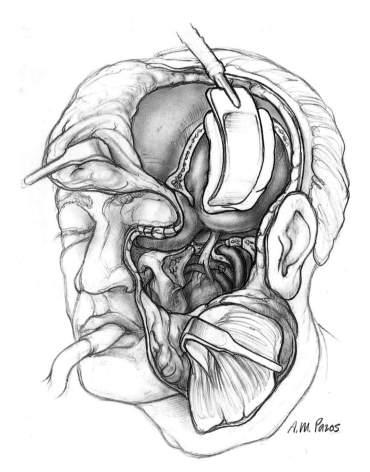

FIGURE 55–12. A subtemporal craniectomy is performed to provide additional exposure and an adequate resection margin of extracranial tumors. Maximal exposure of the infratemporal and central skull base is achieved.

of the orbital tissues posterior to the globe with preservation of the attachments of the orbital soft tissues, including the globe, to the scalp flap. The orbital apex is removed to provide direct anterior access to the cavernous sinus and cavernous ICA. This approach is reserved for patients with benign tumors of the orbita apex and cavernous sinus who have lost vision as a result of tumor growth. It may also be employed for low-grade malignant neoplasms with minimal involvement of the orbital soft apex or optic nerve to obtain complete tumor removal. Extensive involvement of the orbital soft tissues requires an orbital exenteration. The advantages of this approach include improved cosmesis, a result of the preservation of the globe, and excellent anterior and lateral exposure of the cavernous sinus and its associated structures.

A preauricular infratemporal skull base approach is performed, as previously described. The periorbita is elevated from the superior, lateral, and inferior walls of the orbit. The periorbita is then incised and the orbital tissues are transected posterior to the globe using bipolar electrocautery and sharp dissection. A cuff of tissue remains at the orbital apex to provide an adequate tumor margin. The remaining periorbital attachments are then elevated medially to allow complete displacement of the globe from the orbital cavity. Over the medial wall the neurovascular bundles are clipped or cauterized and transected. The lacrimal duct is transected and the sac is marsupialized. Using rongeurs, bone is removed from the lateral wall of the orbit to the superior orbital fissure. The contents of the superior orbital fissure and optic canal are then transected to provide additional exposure of the orbital apex.

Due to the loss of orbital bone, enophthalmos will result unless the orbital defect is reconstructed with bone grafts or titanium mesh. A temporalis transposition or free tissue transfer provides soft tissue augmentation and protection of the carotid artery.

POSTOPERATIVE CARE

Following surgery, the patient is transferred to an intensive care unit for continuous cardiovascular and neurologic monitoring. Laboratory tests to rule out postoperative anemia and electrolyte imbalance are performed. Patients who required multiple blood transfusions should be screened for transfusion-induced coagulation disorders. Mild narcotic analgesia is provided, avoiding sedation that could interfere with a detailed neurologic evaluation.

If the ICA is dissected, ligated, or grafted, close monitoring of the patient's hemodynamic status and fluid balance is essential. When grafting of the ICA is performed, an angiogram is obtained in the early postoperative period to assess the patency of the graft and detect pseudoaneurysm formation. A CT scan of the brain without contrast medium is performed in the first or second postoperative day to screen for intracranial complications such as cerebral contusion, edema or hemorrhage, fluid collections, or pneumocephalus.

A compressive dressing is maintained for 24 to 72 hours. Once the dressing is removed, the wound is cleaned with normal saline solution and covered with antibiotic ointment three to four times a day.

The scalp and other wound drains are kept to bulb suction until the drainage is less than 30 ml per day. The drain is then removed and the wound is closed using an encircling stitch placed at the time of surgery. If the cranial cavity is entered, wall suction is never used because of the risk of direct negative pressure on the central nervous system.

In most cases, the spinal drain is needed only during the surgery and is removed on completion of the procedure. If there is a significant risk of postoperative CSF leak, the spinal drain is kept at the level of the patient's shoulder and 50 ml is removed every 8 to 12 hours. The lumbar drain is removed 3 to 5 days after surgery, and the lumbar puncture site is closed with an encircling stitch (e.g., 2-0 nylon), placed at the time of surgery.

Lagophthalmos, due to weakness or paralysis of the facial nerve may lead to exposure keratoconjunctivitis. Initially, an exposed eye can be protected using artificial tears every 1 to 2 hours, lubrication ointment at bedtime, eye patching, or a moisture chamber. Taping of the eyelids or a temporary tarsorrhaphy is advised if rapid recovery is anticipated. If a prolonged paralysis is expected, we prefer a gold weight implant. This can be performed at the time of the original surgery, using a 0.1 to 0.12 gm weight (No. 10 or 12), or it may be performed during the early postoperative period. Except in selected cases, we favor the latter, because it provides the advantage of being able to establish the exact weight that is needed by the patient.

In most cases, the airway can be secured for a short term using an endotracheal tube (high-volume/low-pressure cuff). Nevertheless, a tracheotomy is indicated for patients in whom significant edema of the upper aerodigestive tract is anticipated or if a prolonged mechanical ventilation is anticipated. A tracheotomy also provides better access to the airway for pulmonary toilet for those patients with an ineffective cough or severe aspiration.

Patients with high vagal lesions or any combination of deficits of cranial nerves IX, X, or XII will suffer severe swallowing difficulty and aspiration. These patients can be assisted with a medialization laryngoplasty, an arytenoid adduction procedure, or an arytenoidpexy with or without a cricopharyngeal myotomy. Patients who continue to aspirate despite all these measures and who develop repeated aspiration pneumonias are managed by a laryngotracheal separation procedure.

PITFALLS AND COMPLICATIONS

The most common morbidity associated with surgery of the infratemporal fossa is related to deficits of the trigeminal nerve. Sacrifice of the third, sometimes second, and rarely the first, divisions of the trigeminal nerve may be necessary for surgical exposure or to obtain adequate clear margins of resection. Facial anesthesia may predispose the patient to self-inflicted injuries, including neurotrophic ulcers.

The loss of corneal sensation, especially in someone with paresis of the facial nerve, greatly increases the risk of a corneal abrasion or exposure keratitis. The loss of motor function of the mandibular nerve causes asymmetry of jaw opening and decreased force of mastication on the operated side. Mastication may be further impaired by resection of the TMJ or mandibular ramus. Whenever feasible, sensory and motor divisions of the trigeminal nerve are repaired or grafted following transection for surgical exposure.

Permanent deficits (accidental) of the facial nerve or its branches are uncommon. The frontal branches of the facial nerve are at risk of injury during elevation of the temporal scalp flap. Injury is usually the result either of a dissection in a plane that is superficial to the superficial layer of the deep temporal fascia or of compression during the retraction of the flap. To avoid a traction injury, a cuff of soft tissue is preserved around the main trunk of the facial nerve when a preauricular approach is employed. The facial nerve can also suffer an ischemic injury that occurs as a result of devascularization on mobilization of its infratemporal or skeletonization of its extratemporal segments. A temporary paresis of the facial nerve is to be expected with mobilization of the mastoid segment of the facial nerve. Close attention to postoperative eye care is necessary in patients with combined deficits of the trigeminal and facial nerves.

In most patients, surgical resection of the TMJ is not a major factor in the development of postoperative trismus or difficulties with mastication. Rather, mastication appears to be most affected by loss of function of the mandibular division of the trigeminal nerve. Nevertheless, every effort is made to preserve the TMJ. If resection of the glenoid fossa is necessary, the capsule of the TMJ is displaced inferiorly. If resection of the TMJ is necessary, no attempt is made to reconstruct the joint. These patients will experience deviation of the jaw to the unaffected side. This is usually of no major consequence, but some patients may need an octussal guide to help them when chewing.

Postoperative trismus is also a common occurrence due to postoperative pain and scarring of the pterygoid musculature and TMJ. Trismus improves dramatically if patients regularly perform stretching exercises for the jaw. Devices such as the Therabite appliance are helpful in stretching the scar tissue and forcefully opening the mouth. In severe cases, a dental appliance may be fabricated that is gradually opened by a screw.

Infectious complications are rare. Predisposing factors include communication with the nasopharynx, seroma or hematoma, and a CSF leak. In general, the dead space should be obliterated to prevent fluid collection that subsequently can be infected, and the cranial cavity should be separated from the sinonasal tract. The use of vascularized tissue flaps is preferred, especially when there has been dissection of the ICA or resection of dura.

Necrosis of the scalp flap is an uncommon occurrence due to its excellent blood supply. Poorly designed incisions, however, may result in areas of ischemia, particularly around the auricle that can make the tissue susceptible to secondary infection. Prolonged use of hemostatic clamps can also lead to necrosis of the wound edges.

Neurovascular complications are of the greatest concern. Postoperative cerebral ischemia may result from surgical occlusion of the ICA, temporary vasospasm, and thromboembolic phenomena. Surgical dissection of the ICA can injure the vessel walls, resulting in immediate or delayed rupture and hemorrhage. The ICA is particularly vulnerable to injury where it enters the cranial base. Injuries to the ICA should be repaired primarily (or using a vein graft). An angiogram is obtained in the early postoperative period to assess the adequacy of the repair. In the event that a repair of the ICA is not possible, it should be permanently occluded by ligation or by the placement of a detachable balloon or vascular coil. When the artery is to be permanently occluded, the occlusion is performed as distal as possible (near the origin of the ophthalmic artery). The potential for thrombus formation is less with a short column of stagnant blood above the level of occlusion. Following occlusion of the ICA, there is a significant risk of immediate and delayed stroke in patients who do not have more than 35 to 40 ml of blood flow per 100 gm of brain tissue per minute by ABOX-CT testing.

Following reconstruction of the ICA with a vein graft, there is a risk of postoperative occlusion due to thrombus formation at the suture line, as well as torsion or kinking of the graft. Pseudoaneurysm formation and delayed blowout of the graft are also a risk, especially in the presence of infection. For this reason, reconstruction of the ICA is usually not indicated in a contaminated field with communication to the upper aerodigestive tract. In such cases, permanent occlusion of the ICA or rerouting of a vein graft posterior to the surgical field is performed. An extracranial-intracranial bypass graft to the middle cerebral artery may be performed prior to tumor resection when sacrifice of the ICA is anticipated. Patients who undergo surgical manipulation of the ICA may also develop cerebral ischemia at the margins of the vascular territories of the cerebral vessels (watershed areas). This is of particular concern when there is sacrifice of extracranial-intracranial collateral blood vessels, which are not routinely assessed by ABOX-CT as part of the surgical approach. Decreased oxygen delivery due to hypoxic postoperative anemia or hypotension can result in a cerebral infarct in these watershed areas.

A watertight dural closure may be difficult to achieve with large infratemporal skull base defects, particularly around nerves and vessels. An epidural fluid collection may result. In most cases, this is contained by the soft tissues and slowly resolves without further intervention. Occasionally, the CSF collection may communicate with the exterior through the external auditory canal, the scalp incision line, or along the eustachian tube to the nasopharynx. Most CSF leaks can be managed nonsurgically by placement of a pressure dressing and a spinal drain to diminish the CSF pressure. Surgical exploration and repair of the dural defect may be necessary if the CSF leak does not resolve within 1 week. A middle ear effusion is often apparent after infratemporal skull base approaches due to dysfunction or interruption of the eustachian tube. However, tympanostomy tubes are not placed for at least 6 weeks postoperatively, because there is always a risk of CSF communication.

We have encountered patients who developed profuse unilateral rhinorrhea in the postoperative period that was misinterpreted as a CSF leak. These cases all were associated with surgical dissection of the petrous ICA and are probably due to loss of the sympathetic fibers that travel along the ICA in their route to the nasal mucosa. This produces vasomotor rhinitis that may be treated with the use of anticholinergic nasal sprays. Testing of the fluid for β_2 transferrin, however, is mandatory to rule out a CSF leak.

Cosmetic deformities may result from the loss of soft tissue and bone. Transposition of the temporalis muscle results in a depression in the temporal area. This can be lessened by placement of a free-fat graft or hydroxyapatite cement in a secondary surgery. If the temporalis muscle is not transposed, the anterior margin of the muscle should be resutured anteriorly and superiorly to prevent its retraction and a resulting depression lateral to the orbital rim. The use of microvascular free muscle flaps, such as the rectus abdominis flap, for reconstruction may necessitate sacrifice of the zygomatic arch to accommodate the additional bulk. As the muscle atrophies, a significant depression may occur. It is important to repair all periosteal and muscle attachments around the maxilla, orbital rim, and zygomatic arch to avoid a "cadaveric" look that occurs when the soft tissues over these areas atrophy or retract. Large muscle flaps, such as a latissimus dorsi flap, may swell and compress the brain if the cranial base is not reconstructed.

References

1. Barbosa JF: Surgery of extensive cancer of paranasal sinuses: Presentation of a new technique. Arch Otolaryngol 73: 129–138, 1961.
2. Terz JJ, Young HF, Lawrence W Jr: Combined craniofacial resection for locally advanced carcinoma of the head and neck: II. Carcinoma of the paranasal sinuses. Am J Surg 140: 618–624, 1980.
3. Fisch U: The infratemporal fossa approach for the lateral skull base. Otolaryngol Clin North Am 17: 513–552, 1984.
4. Biller HF, Shugar JMA, Krespi YP: A new technique for wide-field exposure of the base of the skull. Arch Otolaryngol 107: 698–707, 1981.
5. Sekhar LN, Schramm VL, Jones NF: Subtemporal-preauricular infratemporal fossa approach to large lateral and posterior cranial base neoplasms. J Neurosurg 67: 499, 1987.
6. Cocke EW Jr, Robertson JH, Robertson JT, Crooke JP Jr: The extended maxillotomy and subtotal maxillectomy for excision of skull base tumors. Arch Otolaryngol Head Neck Surg 116: 92–104, 1990.
7. Janecka IP, Sen CN, Sekhar LN, Arriaga M: Facial translocation: A new approach to the cranial base. Arch Otolaryngol Head Neck Surg 103: 413–419, 1990.
8. Catalano PJ, Biller HF: Extended osteoplastic maxillotomy: A versatile new procedure for wide access to the central skull base and infratemporal fossa. Arch Otolaryngol Head Neck Surg 119: 394–400, 1993.
9. Snyderman CH, Carrau RL, de Vries EJ: Carotid artery resection: Update on preoperative evaluation. In Johnson JT, Derkay CS, Mandell-Brown MK, Newman RK (eds): AAO-HNS Instructional Courses, 6. 1993, pp 341–346.
10. Netterville JL, Jackson G, Civantos F: Thyroplasty in the functional rehabilitation of neurotologic skull base surgery patients. Am J Otol 14: 460–464, 1993.
11. Carrau RL, Pou A, Eibling DE, et al: Laryngeal framework surgery for the management of aspiration. Head Neck 21: 139–145, 1999.
12. Pou A, Carrau RL, Eibling DE, Murry T: Laryngeal framework surgery for the management of aspiration in high vagal lesions. Am J Otolaryngol 19: 1–8, 1998.
13. Nuss DW, Janecka IP, Sekhar LN, Sen CN: Craniofacial disassembly in the management of skull-base tumors. Otolaryngol Clin North Am 24: 1465–1497, 1991.
14. Sekhar LN, Sen C, Snyderman CH, Janecka IP: Anterior, anterolateral, and lateral approaches to extradural petroclival tumors. In Sekhar LN, Janecka IP (eds): Surgery of Cranial Base Tumors. New York, Raven Press, 1993, pp 157–223.

56

Petrosal Approach

C. Philip Daspit, M.D. ▪ Robert F. Spetzler, M.D.
Paul W. Detwiler, M.S., M.D.

Surgical approaches through the petrous bone can yield exquisite exposure of posterior fossa lesions, especially those involving the cerebellopontine angle (CPA) and clivus.[1–7] Since Decker and Malis[8] reported their experience with combined posterior fossa and subtemporal approaches to the clivus and medial petrous region in 1970, a variety of transpetrosal approaches have been espoused in the literature.[2, 9–27] Patients considered for surgery at the Barrow Neurological Institute are evaluated by the skull base team, which includes a study nurse, neuropathologist, neuro-otologist, craniofacial/plastic surgeon, neurosurgeon, oncologist, neuro-ophthalmologist, ear-nose-throat specialist, radiation oncologist, neuroradiologists, and a variety of clinical and research fellows. The surgical approach described in this chapter requires a neurosurgeon intimately acquainted with the microsurgical anatomy of the posterior fossa and a neuro-otologist with experience in drilling the petrous bone.

The petrosal approach is essentially a combined subtemporal-presigmoid approach and has three variations[24]: (1) retrolabyrinthine, (2) translabyrinthine, and (3) transcochlear. The retrolabyrinthine approach requires the least amount of drilling of the petrous bone with the goal of preserving hearing. A small window between the sigmoid sinus and labyrinth is created. The translabyrinthine approach requires more petrous bone to be removed, creating a larger and more ventral exposure at the expense of sacrificing hearing.[2] Partial resection of the labyrinth with the preservation of serviceable hearing has been described.[28] Finally, the transcochlear approach provides even more ventral exposure with maximum drilling of the petrous bone, destruction of the cochlear apparatus (sacrifice of hearing), and transposition of the facial nerve. These approaches afford increasing exposure of the clivus and medial petrous region with minimal or no retraction of neurologic structures. The petrosal sinus is sacrificed and the tentorium is completely sectioned. If preoperative angiography or magnetic resonance imaging (MRI) venography reveals stenosis or occlusion of the contralateral sigmoid sinus, the sinus on the side of surgery is preserved.

INDICATIONS

The petrosal approach has been used to treat extremely large lesions that extend above and below the tentorial incisura. Tumors,[26, 27, 29, 30] aneurysms, cavernous malformations, and arteriovenous malformations (AVMs) from the sphenoid region, cavernous sinus, foramen magnum, and anterior cervical spinal cord are amenable to treatment. In a prior report, we reviewed our experience with this approach in 46 patients.[24]

Preoperative MRI with and without contrast agent in the axial, coronal, and sagittal planes has become the diagnostic tool of choice. These studies are usually suggestive of the diagnosis and yield valuable information that can be used to plan the surgical trajectory. When a vascular lesion such as an aneurysm or AVM is suspected, patients undergo conventional cerebral angiography. Computed tomography (CT) with and without contrast agent is less sensitive than MRI for defining lesions around the skull base because resolution is reduced by bony artifact (beam hardening). CT, however, is superior to MRI for defining bony anatomy of the petrous bone. In most cases, the MR images are used in conjunction with a three-dimensional stereotactic image–guided system to localize eloquent brain intraoperatively and to define the borders of the lesion.

Selection of surgical approach is based on the location and size of the lesion, the suspected pathologic diagnosis, and the patient's baseline neurologic examination. Every attempt is made to preserve hearing and facial function in patients with no neurologic deficits. Patients with lesions that have rendered hearing nonfunctional are more likely to be treated with the transcochlear approach than patients with intact hearing.

PATIENT EDUCATION

The risks and benefits of all surgical and nonsurgical options, which are discussed with the patient, typically include embolization, surgical resection, stereotactic radiation, and a conservative approach with follow-up imaging. In patients at risk for cranial nerve injury such as facial palsy, both the risks of and procedures for repair and rehabilitation are discussed. The need for long-term clinical and radiographic follow-up is stressed with patients with skull base tumors such as meningiomas and acoustic neuromas. Follow-up imaging studies and the patient's status are reviewed by the comprehensive skull base team once a month.

NEUROANESTHESIA

After endotracheal anesthesia has been induced, a steroid bolus of intravenous dexamethasone (about 10 mg) is given. Steroids are tapered in the days after surgery depending on the pathologic diagnosis, degree of brain swelling, and degree of surgical manipulation of the cerebellum. A prophylactic dose of intravenous cefuroxime (1.5 g) is given after intubation and three postoperative doses are administered over 24 hours. An arterial line is placed to monitor systemic blood pressure and to evaluate oxygenation and ventilation. A central venous line allows rapid volume replacement if necessary. Compressed spectral analysis (CSA), somatosensory evoked potentials, facial nerve function, and other cranial nerves are monitored as warranted. Brainstem auditory evoked potentials (BAEPs) are monitored bilaterally or only contralaterally if hearing on the side of surgery is sacrificed. Barbiturates (thiopental) are administered intravenously at the time of durotomy and titrated to electroencephalographic burst suppression. This maneuver has two benefits: (1) barbiturate-induced reduction of metabolism provides cerebral protection, and (2) the cerebellum slackens significantly. Another maneuver to slacken the brain involves the drainage of cerebrospinal fluid (CSF) with either a ventriculostomy or lumbar drain. Osmotic agents such as mannitol and furosemide (Lasix) are also helpful.

SURGICAL TECHNIQUE

Patients are transported to the operating room awake and positioned supine on the operating table. General endotracheal intubation with the usual anesthesia monitoring is initiated. Complex monitoring involving BAEPs, CSA, and cranial nerve function is initiated before final positioning. A three-pin Mayfield headholder is attached to the head and rotated to expose the retroauricular area. Essentially, the head is turned parallel to the floor and slightly extended. The degree of neck rotation can be minimized by placing shoulder rolls. The patient is prepared and draped in the routine sterile fashion.

The incision begins over the zygoma approximately 1 cm anterior to the tragus, curves above the ear, and arcs posteriorly to the mastoid tip. If greater exposure is needed,

the posterior arc of the excision can be extended further posteriorly. For maximum inferolateral exposure of the foramen magnum, the incision can be combined with a far-lateral suboccipital approach.[31, 32] The lateral side of the skull is exposed by retracting the scalp flap inferiorly with fishhooks attached to a Leyla bar. This maneuver exposes the zygoma, lateral temporal bone, external auditory meatus, and mastoid region. The transverse sinus, transverse-sigmoid sinus junction, and sigmoid sinus are exposed using an Osteone drill (Hall Surgical, Santa Barbara, CA) and a high-power operating microscope. Continuous suction-irrigation is used during drilling to remove bony debris. The superficial exposure is started with a cutting burr, and finer diamond burrs are used to expose the great sinuses.

In patients with serviceable hearing on the surgical side, an extended retrolabyrinthine approach is favored (Fig. 56–1). The posterior and superior semicircular canals are skeletonized by drilling as far anteriorly as possible both above and below the otic capsule to expose as much dura as possible. After the transverse sigmoid junction is exposed, bone anterior to the sigmoid sinus is removed, exposing the dura of the middle fossa, the superior petrosal sinus, the sinodural angle, and, deeper, the endolymphatic sac. The endolymphatic sac and duct are posterior to the labyrinth and preserved during the exposure.

The neuro-otologist is replaced by the neurosurgeon, and a craniotomy flap is performed from the middle fossa across the transverse sinus into the posterior fossa. We prefer the Midas Rex drill (Midas Rex, Forth Worth, TX) with the B-1 bit and footplate. The stereotactic image–guided system identifies the location of the transverse sinus. Before any sinus is crossed with the drill, microirrigation is used to verify that the drill is in the epidural space and that the dura has not been lacerated. The neurosurgeon needs to be prepared to deal with significant venous hemorrhage if the sinus is injured.

The translabyrinthine approach, which renders the patient deaf (Fig. 56–2), provides greater exposure than the retrolabyrinthine procedure and is similar except that all

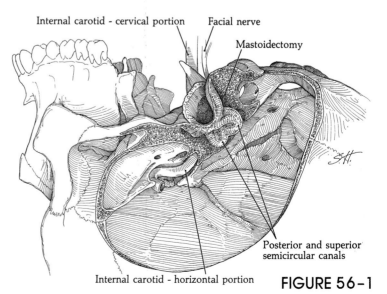

FIGURE 56–1. Artist's rendering of an extended retrolabyrinthine approach on the patient's right side. A mastoidectomy has been performed, and the superior and posterior semicircular canals have been skeletonized. The vertical segment of the petrous carotid artery has been exposed. (Courtesy of Barrow Neurological Institute, Phoenix, AZ.)

Internal carotid - cervical portion

Facial nerve

Mastoidectomy

Posterior and superior semicircular canals

Internal carotid - horizontal portion

FIGURE 56–1

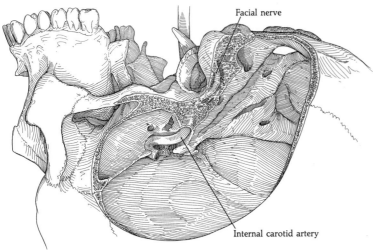

FIGURE 56–2. Right translabyrinthine approach. All three semicircular canals have been resected. The bony portion of the facial nerve in front of the semicircular canals has been exposed. (Courtesy of Barrow Neurological Institute, Phoenix, AZ.)

FIGURE 56-2

three semicircular canals are removed and the posterior half of the internal auditory canal is completely skeletonized. This modification permits greater removal of bone from the face of the petrous pyramid. If the lesion extends to the inferior clivus, bone overlying the sigmoid sinus and jugular bulb can be removed. The posterior external auditory canal and bone overlying the mastoid segment of the facial nerve are thinned. The distal end of the superior vestibular nerve is identified in the vestibule. This anatomic landmark is important because of the proximity to the facial nerve as it exits the internal auditory canal. Drilling over the facial nerve is performed with a diamond burr. A subtemporal-suboccipital craniotomy is performed as described in the retrolabyrinthine approach.

Maximum drilling of the petrous bone via the transcochlear approach sacrifices hearing but yields a very flat angle approach to the clivus (Fig. 56–3). The external auditory canal is transected and oversewn in two layers. The translabyrinthine approach is extended with removal of the facial nerve from its bony canal. The greater superficial petrosal nerve is sectioned and the facial nerve is mobilized

posteriorly. The dura of the internal auditory canal is used to protect the facial nerve. The entire tympanic portion of the temporal bone is removed and the periosteum of the temporomandibular joint is exposed. The internal auditory canal and cochlea are removed. The jugular bulb is exposed by removing the bone that separates it from the internal carotid artery (ICA) at the skull base. Cranial nerves IX, X, and XI are at risk during this maneuver. The bony wall of the carotid is removed to the siphon. The carotid artery can be exposed to allow a petrous ICA-to-subarachnoid ICA saphenous vein bypass, if necessary. The bone medial to the carotid artery is removed, exposing dura to the petrous tip. If direct exposure of the ICA is unnecessary, a thin rim of bone may be left surrounding the vessel. Bone is also removed from the floor of the middle fossa plate down to the horizontal segment of the ICA.

A dural incision is made over the temporal lobe at the anterior limit of the craniotomy (Fig. 56–4). The incision is extended posteriorly to at least 1 cm below the junction of the superior petrosal sinus and sigmoid sinus. Extreme caution must be exercised to avoid injury to the vein of

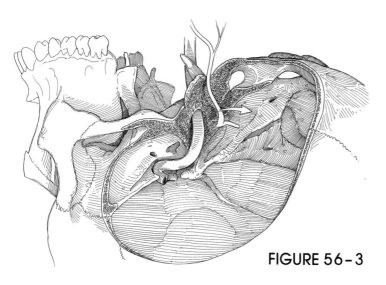

FIGURE 56–3. Transcochlear approach. The facial nerve has been transposed posteriorly to increase exposure. (Courtesy of Barrow Neurological Institute, Phoenix, AZ.)

FIGURE 56-3

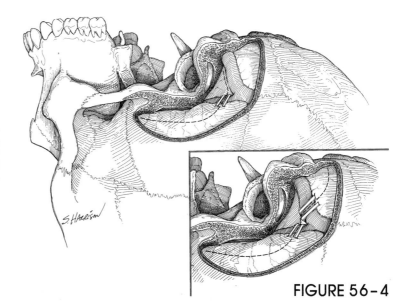

FIGURE 56–4. Translabyrinthine approach and a combined middle fossa–posterior fossa craniotomy. The dural opening *(dashed line)* can include the superior petrosal sinus or both the superior petrosal sinus and sigmoid sinus *(inset)*. (Courtesy of Barrow Neurological Institute, Phoenix, AZ.)

FIGURE 56–4

Labbé. This vein typically has three tributaries and drains into the transverse sinus just proximal to the transverse-sigmoid junction. If the sigmoid sinus is not sacrificed, the dural incision crosses the superior petrosal sinus to join a dural incision in front of the sigmoid sinus. Another incision can be made behind the sigmoid sinus if necessary (Fig. 56–4 *inset*).

The sigmoid sinus on the surgical side can be sacrificed if two criteria are met. First, angiographic verification is needed that both the superior sagittal sinus and straight sinus drain into the contralateral transverse-sigmoid sinus complex. Second, we have developed an intraoperative monitoring technique in which a 25-gauge needle is inserted into the sinus, and pressure is recorded before and after occlusion of the sinus[24] below the proposed side of the occlusion/transection. If pressure increases less than 7 mm Hg, the sinus can be sacrificed. If pressure inside the sigmoid sinus increases by more than 10 mm Hg with temporary occlusion, the sinus is preserved. We have kept the sigmoid sinus intact in one third of our cases based on preoperative angiography or because the additional exposure provided by sectioning the sigmoid sinus was unnecessary.

If the sigmoid sinus is sacrificed, the ipsilateral vein of Labbé drains contralaterally because it reliably enters the lateral sinus above the junction of the superior petrosal and sigmoid sinuses (Fig. 56–5). If the sigmoid sinus is preserved and the superior temporal lobe is elevated, the vein of Labbé is at risk and must be protected.[29] Telfa is placed on the surface of the brain, and retractors are repositioned and optimized to allow exposure of the ipsilateral petrous region, the entire clivus, and the cranial nerves (Figs. 56–6 through 56–13). The lesions are addressed using microsurgical technique with constant attention to minimizing brain retraction.

At the completion of the procedure, the dura is reapproximated using 4-0 braided nylon running sutures. The defect in the temporal bone is obliterated with Gelfoam, abdominal fat graft, and fibrin glue. We are in the process of evaluating the efficacy of reconstructing the bony defect with bone substitutes. It is unclear whether these substitutes will reduce the incidence of delayed CSF leaks and meningitis. Temporary CSF diversion is provided by lumbar drainage titrated to 10 to 15 ml/hr for 3 to 5 days. A routine mastoid head dressing is applied for 2 days. Steroids are tapered over about 6 days. Patients are encouraged to ambulate as soon as possible after removal of the lumbar drain.

SUMMARY

The petrosal approach is a subtemporal-presigmoid sinus operation. Progressively more of the CPA and clivus is exposed as the extent of drilling of the petrous bone increases from the retrolabyrinthine to translabyrinthine to transcochlear approach. The latter two involve the unilateral destruction of hearing. The transcochlear approach also involves mobilization of the facial nerve. CSF leak rates can be as high as 20 per cent and remain a formidable complication (Table 56–1).[11, 33–37]

TABLE 56–1. Complications Associated with the Petrosal Approach

Facial nerve injury
Cerebrospinal fluid leak
Meningitis
Decreased gag reflex
Abducens nerve paresis
Numbness
Aphasia
Sepsis
Hemiparesis
Pneumonia
Intracranial hematoma

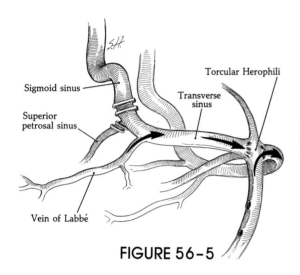

Sigmoid sinus

Transverse sinus

Torcular Herophili

Superior petrosal sinus

Vein of Labbé

FIGURE 56–5

FIGURE 56–5. After the superior petrosal and sigmoid sinuses are sacrificed, the vein of Labbé drains (anterograde) into the transverse sinus (retrograde). (Courtesy of Barrow Neurological Institute, Phoenix, AZ.)

FIGURE 56–6. The temporal lobe and tentorium are elevated with mild retraction without injuring the vein of Labbé. The exposure facilitates access to the ipsilateral petrous region, the entire clivus, and cranial nerves V, VI, VII, VIII, IX, X, and XI. (Courtesy of Barrow Neurological Institute, Phoenix, AZ.)

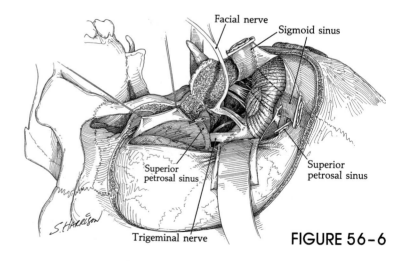

Facial nerve

Sigmoid sinus

Superior petrosal sinus

Superior petrosal sinus

Trigeminal nerve

FIGURE 56–6

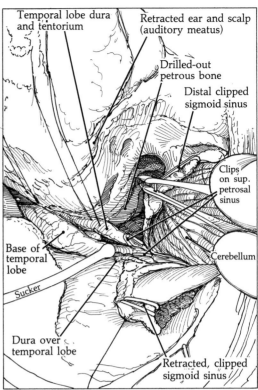

FIGURE 56–7. Translabyrinthine approach. The sigmoid sinus has been sacrificed and divided. The dura of the middle and posterior fossae has been opened (refer to Fig. 56–4). The tentorium is cut starting between the clips on the superior petrosal sinus. (From Spetzler RF, Daspit CP, Pappas CTE: The combined supra- and infratentorial approach for lesions of the petrous and clival regions: Experience with 46 cases. J Neurosurg 76: 588–599, 1992.)

FIGURE 56–7

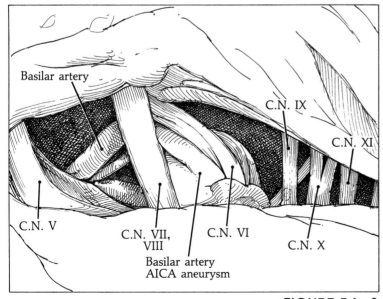

FIGURE 56–8

FIGURE 56–8. Artist's rendering of the petrosal approach to a basilar artery aneurysm. The neck of the aneurysm was well visualized as were cranial nerves (CN) V, VI, VII, VIII, IX, X, and XI. Cranial nerve VI is draped over the dome of the aneurysm. AICA, anteroinferior cerebellar artery. (From Spetzler RF, Daspit CP, Pappas CTE: The combined supra- and infratentorial approach for lesions of the petrous and clival regions: Experience with 46 cases. J Neurosurg 76: 588–599, 1992.)

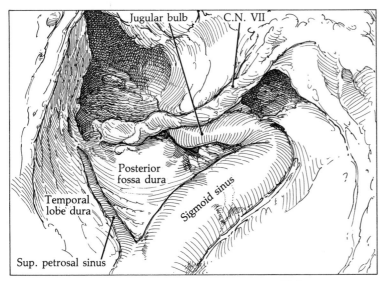

FIGURE 56–9. Transcochlear approach with exposure of the sigmoid sinus and the jugular bulb. The superior (Sup) petrosal sinus courses between the dura of the middle and posterior fossae and enters the proximal sigmoid sinus. The facial nerve has been drilled out and the greater superficial petrosal nerve has been cut to mobilize the facial nerve. CN, cranial nerve. (From Spetzler RF, Daspit CP, Pappas CTE: The combined supra- and infratentorial approach for lesions of the petrous and clival regions: Experience with 46 cases. J Neurosurg 76: 588–599, 1992.)

FIGURE 56-9

FIGURE 56–10. Transcochlear approach with exposure of the ventral brainstem. This approach provides good exposure to lesions involving Meckel's cave. CN, cranial nerve. (From Spetzler RF, Daspit CP, Pappas CTE: The combined supra- and infratentorial approach for lesions of the petrous and clival regions: Experience with 46 cases. J Neurosurg 76: 588–599, 1992.)

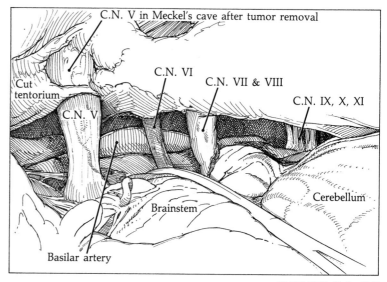

FIGURE 56-10

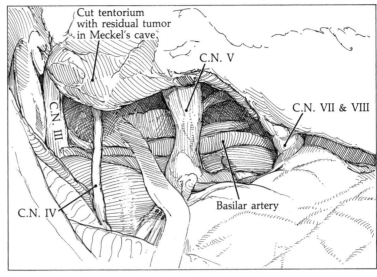

FIGURE 56-11. Schematic drawing demonstrating a more anterior view with exposure of cranial nerves (CN) III through VIII. (From Spetzler RF, Daspit CP, Pappas CTE: The combined supra- and infratentorial approach for lesions of the petrous and clival regions: Experience with 46 cases. J Neurosurg 76: 588–599, 1992.)

FIGURE 56-11

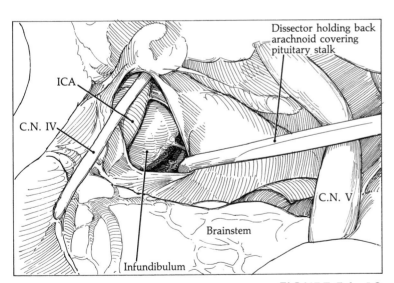

FIGURE 56-12. Artist's rendering after resection of a large clivus meningioma. Note the excellent view of the pituitary stalk. ICA, internal carotid artery; CN, cranial nerve. (From Spetzler RF, Daspit CP, Pappas CTE: The combined supra- and infratentorial approach for lesions of the petrous and clival regions: Experience with 46 cases. J Neurosurg 76: 588–599, 1992.)

FIGURE 56-12

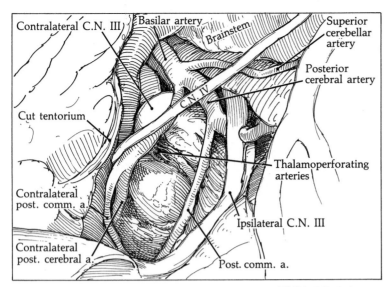

FIGURE 56–13. Schematic view of the ventral brainstem from a different orientation. CN, cranial nerve; post. comm. a., posterior communication artery. (From Spetzler RF, Daspit CP, Pappas CTE: The combined supra- and infratentorial approach for lesions of the petrous and clival regions: Experience with 46 cases. J Neurosurg 76: 588–599, 1992.)

FIGURE 56-13

References

1. Ammirati M, Ma J, Cheatham ML, et al: Drilling the posterior wall of the petrous pyramid: A microneurosurgical anatomical study. J Neurosurg 78: 452, 1993.
2. Briggs RJS, Luxford WM, Atkins JS Jr, et al: Translabyrinthine removal of large acoustic neuromas. Neurosurgery 34: 785, 1994.
3. Glasscock ME III, Miller GW, Drake FD, et al: Surgery of the skull base. Laryngoscope 88: 905, 1978.
4. Maniglia AJ, Fenstermaker RA, Ratcheson RA: Preservation of hearing in the surgical removal of cerebellopontine angle tumors. Otolaryngol Clin North Am 22: 211, 1989.
5. Rhoton ALJ, Tedeschi H: Microsurgical anatomy of acoustic neuroma. Otolaryngol Clin North Am 25: 257, 1992.
6. Sekhar LN, Jannetta PJ, Burkhart LE, et al: Meningiomas involving the clivus: A six-year experience with 41 patients. Neurosurgery 27: 764, 1990.
7. Tator CH, Nedzelski JM: Facial nerve preservation in patients with large acoustic neuromas treated by a combined middle fossa transtentorial translabyrinthine approach. J Neurosurg 57: 1, 1982.
8. Decker RE, Malis LI: Surgical approach to midline lesions at base of skull. J Mt Sinai Hosp 37: 84, 1970.
9. Arriaga MA, Luxford WM, Berliner KI: Facial nerve function following middle fossa and translabyrinthine acoustic tumor surgery: A comparison. Am J Otol 15: 620, 1994.
10. Brackmann DE, Green JD: Translabyrinthine approach for acoustic tumor removal. Otolaryngol Clin North Am 25: 311, 1992.
11. Darrouzet V, Guerin J, Aouad N, et al: The widened retrolabyrinthine approach: A new concept in acoustic neuroma surgery. J Neurosurg 86: 812, 1997.
12. Fagan PA, Sheehy JP, Chang P, et al: The cerebellopontine angle: Does the translabyrinthine approach give adequate access? Laryngoscope 108: 679, 1998.
13. Giannotta SL: Translabyrinthine approach for removal of medium and large tumors of the cerebellopontine angle. Clin Neurosurg 38: 589, 1992.
14. Haddad GF, Al-Mefty O: Approaches to petroclival tumors. In Wilkins RH, Rengachary SS (eds): Neurosurgery, 2nd ed, Vol 2. New York, McGraw-Hill, 1996, p 1695.
15. Hakuba A, Nishimura S, Jang BJ: A combined retroauricular and preauricular transpetrosal-transtentorial approach to clivus meningiomas. Surg Neurol 30: 108, 1988.
16. Hardy DG, MacFarlane R, Baguley DM, et al: Surgery for acoustic neurinoma: An analysis of 100 translabyrinthine operations. J Neurosurg 71: 799, 1989.

17. Hitselberger WE: Translabyrinthine approach to acoustic tumors. Am J Otol 14: 7, 1993.
18. House WF, Belal A Jr: Translabyrinthine surgery: Anatomy and pathology. Am J Otol 1: 189, 1980.
19. King TT, Morrison AW: Translabyrinthine and transtentorial removal of acoustic nerve tumors: Results in 150 cases. J Neurosurg 52: 210, 1980.
20. Lanman TH, Brackmann DE, Hitselberger WE, et al: Report of 190 consecutive cases of large acoustic tumors (vestibular schwannoma) removed via the translabyrinthine approach. J Neurosurg 90: 617, 1999.
21. McElveen JT Jr: The translabyrinthine approach to cerebellopontine angle tumors. In Wilkins RH, Rengachary SS (eds): Neurosurgery, 2nd ed, Vol 1. New York, McGraw-Hill, 1996, p 1107.
22. Roberson JB Jr, Brackmann DE, Hitselberger WE: Acoustic neuroma recurrence after suboccipital resection: Management with translabyrinthine resection. Am J Otol 17: 307, 1996.
23. Shea MC, Robertson JT: Acoustic neuroma removal: A comparative study of translabyrinthine and suboccipital approaches. Am J Otol 1: 94, 1979.
24. Spetzler RF, Daspit CP, Pappas CT: The combined supra- and infratentorial approach for lesions of the petrous and clival regions: Experience with 46 cases. J Neurosurg 76: 588, 1992.
25. Thomsen J, Tos M, Harmsen A: Acoustic neuroma surgery: Results of translabyrinthine tumour removal in 300 patients. Discussion of choice of approach in relation to overall results and possibility of hearing preservation. Br J Neurosurg 3: 349, 1989.
26. Tos M, Thomsen J: The translabyrinthine approach for the removal of large acoustic neuromas. Arch Otorhinolaryngol 246: 292, 1989.
27. Tos M, Thomsen J, Harmsen A: Results of translabyrinthine removal of 300 acoustic neuromas related to tumour size. Acta Otolaryngol (Stockh) 452: 38, 1988.
28. Sekhar LN, Schessel DA, Bucur SD, et al: Partial labyrinthectomy petrous apicectomy approach to neoplastic and vascular lesions of the petroclival area. Neurosurgery 44: 537, 1999.
29. Al-Mefty O, Fox JL, Smith RR: Petrosal approach for petroclival meningiomas. Neurosurgery 22: 510, 1988.
30. Kanzaki J, Shiobara R, Toya S: Acoustic neuroma surgery: Translabyrinthine-transtentorial approach via the middle cranial fossa. Arch Otorhinolaryngol 229: 261, 1980.
31. Heros RC: Lateral suboccipital approach for vertebral and vertebrobasilar artery lesions. J Neurosurg 64: 559, 1986.
32. Spetzler RF, Grahm TW: The far-lateral approach to the inferior

clivus and the upper cervical region: Technical note. BNI Q 6: 35, 1990.

33. Celikkanat SM, Saleh E, Khashaba A, et al: Cerebrospinal fluid leak after translabyrinthine acoustic neuroma surgery. Otolaryngol Head Neck Surg 112: 654, 1995.

34. Hoffman RA: Cerebrospinal fluid leak following acoustic neuroma removal. Laryngoscope 104: 40, 1994.

35. House JL, Hitselberger WE, House WF: Wound closure and cerebrospinal fluid leak after translabyrinthine surgery. Am J Otol 4: 126, 1982.

36. Meyerson LR, Monsell EM, Rock JP: Preventive management of cerebrospinal fluid leakage in translabyrinthine surgery. Laryngoscope 106: 610, 1996.

37. Rodgers GK, Luxford WM: Factors affecting the development of cerebrospinal fluid leak and meningitis after translabyrinthine acoustic tumor surgery. Laryngoscope 103: 959, 1993.

57

Treatment of Bilateral Acoustic Neuromas

Richard T. Miyamoto, M.D., F.A.C.S., F.A.A.P. ▪ Karen L. Roos, M.D.
Robert L. Campbell, M.D.

The presence of bilateral acoustic neuromas is the hallmark of neurofibromatosis type 2 (NF-2) (Fig. 57–1). However, despite this unique hallmark, NF-2 has only recently been recognized as a distinct clinical entity. Prior to 1987, all patients with phenotypic manifestations of neurofibromatosis, that is, café au lait macules or subcutaneous neurofibromas, were considered to be at risk for developing bilateral acoustic neuromas, but extensive screening programs infrequently identified these tumors. The National Institutes of Health Consensus Development Conference on Neurofibromatosis in 1987[1] clarified this inconsistency by identifying two clinically and genetically distinct forms of neurofibromatosis. Clinical criteria differentiating these forms of neurofibromatosis have greatly assisted clinicians in determining which patients are at risk of developing bilateral acoustic neuromas and which are not.

When acoustic neuromas occur bilaterally, initial treatment planning is directed toward the prevention of life-threatening sequelae. Although the preservation of auditory function is of paramount concern, this goal has seldom been documented. With the advent of auditory brainstem response testing, advanced imaging techniques, and new genetic information, bilateral acoustic neuromas can be identified at an early stage when hearing preservation is feasible. Successful surgical intervention that eliminates the inevitable total, bilateral deafness can now be attained in selected patients.[2–11] When surgical removal of the tumors and hearing preservation cannot be accomplished, new technology incorporating electrical stimulation of the auditory system provides a therapeutic option in the aural rehabilitation of these patients.

CLASSIFICATION OF NEUROFIBROMATOSIS (Table 57–1)

Neurofibromatoses primarily affect cell growth of neural tissues and can cause tumors to grow on nerves at any time and at any location. A wide range of expressivity may be seen, even within a family, and variant forms may exist that confound classification in some patients. Resultant manifestations may be innocuous or may be progressive and result in significant morbidity or even mortality.

Neurofibromatosis Type 1

The most common type of neurofibromatosis, NF-1, affects approximately 1 in 4000 individuals. This disorder was previously labeled von Recklinghausen's disease or peripheral neurofibromatosis. Individuals with NF-1 typically have multiple café au lait macules, Lisch nodules, optic nerve gliomas, and dermal, subcutaneous, and plexiform neurofibromas. A diagnosis of NF-1 is made in an individual in whom at least two of the following seven features are found:

1. Six or more café au lait spots larger than 5 mm in children and 15 mm in teenagers and adults
2. Two or more neurofibromas or one plexiform neurofibroma
3. Freckling in the axilla or groin areas
4. Optic nerve glioma
5. Two or more iris hamartomas (Lisch nodules)
6. A distinctive bony lesion, such as sphenoid wing dysplasia or thinning of the long bone cortex, with or without pseudoarthrosis
7. A first-degree relative with NF-1 according to the above criteria

Neurofibromatosis Type 2

NF-2 affects approximately 1 in 40,000 individuals. NF-2 is characterized by bilateral acoustic neuromas, presenile lens opacities, dermal, subcutaneous, and plexiform neurofibromas, and brain and spinal cord tumors. NF-2 has also been referred to as *hereditary bilateral vestibular schwannoma syndrome* to emphasize that the origin of the eighth cranial nerve tumors is the vestibular nerve, not the acoustic nerve, and that the tumors are schwannomas and not true neuromas. The previously applied term "central neurofibromatosis" is no longer used. A diagnosis of NF-2 is made in an individual who has bilateral eighth cranial nerve tumors or a first-degree relative (parent, sibling, or child) with NF-2 and either a unilateral eighth cranial nerve tumor or two of the following:

1. Dermal or subcutaneous neurofibromas
2. Plexiform neurofibroma
3. Schwannoma
4. Glioma
5. Juvenile posterior subcapsular cataract

Although NF-1 and NF-2 are distinctly different disorders, they share many clinical characteristics. Both NF-1 and NF-2 are autosomal dominant disorders; therefore, 50

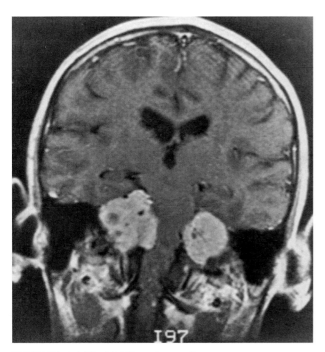

FIGURE 57–1. MRI with bilateral acoustic neuroma.

au lait spots are found predominantly on the trunk and appear within the first year of life in most individuals with NF-1 and are present by age 4 years in most affected children. Neurofibromas appear just before puberty and increase in number and size throughout adulthood. The clinical manifestations of NF-2 are more subtle. Signs of NF-2 may not become apparent until puberty or early adulthood but may appear as late as the seventh decade of life. Therefore, individuals at risk of inheriting the NF-2 gene must be followed up closely for many years for signs of the development of an acoustic neuroma. Although individuals with either disorder may have café au lait spots and neurofibromas, those with NF-2 tend to have a smaller number of café au lait spots and neurofibromas than those with NF-1. Axillary freckling is unique to those with NF-1. An individual who clearly has NF-1 is not at risk for developing an acoustic neuroma.

All individuals with bilateral acoustic neuromas have NF-2 by definition and are at risk for developing other tumors, such as meningiomas, schwannomas, gliomas, ependymomas, and plexiform neurofibromas. Recently, Eldridge and Parry[12] suggested a further subclassification of NF-2. Three broad groupings emerged from a study of families with multiple members affected and individuals representing sporadic cases when age at onset, rate of progression of hearing loss, and presence or absence of associated brain and spinal cord tumors were correlated.

The first type of NF-2, described by Feiling in 1920 and Gardner in 1930, is characterized by onset of hearing loss in the third and fourth decade and few, if any, associated brain and spinal cord tumors. Hearing may be preserved until late in life, especially in males. The second type of NF-2 was described by Wishart in 1822. It is characterized by earlier onset of hearing loss, more rapid progression to spontaneous deafness, and multiple brain and spinal cord tumors. Brain tumors include other cranial nerve schwannomas and meningiomas, which may develop on the optic nerve sheath and may be bilateral in the posterior fossa. Spinal tumors include extramedullary and paraspinal schwannomas and meningiomas, as well as intramedullary

per cent of the offspring of individuals with NF-1 and NF-2 will be affected. Both disorders demonstrate high penetrance but with great variability of expression and severity from one individual to another. Approximately 50 per cent of the cases of NF-1 and NF-2 are the result of sporadic mutations; this mutation rate is the highest for any human genetic disorder described to date. Eighty per cent of the mutations of the NF-1 gene are of paternal origin.

In spite of the similarities, clear distinguishing differences exist between NF-1 and NF-2. The age of onset of signs and symptoms is earlier in NF-1. In fact, the diagnosis may be made at birth or during infancy by examination of the skin. The typical hyperpigmented macules or café

TABLE 57–1. Features of Neurofibromatosis (NF) Types 1 and 2

PARAMETER	NF-1	NF-2
Synonyms	Peripheral NF von Recklinghausen	Central NF Bilateral acoustic NF
Incidence	30/100,000	3/100,000
Age of onset	First decade	Second or third decade
Skin manifestations		
Cutaneous neurofibromas	95% have >2	>30% have >1
>5 café au lait spots	Found in most	Rare
Intertriginous freckles	Usually present	Rare
Eye manifestations		
Lisch nodules	Present in >90%	Rare
Lens abnormalities	Not reported	Posterior capsular cataract in >50%
Bony abnormalities	Common	Not reported
Central nervous system tumors		
Acoustic neuromas	None documented in familial cases	Bilateral in 96%
Other brain tumors	Optic glioma in 2–15%	9–100%, depending on NF-2 type
Spinal cord tumors	Occasional	Common in several types of NF-2

Modified from Ferris NJ, Siu KH: Neurofibromatosis 2: Report of an affected kindred, with a discussion on imaging strategy. Australas Radiol 34:229–233, 1990.

low-grade astrocytomas and ependymomas. Because the clinical course may be rapid, reproduction is often impaired, and cases tend to be sporadic. The third type of NF-2 was described by Lee and Abbott. This form displays variable age at initial hearing loss and at spontaneous deafness. A distinguishing feature is the early morbidity due to associated tumors, which tend to be numerous, especially when they involve the spinal cord. Cerebellopontine angle meningiomas, meningiomatosis en plaque of the falx, and schwannomatosis of spinal nerve roots are common.

The ophthalmologic examination may help distinguish between NF-1 and NF-2 in an individual with café au lait macules and neurofibromas. Both forms of neurofibromatosis may be accompanied by distinct eye changes that can be definitive in diagnosis. Lisch nodules of the iris occur in more than 85 per cent of postpubertal patients with NF-1 but have been reported in only one patient with NF-2.[13] They are melanocytic hamartomas that appear as yellow or brown, raised, dome-shaped lesions on the surface of the iris. Posterior subcapsular opacities of the lens are seen in approximately 40 to 50 per cent of individuals with NF-2 but have not been described in patients with NF-1.[14] This association is of interest because the gene for NF-2 and one of the genes controlling β-B2 lens crystallin are in the same region on the long arm of chromosome 22. Optic gliomas, although seen in NF-1, are not seen in NF-2.

MOLECULAR GENETICS

Neurofibromatosis Type 1

The gene for NF-1 was identified by genetic linkage analysis and found to be on chromosome 17.[15] Subsequently, two unrelated patients with NF-1 were identified who had translocations disrupting chromosome 17 at band 17q11.2. This finding helped localize the NF-1 gene to band 17q on the long arm of chromosome 17 near the centromere.[16]

Neurofibromatosis Type 2

The gene for NF-2 has been localized to the middle of the long arm of chromosome 22. The initial clue for the location of the NF-2 gene was uncovered by the application of a primary mechanism of tumorigenesis in humans that was discovered in embryonal tumors to the formation of tumors associated with NF-2. By this mechanism, tumor growth occurs in a two-step process. The initial event is a primary mutation that results in the formation of an allele—a change in a DNA sequence at a point on a chromosome—that is recessive at the cellular level to the normal allele. The growth of a tumor occurs only after an additional change, such as a loss of a chromosome, allows for expression of the altered allele.[17]

Individuals with NF-2 frequently develop meningiomas as well as acoustic neuromas. The development of a meningioma is associated with a loss of one copy of chromosome 22. As demonstrated by Seizinger and colleagues,[17] the formation of an acoustic neuroma is also specifically associated with loss of genes on chromosome 22, suggesting

that chromosome 22 might contain a locus for a tumor suppressor gene or antioncogene. Loss of this gene allows for malignant transformation of certain cells. These same investigators subsequently demonstrated specific loss of alleles from chromosome 22 in two acoustic neuromas, two neurofibromas, and one meningioma from individuals with NF-2.[18] Only a portion of the long arm of chromosome 22 was deleted in the two acoustic neuromas, narrowing the chromosomal location of the gene causing NF-2 to the region near the center of the long arm of chromosome 22. By linkage analysis of a large kindred with NF-2, Rouleau[19] and Wertelecki[20] and their coworkers were able to pinpoint the locus for this disorder at the center of the long arm of chromosome 22 (22q11.1-22q13.1).

Clinical Manifestations

The initial symptoms of an acoustic neuroma are loss of hearing, tinnitus, or dysequilibrium. The hearing loss is a progressive sensorineural hearing loss, usually with poor discrimination. Although the tumors arise from the vestibular nerves, acute vertigo is uncommon because the slow growth pattern allows the ear to compensate as the tumor enlarges. These tumors may become symptomatic for the first time over a wide age range, from ages 10 to 60 years, although most become symptomatic between ages 20 and 40. The rate of growth of acoustic neuromas in patients with NF-2 is unpredictable. NF-2 should be ruled out in any patient who develops an acoustic neuroma before the age of 40.

The initial evaluation of an individual whose condition is highly suggestive of NF-2 should include pure tone audiometry and a T1W magnetic resonance imaging (MRI) scan with gadolinium. The gadolinium-enhanced MRI scan is the best neuroimaging procedure for detecting small intracanalicular neuromas and can detect these tumors in children before they are symptomatic. Brainstem auditory evoked response and acoustic reflex studies are helpful screening procedures.

Individuals with NF-2 should have annual ophthalmologic evaluations. A posterior subcapsular opacity of the lens is present in 40 to 50 per cent of individuals with NF-2 by age 30 years and may produce progressive visual loss.[21]

Patients with NF-2 are at risk for developing central nervous system tumors, particularly Schwann cell tumors. These tumors develop on spinal nerve roots, within the spinal cord, particularly in the cervical cord area, and on the cranial nerves. The tumors can grow very rapidly. An MRI scan of the entire neural axis in patients with NF-2 is useful in detecting asymptomatic schwannomas along the spinal cord. Individuals with NF-2 are also at risk for meningiomas, spinal ependymomas, and astrocytomas.

All individuals younger than age 40 with a sporadic, unilateral acoustic neuroma should be examined carefully for neurofibromas, café au lait spots, posterior subcapsular cataracts, and abnormalities on neurologic examination that suggest the presence of other central nervous system tumors. Follow-up evaluation with gadolinium-enhanced MRI scan and pure tone audiometry enables early detection of an acoustic neuroma on the contralateral side, if this develops.

MANAGEMENT

When acoustic neuromas occur bilaterally (NF-2), initial treatment planning is influenced by tumor size at the time of diagnosis and their anticipated growth pattern and the patient's age and hearing status. The growth pattern of acoustic neuromas is unpredictable: some tumors grow slowly over many years, whereas others may enlarge rapidly, resulting in deafness, cerebellar dysfunction, or brainstem compression.

Initial treatment planning must be directed toward the prevention of life-threatening sequelae resulting from brainstem compression or increased intracranial pressure. After this concern has been addressed, the preservation of auditory function in at least one ear is of great concern. However, hearing preservation has been an elusive goal in NF-2 patients because bilateral acoustic neuromas have a tendency to invade rather than compress adjacent nerves.[22] This renders difficult the definitive treatment of bilateral acoustic tumors while preserving hearing.

Surgical intervention is currently the only treatment for enlarging acoustic tumors. As a general rule, acoustic tumors of any size should be removed when aidable hearing is not present and the patient is suitable for an elective operation. When serviceable or aidable hearing is present and the tumor does not appear to adhere to the brainstem on preoperative imaging studies, hearing preservation surgery may be appropriate. Because most acoustic neuromas arise from the superior or inferior vestibular nerves, preservation of the cochlear nerve and its blood supply is feasible in some cases through the use of microsurgical techniques. Two surgical approaches have been applied. The middle fossa approach described by William House is appropriate for small intracanalicular tumors or tumors that extend slightly medial to the porus acusticus.[23] The retrosigmoid or suboccipital approach may be applied for intracanalicular tumors or for some slightly larger tumors that extend into the cerebellopontine angle. The intracranial course of the cochlear nerve can be traced from its origin at the pontomedullary junction to the lateral end of the internal auditory canal just proximal to its entrance into the cochlea. Intraoperative monitoring of facial and cochlear nerve function have augmented the current surgical technique.

Although size is only one tumor characteristic influencing hearing preservation, the likelihood of tumor invasion into the cochlear nerve is less if the tumor can be detected early in its course. Current imaging techniques using MRI with gadolinium have greatly enhanced our ability to detect tumors. However, the invasive tendencies of acoustic neuromas cannot be assessed by preoperative imaging. Only by surgical exploration can these properties be determined. If the tumor is invading the cochlear nerve, subtotal removal and decompression of the internal auditory canal may delay progression of hearing loss.[24]

Clinical Approaches

There are seven basic management strategies for patients with bilateral acoustic neuromas. Each has specific indications and disadvantages. Individualization of management is a prerequisite.

Hearing Preservation Surgery—Total Tumor Removal. The two surgical approaches applicable are the middle fossa and retrosigmoid approaches. The indications and limitations discussed in previous chapters for these approaches also apply to bilateral tumors. The difficult decision often involves which side lesion to attempt (larger vs. smaller tumor and better- vs. worse-hearing ear). Usually the larger tumor and poorer-hearing ear are operated on first. If hearing is successfully preserved on one side, the other side may be considered for surgery 6 months following the initial procedure.

Observation Without Surgical Intervention. A small tumor in an only-hearing ear or bilateral tumors too large for hearing preservation are usually managed by observation. Close clinical and MRI follow-up (initially at 6 months and then annually) allows adequate assessment of brainstem compression or hydrocephalus. The patients must understand the importance of notifying the otologist of any symptoms that may signify tumor growth or brainstem compression. Surgery is considered when further hearing loss develops, clinical symptoms increase, or the tumor reaches sufficient size for brainstem compression (usually 3 cm). The observation time is an important opportunity for educational rehabilitation, counseling, signing and lip-reading classes, and family screening.

Middle Fossa Craniotomy—Internal Auditory Canal Decompression Without Tumor Removal. This technique is an option for patients undergoing observation who experience fluctuation or progression of hearing loss. The goal of this strategy is to relieve the constriction on the cochlear nerve and blood supply without subjecting the patient to the increased risk of hearing loss if tumor debulking is initiated. The basic principles of middle fossa tumor surgery apply. The dura of the internal auditory canal and porus acusticus is incised; however, the tumor is not removed or debulked. This technique has been successfully employed to stabilize and even improve hearing in patients with bilateral tumors.[24]

Retrosigmoid Partial Tumor Removal. The theory for partial tumor removal is preservation of the seventh and eighth nerves by removing only those portions of the tumor farthest from the nerves. Although this approach is advocated in some centers,[25] its success has been limited. Debulking the tumor may affect the blood supply along the cochlear nerve, and rapid regrowth of tumor from the well-vascularized capsule is common.

Nonhearing Preservation—Total Removal. When hearing preservation is not an issue, the goal of management is total tumor removal and facial nerve preservation. Translabyrinthine or retrosigmoid techniques are suitable, although distal internal auditory canal exposure of the seventh nerve is often more direct with the translabyrinthine approach. Hearing rehabilitation can be accomplished with a cochlear implant if the cochlear nerve is preserved, or the auditory brainstem implant (see Chapter 58) if the cochlear nerve is transected.

Auditory Brainstem Implant. The auditory brainstem implant is a therapeutic option in cases of bilateral acoustic neuromas. After tumor removal, an electrode array is placed within lateral recess over the cochlear nucleus. Coded electrical signals are presented directly to the brainstem (Figs. 57–2 and 57–3).

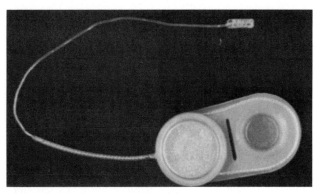

FIGURE 57–2. Auditory brainstem implant electrode and receiver coil.

Stereotactic Radiosurgery (Radiation Therapy). Stereotactic surgery is closed-skull destruction of a precisely definable intracranial tissue through use of ionizing radiation. This technique, which combines a stereotactic delivery device with ionizing radiation, was initially described by Leksell[26] in 1951. In 1968, Larsson and associates[27] designed and applied the first gamma knife stereotactic radiosurgical unit. The dose of radiation in stereotactic radiosurgery is delivered by means of several evenly distributed and precisely collimated beams of ionizing radiation. The radiation dose gradient is extremely sharp at the target tissue, resulting in a radiation lesion that is sharply circumscribed. Tissue adjacent to the target structures sustains little damage.

Stereotactic radiosurgery is a treatment alternative for some NF-2 patients. However, this approach is not without morbidity. Progressive hearing deterioration or deafness has been reported in 64 per cent, transient facial paralysis in 12 per cent, facial hypesthesia in 4 per cent, and progressive tumor growth in 34 per cent. Hydrocephalus has also been reported as a complication of stereotactic radiosurgery.[28]

Additionally, disadvantages of this technique include radiation-induced fibrosis, which complicates tumor removal when surgery becomes necessary owing to continued tumor growth. Similarly, this fibrosis may produce anatomic distortion that prevents successful placement of an auditory brainstem implant. Finally, in larger tumors there is increased risk of radiation necrosis of the adjacent brainstem and cerebellum.

With further refinements and experience with stereotactic radiosurgery, it appears that morbidity has been reduced. In a review of 162 consecutive patients who underwent radiosurgery, tumor control was reported in 98 per cent.[29] Normal facial nerve function was reported in 79 per cent, and 51 per cent reported no hearing change. Thirty-one per cent reported at least one complication, and 3 per cent experienced hydrocephalus.

Other Management Considerations

NF-2 is a heritable disease with significant morbidity; therefore, every patient must be fully educated and the family must be screened to identify other affected or at-risk individuals. Genetic counseling is important, and the geneticist should direct the family screening.

Auditory rehabilitation of all NF-2 patients should anticipate eventual hearing loss. Early training in speechreading, signing, and use of the telephone typewriter (TTY) will provide necessary skills when significant hearing loss occurs.

Other Tumors

Other intracranial and spinous tumors, as well as malignant tumors, occur in NF patients and must be evaluated. The surgical treatment of nonmalignant tumors is selectively introduced when clinically progressive disease is implicated. Ideally, intervention is accomplished without increasing the neurologic deficit.

DISCUSSION

In selected patients, careful observation of the tumors with serial audiometrics and serial MRI scans may be most appropriate. This approach may be advisable in a patient with an apparently stable acoustic neuroma in one ear and no hearing in the opposite ear. The approach may be used in a patient with a family history of the Feiling and Gardner type in which the tumor occurs in the third or fourth decade of life and slow tumor progression has been documented in other family members.

The gamut of possibilities regarding hearing in surgical treatment of bilateral acoustic neuromas ranges from total removal with hearing preservation to removal with the application of sophisticated new technology incorporating electrical stimulation of the auditory system. It is hoped that if newly diagnosed bilateral tumors are treated more aggressively at the outset, hearing preservation surgery will be accomplished more frequently. When total removal and hearing preservation are not possible, cochlear implantation may be feasible if the cochlear nerve can be anatomically preserved. Cohen and colleagues[30] reported on such a patient, in whom total removal of bilateral acoustic neuromas was accomplished but with loss of hearing. The cochlear

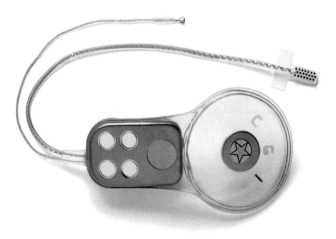

FIGURE 57–3. Nucleus 24 auditory brainstem implant. (Courtesy of Cochlear Corporation, Englewood, CO.)

nerve was preserved on one side, and a cochlear implant was performed in this ear. The patient was able to recognize various environmental sounds and had both closed- and open-set speech discrimination. When total removal of bilateral acoustic neuromas is performed and it is not possible to preserve the cochlear nerve, another treatment option is the auditory brainstem implant.[31] In this approach, an electrode is placed on the cochlear nucleus, and coded electrical signals are presented directly to the brainstem. Ongoing research is being conducted at the House Ear Institute to develop a multichannel brainstem stimulator to improve results over those obtained with the single-channel auditory brainstem implant, which has been under investigation since 1979.[32, 33] Yet another approach that has met with some success is the application of tactile devices that convert sound to tactile displays presented to the skin.[34]

References

1. National Institutes of Health Consensus Development Conference: Conference Report—Neurofibromatosis Conference Statement. Arch Neurol 45: 575–578, 1988.
2. Hitselberger WE, Hughes RL: Bilateral acoustic tumors and neurofibromatosis. Arch Otolaryngol Head Neck Surg 88(Monograph II): 152–711, 1968.
3. Hughes GB, Sismanis A, Glasscock ME III, et al: Management of bilateral acoustic tumors. Laryngoscope 92: 1351–1359, 1982.
4. Malis L: Neurofibromatosis. *In* Cummings CW, Frederickson JM, Harker LE (eds): Otolaryngology—Head and Neck Surgery. St. Louis, CV Mosby, 1986, pp 3449–3456.
5. Tator CH, Nedzelski JM: Preservation of hearing in patients undergoing excision of acoustic neuromas and other cerebellopontine angle tumors. J Neurosurg 63: 168–174, 1985.
6. Dutcher PO, House WF, Hitselberger WE: Early detection of small bilateral acoustic tumors. Am J Otol 8: 35–38, 1987.
7. Piffko P, Pasztor E: Operated bilateral acoustic neurinoma with preservation of hearing and facial nerve function. ORL Otorhinolaryngol Relat Spec 43: 255–261, 1981.
8. Miyamoto RT, Campbell RL, Fritsch M, Lochmueller G: Preservation of hearing in neurofibromatosis 2. Otolaryngol Head Neck Surg 103: 619–624, 1990.
9. Miyamoto RT, Roos KL, Campbell RL, Worth RM: Contemporary management of neurofibromatosis. Ann Otol Rhinol Laryngol 100: 38–43, 1991.
10. Miyamoto RT, Roos KL, Campbell RL: Hearing preservation in neurofibromatosis 2. *In* Tos M, Thomsen J (eds): Acoustic Neuroma. Amsterdam/New York, Kugler Publications, 1992, pp 843–847.
11. Miyamoto RT, Roos KL, Campbell RL: Hearing preservation in neurofibromatosis 2. *In* Samii M (ed): Proceedings of the First International Skull Base Congress. Hannover, Germany, June 14–20, 1992.
12. Eldridge R, Parry D: Neurofibromatosis 2: Evidence for clinical heterogeneity based on 54 affected individuals studied by MRI with gadolinium, 1987–1991. *In* Tos M, Thomsen J (eds): Acoustic Neuroma. Amsterdam/New York, Kugler Publications, 1992, pp 801–804.
13. Lubs ML, Bauer MS, Formas ME, Djokic B: Lisch nodules in neurofibromatosis type 1. N Engl J Med 324: 1264–1266, 1991.
14. Kaiser-Kupfer MI, Freidlin V, Datiles MB, et al: The association of posterior capsular lens opacities with bilateral acoustic neuromas in patients with neurofibromatosis type 2. Arch Ophthalmol Head Neck Surg 107: 541–544, 1989.
15. Goldgar DE, Green P, Parry DM, Mulvihill JJ: Multipoint linkage analysis in neurofibromatosis type 1: An international collaboration. Am J Hum Genet 44: 6–12, 1989.
16. Ledbetter DH, Rich DC, O'Connell P, et al: Precise localization of NF-1 to 17 q 11.2 by balanced translocation. Am J Hum Genet 44: 20–24, 1989.
17. Seizinger BR, Martuza RL, Gusella JF: Loss of genes on chromosome 22 in tumorigenesis of human acoustic neuroma. Nature 322: 644–647, 1986.
18. Seizinger BR, Rouleau G, Ozelius LJ, et al: Common pathogenetic mechanism for three tumor types in bilateral acoustic neurofibromatosis. Science 236: 317–319, 1987.
19. Rouleau GA, Wertelecki W, Haines JL, et al: Genetic linkage of bilateral acoustic neurofibromatosis to a DNA marker on chromosome 22. Nature 329: 246–248, 1987.
20. Wertelecki W, Rouleau GA, Superneau DW, et al: Neurofibromatosis 2: Clinical and DNA linkage studies of a large kindred. N Engl J Med 319: 278–283, 1988.
21. Roos KL, Dunn DW: Neurofibromatosis. CA Cancer J Clin 42: 241–254, 1992.
22. Linthicum FH Jr, Brackmann DE: Bilateral acoustic tumors: A diagnostic and surgical challenge. Arch Otolaryngol Head Neck Surg 106: 729–733, 1980.
23. House WF, Gardner G, Hughes RL: Middle cranial fossa approach to acoustic tumor surgery. Arch Otolaryngol 88: 631, 1968.
24. Gadre AK, Kwartler JA, Brackmann DE, et al: Middle fossa decompression of the internal auditory canal in acoustic neuroma surgery: A therapeutic alternative. Laryngoscope 100: 948–951, 1990.
25. Kemink JL, Langman AW, Niparko JK, Graham MD: Operative management of acoustic neuromas: The priority of neurologic function over complete resection. Otolaryngol Head Neck Surg 104: 96–99, 1991.
26. Leksell L: The stereotaxic method and radiosurgery of the brain. Acta Chir Scand 102: 316–319, 1951.
27. Larsson B, Leksell L, Rexed B, et al: The high-energy proton beam as a neurosurgical tool. Nature 182: 1222–1223, 1968.
28. Thomsen J, Tos M, Borgesen S: Gamma knife: Hydrocephalus as a complication of the stereotactic radiosurgical treatment of acoustic neuroma. Am J Otol 11: 330–333, 1990.
29. Kondziolka D, Lunsford LD, McLaughlin MR, Flickinger JC: Long-term outcomes after radiosurgery for acoustic neuromas. N Engl J Med 339: 1426–1433, 1998.
30. Cohen NL, Ransohoff J, Kohan D, Hoffman R: Cochlear implants in the treatment of acoustic neuromas: A treatment algorithm for bilateral acoustic neuromas (BAN). *In* Tos M, Thomsen J (eds): Acoustic Neuroma. Amsterdam/New York, Kugler Publications, 1992, pp 857–862.
31. Nelson RA: Auditory brainstem implant. *In* Tos M, Thomsen J (eds): Acoustic Neuroma. Amsterdam/New York, Kugler Publications, 1992, pp 869–872.
32. Terr LI, Fayad J, Hitselberger WE, Rizkalla Z: Cochlear nucleus anatomy related to central electroauditory prosthesis implantation. Otolaryngol Head Neck Surg 102: 717–721, 1990.
33. Shannon RV, Otto SR: Psychophysical measures from electrical stimulation of the human cochlear nucleus. Hear Res 47: 159–168, 1990.
34. Miyamoto RT, Myres WA, Wagner M, Punch JL: Vibrotactile devices as sensory aid for the deaf. Otolaryngol Head Neck Surg 97: 57–63, 1987.

58

Auditory Brainstem Implant

Steven R. Otto, M.A. ▪ William E. Hitselberger, M.D.
Fred F. Telischi, M.D. ▪ Derald E. Brackmann, M.D.
Lendra M. Friesen, M.S.

Loss of auditory nerve integrity, as often occurs after removal of vestibular schwannomas in neurofibromatosis type 2 (NF-2), for many years left patients completely deafened. Sign language, lipreading, and vibrotactile aids provided some communication assistance but could not restore useful auditory sensations. The development of the auditory brainstem implant (ABI) provided a means of bypassing the cochlea and auditory nerve to directly stimulate the cochlear nucleus complex, thereby giving sound sensations to otherwise deaf patients.

This chapter updates and discusses the clinical and surgical aspects of ABI electrode array placement and perceptual performance. The techniques are derived from experience in the implantation of 93 patients with various devices since 1979 at House Ear Clinic and Institute (HEI, Los Angeles). Clinical trials of an 8-electrode multichannel ABI are completed and U.S. Food and Drug Administration (FDA) approval was obtained in October 2000. New ABI recipients are being implanted with a 21-electrode ABI. A penetrating electrode array system for the brainstem also has been developed and may proceed to limited use in humans.

General technical and theoretical considerations of central auditory implantation and stimulation have been reviewed elsewhere.[1, 2]

PATIENT SELECTION

Patients have received the ABI under a protocol monitored by the FDA. The criteria for implantation are listed in Table 58–1. Only patients with NF-2 manifesting bilateral vestibular schwannomas may receive the device. At least 90 per cent of NF-2 patients exhibit bilateral eighth nerve neuromas.[3] An unpublished review of patients with NF-2 seen at the House Ear Clinic revealed that two thirds had bilateral internal auditory canal–cerebellopontine angle (CPA) tumors alone or with one other tumor as the only central nervous system manifestation of their disease. The patients were young (average age, 28 years). With improvements in medical care and surgical techniques, the life span of many of these patients has been significantly prolonged. Restoration of even rudimentary auditory function can enhance their quality of life and ability to function in a hearing world. Our results have shown that the multichannel ABI has the potential of offering even greater benefit.

The current protocol allows implantation at the time of first- or second-side acoustic neuroma removal or in patients whose tumors have previously been removed. Implantation during removal of the first tumor has allowed experience with the device and may enhance performance when the patient loses all hearing. Also, implantation on the first side gives the patient two chances at obtaining an optimally functioning system should the procedure in the first side not be successful.

The management of bilateral acoustic neuromas should be highly individualized.[4] Hearing preservation remains an ideal goal in the management of these tumors in patients with NF-2, and early identification and treatment have permitted this in a number of cases. An intact auditory system is highly desirable in preference to an artificial means of restoring hearing. Therefore, preserving as much of the patient's own hearing as possible is paramount. Patients meeting the criteria listed in Table 58–2 may be considered and observed accordingly. The availability of the ABI provides an alternative to a desperate attempt to preserve nonserviceable hearing when large tumors are removed and hearing conservation is unlikely.

Future applications of the ABI and similar devices include bilateral temporal bone fractures and demyelinating diseases affecting the eighth cranial nerve but sparing at least one cochlear nucleus.

PREOPERATIVE EVALUATION AND COUNSELING

The goal of implantation is to place a safe and stable device that provides the patient with some degree of environmental sound awareness and recognition and also improves communication in conjunction with lipreading without side effects. Prospective patients are apprised of the goals, limitations, and risks of the ABI during two or three evaluation and counseling sessions similar to those of cochlear implantation. It is important to impress on the potential candidate that, although the ABI is similar to a

TABLE 58–1. Criteria for Implantation

Evidence of bilateral seventh and eighth cranial nerve tumors involving the internal auditory canal or cerebellopontine angle
Language competency
Age 12 years or older
Psychologic suitability
Willingness to comply with research follow-up protocol
Realistic expectations

TABLE 58–2. Criteria for Observation in Auditory Brainstem Implant Candidacy in Patients with Neurofibromatosis Type 2

Second tumor in an only-hearing ear
Any tumor in a hearing ear that measures >2 cm in the largest diameter (hearing preservation unlikely with removal)
Short life expectancy due to other tumors, medical problems, or advanced age
Serviceable hearing with a tumor that shows no significant growth by sequential magnetic resonance scans and stable hearing by serial audiograms

cochlear implant, it has provided generally lower levels of performance with more gradual improvement over time. The implant candidate's expectations are carefully evaluated, and informed consent is obtained. The importance of an experienced multidisciplinary implant team including the neurotologist, neurosurgeon, audiologist, neuro/auditory physiologist, anatomist, radiologist, and others cannot be overemphasized.

Several factors contribute to a successful result from implantation. Experience of team members can greatly influence outcomes. Chief among these factors are the correct identification of the implantation site and the achievement of a stable placement of the electrode array. This, of course, is essential to obtain auditory sensations from stimulation and to optimize performance. The overall results of tumor removal and postoperative recovery also play a role. For example, factors such as eye dryness related to postoperative facial nerve function may affect lipreading ability and communication using the ABI. General health, social activity level, and presence of a support group also can affect ABI use and benefit. Patient expectations are important and may be influenced by publicity about cochlear implants. Assessing expectations for the ABI and ensuring informed consent prior to implantation are highly important but may be complicated in candidates overwhelmed by a plethora of preoperative concerns. A patient and frank appraisal of the potential benefits, limitations, and requirements for adjusting to the device preoperatively will help increase the likelihood of a satisfied device user in the long run. At this time, the ABI requires a certain level of acceptance, motivation, and commitment from the recipient to maximize benefit; therefore, the device may not be for everyone.

DEVICE

The ABI hardware has evolved through a number of modifications since the original ball electrode was inserted by Drs. William Hitselberger and William House in 1979.[1, 5] Significant design changes have involved transitioning from a percutaneous connector to a transcutaneous coil link to the implant, converting from ribbon electrodes to 1-mm-diameter disk electrodes, and fabrication of a semiflexible silicone electrode carrier (2.5 × 8.5 mm) with a specialized mesh backing to stabilize placement. The first 25 ABI recipients were fitted with a single-channel sound processor and a 2- or 3-electrode array. Since 1992, the electrode array used in most patients has employed eight platinum disks in a perforated silicone and mesh carrier connected to an implantable receiver/stimulator (Cochlear Corporation) (see Fig. 57–2). The external device consists of a postauricular microphone, a transcutaneous transmitter coil, and a sound processor (Spectra Model, Cochlear Corporation). Signal-processing strategies have evolved in an effort to improve performance.[6] Future patients will receive a 21-electrode array (Fig. 58–1A and B) interfaced with a new external sound processor (Sprint Model, Cochlear Corporation). Use of a hybrid ABI array consisting of the present surface electrode and a 6-electrode penetrating array also is pending. Implementation of this system in laboratory animals has shown the capability for improved microstimulation of auditory neurons[7] that may lead to improved perceptual performance in humans.

ANATOMIC CONSIDERATIONS

The target of the ABI electrodes is the cochlear nucleus complex—dorsal and ventral cochlear nuclei. In humans, the cerebellar peduncle that forms the base of the pons covers the auditory nuclei. This means that the nuclei are not visible to the surgeon and must be located from surface

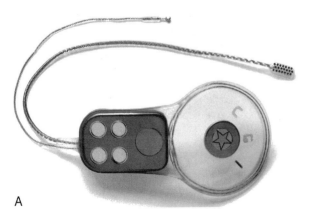
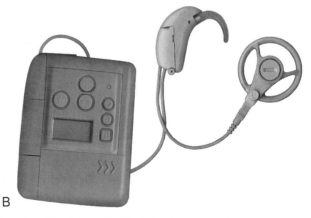

A

B

FIGURE 58–1. *A,* Auditory brainstem implant 24 receiver/stimulator with 21-electrode array and remote ball ground electrode. *B,* Esprit auditory brainstem implant speech processor, postauricular microphone, and transmitter coil. (*A* and *B,* Courtesy of Cochlear Corporation, Englewood, CO.)

landmarks. Figure 58–2 illustrates the major structures of the pontomedullary junction region with the translabyrinthine approach surgical field of view within the dashed lines. The terminus of the sleeve-like lateral recess forms the foramen of Luschka. Just inferior to the foramen is the root of the glossopharyngeal (ninth) nerve. Superior to the foramen lie the root entry and exit zones of the vestibulocochlear and facial nerves. This area is frequently distorted by the tumor, although a computer-assisted three-dimensional (3D) reconstruction of the cochlear nuclei in an acoustic neuroma patient showed the overall shape of the complex unchanged.

The cochlear nuclei come closest to the surface of the brainstem within the superior aspect of the lateral recess.[8, 9] The main target for stimulation is the ventral cochlear nucleus, which forms the main relay for eighth nerve input and the greater part of the ascending auditory pathway.[10] Placement of the electrodes completely within the recess gives the fewest side effects and preserves auditory stimu-

lation even though some part of the electrode array lies adjacent to the dorsal cochlear nucleus.[2] Also, the disadvantage of lack of exposure is partially offset by positional stability provided to the electrode carrier by the limited space in the lateral recess.

SURGICAL CONSIDERATIONS

The surgical approach for tumor removal in ABI cases has been exclusively via translabyrinthine craniotomy (see Chapter 50). The translabyrinthine route has been found to provide the most direct access to the lateral recess and surface of the cochlear nuclei.[11] Until the actual placement of the device, the surgery proceeds as in any other translabyrinthine acoustic neuroma excision, with the following exceptions. Electrodes are placed for recording electrically evoked auditory brainstem responses (EABRs) and for monitoring cranial nerves VII and IX. The routine postau-

FIGURE 58–2

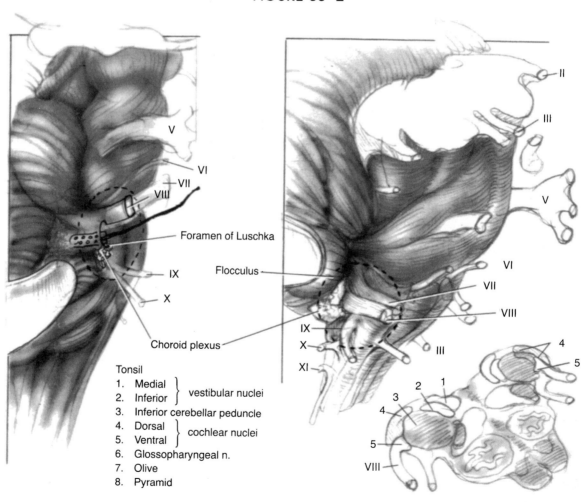

Tonsil
1. Medial ⎱
2. Inferior ⎰ vestibular nuclei
3. Inferior cerebellar peduncle
4. Dorsal ⎱
5. Ventral ⎰ cochlear nuclei
6. Glossopharyngeal n.
7. Olive
8. Pyramid

FIGURE 58–2. Schematic of cochlear nuclei region demonstrating relative location of various landmarks. Dashed area represents approximate surgical view. Electrode is fully inserted into proper position.

ricular incision is used initially but then extended superiorly and posteriorly to create a flap to cover the ABI receiver/stimulator. It is important that the incision not cross the receiver (Fig. 58–3).

Electrophysiologic monitoring is performed during implantation to ensure that the electrode array placement is correct for activating the auditory system and also to assess activation of nonauditory brainstem structures. There may be considerable uncertainty about the correct position for the electrode array when a large tumor has distorted the anatomic landmarks at the brainstem. To aid in placing the electrode array, EABRs are recorded. A repeatable EABR indicates that stimulation of the auditory system is occurring. Intraoperative EABRs obtained with electrical stimulation of the cochlear nucleus differ considerably from brainstem responses routinely recorded with acoustic stimulation (ABRs) in awake individuals.[10] An experienced electrophysiologist interprets these waveforms at the time of implantation based on data collected from previous implants (Fig. 58–4).

For recording EABRs, subdermal needle electrodes are inserted at the vertex of the head, over the seventh cervical vertebra in the neck, and at the hairline of the occiput prior to the draping of the sterile field. After the receiver/stimulator of the implant has been fastened to the skull and the electrode array has been placed on the brainstem, the transmitter coil is placed over the receiver antenna. The stimuli for evoking responses are biphasic current pulses. Scalp-recorded evoked potentials are sampled and averaged by computer following suitable amplification and filtering.

Electrophysiologic monitoring also helps determine the electrode array position that minimizes nonauditory side effects. In addition to monitoring the facial nerve in standard manner,[12] bipolar electrodes are inserted in the ipsilateral pharyngeal (soft palate) muscles to monitor activation of cranial nerve IX. If the electromyographic recordings reveal activation of nonauditory centers during stimulation through the implant, or if a muscle evoked potential is seen in the monitored waveform, the electrode array is repositioned.

IMPLANTATION TECHNIQUE

Tumor dissection proceeds normally via a translabyrinthine craniotomy. After tumor removal and hemostasis, an area of cortical bone posterior to the mastoid is flattened, and a trough to accept the wires from the electrodes to the receiver/stimulator is created in a manner similar to that of cochlear implantation. Using a replica of the receiver/stimulator as a guide, a circular area of bony cortex posterosuperior to the mastoid defect is drilled with cutting burrs (Fig. 58–5). A specially designed butterfly bit or other cylindrical bits associated with newer high-speed

FIGURE 58-3

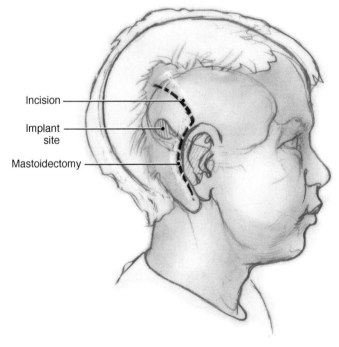

FIGURE 58-4

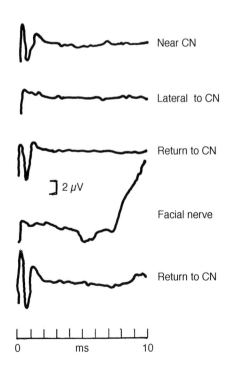

FIGURE 58–3. Location of incision with respect to planned site of receiver coil.

FIGURE 58–4. Electrically evoked auditory brainstem responses. CN, cochlear nucleus.

FIGURE 58-5

FIGURE 58-6

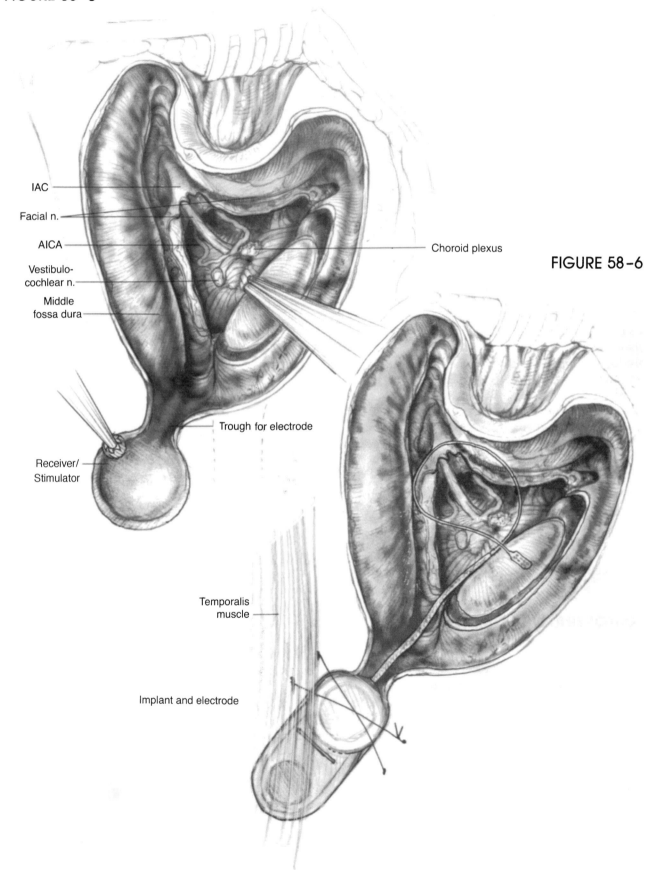

IAC

Facial n.

AICA

Vestibulo-
cochlear n.

Middle
fossa dura

Choroid plexus

Trough for electrode

Receiver/
Stimulator

Temporalis
muscle

Implant and electrode

FIGURES 58–5 and 58–6. *See legends on opposite page*

drills may be employed. Using a replica of the receiver/stimulator as a guide, the surgeon drills four holes into the bone to accept the tiedown suture. The receiver/stimulator is fixed with nylon suture prior to electrode array positioning so that the manipulation of the leads does not alter the electrode placement (Fig. 58–6). Because only bipolar cautery may be used after the electrode array is inserted to minimize the risk of current shunting through the device into the brainstem, meticulous hemostasis of the entire wound and CPA is ensured prior to implantation.

Anatomic landmarks lead the way to the surface of the cochlear nuclei. Normally intact choroid plexus marks the entrance to the lateral recess (foramen of Luschka), and the taenia obliquely traverses the roof of the lateral recess, marking the surface of the ventral cochlear nucleus. These structures may not be clearly visible, however, when a large tumor has significantly distorted the lateral aspect of the pons and medulla. Following the stump of the eighth cranial nerve usually leads to the opening of the lateral recess in these cases. The ninth cranial nerve can also be used as a reference point for the lateral recess. A concavity sometimes visualized between the eighth and ninth nerves should not be confused with the introitus of the recess. The location of the lateral recess may be confirmed by noting the egress of cerebrospinal fluid as the anesthesiologist induces a Valsalva maneuver in the patient. This technique should be reserved as a final check after the opening to the recess has been located by standard landmarks because cerebrospinal fluid will be drained quickly and the advantage of this technique will be lost with multiple Valsalva maneuvers.

After identifying the foramen of Luschka, a Rosen needle is used to insert the electrode array into the lateral recess with the electrodes facing superiorly (Fig. 58–7). With experience, we have found that the system functions better, with fewer side effects, when the electrodes are placed fully within the lateral recess.[2] After placement, selected electrodes in the array are activated to confirm their position over the nucleus. They are tested for the presence of EABRs, stimulation of adjacent cranial nerves (VII and IX), and changes in vital signs. The position of the electrode array usually needs some adjustment to maximize the EABRs and minimize electromyographic responses from the other nerves.

The electrode array is secured by a small piece of Teflon felt packed into the meatus of the lateral recess. Fibrous tissue eventually stabilizes the array in position. The wires are positioned in the mastoid cavity and the bony trough previously drilled (Fig. 58–8). Abdominal fat obliterates the mastoid defect. The incision is closed in three layers, and care is taken not to disturb the wires. The wound is not drained routinely. A large mastoid-type dressing is left in place for 4 days.

POSTOPERATIVE CARE

The postoperative care after implantation shares many of the features of routine translabyrinthine tumor resections (see Chapter 50). A similar schedule for advancing patient activity and decreasing the level of intensity of nursing care is maintained. A mastoid dressing should remain in place for at least 4 days. Careful attention to any moisture on the bandages allows prompt identification of cerebrospinal fluid leak through the postauricular wound. Intravenous antibiotics are administered prophylactically 1 day preoperatively and continued through the fifth day postoperatively.

While we originally attempted testing of ABI recipients' devices within days after surgery, we no longer do so. Swelling of the skin flap covering the receiver/stimulator may prevent an adequate signal from reaching the implant and preventing device power-up. Instead, the device is typically activated for the first time about 4 to 8 weeks after implantation. Because the magnet is typically removed from the receiver/stimulator so that patients may continue to have magnetic resonance imaging (MRI), there may be difficulty in identifying the location of the antenna of the receiver/stimulator at the time of initial stimulation. If the receiver/stimulator cannot be located, the transmitter coil may not be properly positioned at initial stimulation, and it may mistakenly appear that the device is nonfunctional or the patient is nonstimulable. While normally it is possible to palpate the scalp for the location of the receiver, this may not be possible in patients with thicker skin. Therefore, consideration should be given to this potential difficulty at the time of implantation and appropriate steps taken (such as possible thinning of the flap, or otherwise identifying receiver/stimulator location) prior to the initial stimulation session. In actual use, ABI patients must shave this area and apply a thin tape and metal disk to which the magnetic transmitter coil can adhere. The patient, or a companion, must be trained to ensure proper and consistent positioning of the transmitter coil over the implant receiver/stimulator.

POSTOPERATIVE COMPLICATIONS

The most significant complication in the immediate postoperative period is cerebrospinal fluid leak. Unlike routine translabyrinthine surgery, in which the fluid usually takes the nasal route via the eustachian tube, the ABI electrode and wires provide a path along which cerebrospinal fluid can travel beneath the skin flap. We have noted a marked reduction in the rate of leak after transitioning over to the fully implantable receiver from a percutaneous connector used with the single-channel ABI. Prevention of a leak begins with meticulous dural approximation and packing of the eustachian tube and mastoid cavity with various materials. Although the dural opening cannot be closed in a watertight manner, it should be approximated as closely as possible to minimize the opening. A dumbbell-shaped graft of fat will plug the residual space. Muscle and oxidized cellulose (Surgicel) commonly are employed for eustachian tube closure, and autologous fat works well in the

FIGURE 58–5. Surgical view of completed translabyrinthine craniotomy, trough for wires, and coil site being drilled.

FIGURE 58–6. Device secured in place with suture.

FIGURE 58-7

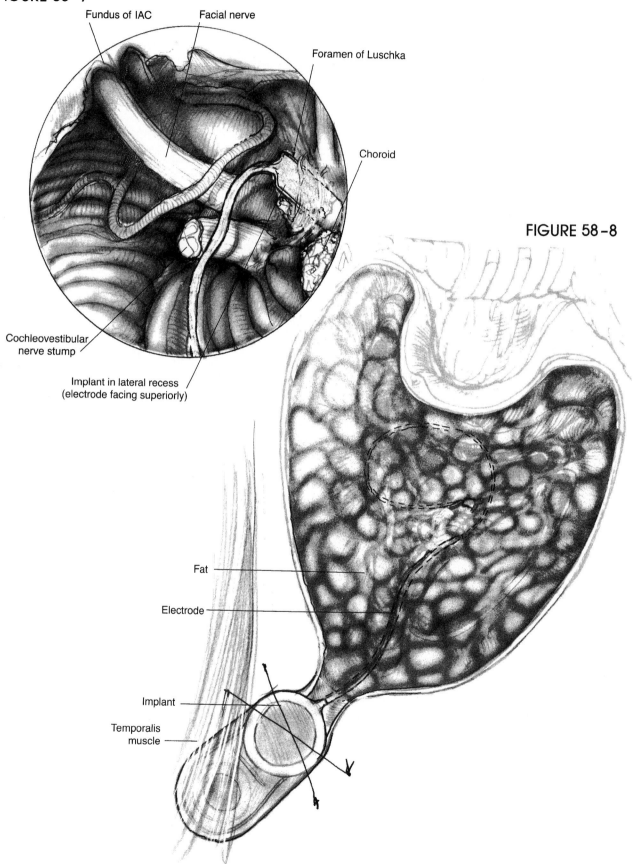

FIGURES 58–7 and 58–8. *See legends on opposite page*

mastoid. Multilayered closure for the wound decreases pathways for cerebrospinal fluid egress.

Despite these precautions, patients with the ABI appear more prone to cerebrospinal fluid leak than do those undergoing translabyrinthine procedures without implantation. Leaks from the nose and wound usually respond to reapplication of mastoid pressure dressing and bed rest. A lumbar-subarachnoid cerebrospinal fluid drain is added for persistent leaks. Finally, surgical exploration and repacking of the wound can be employed for leakage unresponsive to more conservative measures.

Meningitis can occur either spontaneously or as a result of postoperative cerebrospinal fluid leak. This unusual complication, when identified promptly, responds to antibiotics and cessation of the leak.

Normal healing to a stable implant situation usually takes 4 to 6 weeks, after which initial activation of the device occurs. Multichannel ABI recipients now have experienced up to 8 years of trouble-free use of the device. The first patient ever to be implanted with an ABI in 1979 continues to use her single-channel implant with benefit on a daily basis.

RESULTS

Seventy-one patients with NF-2 have been implanted with the Nucleus 8-electrode multichannel ABI system at the HEI between 1992 and the present. These data comprise a large portion of a clinical trials submission to the FDA.[13] Sixty-nine patients at HEI have completed at least the initial stimulation and evaluation session. In this chapter, we present results from speech and environmental sounds testing of 25 patients with at least 2 years of ABI experience. Since performance with the ABI improves more gradually than in cochlear implants, these later results are more representative of the longer term benefit. Early results on a majority of these patients have been presented elsewhere.[6] Even 2 years of experience should not be considered sufficient to reach asymptomatic performance. Although improvements are generally greatest during the first year, several patients have continued to improve even after 7 years of use. All patients used the Nucleus Spectra speech processor with the SPEAK (spectral maxima) speech processing strategy.[14]

Figure 58–9 shows mean scores on a portion of the multichannel ABI perceptual test battery. The lowest scores shown are for the CID and City University of New York (CUNY) sentence tests, which are presented in sound only. These tests are difficult for the majority of ABI recipients, and they reflect the generally limited capability of the ABI in open-set tasks. The CUNY sentence scores in vision alone and in sound plus vision modes are higher than those administered with sound alone because of the visual cues provided. Obviously lipreading cues are highly important in face-to-face communication, and a large average in-crease (39 per cent) in sentence recognition occurs when ABI sound is added to lipreading as indicated by the vision only and sound plus vision CUNY scores.

The Monosyllable, Trochee, Spondee (MTS) test, Sound Effects Recognition Test (SERT), and Northwestern University Children's Perception of Speech (NUCHIPS) test are all closed-set tests in which the individual has to select the correct answer from a limited set of items. Therefore, these tests are somewhat easier than open-set tests, but they nevertheless represent a challenging auditory discrimination task to ABI recipients. In the MTS Word (MTS-W) test and the NUCHIPS test the listener selects a word from a set of alternatives. In the case of NUCHIPS, they are rhyming words. In the SERT, the patient selects the correct sound from a set of four pictured alternatives. The highest mean score on all the perceptual tests occurs on the MTS Stress (MTS-S) test, which is a derived score from the MTS-W test. The patient does not have to correctly identify the word—only the correct stress pattern of the word presented, making it one of the easiest tasks. Tests such as the MTS-S and SERT provide rather immediate evidence to new ABI recipients that the auditory cues they receive from their implants are indeed useful.

With notable exceptions, these results indicate that ABI performance generally has not reached the high levels typically seen with multichannel cochlear implants. At least three patients have shown high levels (≥50 per cent better) of open-set speech recognition ability on sound-only sentence tests, and several others have shown significant (at least 20 per cent correct) ability in this area. There is reason to be hopeful that ABI performance in general will improve. Many ABI recipients experience electrode-specific pitch sensations similar to cochlear implant patients, and it may be possible to increase these cues with improved methods of microstimulation. Capitalizing on these cues by carefully assessing auditory percepts from ABI stimulation can be time consuming but is a necessary part of programming the speech processor to optimize performance.[13]

Perceptual test scores of ABI recipients presently indicate a significant ability to discriminate many environmental sounds as well as enhance sentence recognition ability over lipreading only. Several of the best performers use the telephone with familiar speakers in controlled conditions. Nevertheless, as is true of hearing aids and cochlear implants, the ABI cannot be expected to be highly beneficial for every potential candidate. Because sound from the device is most effective in combination with lipreading cues, patients with limited vision may experience relatively less communication benefit. Patients with limited social contact may find fewer occasions to use the ABI. Also, we have noted generally less satisfactory acceptance and use of the ABI by teenagers. Some patients (7 per cent in our hands) have not received auditory sensations at all, instead experiencing only mild or moderate nonauditory side effects when their device was activated. These cases were

FIGURE 58–7. Surgical view of the electrodes being passed into the lateral recess (magnified view of the dashed area in Figure 58–5).

FIGURE 58–8. Implant, wires, and fat in place prior to skin closure.

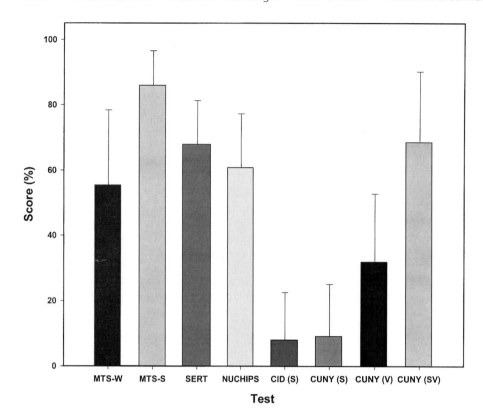

FIGURE 58–9. Mean speech perception test scores of auditory brainstem implant patients with 2 or more years of experience (*N* = 25). MTS-W, Monosyllable, Trochee, Spondee Word Score; MTS-S, Monosyllable, Trochee, Spondee Stress Score; SERT, Sound Effects Recognition Test; NUCHIPS, Northwestern University Children's Perception of Speech Test; CID (S), Central Institute for the Deaf Sentence Test in sound only; CUNY (S), CUNY (V), and CUNY (SV), City University of New York Sentence Tests in sound only, vision only, and sound plus vision, respectively.

noted to involve anatomic difficulties at the time of implantation. Preoperative MRIs may signal potential problems leading to nonstimulation, such as a large lateral recess or tumor damage to the cochlear nucleus region.

OTHER RESEARCH

Niparko and associates[15] demonstrated the feasibility of implanting and stimulating within the substance of the cochlear nucleus in guinea pigs. In a related study, el-Kashlan and colleagues[16] compared the effectiveness of surface electrodes with those placed into the nucleus. They found lower thresholds and a wider dynamic range in animals with penetrating electrodes than in those with surface placement. As mentioned, this more invasive technique has provided a future direction for cochlear nucleus implantation. McCreery and coworkers[7] demonstrated the efficacy of such a system for activating discrete populations

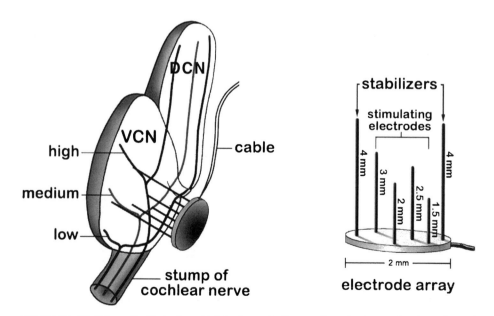

FIGURE 58–10. Schematic illustration *(right)* of penetrating auditory brainstem implant electrode array and implant site *(left)* accessing tonotopic gradient of fibers in ventral cochlear nucleus (VCN). DCN, dorsal cochlear nucleus. (Courtesy of Huntington Medical Research Institute, Pasadena, CA.)

of tonotopically tuned neurons within the substance of the cochlear nucleus. This was achieved without significant risk to tissue or blood supply in longer term preparations with properly constructed and inserted electrodes. Needle-type electrodes with a somewhat blunt-tip configuration (Fig. 58–10) were atraumatically inserted on-axis with a specialized spring-powered tool.

Speech processing for brainstem stimulation has profited from research in cochlear implants. Interestingly, similar strategies used in cochlear implants also have worked well with the brainstem implant.[6] Flexibility of the ABI programming system has been essential to accommodate anatomic variations and the range of auditory and nonauditory sensations that can result from stimulation. Proper assessment and use of this information in configuring ABI speech processors can have a significant effect on speech perception performance. Poor selection or misalignment of frequency bands to electrode channels in speech processor programming can limit performance.[13] Particularly in patients with a greater incidence of nonauditory sensations, experience and flexibility in the clinician's approach can sometimes mean the difference between use and nonuse of a device. Future studies regarding stimulation rates, frequency assignment of channels, and methods of coding speech cues will contribute to improvements in speech processing strategies for the ABI.

SUMMARY

A multiple-electrode array for electrical stimulation can be safely and reliably placed on the brainstem of patients and chronically stimulated to produce useful auditory sensations by selective activation of the cochlear nucleus. Few side effects and minimal morbidity characterize the clinical course of patients with these implants. Speech perception performance varies and, with some exceptions, does not reach the high levels typically seen with modern cochlear implants. In combination with lipreading cues, however, ABI sound has proven to be highly beneficial for the majority of device recipients.

Further research and improvements in the hardware and in sound processing should give patients improved speech understanding in the future.

ACKNOWLEDGMENTS

The authors are grateful to Michael Waring for editorial assistance on electrophysiology, Butch Welch for graphics assistance, and the patients of the House Ear Clinic for their time and effort in laboratory testing.

References

1. Brackmann DE, Hitselberger WE, Nelson RA, et al: Auditory brainstem implant: I. Issues in surgical implantation. Otolaryngol Head Neck Surg 108: 624–633, 1993.
2. Shannon RV, Fayad J, Moore JK, et al: Auditory brainstem implant: II. Postsurgical issues and performance. Otolaryngol Head Neck Surg 108: 634–642, 1993.
3. Riccardi VM: Neurofibromatosis. Neurol Clin North Am 5: 337–349, 1987.
4. Briggs RJ, Popovic EA, Brackmann DE: Recent advances in the treatment of neurofibromatosis type II. Adv Otolaryngol Head Neck Surg 9: 227–245, 1995.
5. Hitselberger N, House WF, Edgerton BS, Whitaker S: Cochlear nucleus implant. Otolaryngol Head Neck Surg 92: 52–54, 1984.
6. Otto SR, Shannon RV, Brackmann DE, et al: The multichannel auditory brainstem implant (ABI): Results in 20 patients. Otolaryngol Head Neck Surg 118: 291–303, 1998.
7. McCreery DG, Shannon RV, Moore JK, et al: Accessing the tonotopic organization of the ventral cochlear nucleus by intranuclear microstimulation. IEEE Trans Rehabil Eng 4: 1–9, 1998.
8. Terr LI, Edgerton BJ: Surface topography of the cochlear nuclei in humans: Two- and three-dimensional. Hear Res 17: 51–59, 1985.
9. Sinha VK, Terr LI, Galey FR, Linthicum FH: Computer-aided three-dimensional reconstruction of the cochlear nerve root. Otolaryngol Head Neck Surg 113: 651–655, 1987.
10. Waring MD: Refractory properties of auditory brainstem responses evoked by electrical stimulation of human cochlear nucleus: Evidence of neural generators. Electroenceph Clin Neurophysiol 108: 331–334, 1998.
11. Monsell EM, McElveen JT, Hitselberger WE, House WF: Surgical approaches to the human cochlear nucleus complex. Am J Otol 8: 450–455, 1987.
12. Niparko JK, Kileny PR, Kemink JL, et al: Neurophysiologic intraoperative monitoring: II. Facial nerve function. Am J Otol 10: 55–61, 1989.
13. Otto SR, Ebinger K, Staller SJ: Clinical trials with the auditory brainstem implant. *In* Waltzman SB, Cohen NL (eds): Cochlear Implants. New York, Thieme, 2000, pp 357–365.
14. McDermott HJ, McKay CM, Vandali AE: A new portable sound processor for the University of Melbourne/Nucleus multielectrode cochlear implant. J Acoust Soc Am 91: 3367–3371, 1992.
15. Niparko JK, Altschuler RA, Xue XL, et al: Surgical implantation and biocompatibility of central nervous system auditory prostheses. Ann Otol Rhin Laryngol 98: 965–970, 1989.
16. El-Kashlan HK, Niparko JK, Altschuler RA, Miller JM: Direct electrical stimulation of the cochlear nucleus: Surface versus penetrating stimulation. Otolaryngol Head Neck Surg 105: 533–543, 1991.

59

Management of Postoperative Cerebrospinal Fluid Leaks

Derald E. Brackmann, M.D. ▪ Grayson K. Rodgers, M.D.

Egress of cerebrospinal fluid (CSF) from the subarachnoid space into surgical wounds often results in leakage of CSF from the wound, the ear canal (if the tympanic membrane is not intact), or the nose (via the eustachian tube). The spinal fluid follows the path of least resistance. Any procedure that encounters the subarachnoid space can be complicated by a postoperative CSF leak. These leaks result from failure to obtain watertight dural closure or from an inadequate seal of dural defects. CSF leaks are a concern because the defect provides a potential portal of entry for infection to seed the leptomeninges. Meningitis in this setting is accompanied by significant morbidity and even mortality. CSF leaks, therefore, should be corrected promptly to avoid more serious complications. This chapter is dedicated to detailing the various techniques for treating postoperative CSF leaks.

PRESSURE DRESSING

For cases in which an abdominal fat graft has been used during closure to plug dural defects, a pressure dressing can be applied to control CSF leaks. The pressure dressing works by pushing the fat back into the dural defect, sealing off the subarachnoid space. In cases in which fat has been used, most leaks stop with a pressure dressing.

Technique

The dressing is applied in similar manner to the initial postoperative dressing. First, a vertical gathering tie is placed in the temporal fossa. Dressing sponges (4 × 4) are folded in half and placed directly over the fat graft and in the postauricular sulcus to support the auricle (Fig. 59–1A). Next, fluffed Kerlix is placed over the 4 × 4 sponges and the auricle (Fig. 59–1B). A tight wrap of roller gauze is then applied (Fig. 59–1C). The direction of the wrap should be from the ear toward the occiput, which ensures that the auricle is not damaged by anterior folding. Also, the vertical tie must be as lateral as possible in the temporal fossa to avoid a pressure point on the forehead. Pressure necrosis of forehead skin can develop easily if attention is not given to this point.

The last layer of this dressing is a 3-inch elastic bandage, which provides the final compression (Fig. 59–1D). The elastic bandage should be wrapped firmly, but patient comfort must be accommodated. Usually, the last several turns can be altered to adjust the exact amount of compression.

Ideally, a pressure dressing should be left in place for 4 or 5 days, which allows time for healing of the CSF leak site to occur. A minimum of 48 hours without leakage must pass before the dressing is removed.

In addition to the pressure dressing, other conservative actions should be undertaken. These measures all are directed at decreasing CSF pressure. Straining (Valsalva maneuver) is strictly avoided, and the patient is kept at bed rest with the head elevated 45 degrees. Limited activity, such as bathroom privileges or brief periods of sitting up in a chair, are at the surgeon's discretion. Stool softeners and cough suppressants can be used. Acetazolamide (Diamox) may be given to decrease CSF production.

LUMBAR DRAIN

The next step in CSF leak treatment is a lumbar subarachnoid spinal fluid drain. By removing CSF from the system at a site away from the dural defect, CSF pressure is decreased, and healing can occur. Some surgeons routinely place a lumbar drain at the time of surgery to assist with intraoperative CSF removal and decompression in the postoperative period.

Technique

To place the catheter, a lumbar puncture is performed at the L4–L5 level. The patient is placed in either a sitting or a lateral decubitus position. The spinous processes are palpated, and L4–L5 is identified at the level of the iliac crest. The patient is asked to flex the back and bring the knees and chin to the chest. A prepared catheter kit contains all the necessary supplies for preparing, draping, and anesthetizing the site. An 18-gauge Touhy needle is introduced in the midline with a slightly superior angle between the spinous processes (Fig. 59–2). The obturator is removed at intervals so the surgeon can look for a flow of CSF. Once a good flow of CSF is established, the epidural catheter is introduced through the needle and threaded into the epidural space. The opened side of the bevel of the needle faces the patient's left or right side on penetrating the spinous ligaments and arachnoid. Before the catheter is threaded, the bevel is turned to open superiorly, thereby facilitating directing the catheter cephalad. With a flow of CSF established, the needle is withdrawn, and the connector is placed on the end of the catheter so that a

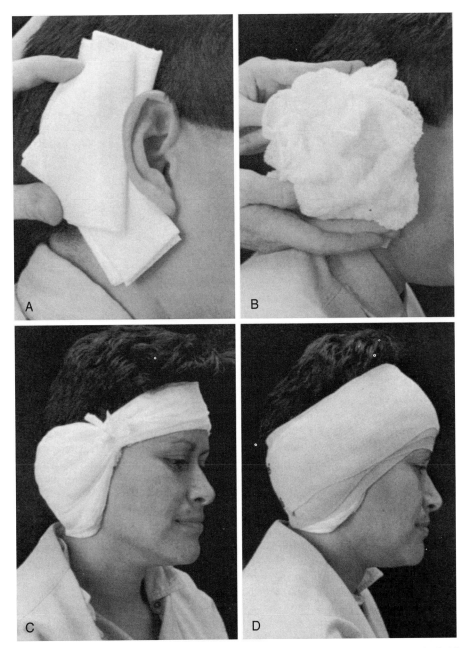

FIGURE 59–1. *A,* Folded 4 × 4 dressing sponges placed over the fat graft site after translabyrinthine acoustic tumor removal. The sponges are also placed in the postauricular crease to support the auricle. *B,* Fluffed Kerlix in place over the 4 × 4 sponges. *C,* Appearance of dressing after the roller gauze wrap. Tape can be applied to secure the position of the dressing. This is especially helpful on the forehead, where the dressing may slide inferiorly onto the brow. Note the laterally placed vertical gathering tie. *D,* Ace wrap in place. Again, tape can be helpful to stabilize the elastic dressing.

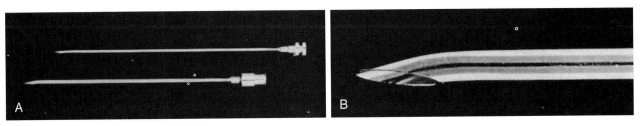

FIGURE 59–2. *A,* Tuohy needle used for lumbar puncture. *B,* Close-up of the end of the Tuohy needle.

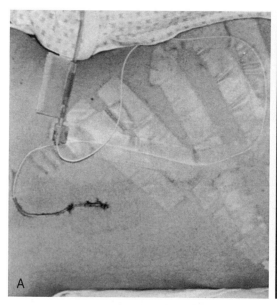

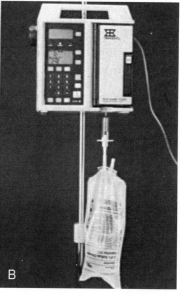

FIGURE 59–3. *A,* Site of the lumbar puncture at L4–L5 with the epidural catheter secured in place by Tegaderm. This provides an occlusive seal over the catheter site and allows for easy inspection of the site. *B,* The IMED pump set up to withdraw cerebrospinal fluid from the patient and into the collection bag.

connection to intravenous tubing can be made. An empty intravenous fluid bag is attached to the tubing, and all connections are secured with tape.

Several methods of regulating CSF output exist. This regulation is important because, if CSF is removed too rapidly, tension pneumocephalus and even brain herniation can occur.[1–3] Alternatively, if an inadequate amount of CSF is removed, the purpose of the drain is defeated. Humans produce approximately 18 ml of CSF per hour. The natural mechanisms of CSF absorption reduce some CSF; therefore, the lumbar drain should remove less than 18 ml of CSF per hour. Common neurosurgical practice is to order 50 ml of CSF removed every 8 hours.

Gravity is the standard method of effecting CSF drainage. The collection bag is placed at the level of the patient's heart or below to create increasing output of CSF as needed. This method requires extremely attentive nursing care to ensure the proper amount of drainage. Drains placed to respond to gravity have highly variable output, and a change in patient position may significantly increase or decrease flow. Establishing an even flow of spinal fluid is difficult, and usually a bolus of fluid is removed, after which the drain is clamped. The system is at risk of occluding during these clamped periods. If flow becomes

impaired, then removing the amount of CSF ordered becomes impossible.

To avoid some of these problems, we place the intravenous tubing in reverse direction through an intravenous infusion pump. The pump is set at 10 ml per hour, and a slow, controlled, continuous flow of CSF is withdrawn from the patient (Fig. 59–3). Because this system is not gravity dependent, patients may move about without fear of a rapid discharge of CSF. Better patency of the catheter system is maintained because the flow is never stopped. Any occlusion of the system or air in the line is sensed, and an alarm is sounded as the pump stops. Other physicians have employed flow-regulated systems,[4, 5] but the system described here is a definite improvement over those described. We have employed this system in a small series of patients and have found it vastly superior to gravity drainage.

While the lumbar drain is in place, the patient must be closely observed for signs of infection. The temperature, surgical wound, lumbar drain site, and white blood cell count must be monitored. Samples of CSF may be examined at any time. Headache during CSF drainage is common, but meningismus should not be present.

As with a pressure dressing, the lumbar drain should be

FIGURE 59–4. *A,* Postauricular approach and transection of the ear canal skin and dissection of cartilage from the canal skin. *B,* Everting stitches placed in the superior and inferior canal skin. These sutures are grasped with a hemostat placed through the canal and then pulled through, thus everting the canal skin. *C,* The everted canal skin is oversewn.

FIGURE 59–5. *A,* A mastoid periosteal flap is developed for a second layer of closure and is pedicled just posterior to the meatus. *B,* This flap is then rotated anteriorly and secured with absorbable sutures.

FIGURE 59–6. Middle fossa exposure with removal of the tegmen tympani and bony eustachian tube (ET) roof. The cochlea, vestibular labyrinth, facial nerve, and internal auditory canal are shown as well.

FIGURE 59–7. *A* and *B,* Obliteration of the bony eustachian tube with bone wax, bone pate, and muscle. Insert *(B)* is a cross-section of the eustachian tube (ET) showing the relationship of the internal carotid artery (ICA), tensor tympani muscle, and greater superficial petrosal nerve.

FIGURE 59-4

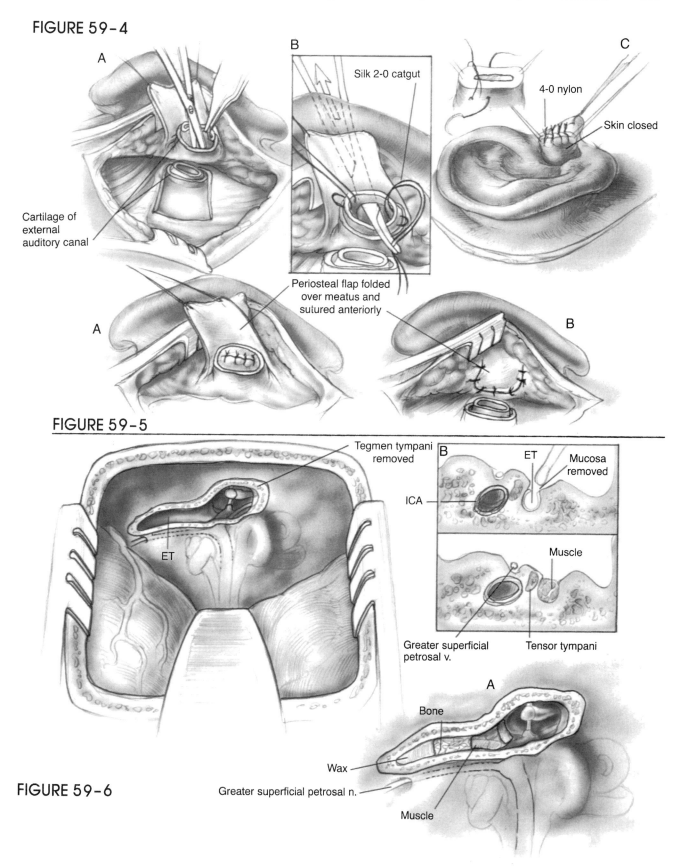

A

Cartilage of external auditory canal

B

Silk 2-0 catgut

C

4-0 nylon

Skin closed

Periosteal flap folded over meatus and sutured anteriorly

FIGURE 59-5

A

B

Tegmen tympani removed

ET

ET

ICA

Mucosa removed

Muscle

Greater superficial petrosal v.

Tensor tympani

FIGURE 59-6

A

Bone

Wax

Greater superficial petrosal n.

Muscle

FIGURE 59-7

FIGURES 59–4 to 59–7. See legends on opposite page

left in place for 4 or 5 days. We often shut the pump off for the last 24 hours so that if the leak recurs, the drainage can be resumed.

WOUND EXPLORATION AND RECLOSURE

When leaks do not resolve within 48 hours with a pressure dressing or lumbar drain, wound exploration with repacking of the abdominal fat and reclosure is indicated. In wounds in which a dural defect was packed with fat, dislodging of the fat from the defect may cause a CSF leak. When the wound is explored, the fat is removed and repacked (with additional fat as required) into the defect, as described in Chapter 50.[6] Some surgeons employ autologous fibrin glue as an adjunct to their closures.[7, 8] This material adds an additional seal to supplement the fat graft or, in other cases, a muscle or pericranial flap. A search should be made for opened mastoid air cells that can serve as pathways for spinal fluid. These air cell tracts can be occluded with bone wax. In cases of severe hearing loss, the eustachian tube should be packed off with Surgicel and temporalis muscle after removal of the incus and cutting of the tensor tympani tendon.

Although a return to the operating room seems aggressive and is accompanied by the small risks brought by further surgery and anesthesia, this course of action has provided the most expedient control of CSF leaks that fail conservative therapy. The expeditious closure of a leak plays an important part in the prevention of infection. The longer a leak remains open, the greater the chance that meningitis has to develop. In a review of CSF leaks after translabyrinthine acoustic tumor removal at the House Ear Clinic, no statistically significant association between postoperative CSF leaks and the development of meningitis was found.[9] One explanation for this is that leaks are aggressively treated and stopped quickly, thus limiting the time available for contamination to occur.

REFRACTORY CEREBROSPINAL FLUID LEAKS

The techniques discussed earlier used separately or in combination stop the vast majority of CSF leaks. Rarely, a leak is refractory to these measures. These leaks involve CSF that tracks through temporal bone cell tracts, finds its way to the middle ear, and subsequently discharges from the nose (eustachian tube) or the ear canal (tympanic membrane not intact). With an intact tympanic membrane, the eustachian tube is the final common pathway of most leaks. Although many methods involving repair of the source of the leakage are described, perhaps an easier and less risky approach is to block the final pathway.

Our management of these difficult leaks depends on the status of the patient's hearing and the tympanic membrane. If no serviceable hearing exists or if the tympanic membrane is not intact, blind sac closure of the ear canal and obliteration of the middle ear and eustachian tube are performed. If the tympanic membrane is intact and the patient has serviceable hearing, middle fossa closure of the eustachian tube is the procedure of choice.

Technique

Ear Canal Closure with Eustachian Tube and Middle Ear Obliteration

Blind sac closure of the ear canal is accomplished through a postauricular incision with transection of the ear canal. The canal skin is separated from the cartilage of the lateral canal and then everted through the external auditory meatus. This everted canal skin is then oversewn with a nonabsorbable suture that is left in place for 10 days postoperatively (Fig. 59–4). A flap of mastoid periosteum is developed on a pedicle just posterior to the external auditory canal. This flap is then rotated anteriorly and secured as a second layer of closure for the meatus (Fig. 59–5). Next, all canal skin, the tympanic membrane, the malleus, and the incus are removed. To ensure complete removal of squamous epithelium and to enlarge the canal, a canalplasty is performed with a cutting burr. The eustachian tube is curetted and then packed with Surgicel and temporalis muscle. Before wound closure, the middle ear and remaining canal are packed with additional muscle. A pressure dressing is placed for 4 postoperative days, and a lumbar spinal fluid drain can also be used in the initial postoperative period.

Middle Fossa Obliteration of the Eustachian Tube

In cases in which the patient has good hearing and the tympanic membrane is intact, closure of the eustachian tube can be accomplished via the middle fossa. This procedure is approached as a middle fossa craniotomy, as outlined in Chapter 49. The bone flap is removed, and the dura is elevated from posterior to anterior. The arcuate eminence, greater superficial petrosal nerve, and middle meningeal artery are identified, and the middle fossa retractor is placed. A diamond burr is used to remove bone from the tegmen tympani and to expose the head of the malleus and the body of the incus (Fig. 59–6). Identification of the tensor tympani tendon and the cochleariform process allows identification of the eustachian tube, which is directly anterior. Also, the eustachian tube is just lateral to the greater superficial petrosal nerve. The bony eustachian tube is unroofed, and the mucosa is carefully curetted from the tube. The surgeon must be aware that the internal carotid artery can be dehiscent in the medial or inferior eustachian tube. The tube is packed first with bone wax, then bone pate, and finally, temporalis muscle (Fig. 59–7). A split-thickness piece of bone from the bone flap is placed over the tegmen defect to avoid fixation of the ossicles against the dura. The wound is closed in the usual manner. In this setting, a pressure dressing is not likely to be helpful, but a lumbar drain could be placed for several postoperative days.

New Strategies

Biomaterials are an important developing adjunct for the prevention and treatment of CSF leaks in neurotologic procedures. Hydroxyapatite compounds such as Bone-Source (Leibinger) are being increasingly applied. A recent consecutive series of 108 translabyrinthine acoustic tumors demonstrated a CSF leak in 2 per cent of the 54 defects closed with hydroxyapatite cement versus 12 per cent of the 54 cases closed with abdominal fat alone (Personal communication, Moises A. Arriaga, M.D., and Douglas A. Chen, M.D., 2000). In that series, a small quantity of abdominal fat was placed over the dural defect, and the mastoid cavity was filled with the hydroxyapatite cement. The ultimate role of these materials will be influenced by success rates, long-term costs, and ease of use.

SUMMARY

Postoperative CSF leak is a potential complication of any cranial base surgical procedure that violates the meninges. Although a CSF leak by itself is not a problem, it provides a portal of entry for bacteria to seed the meninges. Because postoperative meningitis is a serious complication, CSF leaks should be treated aggressively. This chapter discussed the methods for closing CSF leaks in a sequential manner from conservative to aggressive. Using this approach, the skull base surgeon should be able to seal all spinal fluid leaks.

References

1. Snow RB, Kuhel W, Martin SB: Prolonged spinal drainage after the resection of tumors of the skull base: A cautionary note. Neurosurgery 28: 880–883, 1991.
2. Effron MZ, Black FO, Burns D: Tension pneumocephalus complicating the treatment of postoperative CSF otorrhea. Arch Otolaryngol Head Neck Surg 107: 579–580, 1981.
3. Graf CJ, Gross CE, Beck DW: Complication of spinal drainage in the management of cerebrospinal fluid fistula: Report of three cases. J Neurosurg 54: 392–395, 1981.
4. Swanson SE, Kocan MJ, Chandler WF: Flow-regulated continuous spinal drainage: Technical note with case report. Neurosurgery 9: 163–165, 1981.
5. Swanson SE, Chandler WF, Kocan MJ: Flow-regulated continuous spinal drainage in the management of cerebrospinal fluid fistulas. Laryngoscope 95: 104–106, 1985.
6. House JL, Hitselberger WE, House WF: Wound closure and cerebrospinal fluid leak after translabyrinthine surgery. Am J Otol 4: 126–128, 1982.
7. Epstein GH, Weisman RA, Zwillenberg S, Schreiber A: A new autologous fibrinogen-based adhesive for otologic surgery. Ann Otol Rhinol Laryngol 95: 40–45, 1986.
8. Sierra DH, Nissen AJ, Welch J: The use of fibrin glue in intracranial procedures: Preliminary results. Laryngoscope 100: 360–363, 1990.
9. Rodgers GK, Luxford WM: Factors affecting the development of cerebrospinal fluid leak after translabyrinthine acoustic tumor surgery. Laryngoscope 103: 959–962, 1993.

60

Care of the Eye in Facial Paralysis

Robert E. Levine, M.D.

Rehabilitation of the patient with facial paralysis depends on restoration of optimal lid position and function.[1–3] This chapter summarizes techniques that I have found to be most helpful in achieving that goal, based on more than 2000 patients with facial paralysis on whom I have operated during the past 3 decades.

For convenience, the chapter is divided into sections for lid reanimation procedures, lower lid reapposition procedures, and ancillary procedures. In practice, a combination of these techniques may be performed during the same operation. When the procedures are combined, the reanimation procedure is performed first because it is most influenced by the lid swelling that occurs during the course of the surgery. The lower lid reapposition procedure is performed next. Upper lid entropion correction is performed just before the upper lid incision is closed, and brow elevation is performed last. The final section of the chapter explains two useful temporizing procedures.

CRITERIA FOR SURGERY

The following three groups of patients with facial paralysis require lid surgery for functional reasons:

1. Those who are either symptomatic or who show signs of conjunctival or corneal injury, or both, despite maximum tolerated medical therapy.
2. Those who require rapid ocular rehabilitation to resume their usual occupation and responsibilities. For example, keeping the eye full of ointment might protect the cornea adequately but would not be a realistic option for a monocular patient or one who works as a pilot.
3. Those whose ocular status is currently stable but who are at high risk of corneal complications. Patients with diminished corneal sensitivity or totally anesthetic corneas secondary to associated fifth nerve involvement are the prime candidates in this group. If both fifth and seventh nerve deficits are present, even minimal lagophthalmos is a risk factor for corneal breakdown. Poor Bell's phenomenon or the absence of tears may further complicate the picture.

Patients with short-term problems (≤3 months to anticipated recovery of orbicularis oculi function) can usually be treated by conservative means. Patients with significant paralytic deficits who will require 6 months or more to recover, or who are not expected to recover, are generally best served by early surgical intervention.

The group of patients whose prognosis is unclear, for example, those who might improve in 3 months but could conceivably require 6 months or more to recover, poses the greatest challenges in surgical selection. In such patients, criteria such as the reliability of follow-up, the accessibility of medical care, the ability of the patient or family to care for the eye, and the patient's own needs, desires, and lifestyle all play a role in decision making. When it is safe and feasible, a prolonged trial of conservative management may allow the patient and the physician to decide if they are on the correct course.

PREPARATION OF THE PATIENT

The surgery is preferably done on an eye (or head and neck) gurney. Two advantages of this approach are ease of access to the eye area by the surgeon and the assistant and ability to crank up the bed so that the patient is brought to the seated position, thereby enabling the brow and lids to be checked with gravity operative. A doughnut is used to stabilize the head, and a nasal cannula with air is added to provide adequate circulation under the drapes. Some anesthesiologists prefer a carbon dioxide exhaust line as well. Air is used routinely instead of oxygen to eliminate the possibility of an accident resulting from the unhappy mixture of oxygen and cautery. If oxygen is required at any time, cautery is withheld until after the oxygen has been turned off.

ANESTHESIA AND SURGICAL PREPARATION

In lid reanimation procedures, in which the patient's cooperation is required, any medication that might make the patient drowsy and unable to cooperate fully throughout the operation is not used. Rather, short-acting intravenous medication, such as propofol (Diprivan), methohexital (Brevital), or a similar agent is given at the beginning of the surgery in amounts just adequate to cover the discomfort of the local injection. Lidocaine (Xylocaine), 2 per cent, with epinephrine (unless contraindicated by hypertension or cardiac problems) to which sodium bicarbonate, 7.5 per cent, (Neutracain) has been added (one part sodium bicarbonate to nine parts lidocaine with epinephrine) is used at the beginning of the surgery. Bupivacaine (Marcaine), 0.5 per cent, is used at the end of the surgery to reduce pain during the immediate postoperative period. It may also be included in the initial injection, using equal parts of bupivacaine and lidocaine with epinephrine.

Local infiltration is placed in the areas to be operated,

such as along the upper lid fold and along the lateral orbital rim for spring implantations, and at the canthi and brow areas, if surgery is to be performed there. Excessive infiltration should be avoided because it paralyzes the levator, impairs extraocular motility (making it harder to judge lid position), and distorts lid anatomy. The eyelids, both sides of the face above the mouth, and the forehead are prepared with green soap and then with povidone-iodine (Betadine), which is washed off.

DRAPING

The hair is covered with a small drape formed into a turban and secured with a clamp. A second small sheet is incorporated with that drape to cover the superior end of the table. A body sheet is also placed. The eyelids and brow are isolated by means of two No. 1000 Steri-Drapes cut in half (Fig. 60–1). Each of the four drapes forms a

border of the surgical field, which includes both eyes and the forehead area. Before the Steri-Drape is placed over the nose, a thin cloth towel is placed over the nose to avoid the suffocating feeling resulting from plastic over the nose. In addition, the plastic drape over the towel inferior to the adhesive area is excised to prevent moisture accumulation. Care is taken to avoid distorting the lower lid anatomy or brow areas by undue traction from the drapes.

The body drape is fastened to the head drape on both sides with a towel clip so it does not slip down when the patient is brought to the seated position. The patient is secured on the table with a safety belt, and the belt is positioned so as to provide access for loosening it as needed when the patient is brought to the seated position.

The Mayo stand is brought over the drapes for easy access to the instruments. Although the tent effect obtainable by draping over the Mayo stand would be desirable, it does not lend itself readily to moving the stand away when the patient needs to be brought to the seated position.

FIGURE 60-1

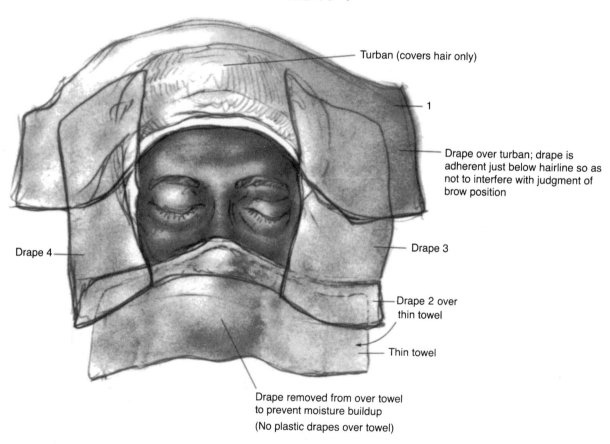

Turban (covers hair only)

1

Drape over turban; drape is adherent just below hairline so as not to interfere with judgment of brow position

Drape 4

Drape 3

Drape 2 over thin towel

Thin towel

Drape removed from over towel to prevent moisture buildup
(No plastic drapes over towel)

FIGURE 60–1. Draping the patient. After the hair has been covered with a turban, which is secured with a towel clip, two No. 1000 Steri-Drapes are cut in half. The first half-drape is placed with the edge as close to the hairline as possible so as not to interfere with judgment of brow position. A thin cloth towel is then placed over the nose, and a half-drape is placed to secure it into position, with the sticky end of the drape bridging the skin and the superior end of the towel. The nonsticky portion of the drape is then cut away and discarded, leaving only the towel over the nose. If the drape is not cut away, excess moisture builds up. A third half-drape is placed laterally, as far lateral to the lateral canthus as is practical, and a fourth half-drape is placed similarly on the contralateral side.

GENERAL CONSIDERATIONS

Procedures are generally performed on an outpatient basis, unless the patient is already hospitalized because of the neurotologic or head and neck surgery. Bipolar or unipolar cautery may be used for hemostasis. Cutting cautery with a fine needle tip is useful for performing the lid dissection. The eye is constantly protected with a scleral shell. At the end of the procedure, antibiotic ophthalmic ointment is applied to the wounds. Ophthalmic ointment is used because it is not irritating if any gets into the eye. The lids are not bandaged. An ice pack is applied to the closed lids and kept in place for 48 hours, after which time warm tap water compresses are used for at least 20 minutes four times a day until the swelling subsides. The antibiotic ointment is applied to the wounds twice a day until they are healed, and appropriate lubricating drops are prescribed for the eye.

UPPER LID REANIMATION PROCEDURES

The four procedures that I believe are the most useful in reanimating paralyzed lids are the following, in order of preference:

1. Enhanced palpebral spring implantation
2. Palpebral spring implantation
3. Gold weight implantation
4. Silicone rod prosthesis implantation

In all of these procedures, the principle is to create an external force that opposes the levator palpebrae superioris, the opening muscle of the lid. The respective forces are spring tension, gravity acting on the gold weight, and elasticity of the silicone band.

The relative merits and limitations of the various procedures are related to how they develop external closing forces and the consequences of increasing those forces. For example, the greater the force required by any device, the greater the pseudoptosis (lid droop in the primary position of gaze that results from the implant). If the palpebral spring, the gold weight, and the silicone rod prosthesis are all adjusted to provide the same closing force in a given patient, the pseudoptosis should be the same with each device. In the enhanced palpebral spring implantation procedure, the levator muscle is strengthened to balance the spring force, and therefore less pseudoptosis is possible with the same closing force, when compared with any of the other three procedures. Similarly, by tightening the levator and therefore using a stronger spring force, the surgeon makes increased blink speed possible.

Because the gold weight is gravity dependent, very large and unsightly gold weights may be required in lids that need a strong closing force. Also, because the gold weight is gravity dependent, lid closure may not be assured when the patient is supine, as in sleep. Further, blink speed is limited with the gold weight. However, the surgeon who does these procedures only infrequently can more easily master the techniques of the gold weight implant and silicone rod prosthesis than the technique of the palpebral spring implant or the enhanced palpebral spring implant.

The silicone rod prosthesis has the advantage of providing support for the lower lid as well. Its major disadvantage is its inevitable loss of elasticity over time, be it months or years. If facial nerve function does not recover before the prosthesis runs out of elasticity, it will need to be replaced. By contrast, a gold weight or palpebral spring can function over many years. A small percentage of springs may fail over time because of fatigue and breakage, thereby necessitating replacement.

An additional advantage of the palpebral spring is that the tension on the wire can be adjusted postoperatively, either externally or through a small incision. This technique allows loosening of the spring when the patient recovers partial function but is not yet well enough to have the spring removed.

All prosthetic devices are subject to the potential hazards of extrusion or infection over the long term. However, with the techniques currently in use, these complications have been sufficiently infrequent as to not limit the usefulness of the devices.

In recent years, since I devised the enhanced palpebral spring procedure, I have used it with increasing frequency instead of nonenhanced spring implantation. The extra surgical effort is usually well rewarded by the diminished pseudoptosis and increased blink speed obtained by this procedure.

In summary, I prefer the enhanced palpebral spring implantation in most cases of significant upper lid closure deficits. When the patient has a strong levator or when the spring is being used only as a short-term remedy, the nonenhanced palpebral spring procedure may be used. Surgeons who are just beginning to undertake palpebral spring implantation should start off with the nonenhanced procedure and then move on to the enhanced procedure.

I find the gold weight of greatest benefit to those patients whose closure problem is relatively minimal but nevertheless just exceeds the limits of conservative management. Patients who require definitive, reliable closure, such as those with coexistent poor Bell's phenomenon or fifth nerve involvement, are better protected with springs than with weights. Patients whose ocular management failed with weights in place have been successfully treated by removing the weights and replacing them with springs. The Silastic elastic prosthesis is most useful in those patients with an excellent prognosis for recovery in about 6 months, in whom significant lower lid lagophthalmos coexists, since stretching of the prosthesis over time may decrease its function after 6 months.

Palpebral Spring Implantation[4-14]

The palpebral spring is built preoperatively either in the office or at the bedside. Building the spring is time consuming, and both the surgeon and the patient should be comfortable during the procedure. Good light must be available, and if possible, the patient should be seated so that lid movement can be best evaluated.

Each spring is constructed from a plain piece of wire that is shaped to conform to the individual lid anatomy of the patient. Generally, a 0.010-inch wire provides suitable tension for most patients. Previously I advocated that pa-

FIGURE 60-2

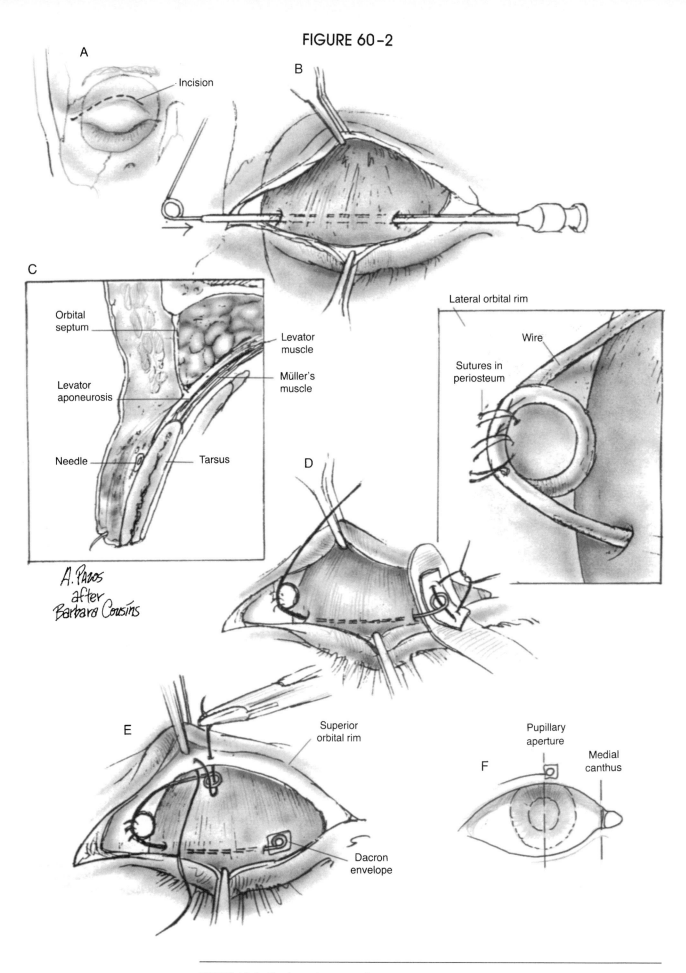

A — Incision

B

C
Orbital septum
Levator aponeurosis
Needle
Levator muscle
Müller's muscle
Tarsus

Lateral orbital rim
Wire
Sutures in periosteum

A. Pazos
after
Barbara Cousins

D

E
Superior orbital rim
Dacron envelope

F
Pupillary aperture
Medial canthus

FIGURE 60–2. *See legend on opposite page*

tients with very strong levators required the use of 0.011-inch or even 0.012-inch wire and that patients with weak levators (when the levator is not going to be tightened) may benefit from the use of 0.009-inch or even 0.008-inch wire. Recently, the same wire used in pacemaker leads, the alloy MP35N, has been made with sufficient tensile strength to replace the previous alloy. With this wire, the 0.010 inch wire diameter need not be varied. Because of its track record in biomechanical applications, it is anticipated to have excellent longevity.

The construction is begun by forming a 5-mm loop at what is to become the fulcrum of the spring. The posterior aspect of that loop should be the superior arm of the spring. Because loosening the spring intraoperatively is easier than tightening it, the two arms should form an angle of about 120 degrees as they leave the fulcrum.

The fulcrum is then placed over the lateral orbital rim and held in position by the surgeon's fingers. Curves are then created in the lower arm to match the patient's lid anatomy. Curvature is also provided to accommodate the fact that the upper eyelid opens up and back, not straight up and down. Slight variations in spring position and curvatures may enhance its effect; therefore, these factors should be varied in the evaluation of the spring preoperatively.

Sometimes, making more than one spring with slightly different curvatures is useful in determining which model will work best. Usually, the fulcrum should be placed as far laterally as possible without lengthening the spring so much that its design and placement are difficult. The completed spring is stored until the day of surgery, when it is placed on a gauze pad to prevent loss and sterilized in a low-temperature chemical unit and not a steam autoclave, to subject the wire to less heat stress.

Surgical Technique

The eye is protected with a scleral shell. An incision is made along the lid fold at the junction of the medial one third and lateral two thirds of the palpebral aperture and is carried across the orbital rim (Fig. 60–2). Dissection is carried superolaterally, in the plane between the septum and orbicularis, to expose the orbital rim. Dissection is carried downward at the medial aspect of the incision to expose the tarsus.

A blunted 22 gauge spinal needle is then passed, beginning in the area of the exposed tarsus, 5 mm superior to the lid margin. The needle passes in the plane between the orbicularis and the tarsus to a point 2 mm above the lid

---

FIGURE 60–2. Palpebral spring implantation. *A,* With a protective scleral shell in place, an incision is made along the lateral two thirds of the lid crease and is carried across the orbital rim laterally. Dissection is carried downward at the medial end of the incision to expose the tarsal plate. Dissection is also carried upward and laterally to expose the orbital rim. *B,* A 22-gauge blunted spinal needle with the stilette in place is passed from the medial end of the dissection to emerge laterally in the plane between the orbicularis and the tarsus. The passage should be carried out overlying the midtarsus, and the needle is angulated slightly downward at its lateral extent. The exit of the needle tract should be close to the lateral orbital rim periosteum. The lid is everted to confirm that the needle has not inadvertently perforated the tarsus. The previously prepared wire spring, sterilized in a low-temperature chemical sterilizer, is passed through the needle, and the needle is withdrawn. *C,* A cross-section of the lid illustrates placement of the needle over the midtarsus in the plane between the tarsus and orbicularis. The wire spring should be resting on the epitarsal surface. *D,* The scleral shell is removed, and the fulcrum of the spring is brought into the desired position along the orbital rim. The spring should be placed in a position in which its curves conform perfectly to the eyelid contour. (*Inset:* The fulcrum of the spring is secured to lateral orbital rim periosteum with three 4-0 Mersilene sutures, and an extra bite of the periosteum is taken with each stitch.) Loops are fashioned at each end, and the spring is cut to size. The loops should be flat and tightly closed to leave no sharp edges. The medial loop is enveloped in 0.2-mm thick polyester (Dacron) patch material, to which it is secured by means of three 8-0 nylon sutures tied internally. The polyester patch is creased in an absorbable gelatin sponge (Gelfoam) press before surgery and is autoclaved with the other instruments. The folded polyester envelope is cut to size at surgery. The crease in the patch material should be directed downward so that the spring and patch together provide a smooth inferior surface. The loop at the end of the inferior arm is directed upward for the same reason. Suturing of the loop to the polyester is facilitated by resting the polyester on a retractor. *E,* The end of the spring with its polyester envelope is replaced into the lid between the tarsus and orbicularis. In time, the end of the spring will become fixed to the tarsus by granulation tissue integrating into the polyester patch. Securing the patch to the tarsus directly with an additional running 8-0 nylon suture helps to provide fixation until connective tissue grows into the polyester. The tension on the spring is checked, with the patient in both the upright and supine positions. The tension can be adjusted by grasping the upper end of the spring with forceps and changing its position. When the correct tension has been determined, the upper loop of the spring is secured to the orbital rim periosteum with a 4-0 Mersilene suture. An extra bite of the periosteum may be taken in the stitch before it is tied. When sutures are placed to secure either the fulcrum or the upper loop of the spring to the orbital rim periosteum, it is safer to sew in the direction away from the globe. Spring tension is again checked with the patient both seated and supine. Additional adjustments can be made by bending the wire or repositioning the loop. When the adjustments are completed, two additional 4-0 Mersilene sutures are placed through the upper loop in a manner similar to that of the initial suture. Deeper tissues overlying the spring are then closed with 5-0 plain gut suture to assure that the spring and Mersilene sutures are well covered. Skin and muscle are closed with running 6-0 plain gut fast-absorbing suture. *F,* The end of the spring should be between the pupillary axis and the medial limbus, with the eyes in the primary position of gaze. (*A–F,* From Tse D, Wright KW (eds): Oculoplastic Surgery. Philadelphia, JB Lippincott, 1992.)

margin at the lateral aspect of the lid. It then continues until it emerges at the anterior aspect of the lateral orbital rim. The stylette is then removed. The undersurface of the lid is inspected to ensure that the needle has not inadvertently perforated the tarsus.

The end of the lower arm of the previously prepared palpebral spring is then passed into the needle, and the needle and spring are withdrawn medially, thereby bringing the spring into the lid. The scleral shell is then removed, and the spring is positioned so that its previously determined curvature conforms to the lid anatomy. The upper arm of the spring is placed in position, and its length is determined. It usually needs to be about 3/4-inch long. A loop is fashioned at the point that is to become the end of the upper arm, and the wire is cut to size. The loop is closed so as to leave no sharp ends. The upper loop is made at a 90° angle to the fulcrum loop, so the upper loop can be tucked under the superior orbital rim. The loop is thus primarily held in place by pushing against the bone, decreasing the role of the sutures and helping to prevent late slippage. The loop at the fulcrum is then held in place with forceps, and the patient is asked to open and close the eye. The position at which the spring curvature best conforms to the lid anatomy is then found, with the eye both opened and closed, and the loop at the fulcrum is sutured in place. The suturing is accomplished with 4-0 Mersilene suture, and an extra bite of periosteum is taken with each stitch. Three such sutures are generally placed for the nonenhanced procedure, and five for the enhanced procedure because of the greater tensions involved.

The lower arm of the spring is cut to size, and a loop (which is also meticulously closed) is formed on its end. The loop should be formed upward to maintain a smooth inferior surface to the spring. The end of the spring should be between the pupillary axis and the medial limbus, with the eyes in the primary position of gaze. In very prominent eyes, terminating the spring slightly sooner, in the pupillary axis, may be preferable. Before the end of the spring is covered with polyester (Dacron) patch material, the angulation of the loop should be checked with the patient's eyes open and closed to ensure that the spring tracks well with lid movement and that the loop stays relatively parallel to the tarsus during opening and closing.

A piece of 0.2 mm polyester patch material, which has been creased by its placement in a press that is used for compressing Gelfoam before it is autoclaved, is cut to size to fit over the inferior loop. This piece is converted into a pouch by closure of the sides with 8-0 nylon sutures tied internally. The creased side is directed downward. The open lateral side is then slipped over the spring, to which it is secured with an 8-0 nylon suture beginning within the pouch. The suture is passed through the spring loop and the posterior end of the pouch and is terminated by passing through the anterior side of the pouch. The knot is tied internally to prevent erosion. The polyester envelope is secured to the tarsus with one or more 8-0 nylon sutures, as needed, to prevent slippage of the polyester until granulation to the tarsus occurs.

Spring tension is then adjusted to just close the eye, by moving the upper arm of the spring closer or farther from the orbital rim. At the desired tension, the upper arm is bent so that the loop can be tucked under the orbital rim;

it is secured with 4-0 Mersilene sutures to periosteum, taking an extra bite of periosteum with each stitch. Tension is checked with the patient seated as well as supine. Additional adjustments can be made by bending the wire of the upper arm to loosen or tighten it.

Bending the wire of the lower arm near the fulcrum should be avoided at this time because such adjustments may be required during the postoperative period, and excess bending of the wire may increase its chance of breakage. Once the final position of the upper loop has been determined in the nonenhanced procedure, two additional 4-0 Mersilene sutures are placed, and an extra bite of periosteum is taken with each stitch. Four additional sutures are used in the enhanced procedure.

The deeper aspect of the wound overlying the orbital rim is closed with 5-0 plain gut suture to cover the spring and Mersilene sutures at the upper loop and fulcrum. The lid fold incision is closed with running 6-0 plain gut suture. The eye is dressed with antibiotic ointment and an ice pack.

Enhanced Palpebral Spring Implantation

The enhancement of the palpebral spring operation consists of tightening of the levator during the same procedure (Fig. 60–3). The spring is prepared similarly, except that wire lighter than 0.010 inch is not used. I use the 0.010 inch MP35N alloy.

A scleral shell is placed. The initial skin fold incision is the same as that described earlier. Dissection is carried upward until preaponeurotic fat can be visualized through the septum. The septum is then opened, and dissection is carried down to expose the levator. Dissection is then carried inferiorly to expose the tarsus centrally. A 5-0 Mersilene suture is then placed through midtarsus where the loop-polyester complex overlies tarsus. The lid's undersurface is inspected to be sure the suture has not perforated tarsus. Both suture arms pass through the polyester, and the medial arm passes through the loop as well, before completing the suture through the levator, to emerge just above the point where aponeurosis ends and levator muscle is visualized. This serves the purposes of directly opposing the maximal force of the spring (at its distal end) with the levator force and of further securing the polyester until granulation tissue fixes it in place. A temporary knot is placed and the patient is asked to open the eye.

The scleral shell is removed and the extent of levator tightening evaluated. If necessary, an additional lateral suture and possibly an additional medial suture are placed in a similar manner to achieve desired lid strengthening and maintenance of proper upper lid curvature. If the surgeon is not sure whether additional sutures are necessary, their placement can be deferred until after the spring has been placed and the overall effect of the spring and the initial suture can be evaluated.

Regardless of how many sutures are used, they are adjusted after the spring is in place, at the same time that the spring itself would otherwise be adjusted. The levator is tightened to a point at which maximum strengthening is achieved without inducing cicatricial lagophthalmos from an overly shortened levator.

FIGURE 60-3

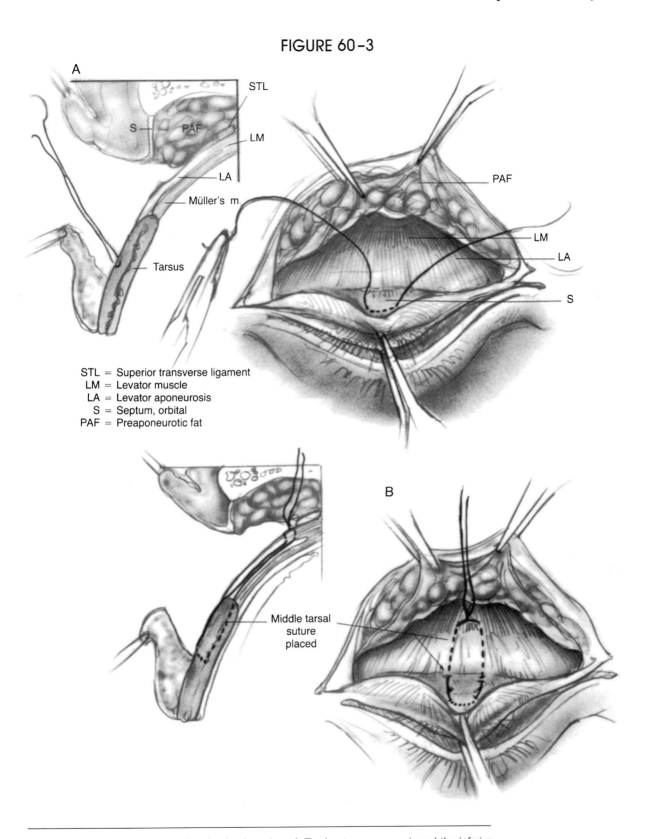

STL = Superior transverse ligament
LM = Levator muscle
LA = Levator aponeurosis
S = Septum, orbital
PAF = Preaponeurotic fat

FIGURE 60–3. Enhanced palpebral spring implantation. *A,* The levator aponeurosis and the inferior aspect of the muscular portion of the levator are exposed. Centrally, the superior portion of the tarsus is also exposed. A double-armed 5.0 Mersilene suture is then placed through midtarsus. *B,* Each arm of the suture is brought superiorly through the levator to emerge just above the point at which the aponeurosis meets the levator muscle. Temporary knots are tied. If necessary, an additional lateral suture and possibly an additional medial suture are placed in a similar manner. *Inset:* The course of the suture is illustrated in cross section. The surgeon should check to be sure that the suture has not perforated either the tarsus or the conjunctiva.

The stronger the levator can be made, the greater the tension possible on the spring and, therefore, the more rapid the blink. The nuances of adjustment of both the levator and the spring can be appreciated only with experience. Nevertheless, once the general principles are understood, excellent results can be obtained (Fig. 60–4).

Gold Weight Implantation[15, 16]

The size of the weight is selected preoperatively. With the patient seated, a gold weight (or the comparable weight from a sizing set) that is estimated to be suitable for the degree of lagophthalmos is selected and is secured to the patient's upper lid with cyanoacrylate glue, double-stick tape, or a temporary lid suture. The patient is then asked to open and close the eye, and the surgeon determines whether the weight of the gold is correct. The evaluation is repeated with the patient supine. Weights in the range of 1.2 to 1.5 g are suitable for use in most patients.

The weight may be fixated either supratarsally (Fig. 60–5) or tarsally. Supratarsal fixation is preferable unless the weight is so large that this is not practical. A scleral shell is placed. An incision is made in the lid fold, and dissection is carried upward to expose the orbital septum. The preaponeurotic fat can be seen through the septum, which is then opened and the weight secured to the levator with a single 5-0 polyester suture placed through the holes in the weight. The knot is buried. The function of the weight is then tested with the patient in the seated and supine positions. If the desired effect is not obtained, a different-sized weight may be tried. Overlying skin muscle is closed with running 6-0 plain gut suture.

Silicone Rod Prosthesis Implantation[17–19]

The prosthesis to be used in silicone rod prosthesis implantation is commercially available as a 1.0-mm diameter rod.

While the eye is protected with a scleral shell, a curvilinear incision is made overlying the medial canthal tendon (Fig. 60–6). The incision should be just lateral to the angular vein to avoid the vein in the course of the dissection. Dissection is then carried posteriorly to expose the origin of the tendon. The prosthesis is threaded on a large, noncutting needle (e.g., #5 Mayo needle), and is sewn

through the tendon twice. The lower arm should emerge from the posterior aspect of the tendon, which facilitates holding the lower lid against the globe.

A second incision is made at the lateral orbital rim, and dissection is carried to the periosteum. By use of sharp dissection, a tunnel is started in the plane between the orbicularis and the tarsus at the lateral aspect of the lower lid. A special introducer is then passed as close to the lid margin as possible across the lid to emerge medially close to where the silicone rod has been sewn through the tendon. The lower arm of the rod is then threaded onto the introducer, and the introducer is withdrawn laterally, thus bringing the rod through the lid. In a similar manner, the upper arm of the prosthesis is brought through the upper lid, except that passage is accomplished over the midtarsus.

The desired point of anchorage for the lower end of the prosthesis is determined, and a suture loop is formed at that point through periosteum by use of a 2-0 Prolene suture sewn through the periosteum twice at the orbital rim. The prosthesis must be secured at the inner aspect of the lateral orbital rim so as to pull the lid posteriorly. The point selected should be just above the horizontal raphe so as to draw the lid upward as well. In a similar manner, the upper arm of the prosthesis is secured just below the horizontal raphe, passing anterior to the lower arm.

With the patient in the seated position, suitable tension is placed on the lower arm to secure the lower lid in the desired position. (For additional discussion on how to best position the lid, see under Assessing Lid Position.) Similarly, the tension on the upper lid is adjusted to permit good opening and closing of the lid, and final knots are tied. Each arm of the prosthesis is further secured with additional suture bites through the lateral rim periosteum. A heavy suture, such as 2-0 Prolene, is selected to avoid cutting through the prosthesis. Deep tissues are closed with 5-0 plain gut suture medially and laterally, and the skin is closed with 6-0 plain gut suture.

LOWER LID REAPPOSITION PROCEDURES

Canthoplasty

Surgery may be performed at either the medial or lateral canthus to tighten and elevate the lower eyelid. Operating

FIGURE 60–4. The patient is a 49-year-old woman with facial paralysis secondary to an acoustic neuroma. She had undergone two tarsorrhaphy procedures before she was first seen for evaluation. A, Eyes open, but eye function is largely blocked by tarsorrhaphy. Note also the brow droop. B, Attempted closure. Note that the tarsorrhaphy, although extensive, fails to protect the cornea well. C, Eyes open. The tarsorrhaphy has been opened and the lid margins reconstructed. The patient also has had enhanced palpebral spring implantation, medial and lateral canthoplasties, correction of upper lid entropion, and elevation of the brow. D, Attempted closure. Note excellent protection of the cornea by the spring.

FIGURE 60–5. Gold weight. The levator is exposed, and the gold weight is secured to it with a single 5-0 polyester suture placed through the holes in the weight. The knot is buried. Larger weights may be placed pretarsally in a similar manner. T, tarsus; see Figure 60–3 for additional abbreviations.

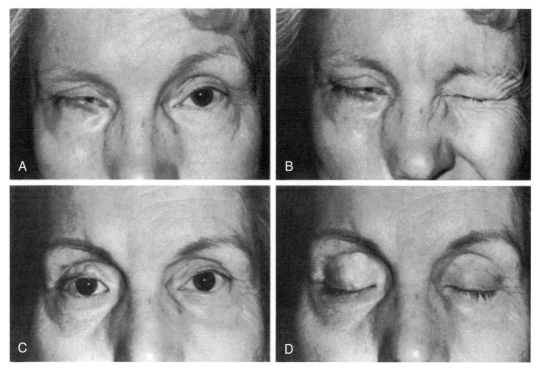

FIGURE 60-4

FIGURE 60-5

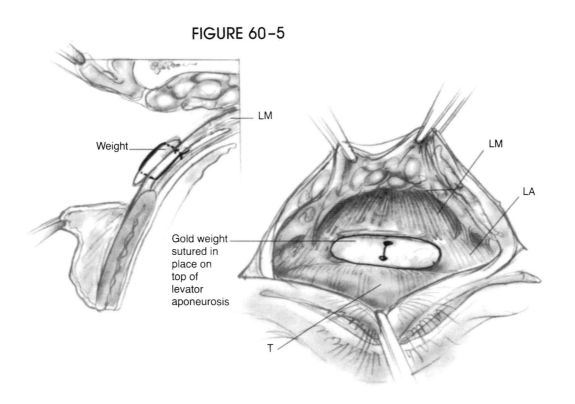

LM

Weight

Gold weight
sutured in
place on
top of
levator
aponeurosis

LM

LA

T

FIGURES 60–4 and 60–5. *See legends on opposite page*

FIGURE 60-6

Silastic
Elastic Prosthesis

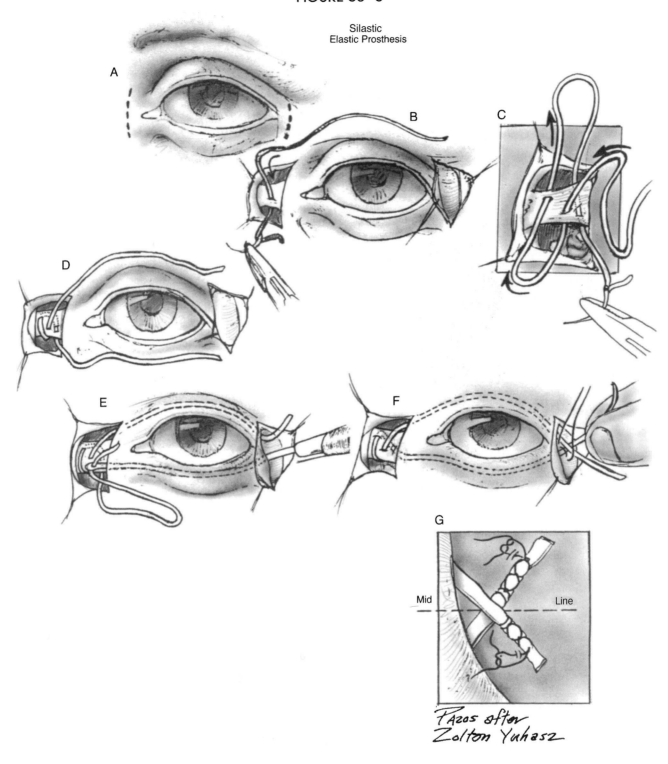

Pazos after
Zolton Yuhasz

FIGURE 60–6. Silicone rod prosthesis. *A,* An incision is made medially just lateral to the angular vein; a second incision is made laterally over the orbital rim. *B,* Laterally, dissection is carried down to expose the orbital rim. Medially, the medial canthal tendon is exposed, and the prosthesis is sewn through it by use of a large noncutting needle. *C,* The prosthesis is further sewn through the tendon so that the lower arm emerges posterior to the tendon, thereby facilitating holding the lower lid against the globe. *D,* Each arm of the prosthesis is ready to be engaged on the introducer. *E,* With a special introducer, the upper arm of the prosthesis has been passed between the orbicularis and tarsus in the upper lid, at the level of midtarsus. The introducer is shown in the lower lid, in preparation for passing the lower lid of the prosthesis. The prosthesis must be as close to the lid margin as possible to prevent ectropion of the lid. *F,* The lower arm of the prosthesis is secured to orbital rim periosteum with 2-0 Prolene suture. *G,* Both arms of the prosthesis are further sutured to the periosteum with 2-0 Prolene. Note that the inferior arm is posterior to the superior arm because the lower lid must be pulled posteriorly.

at the ends of the tarsus has the advantage of not creating an irregular lid margin or interfering with the visual field. Whereas tightening the lid only at the lateral canthus is usually the procedure of choice in patients with nonparalytic lid laxity, the paralyzed lid usually requires medial canthal tightening as well. Otherwise, tightening the lid only laterally may result in either marked displacement of the inferior punctum laterally or failure to elevate the lid. In some cases, tightening the lid only laterally can cause the lid to act as a shorter chord beneath the globe, thus actually lowering the lid rather than raising it. If only a limited amount of lid tightening and elevation is required, medial canthoplasty alone may be the procedure of choice.

Assessing Lid Position

Assuming that extraocular motility has not been impaired by excess local anesthesia infiltration, the position of the lid relative to the limbus (corneoscleral junction) can be used as a guideline in the adjustment of lid position. The gaze of the patient should be directed such that the limbus of the contralateral lid is placed just tangential to the inferior limbus. The lid being operated on can then be tightened to a position in which it, too, is tangential to the limbus, or it can be slightly overcorrected to allow for postoperative loosening. Matching this tangential position is more precise than judging the amount by which the lid crosses the cornea or comes inferior to it, compared with the other eye.

Medial Canthoplasty[20]

Medial canthoplasty consists of exposing the lower arm of the medial canthal tendon and the origin of the common tendon and tightening the lower arm. If additional effect is required, the upper arm of the tendon may also be exposed so that it, too, can be included in the surgical procedure.

Surgical Technique

To expose the medial canthal tendon, the globe is protected with a scleral shell, and the canaliculi are protected with probes. An incision is then made at the mucocutaneous junction, beginning 2 mm medial to the lower punctum, along the mucocutaneous junction to the medial canthus, and for an additional 2 mm beyond the canthus (Fig. 60–7). A skin-muscle flap is then elevated with scissors, and hemostasis is achieved with bipolar cautery. The insertion of the lower arm of the medial canthal tendon is then grasped with forceps and drawn superonasally, thereby permitting the placement of a 5-0 double-armed polyester suture through the insertion. Each arm of the suture is then woven through the tendon and sewn through the origin of the tendon. Temporary knots are tied.

The patient is then brought to the seated position, and the apposition of the lid and position of the punctum are evaluated. If a lateral canthoplasty is also being performed, sitting the patient up can be deferred, and tension on both sets of canthoplasty sutures can be adjusted simultaneously after completion of the lateral canthoplasty. If only a medial canthoplasty is being performed, the tension on the lid is

adjusted, and final knots are tied. In the event that the punctum is not adequately inverted by the suture used to tighten the medial canthal tendon, the canthal tendon is exposed in the upper lid, and a second 5-0 polyester suture is placed. Each arm of that suture starts at the lower edge of the inferior canthal tendon and ends at the upper edge of the superior canthal tendon, further inverting the lower punctum.

The canthoplasty using a suture only in the lower lid is completed by re-forming the mucocutaneous junction with 6-0 plain gut (on a tiny needle) running or interrupted sutures. These may be allowed to dissolve or may be removed in 5 to 7 days. When a second canthal suture is required, the lid flaps are closed to each other with 6-0 plain gut sutures. Since a second canthal suture results in the blunting of the canthal angle and horizontal shortening of the palpebral fissure, such a suture should not be used unnecessarily.

Lateral Canthoplasty[21, 22]

The object of lateral canthoplasty is to pull the lid superoposteriorly against the globe. In lieu of the various lid shortening procedures that have been used in the past, the currently preferred method is to create a new lateral canthal tendon from the tarsus itself and to secure it to the orbital rim.

Surgical Technique

A hemostat is placed across the lateral canthal angle and removed (Fig. 60–8). The clamped area is then cut with scissors, accomplishing a canthotomy. The inferior crux of the lateral canthal tendon is then cut (inferior cantholysis) with scissors. At this point, the lateral aspect of the lower lid is freely movable. The lid is then pulled taut across the globe. If a medial canthoplasty has been performed, suitable tension should be placed on that canthoplasty suture before this maneuver.

The amount of excess lid is marked, and the skin-muscle lamina is separated from the tarsus lateral to this mark. The lid margin in this area is also removed. Some surgeons prefer to remove the conjunctiva at this point, thereby leaving a pure tarsal tongue. I have not found such removal necessary, and the tarsus may be damaged during such attempts. A double-armed 5-0 polyester suture is passed as a mattress suture beginning on the anterior surface of the tarsus, 3 mm from the lateral end, with each needle emerging through the cut end. A second pass of each suture arm is made and each arm of the suture locked. The lower arm of the suture is marked with a marking pen for future reference.

A tunnel is then made underneath the upper arm of the lateral canthal tendon, and a clamp is passed into the tunnel. The sutures are grasped within the clamp and brought through the tunnel. The desired location of the lid is determined, and the sutures are placed appropriately, with care taken to obtain a bite of orbital rim periosteum at the inside aspect of the rim, slightly superior to the desired lid position. In this manner, the lid is drawn up and posteriorly. The previously placed mark on the suture helps

FIGURE 60-7
MEDIAL CANTHOPLASTY

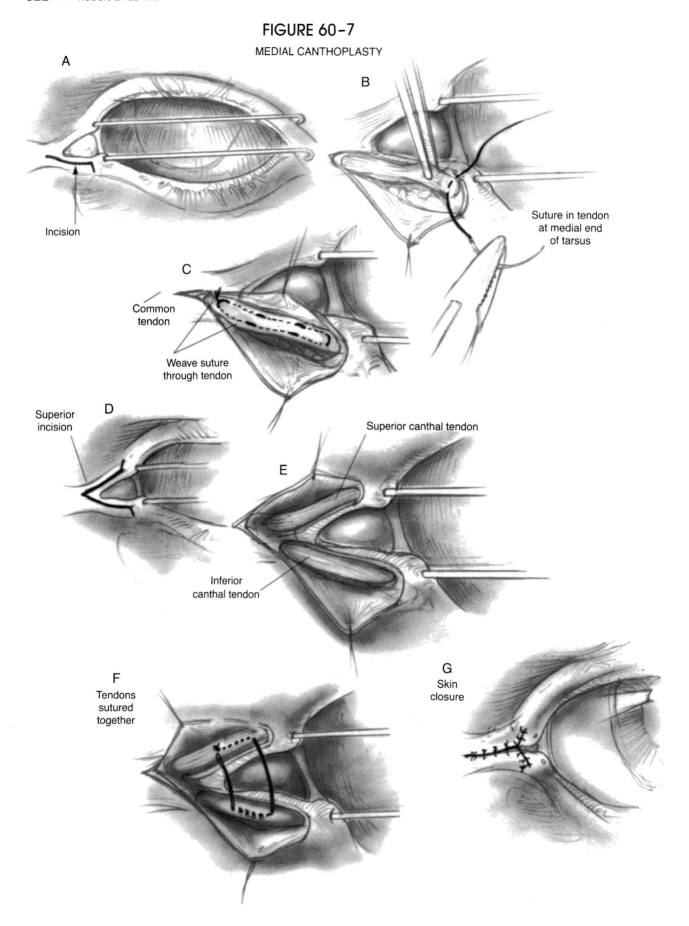

A

Incision

B

Suture in tendon
at medial end
of tarsus

C

Common
tendon

Weave suture
through tendon

D

Superior
incision

E

Superior canthal tendon

Inferior
canthal tendon

F

Tendons
sutured
together

G

Skin
closure

FIGURE 60–7. *See legend on opposite page*

to avoid confusion about the location of the inferior arm of the suture. A temporary knot is tied, and the patient is brought to the seated position. Adjustments in lid position and tension can then be made, and final knots can be tied.

The surgeon completes the canthoplasty by trimming excess skin and muscle, re-establishing the canthal angle with a 5-0 plain gut suture, and closing the skin with 6-0 plain gut suture. In situations in which lateral canthoplasty is combined with palpebral spring implantation and the amount of lid tightening required is not too great, a variant of the technique may be used. In such circumstances, a separate canthal incision is not required. Rather, the upper arm of the lateral canthal tendon may be approached from the existent extended lid fold incision.

A tunnel is made under the upper arm of the tendon. With forceps placed into the tunnel, the lateral aspect of the tarsus of the lower lid is grasped and brought into the tunnel. A 5-0 polyester double-armed suture is then placed in the tarsus. This stitch is used to re-create the lateral canthal tendon in a manner similar to that described previously. However, if a great deal of lid tightening is required, it is not possible to omit the steps of canthotomy and inferior cantholysis and still adequately mobilize the lid to achieve the desired position.

Fascia Lata Suspension of Lower Lid

In patients in whom medial and lateral canthoplasty together are inadequate to elevate the central portion of the lid, the lid may be supported by a fascia lata suspension. In this procedure, the fascia lata is anchored at each end of the lid and acts as a hammock to support the central lid.

Either autologous or banked fascia lata can be used. The preserved fascia lata is more subject to resorption over time; therefore, the autologous fascia lata is more likely to give a reliable long-term result. When autologous fascia lata is used, it is obtained from the leg by a general surgeon while the lid is being prepared for its placement.

Surgical Technique

A strip of fascia 3/16-inch wide and approximately 4 inches long is used. The technique for placing the fascia within the medial canthal tendon and in the lower lid is similar to that described in the section on the silicone rod prosthesis. The medial end of the fascia is anchored by means of a 5-0 polyester suture passed twice through the fascia and the medial canthal tendon (Fig. 60–9). The knot of the suture should be well buried to avoid later erosion.

The lateral end of the tendon is secured to the inner aspect of the lateral orbital rim with 5-0 polyester suture in a manner similar to that described for lateral canthoplasty and is adjusted in a similar way before final knots are tied. The suture, however, should encircle the fascia rather than go through it to avoid tearing it. Once the fascia has been fixed in its position, additional bites through the periosteum and around the fascia are desirable to prevent slippage. Performing canthotomy and inferior cantholysis may be necessary to adequately mobilize the lid so that the fascial suspension holds it in the desired position.

ANCILLARY PROCEDURES

Patients with facial paralysis frequently manifest brow droop and entropion of the upper lid. These problems can be addressed surgically at the same time that upper lid reanimation surgery is undertaken. Elevation of the ptotic brow in a patient with facial paralysis should not be undertaken independent of a procedure to enhance lid closure. The droop of the brow tends to push the lid shut and thereby ameliorates the upper lid lagophthalmos. Therefore, correcting the brow position without concomitantly improving upper lid closure may significantly worsen the patient's lagophthalmos.

Brow Elevation[20]

An eyebrow can be elevated in the following ways:

1. Excising the skin and muscle just above the brow
2. Suspending the brow from the periosteum above it
3. Lifting the forehead by a coronal approach
4. Endoscopically raising the brow

FIGURE 60–7. Medial canthoplasty. *A,* While the globe is protected with a scleral shell and the canaliculi are protected with probes, an incision is made along the mucocutaneous junction and continued downward at a point 2 mm medial to the punctum. *B,* An inferior flap is elevated, which exposes the inferior arm of the medial canthal tendon. The tendon is pulled medially to expose its junction with the lateral aspect of the tarsus (insertion of the tendon), and a 5-0 polyester double-armed suture is placed through the insertion. *C,* Each arm of the suture is woven through the tendon and brought through the origin of the tendon. The two sutures are then tied under appropriate tension, thereby tightening the lower lid. The mucocutaneous junction is then reconstructed with 8-0 Vicryl suture, thereby leaving the medial canthus with a normal appearance. *D,* If additional lower lid inversion is required, a second incision is made in the upper lid along the mucocutaneous junction, directed upward at a point 2 mm medial to the punctum. *E,* A superior flap is elevated, which exposes the superior arm of the canthal tendon. *F,* A 5-0 polyester suture is placed as a horizontal mattress suture. The suture passes near the lower end of the lower tendon and near the upper end of the upper tendon, thus inverting the lids. *G,* The edges of the skin flaps are closed to each other with 6-0 plain gut suture. The steps shown in *D* through *G* may be performed independently when lid inversion is more important than lid tightening, or they may be combined with the steps shown in *A* through *C.* When the steps *D* through *G* are required, the result is a more blunted medial canthal angle, with some shortening of the horizontal fissure. Therefore, if the procedure shown in *A* through *C* suffices, it is preferable. Nevertheless, the additional steps may be required in patients with marked medial lid laxity or eversion.

FIGURE 60–8
LATERAL CANTHOPLASTY

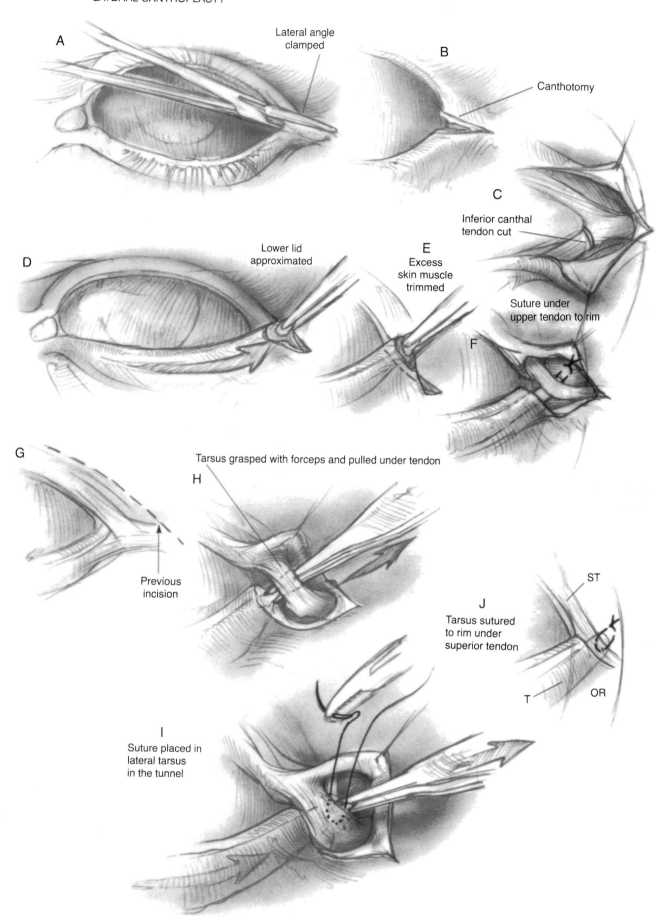

A — Lateral angle clamped

B — Canthotomy

C — Inferior canthal tendon cut
Suture under upper tendon to rim

D — Lower lid approximated

E — Excess skin muscle trimmed

F

G — Previous incision

H — Tarsus grasped with forceps and pulled under tendon

I — Suture placed in lateral tarsus in the tunnel

J — Tarsus sutured to rim under superior tendon
ST
T
OR

FIGURE 60–8 *See legend on opposite page*

The coronal forehead lift requires extensive dissection, does not give as much effect as a direct lift, and may be difficult to control to elevate only one brow. A direct approach to brow elevation is generally preferable in facial paralysis patients. Skin and muscle excision alone is less effective in the paralyzed frontalis than in a normally innervated frontalis. I have found combining skin-muscle excision with brow suspension and simple brow suspension to be the two most useful brow-elevating procedures. Endoscopic brow elevation is more time consuming and therefore may be harder to do in a patient who is undergoing multiple procedures. However, it is an excellent procedure.

The choice of the procedure depends on several factors. First, will frontalis function return? If so, it is best not to excise tissue but only to suspend the brow. The second factor to consider is the effect of raising the brow without tissue excision. In some patients, this process induces a few brow wrinkles, which are actually welcome from an appearance standpoint in a previously abnormally smooth area. In others, only a bulge of tissue is created by elevation of the brow without tissue excision. In such patients skin-muscle excision can be performed.

Elevating the entire brow is not always necessary. The point of maximum brow elevation should be noted on the contralateral side. A line drawn downward through this point usually passes at or near the lateral canthus. The exact position of such an imaginary line should be noted, and a comparable line should be marked on the side to be operated. Some patients have a different brow configuration and require more medial elevation.

Once the point of maximum brow elevation is determined and marked, the brow is raised at that point. How much of the brow must be elevated to obtain a desirable contour can then be seen.

The extent of required brow elevation can also be judged by drawing a line tangential to the point of maximum brow elevation on the contralateral side. This line is drawn perpendicular to a vertical line bisecting the nose. Corresponding points on each brow are marked and measured relative to the horizontal reference line to determine the extent of brow elevation required at each point on the paralyzed side.

If it cannot be determined with certainty whether tissue excision will be required, the extent of the anticipated excision should be marked in advance of lid infiltration, so that the determination is not distorted by the swelling induced by the injection. The brow can then be suspended without tissue excision. If the result is not pleasing, skin-muscle excision can be carried out.

Be sure to assess the role of the ptotic brow in aiding lid closure. If a paretic brow that is assisting closure is raised without simultaneously performing a procedure such as spring implantation to enhance lid closure, the result may be worsened lagophthalmos.

Surgical Technique

The area in which brow elevation, tissue excision, or both, are required is marked as close to the superior extent of the brow as possible (Fig. 60–10), which will help conceal the resultant scar. The skin is incised perpendicular to the skin surface with a scalpel blade until muscle is reached. Blunt dissection is then carried out at each site where a suspension suture is deemed necessary. The brow is elevated during the dissection so that the frontalis periosteum is encountered superior to the brow. A 4-0 Novafil suture on a very curved needle is passed through the periosteum and then through the dermis at the lower aspect of the wound as a horizontal mattress suture. Between one and four such sutures may be required, depending on the contour of the brow.

When all of the planned sutures have been placed and temporary knots have been tied, the patient is brought to the seated position, and the brow contour is adjusted to match that on the contralateral side in the primary position of gaze.

The normally innervated, nonfixated brow moves downward on lid closure—the suspended brow is not capable of doing this. Care must therefore be taken not to elevate the brow so much that a cicatricial lagophthalmos is induced. Especially in patients in whom lid skin is in short supply (e.g., in those who have undergone a previous blepharoplasty), fully elevating the paretic brow may not be possible without adversely affecting lid closure. In such cases, it is better to place the brow slightly lower than the contralateral side rather than induce lagophthalmos. Final knots are then tied. If skin-muscle excision is required, it can then be carried out. The Novafil sutures are rotated to deeply bury the knots.

FIGURE 60–8. Lateral canthoplasty. A, A hemostat is used to clamp the lateral canthal angle for hemostasis. B, The clamp is removed, and a lateral canthotomy is performed. C, The inferior canthal tendon is cut so that the lower lid is freely movable. D, The lower lid is approximated to the desired position with slight overcorrection. E, The excess skin-muscle and mucocutaneous junction tissue are excised, leaving a tarsal tongue. F, A double-armed 5-0 polyester suture is passed through the tarsal tongue, and one arm of the suture is marked with a marking pen for subsequent identification. A tunnel is then created under the superior arm of the lateral canthal tendon. A clamp is passed into the tunnel, and the sutures are grasped and withdrawn laterally. The tarsal tongue is brought into the tunnel and secured under the desired tension to the lateral orbital rim periosteum. By use of the identifying markings previously placed, the superior suture is kept superior, and the inferior suture is kept inferior, preventing twisting of the tarsus. The suture is tied under appropriate tension. The canthoplasty is completed with a 5-0 plain gut suture to re-establish the canthal angle and 6-0 plain gut suture to close skin muscle. G, When lateral canthoplasty is combined with spring implantation and only a moderate amount of lateral canthal tightening is required, the procedure can be accomplished through the prior lid fold incision. H, A tunnel is made under the superior arm of the lateral canthal tendon. A forceps is introduced into the tunnel, and the lateral aspect of the tarsus is grasped. I, The lateral end of the tarsus is drawn into the tunnel, and a doubled-armed 5-0 polyester suture is used to secure it. J, Each arm of the 5-0 polyester suture is secured through orbital rim periosteum under suitable tension (T, tarsus; OR, orbital rim; ST, superior tendon).

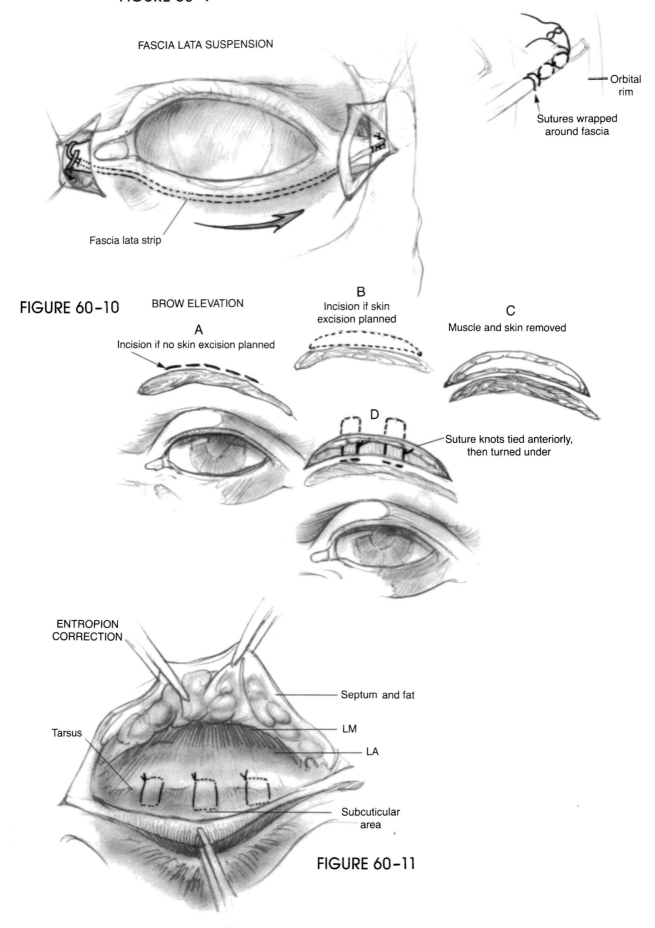

FIGURE 60-9

FASCIA LATA SUSPENSION

Orbital rim

Sutures wrapped around fascia

Fascia lata strip

FIGURE 60-10

BROW ELEVATION

A
Incision if no skin excision planned

B
Incision if skin excision planned

C
Muscle and skin removed

D
Suture knots tied anteriorly, then turned under

ENTROPION CORRECTION

Septum and fat

LM

LA

Tarsus

Subcuticular area

FIGURE 60-11

FIGURES 60–9 to 60–11. *See legends on opposite page*

The brow should be closed in layers to minimize the scar. Depending on the thickness of the tissue, one or two rows of deep 5-0 or 6-0 Vicryl sutures are placed before skin closure with interrupted 5-0 plain gut sutures and a Steri-Strip.

Correction of Upper Lid Entropion

Correction of upper lid entropion is most easily carried out in combination with spring implantation, either enhanced or nonenhanced. This correction can be carried out as a separate procedure by opening the lid in the lid fold or, in combination with gold weight implantation, by extending the lid fold incision across the entire lid.

A series of 6-0 Vicryl sutures is placed across the lid (Fig. 60–11). Each of these sutures begins supratarsally, in the levator, and continues as a horizontal mattress suture through subcuticular tissue just inferior to the lower aspect of the skin incision. Tightening these sutures rotates the lid margin outward, thereby correcting the entropion resulting from the facial paralysis or from the downward pressure from an implanted prosthetic device. Tension on the sutures is adjusted at the time of surgery to give a slight overcorrection. The sutures also create a pleasing lid fold.

TEMPORIZING MEASURES

Two simple techniques are presented to protect the eye before a decision to undertake definitive surgery is made.

Lid Suture Taped to Cheek

A lid suture can easily be placed at the conclusion of a neurotologic or head and neck procedure in which the function of the fifth or seventh cranial nerve is anticipated to be compromised postoperatively. The suture protects the eye during the immediate postoperative period without impairing the ability to check for pupillary or other neurologic signs involving the eye. If the patient subsequently requires temporary eye protection involving less than round-the-clock eye closure, the suture may be taped out of the way (to the forehead) during part of the day and used to close the eye at other times.

The eye is protected with a scleral shell. A 4-0 or 5-0 nonresorbable monofilament suture is passed through the skin and orbicularis, which have been pulled away from the tarsus with forceps (Fig. 60–12). The needle is passed parallel to the tarsus. The two arms of the suture are tied together with multiple knots to prevent slippage underneath the tape and are secured to the cheek with a strip of tape. The suture is then brought upward and locked with a second piece of tape. A third strip further locks the suture and keeps it out of the way. When it is necessary to inspect the eye or to check for pupillary signs, all three pieces of tape can be lifted together with the suture away from the cheek and then replaced. By placing antibiotic ointment at the suture sites in the lid, one can usually maintain a suture in the lid for 2 to 3 weeks without undue lid induration.

Temporary Tarsorrhaphy Suture

Temporary tarsorrhaphy suturing allows the lids to be kept securely closed over a several-week period without damage to the lid margins from the creation of a true tarsorrhaphy. It also permits one to inspect the eye at intervals by untying the suture, inspecting the eye, and retying the suture without having to replace it. It is particularly useful when there is a significant lower lid laxity component to the exposure problem.

The eye is protected with a scleral shell. Each arm of a double-armed, monofilament, nonresorbable suture is passed through the skin and orbicularis of the central third of the upper lid, beginning 5 mm above the lid margin and exiting at the gray line of the lid margin (Fig. 60–13). The sutures continue into the gray line of the lower lid, exiting through the orbicularis and skin 5 mm below the lid mar-

---

FIGURE 60–9. Fascia lata suspension. This technique is analogous to that shown for placing the silicone rod prosthesis. The fascial strip is placed on a large needle and sewn through the medial canthal tendon, emerging behind the tendon. The end is locked with 5-0 polyester suture. With the special introducer, the fascia is brought laterally through the lid, where it is secured to orbital rim periosteum with 5-0 polyester suture in a manner similar to that described under lateral canthoplasty. Excess fascia lata is further secured to the periosteum by continuation of the same sutures after the initial knots are tied. These sutures encircle the fascia rather than perforate it, to avoid tearing it.

FIGURE 60–10. Brow elevation. A, If skin-muscle excision is not planned, an incision is made as close as possible to the brow over the area that needs to be suspended. Usually, this area consists of approximately the central two thirds of the brow. B, When skin-muscle excision is planned, the ellipse to be excised is marked, and skin incision is performed. C, Skin and muscle have been removed. D, Regardless of whether skin-muscle excision is required, suspension sutures are placed in a similar manner. Dissection is carried superiorly to expose periosteum. Sutures of 4-0 Novafil are placed through periosteum and then through subcuticular tissue at the lower end of the wound. After these have been tied under appropriate tension, the brow is closed in layers.

FIGURE 60–11. Correction of upper lid entropion. A series of 6-0 Vicryl horizontal mattress sutures are placed between the lower edge of levator aponeurosis (LA) and subcuticular tissue close to the inferior edge of the wound. Tightening these sutures under appropriate tension rotates the lashes outward and also creates a pleasing lid fold. LM, levator muscle.

FIGURE 60-12

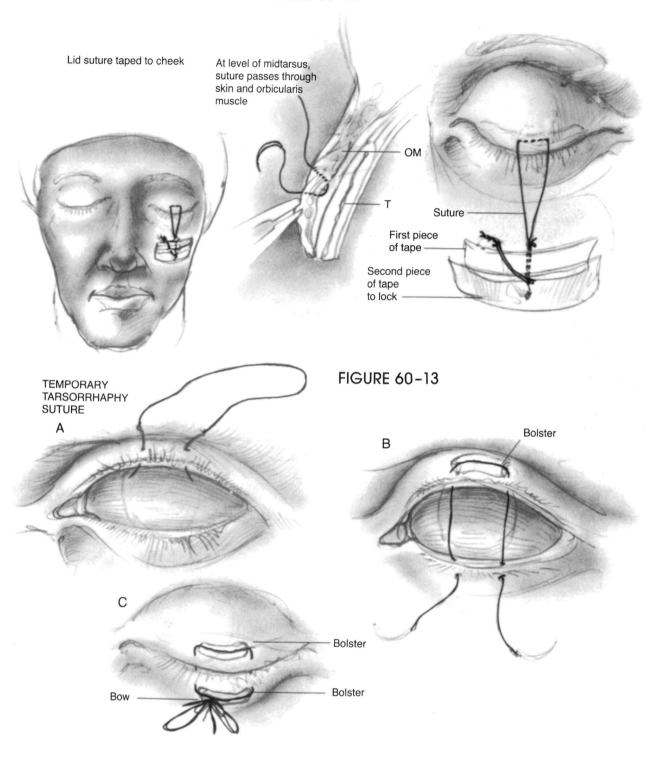

Lid suture taped to cheek

At level of midtarsus, suture passes through skin and orbicularis muscle

OM

T

Suture

First piece of tape

Second piece of tape to lock

TEMPORARY TARSORRHAPHY SUTURE

A

FIGURE 60-13

B

Bolster

C

Bolster

Bolster

Bow

FIGURE 60–12. Lid suture. A 4-0 or 5-0 nonresorbable monofilament suture is passed through skin and orbicularis muscle (OM), which have been pulled away from the tarsus (T) with forceps. The two arms of the suture are tied together with multiple knots to prevent slippage underneath the tape and are secured to the cheek with a strip of tape. The suture is then brought upward and locked with a second piece of tape.

FIGURE 60–13. Temporary tarsorrhaphy suture. *A,* Each arm of a double-armed nonresorbable monofilament suture is passed through the skin and orbicularis of the central third of the upper lid, beginning 5 mm above the lid margin and exiting at the gray line of the lid margin. *B,* The sutures continue to the gray line of the lower lid, exiting through the orbicularis and skin 5 mm below the lid margin. The two arms of the suture are placed 1 cm apart. *C,* Cotton bolsters are placed between the suture and skin before the suture is tied. The suture is tied with a bow, and the ends are left long.

gin. The two arms of the suture are placed 1-cm apart. Cotton bolsters are placed between the suture and skin before the suture is tied. The suture is tied like a shoelace, with a bow (leaving the ends of the suture long), to facilitate untying and retying in the future. The bow and ends of the suture are taped out of the way to the lid. Antibiotic ointment is applied to the suture sites twice daily, thus allowing the suture to be maintained for several weeks without undue induration of the lid.

CONCLUSIONS

By appropriate selection of the procedures presented, most patients with facial paralysis can be helped to obtain markedly improved lid position and function. Because eye problems frequently present major hurdles on the road to recovery, lid surgery greatly advances the patient's chances for successful overall rehabilitation.

The purpose of this chapter is to present procedures as I currently do them. Many of the modifications are my own, and tracing the historical evolution of procedures is not always possible. However, I would be remiss if I did not credit those who initially devised, pioneered, or popularized these procedures. The following is a summary of that information:

Procedure	Author
Palpebral spring	Morel-Fatio and Lalardrie[4, 5] Levine and colleagues[6–14]
Enhanced palpebral spring	Levine[13, 14]
Gold weight	Jobe,[15] May[16]
Silicone rod prosthesis	Arion,[17] Marrone and Soll,[18] Levine[7, 11, 13]
Medial canthoplasty and brow lift	Beard[20]
Lateral canthoplasty	Tenzel and colleagues[21, 22]

References

1. Jelks GW, Smith B, Bosniak S: The evaluation and management of the eye in facial palsy. Clin Plast Surg 6:397–419, 1979.
2. Rosenstock TG, Hurwitz JJ, Nedzelski JM, Tator CH: Ocular complications following excision of cerebellopontine angle tumours. Can Opthalmol 21:134–139, 1986.
3. Seiff SR, Chang J: Management of ophthalmic complications of facial nerve palsy. Otolaryngol Clin North Am 25:669–690, 1992.
4. Morel-Fatio D, Lalardrie JP: Palliative surgical treatment of facial paralysis: The palpebral spring. Plast Reconstr Surg 33:446, 1964.
5. Morel-Fatio D, Lalardrie JP: Le ressort palpebral: Contribution a l'etude de la chirurgie plastique de la paralysie faciale. Neurochirurgie 11:303, 1965.
6. Levine RE, House WF, Hitselberger WE: Ocular complications of seventh nerve paralysis and management with the palpebral spring. Am J Ophthalmol 73:219, 1972.
7. Levine RE: Management of the eye after acoustic tumor surgery. In House WF, Luetje CM (eds): Acoustic Tumors, Vol 2. Baltimore, University Park Press, 1979, pp 105–149.
8. Levine RE: Management of the ophthalmologic complications of facial paralysis. Trans Pac Coast Ophthalmol Otolaryngol Soc 61:85–93, 1980.
9. Levine RE: Protection of the exposed eye. In Brackmann DE (ed): Neurological Surgery of the Ear and Skull Base. New York, Raven Press, 1982, pp 81–87.
10. Levine RE: Protection of the exposed eye in facial paralysis. In Graham MD, House WF (eds): Disorders of the Facial Nerve. New York, Raven Press, 1982, pp 336–375.
11. Levine RE: Eyelid reanimation surgery. In May M (ed): The Facial Nerve. New York, Thieme-Stratton, 1985, pp 681–694.
12. Levine RE: Palpebral spring for lagophthalmos due to facial nerve palsy. In Wesley RE (ed): Techniques in Ophthalmic Plastic Surgery. New York, John Wiley & Sons, 1986, pp 424–427.
13. Levine RE: Management of lagophthalmos with palpebral spring and silastic elastic prosthesis. In Hornblass A (ed): Ophthalmic and Orbital Plastic Reconstructive Surgery, Vol 1. Baltimore, Williams & Wilkins, 1989, pp 384–392.
14. Levine RE: Lid reanimation with the palpebral spring. In Wright K, Tse D (eds): Color Atlas of Ophthalmic Surgery. Philadelphia, JB Lippincott, 1992, pp 231–238.
15. Jobe RP: A technique for lid-loading in the management of lagophthalmos in facial paralysis. Plast Reconstr Surg 53:29–31, 1974.
16. May M: Surgical rehabilitation of facial palsy. In May M (ed): The Facial Nerve. New York, Thieme-Stratton, 1985, pp 695–777.
17. Arion HG: Dynamic closure of the lids in paralysis of the orbicularis muscle. Int Surg 57:48, 1972.
18. Marrone AC, Soll D: Modification of the Arion encircling silicone spring. Thesis for membership in the American Society of Ophthalmic Plastic and Reconstructive Surgery, 1977.
19. Wood-Smith D: Experience with the Arion prosthesis. In Tessier P (ed): Symposium on Plastic Surgery in the Orbital Region. St. Louis, CV Mosby, 1976.
20. Beard C: Canthoplasty and brow elevation for facial palsy. Arch Ophthalmol 71:386–388, 1964.
21. Tenzel RR: Treatment of lagophthalmos of the lower lid. Arch Ophthalmol 81:366–368, 1969.
22. Tenzel RR, Buffam FV, Miller GR: The use of the lateral canthal sling in ectropion repair. Can J Ophthalmol 12:199–202, 1977.

61

Hypoglossal Facial Anastomosis

William M. Luxford, M.D. ▪ James R. House III, M.D.

Facial nerve injury is a debilitating problem, both cosmetically and functionally. During the course of otologic and neurotologic surgery, sacrifice of the facial nerve is sometimes necessary and also may occur inadvertently, no matter how meticulous the technique may be. In these cases, one must be prepared to rehabilitate and restore function as much as possible. Direct repair of the injured nerve is currently the best option available to re-establish facial function. If a direct approximation of the nerve ends is not possible, a graft connecting the two ends is the next best choice. Nevertheless, there are situations in which neither of these options is feasible. Perhaps the most common of these involves the extirpation of cerebellopontine angle tumors, in which the facial nerve is severed at the brainstem and there is no proximal stump in which to splice a graft. There are also cases in which a very attenuated but intact nerve regains no function. In these situations, an alternative to direct repair and nerve grafting is required.

Ideally, facial nerve restoration procedures should provide normal facial tone and symmetry, strong volitional and emotional facial movement, protection of the eye, facilitation of mastication, avoidance of dyskinesias, and no additional motor deficits. Unfortunately, even immediate direct anastomosis cannot fulfill these criteria. Several methods to restore some facial function have been developed that require neither direct repair nor grafting. These include cross-facial nerve grafting, nerve muscle pedicle grafts, and nerve substitutions, such as phrenic, accessory, hypoglossal, and ansa cervicalis.

Connection of a graft with the normal facial nerve followed by redirection of some of these fibers to the paralyzed side known as *crossfacial grafting*. This method provides symmetry of movement, both volitionally and emotionally, while avoiding other motor deficits. However, this procedure partially compromises the normal nerve and provides a scant supply of neural elements to the recipient muscles, leading to inconsistent results.[1–4] As a consequence, this procedure has not met with widespread acceptance.[5–7]

Nerve-muscle pedicle grafts have been used with some success but have also yielded inconsistent results.[8, 9] Because the results of nerve-muscle pedicle grafts and faciofacial crossover grafts have been disappointing, modifications of these procedures have been developed that use combination crossnerve grafting and microvascular free muscle flaps for facial reanimation.[8, 10] Efforts are also being made to use electrical stimulation of nerve pedicle grafts to overcome limitations seen with nerve muscle pedicle grafts.[11]

Nerve substitution procedures have the advantages of providing a large supply of axons to the recipient muscles

and of being technically facile. The results are rather consistent and predictable. The major disadvantages include the loss of emotional facial function and the donor deficit. Because the loss of function of one side of the tongue proves not to be a major debility, and the relationship of tongue movement to facial movement is close, the hypoglossal-facial (XII–VII) anastomosis has proved to be a useful procedure in cases of facial paralysis in which a direct repair or graft is impossible. This chapter focuses on the hypoglossal-facial anastomosis.

PATIENT SELECTION

Patients with facial paralysis must receive a detailed evaluation to determine the etiology of the paralysis. In some cases, the cause is obvious, as in resection of the nerve in the course of removal of a neoplasm. The evaluation of facial palsy of unknown cause is beyond the scope of this chapter. However, careful evaluation should precede any reanimation procedure to avoid missing treatable disease and to avoid destruction of a nerve that has potential for return of function.

In cases of known facial nerve discontinuity in which direct repair or grafting is impossible, the XII–VII anastomosis should be performed as soon as reasonably possible. Muscle atrophy and degeneration proceed rapidly after denervation.[12] Early repair provides axonal growth to the muscles and limits the amount of muscle degeneration.

The severed nerve also begins to experience fibrosis.[13, 14] In early anastomosis, new axons fill the nerve sheath prior to fibrosis and potentially allow a greater supply of axons to the muscles. Although earlier anastomosis gives a better functional result, the XII–VII anastomosis is also effective after a prolonged denervation and should be considered up to 2.5 years after injury.[6] Return of function can occur up to 4.5 years after injury.[15]

In other patients in whom the continuity of the nerve is in question, including those who suffer from trauma, idiopathic palsy, and nerves damaged in surgery, it is prudent to wait at least 1 year to make certain that no return is possible. Electrophysiologic testing is helpful in determining the innervation and viability of facial muscles. A positive response to electroneuronography or evoked electromyography indicates that at least some motor end plates are functional. These patients should be given the longest possible time to show improvement in function. However, some of these patients have so few remaining neural elements that they will never regain any useful function. In this situation, a XII–VII graft helps provide a sufficient amount of neurons to the muscles.

Electromyography helps detect polyphasic action potentials indicative of reinnervation, as well as fibrillation potentials indicative of denervation. In cases of long-standing paralysis (>2.5 years), a muscle biopsy in addition to electromyography may be useful to determine viability, atrophy, and fibrosis. In cases of severe muscle atrophy and neural fibrosis, the results of any reinnervation procedure will be poor, and muscle transfers and other augmentive procedures should be considered.

The clinician should also consider the status of the contralateral twelfth nerve when deciding on the XII–VII crossover. Contralateral hypoglossal paralysis is a contraindication to the XII–VII crossover, as are multiple lower cranial nerve deficits that already compromise swallowing and speech.

SURGICAL TECHNIQUE

In addition to standard head and neck surgical instrumentation, hypoglossal facial anastomosis requires jeweler's forceps to handle the nerve ends, a Castroviejo needle holder, and microforceps for knot tying. A sterile tongue blade is useful to improve visibility when the ends of the nerves are anastomosed under microscopic vision.

After satisfactory general endotracheal anesthesia has been obtained with the patient in the supine position, the neck is extended and the face turned toward the side opposite the paralysis. The ear, face, and neck are prepared and draped in sterile manner. A standard lazy-S parotidectomy incision is made in the preauricular crease and extended behind the lobule and then anteriorly about 2 cm below the angle of the mandible (Fig. 61–1). Skin flaps are raised anteriorly and posteriorly. The parotid is mobilized from the anterior border of the sternocleidomastoid muscle and from the external auditory canal. The angle formed by the cartilage of the anterior external canal, known as the *tragal pointer*, is then followed medially to the stylomastoid foramen, where the facial nerve exits the temporal bone. The nerve is dissected from the parotid gland to expose the pes anserinus and free the main trunk from the gland. The nerve is then transected at the stylomastoid foramen.

The hypoglossal nerve is identified by retracting the sternocleidomastoid muscle posteriorly and exposing the great vessels of the neck. The posterior belly of the digastric muscle is retracted superiorly, and the hypoglossal is found coursing inferiorly with the great vessels and then turning anteriorly as it supplies the ansa cervicalis, which descends in the carotid sheath (Fig. 61–2). The hypoglossal nerve is followed anteriorly and medially as it enters the tongue muscle. The nerve is freed from its fascial attachments in the neck. The network of veins and arteries entering the internal jugular vein and external carotid artery should be controlled during this maneuver. After the nerve is freed from its attachments, it is divided as far anteriorly as is possible to gain sufficient length. The free hypoglossal nerve is then rotated superiorly. Directing the nerve medial to the digastric in this rotation will give the most length but is not necessary for a satisfactory anastomosis.

There are many ways to anastomose the ends of the nerves, including collagen trays and fibrin glue, vein sheaths, laser welding, and various suture techniques. It is beyond the scope of this chapter to describe the various methods; however, several principles are almost universally agreed on. The two ends of the nerves should be free of all tension. This requirement is usually not a problem if the technique described earlier is followed. The ends should be cut sharply to provide a flush connection. The anastomosis should be as atraumatic as possible and yet provide strength to prevent disruption. It is also important to make sure, using frozen section histologic evaluation, that the distal facial nerve has not totally fibrosed in cases of long-standing paralysis. A conventional suture technique that yields reliable results is described as follows:

By use of the operating microscope, the distal end of the facial nerve and proximal end of the hypoglossal nerves are stripped of the epineurium 2 to 3 mm from the cut ends. The ends are freshened with a sharp, clean, perpendicular cut to provide a good flush connection. The perineurium is then approximated with two or three 9-0 nylon sutures (Fig. 61–3). The wound is closed in layers over a Penrose drain. A fluffed, snug parotidectomy dressing is applied, and the drain is removed the next day. Perioperative antibiotics are not necessary.

A modification of the standard XII-VII crossover graft uses a jump graft between the twelfth and seventh nerves. This procedure, as described by May and associates, succeeds in preserving tongue function as well as reinnervating the facial muscles.[16] The exposure of the twelfth and seventh nerves is identical to that described earlier (see Fig. 61–2). In this incision, the great auricular nerve can be seen coursing across the sternocleidomastoid muscle. A 5-cm length of this nerve is harvested (Fig. 61–4). The twelfth nerve is then cut through on half of its diameter in a beveled manner. The incision must be made in a portion of the nerve distal to the divergence of the ansa cervicalis to avoid tapping the fibers that constitute this nerve. Stimulation of the twelfth nerve with a nerve stimulator proximal to the partial transection should confirm preservation of tongue function. The great auricular graft and the distal segment of the facial nerve are then prepared for anastomosis in the manner described for the standard XII–VII crossover. The graft is sutured to the proximal segment of the partially severed twelfth nerve. The other end of the graft is sutured to the prepared distal end of the facial nerve (Fig. 61–5). Two or three sutures are used for this connection. Enough length of graft must be used to avoid tension at the sites of anastomosis. The wound is then closed as in the standard procedure.

The patient is usually kept in the hospital overnight and discharged the following morning after removal of the drain. Although the patient may have some trouble with pooling of food in the ipsilateral oral vestibule, no special diet is necessary.

RESULTS

The patient with facial paralysis who is considered a candidate for the XII–VII crossover procedure should be counseled about the expected results from this procedure. The patient cannot expect normal facial function.[5, 6, 17–21] There are several reasons for this. As in a direct nerve repair, the axons directed to specific muscles find a random path. The

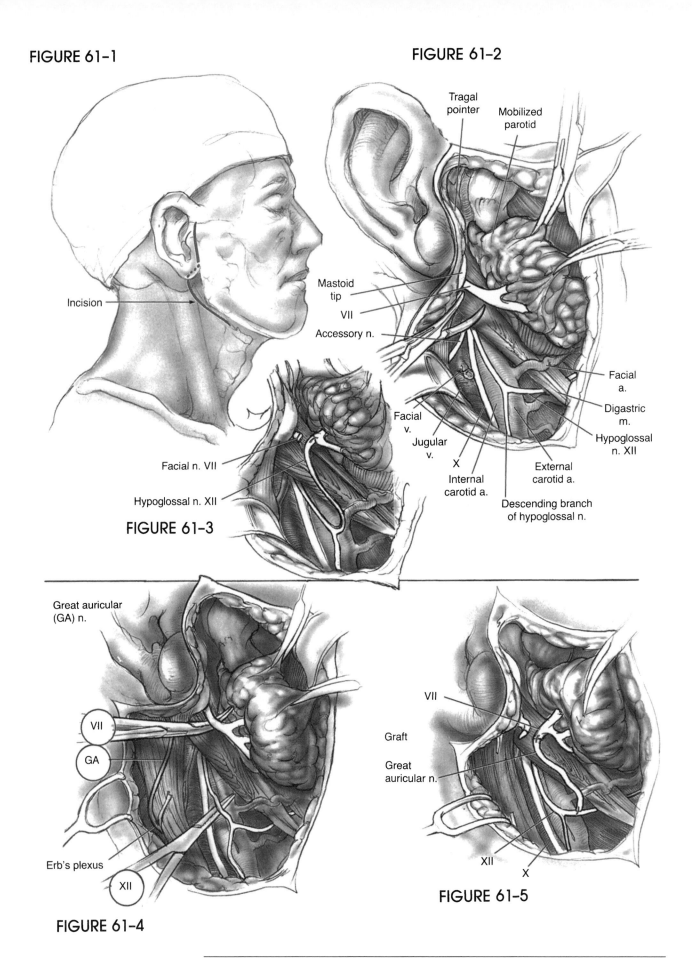

FIGURE 61-1

FIGURE 61-2

Tragal pointer

Mobilized parotid

Mastoid tip

VII

Accessory n.

Facial v.

Jugular v.

X

Internal carotid a.

External carotid a.

Descending branch of hypoglossal n.

Facial a.

Digastric m.

Hypoglossal n. XII

Incision

Facial n. VII

Hypoglossal n. XII

FIGURE 61-3

Great auricular (GA) n.

VII

GA

Erb's plexus

XII

FIGURE 61-4

VII

Graft

Great auricular n.

XII

X

FIGURE 61-5

FIGURES 61-1 to 61-5. *See legends on opposite page*

632

muscles of the face include both agonists and antagonists for various expressions and movements. When agonist and antagonist muscles are simultaneously stimulated, the result is a canceling effect. This effect is similar to that occurring during stimulation of a flexor and extensor muscle at the same time. The hypoglossal nerve obviously controls different muscle groups, thereby allowing training of facial movement as the patient attempts various tongue motions. The training is somewhat successful but is not helpful in emotional facial response. This procedure will not reproduce the blink reflex, even though some investigators have demonstrated a trigeminal-hypoglossal reflex.[17] Therefore, problems with xerophthalmia and exposure keratitis may require adjunctive lid procedures, such as a palpebral spring or gold weight lid implant.

Within 4 to 6 months, the patient will begin to see tone in the muscles and a resting symmetry.[5, 6, 13, 21] With a rehabilitation program, volitional movement is possible, allowing the patient to smile with tongue movement. Electromyographic feedback–enhanced rehabilitation has shown some additional benefits.[1, 13, 22, 23] Because many facial movements are also coordinated with oral function, the XII-VII anastomosis improves the patient's ability to eat by providing tension to the buccal area and keeping the bolus in the oral vestibule. The natural interaction between the facial and hypoglossal nerves in eating, swallowing, and speaking facilitates the rehabilitation seen with this crossover graft as opposed to the accessory or phrenic nerve.

Because of the nonselective nature of reinnervation, movement of the face results in synkinesis and mass movement that varies from patient to patient. Synkinesis can be reduced by exercise and biofeedback early in the course of recovery.[23] Selective section of branches of the facial nerve is also useful in severe cases, as is the use of selective botulinum toxin injections.[24]

Because the function gained by reinnervation procedures cannot compare with normal facial function, a different method of grading facial function is used in evaluation of the results of the XII–VII crossover. A grading system used in a prior analysis of XII–VII crossover patients in our facility is presented in Table 61–1. Although the methods used to evaluate results vary from study to study, we have extrapolated the grading system in Table 61–1 to provide the results from several sizable studies (Table 61–2). This analysis should give the reader a good idea of reasonable expectations from this procedure.

The deficit incurred in the sacrifice of one hypoglossal

TABLE 61–1. Facial Nerve Function After XII–VII Anastomosis: Quality of Return Criteria

Poor	Tone without symmetry or movement
Fair	Tone, symmetry, limited movement
Good	Tone, symmetry, fair movement, moderate synkinesis
Excellent	Tone, symmetry, good movement, mild synkinesis

From Luxford WM, Brackmann DE: Facial nerve substitution: A reivew of 66 cases. Am J Otol (Suppl): 55–57, 1985.

nerve is easily overcome by most patients.[6, 13, 21] Initially, some pooling of food in the lingual sulcus is problematic. As the buccal musculature regains tone, and as the ipsilateral tongue atrophies, this problem lessens. In Conley and Baker's large series, about one fourth of the patients experienced severe or minimal atrophy, respectively, and the remaining half experienced moderate atrophy.[6] Very few patients had trouble with speech. The best results in regaining facial function and overcoming the twelfth nerve deficit were seen with early anastomosis compared with procedures performed on patients with long-standing paralysis.[6]

In patients with bilateral paralysis, May and associates proposed a partial graft of the twelfth nerve to retain function of the tongue.[16] In this procedure, the hypoglossal nerve is partially severed, and a nerve graft is connected between the partially severed nerve and distal facial nerve. This procedure retains tongue function and provides tone and symmetry to the face. In this series, almost all of the patients had adjunctive procedures in addition to the XII–VII jump graft, making the results difficult to compare with those of the traditional XII–VII anastomosis.

Pitfalls to avoid in this surgery include use of the ansa cervicalis branch of the twelfth nerve instead of the twelfth nerve itself. This method has led to a much weaker result. The surgeon should also ensure that the distal facial nerve is not fibrosed and that the facial muscles are still viable.

SUMMARY

The XII-VII crossover graft is a relatively easy and reliable procedure in the rehabilitation of facial paralysis. A thorough preoperative evaluation is required, as is accurate timing. The patient can expect return of tone and symmetry as well as synkinesis and mass movement. The donor deficit is not significant when measured against the benefits gained from the procedure. Patients who are given realistic

FIGURE 61–1. A lazy-S standard parotidectomy incision is used in this procedure. The scar is well hidden in the preauricular crease and in a natural skin crease in the submandibular area.

FIGURE 61–2. The parotid gland is mobilized anteriorly and superiorly as the sternocleidomastoid muscle is retracted posteriorly, thus exposing the facial and hypoglossal nerves.

FIGURE 61–3. The proximal end of the hypoglossal nerve is anastomosed to the distal end of the facial nerve. Care is taken to use the maximal length of each nerve to achieve a tension-free anastomosis.

FIGURE 61–4. In preparation for the XII–VII jump graft, the great auricular nerve is exposed and harvested as it courses superficially across the sternocleidomastoid muscle.

FIGURE 61–5. The great auricular nerve graft is spliced between the hypoglossal and the distal facial nerves at a point distal to the origin of the ansa cervicalis.

TABLE 61–2. Results of XII-VII Anastomosis From Selected Studies

STUDY	*n*	NO FOLLOW-UP	POOR (%)	FAIR (%)	GOOD (%)	EXCELLENT (%)
Sabin et al[19]	134	13	9	48	43	*
Pensak et al[18]	61	0	10	48	39	3
Luxford and Brackmann[21]	54	6	8	32	35	25
Gavron and Clemis[25]	36	6	7	20	33	40
Conley and Baker[6]						
Immediate	94	NA	5	18	77	*
Delayed	43	NA	30	29	41	*

*These studies did not use an "excellent" designation.
NA, not available.

expectations are pleased with the improvement seen from this procedure.

References

1. O'Brien BM, Pederson WC, Khazanchi RK, et al: Results of management of facial palsy with microvascular free-muscle transfer. Plast Reconstr Surg 86: 12–22, 1990.
2. Samii M: Rehabilitation of the face by facial nerve substitution: Panel discussion. *In* Fisch U (ed): Facial Nerve Surgery. Birmingham, AL, Aesculapius, 1977, pp 244–245.
3. May M: Management of cranial nerves I through VII following skull base surgery. Otolaryngol Head Neck Surg 88: 560–575, 1980.
4. Zini C, Sanna M, Gandolfi A: Hypoglosso-facial anastomosis in the rehabilitation of irreversible facial nerve palsies. *In* Portmann M (ed): Facial Nerve. New York, Masson, 1985, pp 519–522.
5. Chuang DCC, Wei FC, Noordhoff, MS: "Smile" reconstruction in facial paralysis. Ann Plast Surg 23: 56–65, 1989.
6. Conley J, Baker DC: Hypoglossal-facial nerve anastomosis for reinnervation of the paralyzed face. Plast Reconstr Surg 63: 63–72, 1979.
7. Tran Ba Huy P, Monteil JP, Rey A: Results of twenty cases of transfacio-facial anastomosis as compared with those of XII-VII anastomosis. *In* Portmann M (ed): Facial Nerve. New York, Masson, 1985, pp 85–87.
8. Tucker HM: Restoration of selective facial nerve function by the nerve-muscle pedicle technique. Clin Plast Surg 6: 293–300, 1979.
9. May M: Surgical rehabilitation of facial palsy. *In* May M (ed): The Facial Nerve. New York, Thieme, 1986, pp 695–777.
10. Harrison DH: The pectoralis minor vascularized muscle graft for the treatment of unilateral facial palsy. Plast Reconstr Surg 75: 206–216, 1985.
11. Broniatowski M, Grundfest-Broniatowski S, Davies CR, et al: Dynamic rehabilitation of the paralyzed face: III. Balanced coupling of oral and ocular musculature from the intact side in the canine. Otolaryngol Head Neck Surg 105: 727–733, 1991.
12. Belal A Jr: Structure of human muscle in facial paralysis: Role of muscle biopsy. *In* May M (ed): The Facial Nerve. New York, Thieme, 1986, pp 99–106.
13. Pitty LF, Tator CH: Hypoglossal-facial nerve anastomosis for facial nerve palsy following surgery for cerebellopontine angle tumors. J Neurosurg 77: 724–731, 1992.
14. Ylikoski J, Hitselberger WE, House WF, et al: Degenerative changes in the distal stump of the severed human facial nerve. Acta Otolaryngol (Stockh) 92: 239–248, 1981.
15. Hitselberger WE: Hypoglossal-facial anastomosis. *In* House WF, Luetje CM (eds): Acoustic Tumors, Vol 2: Management. Baltimore, University Park Press, 1979, pp 97–103.
16. May M, Sobol SM, Mester SJ: Hypoglossal-facial nerve interpositional-jump graft for facial reanimation without tongue atrophy. Otolaryngol Head Neck Surg 104: 818–825, 1991.
17. Stennert E: I. Hypoglossal facial anastomosis: Its significance for modern facial surgery. II. Combined approach in extratemporal facial nerve reconstruction. Clin Plast Surg 6: 471–486, 1979.
18. Pensak ML, Jackson CG, Glasscock ME III, Gulya AJ: Facial reanimation with the VII-XII anastomosis: Analysis of the functional and psychologic results. Otolaryngol Head Neck Surg 94: 305–310, 1986.
19. Sabin HI, Bordi LT, Symon L, Compton JS: Facio-hypoglossal anastomosis for the treatment of facial palsy after acoustic neuroma resection. Br J Neurosurg 4: 313–318, 1990.
20. Chang CGS, Shen AL: Hypoglossofacial anastomosis for facial palsy after resection of acoustic neuroma. Surg Neurol 21: 282–286, 1984.
21. Luxford WM, Brackmann DE: Facial nerve substitution: A review of sixty-six cases. Am J Otol (Suppl): 55–57, 1985.
22. Balliet R, Shinn JB, Gach-Y-Rita P: Facial paralysis rehabilitation: Retraining selective muscle control. Int Rehabil Med 4: 67–74, 1982.
23. Brudny J, Hammerschlag PE, Cohen NL, Ransohoff J: Electromyographic rehabilitation of facial function and introduction of a facial paralysis grading scale for hypoglossal-facial nerve anastomosis. Laryngoscope 98: 405–410, 1988.
24. Dressler D, Schonle PW: Hyperkinesias after hypoglossofacial nerve anastomosis-treatment with botulinum toxin. Eur Neurol 31: 44–46, 1991.
25. Gavron JP, Clemis JD: Hypoglossal-facial nerve anastomosis: A review of forty cases caused by facial nerve injuries in the posterior fossa. Laryngoscope 94: 1447–1450, 1984.

62

Facial Reanimation Techniques

Dieter F. Hoffmann, M.D. ▪ Mark May, M.D.

Numerous surgical techniques have been developed for rehabilitating the paralyzed face. The best procedure is usually one that re-establishes facial nerve continuity and can be performed within 30 days (and no longer than 1 year) after nerve injury. If the proximal facial nerve is unavailable for grafting, a hypoglossal-facial nerve anastomosis or hypoglossal-facial nerve jump graft procedure is preferred.[1, 2] This procedure gives optimal results when performed within 2 years after injury.

Static or other dynamic procedures provide significant improvement in the appearance and function of the paralyzed face, whether or not surgery is performed to re-establish facial nerve function. For example, procedures to reanimate the eye, including implantation of a gold weight or a palpebral spring in the upper lid, and tightening of the lower lid, with or without implantation of cartilage, are usually performed at the time of facial nerve reanimation surgery. Other procedures may also be used if facial nerve reinnervation procedures are inappropriate or have failed, or to provide immediate rehabilitation when reinnervation surgery is not expected to give results for 6 to 12 months. These other procedures are the focus of this chapter.

Dynamic procedures for facial reanimation, in addition to the eye procedures just mentioned, include regional muscle transposition with the temporalis or masseter muscle and reinnervated free muscle flaps. Temporalis muscle transposition, the technique most often used to reanimate the lower face, is discussed at length in this chapter. Free muscle flaps are also reviewed.

Static procedures for facial reanimation include brow lift, adynamic slings, rhytidectomy, and lower lip procedures. These are discussed briefly, as are procedures such as neurolysis and myectomy that may be performed to manage hyperkinesis after facial reinnervation.

DYNAMIC PROCEDURES FOR FACIAL REANIMATION

Temporalis Muscle Transposition

Patient Selection

Patients who may be candidates for temporalis muscle transposition include those (1) who have absent or poor facial function, either with spontaneous recovery 2 years after the onset of paralysis or 2 years after nerve repair or nerve grafting; (2) who are not candidates for or refuse facial nerve repair or grafting or facial-hypoglossal nerve grafting; (3) who have neurofibromatosis, ipsilateral tenth cranial nerve paralysis, or another condition that is a con-

traindication to facial-hypoglossal nerve grafting; and (4) who have undeveloped facial nerves or facial musculature, such as may occur with Möbius' syndrome.[3, 4]

Temporalis muscle transposition has also been used recently in patients undergoing facial nerve repair or grafting. The transposition procedure provides two benefits in these cases: (1) immediate improvement in facial appearance during the 6 to 12 months before recovery can be expected after facial nerve repair or grafting, and (2) augmentation of the results of facial nerve repair or grafting.[5, 6]

Temporalis muscle transposition may also be used in place of a classic facial-hypoglossal nerve anastomosis procedure to reanimate the lower face in combination with separate procedures to reanimate the eyelids and upper face. These multiple reanimation procedures result in separation of eyelid and mouth movement.

Patient Evaluation

When the cause of chronic facial paralysis is in question, a thorough evaluation is indicated before surgical rehabilitation of facial function is planned. The patient must be assessed for the presence of a tumor involving the facial nerve because a tumor takes priority in planning management.

Systematic assessment of facial function in the patient who has elected to undergo temporalis muscle transposition includes evaluation of all areas of the face both at rest and with smiling. First, general facial tone and symmetry at rest are assessed. Next, the upper face is assessed, including brow position, degree of lagophthalmos, lower lid drooping, and ectropion.

The positions of the nasal alae, depths of nasolabial creases, and nasal airway structures are then evaluated. The appearance of nasolabial structures should be considered in the planning for temporal muscle transposition. Airway structures are evaluated because nasal valve collapse may have occurred, and if a nasal septal deformity is also present, nasal obstruction could result. Nasal obstruction may indicate the need for a nasoseptoplasty procedure to be performed at the time of temporalis muscle transposition.

The patient's smile on the unaffected side is classified, as described by Rubin, as (1) corner-of-the-mouth, or "Mona Lisa" (67 per cent of the population); (2) canine, or "Jimmy Carter" (31 per cent of the population); or (3) full-mouth, or "Lena Horne" (2 percent of the population).[7] The appropriate smile can be partly re-created on the affected side by temporalis muscle transposition with careful consideration of how the various muscles of the mouth contract to form each type of smile. Drooping, jowling, and draping of the cervical skin on the affected side of the face are also considered in planning surgery for facial reanimation.

Finally, to make an informed decision for surgery, the patient must understand what is realistically achievable in his or her case. Thus, the surgeon needs to discuss with the patient possible results of facial reanimation surgery. Spontaneous mimetic expression can be restored only with facial nerve reinnervation; however, temporalis muscle transposition can provide significant improvement in appearance and function of the paralyzed face.

Surgical Technique

Temporalis muscle transposition is performed with the patient under general anesthesia. Perioperatively, clindamycin is administered intravenously.

The patient is positioned supine for surgery with the head in a doughnut head holder and turned so that the affected side is exposed. The affected eyelid is protected during this procedure by a suture tarsorrhaphy, which is released at the end of the procedure. The hair is parted along the proposed scalp incision site, which begins superior to the preauricular crease and extends vertically to the temporoparietal region. Hair is trimmed with a scissors on either side of the part (extensive shaving of the scalp is unnecessary); then povidone-iodine solution is applied to the skin of the scalp, face, and neck and blotted dry.

Draping begins with clipping sterile towels along the scalp incision site and around the patient's face and neck. Then, a clear sticky drape is placed over the operative site so that it envelops the endotracheal tube. Ideally, the sticky drape or tape can be used to anchor the tube to the patient's chin and neck without altering lip position.

The scalp and lip-cheek incision sites are infiltrated with a solution of 1 per cent lidocaine with 1:100,000 epinephrine to improve hemostasis. The initial incision is made in the scalp with a blade and continued through subcutaneous tissue and loose aponeurotic tissue with cutting, needle-tip cautery. After the temporalis muscle fascia has been identified, it is widely exposed from the zygomatic arch to just above the superior temporal line. Then a 4-cm-wide segment (about 2 fingerbreadths) of the midportion of the muscle is outlined with the cautery (Fig. 62–1). If necessary, the scalp incision is extended superiorly above the fascial-pericranial border so that the edge of the muscle can be included in the flap. If a facelift is added to the procedure, the temporal incision is extended inferiorly into a standard facelift incision.

A heavy periosteal elevator is used to elevate the muscle off the squamous portion of the temporal bone, beginning superiorly and moving inferiorly to the level of the zygomatic arch (Fig. 62–2). Care must be taken as the medial aspect of the muscle is elevated inferiorly to preserve its neurovascular supply from deep temporal nerves and vessels.

Next, a tunnel is made into which the temporalis muscle will be transposed. The tunnel is begun by developing a plane deep to the hair follicles and superficial to the superficial musculoaponeurotic system (SMAS), in the direction of the corner of the mouth. Remaining superficial to the SMAS protects underlying facial nerve branches, which is particularly important in patients with some intact facial

function or in whom a chance exists for spontaneous recovery or for whom a facial nerve reinnervation procedure is planned. Again, a full facelift flap can be developed if the patient has significant jowling and excessive skin.

The lip-cheek incision is then made near the mouth with a razor blade knife. This incision can be made in the nasolabial crease or in the vermilion-cutaneous border, depending on surgeon preference. The lower face terminus of the tunnel to accept the transposed temporalis muscle is begun by making a pocket off the lip-cheek incision, in the direction of the scalp incision. Fine scissors are used to create this pocket, and, as with the scalp pocket, this pocket is made superficial to the SMAS and facial muscles.

The pockets off the scalp and lip-cheek incisions are connected to form a tunnel large enough to accommodate two of the surgeon's fingers. This tunnel is made with facelift scissors, which have two cutting edges on each blade, and a long bayonet bipolar cautery for hemostasis. Injecting the subcutaneous tissues of the face with saline protects the facial nerve fibers and allows for rapid dissection with less bleeding and trauma. Lighted retractors can aid with visualization of bleeders.

After the tunnel has been made, the temporalis muscle flap is bisected longitudinally, creating two 2-cm-wide pedicles. A 2-0 Prolene suture is placed through each pedicle in a figure 8, and the needle is left on the suture (Fig. 62–3). Then, large clamps are used to pull the needles with sutures and attached muscle pedicles through the subcutaneous tunnel (Fig. 62–4). The pedicles of the temporalis muscle are sutured to facial muscle, if present, and submucosal layers such that one slip is above the oral commissure and one slip below the commissure (Fig. 62–5). Additional sutures are used to secure the muscle such that the corner of the mouth is pulled toward the angle between the two pedicles to create a lateral smile that is overcorrected to show the first molar (Fig. 62–6). Overcorrection is crucial because a certain degree of settling occurs in the first few weeks.

In the past, a prosthetic implant was used to fill the temporal defect. These are now unavailable and occasionally extruded. Currently, the junior author (DFH) uses a separately elevated temporoparietal fascia flap to fill the defect. This flap is pedicled on the superficial temporal artery and vein and elevated before elevation of the temporalis muscle flap. After the temporalis muscle flap has been positioned, the fascia flap is rotated and sutured over the defect created by the transposed muscle. If the patient develops a noticeable defect despite placement of this flap, a dermal fat graft can be successfully used to obliterate the space. Alternatively, a cellular human dermal allograft can be layered into the defect.

At the completion of the procedure, a test tube drain is placed at the corner of the mouth and a Jackson-Pratt drain is positioned in the tunnel alongside the transposed muscle and brought out of the scalp behind the scalp incision. The lip-cheek incision is closed with 4-0 absorbable sutures in the subcutaneous layer, a running subcuticular 5-0 Prolene suture, and a 6-0 fast-absorbing gut suture in the skin. The scalp incision is closed with 3-0 absorbable suture and skin staples. Antibiotic ointment is applied to the incisions, and each is covered with a Telfa pad; then a bulky pressure dressing is placed over the entire operative area.

FIGURE 62-1

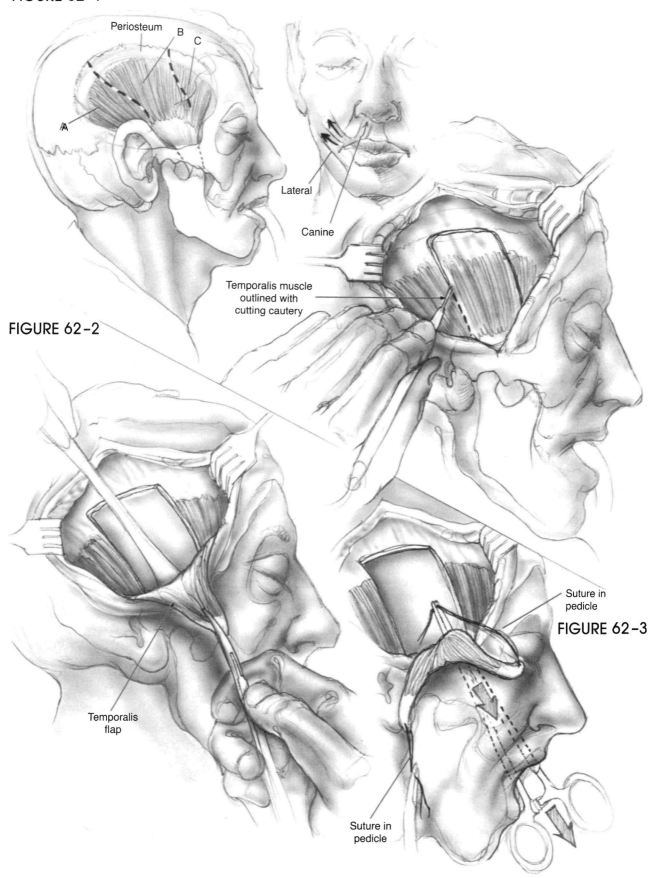

Periosteum

B

C

A

Lateral

Canine

Temporalis muscle
outlined with
cutting cautery

FIGURE 62-2

Temporalis
flap

Suture in
pedicle

FIGURE 62-3

Suture in
pedicle

FIGURE 62-4

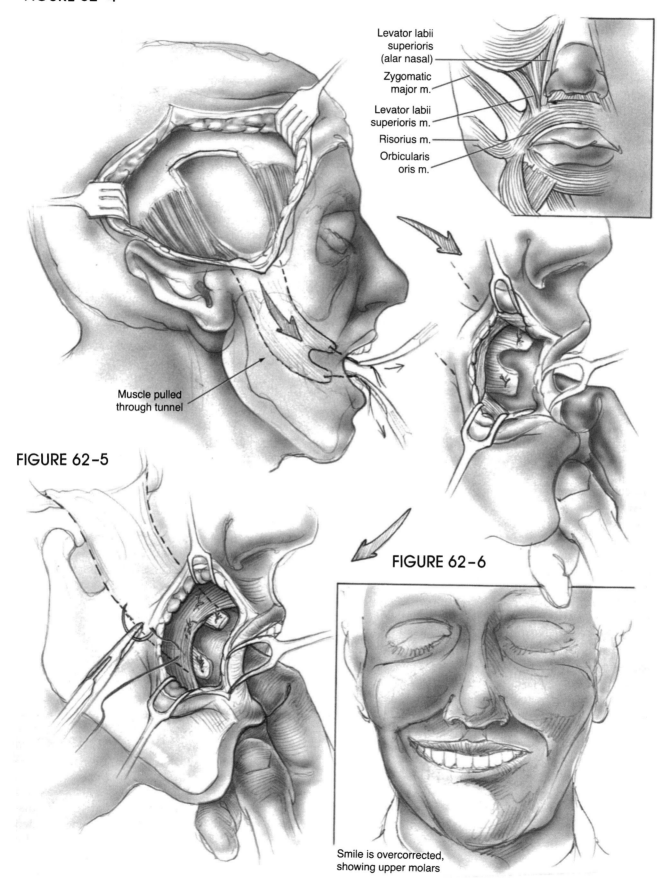

Levator labii
superioris
(alar nasal)

Zygomatic
major m.

Levator labii
superioris m.

Risorius m.

Orbicularis
oris m.

Muscle pulled
through tunnel

FIGURE 62-5

FIGURE 62-6

Smile is overcorrected,
showing upper molars

Postoperatively, most patients have moderate facial edema and ecchymosis for about 10 days. The drains and dressings are removed and intravenous administration of antibiotics is discontinued on the second postoperative day; most patients can be discharged on the third postoperative day. The patient is instructed to follow a soft diet and not to chew vigorously for the first 3 weeks after the operation. Lip sutures are absorbed, and skin staples are removed in 14 days.

Results

The results of temporalis muscle transposition begin to be evident 3 to 6 weeks postoperatively, with the appearance of facial symmetry and resolution of the overcorrected smile.

At 6 weeks postoperatively, patients are instructed to create a smile on the affected side by biting down. They learn to balance this voluntary smile with the smile on the unaffected side by practicing in front of a mirror. In some cases, these efforts can be enhanced by motor sensory re-education, a biofeedback technique in which a therapist uses electromyography to help the patient identify which muscles are being activated by voluntary effort.[8] With time, the amount of conscious effort involved in creating a balanced smile decreases.

The results of temporalis muscle transposition continue to improve for about a year after the procedure. Results are judged to be (1) excellent, if voluntary smiling results in the ability to show teeth; (2) good, if voluntary smiling moves the corner of the mouth; (3) fair, if the face is symmetric at rest; and (4) poor, if no improvement is noted. Good-to-excellent results may be expected in about 85 per cent of patients; 10 per cent of patients actually have some spontaneous emotion movement of the face. In addition, myoneurotization of denervated facial muscles may occur via trigeminal nerve fiber extension. Fair (10 per cent of cases) or poor (5 per cent of cases) results of temporalis muscle transposition may often be improved with revision surgery.

Complications

The complications that occur most frequently after temporal muscle transposition are formation of a hematoma or seroma (2 per cent) and infection (2 per cent). Inflammatory reactions to implant or suture materials may also occur.

A hematoma that forms early in the postoperative period usually must be drained in the operating room. A small seroma can be managed by needle aspiration and application of pressure dressings.

Postoperative infections are rare when prophylactic antibiotic therapy is given perioperatively and two drains are used in the wound. If a wound infection occurs, any abscess present must be incised and drained. A specimen of infectious material should be sent for laboratory culture and sensitivity testing; even before laboratory results are received, however, antibiotic therapy should be instituted with an agent effective against oral pathogens, including anaerobes, and *Staphylococcus aureus*. The antibiotic agent can be adjusted if necessary, based on the results of culture and sensitivity testing.

Extrusion of a silicone sheeting temporal implant has occurred after 3 of 250 procedures in the senior author's (MM) series, and some patients have experienced granuloma formation around Prolene sutures. Suture granulomas are treated by removal of the offending suture. Violation of the parotid duct also occurred in 1 patient, probably during creation of the cheek tunnel to accept the temporalis muscle. A sialocele formed in this patient and subsequently required parotidectomy. This last problem can be avoided by creating the cheek tunnel lateral or superficial to the SMAS.

Other complications of temporalis muscle transposition include separation or slipping of the sutures at the corner of the mouth, resulting in increased drooping of the mouth and loss of ability to create a smile. Surgery can be performed in such cases, through the lip-cheek or vermilion incision, to reattach the temporalis muscle pedicles. Another complication is bulging of the temporalis muscle over the zygomatic arch, usually due to retraction of the transposed muscle's attachment at the lip-cheek crease; occasionally, interposition of fascia lata may be needed to extend and relieve tension on the retracted temporalis muscle. Rarely, the smile may remain overcorrected on the operated side. This condition is relieved by reopening the lip-cheek incision and adjusting the sutures at the corner of the mouth.

Evolution of the Technique

The technique reported here for temporalis muscle transposition was first described by Rubin and modified by Conley (Conley lengthens the muscle by leaving a portion of pericranium attached rather than by using fascial strips, as Rubin described).[3, 7] Temporalis muscle transposition has been used in the past to reanimate the affected eye as well as mouth, but using the technique for mouth reanimation alone, in combination with other techniques to reanimate the eye area, permits separation of eyelid closure and efforts to smile, which is preferred.

The type of temporalis muscle flap raised and its placement affect the results of surgery. Using the midportion of the temporalis muscle is all that is necessary to achieve the desired result, in contrast with the procedure described by Rubin, in which the entire temporalis muscle is used. In addition, using only the middle third of the temporalis muscle and a cheek tunnel 2 fingerbreadths wide has resulted in minimal bulging over the zygomatic arch and in the cheek. The temporal depression left by elevation of the temporal muscle flap is also less prominent when less temporalis muscle is transposed.

Rubin has described attaching *muscle-fascia* strips at specific sites along the vermilion border to recreate a lateral or canine smile. Alternatively, Conley brings *muscle-pericranium* slips through small puncture wounds and sutures them to underlying dermis. The currently described method of placing multiple sutures for direct *muscle-submucosa layer* attachment provides secure attachment and consistently good results. If a nasolabial crease is to be created or exaggerated, this procedure can be performed by placing additional sutures in the dermis underlying the crease.

Use of the masseter muscle for regional facial reanimation, either alone or in combination with temporal muscle transposition, was described by both Rubin and Conley. However, we have found that in most cases, the use of the temporalis muscle alone gives the best results: This muscle provides the upward pull desirable for lifting the corner of the mouth in a smile, and using the masseter muscle is unnecessary and adds more bulk in the cheek. This extra bulk may be desirable, however, if radical parotid or temporal bone surgery has left a large defect in the cheek. In such cases, the masseter muscle may be used to augment facial reanimation by temporal muscle transposition. The masseter muscle is elevated completely from the mandible and attached to the mouth in a manner similar to that used to attach the temporalis muscle.

Free Muscle Flaps

Thompson first described the use of free (non-neurovascularized) autogenous muscle transplants to reanimate the paralyzed face; denervated muscle was placed in direct contact with muscle on the nonparalyzed side of the face. Subsequently, Frielinger introduced the use of free nonvascularized muscle grafts innervated by cross–facial nerve grafting.[9] The techniques described by Thompson and Frielinger had limited success but spurred interest in use of revascularized and innervated free muscle flaps.

Harii and associates reported using a free gracilis muscle graft to reanimate the chronically paralyzed face.[10] The vascular supply to the graft was provided by microvascular anastomosis to the superficial temporal vessels. At first, innervation was supplied by anastomosis of the graft nerve to the deep temporal nerve, but later, cross–facial nerve grafting was performed instead to provide the possibility of symmetric, mimetic facial function.[11]

Numerous donor muscles have been proposed for free muscle graft rehabilitation of the paralyzed face, including the gracilis, rectus abdominis, serratus anterior, latissimus dorsi, and pectoralis minor.[12] Ideally, the donor muscle will have (1) a long neurovascular pedicle, (2) cross-sectional area adequate to provide a flap of the width needed, (3) fiber length suitable to reproduce muscle action on the unaffected side, and (4) anatomy and physiology that permit harvesting with minimal morbidity at the donor site.[13]

Currently, the primary candidate for a free muscle graft procedure is a young person with chronic facial paralysis who is not a candidate for facial nerve repair, nerve grafting, or a muscle transposition procedure. Candidates include those with developmental facial paralysis and those with atrophy or fibrosis of the distal facial nerve or musculature such that standard reinnervation procedures are unlikely to succeed.

The reported results of free muscle grafting to restore facial movement are encouraging. In particular, some patients who have undergone the procedure have achieved a symmetric, mimetic smile.

Free muscle grafting has the disadvantage over muscle transposition of usually requiring several procedures, which also lengthens the time to find results. Recently Harii reported a one-stage procedure using the latissimus dorsi muscle and connecting the thoracodorsal nerve via the upper lip to contralateral facial nerve branches.[14] In general, the results of free muscle grafting are as yet less predictable than temporalis transposition because of limited experience with each of the various donor muscles and techniques. When techniques for this procedure have become standardized so that results are predictable, free muscle grafting may replace regional muscle transposition as the preferred surgical therapy for most patients with facial paralysis.

STATIC PROCEDURE FOR FACIAL REHABILITATION

Brow Lift

Ptosis of a paralyzed eyebrow is a cosmetic and functional problem that occurs frequently with Bell's palsy or herpes zoster oticus, persisting even after spontaneous recovery or surgical correction of other facial function deficits. Patients with brow ptosis complain of a heavy feeling in the upper eyelid and visual field obstruction.

This condition is evaluated by noting the position of the brow on the affected side in relation to the ipsilateral supraorbital rim and contralateral brow, both at rest and with the patient elevating the unaffected brow (if both brows are ptotic, bilateral brow lift procedures may be indicated). Blepharoplasty may also be planned if manual elevation of the affected brow shows significant dermatochalasis or persistent lateral hooding. If orbicularis oculi muscle function is also decreased, an eyelid reanimation procedure, such as implantation of a gold weight or spring, may be indicated. In such patients, the brow lift procedure or blepharoplasty must be planned so as not to worsen lagophthalmos or detract from the success of the reanimation procedure.

The procedure to lift the brow is performed with the patient under local anesthesia so that the surgeon can assess the adequacy of eyelid closure throughout the operation. The choice of technique used depends on whether the patient has prominent forehead wrinkling and whether one or both brows will be operated on. If both brows need to be raised, a mid-forehead lift or coronal lift can be performed.

When one brow is operated on, the incision is made horizontally along the top of the brow hair line. Skin and subcutaneous tissue are excised, and the lower flap is undermined to the level of the orbicularis oculi muscle. The brow is suspended to the frontal periosteum with one or two 4-0 permanent sutures (Fig. 62–7) such that the arch of the brow on the operative side corresponds to that on the normal side. The incision is closed meticulously to minimize postoperative scarring.

Currently, many surgeons recommend endoscopic brow lift in managing unilateral or bilateral brow ptosis. This is particularly applicable in younger patients who prefer to avoid a brow or forehead scar.

Static Slings

A static sling (muscle plication procedure) may be performed to elevate paralyzed lower face tissues. Although it does not affect facial function, plication of the angular elevator muscles of the mouth may improve facial symme-

FIGURE 62-7

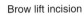

Brow lift incision

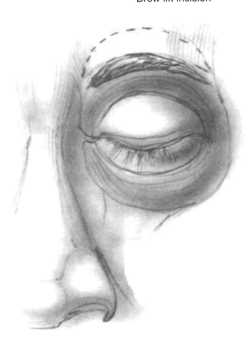

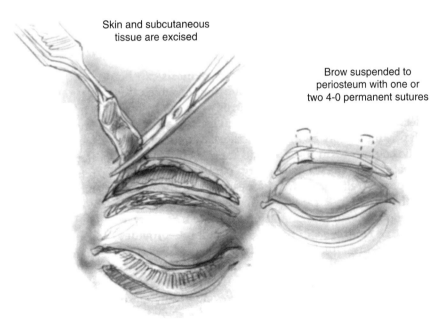

Skin and subcutaneous
tissue are excised

Brow suspended to
periosteum with one or
two 4-0 permanent sutures

try at rest. Patients who may be candidates for such a procedure are those in whom a facial reinnervation or other facial reanimation procedure has failed and those who are not candidates for a dynamic procedure.

A lower face muscle plication procedure is performed through a nasolabial or vermilion-cutaneous incision. Fascia lata grafts or palmaris longus muscle tendon are used to suspend the corner of the mouth and collapsed nasal ala from the zygomatic arch in a procedure similar to that for temporalis muscle transposition. We have also used Gore-Tex patch for static facial suspension but have found an extrusion rate of 10 to 30 per cent. The grafts are first fixed to the muscle and submucosal tissue around the mouth, and the mouth or ala is elevated and slightly overcorrected by pulling the grafts toward the malar bone. The tendon or fascia grafts are then fixed to the zygomatic arch with a miniplate and screws. In addition to this technique to suspend deeper muscles, a standard rhytidectomy procedure is usually performed to suspend sagging skin.

Lower Lip Rehabilitation

Many procedures have been developed to depress the lower lip during smiling to create a "full-mouth" smile. Patients who have complete facial paralysis are not candidates for such a procedure, because depression of the lower lip would decrease oral competence, particularly if a procedure was also performed to elevate the corner of the mouth. Rehabilitation of the paralyzed lower lip is appropriate, however, when this is an isolated problem.

One method for rehabilitating the lower lip is to transpose the tendon of the anterior belly of the digastric muscle to the paralyzed orbicularis oris muscle.[15] A tunnel is created between the tendon of the anterior belly of the digastric muscle and the lower lip depressor muscles. Then, the anterior belly of the digastric muscle is left attached to the mandible, and the tendon is brought through the tunnel and attached to the lip depressor muscles. This procedure provides a symmetric smile in the patient with isolated lower lip paralysis because downward pull of the digastric muscle tendon counteracts upward pull of muscles elevating the lips.

In patients with oral incompetence, a procedure to reduce the size of the oral sphincter and transpose innervated muscle from the normal side to the denervated side can improve oral sphincter function. One such cheiloplasty procedure is V-wedge excision of a portion of the paralyzed lower lip; another is commissure Z-plasty. Others have been described.

Surgical Management of Hyperkinesis

Some degree of synkinesis, hypokinesis, and hyperkinesis accompanies reinnervation of the face, whether nerve regeneration occurs with nerve grafting or nerve substitution techniques or with spontaneous recovery from a denervating injury. Synkinesis can be improved by sensorimotor re-education in which the patient practices in front of a mirror, with the help of electromyography, to separate facial muscle activities. Hyperkinesis may be treated medically or

surgically.[16] Botulinum toxin injected into muscles involved in hyperkinesis causes temporary paralysis and thus temporary relief from hyperkinesis. When the effects of the toxin dissipate (3 to 6 months after injection), botulinum toxin injection can be repeated. Surgically selective neurolysis or regional myectomy can provide longer-lasting treatment for hyperkinesis. Selective neurolysis involves weakening or paralyzing innervation to the hyperkinetic muscle. The results of neurolysis are difficult to predict, however, and hyperkinesis may return, even after excision of a segment of nerve. For these reasons, regional myectomy is the currently preferred surgical technique for management of hyperkinesis.

Hyperkinesis of muscles around the eye, which results in squinting and diminished vision, can be treated by excision of a portion of the orbicularis oculi muscle. A large part of this muscle can be excised, through standard upper and lower blepharoplasty incisions, without compromising eyelid closure as long as a strip of pretarsal muscle is left intact. Additional plastic surgery procedures, such as a brow lift procedure, blepharoplasty, and lower lid–tightening procedure, may be performed simultaneously with myectomy to treat orbital muscle hyperkinesis. Excision of a portion of the orbicularis oculi muscle may also be performed to treat blepharospasm and hemifacial spasm.

Hyperkinesis of the oral levator muscles, which results in pulling of the mouth to the affected side, can be improved by selective resection of the zygomaticus and levator labii superioris muscles. The problem with paralyzing or resecting these muscles is oral commissure drooping; therefore, such a resection must be done conservatively. Chin spasm may be improved by mentalis myectomy, which is performed through a submental incision. Platysma hyperkinesis, which results in unsightly cords being evident in the neck, can usually be treated satisfactorily by excision of a portion of this muscle through a horizontal cervical incision.

SUMMARY

Surgical rehabilitation of the paralyzed face is a challenging, yet rewarding, area of specialization. When the patient is not a candidate for a standard facial reinnervation procedure or when such a procedure has failed, a combination of static and dynamic procedures may successfully improve the appearance and function of the face. Facial symmetry, eyelid closure, and balanced smile can usually be restored by standard techniques, and recent innovations as well as future developments in this field promise the possibility of re-establishing spontaneous mimetic motion of the face.

References

1. May M, Sobol SM, Mester SJ: Hypoglossal-facial nerve interpositional jump graft for facial reanimation without tongue atrophy. Otolaryngol Head Neck Surg 204: 818–826, 1991.
2. Hammerschlag P: Facial reanimation with jump interpositional graft hypoglossal facial anastomosis: Evolution in management of facial paralysis. Laryngoscoope 109(Suppl 90): 1–23, 1999.
3. May M (ed): The Facial Nerve. New York, Thieme, 1986.
4. May M: Muscle transposition for facial reanimation. Arch Otolaryngol Head Neck Surg 110: 184–189, 1984.

5. Sobol SM, May M, Mester S: Early facial reanimation following radical parotid and temporal bone tumor resections. Am J Surg 160: 382–386, 1990.
6. Cheney ML, McKenna MJ, Megerian CA, Ojemann RG: Early temporalis muscle transposition for the management of facial paralysis. Laryngoscope 105: 993–1000, 1995.
7. Rubin L: Reanimation of the paralyzed face. St. Louis, CV Mosby, 1977.
8. Diels HJ: New concepts in nonsurgical facial nerve rehabilitation. *In* Advances in Otolaryngology/Head and Neck Surgery. Mosby–Year Book, 1995, pp 289–315.
9. Frielinger G: A new technique to correct facial paralysis. Plast Reconstr Surg 56: 44–48, 1975.
10. Harii K, Ohmori K, Torii S: Free gracilis muscle transplantation with microneurovascular anastomoses for the treatment of facial paralysis. Plast Reconstr Surg 57: 133–143, 1976.
11. Harii K: Microneurovascular free muscle transplantation for reanimation of facial paralysis. Clin Plast Surg 6: 361–375, 1979.
12. O'Brien BM, Pederson WC, Khazanchi RK, et al: Results of management of facial palsy with microvascular free-muscle transfer. Plast Reconstr Surg 86: 12–22, 1990.
13. Wells MD, Manktelow RT: Surgical management of facial palsy. Clin Plast Surg 17: 645–653, 1990.
14. Harii K, Asato H, Yoshimura K, et al: One-stage transfer of the latissimus dorsi muscle for reanimation of a paralyzed face: A new alternative. Plast Reconstr Surg 102: 941–951, 1998.
15. Conley J, Baker DC, Selfe TW: Paralysis of the mandibular branch of the facial nerve. Plast Reconstr Surg 70: 569–576, 1982.
16. May M, Croxson GR, Klein SR: Bell's palsy: Management of sequelae using EMG rehabilitation, botulinum toxin, and surgery. Am J Otol 10: 220–229, 1981.

63

Intraoperative Neurophysiologic Monitoring

Aage R. Møller, Ph.D. (D.Med.Sci.)

Progress in surgical and anesthesia techniques has reduced the risk of death to very small numbers in neurosurgical operations such as operations for acoustic tumors. The focus is now on maintaining quality of life postoperatively, and it has therefore become essential to reduce the risk of surgically induced neurologic deficits in such operations.

The use of relatively standard electrophysiologic techniques can help reduce neurologic deficits in many types of operations. The use of evoked potentials in intraoperative monitoring is based on the fact that changes in function occur before cell integrity is in jeopardy and before permanent neurologic deficit results. Such monitoring can be used to guide interventions to reverse surgically induced injuries. A rationale for using neurophysiologic intraoperative monitoring to reduce the risk of permanent postoperative neurologic deficits is that the injury can be reversed.[1]

Progress in the diagnostics of acoustic tumors has made it possible to identify very small tumors. Many of such patients have useful hearing and that has made preservation of hearing important in operations for acoustic tumors. Intraoperative monitoring of neural conduction in the auditory nerve using recordings of auditory evoked potentials has helped preserve hearing during removal of acoustic tumors in such patients. Preservation of hearing is particularly important in patients who have bilateral tumors from neurofibromatosis type 2 or in patients in whom it is suspected that tumors may develop later on the side opposite to that being operated on. In addition, the vestibular nerve is at risk of being injured during such operations, and it has been shown that patients operated for acoustic tumors often have postoperative vestibular disturbances.[2] So far, no method has been devised that can monitor vestibular function, but the proximity between the vestibular and the auditory portions of the eighth cranial nerve suggests that avoiding surgical manipulations that impair the function of the auditory nerve will also reduce the risk of impairment of the vestibular nerve. Monitoring auditory function can also help reduce the risk of hearing loss in other operations of the cerebellopontine angle such as microvascular decompression (MVD) operations to relieve hemifacial spasm, trigeminal neuralgia, or disabling positional vertigo and operations of other kinds of tumors in the cerebellopontine angle.

Loss of facial function following operations to remove acoustic tumors was almost inevitable in the past, but it is now possible to preserve facial function in the majority of acoustic tumor operations. The introduction of neurophysiologic monitoring has contributed to that achievement, as

has the introduction of microsurgical techniques. Neurophysiologic techniques make it possible to identify neural tissue that is not identifiable by visual observation so that the risk from surgically induced injury can be reduced. Introduction of neurophysiologic techniques in the operating room has made it possible to identify the anatomic location of the facial nerve even when it is not visible in the surgical field. That has contributed to reducing the risks of injuring the facial nerve during tumor removal.[3–15]

Intraoperative neurophysiologic monitoring of several cranial motor nerves can decrease the risk of postoperative neural deficits in operations on skull base tumors.[7, 8, 16–19] Intraoperative monitoring of the nerves that innervate the extraocular muscles is useful in many skull base operations, particularly those operations involving the cavernous sinus, where these nerves are often at risk of being injured due to surgical manipulations.[7, 8, 16] The motor portion of the fifth cranial nerve may also be involved in skull base tumors and intraoperative recordings of electromyographic (EMG) potentials from the masseter or temporal muscles can reduce the risk of injuries to this nerve.[8] When tumors that involve the caudal skull base are removed, intraoperative monitoring of the eleventh and twelfth cranial nerves can be useful in preserving the function of these nerves.[8, 17–20]

Monitoring of auditory evoked potentials can also be of value in operations on the ear,[21–24] and intraoperative neurophysiologic monitoring of the facial nerve can be useful in preserving the peripheral portion of the facial nerve in operations on the face, such as in trauma cases or in operations to remove parotid tumors.[25]

In this chapter, techniques for intraoperative neurophysiologic monitoring are described and interpretations of the obtained results are discussed.

TECHNIQUES OF INTRAOPERATIVE NEUROPHYSIOLOGIC MONITORING

The electrophysiologic techniques of recording sensory evoked potentials and EMG potentials used intraoperatively are similar to the techniques that have been used clinically for many years, but there are certain important differences in the application of these methods in the operating room. Time is an important factor when monitoring intraoperatively. Interpretable records must be obtained in as short a time as possible, and the interpretation of the recordings obtained must be done promptly to detect changes in function with the smallest possible delay. This has implications regarding choice of technique and equipment used for intraoperative monitoring. It also requires that the personnel who perform intraoperative monitoring are capable of interpreting the results.

The equipment selected for intraoperative monitoring must be of good quality to ensure a high degree of reliability, and it must be easy to operate. Most intraoperative neurophysiologic monitoring tasks are relatively simple, consisting of recording, averaging, and displaying neuroelectric potentials. That can be done by standard basic equipment, but there is a trend to make equipment universal and provide many options. In the operating room it is better to use equipment with only the options that are necessary because equipment that can perform many different functions involves a higher risk of mistakes than does equipment with fewer functions. Setting up of complex equipment can also be more time consuming than setting up simpler equipment.

The environment in the operating room is different from that of the clinic. The operating room is noisy and electrical interference is abundant. The first action to reduce the electrical interference that reaches the input of amplifiers used to record evoked potentials should be to reduce the emission of interference signals. For that, the sources of the electrical interference must be identified. Surveying an operating room for sources of electrical interference can best be done late in a day when no operations are scheduled and when equipment can be switched on and off freely. Examples of equipment that often cause electrical interference are blood warmers and electrical operating tables, but any electrical equipment that is faulty is a common source of electrical interference. There are no established standards for emission of electrical interference from equipment used in an operating room. Equipment is often purchased based on cost, and inexpensive equipment is more likely to emit interference signals than is more expensive equipment. When reduction of electrical interference at the source has been exhausted, rearrangement of equipment that emits electrical interference is helpful. Moving equipment that emits electrical interference away from the patient and the recording electrodes is effective in reducing the effect of electrical interference. Twisting or braiding electrode leads is effective in reducing the electrical interference that reaches the input of the amplifiers (for more details, see Møller[8]).

Subdermal needle electrodes (e.g., type E2, Grass Instrument Co., Quincy, MA) are the most practical type of electrodes for recording evoked potentials (brainstem auditory evoked potentials [BAEP]) and for recording EMG potentials in the operating room. When such electrodes are held in place with a good-quality adhesive tape that will not be affected by moistening of the skin (e.g., Blenderm), they provide a stable recording condition for many hours. Surface electrodes take longer to place and tend to provide less stable recordings than do needle electrodes, especially during operations that last many hours. Insert earphones are the most suitable earphones for delivering sounds for recordings of auditory evoked potentials.

In clinical testing, malfunctions in equipment or other technical problems do not have any major impact on the test results, and its only effect may be inconvenience to the personnel and the patient. It is almost always possible to repeat a test in the clinic if the results should not be satisfactory, for one reason or another. In the operating room, neurophysiologic recordings are worthless if they are not interpreted immediately, and technical problems that cannot be corrected promptly can eliminate the gain from intraoperative monitoring. To minimize the likelihood of technical problems, only high-quality equipment should be used. The personnel who perform intraoperative monitoring must be present in the operating room well in advance of the beginning of the operation to make certain that all equipment is functioning properly and that electrodes and other needed items are available and prepared for use. The use of a checklist that includes everything to be taken to the operating room; that details how to set amplification, filters, and stimulus parameters; and that describes computer start-up routines and the necessary parameters to be entered can reduce the number of mistakes.[8] The use of such a checklist makes it possible to concentrate on important matters rather than trivial ones.

Psychologically, and indeed practically, it is important that preparation for intraoperative neurophysiologic monitoring does not delay other activities in the operating room. Earphones and recording and stimulating electrodes must be placed on the patient at a time when it does not interrupt the normal routine in the operating room. It can usually be done when the patient is being shaved or when other activities are in progress.

The purpose of intraoperative monitoring of sensory evoked potentials is to detect changes in the recorded potentials. The recorded potentials should therefore be compared with a baseline recording obtained in the patient before the beginning of the operation. Such a baseline recording is best obtained after the patient is brought to sleep but before the operation begins. When evoked potentials such as the BAEP are to be monitored, preoperative recordings of the same kind of evoked potentials should be obtained in the clinic before the operation. If it is not possible to obtain a satisfactory recording before the operation, then there is little chance that it will be possible to obtain one in the operating room. Similarly, if reproducible recordings could be obtained from the patient preoperatively but not intraoperatively, the most likely reason is technical problems in the operating room, and those should be corrected.

Patients in whom injury to the ear or the auditory nerve may occur intraoperatively should have a complete hearing test in the clinic before the operation. Without preoperative tests of a patient's hearing threshold and speech discrimination, it is not possible to determine quantitatively if the patient's hearing status has changed as a result of an operation. Relying on the patient's own assessment of changes in hearing is not satisfactory. Likewise, if facial nerve monitoring is to be done, the status of the patient's preoperative facial function should be checked.

Although commonly used anesthesia regimens have minimal effect on BAEP or other short-latency auditory evoked potentials,[26–29] the use of muscle relaxants during monitoring of motor nerves makes it impossible to record muscle contractions, regardless of the method used. Muscle relaxants are components of common anesthesia regimens, and the anesthesia therefore often has to be changed whenever muscle responses are to be recorded. Anesthesia without muscle-relaxing drugs has been in general use for many years with no known adverse effects during operations in which monitoring of EMG potentials is done. If short-acting muscle endplate blocking (or depolarizing) agents are used during intubation, it must be confirmed that the effect of the muscle-relaxing drug has disappeared when responses from muscles are to be recorded intraoperatively.

It has recently been suggested that an appropriately adjusted, low level of muscle relaxation can allow recordings of muscle responses while still protecting the patient from moving during an operation. To achieve that, the paralyzing agent is administered through servo-controlled infusion.[30] However, experience has shown that it is difficult to maintain an adequate level of paralysis while still making it possible to record muscle responses satisfactorily. Partial muscle relaxation causes rapid fatigue of a muscle, and although the amplitude of the response to the first stimulus may be normal, the following stimuli will evoke responses of much smaller amplitudes. Continuous muscle activity, such as that elicited from surgical manipulation of a motor nerve, may not be detectable if the muscle is still being affected by the muscle endplate blocking agent. Furthermore, the lowest level of paralysis that allows satisfactory recordings of muscle responses probably does not provide satisfactory protection against inadvertent patient movements during an operation. These are some of the reasons that partial muscle relaxation is not suitable and the method has not gained common use.

MONITORING AUDITORY EVOKED POTENTIALS

The most common reason for monitoring auditory evoked potentials is to reduce the risk of injuries to the auditory nerve in operations in the cerebellopontine angle. Other reasons for recordings of auditory evoked potentials intraoperatively are for monitoring neural conduction in the ascending auditory pathways, which is useful in operations in which the brainstem may be manipulated. Recordings of auditory evoked potentials are also used to monitor the function of the cochlea. Intraoperative recordings of evoked potentials directly from the auditory nerve are in use in operations for vestibular nerve section. Monitoring of auditory evoked potentials from the ear (electrocochleographic [ECoG] potentials) is in use for monitoring decompression operations of the endolymphatic system (endolymphatic shunt operations).

Monitoring Neural Conduction in the Auditory Nerve

Neural conduction in the auditory nerve can be monitored mainly in three ways: (1) by recording BAEPs, (2) by recording evoked potentials directly from the exposed intracranial portion of the eighth cranial nerve, and (3) by recording directly from the surface of the cochlear nucleus.

Recording of BAEP is the most common method for monitoring the auditory nerve intraoperatively. When the intracranial portion of the eighth cranial nerve is exposed, recordings of the responses directly from the exposed auditory nerve or from the cochlear nucleus are better suited than BAEP to detect injuries of the auditory nerve. This is because these potentials have larger amplitudes than the BAEP and therefore only a few responses need to be added to obtain an interpretable record,[8, 31] which makes it possible to obtain interpretable records in a few seconds. It takes at least 30 seconds and commonly 1 to 2 minutes to obtain an interpretable record of the BAEP because its small amplitude makes it necessary to average 1000 to 2000 responses.

Brainstem Auditory Evoked Potentials

BAEPs consist of 5 to 7 vertex-positive peaks. The BAEPs recorded from electrodes placed on the scalp represent the electrical activity of the auditory nerve and the nuclei and fiber tracts of the ascending auditory pathway. The BAEP is sometimes shown with the vertex-positive peaks as upward deflections and sometimes as downward deflections, and different types of filtering will affect the waveform of these potentials (Fig. 63–1). The first five peaks can be identified in most individuals who have normal hearing and no neurologic pathologies affecting the ascending auditory nervous system.

The time it takes to obtain interpretable records of evoked potentials depends on their amplitude in relation to the background noise, the repetition rate of the stimulation, and the method used for quality control. The following factors can reduce the time it takes to obtain an interpretable BAEP:

1. Reduction of the electrical interference that reaches the recording electrodes
2. Use of optimal filtering of the recorded potentials so that the background noise is attenuated the most while the features of importance for interpretation are preserved
3. Use of optimal stimulus repetition rate and stimulus strength
4. Optimal electrode placement of recording electrodes and low electrode impedance
5. Use of methods for quality control that do not require replication of records

It is not only electrical interference that increases the number of responses that must be added to obtain an interpretable record of a BAEP but also biologic potentials such as ongoing brain activity (electroencephalographic potentials) and EMG potentials generated by muscles. When the patient is paralyzed, noise from muscle activity is abolished but muscle relaxants cannot be used in operations where EMG potentials are to be recorded.

Appropriate filtering of the recorded evoked potentials can reduce the number of responses that must be collected to obtain an interpretable record. The filters should be designed so that they attenuate background noise more than the components of the evoked potentials that are important for their interpretation. Digital filters are more flexible than electronic filters[8, 32–34] (see Fig. 63–1). Spectral filtering using conventional electronic filters can be used,

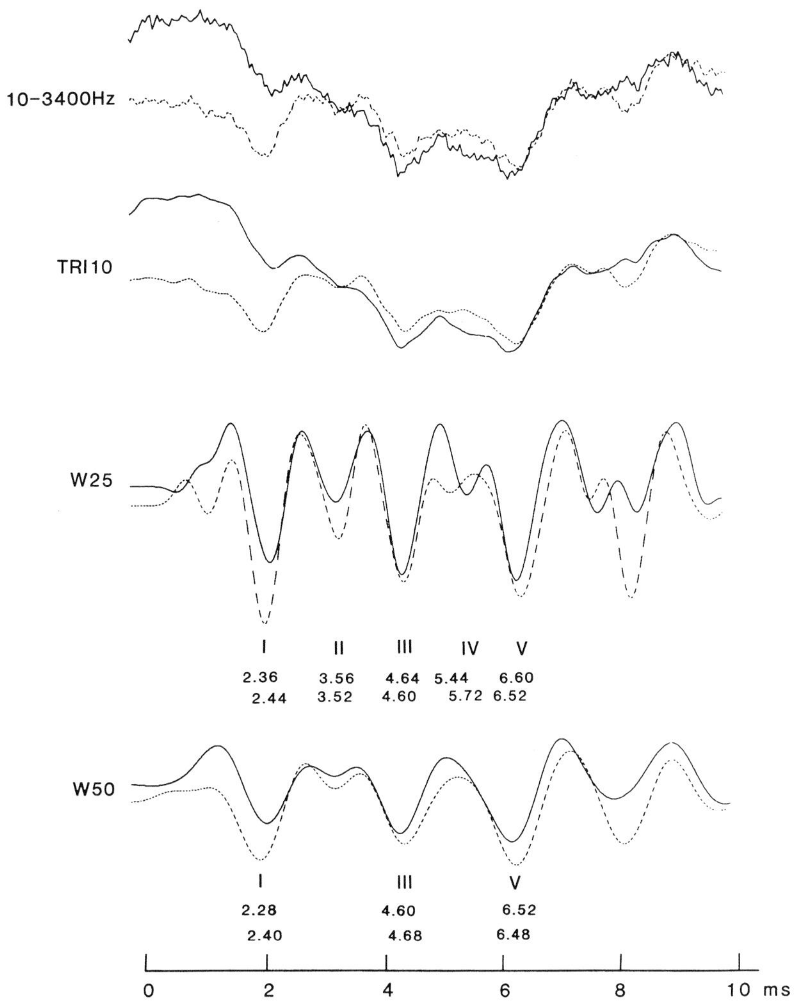

FIGURE 63–1. Brainstem auditory evoked potentials (BAEPs) recorded in the traditional way (differentially between vertex and mastoid) obtained from a person with normal hearing while the background noise was low to show the effects of different types of digital filtering. Note that the vertex-positive peaks (indicated by Roman numerals I to V) are shown as downward deflections, in accordance with common practice for displaying neuroelectric potentials. Some investigators, however, prefer to display the BAEP with the vertex-positive peaks as upward deflections. The upper tracings were averaged responses to 2048 stimulus presentations (rarefaction clicks, *solid lines*; condensation clicks, *dashed lines*) and filtered only by traditional electronic filters (10 to 3400 Hz). The other tracings represent the same data as the upper tracings, but after different kinds of zero-phase digital filtering and after removal of the stimulus artifact. The TRI10 filter is a low-pass filter, whereas the W25 and W50 filters are band-pass filters. The data were obtained in a patient with normal hearing who was undergoing a microvascular decompression operation.

but it will shift the peaks of the BAEP, depending on the waveform of the peaks.

Increasing the repetition rate of the stimulation increases the number of responses collected per unit time and thereby shortens the time it takes to average a certain number of responses. However, the effect on the time it takes to obtain an interpretable record is counteracted by the decrease in amplitude of the responses that occurs when the stimulus rate is increased above a certain value. When the decrease in the amplitude equals the gain of getting more response per unit time, the optimal rate has been reached. For peaks I, II and III of the click-evoked BAEP, that rate is higher than 50 pulses per second (pps). Peak V is less affected by the stimulus rate than the earlier peaks, and the optimal rate for peak V is approximately 80 pps.[5, 8, 35] That is much higher than the commonly used stimulus rates of 10 to 20 pps. The optimal stimulus rate may be lower in individuals with hearing loss from injury to the auditory nerve, but it is little affected by cochlear hearing loss.[35]

The stimulus intensity should be chosen to be approximately 65 dB above normal hearing threshold determined at a repetition rate of 20 pps (approximately 105 dB peak equivalent sound pressure level [Pe SPL]). Use of high stimulus rates together with a high stimulus intensity may involve risk of hearing loss when continuous exposure occurs for many hours.

The method used for quality control should not require replication of records because that increases the time it takes to obtain an interpretable record twofold.[8]

Recording Technique. In the clinic, recording of the BAEP is traditionally done differentially between one electrode placed on the vertex and one placed on the ipsilateral earlobe (or mastoid). In the operating room, it is more practical to record BAEP in two channels: one recording between the vertex and upper neck and the other between electrodes placed on each earlobe.[8]

Digital filtering is usually implemented on the averaged waveform, which has the same effect as implementing filtering before signal averaging is performed. If digital filtering is available, the electronic filters that are integral parts of physiologic amplifiers should be set at 10 to 3000 Hz, but if digital filtering is not available, settings such as 150 to 1500 Hz are more suitable.

The aggressive filtering that zero-phase digital filtering provides also makes the records sufficiently clean so that automatic computer programs can be used to identify the individual peaks and to measure the latencies without any human intervention.[8] Several schemes have been described for quality control that does not necessitate replication.[36, 37]

Sound Stimulation. BAEP can be elicited by different kinds of transient sounds, but the most suitable stimuli for use in the operating room are clicks. The stimulus repetition rate should be at least 40 pps.[5, 8, 35] A stimulus intensity of about 105 dB Pe SPL (65 to 70 dB above normal threshold) is appropriate. Standard audiometric earphones are not suitable for intraoperative monitoring of BAEP. For many years, we have used miniature stereo earphones (Realistic, Radio Shack, Ft. Worth, Texas) that are normally used in conjunction with the "Walkman" type of sound equipment.[8] Now, many other types of earphones that are suitable for use in the operating room (such as the Tube-phone, Etymotic Research, Elk Grove Village, IL) are available. The use of miniature stereo earphones or insert earphones eliminates the need for contralateral masking in most instances because of the low contralateral sound stimulation by such earphones. Only when the hearing loss on the tested ear is excessive is it necessary to use contralateral masking when such earphones are used.

Interpretation of BAEP. It is changes in the recorded BAEP that occur during the operation that are important in intraoperative monitoring. It is therefore the deviation of the BAEP from a baseline recording obtained in the same patient that is of interest. A preoperative recording of the BAEP made in the clinic can be used as the baseline recording, but the best time to obtain a baseline recording is just after the patient has been anesthetized but before the operation begins, using the same equipment and electrode placements that are to be used during the operation. Changes in neural conduction of the auditory nerve such as may occur as a result of surgical manipulations cause increased latencies of all the peaks of the BAEP except peak I. Peak V is usually monitored because it has the largest amplitude. However, the latency of peak V can change because of reasons other than increased conduction time in the auditory nerve. Peak III may be better suited as an indicator of changes in conduction velocity of the auditory nerve, or the negative peak between peak III and peak IV–V. Change in neural conduction of the auditory nerve also causes change in the amplitude of the BAEP, but that is seldom used in monitoring. Although stretching the auditory nerve mainly results in prolongation of the conduction time in the auditory nerve, a recent study in dogs[38] has shown that compression of the auditory nerve causes a decrease in the amplitude of the peaks of the BAEP, except peak I. In another study[39] it was found that increased latency of peak V of the BAEP in patients undergoing MVD operations of cranial nerves was always accompanied by a decrease in the amplitude of peak V and that the decrease in the amplitude was greater in the patients with postoperative hearing loss than in the patients with unchanged hearing. That means that changes in the amplitude of peak V of the BAEP may be a better indicator of injury to the auditory nerve that may cause hearing loss than prolongation of the latency of peak V. However, the large variability of the amplitude of peak V has detracted from its use as an indicator of injury of the auditory nerve. Decrease of 50 per cent or more in the amplitudes of the peaks of the BAEP should, however, be taken as a strong indication of injury to the auditory nerve.

Recording Directly from the Intracranial Portion of the Eighth Nerve

Compound action potentials (CAPs) recorded by an electrode placed directly on the exposed intracranial portion of the exposed eighth nerve[8, 31] have much larger amplitudes than the BAEP; therefore, fewer responses need to be averaged to obtain an interpretable record. Such recordings reflect neural activity in the auditory nerve distal to the recording electrode and can be used to detect changes in neural conduction in the portion of the auditory nerve that is located peripherally to the recording electrode. This technique was developed to detect injuries to the auditory nerve from surgical manipulations during MVD operations,[31] and it is also used in operations on acoustic tumors.[5, 40]

Recording Technique. The CAP generated in the intracranial portion of the auditory nerve is recorded by placing a monopolar recording electrode in contact with the exposed nerve (Fig. 63–2). A fine, malleable, multistrand, Teflon-coated, silver wire with a cotton wick sutured to its uninsulated tip is a suitable electrode for such recordings[8, 31] (Fig. 63–3). The reference electrode should be placed on the opposite earlobe or in the wound.

Whenever recordings are made directly from the exposed auditory nerve, the BAEP should be recorded simultaneously on a second recording channel so that BAEP can be recorded before the eighth nerve is exposed and during closing. It is also important to have a recording of the BAEP available if the direct eighth nerve recording electrode should become dislodged.

Sound Stimulation. The same sound stimulation that is used to record BAEP can be used for eliciting the CAP recorded directly from the auditory nerve.

Interpretation of Results. The CAP recorded directly from the exposed auditory nerve reflects the discharge pattern of the auditory nerve fibers and it provides more detailed information about injury to the auditory nerve than the BAEP. The CAP elicited by click stimulation has a triphasic waveform as is typical for the potentials recorded with a monopolar electrode from a long nerve in which an area of depolarization propagates.[41] The initial positive deflection occurs as a sign that the area of depolarization is approaching the recording electrode. The following large negative deflection is generated when the depolarization is located under the recording electrode and the following small positive deflection is generated when the depolarization is leaving the site of the recording electrode.

If the eighth nerve is stretched, such as in retraction of the cerebellum, the neural conduction velocity decreases. That causes prolongation of the latency of the negative peak in the CAP, and that peak may also become broader because the decrease in conduction velocity is different for different auditory nerve fibers. A total neural conduction block in the auditory nerve distal to the recording electrode results in a single positive deflection because the volley of neural activity approaches the recording electrode but never reaches the location of the recording electrode. A partial conduction block results in a CAP that has a large initial positive deflection and a smaller than normal negative peak (see Fig. 63–3B). The waveform of the CAP in individuals with hearing loss of the cochlear type is often more complex than that shown in Figure 63–3A.[42]

Recordings from the Surface of the Cochlear Nucleus

The floor of the lateral recess of the fourth ventricle is the surface of the ventral and the dorsal cochlear nucleus.[43]

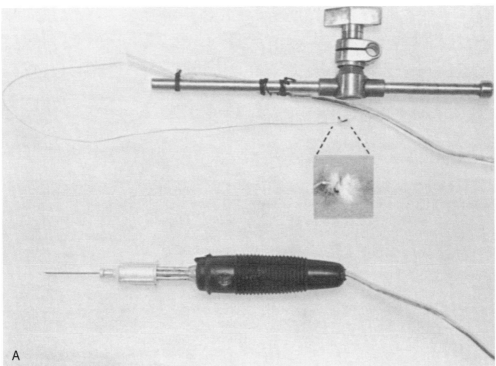

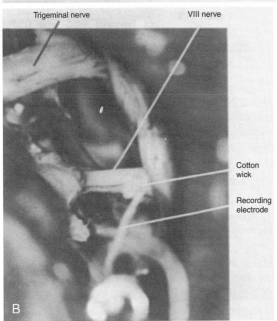

FIGURE 63–2. *A*, Electrode used to record compound action potentials from the eighth nerve. *B*, Electrode in place on the exposed eighth nerve. (From Møller AR: Evoked Potentials in Intraoperative Monitoring. Baltimore, Williams & Wilkins, 1988.)

Recordings from the surface of the cochlear nucleus can therefore be made by placing an electrode in the lateral recess of the fourth ventricle. The responses have approximately the same amplitude as the potentials recorded directly from the auditory nerve, and such recordings thus provide similar advantages as recordings from the auditory nerve.[44, 45] It is a further advantage that the recording electrode is less likely to be dislocated by surgical manipulations in operations that involve the eighth cranial nerve, such as those for acoustic tumors.[8, 43] Recordings from the surface of the cochlear nucleus is also advantageous in operations such as MVD of the seventh and eighth cranial nerves.

Recording Technique. The same monopolar electrode as described for recordings from the auditory nerve can be used for recordings from the cochlear nucleus. The recording electrode is gently pushed into the foramen of Luschka to reach the lateral recess of the fourth ventricle.[43, 45] The foramen of Luschka is located just above the entrance of cranial nerves IX and X into the brainstem when viewed through a retromastoid craniectomy (Fig. 63–4).

Often tufts of the choroid plexus can be seen protruding from the foramen of Luschka, and if excessive, it may have to be shrunk by electrocoagulation. In operations in the cerebellopontine angle such as removal of acoustic

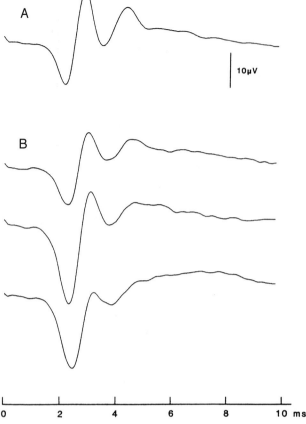

FIGURE 63–3. Recordings from the eighth nerve before *(A)* and after *(B)* the eighth nerve was subjected to heat from electrocoagulation. The results were obtained in a patient with normal hearing who was undergoing a microvascular decompression operation to relieve disabling positional vertigo. *(From Møller AR: Evoked Potentials in Intraoperative Monitoring. Baltimore, Williams & Wilkins, 1988.)*

tumors, the electrode wire is placed along the caudal wall of the wound and tugged under the dura sutures (see Fig. 63–4). In that way the electrode is far from the operative field and its position will not be disturbed by the operation. Recordings directly from the surface of the cochlear nucleus thus provide stable recordings for many hours that are suitable for monitoring neural conduction in the auditory nerve. If it is difficult to place the recording electrode in the lateral recess, satisfactory recordings can be achieved by placing the recording electrode on the cranial nerves IX and X where they enter the brainstem.

Sound Stimulation. The same sound stimulation that was used to record CAP from the auditory nerve and BAEP can be used to elicit responses from the cochlear nucleus.

Interpretation of Results. The click evoked potentials recorded from the surface of the cochlear nucleus have the characteristic waveform of recordings from a sensory nucleus, that is, an initial positive-negative deflection followed by a broad deflection that may be positive or negative, depending on the location from which the recording is made (Fig. 63–5). The initial deflections are generated when the area of depolarization of auditory nerve reaches the cochlear nucleus. These early components of the recorded potentials are probably the most useful for monitor-

ing purposes because they change in a manner similar to recordings from the most central portion of auditory nerve after injury. These early components can be enhanced by suitable filtering.

Use of ECoG Potentials in Monitoring the Auditory Nerve

Recording of ECoG potentials has limited use in intraoperative monitoring of the auditory nerve but may be used in operations for decompression of the endolymphatic sac (see section on Electrocochleography). ECoG potentials consist of the cochlear microphonics, the summating potential (SP), and the CAP of the auditory nerve. ECoG potentials are traditionally recorded from an electrode that is passed through the tympanic membrane to rest on the promontorium,[21, 22] but ECoG potentials can also be recorded noninvasively by placing an electrode in the ear canal near the tympanic membrane.[46]

The fact that ECoG potentials have much larger amplitudes than BAEP has led some investigators to promote the use of ECoG to monitor hearing in operations on acoustic tumors.[24, 47, 48] However, the ECoG potentials include only potentials that are generated in the ear, and ECoG potentials are therefore not affected by changes in neural conduction in the intracranial portion of the auditory nerve, which is the most common reason for hearing impairment in operations for acoustic tumors. The neural component of the ECoG response (AP) is affected by compromise to the cochlear blood supply, but that it is seldom reversible means that monitoring of ECoG is of little use in preservation of hearing during removal of acoustic tumors. Its use may in fact induce a false impression of security.

Changes in Auditory Evoked Potentials from Nonsurgical Factors

Several factors that are not directly related to surgical manipulations may affect recorded auditory evoked potentials. A fall in the patient's body temperature may produce prolongation of the latency of peak V of the BAEP similar to that caused by surgical manipulations of the eighth nerve.[49, 50] Irrigation around the eighth nerve with a solution the temperature of which is lower than normal body temperature will result in changes in all peaks of the BAEP except peak I. Commonly used anesthesia regimen, on the other hand, has little effect on the BAEP,[26–29] but if the blood pressure falls below a certain value, the latency of peak V increases and its amplitude decreases.

Recordings of Auditory Evoked Potentials that Can Guide the Surgeon in an Operation

Recording the CAP from the exposed eighth nerve can also be of help to identify the demarcation line between the superior vestibular nerve and the auditory nerve,[51] which is important in operations in which the vestibular portion of the eighth nerve is to be severed to treat vestibular disorders. Recordings of ECoG may help ascertain whether

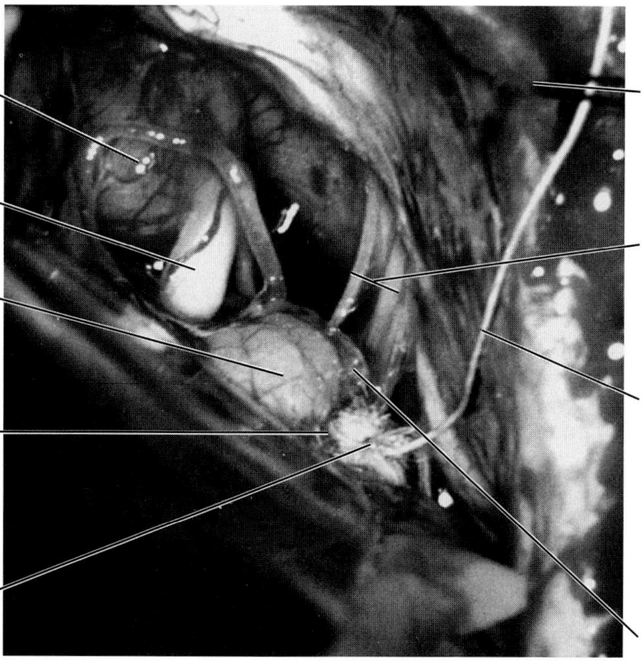

FIGURE 63–4. Placement of the electrode for recording directly from the surface of the cochlear nucleus in an operation for an acoustic tumor. (Modified from Møller AR, Jho HD, Jannetta PJ: Preservation of hearing in operations on acoustic tumors: An alternative to recording BAEP. Neurosurgery 34: 688–693, 1994.)

the therapeutic goal of decompression operations of the endolymphatic sac has been achieved.

Recording of CAP from the Exposed Cranial Nerve

It is often difficult to determine the demarcation between the vestibular (superior) nerve and the auditory nerve through visual observation. Recording of click-evoked CAP from the exposed intracranial portion of the eighth nerve is helpful in that task, but it requires a high degree of spatial selectivity of the recording electrode. The spatial selectivity of a monopolar recording electrode is insufficient for that purpose and a bipolar recording electrode is more suitable.

Recording Techniques. A bipolar recording electrode that is suitable for identifying the demarcation line between the auditory and the vestibular nerve can be made from two insulated wires of the same type used for making of the monopolar electrode described earlier, but without cotton wicks. Both wires are cut so that their tips are equal in length and about 1 mm apart. The electrode must be placed on the eighth nerve so that a line through the tips is parallel to the longitudinal axis of the nerve.[52] Such a bipolar electrode should be used with caution because its metal tips are not protected by a cotton wick, as is the tip of the monopolar recording electrode described earlier.

Stimulation. Click stimulation at much lower sound level than used for monitoring neural conduction in the auditory nerve should be used for finding the demarcation line between the vestibular and the auditory nerve. Approximately 25 dB above normal hearing threshold is suitable.[51]

Interpretation of Results. Identification of the demarcation line between the auditory nerve and the superior vestibular nerve using a bipolar electrode is based on the amplitude of the recorded CAP. The amplitude is greatest when the electrode is placed on the auditory nerve and

becomes small when located on the vestibular nerve (Fig. 63–6).

Electrocochleography

Recording of ECoG potentials is used during endolymphatic sac shunt operations in patients with Ménière's disease. It is the SP of the ECoG potentials that is monitored in such operations.

Recording Technique. ECoG potentials are recorded from the surface of the promontorium by penetrating the tympanic membrane with the recording electrode.[21] It is, however, possible to record ECoG noninvasively by placing a suitable electrode close to the tympanic membrane.[22, 46] Such an electrode records potentials with similar wave shape as the potentials recorded from the promontorium, but with much lower amplitudes.

Sound Stimulation. The most commonly used sound stimulation is click sounds, similar to those used in connection with recording of BAEP. Click stimulation is adequate for monitoring the neural (AP) component; however, tone bursts are more suitable for monitoring the SP component. Tone burst stimulation makes it possible to measure the amplitude of the SP component without interference from the AP component.[53] The SP component of the click-evoked ECoG response occurs without latency, thus earlier than the AP component, but it often appears as a shoulder on the AP responses, which cannot be distinguished from the cochlear microphonics component elicited by click sounds.

Interpretation of Results. Monitoring the amplitude of the SP components during shunting of the endolymphatic system has been advocated as a means to ensure that the goal of such operations has been achieved before the operation is ended.[54, 55] The amplitude of the SP component of the ECoG is assumed by some investigators to be elevated in patients with Ménière's disease,[56] whereas oth-

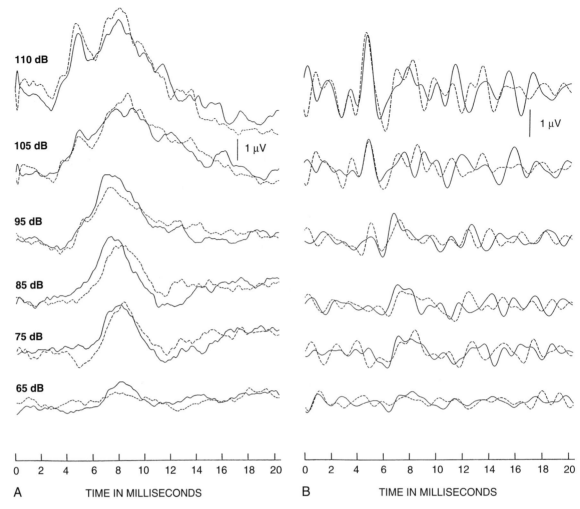

110 dB

105 dB

95 dB

85 dB

75 dB

65 dB

1 µV

1 µV

0 2 4 6 8 10 12 14 16 18 20

A   TIME IN MILLISECONDS

0 2 4 6 8 10 12 14 16 18 20

B   TIME IN MILLISECONDS

FIGURE 63–5. Typical recordings from the cochlear nucleus obtained using the electrode placement shown in Figure 63–4. Unfiltered responses are shown in A, and band-pass filtered responses using a zero-phase digital filter are shown in B. (From Møller AR, Jho HD, Jannetta PJ: Preservation of hearing in operations on acoustic tumors: An alternative to recording BAEP. Neurosurgery 34: 688–693, 1994.)

ers have failed to find significant abnormalities in the ratio between the amplitude of the SP and the AP components of the ECoG.[57] The large intersubject variability has been an obstacle in the use of the SP:AP ratio in clinical diagnosis, but that is not a factor when used in intraoperative monitoring because the SP is compared with the patient's own values. The use of monitoring of ECoG potentials to determine when the shunting has been successfully accomplished is based on the assumption that the SP potentials normalize when the pressure imbalance in the cochlea has been eliminated. Normalization of the SP component of the ECoG during the operation is thus assumed to be an indication that the operation has been successful.

MONITORING CRANIAL MOTOR NERVES

One of the earliest attempts to improve the preservation of cranial motor nerves through intraoperative monitoring was applied to the facial nerve in operations to remove acoustic

tumors.[58] However, it was not until the early 1980s that intraoperative monitoring of facial function during neurosurgical operations became routine practice.[5, 6, 8, 9, 12, 13, 59]

Intraoperative monitoring of other cranial motor nerves, such as those that innervate the extraocular muscles and the muscles of the shoulder and tongue, are important when these nerves are involved in a tumor and if surgical manipulation may involve manipulation of these nerves.[7, 8, 16] Monitoring of cranial motor nerves is now in routine use in many institutions in operations of skull base tumors.[8, 19, 20]

Preserving the Facial Nerve in Operations on Acoustic Tumors

Monitoring the facial nerve to reduce surgically induced injury has been used successfully for some time. Monitoring of the facial nerve is based on recordings of facial muscle contractions elicited by probing the surgical field with a electrical stimulating electrode, by surgical stimula-

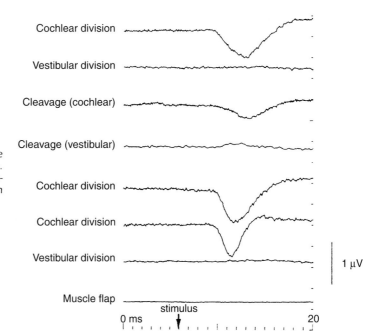

FIGURE 63–6. Recordings from different locations on the eighth cranial nerve using a bipolar recording electrode. (From Rosenberg SI, Martin WH, Pratt H, et al: Bipolar cochlear nerve recording technique: A preliminary report. Am J Otol 14: 362–368, 1993.)

tion of the facial nerve, and by observing facial muscle activity that is a result of injuries to the facial nerve. One of the first electronic methods to detect facial movements in acoustic tumor operations described almost two decades ago made use of mechanical sensors (accelerometers).[59] That was followed by description of several similar methods of recording movements of the face.[11, 60] Recording of EMG potentials from facial muscles[4] is now the most common way to detect facial muscle contractions.[5, 6, 8, 9, 11–14]

Recording EMG Potentials. Subdermal needle electrodes are suitable for recording EMG potentials. One of these can be placed in the upper face and one in the lower face so that contractions of any of the facial muscles on one side will contribute to the recorded response in one single channel. We have found this to be a convenient and practical way to monitor facial muscle activity.[6, 8] Other authors have preferred to use two channels, one recording EMG potentials from the upper face and one from the lower face. To accomplish that, two electrodes are placed in each of these muscles and connected to the amplifiers of the two recording channels.

The recorded EMG potentials should be displayed on an oscilloscope, in addition to being made audible so that not only the person who is performing the monitoring can observe the responses but also the surgeon can directly hear when the muscles contract.[5, 6, 12, 13] Some equipment can produce tone signals when the EMG potentials have reached a set threshold instead of making the raw EMG signal audible. The EMG signal contains much important information that can be appreciated when the EMG signal is made audible but most of which is lost when converted to tone signals. Most equipment includes muting of the sound from the stimulus artifact.[6]

Stimulation. Short (0.1 msec) rectangular electrical impulses delivered by a monopolar, handheld, stimulating electrode provide suitable electrical stimulation for probing the surgical field to find the facial nerve. The same stimulation can be used to identify areas of a tumor in which no

parts of the facial nerve are present. The use of a constant (or rather a semi-constant) voltage stimuli is preferred over the constant current type commonly used for stimulation of peripheral nerves through the skin.[6, 15] Shunting of electrical current varies when the surgical field changes from being relatively dry to becoming wet from cerebrospinal fluid covering the stimulating electrode. If constant current stimulation is used intracranially, the effectiveness of the stimulation of a nerve will change when the shunting of current varies. Some authors[61] have advocated the use of constant current when stimulating with an electrode that is insulated except at the tip (flush tip).

Some investigators advocate the use of a bipolar stimulating electrode for preservation of facial function in connection with acoustic tumor operations.[62] A bipolar electrode stimulates a smaller area of tissue than does a monopolar electrode, and it is thus more spatially selective. Unfortunately, a bipolar electrode is also more difficult to use because its ability to stimulate nervous tissue depends on its orientation. The high spatial selectivity of a bipolar stimulating electrode is, however, of value for distinguishing between two nerves that are located close to each other, but it should not be used to identify portions of a tumor in which no motor nerve is present.[6, 8] It may be convenient to have a choice of using bipolar and monopolar stimulating electrodes in an operation. The bipolar stimulating electrode could then be used to distinguish between the facial nerve and the eighth cranial nerve because they are located close to each other while a monopolar stimulating electrode should be used to probe a tumor to find portions with no parts of the facial nerve present.

In all use of electrical stimulation it is important that the correct stimulus strength is used. Too strong stimulation used to find areas with no facial nerve present will give the impression that larger regions of a tumor contain the facial nerve than what actually is the case. If the stimulation is too weak, it may show that a region of a tumor can safely be removed when it in fact contains the facial nerve or parts of it. The spacial selectivity of bipolar stimulating electrodes is also impaired from too strong electrical stimulation.

Interpretation of Results. Intraoperative recordings of facial EMG activity are done while probing the surgical field with a handheld stimulating electrode to find the facial nerve in the surgical field when it is not visible. Perhaps more important, such probing of a tumor can also be used to find regions of a tumor where no part of the facial nerve is present, making it possible to remove large portions of tumors with little risk of injuring the facial nerve.[5, 6, 8] When probing a tumor with a handheld stimulating electrode using a stimulus intensity that is properly set, the amplitude of the EMG potentials recorded from facial muscles is related to the distance between the stimulating electrode and the facial nerve. If the amplitude of the EMG potentials decreases when the stimulating electrode is moved, it is a sign that the electrode is moved away from the facial nerve; conversely, if the amplitude of the EMG potentials increases, it is a sign that the stimulating electrode is moved toward the location of the facial nerve. Proper interpretation of the EMG potentials elicited when the surgical field is probed by a stimulating electrode can thus provide important information about the location of the facial nerve. When the facial nerve has been identified stimulation at different locations can be used to assess the neural conduction in the facial nerve by observing the latency of the response obtained when stimulating at different locations along the facial nerve.

When using a single EMG recording channel, contraction of the muscles of mastication will contribute to the recorded EMG potentials. Electrical stimulation of the motor portion of the fifth cranial nerve that elicits contractions of the mastication and temporalis muscles gives rise to EMG potentials that are picked up by the recording electrodes placed in the upper and lower face muscles. The latency in the response from the mastication muscles to electrical stimulation of the trigeminal nerve is much shorter than that of the facial muscles in the response elicited by stimulation of the facial nerve (1.5 to 2.0 msec vs. 5 to 6 msec).[8] That difference in latency makes it possible to distinguish between an EMG response elicited by stimulation of the motor portion of the fifth nerve and that elicited by stimulation of the facial nerve (Fig. 63–7). The sounds of these EMG potentials are indistinguishable from each other, and that is one reason why it is important to have an oscilloscopic display or the recorded EMG potentials from which their latencies can be estimated.

It is not only EMG activity elicited by electrical stimulation of the facial nerve that is important in monitoring facial function during operations. Continuous monitoring of facial muscle activity is also valuable for identifying surgical manipulations that imply risks for permanent facial deficits. Surgical manipulations of the facial nerve that may occur during removal of acoustic tumors may elicit EMG potentials that have the form of short bursts or more continuous repetitive or nonrepetitive activity.[13] Heat being transferred to the facial nerve from electrocoagulation can also elicit such EMG potentials in the respective muscles. If such activity occurs many times during an operation or during more than a few seconds, it is an indication of a high risk of postoperative facial deficit. The operation should therefore be halted when such EMG activity occurs

and not continued until the activity has stopped. Similar EMG activity can be elicited by probably harmless events, such as irrigation with fluid, the temperature of which is below normal body temperature.

Surgically induced EMG activity from facial and mastication muscles can thus not be distinguished from each other using recordings between electrodes placed in the upper and lower face. If a second recording channel equipped with EMG amplifiers is available, it is helpful to record EMG potentials from the masseter muscle in addition to recording EMG potentials from facial muscles. In that way, it is possible to distinguish between all kinds of activation of the facial and trigeminal nerves.

The use of intraoperative monitoring of the facial nerve not only reduces the risk of postoperative deficits in facial function but it also reduces the operating time and it can give the surgeon an increased feeling of security.

Monitoring Other Cranial Motor Nerves

Tumors of the skull base may involve many cranial nerves, and these nerves are at risk of being injured in operations for such tumors. It is especially the third, fourth, and sixth cranial nerves, which control the extraocular muscles, that are at risk in operations of tumors involving the cavernous sinus. The motor portion of the fifth cranial nerve may also be involved in skull base tumors and the ninth, tenth, eleventh, and twelfth cranial nerves may be involved in skull base tumors that extend far caudally. Loss of function of the extraocular muscles, particularly of those innervated by the third cranial nerve, has severe consequences and can essentially result in loss of function in the eye that is affected. The risk of loss of the twelfth nerve is high in operations to remove tumors that affect the medulla and upper spinal cord in the area of the foramen magnum.

The cranial motor nerves are often difficult to identify visually, especially when a tumor has altered the anatomy. However, it is rather easy to localize these nerves by using a technique similar to that described for monitoring the facial nerve during operations on acoustic tumors. Thus, electrical stimulation of the area where these nerves are assumed to be located in connection with recording EMG potentials from muscles that are innervated by these cranial nerves is effective in reducing the risk of postoperative deficits related to cranial motor nerves that are often at risk in skull base operations.

Recording Technique. Monitoring of the nerves that innervate the extraocular muscles is done by placing needle electrodes (such as type E2 subdermal) percutaneously in the extraocular muscles that are innervated by a respective cranial motor nerve (as shown in Fig. 63–8). Usually only the extraocular muscles of one eye are monitored because operations are normally limited to one side of the skull. Naturally, great care should be exercised when inserting such needle electrodes so that they do not injure the eyeball. Reaching the lateral rectus muscle for monitoring the sixth cranial nerve or the medial rectus muscle for monitoring the third cranial nerve is usually not difficult, but it may take some practice to reach the superior oblique muscle or its close vicinity for satisfactory monitoring of the fourth

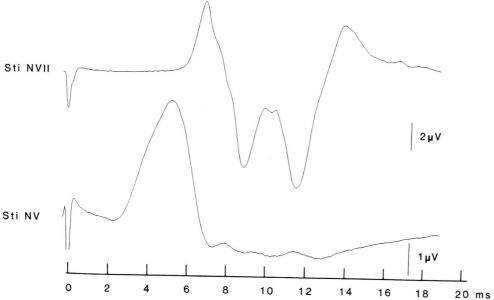

FIGURE 63–7. *Upper recording,* Electromyographic activity typical of those obtained from a set of electrodes, one placed in the upper face and one in the lower face, while the intracranial portion of the facial nerve is being stimulated electrically with rectangular impulses of 100-μS duration set at about 0.8 V using a hand-held monopolar stimulating electrode. *Lower recording,* Similar recording obtained when the intracranial portion of the trigeminal nerve (portio minor) is being stimulated using a hand-held monopolar stimulating electrode. (From Møller AR: Evoked Potentials in Intraoperative Monitoring. Baltimore, Williams & Wilkins, 1988.)

cranial nerve. It is important to secure the electrodes with a good-quality adhesive tape so that the location of the electrodes is not altered if the patient is moved, and for this reason the electrodes should always be secured to the face of the patient by adhesive tape at a distance from the electrodes.

Since only one electrode can be placed in each muscle, one reference electrode for each of the recording electrodes must be placed in a different location. The forehead on the opposite side is a suitable position that avoids contamination of the recorded potentials by EMG potentials from the facial muscles on the operated side.

Some investigators have recorded EMG potentials from the extraocular muscles after surgically exposing the muscles and placing recording electrodes directly on these muscles.[63] A noninvasive method for recording EMG potentials from the extraocular muscles using electrodes that have the shape of wire loops has been described.[64] These electrodes are placed under the eyelids and provide satisfactory recordings of EMG potentials from extraocular muscles,[64] although of a smaller amplitude than what is obtained from needle electrodes placed in or close to the extraocular muscles.

Recording of the EMG potentials from the soft palate and from the tongue are convenient ways to monitor the ninth and twelfth cranial nerves.[19, 20] Recording from electrodes placed in the false vocal cords can be used to monitor the tenth cranial nerve[8, 20] or from needles inserted percutaneously in laryngeal muscles.[65] Recording from the sternocleidomastoid muscle or the trapezoid muscle is a suitable way to monitor the eleventh cranial nerve. Monitoring of the twelfth cranial nerve can be done by placing two recording electrodes in the lateral side of the tongue about 1 cm apart.[66]

Recording of EMG potentials from muscles that are innervated by these cranial motor nerves should be done on separate channels so that the responses from different muscles can be viewed separately. Simultaneous recording and watching many channels of EMG recordings, in addition to monitoring sensory evoked potentials is a challenge in addition to organizing equipment and connecting electrodes to respective amplifiers without making mistakes. Although several channels on an oscilloscope can be watched simultaneously, it is not easy to listen to the sound of more than one channel at a time. The loudspeaker in the operating room must therefore be switched to the channel that is at any given time most important to listen to while all channels are watched on the oscilloscope.

Interpretation of Results. Recorded in the way shown in Figure 63–8, the EMG potentials from the extraocular muscles are large and can easily be viewed on an oscilloscope without averaging (Fig. 63–9). EMG potentials from all other muscles described earlier, including the laryngeal muscles, are large and can be observed directly on an oscilloscope. The response elicited by electrical stimulation of respective motor nerves provides information about the location and identity of a respective nerve. Continuous monitoring of activity in the muscles that are innervated by these nerves provides important information about surgical manipulations that may place the respective nerve at risk for permanent injury.

MONITORING OF THE ASCENDING AUDITORY PATHWAYS

Several auditory relay nuclei are located in the brainstem together with fiber tracts of the ascending auditory pathways. Since the neural conduction in both nuclei and fiber tracts is likely to change from mechanical deformations of

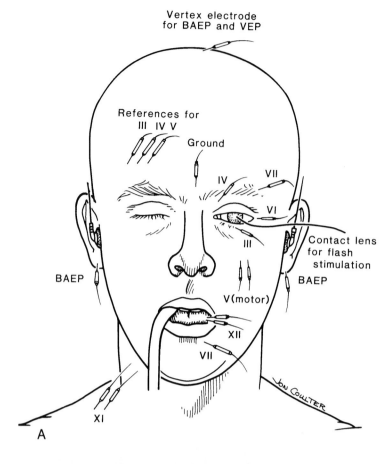

Vertex electrode
for BAEP and VEP

References for
III IV V

Ground

IV

VII

VI

III

Contact lens
for flash
stimulation

BAEP

BAEP

V(motor)

XII

VII

XI

JON COULTER

A

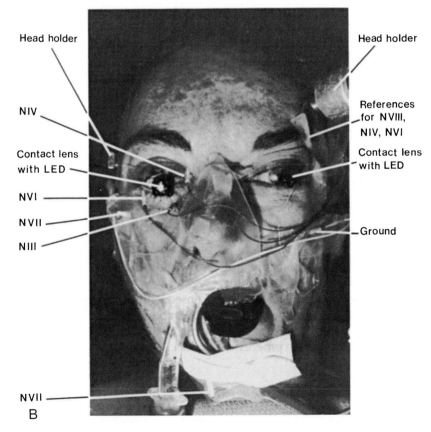

Head holder

Head holder

NIV

References
for NVIII,
NIV, NVI

Contact lens
with LED

Contact lens
with LED

NVI

NVII

NIII

Ground

NVII

B

FIGURE 63–8. *A,* Schematic illustration of the placement of electrodes for recording electromyographic activity from the extraocular muscles as well as from the facial muscles, the masseter muscle, and the tongue. *B,* Illustration of the placement of the electrodes shown in *A* in a patient undergoing an operation to remove a skull base tumor. (*A,* From Møller AR: Intraoperative monitoring of evoked potentials: An update. *In* Wilkins RH, Rengachary SS (eds): Neurosurgery Update I: Diagnosis, Operative Technique, and Neuro-Oncology. New York, McGraw-Hill, 1990, pp 169–176. *B,* From Møller AR: Evoked Potentials in Intraoperative Monitoring. Baltimore, Williams & Wilkins, 1988.)

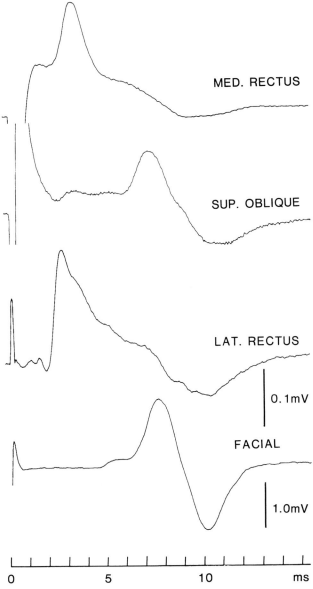

FIGURE 63–9. Recordings typical of those obtained from the extraocular muscles and facial muscles in response to electrical stimulation of the respective motor nerves intracranially. The stimuli were rectangular impulses of 150-μS duration set at 0.8 to 1.5 V. Stimulation of the respective cranial nerves intracranially was performed with a hand-held electrode. (From Møller AR: Evoked Potentials in Intraoperative Monitoring. Baltimore, Williams & Wilkins, 1988.)

the brainstem, monitoring of the ascending auditory pathway can be useful in operations where the brainstem may be manipulated. Changes in heart rate and blood pressure have traditionally been used to detect manipulations of the brainstem, but recent studies have shown that changes in the BAEP are more consistent and tend to occur before cardiovascular changes occur.[67] To fully utilize the BAEP for that purpose, it is important to consider the origin of the various components of the BAEP.

Neural Generators of the BAEP

The different components of the BAEP are generated by the auditory nerve and the nuclei and fiber tracts of the ascending auditory pathway. The distal portion of the auditory nerve in humans is the generator of peak I, and the central portion is the generator of peak II.[68–70] Peak III of the BAEP is mainly generated by the cochlear nucleus, and peak V is generated by the termination of the lateral lemniscus in the inferior colliculus. The slow potential that sometimes can be seen to follow peak V (SN_{10})[71] is probably generated by the inferior colliculus.[72, 73] Peak IV is rather variable, even in patients with normal hearing, and the neural generator of this peak is unknown. Whereas it is almost certain that peaks I and II are exclusively generated by the auditory nerve, peaks III, IV and V most certainly have multiple generators and the same nucleus or fiber tract may contribute to more than one peak. Not all of the nuclei of the ascending auditory pathway are represented in the BAEP, however, because some nuclei have an internal organization that makes the electrical field decrease rapidly with distance.[8, 70, 74–76] A schematic and simplified illustration of the neural generators of the BAEP is seen in Figure 63–10.

Recording Technique. For the purpose of monitoring the brainstem, BAEP is elicited from the ear opposite the side where the operation is performed. Similar electrode

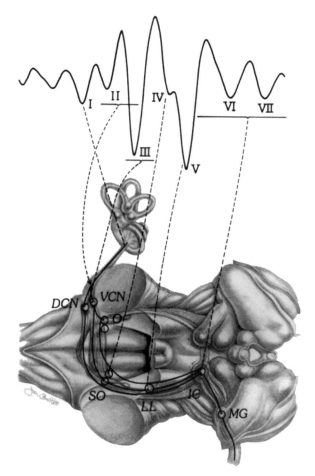

FIGURE 63–10. Simplified illustration of the neural generators of the brainstem auditory evoked potentials based on the results of intracranial recordings in patients undergoing neurosurgical operations. (From Møller AR, Jannetta PJ: Neural generators of the auditory brainstem response. In Jacobson JT [ed]: The Auditory Brainstem Response. San Diego, College-Hill Press, 1984, pp 13–31.)

placements and stimulus parameters as used for other kinds of intraoperative recordings of the BAEP can be used (see Techniques of Intraoperative Neurophysiologic Monitoring).

Interpretation of Results. An increase of the latency of only peak V (increased interpeak latency [IPL] III–V) and/or a decrease in the amplitude of peak V with no change in the amplitude of peak III is taken as an indication that the brainstem has been manipulated in one way or another (Fig. 63–11). Changes in the IPL I–III are an indication of stretching or compression of the auditory nerve.

Changes in the BAEP caused by brainstem manipulations were detectable an average of 15 minutes before cardiovascular changes, such as changes in heart rate and blood pressure, could be detected.[67] The latency of peak V may change (become prolonged) as a result of a decrease in blood pressure.

WHICH CHANGES IN RECORDED POTENTIALS SHOULD BE COMMUNICATED TO THE SURGEON?

It has been debated how much the recorded potentials must change before the surgeon is informed. The answer to this question depends on whether the purpose of intraoperative monitoring is to provide warnings (only) regarding a presumed noticeable increase in risk of postoperative neurologic deficits or to furnish information about surgical manipulations of neural tissue without assuming that the change in function revealed is an indication of an increased risk of postoperative deficits. However, this question cannot be adequately answered because of a lack of data. The change in evoked potentials that indicates a risk of neurologic deficit is generally unknown and it is therefore not possible to set a limit for how much evoked potentials can be allowed to change.

Because of this we have taken the approach to routinely inform the surgeon about any change in evoked potentials as soon as these changes reach a magnitude that is larger than normal spontaneous variations and about any abnormalities in EMG potentials. Although we do not believe that all small changes indicate a noticeable risk of postoperative deficit, informing the surgeon immediately when these changes occur has several advantages: (1) it makes it possible for the surgeon to precisely identify what caused a certain change in the recorded potentials; (2) it leaves the surgeon with the option of either intervening immediately or waiting to see if the changes increase to values that the surgeon might regard as a sign of a noticeable risk of permanent postoperative deficit; and (3) it relieves the surgeon from being concerned about the possible risk of postoperative deficits.

If the surgeon is not informed until the changes have reached a level that may be regarded to indicate a noticeable risk of permanent neurologic deficit, he or she may not be able to identify which surgical manipulations caused the change in function. Consequently, it would be difficult to reverse the manipulation. If on the other hand the surgeon is informed promptly when a change first occurs and

decides to wait, he or she can always reverse the manipulation later if the changes progress because it would then be obvious which specific manipulation caused the injury. We do, however, find it much more satisfactory to reverse the manipulation as soon it is detected than to take the "wait and see" stance.

The best use of intraoperative monitoring of evoked potentials is therefore not as warnings of imminent disasters but rather as a support system to the surgeon, providing information about the specific neural tissue that he or she has manipulated. Such information is important for carrying out an operation with the least risk of postoperative neurologic deficits. The key element is that the reversal of the manipulation can reverse the injury so that it most likely does not result in a permanent postoperative neurologic deficit. In fact, comparison between the postoperative deficits experienced by different surgeons favors early intervention as by far the most effective way to reduce the occurrence of postoperative neurologic deficits.

The surgeon must make decisions regarding how to respond to changes in the recorded potentials. To facilitate such decision making, the information must be given in a form that the surgeon can use, considering that the surgeon is occupied mentally by the operation. If only raw data, such as the size of the prolongation of latencies of evoked potentials, are conveyed, the surgeon's full mental attention may be required and he or she would have to recall knowledge in the field of neurophysiology to interpret and understand the implications of the information provided. This is obviously not an ideal situation. Optimal utilization of results from intraoperative monitoring requires the person who conducts the monitoring to interpret the acquired data before the information is conveyed to the surgeon.

DOCUMENTATION OF THE BENEFITS OF INTRAOPERATIVE NEUROPHYSIOLOGIC MONITORING

Although most surgeons who have been introduced to the use of intraoperative neurophysiologic monitoring agree that these techniques are valuable in reducing neurologic deficits and in some cases help to achieve the therapeutic goals of an operation, it has been difficult to prove that the use of intraoperative neurophysiologic monitoring has reduced the incidence of postoperative neurologic deficits in a strictly statistical sense. One of the reasons is that it has not been possible to apply traditional methods for testing of the efficacy, such as the double-blind method, of intraoperative neurophysiologic monitoring. Except in a few instances it has not been possible to determine the efficacy of intraoperative neurophysiologic monitoring of BAEP using statistical methods.[77] A few published studies, based on historical data, have shown a clear reduction in postoperative permanent hearing loss following MVD operations for hemifacial spasm, trigeminal neuralgia, disabling positional vertigo, and glossopharyngeal neuralgia.[78] With regard to the benefits of facial nerve monitoring during acoustic tumor operations as well as during operations on skull base tumors, studies have shown a clear

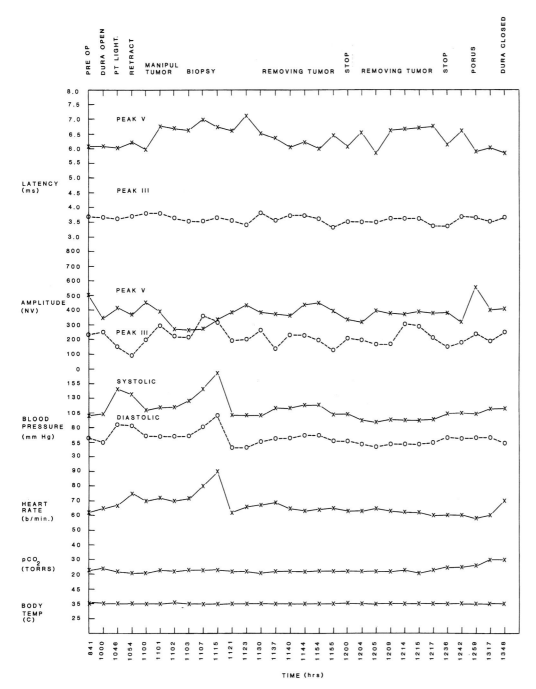

FIGURE 63–11. Changes in the latencies and amplitudes of peaks III and V of the brainstem auditory evoked potential (BAEP) as a function of time, displayed together with cardiovascular changes during an operation to remove a large acoustic tumor. The BAEPs were elicited by stimulating the ear opposite the side of the tumor. (From Angelo R, Møller AR: Contralateral evoked brainstem auditory potentials as an indicator of intraoperative brainstem manipulation in cerebellopontine angle tumors. Neurol Res 18: 528–540, 1996.)

improvement in outcome as a result of intraoperative monitoring of facial function.[9–11, 79] However, different ways to evaluate results hamper comparison of facial nerve preservation in different hospitals, but the increased utilization of common classification methods, such as the House-Brackmann classification,[80] has improved the possibilities of comparing results from different institutions. However, it still can be argued that improvements in techniques during the same period have contributed to the observed improvement in results.

It is also generally recognized that the introduction of neurophysiologic methods for intraoperative monitoring in the operating room has fostered better operating methods and that it has had an important function in teaching residents.

References

1. Grundy BL: Evoked potentials monitoring. *In* Blitt CD (ed): Monitoring in Anesthesia and Critical Care Medicine. New York, Churchill Livingstone, 1985, pp 345–411.

2. Sekiya T, Iwabuchi T, Hatayama T, Shinozaki N: Vestibular nerve injury as a complication of microvascular decompression. Neurosurgery 29: 773–775, 1991.

3. Kartush JM, Bouchard KR: Intraoperative facial monitoring: Otology, neurotology, and skull base surgery. In Kartush JM, Bouchard KR (eds): Neuromonitoring in Otology and Head and Neck Surgery. New York, Raven Press, 1992, pp 99–120.

4. Delgado TE, Buchheit WA, Rosenholtz HR, Chrissian S: Intraoperative monitoring of facial muscle evoked responses obtained by intracranial stimulation of the facial nerve: A more accurate technique for facial nerve dissection. J Neurosurg 4: 418–421, 1979.

5. Linden RD, Tator CH, Benedict C, et al: Electrophysiological monitoring during acoustic neuroma and other posterior fossa surgery. J Sci Neurol 15: 73–81, 1988.

6. Møller AR, Jannetta PJ: Preservation of facial function during removal of acoustic neuromas: Use of monopolar constant-voltage stimulation and EMG. J Neurosurg 61: 757–760, 1984.

7. Møller AR: Electrophysiological monitoring of cranial nerves in operations in the skull base. In Sekhar LN, Schramm V (eds): Tumors of the Cranial Base: Diagnosis and Treatment. Mt. Kisco, NY, Futura Publishers, 1987, pp 123–132.

8. Møller AR: Intraoperative Neurophysiologic Monitoring. Luxembourg, Harwood, 1995.

9. Harner SG, Daube JR, Ebersold MJ, Beatty CW: Improved preservation of facial nerve functions with use of electrical monitoring during removal of acoustic neuromas. Mayo Clin Proc 62: 92–102, 1987.

10. Harner SG, Daube JR, Beatty CW, Ebersold MJ: Intraoperative monitoring of the facial nerve. Laryngoscope 98: 209–212, 1988.

11. Dickins JRE, Graham SS: A comparison of facial nerve monitoring systems in cerebellopontine angle surgery. Am J Otol 12: 1–6, 1991.

12. Prass RL, Lueders H: Acoustic (loudspeaker) facial electromyographic monitoring: I. Neurosurgery 19: 392–400, 1986.

13. Prass RL, Kinney SE, Hardy RW, et al: Acoustic (loudspeaker) facial electromyographic monitoring: II. Use of evoked EMG activity during acoustic neuroma resection. Otolaryngol Head Neck Surg 97: 541–551, 1987.

14. Benecke JE, Calder HB, Chadwick G: Facial nerve monitoring during acoustic neuroma removal. Laryngoscope 97: 697–700, 1987.

15. Yingling CD, Gardi JN: Intraoperative monitoring of facial and cochlear nerves during acoustic neuroma surgery. Otolaryngol Clin North Am 25: 413–448, 1992.

16. Sekhar LN, Møller AR: Operative management of tumors involving the cavernous sinus. J Neurosurg 64: 879–889, 1986.

17. Daube JR: Intraoperative monitoring of cranial motor nerves. In Schramm J, Møller AR (eds): Intraoperative Neurophysiologic Monitoring in Neurosurgery. Heidelberg, Germany, Springer-Verlag, 1991, pp 246–267.

18. Daube JR, Harper CM: Surgical monitoring of cranial and peripheral nerves. In Desmedt JE (ed): Neuromonitoring in Surgery. Amsterdam, Elsevier, 1989, pp 115–138.

19. Yingling CD: Intraoperative monitoring in skull base surgery. In Jackler RK, Brackmann DE (eds): Neurotology. St. Louis, Mosby–Year Book, 1994, pp 967–1002.

20. Lanser MJ, Jackler RK, Yingling CD: Regional monitoring of the lower (ninth through twelfth) cranial nerves. In Kartush J, Bouchard K (eds): Intraoperative Monitoring in Otology and Head and Neck Surgery. New York, Raven Press, 1992, pp 131–150.

21. Eggermont JJ: Electrocochleography. In Keidel WD, Neff WD (eds): Handbook of Sensory Physiology, Vol III. New York, Springer-Verlag, 1976, pp 625–705.

22. Ferraro JA, Murphy GB, Ruth RA: A comparative study of primary electrodes used in extratympanic electrocochleography. Semin Hear 7: 279–287, 1986.

23. Lambert PR, Ruth RA: Simultaneous recording of noninvasive ECoG and ABR for use in intraoperative monitoring. Otolaryngol Head Neck Surg 98: 575–580, 1988.

24. Levine RA, Ojemann RG, Montgomery WW, McGaffigan PM: Monitoring auditory evoked potentials during acoustic neuroma surgery: Insights into the mechanism of the hearing loss. Ann Otol Rhinol Laryngol 93: 116–123, 1984.

25. Schwartz DM, Rosenberg SI: Facial nerve monitoring during parotidectomy. In Kartush J, Bouchard K (eds): Intraoperative Monitoring in Otology and Head and Neck Surgery. New York, Raven Press, 1992, pp 121–130.

26. Smith DI, Mills JH: Anesthesia effects: Auditory brainstem response. Electroencephalogr Clin Neurophysiol 72: 422–428, 1989.

27. Duncan PG, Sanders RA, McCullough DW: Preservation of auditory brainstem responses in anesthetized children. Can Anaesth Soc J 26: 492–495, 1979.

28. Sanders RA, Duncan PG, McCullough DW: Clinical experience with brainstem audiometry performed under general anesthesia. J Otolaryngol 8: 24–32, 1979.

29. Sloan T: Evoked potentials. In Albin MS (ed): A Textbook of Neuroanesthesia with Neurosurgical and Neuroscience Perspectives. New York, McGraw-Hill, 1996, pp 221–276.

30. O'Hara DA, Derbyshire GJ, Overdyk FJ, et al: Closed-look infusion of atracurium with four different anesthetic techniques. Anesthesiology 74: 258–263, 1991.

31. Møller AR, Jannetta PJ: Monitoring auditory functions during cranial nerve microvascular decompression operations by direct recording from the eighth nerve. J Neurosurg 59: 493–499, 1983.

32. Doyle DJ, Hyde ML: Analogue and digital filtering of auditory brainstem responses. Scand Audiol (Stockh) 10: 81–89, 1981.

33. Sgro JAS, Emerson RG, Pedley TA: Methods for steadily updating the averaged responses during neuromonitoring. In Desmedt JE (ed): Neuromonitoring in Surgery. Amsterdam, Elsevier, 1989, pp 49–60.

34. Møller AR: Evoked Potentials in Intraoperative Monitoring. Baltimore, Williams & Wilkins, 1988.

35. Campbell KCM, Abbas PJ: The effect of stimulus repetition rate on auditory brainstem response in tumor and nontumor patients. J Speech Hear Res 30: 494–502, 1987.

36. Hoke M, Ross B, Wickesberg R, Luetkenhoener B: Weighted averaging: Theory and application to electrical response audiometry. Electroencephalogr Clin Neurophysiol 57: 484–489, 1984.

37. Schimmel H: The (+/−) reference: Accuracy of estimated mean components in average response studies. Science 157: 92–94, 1967.

38. Hatayama T, Sekiya T, Suzuki S, Iwabuchi T: Effect of compression on the cochlear nerve: A short- and long-term electrophysiological and histological study. Neurol Res 21: 599–610, 1999.

39. Hatayama T, Møller AR: Correlation between latency and amplitude of peak V in brainstem auditory evoked potentials: Intraoperative recordings in microvascular decompression operations. Acta Neurochir (Wien) 140: 681–687, 1998.

40. Silverstein H, Norrell H, Hyman S: Simultaneous use of CO_2 laser with continuous monitoring of eighth cranial nerve action potential during acoustic neuroma surgery. Otolaryngol Head Neck Surg 92: 80–84, 1984.

41. Lorento de No R: Analysis of the distribution of action currents of nerve in volume conductors. Stud Rockefeller Inst Med Res 132: 384–482, 1947.

42. Møller AR, Møller MB, Jannetta PJ, Jho HD: Auditory nerve compound action potentials and brainstem auditory evoked potentials in patients with various degrees of hearing loss. Ann Otol Rhinol Laryngol 100: 488–495, 1991.

43. Kuroki A, Møller AR: Microsurgical anatomy around the foramen of Luschka with reference to intraoperative recording of auditory evoked potentials from the cochlear nuclei. J Neurosurg 82: 933–939, 1995.

44. Møller AR, Jannetta PJ: Auditory evoked potentials recorded from the cochlear nucleus and its vicinity in man. J Neurosurg 59: 1013–1018, 1983.

45. Møller AR, Jho HD, Jannetta PJ: Preservation of hearing in operations on acoustic tumors: An alternative to recording BAEP. Neurosurgery 34: 688–693, 1994.

46. Coats AC: Human auditory nerve action potentials and brainstem evoked responses: Latency-intensity functions in detection of cochlear and retrocochlear pathology. Arch Otolaryngol 104: 709–717, 1978.

47. Ojemann RG, Levine RA, Montgomery WM, McGaffigan PM: Use of intraoperative auditory evoked potentials to preserve hearing in unilateral acoustic neuroma removal. J Neurosurg 61: 938–948, 1984.

48. Sabin HI, Bentivoglio P, Symon L, et al: Intraoperative electrocochleography to monitor cochlear potentials during acoustic neuroma excision. Acta Neurochir (Wien) 85: 110–116, 1987.

49. Markand ON, Lee BI, Warren C, et al: Effects of hypothermia on brainstem auditory evoked potentials in humans. Ann Neurol 22: 507–513, 1987.

50. Sohmer H, Gold S, Cahani M, Attias J: Effects of hypothermia on auditory brainstem and somatosensory evoked response: A model of a synaptic and axonal lesion. Electroencephalogr Clin Neurophysiol 74: 50–57, 1989.

51. Rosenberg SI, Martin WH, Pratt H, et al: Bipolar cochlear nerve recording technique: A preliminary report. Am J Otol 14: 362–368, 1993.

52. Møller AR, Colletti V, Fiorino F: Click evoked responses from the exposed intracranial portion of the eighth nerve during vestibular nerve section: Bipolar and monopolar recordings. Electroencephalogr Clin Neurophysiol 92: 17–29, 1994.

53. Sass K, Densert B, Arlinger S: Recording techniques for transtympanic electrocochleography in clinical practice. Acta Otolaryngol (Stockh) 118: 17–25, 1998.

54. Ferraro JA, Best LG, Arenberg IK: The use of electrocochleography in the diagnosis, assessment, and monitoring of endolymphatic hydrops. Otolaryngol Clin North Am 16: 69–82, 1983.

55. Kanzaki J, Ouchi T, Yokobbori H, Ino T: Electrocochleographic study of summating potentials in Ménière's disease. Audiology 21: 409–424, 1982.

56. Coats AC: The summating potential and Ménière's disease: I. Summating potential amplitude in Ménière and non-Ménière ears. Arch Otolaryngol 107: 199–208, 1981.

57. Campbell KCM, Harker LA, Abbas PJ: Interpretation of electrocochleography in Ménière's disease and normal subjects. Ann Otol Rhinol Laryngol 101: 496–500, 1992.

58. Rand RW, Kurze TL: Facial nerve preservation by posterior fossa transmeatal microdissection in total removal of acoustic tumours. J Neurol Neurosurg Psychiatry 28: 311–316, 1965.

59. Sugita K, Kobayashi S: Technical and instrumental improvements in the surgical treatment of acoustic neurinomas. J Neurosurg 57: 747–752, 1982.

60. Silverstein H, Smouha E, Jones R: Routine identification of facial nerve using electrical stimulation during otological and neurotological surgery. Laryngoscope 98: 726–730, 1988.

61. Prass RL, Lueders H: Constant-current versus constant-voltage stimulation. J Neurosurg 62: 622–623, 1985.

62. Babin RM, Jai HR, McCabe BF: Bipolar localization of the facial nerve in the internal auditory canal. In Graham MD, House WF (eds): Disorders of the Facial Nerve: Anatomy, Diagnosis, and Management. New York, Raven Press, 1982, pp 3–5.

63. Sekiya T, Iwabuchi T, Suzuki S, et al: Recordings of evoked electromyographic response from the extraocular muscle to monitor the oculomotor, trochlear, and abducens nerve function during skull base and orbital surgery. No Shinkei Geka 18: 447–451, 1990.

64. Sekiya T, Hatayama T, Iwabuchi T, Maeda SH: A ring electrode to record extraocular muscle activities during skull base surgery. Acta Neurochir (Wien) 117: 66–69, 1992.

65. Stechison MT: Vagus nerve monitoring: A comparison of percutaneous versus vocal fold electrode recording. Am J Otol 16: 703–706, 1995.

66. Møller AR: Intraoperative monitoring of evoked potentials: An update. In Wilkins RH, Rengachary SS (eds): Neurosurgery Update I: Diagnosis, Operative Technique, and Neuro-Oncology. New York, McGraw-Hill, 1990, pp 169–176.

67. Angelo R, Møller AR: Contralateral evoked brainstem auditory potentials as an indicator of intraoperative brainstem manipulation in cerebellopontine angle tumors. Neurol Res 18: 528–540, 1996.

68. Møller AR, Jannetta PJ, Møller MB: Neural generators of brainstem evoked potentials: Results from human intracranial recordings. Ann Otol Rhinol Laryngol 90: 591–596, 1981.

69. Møller AR, Jannetta PJ, Sekhar LN: Contributions from the auditory nerve to the brainstem auditory evoked potentials (BAEPs): Results of intracranial recording in man. Electroencephalogr Clin Neurophysiol 71: 198–211, 1988.

70. Hashimoto I, Ishiyama Y, Yoshimoto T, Nemoto S: Brainstem auditory evoked potentials recorded directly from human brainstem and thalamus. Brain 104: 841–859, 1981.

71. Davis H, Hirsh SK: A slow brainstem response for low-frequency audiometry. Audiology 18: 445–461, 1979.

72. Møller AR, Jannetta PJ: Evoked potentials from the inferior colliculus in man. Electroencephalogr Clin Neurophysiol 53: 612–620, 1982.

73. Møller AR, Jho HD, Yokota M, Jannetta PJ: Contribution from crossed and uncrossed brainstem structures to the brainstem auditory evoked potentials (BAEP): A study in humans. Laryngoscope 105: 596–605, 1995.

74. Møller AR, Burgess JE: Neural generators of the brainstem auditory evoked potentials (BAEPs) in the rhesus monkey. Electroencephalogr Clin Neurophysiol 65: 361–372, 1986.

75. Legatt AD, Arezzo JC, Vaughn HG: Short-latency auditory evoked potentials in the monkey: II. Intracranial generators. Electroencephalogr Clin Neurophysiol 64: 53–73, 1986.

76. Møller AR: Neural generators of auditory evoked potentials. In Jacobson JT (ed): Principles and Applications in Auditory Evoked Potentials. Boston, Allyn & Bacon, 1994, pp 23–46.

77. Radtke RA, Erwin W, Wilkins RH: Intraoperative brainstem auditory evoked potentials: Significant decrease in postoperative morbidity. Neurology 39: 187–191, 1989.

78. Møller AR, Møller MB: Does intraoperative monitoring of auditory evoked potentials reduce incidence of hearing loss as a complication of microvascular decompression of cranial nerves? Neurosurgery 24: 257–263, 1989.

79. Leonetti JP, Brackmann DE, Prass RL: Improved preservation of facial nerve function in the infratemporal approach to the skull base. Otolaryngol Head Neck Surg 101: 74–78, 1989.

80. House JW, Brackmann DE: Facial nerve grading system. Otolaryngol Head Neck Surg 93: 146–167, 1985.

Index

Note: Page numbers in *italics* indicate illustrations; those followed by t indicate tables.

ISBN 0-7216-8976-0

90038